Contemporary Therapy in
OBSTETRICS
and
GYNECOLOGY

Contemporary Therapy in
OBSTETRICS
and
GYNECOLOGY

Editors

Scott B. Ransom, DO, MBA, MPH
Senior Vice President/Chief Quality Officer
  Detroit Medical Center
Chief, Section of Gynecology
  John D. Dingell VA Medical Center
Associate Professor in Obstetrics and Gynecology
  Wayne State University School of Medicine
  Detroit, Michigan
Adjunct Associate Professor in Health Management
    and Policy
  University of Michigan
  Ann Arbor, Michigan

Mark I. Evans, MD
Professor and Chairman of Obstetrics and
    Gynecology
  Department of Obstetrics and Gynecology
  MCP-Hahnemann School of Medicine
  Philadelphia, Pennsylvania

Mitchell P. Dombrowski, MD
Professor in Obstetrics and Gynecology
  Wayne State University School of Medicine
Staff Physician
  Division of Maternal-Fetal Medicine
  St. John Hospital and Medical Center
  Detroit, Michigan

Kenneth A. Ginsburg, MD
Associate Professor in Obstetrics and Gynecology
Assistant Dean for Clinical Education
  Wayne State University School of Medicine
Department of Obstetrics and Gynecology
  Division of Reproductive Endocrinology and
    Infertility
  Hutzel Hospital
  Detroit, Michigan

W.B. SAUNDERS COMPANY
An Imprint of Elsevier Science
Philadelphia London New York St. Louis Sydney Toronto

W.B. SAUNDERS COMPANY
An Imprint of Elsevier Science

The Curtis Center
Independence Square West
Philadelphia, Pennsylvania 19106

Library of Congress Cataloging-in-Publication Data

Contemporary therapy in obstetrics and gynecology/Scott B. Ransom . . . [et al.].

p.   cm.

ISBN 0–7216–9286–9

1. Generative organs, Female—Diseases—Treatment.
    2. Obstetrics—Complications—Treatment.   I. Ransom, Scott B.
    [DNLM: 1. Pregnancy Complications—therapy.   2. Genital Diseases,
    Female—therapy.
WQ 240 C7617 2002]
RG125 .C66 2002
618′.046—dc21   2001031121

Editor-in-Chief: Richard Zorab
Acquisitions Editor: Judy Fletcher
Production Editor: Mimi McGinnis
Production Manager: Mary B. Stermel
Book Designer: Steven Stave
Illustrators: Karen Giacomucci, John Dzedzy
Indexer: Dennis Dolan

CONTEMPORARY THERAPY IN OBSTETRICS AND GYNECOLOGY   ISBN 0–7216–9286–9

Printed in the United States of America.

Last digit is the print number: 9   8   7   6   5   4   3   2   1

To our mentors and students from whom we continue to learn

To our families who have supported us with patience and understanding—
Elizabeth, Kelly, Christopher, Sarah, Jocelyn,
Michael, Jacqueline, David, Lizzy, Kiera, Shara, Bonnie, Kate, and Kevin

Contributors

Huda B. Al-Kouatly, MD
Fellow in Obstetrics and Gynecology, Cornell University Joan and Sanford I. Weill Medical College and Graduate School of Medical Sciences; Clinical Fellow in Obstetrics and Gynecology, New York and Presbyterian Hospital, New York, New York
Ultrasound in Pregnancy: Routine or by Indication?

William W. Andrews, PhD, MD
Bruce Harris, M.D. Professor, Director, Division of Obstetrics, University of Alabama at Birmingham, Birmingham, Alabama
Herpes Infections in Pregnancy

Rodney A. Appell, MD
Professor, Department of Urology, Baylor College of Medicine; F. Brantley Scott Chair, St. Luke's Episcopal Hospital, Houston, Texas
Periurethral Injectables

David F. Archer, MD
Professor of Obstetrics and Gynecology, Eastern Virginia Medical School; Director, Clinical Research Center, Jones Institute for Reproductive Medicine, Norfolk, Virginia
Management of Iatrogenic Bleeding in Postmenopausal Women

Howard R. Belkin, MD, DDS, JD
Resident Physician, Department of Psychiatry and Behavioral Neurosciences, Wayne State University School of Medicine, Detroit, Michigan
Some Legal Issues in Infertility Therapy

Ross S. Berkowitz, MD
William H. Baker Professor of Gynecology, Harvard Medical School; Co-director, New England Trophoblastic Disease Center and Director of Gynecologic Oncology, Brigham and Women's Hospital, Dana Farber Cancer Institute, Boston, Massachusetts
What Is New in the Management of Gestational Trophoblastic Disease

Marilyn R. Bernstein, MHP
Administrative Assistant, New England Trophoblastic Disease Center, Brigham and Women's Hospital, Dana Farber Cancer Institute, Boston, Massachusetts
What Is New in the Management of Gestational Trophoblastic Disease

Stanley M. Berry, MD
Associate Professor of Obstetrics and Gynecology, Wayne State University School of Medicine; Director of Maternal Fetal Medicine Fellowship Program, Hutzel Hospital, Department of Obstetrics and Gynecology, Detroit, Michigan
Updates in Red Cell Isoimmunization

Charla M. Blacker, MD
Assistant Professor, Department of Obstetrics and Gynecology, Division of Reproductive Endocrinology and Infertility, Wayne State University School of Medicine; Director, Assisted Reproductive Endocrinology, Hutzel Hospital, Detroit, Michigan
Perinatal Outcome after Assisted Reproductive Techniques; Tubal Surgery versus In Vitro Fertilization: Where Do We Draw the Line?

Sean C. Blackwell, MD
Assistant Professor, Division of Maternal-Fetal Medicine, Department of Obstetrics and Gynecology, Hutzel Hospital, Wayne State University School of Medicine, Detroit, Michigan
Antenatal Magnesium Sulfate Exposure and the Risk of Cerebral Palsy in Preterm Neonates: An Update

Steven L. Bloom, MD
Assistant Professor, Department of Obstetrics and Gynecology, University of Texas Southwestern Medical Center; Associate Medical Director of Obstetrics, Parkland Health and Hospital System, Dallas, Texas
Walking during Labor: Myths and Realities

Renee A. Bobrowski, MD
Assistant Professor, Department of Obstetrics and Gynecology, Division of Maternal-Fetal Medicine, University of Connecticut, Farmington; Attending Perinatologist, Division of Maternal-Fetal Medicine, Hartford Hospital, Hartford, Connecticut
Anticoagulation

Catherine S. Bradley, MD
Clinical Instructor, University of Pennsylvania School of Medicine; Fellow in Urogynecology and Reconstructive Pelvic Surgery, Department of Obstetrics and Gynecology, University of Pennsylvania Medical Center, Philadelphia, Pennsylvania
Nonsurgical Treatments for Female Urinary Incontinence

Wendy R. Brewster, MD, PhD
Assistant Professor, Department of Obstetrics and Gynecology, University of California, Irvine, Irvine, California
Hormone Replacement Therapy in Breast Cancer Survivors

David W. Britt, PhD
Research Professor of Obstetrics and Gynecology, MCP-Hahnemann School of Medicine, Philadelphia, Pennsylvania
Emerging Psychosocial Issues in Prenatal Diagnosis

Richard Bronsteen, MD
Assistant Professor of Obstetrics and Gynecology, Wayne State University, Detroit; Divisions of Fetal Imaging and Maternal-Fetal Medicine, William Beaumont Hospital, Royal Oak, Michigan
Shoulder Dystocia

Cynthia A. Brown
Director, Health Policy, American College of Surgeons, Washington, D.C.
The History, Impact, and Future of the Medicare Fee Schedule

Peter Bryant-Greenwood, MD
Clinical Associate, Molecular Diagnostics, Laboratory of Pathology, National Cancer Institute, National Institutes of Health, Bethesda, Maryland
Molecular Diagnostics in Obstetrics and Gynecology

Ronald T. Burkman, MD
Deputy Chair and Professor, Department of Obstetrics and Gynecology, Tufts University School of Medicine, Boston; Chairman, Department of Obstetrics and Gynecology, Baystate Medical Center, Springfield, Massachusetts
The Contraceptive and Noncontraceptive Health Benefits of Oral Contraceptives: An Update

Byron C. Calhoun, MD
Adjunct Associate Professor in Obstetrics and Gynecology, Uniformed Services University of the Health Sciences F. Edward Hébert School of Medicine, Bethesda, Maryland; Attending Faculty, Department of Obstetrics and Gynecology and Program Director, Maternal-Fetal Medicine, Madigan Army Medical Center, Tacoma, Washington
Prevention of Group B Streptococcus Disease; Adolescent Pregnancy: Improving Outcomes through Focused Multidisciplinary Obstetric Care; Teratology

Bruce R. Carr, MD
Professor and Director, Division of Reproductive Endocrinology and Infertility; Holder, Paul C. MacDonald Distinguished Chair in Obstetrics and Gynecology, The University of Texas Southwestern Medical Center at Dallas; Senior Attending Staff, Zale Lipshy University Hospital, Parkland Health and Hospital System, and St. Paul University Medical Center, Dallas, Texas
Selective Estrogen Receptor Modulators

Stephen T. Chasen, MD
Assistant Professor of Obstetrics and Gynecology, and Director of High-Risk Obstetrics, Cornell University Joan and Sanford I. Weill Medical College and Graduate School of Medical Sciences, New York, New York
Ultrasound in Pregnancy: Routine or by Indication?

Frank A. Chervenak, MD
Professor and Chairman of Obstetrics and Gynecology, Cornell University Joan and Sanford I. Weill Medical College and Graduate School of Medical Sciences; Obstetrician and Gynecologist-in-Chief, New York and Presbyterian Hospital, New York, New York
Ultrasound in Pregnancy: Routine or by Indication?; Principles of Screening

Gregory E. Chow, MD
Assistant Professor, Department of Obstetrics and Gynecology, University of Washington, Seattle; Associate Program Director, Obstetrics and Gynecology Residency Program, Madigan Army Medical Center, Tacoma, Washington; Assistant Professor, Uniformed Services University of the Health Sciences, Bethesda, Maryland
Obstetric and Gynecologic Infections

Jeffrey B. Clark, MD, MPH
Department Chief, Department of Obstetrics and Gynecology, Womack Army Medical Center, Fort Bragg, North Carolina
Unintended Pregnancy

Christine H. Comstock, MD
Associate Professor, Department of Obstetrics and Gynecology, Wayne State University, Detroit; Director, Fetal Imaging, William Beaumont Hospital, Royal Oak, Michigan
Universal Ultrasound Screening—Useful or a Waste?

Deborah L. Conway, MD
Assistant Professor, Division of Maternal-Fetal Medicine, Department of Obstetrics and Gynecology, University of Texas Health Science Center, San Antonio, Texas
Management of Isolated Oligohydramnios at Term

John L. Currie, MD
Professor, Department of Obstetrics and Gynecology, Dartmouth Medical School, Hanover, New Hampshire
Management of Ovarian Cancer

Vanessa D. Dance, MD
Chairperson, Department of Obstetrics and Gynecology, William Beaumont Army Medical Center, El Paso, Texas
Breast Disease

Kristin Dardano, MD
Assistant Professor, Department of Obstetrics and Gynecology, Tufts University School of Medicine, Boston; Baystate Medical Center, Springfield, Massachusetts
The Contraceptive and Noncontraceptive Health Benefits of Oral Contraceptives: An Update

Leslie R. DeMars, MD
Assistant Professor, Department of Obstetrics and Gynecology, Dartmouth Medical School and Dartmouth Hitchcock Medical Center, Lebanon, New Hampshire
Management of Ovarian Cancer

Lawrence D. Devoe, MD
Brooks Professor and Chair, Department of Obstetrics and Gynecology; Chief of Obstetrics and Gynecology Service, Medical College of Georgia, Augusta, Georgia
Issues in Cervical Ripening/Labor Induction

Peter Dews
Assistant Professor of Internal Medicine, Wayne State University School of Medicine, Detroit, Michigan
What Are Employers and Payers Looking at in Obstetric and Gynecologic Practice?

Michael P. Diamond, MD
Kamran S. Moghissi Professor and Associate Chairman, Department of Obstetrics and Gynecology; Director, Division of Reproductive Endocrinology and Infertility, Wayne State University School of Medicine, Detroit, Michigan
Prevention and Management of Adhesions

Philip J. DiSaia, MD
Professor, University of California, Irvine, Irvine; Director, Division of Gynecologic Oncology, University of California, Irvine, Medical Center, Orange, California
Hormone Replacement Therapy in Breast Cancer Survivors

Lucia DiVenere, MA
Manager, Federal Policy and Outreach, Department of Government Relations, American College of Obstetricians and Gynecologists, Washington, District of Columbia
Your Practice and the United States Congress

Michelle M. DiVito, MSN
Perinatal Research Coordinator, Thomas Jefferson University, Philadelphia, Pennsylvania
Controversies Involving Antenatal Corticosteroids

Donna Dizon-Townson, MD
Assistant Professor, Department of Obstetrics and Gynecology, University of Utah School of Medicine, Salt Lake City; Co-Director, Maternal-Fetal Medicine, Utah Valley Regional Medical Center, Intermountain Health Care, Provo, Utah
Recently Described Hereditary Thrombophilias and Obstetric Outcome

Michael Dombrowski
Computer Consultant, Grosse Point Farms, Michigan
Benefits and Perils of Computers in Medical Care

Mitchell P. Dombrowski, MD
Professor in Obstetrics and Gynecology, Wayne State University School of Medicine; Staff Physician, Division of Maternal-Fetal Medicine, St. John Hospital and Medical Center, Detroit, Michigan
Operative Vaginal Delivery; Management of Asthma in Pregnancy; Benefits and Perils of Computers in Medical Care

Arie Drugan, MD
Associate Professor, Department of Obstetrics and Gynecology, Wayne State University School of Medicine, Detroit, Michigan; Director, Labor and Delivery, Rambam Medical Center, Haifa, Israel
Invasive Procedures for Perinatal Diagnosis

Donald J. Dudley, MD
Professor, Department of Obstetrics and Gynecology, University of Texas Health Sciences Center at San Antonio, San Antonio, Texas
Controversies Involving Antenatal Corticosteroids

Jeffery S. Dzieczkowski, MD
Hospitalist, Internal Medicine, Eastern Connecticut Health Network, Manchester General Hospital, Manchester, Connecticut
Anticoagulation

Philip N. Eskew, Jr., MD
Medical Director, Women and Infant Services, St. Vincent Hospital, Indianapolis, Indiana
Coding in Obstetrics and Gynecology

Mark I. Evans, MD
Professor and Chairman of Obstetrics and Gynecology, Department of Obstetrics and Gynecology, MCP-Hahnemann School of Medicine, Philadelphia, Pennsylvania
Invasive Procedures for Prenatal Diagnosis; New Genetic Concepts; Principles of Screening; Second Trimester Screening; Multifetal Pregnancy Reduction; Multifetal Pregnancy Reduction: Psychosocial and Family Issues

Mary P. Fairchok, MD
Clinical Assistant Professor of Pediatrics, University of Washington, Seattle; Chief, Pediatric Infectious Diseases, Madigan Army Medical Center, Tacoma, Washington; Associate Professor, Pediatrics, Uniformed Services University of the Health Sciences, Bethesda, Maryland
Obstetric and Gynecologic Infections

Sebastian Faro, MD, PhD
Professor, Department of Obstetrics and Gynecology, The University of Texas Health Science Center at Houston; Department of Obstetrics and Gynecology, Woman's Hospital of Texas, Houston, Texas
Postpartum Endometritis

Charles W. Fisher, JD
Principal, Kitch, Drutchas, Wagner, DeNardis, and Valitutti,
P.C., Detroit, Michigan
Medical Legal Risk Management in Obstetrics

Diane M. Flynn, MD, ScM
Adjunct Assistant Professor of Family Medicine, Uniformed Services University of the Health Sciences, Bethesda, Maryland; Staff Physician, Faculty Development Fellow, Madigan Army Medical Center, Tacoma, Washington
Unintended Pregnancy

Michael L. Freeman, MD
Fellow, Division of Reproductive Endocrinology and Infertility, Department of Obstetrics and Gynecology, Hutzel Hospital, Wayne State University School of Medicine, Detroit, Michigan
Tubal Surgery versus In Vitro Fertilization: Where Do We Draw the Line?

Francisco A. R. Garcia, MD, MPH
Assistant Professor of Obstetrics and Gynecology, and Director, Division of Gynecology, University of Arizona, Tucson, Arizona
Emergent Postcoital Contraception

Kenneth A. Ginsburg, MD
Associate Professor in Obstetrics and Gynecology, and Assistant Dean for Clinical Education, Wayne State University School of Medicine, Detroit; Department of Obstetrics and Gynecology, Division of Reproductive Endocrinology and Infertility, Hutzel Hospital, Ann Arbor, Michigan
Induction of Ovulation; Male Infertility: Interpreting and Using the Semen Analysis

Steven H. Golde, MD
Associate Professor, Department of Obstetrics and Gynecology; Active Medical Staff Physician, Medical College of Georgia, Augusta, Georgia
Issues in Cervical Ripening/Labor Induction

Donald P. Goldstein, MD
Professor of Obstetrics and Gynecology, Harvard Medical School; Co-Director, New England Trophoblastic Disease Center, Brigham and Women's Hospital, Dana Farber Cancer Institute, Boston, Massachusetts
What Is New in the Management of Gestational Trophoblastic Disease

Bernard Gonik, MD
Professor and Associate Chairman, Department of Obstetrics and Gynecology, Wayne State University School of Medicine, Detroit, Michigan
Shoulder Dystocia

David M. Gorenberg, MD
Clinical Instructor, Department of Obstetrics and Gynecology, University of California, Irvine, School of Medicine; Clinical Instructor in Obstetrics and Gynecology, Division of Maternal-Fetal Medicine, University of California Medical Center, Irvine, Orange, California
Urinary Tract Infections in Pregnancy

Laura A. Gorski, DO
Instructor and Maternal-Fetal Medicine Fellow, Department of Obstetrics and Gynecology, Thomas Jefferson University, Philadelphia, Pennsylvania
Diagnosis and Management of Premature Rupture of the Membrane

Rivka Greenberg, PhD
Adjunct Assistant Professor, Wayne State University School of Medicine, Detroit, Michigan; Research Coordinator, Pharmaceutical Research Unit, Haight Ashbury Free Clinics, Inc., San Francisco, California
Contemporary Options in Substance Abuse Treatment for Women

Naomi H. Greene, MPH, RDMS, RDCS
Clinical Project Associate, Cedars Sinai Medical Center, Department of Obstetrics and Gynecology, Los Angeles, California
Screening for Ovarian Cancer

George Grunberger, MD
Henry L. Brasza Professor, Department of Internal Medicine, Center for Molecular Medicine and Genetics, Wayne State University School of Medicine; Medical Director, Morris Hood Jr. Comprehensive Diabetes Center, Wayne State University, Detroit, Michigan
Diabetes Mellitus

Debra A. Guinn, MD
Assistant Professor, Division of Maternal-Fetal Medicine, University of Colorado Health Sciences Center, Denver Health Medical Center, Denver, Colorado
Acute Therapy for Preterm Labor; Maintenance Therapy following Successful Arrest of Preterm Labor

Jennifer Gunter, MD
Assistant Professor, Department of Obstetrics and Gynecology, The University of Colorado, Denver, Colorado
Trauma in Pregnancy

Terrence W. Hallahan, PhD
Director, Research and Development Division, and Assistant Laboratory Director, NTD Laboratories, Inc., Huntington Station, New York
First Trimester Screening

Elizabeth Golladay Hancock, MD
Adjunct Associate Professor, Clinical Obstetrics and Gynecology, Uniformed Services University of the Health Sciences F. Edward Hébert School of Medicine, Bethesda, Maryland; Fellow, Maternal-Fetal Medicine, Madigan Army Medical Center, Tacoma, Washington
Adolescent Pregnancy: Improving Outcomes through Focused Mutidisciplinary Obstetric Care

Margaret A. Harper, MD
Associate Professor, Department of Obstetrics and Gynecology, Wake Forest University School of Medicine, Winston-Salem, North Carolina
Rescue Cerclage for the Incompetent Cervix

Harry Harrison, MD
University of Arizona College of Medicine, Department of Pathology, Tucson; Southwest Genetics and Laboratory Medicine, Scottsdale, Arizona
Second Trimester Screening

Barbara R. Herzig, MD
Resident Physician, Department of Psychiatry and Behavioral Neurosciences, Wayne State University School of Medicine, Detroit, Michigan
Some Legal Issues in Infertility Therapy

Sharon L. Hillier, PhD
Professor, Department of Obstetrics, Gynecology, and Reproductive Sciences, Magee-Women's Hospital, University of Pittsburgh School of Medicine, Pittsburgh, Pennsylvania
Implications of Bacterial Vaginosis in Obstetrics

Bobby C. Howard, MD
Fellow in Maternal-Fetal Medicine, Department of Obstetrics and Gynecology, Madigan Army Medical Center, Tacoma, Washington
Obstetric and Gynecologic Infections

George R. Huggins, MD
Professor, Department of Obstetrics and Gynecology, University School of Medicine, Baltimore, Maryland
Emergent Postcoital Contraception

Roderick F. Hume, Jr., MD
Associate Professor of Clinical Obstetrics and Gynecology, Uniformed Services University of the Health Sciences F. Edward Hébert School of Medicine, Bethesda, Maryland; Chairman, Clinical Investigation, Madigan Army Medical Center, Tacoma, Washington
Prevention of Group B Streptococcus Disease; Adolescent Pregnancy: Improving Outcomes through Focused Multidisciplinary Obstetric Care; Unintended Pregnancy; Teratology

Steven R. Inglis, MD
Associate Professor of Clinical Obstetrics and Gynecology, Cornell University Joan and Sanford R. Weill Medical College and Graduate School of Medical Sciences, New York; Network Chief of Obstetrics and Gynecology, St. Barnabas Hospital, Bronx, New York
Management of HIV in Pregnancy

Mark Paul Johnson, MS, MD
Associate Professor, Departments of Obstetrics-Gynecology and Surgery, University of Pennsylvania School of Medicine; Director of Obstetrical Services, Center for Fetal Diagnosis and Treatment; Associate Professor, Divisions of Maternal-Fetal Medicine, Pediatric Surgery, and Medical Genetics, Children's Hospital of Philadelphia and the University of Pennsylvania School of Medicine, Philadelphia, Pennsylvania
New Genetic Concepts

Theodore B. Jones, MD
Associate Professor of Obstetrics and Gynecology, Wayne State University, Detroit, Michigan
Vaccines in Pregnancy

Beth Y. Karlan, MD
Professor, Obstetrics and Gynecology, University of California, Los Angeles, School of Medicine; Board of Governors Endowed Chair in Gynecologic Oncology; Director, Division of Gynecologic Oncology, Cedars-Sinai Medical Center, Los Angeles, California
Screening for Ovarian Cancer

Vern L. Katz, MD
Clinical Assistant Professor, Department of Obstetrics and Gynecology, Oregon Health Sciences University School of Medicine, Portland; Director, Perinatal Services, Sacred Heart Medical Center, Eugene, Oregon
Selective Arterial Embolization in the Management of Obstetric Hemorrhage

Helen H. Kay, MD
Professor and Director of Maternal-Fetal Medicine, Department of Obstetrics and Gynecology, University of Wisconsin Medical School, Madison, Wisconsin
Fetal Macrosomia: Antenatal Diagnosis and Management

Moon H. Kim, MD
Professor and Director, Division of Reproductive Endocrinology and Infertility, Department of Obstetrics and Gynecology, University of California, Irvine, Medical Center, Orange, California
Unexplained Infertility: Management Options

Debora F. Kimberlin, MD
Assistant Professor, Department of Obstetrics and Gynecology, University of Alabama at Birmingham, Birmingham, Alabama
Herpes Infections in Pregnancy

Christine M. Kovac, MD
Fellow in Maternal-Fetal Medicine, Department of Obstetrics and Gynecology, Madigan Army Medical Center, Tacoma, Washington
Teratology

S. Robert Kovac, MD
John D. Thompson Professor of Gynecologic Surgery, Department of Obstetrics and Gynecology, Emory University School of Medicine, Atlanta, Georgia
Guidelines for Determining the Route of Hysterectomy

Carole L. Kowalczyk, MD
Assistant Professor and Associate Residency Director, Wayne State University School of Medicine; Department of Obstetrics and Gynecology, Hutzel Hospital, Division of Reproductive Endocrinology/Infertility, Detroit, Michigan
Adolescent Eating Disorders

Robert A. Kozol, MD
Professor of Surgery, University of Connecticut School of Medicine, Farmington; Chief of Surgery, University of Connecticut Health Center, Farmington, Connecticut
Advances in Surgical Technology

Ralph L. Kramer, MD
Attending Physician, Department of Obstetrics and Gynecology, Patrick Community Memorial Hospital, Stuart, Virginia
New Genetic Concepts

David A. Krantz, BS
Director, Division of Biostatistics, NTD Laboratories, Inc., Huntington Station, New York
First Trimester Screening

Eric L. Krivchenia, MS
Research Coordinator, Department of Obstetrics and Gynecology, MCP-Hahnemann University, Philadelphia, Pennsylvania
Principles of Screening

Mary V. Krueger, DO
Faculty Development Fellow, Madigan Army Medical Center, Tacoma, Washington
Breast Disease

Kristine Y. Lain, MD
Assistant Professor, Department of Obstetrics and Gynecology, University of Pittsburgh School of Medicine, Pittsburgh, Pennsylvania
Management of Preeclampsia

Michael E. Lantz, MD
Assistant Professor, Department of Gynecology and Obstetrics, Johns Hopkins University School of Medicine, Baltimore; Director, Department of Obstetrics and Gynecology, Shore Perinatal Centers, Stevensville, Maryland
Current Therapy for Ectopic Pregnancy

John W. Larsen, MD
Oscar I. and Mildred S. Dodek Professor and Interim Chairman, Department of Obstetrics and Gynecology, The George Washington University; Chairman, Department of Obstetrics and Gynecology, The George Washington University Hospital, Washington, District of Columbia
Urinary Tract Infections in Pregnancy

Michele R. Lauria, MD
Assistant Professor, Dartmouth Medical School, Hanover; Division of Maternal-Fetal Medicine, Department of Obstetrics and Gynecology, Dartmouth Hitchcock Medical Center, Lebanon, New Hampshire
Fetal Lung Maturity Testing

Robert P. Lorenz, MD
Associate Professor, Department of Obstetrics and Gynecology, Wayne State University, Detroit; Director, Maternal Fetal Medicine; Vice Chief, Obstetrics, William Beaumont Hospital, Royal Oak, Michigan
Cervical Length

Wendy Ma, MD, FACOG
Chief, Ambulatory Care Service, Obstetrics and Gynecology, Madigan Army Medical Center, Tacoma, Washington
Breast Disease

William C. Mabie, MD
Professor of Obstetrics and Gynecology, University of Tennessee, Memphis, College of Medicine, Memphis, Tennessee
Management of Epilepsy

James N. Macri, PhD
Laboratory Director and President, NTD Laboratories, Inc., Huntington Station, New York
First Trimester Screening

Paul Makela, MD
Assistant Professor, Department of Obstetrics and Gynecology, Wayne State University School of Medicine, Detroit, Michigan
Intraoperative Hemorrhage

John M. Malone, Jr., MD
Professor and Chairman, Department of Obstetrics and Gynecology, and Associate Dean, Wayne State University School of Medicine, Detroit, Michigan; Senior Vice President for Academic Affairs, Detroit Medical Center, Detroit, Michigan
HIV and AIDS in Cervical Neoplasia

Brian A. Mason, MD
Assistant Professor, Department of Obstetrics and Gynecology, Wayne State University School of Medicine; Division of Maternal-Fetal Medicine, St. John Hospital and Medical Center, Detroit, Michigan
Peripartum Pulmonary Edema

Judith Fry McComish, BSN, MSN, PhD
Assistant Professor, Wayne State University School of Medicine and College of Nursing, Detroit, Michigan
Contemporary Options in Substance Abuse Treatment for Women

Kevin T. McGinnis, MD
Clinical Instructor, Department of Obstetrics and Gynecology, Wayne State University School of Medicine, Detroit, Michigan
Induction of Ovulation

James A. McGregor, MD, CB
Professor, Department of Obstetrics and Gynecology, University of Colorado School of Medicine; Technical Physician, Denver Health Medical Center, Denver, Colorado
Diagnostic Strategies for "Threatened Preterm Labor"

Brian M. Mercer, MD
Professor of Reproductive Biology, Case Western Reserve University; Director, Maternal Fetal Medicine, MetroHealth Medical Center, Cleveland, Ohio
Diagnosis and Management of Premature Rupture of the Membrane

Ira H. Mickelson, MD, MBA
Clinical Instructor, University of Michigan Medical School, Ann Arbor; Attending Physician, William Beaumont Hospital, Royal Oak; William Beaumont Hospital, Troy; Huron Valley-Sinai Hospital, Commerce Township, Michigan
Selective Estrogen Receptor Modulators in the Long-term Management of Postmenopausal Women; Cost-Benefit and Decision-Making Analyses in Obstetrics and Gynecology

Virginia L. Miller, DrPH
Assistant Professor, Department of Obstetrics and Gynecology, Wayne State University School of Medicine, Detroit, Michigan
Family Decision-Making in Prenatal Genetic Testing; Multifetal Pregnancy Reduction: Psychosocial and Family Issues

Debra A. Minjarez, MD
Staff Physician, Colorado Reproductive Endocrinology, Denver, Colorado
Selective Estrogen Receptor Modulators

Menachem Miodovnik, MD
Professor and Vice Chairman of Obstetrics and Gynecology, St. Luke's Roosevelt Hospital Center; Vice-Chairman, Department of Obstetrics and Gynecology, St. Luke's Roosevelt Hospital Center, University Hospital of Columbia, and University College of Physicians and Surgeons, New York, New York
Pregnancy and Medical Complications of Diabetes

Kamran S. Moghissi, MD
Professor of Obstetrics and Gynecology, Division of Reproductive Endocrinology and Infertility, Wayne State University School of Medicine, Detroit, Michigan
New Advances in the Management of Endometriosis; Efficient and Effective Evaluation of Infertility

Robert T. Morris, MD
Assistant Professor, Department of Obstetrics and Gynecology, Wayne State University School of Medicine; Assistant Professor, Department of Molecular Biology and Genetics, The Barbara Ann Karmanos Cancer Institute, Detroit, Michigan
Human Papillomavirus and Genital Neoplasia

Joseph P. Muldoon, MD
Assistant Clinical Professor of Surgery, Northwestern University Medical School; Colon Rectal Surgeon, Evanston-Northwestern Healthcare, Evanston, Illinois
Evaluation and Treatment of Anal Incontinence

Adnan R. Munkarah, MD
Director of Gynecologic Oncology and Associate Professor of Obstetrics and Gynecology, Wayne State University School of Medicine, Detroit, Michigan
Premalignant Diseases of the Vulva and Vagina

Joseph E. O'Brien, MD
Quest Diagnostics, Teterboro, New Jersey
Second Trimester Screening

Avi Orr-Urtreger, MD, PhD
Senior Lecturer, Sackler Faculty of Medicine, Tel Aviv University; Director, Genetic Institute, Tel Aviv Sourasky Medical Center, Tel Aviv, Israel
Fetal Gene Therapy Update

Barbara V. Parilla, MD
Associate Professor, Department of Obstetrics and Gynecology, Northwestern University Medical School, Chicago; Director of Fetal Diagnostics, Evanston-Northwestern Healthcare, Evanston, Illinois
Acute Therapy for Preterm Labor

Alan M. Peaceman, MD
Associate Professor, Department of Obstetrics and Gynecology, Northwestern University Medical School, Chicago, Illinois
Vaginal Birth after Cesarean: A Re-evaluation

Brian Thomas Pierce, MD
Adjunct Instructor in Obstetrics and Gynecology, Uniformed Services University of the Health Sciences F. Edward Hébert School of Medicine, Bethesda Maryland; Attending Faculty, Department of Obstetrics and Gynecology, and Fellow, Maternal-Fetal Medicine, Madigan Army Medical Center, Tacoma, Washington
Prevention of Group B Streptococcus Disease

James M. Pivarnik, PhD
Professor of Kinesiology and Osteopathic Surgical Specialties, Michigan State University, East Lansing, Michigan
Exercise in Pregnancy

Lawrence D. Platt, MD
Professor, Department of Obstetrics and Gynecology, University of California, Los Angeles, School of Medicine, Los Angeles, California
Screening for Ovarian Cancer

Peter G. Pryde, MD
Associate Professor and Director of Prenatal Diagnosis, Department of Obstetrics and Gynecology, Division of Maternal-Fetal Medicine, University of Wisconsin Medical School, Madison, Wisconsin
Fetal Macrosomia: Antenatal Diagnosis and Management

Raymond Rackley, MD
Co-Head, Section of Voiding Dysfunction and Female Urology, and Staff, Urological Institute, Cleveland Clinic Foundation, Cleveland, Ohio
Office Evaluation of Urinary Incontinence

Scott B. Ransom, DO, MBA, MPH
Senior Vice President/Chief Quality Officer, Detroit Medical Center; Chief, Section of Gynecology, John D. Dingell VA Medical Center; Associate Professor in Obstetrics and Gynecology, Wayne State University School of Medicine, Detroit; Adjunct Associate Professor in Health Management and Policy, University of Michigan, Ann Arbor, Michigan
Benefits and Perils of Computers in Medical Care; Implementing Quality Improvement in Obstetric and Gynecologic Practice; What Are Employers and Payers Looking at in Obstetric and Gynecologic Practice?; Cost-Benefit and Decision-Making Analyses in Obstetrics and Gynecology

Mark E. Redman, MD
Clinical Instructor, Department of Obstetrics and Gynecology, Wayne State University School of Medicine; Maternal-Fetal Medicine Fellow, Hutzel Hospital, Detroit, Michigan
Updates in Red Cell Isoimmunization; Thyroid Disease in Pregnancy

Robert L. Reid, MD
Professor of Obstetrics and Gynecology and Head, Division of Reproductive Endocrinology and Infertility, Queen's University Faculty of Health Sciences; Deputy Head, Department of Obstetrics and Gynecology, Kingston General Hospital, Kingston, Ontario, Canada
Current Issues in Premenstrual Syndrome

John T. Repke, MD
Chris J. and Marie A. Olson Professor of Obstetrics and Gynecology; Chairman, Department of Obstetrics and Gynecology, University of Nebraska Medical Center, Omaha, Nebraska
Medication Use during Pregnancy

Spencer S. Richlin, MD
Division of Reproductive Endocrinology and Infertility, Emory University School of Medicine, Atlanta, Georgia
Update on Endometrial Ablation and Related Techniques

Juanita Maria Rivera, BS
CMD-MS student, Department of Physiology, College of Human Medicine, Michigan State University, East Lansing, Michigan
Exercise in Pregnancy

James M. Roberts, MD
Professor and Vice Chair (Research), Department of Obstetrics, Gynecology, and Reproductive Sciences; Professor of Epidemiology, Graduate School of Public Health, University of Pittsburgh; Vice President for Research, Magee Women's Hospital and Director, Magee Women's Research Institute, Pittsburgh, Pennsylvania
Managment of Preeclampsia

John A. Rock, MD
James Robert McCord Professor of Gynecology and Obstetrics, and Chairman, Emory University School of Medicine, Atlanta, Georgia
Update on Endometrial Ablation and Related Techniques

Barak M. Rosenn, MD
Director of Obstetric and Maternal-Fetal Medicine, Department of Obstetrics and Gynecology, St. Luke's Roosevelt Hospital Center, New York, New York
Pregnancy and Medical Complications of Diabetes

Philip Samuels, MD
Associate Professor in Obstetrics and Gynecology; Director, Obstetrics and Gynecology Residency Program; Director, Maternal Fetal Medicine Program, Ohio State University Hospital, Columbus, Ohio
Thrombocytopenia

Veronica L. Schimp, DO
Fellow in Gynecologic Oncology, The University of Texas M. D. Anderson Cancer Center, Houston, Texas
HIV and AIDS in Cervical Neoplasia

John O. Schorge, MD
Clinical Fellow in Gynecologic Oncology, Harvard Medical School; Division of Gynecologic Oncology, Brigham and Women's Hospital, Dana Farber Cancer Institute, Boston, Massachusetts
What Is New in the Management of Gestational Trophoblastic Disease

David E. Seubert, MD, MBA
Assistant Professor of Obstetrics and Gynecology, Tufts University School of Medicine, Boston; Department of Obstetrics and Gynecology, Division of Maternal Fetal Medicine, Baystate Medical Center, Springfield, Massachusetts
Operative Vaginal Delivery

Seetha Shankaran, MD
Professor of Pediatrics, Wayne State University School of Medicine; Director, Neonatal-Perinatal Medicine, Children's Hospital of Michigan; Director, Detroit Medical Center Nurseries, Hutzel Hospital, Detroit, Michigan
Severe Prematurity: Implications and Counseling

Kimberley Shewmaker, MSW
Director, Children's Therapeutic Services, Flint Odyssey House, Flint, Michigan
Contemporary Options in Substance Abuse Treatment for Women

Robert M. Silver, MD
Associate Professor, Department of Obstetrics and Gynecology, University of Utah School of Medicine; Division Head, Maternal Fetal Medicine; Residency Director, Obstetrics and Gynecology, University of Utah, Salt Lake City, Utah
Management of Antiphospholipid Syndrome

Jack D. Sobel, MD
Professor of Medicine, Wayne State University School of Medicine; Chief, Division of Infectious Diseases, Detroit Medical Center, Detroit, Michigan
Recent Advances in the Treatment of Vulvovaginal Candidiasis

Yoram Sorokin, MD
Professor, Department of Obstetrics and Gynecology, Wayne State University; Director, Divisions of Obstetrics/Maternal Fetal Medicine, Hutzel Hospital, Detroit, Michigan
Antenatal Magnesium Sulfate Exposure and the Risk of Cerebral Palsy in Preterm Neonates: An Update

Carol A. Stamm, MD
Assistant Professor in Obstetrics and Gynecology, University of Colorado Health Sciences Center; Staff Obstetrician/Gynecologist, Denver Health Medical Center, Denver, Colorado
Diagnostic Strategies for "Threatened Preterm Labor"

Andrea L. Stein, MD
Clinical Instructor, Department of Obstetrics and Gynecology, University of Southern California School of Medicine, Los Angeles, California
Alternatives to Hysterectomy for Abnormal Uterine Bleeding

Carol Ann Tarnowsky, JD
Associate General Counsel, Detroit Medical Center, Detroit, Michigan
Medical Legal Risk Management in Obstetrics

Maida Taylor, MD, MPH
Associate Clinical Professor, Department of Obstetrics and Gynecology, University of California, San Francisco, San Francisco, California
Alternatives to Conventional Hormone Replacement

Rafael F. Valle, MD
Professor, Department of Obstetrics and Gynecology, Northwestern University Medical School; Attending Physician, Northwestern Memorial Hospital, Chicago, Illinois
Complications of Hysteroscopy: Prevention, Recognition, and Management

Nikos F. Vlahos, MD
Assistant Professor of Gynecology, Department of Gynecology and Obstetrics, Johns Hopkins University School of Medicine, Baltimore, Maryland
Contemporary Management of Leiomyomas

Elizabeth Wagner, DO
Department of Obstetrics and Gynecology, Phoenix Indian Medical Center, Phoenix, Arizona
Premalignant Diseases of the Vulva and Vagina

Catherine A. Walla, MA, MN
Coordinator of Clinical Research, Department of Obstetrics and Gynecology, Cedars-Sinai Medical Center, Los Angeles, California
Screening for Ovarian Cancer

Edward E. Wallach, MD
V. Donald Woodruff Professor of Gynecology, Department of Gynecology and Obstetrics, Johns Hopkins University School of Medicine, Baltimore, Maryland
Contemporary Managment of Leiomyomas

Ronald J. Wapner, MD
Professor in Obstetrics and Gynecology, MCP-Hahnemann School of Medicine; Vice-Chairman, Obstetrics and Gynecology, and Director, Maternal-Fetal Medicine and Reproductive Genetics, MCP-Hahnemann University, Philadelphia, Pennsylvania
Controversies Involving Antenatal Corticosteroids

Louis Weinstein, MD
Professor, Chairperson, and Clinical Service Chief, Department of Obstetrics and Gynecology, Medical College of Ohio, Toledo, Ohio
How to Give a Deposition

Marsha Wheeler, MD
Assistant Professor, Obstetric Genetics, Department of Obstetrics and Gynecology, University of Colorado Health Sciences Center, Denver Health Medical Center, Denver, Colorado
Maintenance Therapy following Successful Arrest of Preterm Labor

Joseph G. Whelan III, MD
Clinical Instructor of Gynecology, Department of Gynecology and Obstetrics, Johns Hopkins University School of Medicine, Baltimore, Maryland
Contemporary Management of Leiomyomas

Kristene E. Whitmore, MD
Clinical Associate Professor of Urology, MCP-Hahnemann University; Chief, Division of Urology, Graduate Hospital, Philadelphia, Pennsylvania
Nonsurgical Treatments for Female Urinary Incontinence

Paul T. Wilkes, MD
Instructor/Fellow, Department of Obstetrics and Gynecology, University of Colorado Health Sciences Center, Denver, Colorado; Instructor, Department of Obstetrics and Gynecology, University of Nevada School of Medicine, Las Vegas, Nevada
Diagnostic Strategies for "Threatened Preterm Labor"

R. Stan Williams, MD
Harry Prystowsky Professor of Reproductive Medicine, and Chief, Reproductive Endocrinology and Infertility, University of Florida College of Medicine, Gainesville, Florida
New Methods of Giving Progesterone: Are They Better?

J. Christian Winters, MD
Chief, Section of Female Urology, Ochsner Clinic, New Orleans, Louisiana
Periurethral Injectables

Honor M. Wolfe, MD
Associate Professor in Maternal-Fetal Medicine, Department of Obstetrics and Gynecology, University of North Carolina at Chapel Hill, Chapel Hill, North Carolina
Selective Arterial Embolization in the Management of Obstetric Hemorrhage

Yuval Yaron, MD
Senior Lecturer, Department of Obstetrics and Gynecology, Sackler Faculty of Medicine, Tel Aviv University; Director, Prenatal Diagnosis Unit, Tel Aviv Sourasky Medical Center, Tel Aviv, Israel
New Genetic Concepts; Fetal Gene Therapy Update

Preface

Contemporary Therapy in Obstetrics and Gynecology was written to provide a concise update of current clinical practices and issues for selected topics in obstetrics and gynecology. As research and improved methodologies are developed in our profession, physicians who manage their patients in the highest quality and current manner will be in a superior position to care for their patients. Whereas many of the principles of obstetrics and gynecology have existed for many years, new research findings and clinical practices have dramatically changed the contemporary physician's approach for many patient complaints. The book's focus on a concise update may leave the reader with a desire to learn more; in these cases, each chapter provides the best and most current references for further investigation of the subject. This book is devoted to presenting an update of selected contemporary issues in obstetrics and gynecology for the practicing physician.

We are fortunate to have recruited top individuals to serve as contributors for each of the chapters in this book. Each chapter offers the most current evidence-based approach for the subject addressed. The editor appreciates the commitment to excellence provided by each of the contributors. I am indebted to all the chapter contributors for taking the time from their families, patients, research, teaching, and administrative tasks to contribute to this book. I am especially appreciative of the assistance, expertise, and guidance of the other editors: Mitchell P. Dombrowski, MD, Kenneth A. Ginsburg, MD, and Mark I. Evans, MD. The editorial support from W.B. Saunders was outstanding through all phases of this book. I would like to extend special thanks to William Schmitt, Heather Krehling, and Judith Fletcher for their expertise in editing and publishing this book. This book could not have been produced with such quality in a timely fashion without the hard work and dedication of all those who contributed to this effort. Thanks for all your help.

Scott B. Ransom

Contents

xix

Walking during Labor: Myths and Realities

Steven L. Bloom

During the first stage of labour the patient usually prefers to move about her room, and frequently is more comfortable when occupying a sitting position. During this period, therefore, she should not be compelled to take to her bed unless she feels so inclined.

J. Whitridge Williams (1903)

At the beginning of the 20th century, J. Whitridge Williams,[1] in the first edition of his textbook on obstetrics, observed that the choice of optimal position during labor was best left to the discretion of the mother. Such early observations, however, later gave way to the opinion that recumbency during labor should be the norm, and it continues to be required by many of the professionals who provide care during labor.[2, 3] This requirement has sometimes placed them at odds with the woman who is attempting to discover the most comfortable position possible during labor.

A principal concern of those who advocate recumbency during labor is safety. Clearly, the risk of a laboring woman falling is negated if she remains recumbent. In addition, the ability to continuously monitor the well-being of the fetus is potentially more problematic while a mother ambulates. On the other hand, proponents of walking have argued that such activity is associated with several advantages, including shorter labors and greater maternal comfort. Until recently, there has been little research to assess the validity of the various strongly held opinions that exist about maternal position during labor.[2] Indeed, it is nearly a century after J. Whitridge Williams' observations were first published that scientific research addressing walking during labor has begun to emerge that permits a more objective evaluation. The results of this research are reviewed in this chapter in an effort to clarify the myths and realities regarding walking during labor.

EFFECTS OF WALKING DURING LABOR

Remarkably few randomized trials designed to measure the effects of walking during labor have been published, especially given that an understanding of how maternal activity influences labor is seemingly so fundamental. Further contributing to our limited understanding is the reality that the few randomized studies that have been published have produced disparate results (Table 1–1). The recent publication of larger randomized trials and more comprehensive reviews, however, has provided greater insight into the influence of walking on the length of labor, uterine contractility, and maternal satisfaction.

Length of Labor

There has been considerable controversy regarding the effect of walking on the length of labor. Whereas several observational studies have suggested that walking shortens labor, there have been conflicting results among the few randomized trials. Lupe and Gross[4] attempted to evaluate objectively the effect of walking on the length of labor by reviewing the available literature (a total of 16 reports). Because of significant variations in study designs and small sample sizes, however, the authors concluded that "the question of whether or not maternal ambulation during labor shortens labor length remains unanswered."

Similar uncertainty stemmed from the results of a large randomized trial conducted in Finland.[5] In this study, 630 laboring women with uncomplicated pregnancies were randomly assigned to either an ambulation or a control group. The investigators found no significant differences in the total length of labor or the length of the second stage between the two groups. After adjusting for parity, however, they found that the labors of primiparous women who ambulated were actually 1 hour longer than those in the comparison group.

In 1998, Bloom and colleagues[6] completed the most extensive randomized investigation designed to measure the effect of walking on the length of labor. In this trial, 1067 women with uncomplicated pregnancies were randomly assigned to either walking or recumbency during the active phase of labor. The women assigned to the recumbency group were permitted to assume their choice of supine, lateral, or sitting position during labor. The women assigned to the walking group were encouraged to ambulate but were instructed to return to their beds when they needed intravenous or epidural analgesia, when they had an indication for continuous electronic fetal monitoring, or when the second stage of labor began. Pedometers were used to quantify walking. After adjusting for parity, and using both intent-to-treat and as-treated analyses, the investigators found that the lengths of the first and second stages of labor were virtually identical between the 536 women assigned to walk and the 531 who labored in bed. Additional results of the investigation are summarized in Table 1–2.

Dysfunctional Labor

It has been suggested that walking during labor may lead to a decreased need for oxytocin and may serve as a

Table 1–1. Summary of the Effect of Walking during Labor on Selected Outcomes in Recent Randomized Trials

	Bloom et al, 1998[6]	Hemminki & Saarikoski, 1983[5]	Read et al, 1981[7]	Flynn et al, 1978[8]	McManus & Calder, 1978[12]
Sample size	1067	630	14	68	40
Length of labor	No effect	Increased	Decreased	Decreased	No effect
Use of oxytocin	No effect	No effect	—	Decreased	No effect
Operative delivery	No effect	No effect	No effect	Decreased	No effect
Use of analgesics	No effect	No effect	—	Decreased	No effect

treatment for dysfunctional labor. In addition to walking's possibly taking better advantage of gravity, several investigators, using randomized study designs, have reported that uterine contractility is increased in the upright position.[3, 7, 8] For example, Read and associates[7] published a preliminary report in which 14 women with an indication for labor augmentation were randomized to either a walking or an oxytocin group. Although the investigators were unable to measure any statistically significant differences in labor outcome, they did observe that walking produced a more immediate increase in uterine contractions compared to oxytocin.

Expanding on the Read study, Hemminki and coworkers[9] conducted the largest randomized study published to date that was designed specifically to address the effect of walking on dysfunctional labor. In this investigation, 57 women with protracted labor were randomly assigned to either oxytocin augmentation or ambulation as the treatment for abnormal labor. *Protracted labor* was defined as

active phase arrest of dilatation or descent for at least 2 hours. If the membranes were intact at the time protracted labor was diagnosed, amniotomy was performed and an additional 2 hours had to elapse without progress in order to be eligible for randomization. These investigators found no significant difference in the length of labor between the two groups. In addition, whereas the incidence of cesarean delivery was higher in the walking group (10% compared with no cesareans in the oxytocin group), the difference was not statistically significant ($P = .09$). Of note, however, 17 (57%) of the 30 women assigned to ambulation spontaneously delivered without being treated with oxytocin; this prompted the authors to conclude "that ambulation deserves further attention as a possible treatment of protracted labor in the active phase."[9] Although intriguing, these preliminary observations clearly require validation in larger investigations before it can be concluded that ambulation alone is an effective treatment for abnormal labor.

Table 1–2. Selected Outcomes from the Largest Randomized Investigation of Walking Compared with Recumbency during Active Labor

Outcome	Walking Group N = 536 (%)	Recumbent Group N = 531 (%)	P Value
Duration of labor (hr)			
First stage	6.1 ± 3.6	6.1 ± 3.5	.83
Second stage	0.6 ± 0.8	0.6 ± 0.7	.80
Labor augmentation (%)	122 (23)	137 (26)	.25
Analgesia (%)			.92
None	84 (16)	76 (14)	
Intravenous only	285 (53)	271 (51)	
Epidural only	29 (5)	31 (6)	
Both	138 (26)	153 (29)	
Episiotomy (%)	122 (23)	124 (23)	.86
Spontaneous delivery (%)	490 (91)	483 (91)	.39
Forceps delivery (%)	23 (4)	17 (3)	.35
Cesarean delivery (%)			
Total	23 (4)	31 (6)	.25
Dystocia	17 (3)	17 (3)	.98
Fetal distress	5 (1)	12 (2)	.08
Prolapsed cord	0 (—)	1 (0.2)	.32
Breech presentation	1 (0.2)	1 (0.2)	.99

Table adapted from data published in Bloom SL, McIntire DD, Kelly MA, et al: Lack of effect of walking on labor and delivery. N Engl J Med 1998;339:76–79.

Maternal Satisfaction

The results of earlier randomized studies have suggested that women who walk during labor require less analgesia and report greater satisfaction compared with those who labor in bed.[3, 8] In contrast, the much larger, later studies found no such reduction in analgesia requirements attributable to ambulation. In the 1998 study by Bloom and associates,[6] for example, there were no significant differences in the rates of requests for intravenous or epidural analgesia between the walking and the recumbent groups (see Table 1–2). In addition, the actual doses of analgesia required were virtually identical. As shown in Table 1–1, other investigators have found similar results.

Although objective analyses do not indicate that walking is associated with reduced analgesia requirements during labor, virtually all studies have found greater maternal satisfaction associated with the opportunity to ambulate.[4] As a counterpoint, it must also be recognized that a significant percentage of women prefer not to walk during labor. For example, Bloom and associates[6] found that 22% of the women randomly assigned to the walking group did not, in fact, choose to walk during labor. These women were found to have had significantly faster labors, which was speculated to have precluded walking. Similar findings were reported by Calvert and colleagues[10] in a randomized study of conventional fetal monitoring versus radiotelemetry. Among the 100 women randomly assigned to radiotelemetry, and who were told they could ambulate as much as they desired, 45 chose to remain in bed. Moreover, the mean duration of labor was significantly shorter (by approximately 1½ hours) for those women who opted to remain in bed compared with those who walked.

Safety

One of the most important considerations with respect to walking during labor is safety—for both the mother and the fetus. For the mother, the most obvious theoretical safety concern—falling—has not been reported in the studies addressing walking during labor. Because of this concern, however, ambulating women in the largest randomized trial, that of Bloom and colleagues,[6] were not permitted to walk unattended and were asked to return to bed if they required analgesia.

Potential safety concerns associated with walking during labor for the fetus have included a greater risk of umbilical cord prolapse and uncertainty regarding the effect of ambulation on fetal well-being. Ironically, the only case of umbilical cord prolapse reported among the randomized trials occurred in a woman assigned to bed rest.[6]

Walking does not appear to elicit abnormal fetal heart rate patterns.[11] Furthermore, among the randomized trials summarized in Table 1–1, maternal ambulation was not reported to be associated with any adverse neonatal outcomes. Lupe and Gross[4] concluded "that if ambulant patients are carefully monitored in labor according to standard protocols and if patients at risk for cord prolapse are not permitted to ambulate, ambulation does not pose risk to the fetus." Based on the bulk of recent literature, it seems reasonable to conclude that maternal ambulation poses little risk to the fetus.

SUMMARY

The preponderance of objective evidence indicates that walking has no salutary or deleterious effect on the duration of labor, the frequency of operative delivery, or the need for analgesia. Whereas the majority of women studied have reported increased satisfaction with the opportunity to ambulate, a significant percentage prefer to labor in bed. In addition, it appears that if ambulating women are carefully monitored in labor according to standardized protocols, walking does not pose a significant threat to the fetus. It must be concluded that the notion that walking enhances labor in any way or, alternatively, harms the mother or her infant is a myth not supported by the realities of evidence-based medicine. Thus, we seem to have come full circle to the conclusion reached by J. Whitridge Williams in 1903,[1] that during labor a woman "should not be compelled to take to her bed unless she feels so inclined."

Suggestions for Future Reading

Bloom SL, McIntire DD, Kelly MA, et al: Lack of effect of walking on labor and delivery. N Engl J Med 1998;339:76–79.

Lupe PJ, Gross TL: Maternal upright posture and mobility in labor: A review. Obstet Gynecol 1986;67:727–734.

Roberts J: Maternal position during the first stage of labour. In Chalmers I, Enkin M, Keirse MJNC (eds): Effective Care in Pregnancy and Childbirth, vol 2. Childbirth. Oxford, Oxford University Press, 1991, pp. 883–892.

References

1. Williams JW: Obstetrics: A Text-Book for the Use of Students and Practitioners. New York, D Appleton, 1903, p. 282.
2. Roberts J. Maternal position during the first stage of labour. In Chalmers I, Enkin M, Keirse MJNC (eds): Effective Care in Pregnancy and Childbirth, vol 2. Childbirth. Oxford, Oxford University Press, 1991, pp. 883–892.
3. Mitre IN: The influence of maternal position on duration of the active phase of labor. Int J Gynaecol Obstet 1974;12:181–183.
4. Lupe PJ, Gross TL: Maternal upright posture and mobility in labor—a review. Obstet Gynecol 1986;67:727–734.
5. Hemminki E, Saarikoski S. Ambulation and delayed amniotomy in the first stage of labor. Europ J Obstet Gynecol Reprod Biol 1983;15:129–139.
6. Bloom SL, McIntire DD, Kelly MA, et al: Lack of effect of walking on labor and delivery. N Engl J Med 1998;339:76–79.
7. Read JA, Miller FC, Paul RH: Randomized trial of ambulation versus oxytocin for labor enhancement: A preliminary report. Am J Obstet Gynecol 1981;139:669–672.
8. Flynn AM, Kelly J, Hollins G, Lynch PF: Ambulation in labour. BMJ 1978;2:591–593.
9. Hemminki E, Lenck M, Saarikoski S, Henriksson L: Ambulation versus oxytocin in protracted labour: A pilot study. Eur J Obstet Gynecol Reprod Biol 1985;20:199–208.
10. Calvert JP, Newcombe RG, Hibbard BM: An assessment of radiotelemetry in the monitoring of labour. Br J Obstet Gynaecol 1982;89:285–291.
11. Devoe LD, Arthur M, Searle N: The effects of maternal ambulation on the nonstress test. Am J Obstet Gynecol 1987;157:240–244.
12. McManus TJ, Calder AA: Upright posture and the efficiency of labour. Lancet 1978;1:72–74.

Diagnostic Strategies for "Threatened Preterm Labor"

James A. McGregor, Paul T. Wilkes,

and Carol Stamm

Spontaneous preterm labor continues as the leading cause of preterm birth and low birth weight. Preterm birth occurs in approximately 1 in 10 births in the United States. *Preterm labor* is defined as labor occurring before the completion of 37 weeks (<259 days from the last menstrual period).[1] Primary and secondary prevention of preterm birth are the preeminent challenges facing modern obstetric care providers, as well as the families they serve. Primary prevention is elimination or mitigation of original causes; secondary prevention is accurate diagnosis and effective treatment. Preterm labor syndrome has multiple, separate causes. Inaccurate diagnosis of preterm labor continues as a major obstacle to improving obstetric outcomes and providing clinically and cost-effective, etiology-based interventions.

Because fully one half of women treated are not in preterm labor, we analyze advances in accurate and cost-effective identification of women in early preterm labor. Timely identification of true preterm labor ("contractions" vs. "contractures") powerfully affects the potential efficacy of treatments such as tocolysis, corticosteroid treatment, and antimicrobial treatment or prophylaxis, as well as need for maternal transport, and so on. Avoidance of unnecessary, as well as costly and potentially harmful, treatments can be associated with reduction of costs and liabilities.[2]

Clinical preterm labor is defined as progressive cervical dilatation and/or effacement with regular contractions (usually at <10-minute intervals) leading to birth before 37 weeks' gestation, in the absence of effective treatment.[3] In the United States, the definition of preterm labor and preterm birth usually assumes a lower gestational age limit of 20 weeks from the last menses. The standard definitions of low birth weight (<2500 g), very low birth weight (<1500 g), and extremely low birth weight (<1000 g) imprecisely correlate with gestation length–based definitions: mildly preterm (32–36 weeks), very preterm (<32 weeks), and extremely preterm (<28 weeks).[4]

Extremely low birth weight or extremely preterm infants represent about 1% of American births but account for over 50% of perinatal mortality and morbidity.[1] Conversely, preterm birth at later gestational ages is less dangerous, but similarly costly, because many more preterm births occur at greater birth weights and gestational ages.[5]

Use of preterm labor diagnostic technologies, as well as clinical decision-making strategies regarding preterm labor, is influenced by knowledge of local circumstances regarding (1) probabilities for survival and morbidity, (2) likely etiologic mechanisms, and (3) potential liabilities and costs. Desirable bayesian performance characteristics of means to identify preterm labor depend on gestational age and available resources to safely prevent or mitigate the consequences of prematurity. For instance, enhanced sensitivity is more desirable if the consequences of prematurity are "costly" and treatments are available, effective, and safe. Conversely, specificity is more desirable if the consequences are not so "costly" or if treatments are ineffective, expensive, or potentially harmful. Positive predictive values are determined by the prevalence of the causative condition(s) in the population being served. Negative predictive values of preterm labor detection modalities frequently have been undervalued by clinicians. Tests with high negative predictive values can assist in identifying women who may safely avoid being exposed to unnecessary treatment-associated risks and costs.[5] Future research on diagnosis of preterm labor should usefully provide receiver operating characteristic (ROC) curves and other clinically relevant means to evaluate performance parameters at different gestational ages and birth weight categories in different model populations.

Other desirable features of diagnostic strategies for early or threatened preterm labor include information regarding (1) interobserver reliability, (2) accuracy in different populations, (3) putative pathologic mechanisms, (4) ease of use, and (5) cost-saving abilities. Pertinent clinical questions include (1) can early detection of preterm labor lead to beneficial interventions? (2) Is prompt delivery needed? (3) Is maternal transport or referral necessary? (4) Are treatable causes of preterm labor present? (5) Are treatments (e.g., tocolytics, corticosteroids, antimicrobials), indicated and safe?

"TRADITIONAL DIAGNOSIS"

The classic textbook diagnosis of true preterm labor (i.e., it would progressively lead to birth if untreated) is commonly defined as clinical detection of regular uterine contractions accompanied by cervical change (effacement or dilatation). The frequency of contractions is commonly

Table 2–1. Selected Studies of Fetal Fibronectin Test Positivity as a Predictor of Preterm Delivery in Patients with Intact Membranes

Study	Sensitivity (%)	Specificity (%)	PPV	NPV
Fetal Fibronectin				
Preterm delivery				
Iams[9]	44	86	60	76
Bartnicki[7]	68	90	79	83
Malak[8]	63	96	44	98
Delivery < 7 days				
Iams[9]	93	82	29	95
Bartnicki[7]	100	71	6	96
Malak[8]	80	90	44	98
Salivary Estriol				
Heine[10]				
1.4 μg/mL	61	76	88	42
2.1 μg/mL	29	92	44	94

NPV, negative predictive value; PPV, positive predictive value.

set at at least one every 10 minutes, with cervical length less than 1 cm and cervical dilatation of 2 cm or more. Meta-analysis shows that these criteria are only 50% predictive of preterm birth. Meta-analysis also shows that diagnosis of preterm labor primarily by assessment of uterine contractions is sensitive *but* not specific—that is, preterm birth occurs in 40% to 50% of mothers in controlled trials of tocolytics.[6] Assessment of contraction frequency, regularity, duration, and painfulness does not reliably distinguish preterm labor.[6]

Although sometimes dismissed by care providers, the mother's own "diagnosis" of preterm labor is frequently useful. In one study, 75% of women were correct in their estimation that "something was wrong" in that they either delivered preterm or were hospitalized for more than 48 hours for diagnostic or therapeutic measures. Multiparas were better than nulliparas in identifying preterm labor, which reinforces the importance of preterm labor detection education among all pregnant women.

Biomarkers of Preterm Labor

Improved methods of early diagnosis of preterm labor are clearly desirable. Since about 1990, multiple biomarkers of preterm labor have been evaluated. Several of these are approved by the U.S. Food and Drug Administration and are commercially available as laboratory, "bed side," or point-of-care tests,—that is, fetal fibronectin and salivary estriol. Other less thoroughly evaluated biomarkers include evidence of (1) cervical inflammation (e.g., white blood cells, interleukin-6 [IL-6] and -1, matrix metalloproteinase-8) [MMP-8], (2) bacterial vaginosis (pH > 4.5), and (3) decidual proteins (insulin-like growth factor 1, prolactin), as well as other endocrine/paracrine markers (corticotropin-releasing hormone [CRH], CRH-binding protein).

Preterm birth is preceded by separation of the maternal decidua and the fetal chorion, with subsequent increased cervical levels of the fetal isoform of fibronectin: fetal fibronectin (fFN). Separation can be caused by infection or inflammation, hemorrhage, overdistention, or contractions. Multiple controlled studies establish that increased fFN concentrations (>50 ng/mL) accurately and usefully identify symptomatic women who are at risk for preterm delivery or delivery within 7, 14, or 21 days (Table 2–1). Separate studies by Bartnicki and associates[7] and Malak and coworkers[8] specifically evaluated for early preterm labor in patients between 24 and 34 weeks' gestation who had little cervical dilatation (<2 cm) (see Table 2–1).

fFN is available as a rapid (60-min) test, whose accuracy is comparable to that of a centralized laboratory. Studies by Lopez and colleagues[11] and Joffe and associates[12] have evaluated fFN in actual use. Lopez and colleagues found the positive predictive value to be greater for delivery (P < .002) within 7 days than had been published in controlled trials. Emphasizing the usefulness of high negative predictive values (>96%), Joffe and associates were able to reduce preterm labor admissions, length of stay, and use of tocolysis, with estimated savings of $486,000 during the study period.

Researchers stress the importance of fFN collection before digital cervical examination. Samples can be set aside in a refrigerator and processed after the initial clinical evaluation is completed. Similar strategies are suggested for performance of cervicovaginal wet preparation, Gram stain, and pH, as well as collection of cervical inflammatory mediators or proteinase (MMP-8) and tests for bacterial vaginosis, *Chlamydia trachomatis*, other prevalent sexually transmitted infections, and bacteriuria or urinary tract infection.

Studies are under way to evaluate the efficacy of antimicrobial (metronidazole/erythromycin) and other interventions for the treatment of preterm labor in fFN-positive women. Therapeutic or preemptive antimicrobial treatment is likely to be most effective when administered before clinically detectable intrauterine infection or activation of labor mechanisms.

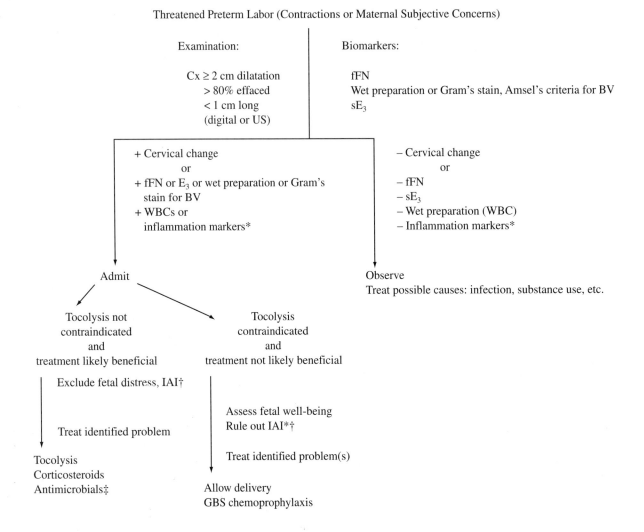

*IL-1, IL-6, MMP-8, if available.

†IAI (glucose <16 mg/dL), WBC (>50 cells/μL), interleukin-6 >11.3 ng/mL,
 Gram's stain positive bacteria.

‡GBS chemoprophylaxis, adjunctive erythromycin, clindamycin, or
 ampicillin plus metronidazole.

Figure 2–1. Author's recomended approach to "threatened preterm labor." BV, bacterial vaginosis; Cx, cervix; E_3, estriol; fFN, fetal fibronectin; GBS, group B streptococcus; IAI, intra-abdominal infection; IL, interleukin; MMP-8, matrix metalloproteinase–8; sE_3, salivary estriol; US, ultrasound; WBC, white blood cell.

FETAL ENDOCRINE/PARACRINE MARKERS OF PARTURITION

Salivary estriol (sE_3) testing is commercially available and measures tissue levels of estriol produced (<90%) in the placenta. Elevated sE_3 levels (as well as serum E_3) indicate fetal signaling for the onset of labor.[10] Heine and Robertson[10] demonstrated predictive values similar to those of fFN (see Table 2–1), despite not taking diurnal variation (estriol elevated at night) into account. Saliva is easy to obtain (no vaginal examination) and is stable (72 hr) without refrigeration. Saliva samples can be mailed by patients or refrigerated at home before laboratory testing. Cortico-

tropin-releasing factor (CRF) or CRH produced in the placenta and fetus drives estriol production in the placenta, but testing is not yet commercially available.

INFLAMMATION BIOMARKERS, PROTEASES, AND MARKERS OF DECIDUAL ACTIVATION

Preliminary studies show that combinations of cervicovaginal bacterial vaginosis (Amsel's criteria), cervical neutrophils (on wet preparation or Gram stain), or increased IL-6 are comparably predictive of progress in labor and preterm labor birth as well as fFN or sE_3. Others have shown that cervical MMP-8 or -9 are also highly predictive. Amniocentesis evidence of intra-abdominal infection (IAI) (increased IL-1, IL-6, tumor necrosis factor-α, MMP-8, neutrophils, positive Gram stain, culture) is also predictive of impending preterm birth. Identification of IAI should prompt urgent consideration of delivery and nursery treatment for perinatal infection if evidence of chorioamnionitis is confirmed. All women who are evaluated for preterm labor should receive evaluation and indicated treatment for locally common causes of preterm labor, including cervicitis, urinary tract infection/asymptomatic bacteriuria (UTI/ ASB), and substance use/abuse. Many at-risk mothers benefit from frequent phone call assessment and support or by receiving commercially available preterm labor surveillance services. We recommend selective media screening for group B streptococcus and evaluation and treatment of cervicitis (wet preparation microscopy) and UTI/ASB during all preterm labor evaluations (Fig. 2–1).

Other biomarkers of parturition (preterm or term) are being actively investigated but have not yet found a place in clinical practice for diagnosis of preterm labor. These include (1) cervical factors: intercellular adhesion molecule-1, IL-1, IL-8, tumor necrosis factor α, neopterin, prolactin, α-fetoprotein, and leukocyte esterase; (2) maternal serum markers: C-reactive protein, fFN, and multiple interleukins, and (3) amniotic fluid substances: multiple cytokines. Uterine electromyography is also being investigated.[13] Models have been constructed using a combination of clinical findings and multiple diagnostic tests. In preliminary studies, use of multidimensional "scoring" systems appears more accurate than do single-test diagnostic schemes.

Use of evidence-based diagnostic strategies (see Fig. 2–1) is intended to improve perinatal and maternal outcomes. Ongoing, local assessment of performance is imperative to ensure optimized care of women and children at risk from preterm birth. Increasingly accurate detection of preterm labor can be expected to enhance perinatal outcomes, improve timeliness of evidence-based, etiologically directed treatments, and reduce short- and long-term costs and liabilities.

References

1. American College of Obstetricians and Gynecologists: Preterm Labor (Technical Bulletin No. 206). Washington, DC, ACOG, June 1995.
2. American College of Obstetricians and Gynecologists: Fetal Fibronectin Preterm Labor Risk Test (Committee Opinion No. 187). Washington, DC, ACOG, September 1997.
3. McNamara HM, Vintzileos AM: The clinical approach to preterm labor. In Elder MG, Romero R, Lamont RF (eds): Preterm Labor, Churchill Livingstone, New York, 2000, pp 207–242.
4. Aylward GP, Pfeiffer SI, Wright A, et al: Outcome studies of low birth weight infants published in the last decades: A meta-analysis. J Pediatr 1989;115:515–520.
5. Nicholson WK, Frick KD, Powe NR: Economic burden of hospitalizations for preterm labor in the United States. Obstet Gynecol 2000;96:95–101.
6. King JF, Grant A, Keirse MJ, et al: Beta-mimetics in preterm labour: An overview of the randomised trials. Br J Obstet Gynaecol 1988;5:211–222.
7. Bartnicki J, Casal D, Kreaden US, et al: Fetal fibronectin in vaginal specimens predict preterm delivery and very low birth weight infants. Am J Obstet Gynecol 1996;174:971–974.
8. Malak TM, Sizmur F, Bell SC, et al: Fetal fibronectin in cervicovaginal secretions as a predictor of preterm birth. Br J Obstet Gynaecol 1996;103:648–653.
9. Iams JD, Casal D, McGregor JA, et al: Fetal fibronectin improves the accuracy of diagnosis of preterm labor. Am J Obstet Gynecol 1995;173:141–145.
10. Heine RP, McGregor JA, Goodwin TM, et al: Serial salivary estriol to detect increased risk of preterm birth. Obstet Gynecol 2000;96:4907.
11. Lopez RL, Francis JA, Garite TJ, et al: Fetal fibronectin detection as a predictor of preterm birth in actual practice. Am J Obstet Gynecol 2000;182:1103–1106.
12. Joffe GM, Jacques D, Bemis-Heys R, et al: Impact of fetal fibronectin assay on admission for preterm labor. Am J Obstet Gynecol 1999;180:581–586.
13. Garfield RE, Chwalisz K, Shi L, et al: Instrumentation for the diagnosis of term and preterm labour. J Perinat Med 1998;26:413–436.

Suggestions for Future Reading

Burrus DR, Ernest JM, Veille JC: Fetal fibronectin, interleukin-6, and C-reactive protein are useful in establishing prognostic subcategories of idiopathic preterm labor. Am J Obstet Gynecol 1995;173:1258–1262.
Gonzalez-Bosquet E, Cerqueira MJ, Dominguez C, et al: Amniotic fluid glucose and cytokine values in the early diagnosis of amniotic infection in patients with preterm labor and intact membranes. J Matern Fetal Med 1999;8:155–158.
Hitti J, Hillier SL, Agnew KJ, et al: Vaginal indicators of amniotic fluid infection among women in preterm labor. Obstet Gynecol 2001;97:211–219.
Macones GA, Segel SY, Stamilio Morgan MA: Prediction of delivery among women with early preterm labor by means of clinical characteristics alone. Am J Obstet Gynecol 1999;181:1414–1418.
McGregor JA, Jackson GM, Lachelin GC, et al: Salivary estriol as risk assessment for preterm labor: A prospective trial. Am J Obstet Gynecol 1995;173:1337–1342.
Tsatsaris V, Carbonne B, Cabrol D: The place of amniocentesis in the assessment of preterm labour. Eur J Obstet Gynecol Reprod Biol 2000;93:19–25.

Management of HIV in Pregnancy

Steven R. Inglis

HIV infection during pregnancy is regarded as an emergency that requires immediate attention to prevent serious consequences. Intensive patient education and cooperation must be coupled with time and attention from numerous providers. The effort must continue until delivery. The stakes are high because of the risk of vertical transmission, and the consequences for the infected newborn cannot be overstated. As success in the treatment of this infection continues and life spans are increased, vertical transmission from women to their offspring has taken on increasing importance. The proliferation of medications and paucity of research in pregnancy make recommendations for antiretroviral therapy during pregnancy increasingly complex. Management of HIV infection in pregnancy includes prevention of vertical transmission by stabilization of HIV disease and reduction of the viral load and prevention of opportunistic diseases. Assessment of social and medical risk factors in pregnancy is also important. This chapter begins with a discussion of the current status of HIV treatment in general and in pregnancy. This is followed with our current protocol for the management of HIV in pregnancy.

IS HIV DISEASE THE SAME IN MEN AND WOMEN?

In February of 1997, the U.S. Centers for Disease Control and Prevention (CDC) first released statistics for HIV and AIDS for the United States showing that deaths from AIDS had decreased by 14% for the first half of 1996.[1] New York State had previously reported the same trend, but it was thought to be a statistical aberration. This was hailed as the first proof of improved therapy and outcome for patients with HIV infection. Hidden in this report, and perhaps more importantly, the data showed much less improvement for women.

In fact, AIDS deaths increased by 4% for the same period for women. Why would women not be benefiting from the new therapies that were so successful in men? Possible explanations include delays in diagnosis or differences in treatment. Women might be treated differently secondary to intervening pregnancies or they might have an inherently different immune response. In fact, more recently a study was released on this question of a gender difference.[2] The Johns Hopkins School of Public Health studied 650 patients who had participated in research studies since 1988. These patients all had frozen samples of blood that were available for study, and the long-term outcome of these patients was available. The study found that those women with the same viral load as a man had a 60% higher risk of developing AIDS. At a given stage of disease, a woman's viral load was lower than a man's, even though her immune system had sustained similar damage. These researchers warned that those using the viral load as a benchmark may be misled into thinking that a woman is healthier than she really is. This difference is likely to be confirmed because others are reporting similar findings. These findings will likely add fuel to the debate regarding the best time for patients with HIV infection to initiate antiretroviral therapy. Most importantly, such findings bring into question whether guidelines for the general population are appropriate for women or their pregnancies.

TO TREAT OR NOT TO TREAT?

For the nonpregnant population, there is debate on when therapy should be started. Essentially, it depends on whether one feels it is acceptable for a patient to have detectable virus in the circulation and not treat it. It is possible to treat early before the immune system undergoes injury, but run the risk of inducing later viral resistance. Experts in the field differ widely on this question; some begin therapy early in the disease whereas others would not begin therapy if the CD4 count is between 350 and 500 as long as the viral load remains below 10,000 (bDNA) or below 20,000 (reverse transcriptase-polymerase-chain reaction [RT-PCR]). Table 3–1 summarizes the points of the debate regarding the risks and benefits of early intervention with antiretroviral therapy.

During pregnancy, treatment has a defined benefit for the unborn fetus by reducing the risk of vertical transmission. All patients should be offered zidovudine (ZDV) at 14 weeks' gestation. For pregnant women with HIV infection, management has been based on the Pediatric AIDS Clinical Trial Group (PACTG) 076 trial. In this trial, patients were randomized to oral ZDV or placebo starting at 14 weeks in the antepartum period, intravenous ZDV in the intrapartum period, and oral ZDV syrup for the neonate. The risk of vertical transmission may be reduced to as low as 8% with the use of ZDV.[3] As such, oral ZDV is recommended

Table 3–1. Risks and Benefits of Early Treatment of HIV for Nonpregnant Patients

Potential Benefits of Early Intervention with Antiretroviral Therapy
Control of viral replication and mutation, reduction of viral burden
Prevention of progressive immune system injury
Delay progression to AIDS and prolongation of life
Decrease risk of selection of resistant virus
Decrease risk of drug toxicity

Potential Risks of Early Intervention with Antiretroviral Therapy
Reduction in quality of life from adverse drug effects and the inconvenience of taking medications
Earlier development of drug resistance
Limitation in future choices of antiretroviral agent due to development of resistance
Unknown long-term toxicity of antiretroviral drugs
Unknown duration of effectiveness of current antiretroviral therapies

between 14 weeks of gestation and term and intravenous ZDV is recommended with a 2 mg/kg load and 1 mg/kg/hr continuous intravenous infusion during labor. Standard therapy also dictates that the neonate be treated with ZDV syrup in the postnatal period.

The prevailing wisdom for women on antiretrovirals when they become pregnant is that therapy continues during early pregnancy if their disease is controlled. Although many patients and their providers stop their medications during early pregnancy, we restart them either immediately or by 14 weeks' gestation.

SELECTION OF ANTIRETROVIRALS DURING PREGNANCY

At present, three main classes of antiretroviral medications are available. Nucleoside analogues were the first group and are similar to the nucleosides that make up DNA. Once the nucleoside analogue is bound by reverse transcriptase, the enzyme is blocked and unable to continue taking up nucleosides; hence, the name *chain terminator*. Production of new virus is blocked at an early stage of the reproductive cycle. Non-nucleoside reverse transcriptase inhibitors work at the level of the reverse transcriptase. They bind near the catalytic site of reverse transcriptase and inhibit the enzyme. Protease inhibitors work later in the viral reproductive cycle by preventing protease enzyme in the cell from cutting newly produced viral proteins into the smaller pieces used to make the viral capsule. The new viral particles are unable to be released because of a lack of viral proteins to make the viral capsule. Most recently, a new class of medications has been developed that blocks viral entry into the CD4 cells by interfering with binding to the cell wall. Table 3–2 gives the U.S. Food and Drug Administration's (FDA) Use-In-Pregnancy categories for the more commonly used antiretroviral agents. Table 3–3 lists the common side effects of these medications.

It is clear that combination therapy in nonpregnant patients leads to prolonged effectiveness as measured by lower viral loads and nonprogression to AIDS.[4–6] It is likely that combination therapy is successful because it more effectively shuts down viral turnover and therefore development of mutations. As such, the International AIDS Society has recommended that combination therapy be used as initial therapy in all cases. The future of triple and even quadruple therapy including a protease inhibitor looks promising. Long-term studies are addressing metabolic problems and possible solutions for these.

In pregnant women, the primary objectives are stabilizing HIV disease, preventing vertical transmission, and reducing the viral load. For pregnant women, antiretroviral therapy has historically centered on monotherapy with ZDV. This medication is well tolerated during pregnancy, but there is much concern regarding the development of resistance to ZDV. Minkoff and Augenbraun[7] recommended the use of combination therapy in pregnant women. The FDA categorization for each of the antiretroviral agents in Table 5–2 does not suggest undue risk from these medications.

The selection of which combination therapy to employ is complex in any patient and no less so for a pregnant woman. With the goal of avoiding vertical transmission, aggressive therapy and serial monitoring of viral loads are

Table 3–2. U.S. Food and Drug Administration Use-In-Pregnancy Ratings Antiretroviral Agents

Category	Interpretation	Antiretroviral Agent
A	Controlled studies show no risk. Adequate, well-controlled studies of pregnant women have failed to demonstrate risk to the fetus.	
B	No evidence of risk in humans. Either animal findings show risk, but human findings do not, or, if no adequate human studies have been done, animal findings are negative.	Didanosine* Saquinavir Ritonavir Nelfinavir
C	Risk cannot be ruled out. Human studies are lacking, and animal studies are either positive for fetal risk or lacking as well. However, potential benefit may justify potential risk and animal studies lacking.	ZDV Lamivudine Zalcitabine Stavudine* Nevirapine Delavirdine Indinavir Abacavir
D	Positive evidence of risk. Investigational or postmarketing data show risk to fetus. Nevertheless, potential benefits may outweigh potential risk.	
X	Contraindicated in pregnancy. Studies in animals or human or investigational or postmarketing reports have shown fetal risk that clearly outweighs any possible benefit to the patient.	

*Caution: Pregnant women using d4T (stavudine [Zerit]) and ddI (didanosine) may be at increased risk of severe lactic acidosis and liver toxicity. Avoid in pregnancy whenever possible.
ZDV, zidovudine.

indicated. The main factors involved in the selection of agents are the patient's previous and/or present use of antiretrovirals; viral load; CD4 count; the presence of AIDS, thrush, unexplained fevers or wasting; and patient motivation. The viral load is the most important predictor of vertical transmission, with the risk approaching zero as viral loads become undetectable.

For the antiretroviral-experienced pregnant woman, the selection of agents is individualized. Generally, we utilize the same regimen if it was well tolerated and effective in terms of viral suppression. ZDV is always incorporated into the combination. Table 3–4 contains our protocol for initiation of antiretroviral agents to antiretroviral-naïve women during pregnancy. It was formulated using outcome data from nonpregnant women.[8] ZDV remains the primary antiretroviral agent because of its significant effects on perinatal transmission of the virus. Lamivudine (3TC) is commonly the second agent and a protease inhibitor the third because of their excellent safety, side effect profile, patient acceptability, and proven efficacy in combination with ZDV.[5, 6] We find that this simple combination is well tolerated by HIV-positive pregnant women. Commonly, a profound drop in the viral load to "none detected" and an improved CD4 count are seen. The main benefit of adding this combination during pregnancy is the prolonged interval until the development of resistance with complete suppres-

Table 3–4. Guidelines for Antiretroviral Therapy in Pregnancy (Antiretroviral Naïve Patients)

Symptomatic (AIDS, thrush, unexplained fever), acute HIV infection, or within 6 mo of seroconversion, any value for tests	Immediate triple medication therapy including a protease inhibitor

CD4 Count	Viral Load	Recommended Therapy
Any	>10,000 copies/mL	Immediate triple medication therapy including a protease inhibitor
Any	<10,000 copies/mL	Delay until 14 wk of gestation; then initiate triple medication therapy including a protease inhibitor

sion of the virus. Development of resistance to ZDV with monotherapy after 6 months is very concerning, and ZDV resistance mutations can now be found during primary infections in 8% to 26% of cases. Triple combination therapies with the addition of protease inhibitors should be employed if there is failure of the initial antiretroviral regimen.

ZDV should be used as part of combination therapy during pregnancy almost without exception. This includes women with a virus known to be resistant to ZDV. If the patient had been on another nucleoside analogue, it can frequently be interchanged with ZDV, or ZDV can be added to the regimen. If the patient has failed to respond to a combination of medications, two other medications should be added and the ZDV continued. The dosage would optimally replicate the PACTG 076 trial of 100 mg five times per day. In the real world, this dosage schedule is close to impossible to maintain. We suggest using 200 mg three times a day or 300 mg twice a day. There is evidence that serum levels are sustained with the twice-daily dosing.

The viral load measurement has become the most important tool in terms of assessment of antiretroviral therapy. We expect a significant decrease in viral load after 1 to 2 months of antiretroviral therapy. If no decrease in the viral load is documented, either patient adherence (compliance) or a therapeutic failure secondary to resistance is considered. If a change in therapy is considered, two different agents are started. The goal of this therapy is to have a none-detected viral load.[9–11]

Table 3–3. Antiretroviral Classification and Side Effects

	Antiretroviral Agent	Toxicity/Side Effects
Nucleoside Analogues	Zidovudine (ZDV)	Anemia, neutropenia, GI upset, headache, myopathy
	Lamivudine (3TC)	Minimal toxicity
	Didanosine (ddl)	Pancreatitis, diarrhea, peripheral neuropathy
	Zalcitabine (ddC)	Peripheral neuropathy, pancreatitis, diarrhea
	Abacavir	Hypersensitivity reaction: malaise, low-grade fever, and rash
	Stavudine (d4T)	Peripheral neuropathy, pancreatitis
Non-Nucleoside Reverse Transcriptase Inhibitors	Nevirapine	Numerous drug interactions, severe rash
	Delavirdine	Numerous drug interactions, severe rash
Protease Inhibitors	Indinavir	Nephrolithiasis, numerous drug interactions, hyperbilirubinemia, metabolic abnormalities
	Saquinavir	Numerous drug interactions, GI disturbances, metabolic abnormalities
	Nelfinavir	Numerous drug interactions, severe diarrhea, metabolic abnormalities
	Ritonavir	Numerous drug interactions, GI disturbances, metabolic abnormalities, paresthesias

GI, gastrointestinal.

Special Considerations for HIV-Positive Pregnancies

Hyperemesis gravidarum deserves special mention because it is so common. In HIV-positive women, it is especially troublesome because of poor drug absorption, drug intolerance, and the development of viral resistance. In such cases, we stop all antiretroviral drugs until the patient is able to tolerate oral medications.

The choice of cesarean delivery is perhaps one of the most common questions raised relating to HIV in pregnancy. There is evidence that cesarean delivery can reduce the rate of vertical HIV transmission. In a prospective trial in Europe,[12] 188 women were randomized to cesarean delivery and had a significantly lower rate of vertical transmission (1.8%) compared with the 182 women randomized to vaginal delivery (10.5%, $P < .001$). However, among the 236 receiving ZDV prophylaxis, the reduction in transmission rate was smaller and not statistically significant. Further, the risk of vertical transmission may be lower with combination antiviral therapy. In a recent study using combination therapy including protease inhibitors,[13] there was no case of vertical transmission among the first 178 subjects, with a 95% confidence interval of 0% to 2%.

There is no evidence to support performing cesarean delivery for a woman who has an undetectable viral load.[13, 14] Ideally, counseling should be individualized and should be based on viral load and treatment. The American College of Obstetricians and Gynecologists has recently amended their recommendations.[15] The new recommendations are that women with greater than 1000 copies per milliliter should be counseled regarding the potential benefit of scheduled cesarean delivery to further reduce the risk of vertical transmission. Women who have not received antiviral therapy should be counseled that ZDV therapy alone reduces the risk of vertical transmission to 5% to 8%. Combined with ZDV therapy, a scheduled cesarean delivery reduces the risk to approximately 2%.

Expedited HIV testing in women in labor was mandated by state law in New York beginning in August 1999. Under the mandate, all women lacking a documented HIV test during the antenatal period were to be offered expedited HIV testing while in labor in order to obtain a preliminary (not confirmed with Western blot) result. If the result returned positive, the mother if still in labor was offered intrapartum ZDV and instructed to refrain from breastfeeding. Additionally, the newborn is offered ZDV to reduce the risk of vertical transmission. Thus far, this scheme has identified many HIV-positive mothers. The significant (and well-publicized) downside of the testing so far is that being told that the preliminary test was positive when the final result later returned negative traumatized many women. These mothers suffered extreme anxiety and distress during childbirth and had their babies treated with medications that were not needed and had unknown consequences. At this point, some hospitals in New York are trying different testing schemes to reduce the risk of false-positive results.

Conclusion

Identification of the HIV-positive pregnant woman remains the most important goal in this epidemic. In order to achieve this, all women must have prenatal care. Although access to prenatal care is generally available, many gravidas do not go for financial reasons, because of illegal alien status, because of lack of information regarding the importance of prenatal care, or because of difficulty negotiating the bureaucracy to obtain care. These women need to be brought into the health care system as early in pregnancy as possible. Further study into how to attract these women is needed and also into other ways to reduce the rate of vertical transmission in this country.

PROTOCOL FOR MANAGEMENT OF HIV IN PREGNANCY

Goals

- Prevention of vertical transmission of the infection
- Stabilization of HIV disease
- Reduction of viral load
- Prevention of opportunistic diseases
- Assessment of other social and medical risk factors for poor outcome

Assessment in Pregnancy

Comprehensive History

- *HIV history*—duration, symptomatology, CD4 count, viral load, current medications, current care (where and by whom), risk behaviors
- *Sexual history*—type of activity, number of partners, partners' HIV status, partner contact notification, use of condoms, other contraceptives, knowledge of safer sex, history of sexually transmitted diseases
- *Substance abuse history*—types of drug(s), route(s) of administration, frequency, amount, needle-sharing practices
- *Psychosocial status/support systems*—partner support, others with knowledge of serostatus, support from family and friends, history of physical and/or sexual abuse, coping skills, stage of acceptance of HIV infection, evidence of depression, suicidal ideation and/or attempts, history of psychiatric illness, history and risk assessment for physical and mental abuse, financial resources, health and life insurance

Review of Systems and Physical Examination

- *Constitutional*—fatigue, malaise, anorexia, weight loss, fever, night sweats
- *Dermatologic*—rash, sores (skin or mucosal), lesions (molluscum, Kaposi's), herpes, shingles, pruritus
- *Lymph nodes*—enlargement
- *Ophthalmologic*—decreases in vision, photophobia, pain, retinitis

- *Ear, nose, and throat*—sinusitis, oral lesions (thrush, oral hairy leukoplakia), gingivitis, bleeding, dentition, dysphagia and/or odynophagia
- *Respiratory*—cough, discolored sputum, shortness of breath, pain
- *Gastrointestinal*—diarrhea, nausea and/or vomiting, pain, hepatosplenomegaly
- *Genitourinary*—vaginal/vulvar irritation, genital lesions (ulcers, blisters, warts), abnormal vaginal discharge, pelvic pain, bleeding
- *Musculoskeletal*—myalgia, weakness, arthralgia
- *Neurologic*—memory impairment, cognitive changes, difficulty sleeping, headache, neuropathy (sensory and/or motor), balance, gait

Consultants

Maternal-fetal medicine, infectious disease, addiction medicine, hematology, ophthalmology, neurology, social work, nutrition and/or dietary

Initial Laboratory Screening

- If no documentation, repeat HIV serology testing.
- Viral load and CD4 count.
- Complete blood count (CBC) with differential and platelet counts.
- Rapid plasma reagin (RPR), hepatitis B surface antigen and antibody, hepatitis C antibody.
- Immunoglobulin G titers to cytomegalovirus and *Toxoplasma,* liver and renal profile.
- Drug screen.
- Cultures for *Chlamydia, Neisseria gonorrhoeae.*
- Wet mount for *Trichomonas,* possible evaluation for bacterial vaginosis.
- Pap smear.
- Genotype antiretroviral resistance testing if needed.

Repeat Laboratory Screening

- Drug screens monthly or more often in those with history of substance abuse or presently on a "program."
- CBC with platelets and liver profile monthly to monitor effects of antiretroviral therapy.
- Viral load and CD4 count every 2 to 3 months
- Tables 3–5 and 3–6 have laboratory data and flow sheets for monitoring HIV-positive women in pregnancy.

Tuberculosis Screening

- Purified protein derivative (PPD) intradermal screening used unless the patient is known to be PPD positive.
- Routine anergy testing is no longer recommended because false-positive anergy tests occur in patients with known tuberculosis infection and negative PPD skin tests.
- Read in 48 to 72 hours. Induration greater than 5 mm is positive; the patient is symptomatic or has been exposed to active tuberculosis.
- If chest x-ray is negative, some elect to postpone treatment until postpartum. Consider consulting infectious disease specialist if concerns arise. Alternatively, after the first trimester treat patients with isoniazid (INH), 300 mg PO every day, and pyridoxine, 50 mg PO every day, for 9 months.
- Active tuberculosis requires consultation with a specialist, because isolation may be required.

Immunizations and Behavioral Modification

- Obtain the CD4 count and viral load before any vaccinations.
- We routinely give pneumococcal and flu vaccines (when appropriate) in pregnancy. At present, we are not routinely using the hepatitis vaccine and tetanus vaccines. There are data suggesting that the viral load will show a rise in viral burden for a few weeks after vaccination.
- Risk behaviors such as unprotected intercourse, smoking, substance abuse, and increased stress should all be avoided because of the likelihood of increasing the viral load, speeding the disease process, and increasing the risk of vertical transmission.
- Counseling regarding substance abuse, with an emphasis on not using cocaine, is recommended.
- For those with negative *Toxoplasma* titers, counsel regarding keeping work areas and implements clean when working with raw or undercooked meats, avoiding cat litter and cat feces, avoiding work in gardens with cats in the vicinity.
- For those with negative cytomegalovirus titers, counsel regarding nurseries and preschool children, kissing of such children, and careful hand washing.
- Pneumococcal vaccine may be considered for patients who have never received the vaccine.
- Hepatitis B vaccine is given if there is a history of injection drug use, sexually transmitted diseases, or multiple partners.
- Nutrition is a variable that may be used to advantage. Nutrition counseling and consultation may offer suggestions regarding ways to enhance adequate weight gain and oral intake.
- Immune modulation in patients with HIV infection in pregnancy has not been well studied. For this reason, the use of interleukin-2, Remune vaccination, and strategic treatment interruptions to improve immune function and antibody response are avoided during pregnancy at this time.

Prophylaxis for Opportunistic Infections in Pregnancy

- There are increasing data regarding the safety of stopping prophylaxis for patients who have had improvement in

Table 3–5. Maternal-Fetal Medicine
HIV-Positive Pregnancy

DATA SHEET

Allergies:			
LMP:	EDD:		
Gr:	P:	Abortion:	Miscarriage:
TEST	DATE DONE	RESULTS	TREATMENT DATE
RPR	_____	_____	_____
GC/Chlamydia	_____	_____	_____
Hepatitis	_____	_____	_____
WBC	_____	_____	_____
Hb	_____	_____	_____
Hematocrit	_____	_____	_____
Blood Type	_____	_____	_____
Rh and Ab Screen	_____	_____	_____
U/A	_____	_____	_____
Rubella	_____	_____	_____
Glucose	_____	_____	_____
OTHER	_____	_____	_____

Sonogram Date	Weeks Gest:

MEDICATION Hx: _____

_____

OBSTETRIC Hx: _____

_____

COMMENTS: _____

_____

_____

_____

their CD4 counts above 200. At this point, it is not clear that these data apply to pregnant women as well.

- Decisions regarding prophylaxis are based on the lowest CD4 value obtained.
- *Pneumocystis carinii* pneumonia (PCP)

  Initiate prophylaxis when CD4 count is below 200, or with a previous history of PCP, unexplained fever (>100°F for more than 2 weeks), or oral candidiasis.

  Dosage: trimethoprim-sulfamethoxazole (TMP-SMX), 1 double-strength tablet PO every other day (e.g., Monday, Wednesday, Friday).

  Alternative dosage: TMP-SMX, 1 double-strength tablet PO every day.

  Dapsone, 100 mg PO every day.

  Aerosolized pentamidine, 300 mg every month via nebulizer.

- *Toxoplasma* infection

  Initiate prophylaxis when CD4 count is less than 100. Use TMP-SMX double strength, 1 tablet PO every day. Continue until delivery. Concerns regarding bilirubin and kernicterus in the neonate are unwarranted.

- *Mycobacterium avium* complex

  Initiate prophylaxis when CD4 count is less than 50. Use azithromycin (Zithromax), 1200 mg PO once a week.

Patient Counseling Regarding Antiretroviral Therapy in Pregnancy

- ZDV is indicated for all women, regardless of disease status, regardless of resistance, for the prevention of vertical transmission.
- Triple therapy is now commonly used as initial therapy, and, as such, it is reviewed with patients.

**Table 3–6. Maternal-Fetal Medicine
            HIV-Positive Pregnancy**

FLOW SHEET

PATIENT BASELINE DATA		
NAME:	DATE:	

FINDING	YES / NO	FINDING	YES / NO	FINDING
Thrush	Y N	Crypto	Y N	CD4 by Hx_____
Esophagitis	Y N	Toxoplasma	Y N	Toxo/CMV Titer_____
TB	Y N	CMV	Y N	Hep B Ag_____
Pneumonia	Y N	Hepatitis	Y N	Hep B Ab_____
PCP	Y N	Anergic	Y N	Hep C Ab_____
ITP	Y N	G6PD NL	Y N	Year Dx_____
Syphilis	Y N	PPD_____		Year First Rx_____
Zoster	Y N	CXR_____		Pneumovax_____

OTHER: **MEDS:**

DATE	Meds	Hb Hct	WBC GRAN	PLT CT	AST ALT	BILI	BUN Cr	CD4	V.L.	COMMENT

Medication Abbreviations:
A: Retrovir   V: Saquinavir
B: Bactrim   S: Dapsone
C: ddC   T: 3TC
D: ddI   X: Indinavir
F: Fluconazole   Z: Stavudine
P: Pentamidine   M: Zithromax
N: Ritonavir

- Drug adherence is essential for all antiretroviral therapies.
- For women already on antiretrovirals in early pregnancy, we usually continue the previous regimen.
- If any antiretroviral is stopped in early pregnancy, then all antiretrovirals should be stopped.
- Antiretrovirals can be restarted immediately or at 12 to 14 weeks' gestation.
- Add ZDV to all combination regimens.

Guidelines for Antiretroviral Therapy in Pregnancy

- ZDV monotherapy is avoided.
- Antiretroviral therapy is generally started at 14 weeks' gestation, although it may be initiated at any time.
- All patients, regardless of CD4 count or viral load, are candidates for ZDV therapy.

- Document informed consent regarding the antiretroviral therapy planned.
- Monthly CBC with differential to assess bone marrow suppression (macrocytosis is an indication of compliance).
- Monthly liver profile to assess for toxicity.
- CD4 count and viral load every 2 to 4 months.
- Consider discontinuing ZDV if hemoglobin is less than 8 g/dL or absolute neutrophil count is less than 750 cells/μL.
- Therapy options for ZDV-induced anemia
    Start erythropoietin (EPO), 100 to 200 units/kg three times a week SC, and continue ZDV.
    Await bone marrow recovery, then reinstate ZDV therapy.
    Transfuse and continue ZDV.
    Switch to alternative antiretroviral therapy.
- Goal is no detectable virus at 3 to 4 months using an assay with a threshold of less than 500 copies/mL and less than 50 copies/mL if possible.
- Tables 3–5 and 3–6 have laboratory data and flow sheets for monitoring HIV-positive women in pregnancy.

Changing an Antiretroviral Regimen for Suspected Drug Failure in Pregnancy

- Criteria for a change in therapy
    Detectable viral load after 3 to 4 months of therapy.
    Reappearance of viremia after suppression to an undetectable level.
    Significant increases in plasma viremia from the nadir of suppression.
- When the decision to change therapy is based on viral load determination, it is preferable to confirm the viral load with a second specimen.
- Distinguish between the need to change a regimen owing to drug intolerance or inability to comply with regimen and drug failure.
- In the event of drug failure, add at least two new agents.
- Consider the use of genotype antiretroviral resistance testing.
- Protease inhibitors should be used in combination therapy, in full dose, and with good drug compliance.
- Avoid changing from ritonavir to indinavir or vice versa for drug failure, because high level cross-resistance is likely.
- Avoid changing from nevirapine to delavirdine or vice versa for drug failure, because high level cross-resistance is likely.
- Do not measure viral load within 1 month of an acute illness or immunization.
- Possible alternative regimens if maternal status warrants
    ZDV + didanosine (ddI)
    ZDV + 3TC
    ZDV + 3TC + nevirapine
    ZDV + 3TC + protease inhibitor

Therapy during Labor and Delivery

- During labor, continue oral antiretrovirals with sips of water, except change the ZDV to intravenous therapy at 2 mg/kg loading dose, then 1 mg/kg/hr.
- When the infusion is stopped after the delivery, oral antiretroviral therapy is resumed.
- Avoid amniocentesis, prolonged rupture of the membranes, artificial rupture of membranes, long labors, fetal scalp sampling, internal scalp electrodes, intrauterine pressure monitors, instrumental delivery, and episiotomy because they appear to increase vertical transmission of the virus.
- Cesarean delivery during labor is inadequately studied to be offered as a means to reduce the risk of vertical transmission (see Special Considerations for HIV-Positive Pregnancies section).
- Use wall suction for meconium.
- Obtain cord blood samples by draining the cord.

Postpartum Management

- Breastfeeding is contraindicated; rubella vaccine is given if indicated.
- Sterilization is performed if requested.
- Contraception counseling should have no major alterations from standard recommendations. Encourage use of latex condoms, levonorgestrel (Norplant), and medroxyprogesterone acetate (Depo-Provera). An intrauterine device (IUD) appears safe. Some protease inhibitors may reduce efficacy of oral contraceptives.
- Arrange for ongoing maternal and pediatric medical care and social services.
- Arrange for ongoing infectious disease management of HIV disease.

References

1. U.S. Centers for Disease Control and Prevention: Update: Trends in AIDS incidence, deaths, prevalence—United States, 1996. MMWR Morb Mortal Wkly Rep 1997;46:165–173.
2. Farzadegan H, Hoover DR, Astemborski J, et al: Sex differences in HIV-1 viral load and progression to AIDS. Lancet 1998;352:1510–1514.
3. Connor EM, Sperling RS, Gelber R, et al: Reduction of maternal-infant transmission of human immunodeficiency virus type 1 with ZDV treatment. N Engl J Med 1994;331:1173–1180.
4. Delta: A randomized double-blind controlled trial comparing combinations of ZDV plus didanosine or zalcitabine with ZDV alone in HIV infected individuals: Delta Coordinating Committee. Lancet 1996;348:283–291.
5. Eron JJ, Benoit SI, Jemsek J, et al: Treatment with lamivudine, ZDV or both in HIV-positive patients 200–500 per cubic millimeter: North America HIV Working Party. N Engl J Med 1995;333:1662–1669.
6. Hammer SM, Katzenstein DA, Hughes MD, et al: A trial comparing nucleoside monotherapy with combination therapy in HIV-infected adults with CD4 cell counts from 200–500 per cubic millimeter: AIDS Clinical Trials Group Study 175 Study Team. N Engl J Med 1996;335:1081–1090.
7. Minkoff H, Augenbraun M: Antiretroviral therapy for pregnant women. Am J Obstet Gynecol 1997;176:478–489.
8. Carpenter CC, Fischl MA, Hammer SM, et al: Antiretroviral therapy

for HIV infection in 1997: Updated Recommendations of the International AIDS Society—USA panel. JAMA 1997;277:1962–1969.

9. O'Brien WA, Hartigan PM, Martin D, et al: Changes in plasma HIV-1 RNA and CD4 + lymphocyte counts and the risk of progression to AIDS: Veterans Affairs Cooperative Study Group. N Engl J Med 1996;334:426–431.

10. Mellors JW, Kingsley LA, Rinaldo CR Jr, et al: Quantitation of HIV-1 RNA in plasma predicts outcome after seroconversion. Ann Intern Med 1995;122:573–579.

11. Saksela K, Stevens CE, Rubinstein P, et al: HIV-1 messenger RNA in peripheral blood mononuclear cells as an early marker of risk for progression to AIDS. Ann Intern Med 1995;123:641–648.

12. Parazzini F, for the European Mode of Delivery Collaboration: Elective cesarean section versus vaginal delivery in the prevention of vertical HIV-1 transmission: A randomized controlled trial. Lancet 1999;353:1035–1039.

13. Stringer JSA, Rouse DJ, Goldenberg RL: Prophylactic cesarean delivery for the prevention of perinatal human immunodeficiency virus transmission: The case for restraint. JAMA 1999;281:1946–1949.

14. Star J, Powrie R, Cu-Uvin S, Carpenter CCJ: Should women with human immunodeficiency virus be delivered by cesarean? Obstet Gynecol 1999;94:799–801.

15. The American College of Obstetricians and Gynecologists: Scheduled cesarean delivery and the prevention of vertical transmission of HIV infection (Committee Opinion No. 234). Washington, DC, American College of Obstetricians and Gynecologists, May 2000.

Four

Implications of Bacterial Vaginosis in Obstetrics

Sharon L. Hillier

The role of bacterial vaginosis (BV) in complications of pregnancy has been the subject of over 25 publications since about 1980. This common vaginal syndrome has been associated with spontaneous abortion, preterm delivery, histologic chorioamnionitis, intra-amniotic infection, and postpartum endometritis. Although the data linking BV with adverse outcomes of pregnancy are very consistent, the results of treatment trials evaluating the effectiveness of antibiotic therapy in preventing these outcomes have been much more variable. In this chapter, the data linking BV with adverse outcomes of pregnancy are reviewed briefly, the results of published clinical trials are summarized, and the implications of these data in management of pregnant women with BV are discussed.

BV is a very common type of vaginal infection in pregnant women. In large cross-sectional studies evaluating thousands of American women seeking prenatal care, it has been found that between 8% and 20% of women have this condition.[1-4] The cause of BV is thought to be due to the replacement of vaginal lactobacilli with a mixed flora consisting of *Gardnerella vaginalis*, obligately anaerobic gram-negative rods, and genital mycoplasmas. Longitudinal studies have found that women are more likely to acquire BV when they douche routinely for hygiene or have exposure to multiple sexual partners.[5, 6] However, many women who are in monogamous relationships and who do not practice douching still acquire BV. The primary biologic risk factor for acquisition of BV appears to be the absence of lactobacilli that produce H_2O_2. Because H_2O_2-producing strains of lactobacilli are better able to sustain themselves in the vaginal ecosystem, women colonized by these strains are more resistant to infection.

BV can be diagnosed in pregnant women in a number of different ways. The most widely accepted clinical criteria for diagnosis include vaginal pH greater than 4.5, detection of clue cells on wet mount, and the release of an amine (fishy odor) after addition of 10% potassium hydroxide to the discharge. There are two commercially available point-of-care tests that can be used to screen for BV. One of these tests relies on detection of elevated pH and the presence of amine in a colorimetric card format (Fem Exam Testcard, Cooper Surgical, Shelton, Conn.). A second point-of-care test is a rapid colorimetric test to detect proline iminopeptidase, an enzyme produced by *G. vaginalis*. This test is produced by Litmus Concepts, Santa Clara, Calif.

Laboratory testing for BV can be conducted most simply through the evaluation of Gram-stained vaginal smears. A method for interpretation of vaginal smears for diagnosis of BV was developed by Nugent and colleagues.[7] This standardized method has now been widely used in laboratories throughout the world. Although this method is reproducible, it is usually performed in clinical laboratories and is therefore not an optimal point-of-care test. There is one DNA probe–based test for diagnosis of vaginitis in clinical laboratories (Affirm VP III, Becton Dickinson Corp., Sparks, Md). This automated system detects high concentrations of *G. vaginalis* while simultaneously incorporating probes for detection of yeast and *Trichomonas vaginalis*. This test is available generally in commercial laboratories and would have a turnaround time similar to that of the Gram stain. Vaginal cultures are not recommended as a method for diagnosis of BV for either pregnant or nonpregnant women because of their low specificity.

Many researchers have focused on evaluating the association between BV and preterm delivery. As shown in Table 4–1, a wide variety of studies have been conducted by investigators from around the world. Several of the early studies evaluated whether or not women delivering preterm were more likely to have BV than women delivering at term. One valid criticism of these cross-sectional studies was that there was no evidence that the presence of BV preceded development of preterm labor. However, later studies did document that women who had BV diagnosed in the first or second trimester of pregnancy were more likely to deliver preterm. These studies came from a wide variety of women living under very different conditions, having different diets and different cultural backgrounds. For example, the study by Kurki and associates[12] evaluated low-risk primigravidas attending a prenatal clinic in Finland, whereas the study by Riduan and coworkers[13] focused entirely on a low-income group of women in Jakarta, Indonesia. The consistency of the relationship between BV and preterm birth in women having very different lifestyles, races, and exposure to other risk factors for preterm delivery suggests that BV was not a marker for another lifestyle characteristic.

The first studies of BV treatment used intravaginal clindamycin cream versus placebo in women with BV[17-20] (Table 4–2). The hypothesis for all of the studies was that women who received clindamycin cream treatment in the second trimester of pregnancy would be more likely to

Table 4–1. Epidemiologic Data on Bacterial Vaginosis and Increased Risk of Preterm Delivery

Author	Year	Country	Women (N)	Enrollment (wk)	OR (95% CI)
Eschenbach et al[8]	1984	U.S.	171	Delivery	3.1 (1.6–6.1)
Gravett et al[9]	1986	U.S.	534	13–41	2.0 (1.1–3.5)
Gravett et al[9]	1986	U.S.	88	Delivery	3.8 (1.2–11.6)
Martius et al[10]	1988	U.S.	212	Delivery	2.3 (1.1–5.0)
McGregor et al[11]	1990	U.S.	202	24	1.5 (0.2–14.2)
Kurki et al[12]	1992	Finland	790	8–17	6.9 (2.5–18.8)
Riduan et al[13]	1993	Indonesia	490	16–20	2.0 (1.0–3.9)
Holst et al[14]	1994	Sweden	87	Delivery	2.1 (1.2–3.7)
Hay et al[4]	1994	U.K.	461	<16	5.5 (2.3–13.3)
Meis et al[15]	1995	U.S.	2929	28	1.8 (1.2–2.3)
Hillier et al[16]	1995	U.S.	10,397	23–26	1.4 (1.1–1.8)

CI, confidence interval; OR, odds ratio.

deliver at term than placebo-treated women. In these studies, clindamycin cream treatment was found to be effective in eradicating the abnormal flora associated with bacterial vaginosis. However, these four studies failed to document a reduction in the incidence of preterm birth in the women who received clindamycin cream. Surprisingly, in two of the studies there was a trend toward an *increased* incidence of low birth weight among women who received the active agent.[18, 20] In 1995, McGregor and coworkers[1] published a prospective two-phase study evaluating the effect of oral clindamycin therapy on prevention of preterm birth. In this study, women who were not routinely treated for BV had an incidence of preterm delivery of 19% compared with 10% in women given oral clindamycin at a dosage of 300 mg twice daily for 7 days. These studies were interpreted as suggesting that oral but not vaginal clindamycin prevented preterm delivery. One hypothesis proposed to explain the apparent discrepancy in these trials was that upper tract infection could be the mechanism by which BV caused preterm birth. Thus, vaginal therapy would be likely to be less successful than oral therapy in preventing preterm birth.

Oral metronidazole has been evaluated for its effect on prevention of preterm delivery in four published studies

(Table 4–3). Morales and associates[21] evaluated a group of 80 women who had previously delivered preterm and found that women who were treated with oral metronidazole had a 50% decreased incidence of repeat preterm birth compared with the placebo-treated women. McDonald and coworkers[22] conducted a study in relatively low-risk women in Adelaide, Australia, and found that there was no significant decrease in the incidence of preterm birth in women receiving metronidazole. These data are similar to those of a recent large, randomized, placebo-controlled study by Carey and colleagues[2] of oral metronidazole, 2 g given twice 2 days apart in the second trimester and again 1 month later. Although BV resolved in 77.8% of the cohort treated with metronidazole compared with 37.4% receiving placebo, there was no effect on the incidence of preterm delivery, even among women who had previously delivered preterm. In 1995, Hauth and coworkers[3] compared treatment with both metronidazole and erythromycin to placebo. They found that treatment with a combination of antibiotics did reduce the incidence of preterm birth among women at high risk.

The inconsistency of the BV treatment studies has led many clinicians to conclude that BV is not a cause of preterm delivery. Others have speculated that many of the trials had been flawed in their design or execution. Some investigators have speculated that metronidazole alone is insufficient to eradicate the organisms that can ascend to cause upper genital tract infection in women. Others have speculated that the dosage of metronidazole or clindamycin used was adequate to treat local vaginal infection, but inadequate to eradicate organisms from the upper genital tract. Other investigators have argued that treatment would have been more successful had it been provided earlier in pregnancy. These researchers have argued that treatment in the second trimester is simply too little, too late, to prevent adverse pregnancy outcomes. Whatever the reasons accounting for the discrepancy of results in these studies, it has left an area of great confusion among physicians who care for pregnant women.

If BV causes preterm delivery through the mechanism of silent upper genital tract infection, then one might expect

Table 4–2. Clindamycin for Prevention of Preterm Birth among Women with Bacterial Vaginosis

Author	Year	Preterm Birth	
		Treatment Group	*Comparison Group**
Intravaginal			
McGregor et al[17]	1994	9/60 (15%)	5/69 (7%)
Joesoef et al[18]	1995	51/340 (15%)	46/341 (14%)
Vermuelen and Bruinse[19]	1999	23/83 (28%)	18/85 (21%)
Kurkinen-Raty et al[20]	2000	7/51 (14%)	3/50 (6%)
Oral			
McGregor et al[1]	1995	19/194 (10%)	31/165 (19%)

*All studies except McGregor et al[1] included a placebo control.

Table 4–3. Oral Metronidazole for Prevention of Preterm Birth among Women with Bacterial Vaginosis

| Author | Year | Dosage | Enrollment Gestation (wk) | Preterm Birth | | P Value |
				Treatment Group	Placebo Group	
Morales et al[21]	1994	250 mg tid × 7 days	3–20	8/44 (18%)	14/36 (39%)	<.05
McDonald et al[22]	1997	400 mg bid × 2 days	24	11/242 (5%)	15/238 (6%)	NS
Carey et al[2]	2000	2 g × 2 days, 2 days apart	16–24	116/953 (12%)	121/966 (13%)	NS
Hauth et al[3]	1995	250 mg tid × 7 days plus erythromycin × 14 days	<24	54/172 (31%)	42/86 (49%)	.006

NS, not significant.

to see that pregnant women with BV would be more likely to have an increased incidence of spontaneous abortion and late miscarriage. In fact, there is a growing body of data suggesting that women with BV are substantially more likely to suffer a pregnancy loss compared with women with normal vaginal microflora. Three studies have shown an association between BV and second trimester spontaneous abortion. Hay and colleagues[4] found that the frequency of late miscarriage was 6% among women with BV and 1% among women with normal vaginal flora ($P < .008$). McGregor and his coworkers[1] similarly found that 4.4% of 305 women with BV had a second trimester spontaneous abortion compared with 1.4% of women negative for BV. Finally, Llahi-Camp and associates[23] conducted a retrospective study of women attending a recurrent miscarriage clinic. Women who had never had a term pregnancy but who had at least three previous second trimester spontaneous abortions were more likely to have BV (26%) than were women who were having a first trimester spontaneous abortion (8%). Most recently, a study conducted in women undergoing in vitro fertilization found that pregnancy rates were similar for women without bacterial BV, but that spontaneous pregnancy loss was substantially higher among women with BV than in those having normal vaginal flora.[24]

Other data supporting upper genital tract infection in BV in the second trimester have also been provided by studies evaluating the association between BV and histo-

logic chorioamnionitis and amniotic fluid infection (Table 4–4). In 1988, Hillier and colleagues[25] reported that women with BV were significantly more likely to have histologic evidence of chorioamnionitis in the placentas at delivery. Later studies documented that the organisms recovered from the chorioamnion of women with chorioamnionitis were frequently those recovered from women having BV.[29] Further, these studies, conducted among women in preterm labor with intact fetal membranes, demonstrated that organisms found in the vagina of women with BV were able to infect the amniotic fluid and invite production of inflammatory cytokines that can induce labor.[29] Taken together, these studies suggest that the pathogens found in the vagina of women with BV can and do ascend into the upper genital tract.

The consistency of data linking BV with adverse outcomes of pregnancy would suggest that treatment of BV should prevent a sizable proportion of this morbidity. However, the conflicting results of the treatment trials performed to date suggest that simple treatment of BV is inadequate to prevent the sequelae of this condition. The conflicting studies have demonstrated that our understanding of the pathophysiology and the mechanisms by which infection causes preterm birth is too rudimentary to guide the design of interventional trials. Clearly, additional research is needed to clarify the best time to detect and treat BV, the appropriate medication for treatment in pregnancy, and the mechanisms by which these organisms incite pre-

Table 4–4. Bacterial Vaginosis Linked to Upper Genital Tract Infections Known to Be Associated with Preterm Birth

Author	Year	Outcome	OR (95% CI)
Gravett et al[9]	1986	Amnionitis*	2.1 (1.1–3.9)
Hillier et al[25]	1988	Chorioamnionitis†	2.6 (1.0–6.6)
		Chorioamnion infection‡	3.2 (1.1–6.6)
Silver et al[26]	1989	Intra-amniontic infection§	2.6 (1.1–6.6)
Watts et al[27]	1990	Intra-amniotic infection§	6.8 (3.6–12.7)
Krohn et al[28]	1995	Intra-amniotic infection§	1.5 (1.1–2.2)
Hillier et al[29]	1995	Amnionitis* (intact membranes)	1.9 (1.1–3.3)

*Presence of bacteria in amniotic fluid obtained by transabdominal amniocentesis.
†Histologic chorioamnionitis.
‡Bacteria recovered from between the chorion and the amnion.
§Fever during labor and other clinical signs of amniotic fluid infection during labor.
CI, confidence interval; OR, odds ratio.

term labor. There is a complex interaction between the maternal immune system and the infectious insult presented in women with BV. Whereas most women with BV deliver at term, a small subset develops obstetric complications. Having a clear understanding of the women who are truly at risk for these complications will suggest how studies should be designed and interventions targeted to those women at greatest risk.

What should clinicians do today in their care of pregnant women with BV? There are no clear answers, and different experts recommend different strategies. Some practitioners have argued that we do not know how to prevent preterm birth due to BV, and therefore should treat BV in pregnant women primarily to relieve symptoms. Therefore, these authorities would suggest that only women complaining of symptoms should be evaluated and treated for BV. Other experts have argued that treatment of BV in asymptomatic women at high-risk for preterm delivery has been shown to be effective in some studies. Therefore, these practitioners could argue that treatment should be offered to all high-risk women having BV in addition to low-risk women having symptoms. Finally, some experts have argued that women should be informed if they have BV, even those at low risk, and that women should be offered the opportunity to request therapy if they choose to do so. In the absence of compelling data supporting one treatment strategy over another, providers of obstetric care may have to develop practice recommendations based on the characteristics of the populations they serve.

References

1. McGregor JA, French JI, Parker R, et al: Prevention of premature birth by screening and treatment for common genital tract infections: Results of a prospective controlled evaluation. Am J Obstet Gynecol 1995;173:157–167.
2. Carey JC, Klebanoff MA, Hauth JC, et al: Metronidazole to prevent preterm delivery in pregnant women with asymptomatic bacterial vaginosis. N Engl J Med 2000;342:534–540.
3. Hauth JC, Goldenberg RL, Andrews WW, et al: Reduced incidence of preterm delivery with metronidazole and erythromycin in women with bacterial vaginosis. N Engl J Med 1995;333:1732–1736.
4. Hay PE, Lamont RF, Taylor-Robinson D, et al: Abnormal bacterial colonization of the genital tract and subsquent preterm delivery and late miscarriage. BMJ 1994;308:295–298.
5. Hawes E, Hillier SL, Benedetti J, et al: Hydrogen peroxide–producing lactobacilli and acquisition of vaginal infections. J Infect Dis 1996;174:1058–1063.
6. Borbone F, Austin H, Louv WC, Alexander WJ: A follow-up study of methods of contraception, sexual activity, and rates of trichomoniasis, candidiasis, and bacterial vaginosis. Am J Obstet Gynecol 1990;163:510–514.
7. Nugent RP, Krohn MA, Hillier SL: The reliability of diagnosing bacterial vaginosis is improved by a standardized method of Gram stain interpretation. J Clin Microbiol 1991;29:297–301.
8. Eschenbach DA, Gravett MG, Chen K, et al: Bacterial vaginosis during pregnancy: An association with prematurity and postpartum complications. Scand J Urol Nephol 1985;86:213–222.
9. Gravett MG, Nelson HP, DeRouen T, et al: Independent associations of bacterial vaginosis and Chlamydia trachomatis infection with adverse pregnancy outcome. JAMA 1986;256:1899–1903.
10. Martius J, Krohn MA, Hillier SL, et al: Relationships of vaginal Lactobacillus species, cervical Chlamydia trachomatis, and bacterial vaginosis to preterm birth. Obstet Gynecol 1988;71:89–95.
11. McGregor JA, French JI, Richter R, et al: Antenatal microbiologic and maternal risk factors associated with prematurity. Am J Obstet Gynecol 1990;163:1465–1473.
12. Kurki T, Sivonen A, Renkonen OV, et al: Bacterial vaginosis in early pregnancy and pregnancy outcome. Obstet Gynecol 1992;80:173–177.
13. Riduan JM, Hillier SL, Utoma B, et al: Bacterial vaginosis and prematurity in Indonesia: Association in early and late pregnancy. Am J Obstet Gynecol 1993;169:175–178.
14. Holst E, Goffeng AR, Andersch B: Bacterial vaginosis and vaginal microorganisms in idiopathic premature labor and association with pregnancy outcome. J Clin Microbiol 1994;32:176–186.
15. Meis P, Goldenberg R, Iams J, et al: Vaginal infections and spontaneous preterm birth [abstract]. Am J Obstet Gynecol 1995;172:410.
16. Hillier SL, Nugent RP, Eschenbach DA, et al: The association between bacterial vaginosis and preterm delivery of a low-birth-weight infant. N Engl J Med 1995;333:1732–1736.
17. McGregor JA, French JI, Jones W, et al: Bacterial vaginosis is associated with prematurity and vaginal fluid mucinase and sialidase: Results of a controlled trial of topical clindamycin cream. Am J Obstet Gynecol 1994;170:1048–1060.
18. Joesoef MR, Hillier SL, Wiknjosastro G, et al: Intravaginal clindamycin treatment for bacterial vaginosis: Effects on preterm delivery and low birth weight. Am J Obstet Gynecol 1995;173:1527–1531.
19. Vermeulen GM, Bruinse HW: Prophylactic administration of clindamycin 2% vaginal cream to reduce the incidence of spontaneous preterm birth in women with an increased recurrence risk: A randomised placebo-controlled double-blind trial. Br J Obstet Gynecol 1999;106:652–657.
20. Kurkinen-Raty M, Vuopala S, Koskela M, et al: A randomised controlled trial of vaginal clindamycin for early pregnancy bacterial vaginosis. Br J Obstet Gynecol 2000;107:1427–1432.
21. Morales WJ, Schorr S, Albritton J: Effect of metronidazole in patients with preterm birth in preceding pregnancy and bacterial vaginosis: A placebo-controlled, double-blind study. Am J Obstet Gynecol 1994;171:345–349.
22. McDonald HM, O'Loughlin JA, Vigneswaran R, et al: Impact of metronidazole therapy on preterm birth in women with bacterial vaginosis flora (Gardnerella vaginalis): A randomized, placebo controlled trial. Br J Obstet Gynaecol 1997;104:1391–1397.
23. Llahi-Camp JM, Rai R, Ison C, et al: Association of bacterial vaginosis with a history of second trimester miscarriage. Hum Reprod 1996;11:1575–1578.
24. Ralph SG, Rutherford AJ, Wilson JD: Influence of bacterial vaginosis on conception and miscarriage in the first trimester: Cohort study. BMJ 1999;319:220–223.
25. Hillier SL, Martius J, Krohn MA, et al: A case controlled study of chorioamnioic infection and histologic chorioamnionitis in prematurity. N Engl J Med 1988;319:972.
26. Silver HM, Sperling RS, St. Clair PJ, Gibbs RS: Evidence relating bacterial vaginosis to intraamniotic infection. Am J Obstet Gynecol 1989;161:808–812.
27. Watts DH, Krohn MA, Hillier SL, Eschenbach DA: Bacterial vaginosis as a risk factor for postcesarean section endometritis. Obstet Gynecol 1990;75:244–248.
28. Krohn MA, Hillier SL, Nugent RP, et al: The genital flora of women with intraamniotic infection. J Infect Dis 1995;171:1475–1480.
29. Hillier SL, Krohn MA, Cassen E, et al: The role of bacterial vaginosis and vaginal bacteria in amniotic fluid infection in women in preterm labor with intact fetal membranes. Clin Infect Dis 1995;20(Suppl 2):S276–S278.

FIVE

Controversies Involving Antenatal Corticosteroids

Ronald J. Wapner, Donald J. Dudley, and

Michelle M. DiVito

Since the initial observations of Liggins and Howie in the late 1960s,[1] the maternal administration of antenatal steroids to minimize the effects on the neonate of preterm birth has become an accepted intervention. Corticosteroid-exposed neonates born between 24 and 34 weeks' gestation demonstrate significant reductions in mortality (odds ratio [OR] = 0.6), respiratory distress syndrome (RDS; OR = 0.5), and intraventricular hemorrhage (IVH; OR = 0.4). Reductions in the frequency of necrotizing enterocolitis (NEC) and hyperbilirubenemia have also been described. This dramatic improvement has been accomplished with minimal to no maternal or fetal short- or long-term complications when a single course of either betamethasone or dexamethasone is administered within 7 days of birth. These observations led a National Institutes of Health (NIH) consensus panel to conclude in 1994[2] that the benefits of antenatal corticosteroids to fetuses at risk of preterm delivery vastly outweigh the potential problems.

What is unclear is whether repeat doses of corticosteroids are required and safe when an at-risk pregnancy remains in utero more than 1 week after the initial course. In these women, it has become common practice to readminister corticosteroids every 7 to 10 days until approximately 34 weeks' gestation, when the hazards of preterm birth become less. A recent survey of United States maternal fetal medicine specialists revealed that over 90% administered repeated courses of steroids on a weekly basis, 28% doing so even after preterm labor has abated. Almost 60% of respondents would administer more than six courses if required.[3] A 1997 survey of Australian obstetricians revealed that 85% prescribed repeated courses when the risk of preterm birth persisted.[4] Seventy-four percent of United Kingdom maternity units give repeated doses on a weekly basis to such women. This practice appears to have arisen based both on in vitro observations and clinical trials that have been interpreted to suggest that the beneficial effects of corticosteroid treatment may be short-lived.

To evaluate the evidence suggesting that the effects of corticosteroids are reversible, it is necessary to understand their effects on fetal lung development. These steroid-induced changes are commonly referred to as either induction or maturation of fetal lung development, but it is unclear whether the pharmacologically induced events completely mimic the normal maturational sequence. Although it is possible that exogenous corticosteroids simply trigger the normal maturational process prematurely, it is more likely that they accelerate certain aspects of lung development, resulting in changes that are somewhat advanced for gestational age. Some changes persist until further maturation is triggered near term. For other components, however, antenatal steroids induce only a temporary response, which reverts if exposure is not continued. Present evidence suggests that the steroid-induced production of surfactant is reversible once steroids are removed, whereas the maturational effects on the developing interstitium and epithelium, as measured by improved lung volume, gas exchange, and compliance, are maintained. This dichotomous effect may have clinical implications, because the biochemical deficit that occurs when steroids are removed could be adequately treated with postnatal surfactant if the structural changes are sufficiently advanced.

There are currently inadequate clinical data to quantify the duration of the effects of antenatal corticosteroids. The original suggestion of a diminishing effect over time came from the studies of Liggins and Howie.[1] These prospective randomized trials compared pregnant women at risk for preterm birth treated with 12 mg betamethasone every 24 hours for two doses with women administered a placebo. Whereas a beneficial effect was evident for women receiving steroids more than 24 hours but less than 7 days prior to birth, a subgroup analysis of women delivering more than 7 days after drug administration demonstrated no improvement in RDS in the steroid-treated group compared with the controls, suggesting a dissipated effect of the betamethasone. However, detailed review of this study demonstrates the inability of this subgroup analysis to adequately evaluate the remaining benefit of steroids after 7 days. Because 82% of the patients in the subgroup who were undelivered at 1 week remained undelivered for more than 3 weeks, this advancement in gestational age resulted in an incidence of RDS of only 3.3% in the placebo group, making any lingering benefit of corticosteroids statistically undetectable. The large placebo-controlled evaluation of corticosteroids, performed under the auspices of the NIH, was similarly confounded by the effect of advancing gestational age and was unable to demonstrate any beneficial effects of antenatal steroids in patients more than 7 days after initial drug administration. However, in a subgroup of neonates delivering 7 days after treatment but at less than 34 weeks' gestation, a 30% decrease in the frequency of RDS was seen in the corticosteroid-treated group, suggesting that the most "at-risk" babies may continue to benefit from the initial dose of steroids.

Crowley, in 1995,[5] performed a meta-analysis in which seven randomized controlled studies were analyzed to evaluate the effect of corticosteroids more than 7 days after initial administration. This analysis demonstrated an overall reduction in RDS in the steroid-exposed group (OR = 0.63). However, because of the low frequency of RDS in this group, there were insufficient patients to reach statistical significance. In the only other controlled study of significant size, the United Kingdom Multicenter Trial suggested that the beneficial effects of corticosteroids may persist up to 18 days after initial treatment.[6]

Only in recent years have animal and human studies attempted to evaluate the additive effect of repetitive steroid dosing. In sheep studies, Ikegami and colleagues[7] showed a sequential improvement in lung function with increasing numbers of weekly courses. Prematurely delivered lambs showed a 150% increase in lung compliance and a threefold increase in lung volume after four doses.

To date, no prospective human studies have compared single- with multiple-course treatment protocols, leaving the clinician only retrospective, observational data to guide management. There are currently four published retrospective studies[8–11] evaluating the efficacy of repetitive doses of corticosteroids (Table 5–1). Two of these studies have shown no reduction in RDS, IVH, chronic lung disease, or mortality with repeat dosing, whereas two others have demonstrated a significant reduction in RDS. Published abstracts have shown similarly inconsistent results, with four showing a reduction in the frequency of RDS with multiple doses and two revealing no improvement.

The confusion seen in the retrospective series is not surprising because a number of potential confounders are obvious. For example, the group receiving multiple doses is likely to have had initial treatment at an earlier gestational age and to have had a longer latency period from the initial dose until delivery than the group in which only one dose was able to be given. The studies also contain varying indications for steroid use.[8–11] For example, approximately one third of the patients evaluated had preterm

premature rupture of the membranes (pPROM) as the indication for steroid administration. Fetuses treated for this indication may not demonstrate an equivalent effect to those with intact membranes and are also much more likely to deliver before multiple doses are administered. Vermillion and colleagues[12] recently suggested that multiple steroid courses in patients with pPROM may actually increase the risk of RDS, NEC, and IVH compared with the result with a single dose. Likewise, many of these studies contain a larger proportion of twin gestations in the multiple-course group, when efficacy of even one course of corticosteroids in multiple gestations is unproved.[8–11] Other indications, such as intrauterine growth restriction and preeclampsia, have been included despite evidence of diminished response to corticosteroids.

Until prospective randomized trials are completed, the benefits of repetitive steroid dosing remain uncertain. Such trials are currently under way in the United States, Canada, Great Britain, and Australia. An interim analysis from one of the United States trials was recently presented and demonstrated no difference in the frequency of a composite outcome, including RDS, mortality, IVH, periventricular leukomalacia, chronic lung disease, sepsis, and necrotizing enterocolitis between a group receiving only a single course and one receiving multiple courses.[13] There was, however, a 30% reduction in RDS in one group and an increase in severe IVH in the other. There was also a significant difference in the latency time from initial treatment to delivery between groups. Unfortunately, because this was an interim analysis, the specific group designation was not divulged.

Data on the safety of repetitive antenatal steroid dosing are limited to animal and retrospective human studies (Table 5–2). Both small and large animals have demonstrated a symmetrical decrease in fetal size after repetitive doses of corticosteroids. In addition to decreased overall growth, specific organ systems, including the brain, have been involved. Most recently, a significant dose-dependent decrease in the birth weight of fetal lambs receiving repeti-

Table 5–1. Retrospective Studies of the Efficacy of Repeat-Dose Corticosteroids

	RDS Incidence (%) No. of Courses			IVH Incidence (%) No. of Courses			Mortality (%) No. of Courses			CLD Incidence (%) No. of Courses		
	1	2	≥3	1	2	≥3	1	2	≥3	1	2	≥3
French et al[8]	34	22	23				11	5	9	24	15	26
Banks et al[9]												
25–28 wk	82	83	83	No difference			13	11	26*	No difference		
28–32 wk	48	38	39				OR = 2.8					
Abassi et al[10]	45	34	29	No difference			2.2	3.1		No difference		
1 course vs. ≥ 2 courses	OR = 0.44 (0.25–7.79)											
1 course vs. ≥ 3 courses	OR = 0.37 (0.2–0.7)						11		5			
Elimian et al[11]												
1 course vs. ≥ 3 courses	41		18	No difference								
	OR = 0.35 (0.18–0.7)											

*Fifty-four percent from multiple gestations, 5% had pulmonary hypoplasia.
CLD, chronic lung disease; IVH, grade III and IV intraventricular hemorrhage; OR, odds ratio (95% confidence interval); RDS, respiratory distress syndrome.

Table 5–2. Retrospective Studies of the Safety of Repetitive Steroids

	Birth Weight No. of Courses			Head Circumference No. of Courses		
	1	*2*	*≥3*	*1*	*2*	*≥3*
French et al[8]						
BW ratio/HC difference (cm)	0.99	0.93	0.87	−0.42 cm	−0.74 cm	−1.02 cm
BW < 10th percentile	17%	15%	36%			
Mean (cm)				28	28	29
Banks et al[9]						
1 course vs. ≥ 2 courses < 32 wk		−39 g (P = .02)			No difference	
1 course vs. ≥ 2 courses > 32 wk		−80 g (P = .09)			No difference	
Abassi et al[10]						
24–≤34 wk	1626	No difference	1687 (P = NS)		−0.46 cm (P < .005)	
35–42 wk		No difference			No difference	
All births		No difference			−0.23 cm (P = NS)	
Elimian et al[11]						
Percentile (mean)	39.2		36.7	40	40.1	

BW, birth weight; HC, head circumference; NS, not significant.

tive, prolonged steroid exposure was reported, with a 27% reduction in weight in lambs receiving three or more weekly courses.[14] Fetal treatment did not cause growth failure when initiated later in gestation, suggesting a critically sensitive period for the growth-altering effects of steroids. Specific defects of myelination after repetitive steroid doses in sheep have also been suggested. However, despite these suggestions from animal studies, there is no conclusive evidence of a long-term harmful effect of repetitive doses of steroids on the human fetus.

A potential alteration of fetal growth in humans was initially described by French and coworkers[8] in their review of the Australian experience with antenatal steroids from 1990 to 1992. In this evaluation, 35% of preterm neonates receiving three or more courses of corticosteroids had birth weights below the 10th percentile. There was also a significant and progressive association between increasing courses of steroids and reduced head circumference. Whereas these observations are of concern, the study suffers from its retrospective nature and limited sample size because only 23 infants received three or more courses. The group receiving three or more courses also received their initial course 4 weeks earlier than the single-course group and remained in utero more than 4 weeks longer. There was an independent decrease in birth weight based on the interval from first dose to delivery. Therefore, the observed alterations in growth could be related to the early exposure to steroids rather than the number of courses. Likewise, the prolonged retention in utero after the initial episode of preterm labor may have an impact on fetal growth. Unfortunately, it remains unclear whether multiple courses of steroids independently affect fetal growth or are perhaps a marker for other perinatal events. Three other retrospective series have been published[9–11] and a number of abstracts have been presented that have attempted to evaluate the impact of multiple-dose steroids on fetal growth. Of the three published series, only one demonstrated a significant reduction in fetal weight.[9] Likewise,

no consistent effect on birth weight was seen in the abstracts. Only the Australian study[8] has shown a decrease in head circumference.

Whereas in utero exposure to a single course of corticosteroids results in only transient and clinically insignificant alterations of the fetal hypothalamic-pituitary axis, repetitive exposure may result in more prolonged suppression. Fortunately, despite laboratory evidence of hypothalamic suppression, neonates exposed to repetitive courses continue to respond appropriately to both ACTH stimulation and clinical stress.[9]

Because prolonged use of corticosteroids has an immunosuppressive effect, there is concern that infants exposed to repetitive antenatal doses may have a greater risk of chorioamnionitis or fetal sepsis. Whereas it is reassuring that the effects on maternal immune function of a single course are short-lived, rarely lasting longer than 72 hours, the risk from repetitive dosing has not been adequately evaluated. Repetitive use of antenatal steroids may alter the expression of pro- and anti-inflammatory cytokines in both the fetus and the mother. Because the inflammatory process may play a role in the pathophysiology of up to 30% of cases of preterm labor, and possibly cerebral palsy, the impact of steroids on this effect needs to be studied. Recently, it has been reported that repetitive exposure to steroids with pPROM may be associated with an increased incidence of chorioamnionitis and fetal sepsis compared with a single dose.[12] Although this study was retrospective, inasmuch as the efficacy of steroids in pPROM is uncertain it seems reasonable to limit these patients to a single course.

Recently, corticosteroids have been implicated in the initiation of human parturition through a number of mechanisms, including stimulation of corticotropin-releasing hormone, raising the issue of whether their repetitive use could increase the likelihood of preterm birth. Chronic use of prednisone from early in gestation to treat recurrent pregnancy loss has been associated with an increased risk of premature labor, pPROM, and preterm delivery. Although the effect of bolus courses of beta- or dexamethasone later in gestation on the incidence of preterm birth has not been studied, the decreased latency period reported in some studies of multiple courses of steroids needs further evaluation.

In addition to the acute effects on the neonate of repetitive courses of steroids, the impact on long-term development is equally important. French and coworkers[5] have continued to follow the neonates from the Australian cohort through age 3 years. The dose-related differences in weight and head circumference seen at birth were no longer detectable at this age. Equally reassuring was the fact that there was no increase in cerebral palsy or developmental disabilities in the multiple-dose group. On the contrary, the multiple-dose–exposed neonates had a lower incidence of these long-term complications. In 2000, Esplin reported a 21-month follow-up of preterm infants exposed to either zero, one, or two or more courses of antenatal steroids.[15] No difference in weight was seen nor was there a difference in the motor component of the Baley developmental examination. However, the infants exposed to two or more courses showed a decrease in the psychomotor component. Unfortunately, the severity of the neonatal course and the incidence of perinatal mortality was not taken into consideration, leaving the possibility that improved survival of sicker neonates among those exposed to multiple courses could result in a higher proportion of impaired infants in that group.

The risks to the mother of repetitive steroids cannot be ignored. Whereas a single course may cause an acute rise in blood sugar or initiate pulmonary edema when utilized with tocolytics, no long-term sequelae have been described. Repetitive dosing, however, may have more significant effects, especially in women receiving four or more courses. A maternal cushingoid appearance is frequently seen with multiple doses. Other potential risks include hypertension, increased susceptibility to infection, and gestational diabetes. Of special concern is the effect on calcium metabolism leading to osteoporosis, especially when compounded by bed rest and heparin, which are frequently prescribed for patients at risk of preterm birth. Spontaneous fractures, including of the vertebrae, have been reported in such patients.

At present, neither the efficacy nor the safety of repetitive doses of steroids has been quantified, leaving the clinician without a clear treatment approach. Until multicentered, prospective, randomized trials can be completed, no evidence-based paradigm can be developed. In August of 2000, the NIH organized a 1½-day conference at which investigators presented research on antenatal corticosteroid therapy and the audience was invited to participate in discussion.[16] The panel, consisting of the original members from the 1994 conference, weighed the scientific evidence and made the following conclusions:

1. The collective international data continue to strongly support the use and efficacy of a single course of antenatal corticosteroids, using the dosage and interval of administration specified in the 1994 Consensus Development Conference report.
2. The current benefit and risk data are insufficient to support the routine use of repeat or rescue courses of antenatal corticosteroids in clinical practice.
3. Clinical trials are in progress to assess potential benefits and risks of various regimens of repeat corticosteroids. Until data establish a favorable benefit-to-risk ratio, repeat courses of antenatal corticosteroids, including rescue therapy, should be reserved for patients enrolled in clinical trials.

THE UTILIZATION OF CORTICOSTEROIDS IN PREGNANCIES COMPLICATED BY PRETERM RUPTURED MEMBRANES

Premature rupture of the membranes accounts for approximately one third of all preterm births. Although the complication is identified in only 1.7% of all pregnancies, it contributes to 20% of all perinatal deaths. Standard management at present is to delay delivery until labor ensues or chorioamnionitis develops, because the risks of prematurity are greater than those of sepsis. However, controversy still exists on the utilization of corticosteroids in these patients. The NIH consensus development panel concluded that the use of antenatal corticosteroids in the presence of ruptured membranes remains controversial.[2] They suggested, however, that in pPROM at less than 30 to 32 weeks' gestation, in the absence of clinical chorioamnionitis, antenatal corticosteroid use is recommended because of the high risk of IVH at this gestational age.[2] Despite this recommendation, concerns about the immunosuppressive effects of corticosteroids, the potential for maternal or neonatal infection, and the fetal and neonatal effects of the biochemical products resulting from microbial infection have added to the controversy.

The predominant work justifying the utilization of steroids with pPROM is the meta-analysis of Crowley.[17] This involved the compilation of 15 randomized studies, of which 11 specifically addressed the efficacy of steroids in reducing RDS in the setting of pPROM. The pooled OR for these 11 studies suggested that treatment with corticosteroids would reduce RDS by approximately 50%. However, two of the studies have undergone considerable scrutiny because of perceived flaws in the study design. Removal of these studies from the meta-analysis would reduce the OR to 0.73 and eliminate the statistical significance of the overall conclusion (95% CI: 0.5, 1.08).

In December 1994, the ACOG Committee on Obstetric Practice (No. 147) offered a statement refuting the consensus panel's opinion that corticosteroids should be used in pPROM, suggesting instead that further research is needed to evaluate the risks and benefits. However, in June 1998, an ACOG practice bulletin (No. 1) recommended that antenatal steroids should be utilized with pPROM prior to 32 weeks' gestation. Since this opinion, subsequent studies have failed to resolve the issue.

In addition to RDS, corticosteroids have been reported to reduce the risk of IVH. Of the 15 studies included in the meta-analysis of Crowley,[17] six specifically address IVH, although not exclusively in the setting of pPROM. These studies show that antenatal treatment with corticosteroids reduces the risk of IVH by 50%. Unfortunately, little scientific evidence is available addressing their efficacy in the prevention of IVH complicated by pPROM.

It is unlikely that a prospective study evaluating steroids in patients with pPROM will be performed, because the present consensus is that the benefits of administration outweigh the theoretical risks. For this reason, we concur with the ACOG opinion that steroids should be part of the treatment protocol with pPROM. However, based on the data presented herein, we believe that treatment should be limited to only one course.

References

1. Liggins GC, Howie RN: Prevention of respiratory distress syndrome in premature infants by antepartum glucocorticoid treatment. In Villee CA, Villee DB, Suckerman J (eds): Respiratory Distress Syndrome. London, Academic, 1973, pp. 369–380.
2. National Institutes of Health Consensus Development Conference Statement: Effect of corticosteroids for fetal maturation on perinatal outcomes, February 28–March 2, 1994. Am J Obstet Gynecol 1995;173:246–252.
3. Quinlivan JA, Evans SF, Dunlop SA, et al: Use of corticosteroids by Australian obstetricians—a survey of clinical practice. Aust N Z J Obstet Gynaecol 1998;38:1–7.
4. Planer BC, Ballard RA, Ballard PL, et al: Use of antenatal corticosteroids (ANCS) in USA. Am J Obstet Gynecol 1996;174:A576, SPO.
5. Crowley PA: Prophylactic corticosteroids for preterm delivery. In Cochrane Collaboration. Cochrane Library, Issue 3. Oxford, Update Software, 1999.
6. Gamsu H, Mullinger B, Donnai P, Dash C: Antenatal administration of betamethasone to prevent respiratory distress syndrome in preterm infants: Report of a UK multicenter trial. Br J Obstet Gynecol 1989;96:401–410.
7. Ikegami M, Jobe AH, Newnham J, et al: Repetitive prenatal glucocorticoids improve lung function and decrease growth in preterm lambs. Am J Respir Crit Care Med 1997; 156:178–184.
8. French H, Hagan R, Evans S, et al: Repeated antenatal corticosteroids: Size at birth and subsequent development. Am J Obstet Gynecol 1999;180:114–121.
9. Banks BA, Cnaan A, Morgan MA, et al for the the North American Thyrotropin-Releasing Hormone Study Group: Multiple courses of antenatal corticosteroids and outcome of premature neonates. Am J Obstet Gynecol 1999;181:709–717.
10. Abassi S, Hirsch D, Davis J, et al: Effect of single vs. multiple courses of antenatal steroids on maternal and neonatal outcome. Am J Obstet Gynecol 2000; 182:1243–1249,
11. Elimian A, Verma U, Visintainer P, Tejani N: Effectiveness of multi-dose antenatal steroids. Obstet Gynecol 1999;95:34–36.
12. Vermillion ST, Soper DE, Chasedunn-Roark J: Neonatal sepsis after betamethasone administration to patients with preterm premature rupture of membranes. Am J Obstet Gynecol 1999;181:320–327.
13. Guinn DA, and the BMZ Study Group: Multicenter randomized trial of single or weekly courses of antenatal corticosteroids: Interim analysis [abstract 3]. Am J Obstet Gynecol 2000;182(1):512.
14. Ikegami M, Jobe AH, Newnham J, et al: Repetitive prenatal glucocorticoids improve lung function and decrease growth in preterm lambs. Am J Respir Crit Care Med 1997;156:178–184.
15. Esplin MS, Fausett MB, Smith S, et al: Multiple courses of antenatal steroids are associated with a delay in psychomotor development in children with birth weights less than or equal to 1500 grams [abstract 27]. Am J Obstet Gynecol 2000;182(1):524.
16. Antenatal Corticosteroids Revisited: Repeat Courses (NIH Consensus Statement 112). Aug 17–18, 2000;17(2):1–10.
17. Crowley PA: Antenatal corticosteroid therapy: A meta-analysis of the randomized trials, 1972 to 1994. Am J Obstet Gynecol 1995;173:322–335.

Six

Rescue Cerclage for the Incompetent Cervix

Margaret A. Harper

Management of the patient presenting in the middle trimester with painless cervical dilatation and prolapsing but intact fetal membranes presents a major challenge. The management of this precarious situation must be individualized. Careful evaluation for intra-amniotic infection (IAI), labor, and fetal anomalies is essential prior to an attempt at rescue cerclage placement. Success in prolonging pregnancy is inversely related to the degree of cervical dilatation and the extent of prolapse of the fetal membranes.

Iams and coworkers[1] suggested that cervical competence may be a continuum rather than a dichotomous characteristic. They and others[2] have reported the association between a shortened cervix on endovaginal ultrasound and preterm birth. These findings have stimulated an interest in assessing the cervix for shortening and funneling in gravidas considered at risk. However, not all women destined to preterm delivery can be identified by risk screening. Therefore, it is likely that women in the midtrimester with painless cervical dilatation and herniating membranes will continue to be encountered in the practice of obstetrics.

Most often, gravidas are not suspected of having an incompetent cervix until they present with pelvic pressure or increased vaginal discharge. The possible findings on speculum examination are a continuum from minimal cervical dilatation with fetal membranes visible through the os to hourglassing fetal membranes that completely fill the vagina. Therapeutic options include bed rest and expectant management or an attempt to replace the membranes and placement of a cervical cerclage—a rescue or emergency cerclage.

EVIDENCE THAT RESCUE CERCLAGE IMPROVES PREGNANCY OUTCOME

The three components that can be brought to bear on the management of any clinical problem include research evidence, clinical expertise, and patient preference. Evidence-based medicine focuses on systematic studies to determine the clinical efficacy of an intervention. The best evidence comes from randomized trials, a study design that ensures equal distribution of both recognized and unrecognized confounders among the study groups. There are few randomized trials of rescue cervical cerclage versus expectant management for midtrimester cervical incompetence.

Recently, Rust and colleagues[3] reported no improvement in perinatal outcome among 113 gravidas between 16 and 24 weeks with funneling of membranes into the endocervical canal but without prolapse beyond the external os. They offered a rescue cerclage to 8 who later developed prolapsing membranes. A randomized trial from the Netherlands[4] of cerclage and bed rest versus bed rest alone for 35 gravidas with a cervical length less than 2.5 cm at less than 27 weeks reported higher birth weights, later gestational age at delivery, and less perinatal morbidity in the cerclage group.

From an observational study, Heath and coworkers[5] reported a rate of preterm delivery before 32 weeks of 52% in 21 women managed expectantly, but in only 5% of 22 women who underwent Shirodkar cerclage, after a 23-week ultrasound indicated a cervical length less than 1.5 cm.

Olatunbosun and associates[6] published a nonrandomized, prospective study of rescue cerclage versus bed rest and expectant management. The 37 women in the study were between 20 and 27 weeks of gestation; 22 agreed to rescue cerclage. The remaining 15 either refused or were not offered the procedure. There was a significantly higher rate of preterm premature rupture of the fetal membranes (pPROM) in the noncerclage group, 60% versus 22.7%. However, after pPROM, the latency period was longer in the noncerclage group, 16.4 versus 1.6 days. The difference in neonatal survival between the two groups was not statistically significant ($P = .3$). It should be noted that this study had only 20% statistical power to show a significant difference in the proportion with neonatal survival and, therefore, should be considered inconclusive.

Other evidence comes from published case series. Aarts and associates[7] reviewed 12 studies published between 1980 and 1992 for a total of 249 patients. The success of rescue cerclage in significantly prolonging pregnancy varies with the findings on ultrasound and/or physical examination and the presence or absence of IAI. The degree of cervical dilatation and station of the fetal membranes at the time of cerclage placement has been reported to significantly affect pregnancy outcome in three case series.[8–10] The results are summarized in Tables 6–1 to 6–3. It is unclear whether rescue cerclage is effective in prolonging pregnancy for a sufficient period to improve perinatal survival in the midtrimester with a cervix more than 3 cm dilated with membranes herniating through the cervical os. Reports of large case series of similar patients managed

Table 6–1. Results from Treadwell and Associates' Case Series

Cervical Dilatation (cm)	N	Interval to Delivery (wk)	GA at Delivery (wk)
0	410	19.2 ± 6.6	35.6 ± 6.3
1	41	12.6 ± 7.5	33.3 ± 7.1
2	19	8.8 ± 8.2	28.7 ± 9.4
≥3	12	1.2 ± 2.1	23.5 ± 4.1

GA, gestational age.
From Treadwell M, Bronsteen R, Bottoms S: Prognostic factors and complication rates for cervical cerclage: A review of 482 cases. Am J Obstet Gynecol 1991;165:555–558.

Table 6–3. Results from Schorr and Morales' Case Series

Cervical Examination	Mortality	Normal Development (%)
<4 cm	20% (3/15)	75
≥4 cm	57% (4/7)	33

From Schorr SJ, Morales WJ: Obstetric management of incompetent cervix and bulging fetal membranes. J Reprod Med 1996;41:235–238.

expectantly without cerclage are lacking, and randomized trials have not been conducted. With a smaller degree of cervical change, such as shortening found on routine transvaginal ultrasound, cerclage is more likely to be of benefit.

THE ROLE OF INTRA-AMNIOTIC INFECTION IN PATIENTS WITH SUSPECTED CERVICAL INCOMPETENCE

A significant number of women will have microbial invasion of the amniotic cavity at the time of diagnosis of previously unsuspected incompetent cervix. It is unclear whether subclinical IAI precedes cervical dilatation, or, more likely, if exposure of the fetal membranes to vaginal flora leads to an ascending infection. Treadwell and associates[8] found an association between the degree of cervical dilatation and IAI with an infection rate of 41.7% for those with a cervix dilated more than 2 cm but only 6.2% for those with a cervix dilated 2 cm or less.

In a case series of 33 women at 24 or fewer weeks' gestation with cervical dilatation of 2 cm or more, intact membranes without uterine contractions, and no clinical signs of chorioamnionitis, Romero and colleagues[11] found that 51.5% had positive amniotic fluid cultures. *Ureaplasma urealyticum* was the single most common isolate.

The pregnancy outcome is uniformly dismal in patients with IAI. Rupture of the fetal membranes, onset of active labor, maternal pyrexia, and sepsis after cerclage placement may be considered complications of the surgical procedure when, in fact, these are complications of preexisting IAI. It appears reasonable to recommend amniocentesis to rule out subclinical chorioamnionitis in all patients being considered for rescue cerclage. The fluid should be analyzed for glucose content and evidence of bacteria on Gram stain. A glucose level less than 10 mg/dL or organisms on Gram stain can be considered a contraindication to cerclage placement. Culture of the fluid should also be requested, but it is not feasible to await results that may take 24 to 72 hours. If there is any question of rupture of the fetal membranes, 5 to 10 mL of indigo carmine can be instilled at the time of amniocentesis.

TECHNIQUE OF RESCUE CERCLAGE

Prophylactic Tocolysis

Endogenous prostaglandins have been found to be elevated in patients undergoing cerclage procedures. Most patients have some uterine activity after cerclage placement. Indomethacin, a prostaglandin synthetase inhibitor, has been shown to be an effective tocolytic in randomized controlled trials. Prostaglandin synthetase inhibitors are well tolerated and, with duration of treatment of less than 48 hours, have little side effects for the fetus. Theoretically, the prophylactic use of indomethacin in the perioperative period could be of benefit, but this has not been examined in prospective trials.

Table 6–2. Results from Wong and Colleagues' Case Series

Group*	N	Median GA at Cerclage (wk)	Mean GA at Delivery (wk)	Pregnancy Prolongation (wk)	Perinatal Mortality (%)	Handicap at Discharge
I	15	22	39	16	0	0
II	18	23.2	25.8	1.8	50	3
III	18	22.5	24.1	1.0	55.6	3

*Group I: Beaking and funneling or a cervical length < 3 cm by ultrasound.
 Group II: Cervical dilatation < 3 cm. Membranes were prolapsed through the os in 12 of 18 patients.
 Group III: Cervical dilatation ≥ 3 cm. Membranes were prolapsed through the os in 14 of 18 patients.
GA, gestational age.
From Wong GP, Farquharson DF, Dansereau J: Emergency cervical cerclage: A retrospective review of 51 cases. Am J Perinatol 1993:10:341–347.

Prophylactic Antibiotics

Perioperative broad-spectrum antibiotics have been recommended for rescue cerclage. However, there is no evidence that prophylactic antibiotics are of benefit. Mitra and coworkers[12] examined retrospectively the pregnancy outcomes of 20 women undergoing rescue cerclage who received prophylactic antibiotics and 20 others who had a rescue cerclage but no antibiotics. There was no difference in postoperative complications or infant survival between the two groups.

Anesthesia for Rescue Cerclage

Although some experienced in rescue cerclage placement have recommended deep general anesthesia to relax the uterus at the time of surgery, this does not appear to have any advantage over the preoperative use of uterine relaxants and/or tocolytics. The choice of anesthetic technique does not significantly alter the success of the procedure and should be chosen on the basis of patient safety and preference.

Replacing the Fetal Membranes

Several different approaches have been described for replacing the fetal membranes before cerclage placement. In a series of 15 patients, Barth[13] reported good results with most methods except the use of a moistened sponge stick. This technique was associated with intraoperative rupture of the membranes in two of three patients, and he recommended abandoning its use.

Distention of the urinary bladder with 1 to 1.5 L of sterile saline solution does help to displace the herniated sac up into the uterus, decreasing the risk of iatrogenic rupture. However, it also causes a displacement of the cervix cephalad. This can make it more difficult to place the cerclage high enough at the level of the internal os. Nevertheless, this remains an excellent method for a "no touch" technique for rescue cerclage.

The use of a sterile urinary catheter with a 30-mL balloon has also been described. The balloon is inflated to hold the membranes in the lower uterine segment and out of harm's way as the cerclage is placed (Fig. 6–1). The balloon can then be deflated and removed after the cerclage is tied down. If a double cerclage is placed, the more cephalad suture is tied down before the catheter is removed and the more caudal suture is tied after the catheter is removed. This technique allows for good closure without trapping the membranes in the cerclage.

Other techniques that have been reported include preoperative reduction amniocentesis, intravenous nitroglycerin, and deep Trendelenburg position. Another approach is the use of five to eight small-gauge (such as 00 silk) simple sutures in the edge of the cervix to facilitate pulling the cervix down over the membranes, as shown in Figure 6–2.

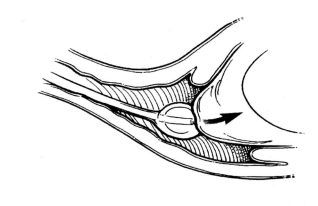

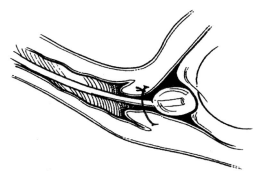

Figure 6–1. A catheter with a 30-mL balloon can be used to reduce the fetal membranes and facilitate placement of a rescue cervical cerclage.

These sutures are used only for traction and are removed after the cerclage is in place.

Surgical Technique

The McDonald procedure is most commonly used for emergency cervical cerclage. Harger[14] compared the McDonald and Shirodkar techniques in 202 elective and 42

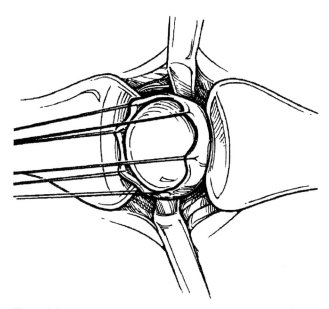

Figure 6–2. Simple sutures are placed to allow for traction on the cervix.

rescue procedures and could not demonstrate that one method was superior to the other. With more advanced cervical changes, the Shirodkar technique is technically more difficult than the McDonald procedure.

The Shirodkar procedure places a wide suture, such as a 5-mm Mersilene band, submucosally at the cervicovaginal junction. A 1- to 2-cm transverse incision is made in the vaginal mucosa at the level of the internal cervical os anteriorly and posteriorly. If necessary, the bladder is dissected up out of the way. The suture is passed on an atraumatic needle beneath the mucosa between the two incisions and tied. The band can be sutured to the cervix to prevent slippage. The mucosal incisions are then closed with interrupted absorbable suture. The Shirodkar cerclage can be removed to allow for vaginal delivery by incising a small area of vaginal mucosa to expose the knot.

The McDonald cerclage utilizes a circumferential non-absorbable suture, such as No. 2 silk, Mersilene, Ticron, or Prolene, placed with four to five sequential bites in a purse-string fashion. The cervical edge is best grasped with a ring thumb forceps. The suture is usually started anteriorly and should be placed at the level of the internal os, being careful to avoid the endocervical canal and fetal membranes. With advanced cervical changes, difficulty may be encountered in placing the suture high enough. In this case, the first cerclage suture can be used as traction before it is tied to pull the cervix down, allowing for the placement of a second suture more cephalad. With either a Shirodkar or a McDonald cerclage, the surgeon must take great care to ensure the membranes are reduced sufficiently to avoid their strangulation within the cervical canal as the sutures are cinched and tied. This can be facilitated by a 30-mL catheter balloon, as described previously. The balloon is deflated and the catheter withdrawn after the sutures are tied. The ears of the sutures should be left long enough to be easily identified. Tying the ears together in a 2-cm loop, which can be easily grasped and used to elevate the knot above the vaginal mucosa, facilitates removal.

Complications of Rescue Cerclage

pPROM, chorioamnionitis, and preterm labor occur frequently after prolapse of the fetal membranes. Whether these complications are more or less frequent after placement of a rescue cerclage is unclear. Other less common complications of rescue cerclage include cervical lacerations, septic shock, cervicovaginal fistula, and even one report of a maternal death. The potential for these complications must be considered in the decision to attempt rescue cerclage placement. In order to minimize risk, preexisting IAI should be ruled out.

Preterm Premature Rupture of the Membranes and Cervical Cerclage

Cervical cerclage, whether placed prophylactically in the late first trimester or emergently after cervical changes in the midtrimester, is a risk factor for pPROM. This has been demonstrated in prospective series as well as case control studies. When pPROM occurs, the obstetric provider must decide whether or not to remove the cerclage. One study by Yeast and Garite[15] and a second by Blickstein and associates,[16] for a combined total of 64 cerclage patients, demonstrated no significant difference in perinatal outcomes in pregnancies without a cerclage and pPROM versus pregnancies with a cerclage and pPROM when the cerclage was removed immediately after the membranes ruptured. In a study in which the cerclage was not removed, Goldman and coworkers[17] reported a significantly shorter latency period, lower gestational age at delivery, increased maternal infectious morbidity, perinatal morbidity, and mortality for pregnancies complicated by cerclage and pPROM compared with matched controls with pPROM and no cerclage. Similarly, Ludmir and colleagues[18] found significantly increased rates of neonatal mortality and sepsis among 20 pregnancies with retained cerclage and pPROM compared with a group of 10 pregnancies with pPROM and immediate removal of the cerclage or a group of 33 controls with pPROM and no cerclage. It would, therefore, seem advisable to remove the cerclage after membranes rupture.

Summary

The evidence regarding emergency cervical cerclage for painless cervical dilatation and effacement in the midtrimester relies primarily on case series. It is likely that unsuccessful cases are underreported. Whereas some reports offer enthusiastic support for this procedure regardless of the degree of cervical dilatation or station of the fetal membranes, most are cautious in recommending emergency cerclage in those with a cervix more than 3 cm dilated and/or membranes prolapsing well beyond the external os. Although it is technically feasible to place a cerclage in this setting, the proof of benefit of this intervention awaits randomized clinical trials.

References

1. Iams JD, Johnson F, Sonek J, et al: Cervical competence as a continuum: A study of ultrasonographic cervical length and obstetric performance. Am J Obstet Gynecol 1995;172:1097–1106.
2. Wong G, Levine D, Ludmir J: Maternal postural challenge as a functional test for cervical incompetence. J Ultrasound 1997;16:169–175.
3. Rust O, Atlas R, Reed J, et al: Revisiting the clinical efficacy of cerclage in the treatment of second-trimester sonographically detected premature dilation of the internal os. (Abstract 6) Twenty-first Annual Meeting of the Society for Maternal-Fetal Medicine. Reno. February 5–10, 2001.
4. Althuisius S, Dekker G, Hummel P, et al: CIPRAT: Therapeutic cerclage with bedrest versus bedrest, final results. (Abstract 2) Twenty-first Annual Meeting of the Society of Maternal-Fetal Medicine. Reno. February 5–10, 2001.
5. Heath VCF, Souka AP, Erasmus I, et al: Cervical length at 23 weeks of gestation: The value of Shirodkar suture for short cervix. Ultrasound Obstet Gynecol 1998;12:318–322.

6. Olatunbosun OA, Al-Nuaim L, Turnell RW: Emergency cerclage compared with bed rest for advanced cervical dilatation in pregnancy. Int Surg 1995;80:170–174.

7. Aarts JM, Brons JTJ, Bruinse HW: Emergency cerclage: A review. Obstet Gynecol Surv 1995;50:459–469.

8. Treadwell M, Bronsteen R, Bottoms S: Prognostic factors and complication rates for cervical cerclage: A review of 482 cases. Am J Obstet Gynecol 1991;165:555–558.

9. Wong GP, Farquharson DF, Dansereau J: Emergency cervical cerclage: A retrospective review of 51 cases. Am J Perinatol 1993;10:341–347.

10. Schorr SJ, Morales WJ: Obstetric management of incompetent cervix and bulging fetal membranes. J Reprod Med 1996;41:235–238.

11. Romero R, Gonzales R, Sepulveda W, et al: Microbial invasion of the amniotic cavity in patients with suspected cervical incompetence: Prevalence and clinical significance. Am J Obstet Gynecol 1992;167:1086–1091.

12. Mitra AB, Katz VL, Bowes WA Jr, Carmichael S: Emergency cerclages: A review of 40 consecutive procedures. Am J Perinatol 1992;9:142–145.

13. Barth WH Jr: Cervical incompetence and cerclage: Unresolved controversies. Clin Obstet Gynecol 1994;37:831–841.

14. Harger JH: Comparison of success and morbidity in cervical cerclage procedures. Obstet Gynecol 1980;56:543–548.

15. Yeast JD, Garite T: The role of cervical cerclage in the management of preterm premature rupture of the membranes. Am J Obstet Gynecol 1988;158:106–110.

16. Blickstein I, Katz Z, Lancet M, Mogilner BM: The outcome of pregnancies complicated by preterm rupture of membranes with and without cerclage. Int J Gynaecol Obstet 1989;28:237–242.

17. Goldman JM, Greene MF, Tuomala RE: Outcome of expectant management in preterm premature rupture of the membranes with cervical cerclage in place (abstract 139). Tenth Annual Meeting of the Society of Perinatal Obstetricians, Houston. Jan 23–27, 1990.

18. Ludmir J, Bader T, Chen L, et al: Poor perinatal outcome associated with retained cerclage in patients with premature rupture of membranes. Obstet Gynecol 1994;84:823–826.

Acute Therapy for Preterm Labor

Debra A. Guinn and Barbara V. Parilla

Preterm labor is defined as uterine contractions resulting in progressive cervical dilatation and effacement prior to 37 weeks' gestation. Management decisions regarding treatment are influenced greatly by the gestational age and cervical dilatation at presentation. Early gestational age and advanced cervical dilatation are associated with the highest risk of preterm delivery. In an effort to decrease uterine contractions and prolong the time to delivery, tocolytic agents are widely used in women with suspected preterm labor and intact membranes. A variety of agents have been studied for tocolysis, including hormonal replacement, alcohol, beta-mimetics, magnesium sulfate, prostaglandin synthetase inhibitors, calcium channel blockers, and nitroglycerin.

BETA-MIMETICS

The beta-mimetics have been the most thoroughly investigated tocolytic agents and have consistently demonstrated an ability to prolong gestation by 24 to 48 hours when compared with similarly administered placebo.[1] Unfortunately, both maternal and fetal side effects are common with therapy and limit their use. The most serious maternal complication of beta-mimetic therapy is pulmonary edema, complicating 1 in 400 exposures. This complication is potentially avoidable by limiting the use of hydration with dilute solutions and careful observation. In the majority of cases of pulmonary edema, patients respond to fluid restriction and diuretic therapy. However, maternal deaths have been associated with therapy.[1a] In addition, the beta-mimetics have been associated with neonatal intraventricular hemorrhage.[2] As a result, in the United States intravenous treatment with the beta-mimetics has fallen out of favor.

MAGNESIUM SULFATE

Magnesium sulfate is a nonspecific calcium antagonist. Macones and colleagues in 1997[3] and Gyetvai and coworkers in 1999[4] evaluated the efficacy of magnesium sulfate and tocolysis using meta-analysis. A limited number of studies were identified that evaluate the efficacy of magnesium sulfate when compared with either placebo or other tocolytic agents. In both meta-analyses, when magnesium sulfate was compared with placebo, there were no significant differences in time gained in utero or delay in delivery. Macones and colleagues also compared the outcomes of women who received magnesium sulfate or other tocolytic agents. Magnesium sulfate was equivalent to ritodrine or other beta-mimetics in prolonging delivery 24 to 48 hours with fewer maternal side effects.[3]

Regardless of the lack of data to support its use, magnesium sulfate is the primary tocolytic agent used in North America. As its use has become more widespread, there have been reports of adverse reactions to magnesium sulfate. Rare serious maternal complications include respiratory depression, pulmonary edema, and death. In addition, fetal hypermagnesemia and depression have been reported. Of particular concern is the MAGnet trial.[5] This trial was designed to evaluate the neuroprotective effect of magnesium sulfate exposure in preterm fetuses. Previous retrospective reviews have suggested that magnesium sulfate exposure prior to preterm delivery of a very-low-birth-weight neonate reduced cerebral palsy.[6] In the MAGnet trial, women were randomized to receive magnesium sulfate or other tocolytic agents, or placebo if they presented with advanced cervical dilatation. However, the study was halted after only 75 subjects were enrolled in each arm. An interim safety analysis revealed a significantly increased rate of pediatric deaths among the 75 mothers in the magnesium sulfate–treated group compared with subjects randomized to receive other tocolytics or saline placebo. Several large, randomized, controlled trials are now in progress to evaluate the impact of antenatal magnesium sulfate exposure on neonatal morbidity and mortality. To our knowledge, none of these trials has been stopped for safety concerns.

PROSTAGLANDIN SYNTHETASE INHIBITORS

Indomethacin, a prostaglandin synthetase inhibitor, is an effective tocolytic agent in delaying delivery. Its ease of administration, maternal safety, and low cost offer substantial advantages over other agents. The use of indomethacin as a primary tocolytic agent is reviewed later in this chapter.

OTHER AGENTS

Calcium channel blockers (nifedipine and nicardipine) and nitroglycerin (intravenous and patch) have been tested as potential tocolytic agents.[7] The rate-limiting factors with these agents are maternal vasodilatation and hypotension. There has been a report of maternal myocardial infarction after administration of nifedipine for tocolysis.[8] Both classes of agents offer promise. Further studies need to identify the agent with the highest level of uterospecificity and effectiveness. These agents need to be tested in properly designed randomized, placebo-controlled trials using neonatal outcome as the primary end point. Finally, antosiban, an oxytocin antagonist, was tested in clinical trials in the United States. It was highly effective in reducing uterine contractions and appeared to be promising in prolonging gestation.[4] However, the Food and Drug Administration (FDA) did not approve its use in the United States and at this time it is not available.

JUSTIFICATION FOR USE OF TOCOLYTIC AGENTS

Regardless of which agent is used, tocolytic therapy has not influenced the rate of preterm birth or resulted in a decrease in neonatal morbidity or mortality, the primary goal of prolonging pregnancy.[4, 9] However, in the majority of tocolytic trials, the concomitant use of antenatal corticosteroids was low. Antenatal corticosteroids reduce the incidence of respiratory distress syndrome, intraventricular hemorrhage, and death in premature infants. The American College of Obstetricians and Gynecologists recommends antenatal corticosteroids for all women at risk for preterm delivery prior to 34 weeks' gestation. It is possible that the time gained with tocolytic exposure will allow the physician to treat the mother with antenatal corticosteroids, thus reducing neonatal morbidity and mortality. If this supposition is confirmed in properly designed randomized, controlled trials, it could justify the potential risk to the mother of being treated with tocolytic therapy.

Another potential benefit of the 24- to 48-hour window with tocolytic therapy is to allow for the transfer of the mother to a suitable tertiary care center. Babies born in tertiary care centers between 26 and 34 weeks' gestation have significantly higher rates of survival and decreased rates of intraventricular hemorrhage when compared with neonatal transfers.

Finally, the 24 to 48 hours gained with tocolysis may allow for a thorough evaluation of the pregnancy, including gestational age, number of fetuses, presence of congenital anomalies, fetal lie, and placental position. This information is important in determining appropriate interventions, including mode of delivery, operative delivery for fetal distress, and planned neonatal resuscitation.

INDOMETHACIN

Rationale for Use

Based on our review of the literature, we believe that indomethacin is an ideal primary tocolytic agent in pregnancies complicated by preterm labor of less than 32 weeks' gestation. We have reached this conclusion because we believe that indomethacin poses the least amount of risk to the mother while achieving the desired goal of prolonging pregnancy to allow for administration of tocolysis, arrange transport to a tertiary care facility, and thoroughly evaluate the pregnancy.

Efficacy

Indomethacin has been reported to be effective in two small randomized, placebo-controlled trials. Niebyl and colleagues[10] found indomethacin superior to placebo in delaying delivery for 48 hours (80% vs. 33%). Zuckerman and associates[11] reported sustained delay in delivery for patients treated with indomethacin (95% at 48 hours and 83% at 7 days) compared with placebo (23% at 48 hours and 16% at 7 days). Additional prospective, randomized trials have found indomethacin to be comparable to ritodrine and magnesium sulfate, and superior to nifedipine for tocolysis. There are additional reports that describe indomethacin tocolysis favorably, but many utilized other tocolytic agents simultaneously or sequentially.

Protocol for Indomethacin Tocolysis

Our recommended protocol for indomethacin tocolysis involves the administration of a 100-mg loading dose given as a suppository per rectum. If regular uterine contractions persist 1 to 2 hours after the initial 100-mg suppository, an additional 50 to 100 mg may be given. Oral therapy is then instituted at 50 mg every 6 hours for 48 hours while betamethasone is dispensed. Magnesium sulfate is added as a second agent if there is continued cervical change or no decrease in uterine activity after two loading doses of indomethacin. If preterm labor recurs before 7 days after the first course of indomethacin, magnesium sulfate is utilized. Penicillin prophylaxis for group B beta streptococcus is administered intrapartum to all gestations prior to 37 completed weeks. Fetal echocardiography is not considered necessary when administering indomethacin as outlined previously. In fact, we do not believe the risk-benefit ratio is ever in favor of prolonged indomethacin use for preterm labor. The primary goal of tocolysis is to delay delivery for 48 hours in order to administer corticosteroids. Fetal contraindications to the use of indomethacin include growth restriction, renal anomalies, chorioamnionitis, oligohydramnios, ductal-dependent cardiac lesions, and twin-twin transfusion syndrome.

Maternal Side Effects

Indomethacin is very well tolerated in the gravida in comparison to other tocolytic agents. Serious maternal side effects are rare when the agent is used in a brief course of tocolysis. As with any nonsteroidal anti-inflammatory drug (NSAID), mild gastrointestinal upset may occur. More serious potential complications include gastrointestinal bleeding, alterations in coagulation, thrombocytopenia, and asthma in aspirin-sensitive patients. Lunt and coworkers[12] reported normal prothrombin and activated partial thromboplastin times, but found abnormal prolonged bleeding times in 65% of women treated for 48 hours.

Prolonged treatment can lead to renal injury, especially when nephrotoxic drugs such as aminoglycosides are employed. Drugs of this class are antipyretic agents and may obscure a clinically significant fever. Maternal contraindications to indomethacin tocolysis include renal or hepatic disease, active peptic ulcer disease, poorly controlled hypertension, asthma, and coagulation disorders.

Fetal and Neonatal Side Effects

In contrast to the generally favorable maternal side effect profile, the potential for fetal and neonatal complications of indomethacin tocolysis is worrisome. In actuality, serious complications are rare when treatment is limited to short courses and established protocols are adhered to.

The principal side effects of indomethacin tocolysis have been constriction of the ductus arteriosus, oligohydramnios, and neonatal pulmonary hypertension. The ductal constriction occurs because formation of prostacyclin and prostaglandin E_2, which maintain ductal vasodilatation, is inhibited by indomethacin. In 1988, Moise and colleagues[13] reported Doppler evidence of ductal constriction in 7 of 14 fetuses exposed to indomethacin between 27 and 31 weeks' gestation. Tricuspid regurgitation occurred in 3 fetuses. All ductal abnormalities resolved within 24 hours of discontinuation of indomethacin and none of the neonates had pulmonary hypertension. In 1993 Moise and colleagues[14] reported the effect of advancing gestational age on ductal constriction in association with indomethacin and stated that "a dramatic increase in constriction was noted at 32 weeks' gestation when the rate of compromise approached 50%." However, ductal constriction was noted as early as 24 weeks, and occurred in 11 of the 23 fetuses prior to 30 weeks. This was a retrospective analysis of echocardiograms performed on 44 patients with premature labor or hydramnios treated with indomethacin. Although it was never clearly stated, these patients appeared to be on courses of therapy for greater than 48 hours, and indomethacin was the "third-line agent" in premature labor unresponsive to terbutaline or magnesium sulfate.

Oligohydramnios associated with indomethacin tocolysis is common, dose-related, and reversible. The oligohydramnios is a consequence of reduced fetal urine production due in turn to reduction by indomethacin of the normal prostaglandin inhibition of antidiuretic hormone and by direct effects on the renal blood flow. That is why it can be an effective therapy for hydramnios, especially that complicated by preterm labor.

Primary pulmonary hypertension in the neonate is a serious condition that has also been reported with prolonged (more than 48 hours) indomethacin therapy. Primary neonatal hypertension has not been reported with 24 to 48 hours of therapy, but the incidence may be as high as 5% to 10% with long-term therapy.[15]

Necrotizing enterocolitis[16, 17] and intraventricular hemorrhage[18] have been observed in the low-birth-weight neonate exposed to indomethacin in utero when it was used outside of standardized protocols that did not limit the duration of treatment or was the second or third agent added to recalcitrant preterm labor. Because such patients have an increased risk of subclinical intra-amniotic infection, and because intra-amniotic infection is associated with a greater risk of such complications, it is not clear that indomethacin incurs independent risk for these mobidities. Follow-up studies of children treated in utero with indomethacin by Niebyl and Witter[19] and Dudley and Hardie[20] have not found significant long-term effects, although they did not specifically target the low-birth-weight neonate. Gardner and associates[21] performed a matched cohort study of indomethacin exposure (62 cases and 62 controls) between 24 and 31 5/7 weeks' gestation and found no increase in neonatal morbidities. In 1997, Vermillion and colleagues[22] performed a cohort study of neonates delivered between 24 and 32 weeks' gestation after recent indomethacin tocolysis and found no association with increased neonatal complications. We also recently performed a case-control study and found that tocolysis with indomethacin as a single agent was not associated with necrotizing enterocolitis.[23]

Indomethacin is an effective tocolytic agent that is well tolerated by the mother and appears to be tolerated by the fetus when used appropriately. We do not use the drug for longer than 48 consecutive hours, but occasionally repeat a course of treatment after a 5-day drug-free interval. Because of the abundance of prostaglandin-mediated physiologic functions, it is not surprising that prostaglandin inhibition may have multiple and diverse side effects, especially with prolonged use. Cyclooxygenase (COX) inhibition with indomethacin is nonspecific and affects COX throughout the body. Interestingly, it was recently found that COX activity is contributed by two separate isoenzymes, COX-1 and COX-2. Evidence suggests it is the COX-2 isoform that is primarily involved in the production of prostaglandins within the fetal membranes and uterus, whereas the adverse fetal side effects that limit its use to only 48 hours may be a result of COX-1 inhibition. Highly selective COX-2 inhibitors are presently being studied as tocolytic agents and hold promise.

References

1. King JF, Grant A, Kierse MJ, Chalmers I: Beta-mimetics in preterm labor: An overview of the randomized controlled trials. Br J Obstet Gynaecol 1988;95:211–222.
1a. Hudgens DR, Conradi SE: Sudden death associated with terbutaline sulfate administration. Am J Obstet Gynecol 1993;169:120–121.
2. Groome LJ, Goldenberg RL, Cliver SP, et al, for the March of Dimes Multicenter Study Group: Neonatal periventricular-intraventricular hemorrhage after maternal beta-sympathomimetic tocolysis. Am J Obstet Gynecol 1992;167:873–879.
3. Macones GA, Sehdev HM, Berlin M, et al: Evidence for magnesium sulfate as a tocolytic agent. Obstet Gynecol Surv 1997;52:652–658.

4. Gyetvai K, Hannah ME, Hodnett ED, Ohlsson A: Tocolytics for preterm labor: A systematic review. Obstet Gynecol 1999;94:869–877.

5. Mittendorf R, Covert R, Boman J, et al: Is tocolytic magnesium sulphate associated with increased total paediatric mortality. Lancet 1997;250:1517–1518.

6. Schendel DE, Berg CJ, Yeargin-Allsopp M, et al: Prenatal magnesium sulfate exposure and the risk for cerebral palsy or mental retardation among very low-birth-weight children aged 3 to 5 years. JAMA 1996;276:1805–1810.

7. Lockwood CJ: Calcium-channel blockers in the management of preterm labour. Lancet 1997;35:1339–1340.

8. Oei SG, Oei SK, Brolmann H. Myocardial infarction during nifedipine therapy for preterm labor. N Engl J Med 1999;340:154.

9. Ventura SJ, Martin JA, Mathews TJ, Clarke SC: Advance report of final natality statistics, 1994. Mon Vital Stat Rep 1996;44:75.

10. Niebyl JR, Blake DA, White RD, et al: The inhibition of premature labor with indomethacin. Am J Obstet Gynecol 1980;136:1014–1019.

11. Zuckerman H, Reiss U, Rubinstein I: Inhibition of human premature labor by indomethacin. Obstet Gynecol 1974;44:787–792.

12. Lunt CC, Satin AJ, Barth WH: The effect of indomethacin tocolysis on maternal coagulation status. Obstet Gynecol 1994;84:820.

13. Moise KJ, Huhta JC, Sharif DS: Indomethacin in the treatment of premature labor: Effects on the fetal ductus arteriosus. N Engl J Med 1988;319:327–331.

14. Moise KJ: Effect of advancing gestational age on the frequency of fetal ductal constriction in association with maternal indomethacin use. Am J Obstet Gynecol 1993;168:1350–1353.

15. Iams JD: Preterm birth. In Gabbe SG NJ, Simpson JL (eds): Obstetrics: Normal and Problem Pregnancies. New York, Churchill Livingstone, 1996, pp. 774–776.

16. Norton ME, Merrill J, Cooper AB, et al: Neonatal complications after the administration of indomethacin for preterm labor. N Engl J Med 1993;329:1602–1607.

17. Major CA, Lewis DF, Harding JA, et al: Tocolysis with indomethacin increases the incidence of necrotizing enterocolitis in the low-birth-weight neonate. Am J Obstet Gynecol 1994;170:102–106.

18. Ianucci TA, Besinger RE, Fisher SG: The effect of dual tocolysis on the incidence of severe intraventricular hemorrhage among extremely low-birth-weight infants. Am J Obstet Gynecol 1996;175:1043–1046.

19. Niebyl JR, Witter FR: Neonatal outcome after indomethacin treatment for preterm labor. Am J Obstet Gynecol 1986;155:747–749.

20. Dudley DK, Hardie MB: Fetal and neonatal effects of indomethacin used as a tocolytic agent. Am J Obstet Gynecol 1985;151:181–184.

21. Gardner MO, Skelly S, Hauth JC: Preterm delivery after indomethacin: A risk factor for complications? J Reprod Med 1996;41:903–906.

22. Vermillion ST, Scardo JA, Lashus AG, Wiles HB: The effect of indomethacin tocolysis on fetal ductus arteriosus constriction with advancing gestational age. Am J Obstet Gynecol 1997;177:256–271.

23. Parilla BV, Grobman WA, Holtzman RB, et al: Indomethacin tocolysis and risk of necrotizing enterocolitis. Obstet Gynecol 2000;96:120–123.

Management of Isolated Oligohydramnios at Term

Deborah L. Conway

The finding of diminished amniotic fluid has long held an association with fetal compromise and adverse outcomes, even before the advent of sonography and semi-quantitative measures for assessing amniotic fluid volume. Oligohydramnios can serve as a marker for fetal structural abnormalities (particularly of the kidneys and urinary tract), result from placental dysfunction and represent shunting of fetal blood away from the kidneys, and beget further fetal compromise due to umbilical cord compression. There is good evidence that, in specific settings, the presence of oligohydramnios worsens the prognosis for the fetus.

It is not clear, however, what a "low" amniotic fluid volume means in a pregnancy that otherwise appears normal. The body of literature on oligohydramnios consists almost exclusively of studies in high-risk pregnancies. Despite this, data obtained from high-risk pregnancies with oligohydramnios have been extrapolated to low-risk pregnancies, perhaps inappropriately. Like their high-risk counterparts, women with "isolated" oligohydramnios undergo tests of fetal well-being and labor induction in the name of potential fetal compromise. If such intervention proves to be unnecessary, we are exposing our patients to added expense and inconvenience, at best, and to increased risk for maternal morbidity, at worst. Based on emerging evidence, this may indeed be the case.

WHEN IS INTERVENTION WARRANTED?

Specific conditions have been identified that exhibit worse fetal outcome when oligohydramnios is also present. In the setting of prolonged pregnancy or suspected fetal growth restriction, women with decreased amniotic fluid volume show higher rates of complications such as fetal distress, meconium-stained amniotic fluid, low Apgar scores, neonatal intensive care unit admission, and actual birth weight below the 10th percentile for gestational age compared with women with the same pregnancy complications but with normal amniotic fluid volume.[1–3] Thus, delivery is justified in such circumstances in pregnancies at or beyond 37 weeks' gestation.

On the other hand, diagnoses typically associated with placental insufficiency or vascular disease, such as hypertensive disorders and diabetes mellitus, show a surprising lack of direct correlation between low amniotic fluid volume and adverse fetal outcome. In a group of women hospitalized for hypertension in pregnancy (exacerbation of chronic hypertension, transient hypertension, or preeclampsia), detection of oligohydramnios at any point in the hospitalization did not predict fetal distress or cesarean delivery. However, when oligohydramnios was present at admission, fetal growth restriction was also present in 86% of cases.[4] Thus, when the term pregnancy is complicated by both hypertension and decreased amniotic fluid, fetal growth restriction is likely, and delivery might be considered for this reason.

In a large cohort of pregnant diabetic women undergoing outpatient antepartum surveillance, fetal nonstress testing was performed and amniotic fluid volume was measured twice weekly. Whereas abnormalities of the nonstress test (decelerations and/or absence of accelerations) carried an increased risk for cesarean delivery for fetal distress, neither the amniotic fluid index (AFI) nor the largest vertical pocket measurement predicted this outcome. Multivariate analysis of the combination of nonstress testing and amniotic fluid assessment to predict cesarean delivery for fetal distress revealed that amniotic fluid assessment added nothing to the predictive value of nonstress testing alone.[5] Although routine amniotic fluid assessment should not be included in the surveillance plan for diabetic women, we do not yet know whether expectant management is safe once oligohydramnios is identified in such patients.

ISOLATED OLIGOHYDRAMNIOS AT TERM

Is Delivery Necessary?

When oligohydramnios occurs in the absence of other identifiable pregnancy complications, is perinatal outcome adversely affected? In other words, what is the meaning of oligohydramnios (typically diagnosed when the AFI is below 5.0 cm or below the 5th percentile for gestational age) found in a woman between 37 and 41 weeks, with no medical problems, and an appropriately grown fetus with otherwise normal biophysical parameters? Very little information exists regarding this type of patient. However, women fitting this description undergo labor induction on a regular basis. In our teaching hospital in San Antonio, *oligohydramnios* is given as an indication in about 20% of labor inductions performed at term, and is the sole indication in approximately 40% of those.

In a retrospective study, a cohort of women who underwent labor induction for the sole indication of an AFI of 5.0 cm or lower were compared with women who presented in spontaneous labor with normal amniotic fluid measurements. The groups were compared in terms of perinatal outcome and mode of delivery (Table 8–1). No difference

Table 8–1. Perinatal Outcomes in Women with and without Isolated Oligohydramnios at Term

Outcome Measure	AFI ≤ 5 cm (N = 183)	AFI > 5 cm (N = 183)	P Value
Meconium (%)			
All	24.0	23.5	.88
Moderate/thick	12.6	12.0	.88
Birth weight (g)*	3398 ± 453	3421 ± 483	.54
Ponderal index*	2.48 ± 0.24	2.51 ± 0.23	.15
Arterial cord pH < 7.15 (%)	10.4	7.1	.35
Apgar score (5 min) < 7 (%)	1.1	0.6	.44
NICU admission (%)	16.4	11.5	.22

*Expressed as mean ± SD.

AFI, amniotic fluid index; NICU, neonatal intensive care unit.

Data from Conway DL, Adkins WB, Schroeder B, Langer O: Isolated oligohydramnios in the term pregnancy: Is it a clinical entity? J Matern Fetal Med 1998;7:197–200.

in any marker of adverse perinatal outcome could be identified, including growth abnormalities, meconium, Apgar scores, and arterial cord pH. However, women undergoing induction of labor for oligohydramnios had more than twice the rate of cesarean delivery as women in spontaneous labor (relative risk, 2.4; 95% confidence interval, 1.3–4.6), but no difference in the rate of cesarean delivery owing to fetal distress.[6] It is possible, however, that comparable perinatal outcomes between the women with oligohydramnios and those with normal amniotic fluid volume occurred because delivery was effected in the group with decreased amniotic fluid volume.

Is Expectant Management Safe?

The alternative to intervention for the finding of isolated oligohydramnios is expectant management, or monitoring the fetal status while awaiting spontaneous labor. Unfortunately, we currently lack a prospective study designed specifically to compare these two management schemes. However, we can find information in the existing literature to support an expectant management strategy in women with isolated oligohydramnios. The logic for such an approach is based on three findings: (1) that commonly used sonographic definitions for oligohydramnios lack specificity for adverse outcome, even in "high-risk" pregnancies; (2) that amniotic fluid measurements fluctuate over time; and (3) that the decrease in amniotic fluid volume may signal the approach of spontaneous labor.

Two recent studies point out the poor performance of amniotic fluid volume measurement as a predictor of adverse perinatal outcome. In the first, a prospective study of 1001 women undergoing antenatal fetal surveillance was divided according to results from two methods of amniotic fluid volume determination (AFI ≤ 5 cm vs. > 5 cm; two-dimensional pocket measurement ≤ 15 cm² vs. > 15 cm²).[7] Oligohydramnios did not carry a significant risk for any perinatal outcome measure studied. Abnormally low amniotic fluid volume was diagnosed in 21% of cases by AFI

and in 46% by two-dimensional pocket criteria. With rates of most adverse events ranging from 10% to 15%, it is clear that these definitions for abnormality lack specificity and positive predictive value. In the second study, high-risk women who underwent labor induction for an AFI of 5 cm or lower were matched by indication for antenatal testing to women with normal amniotic fluid volume.[8] Again, no differences were noted between the groups in any category of perinatal outcome (Table 8–2).

The control of amniotic fluid volume is complex and not well characterized, and the transient nature of sonographic estimates of amniotic fluid measurements has been noted repeatedly. Volume increases in response to hydration both in the pregnancy with normal amniotic fluid volume[9] and in women with oligohydramnios.[10] Furthermore, amniotic fluid estimates change with time. When serial AFI determinations are performed over time, oligohydramnios (by various definitions) reverts to normal in 40% to 50% of cases.[11, 12]

When amniotic fluid volume is plotted against gestational age, decreasing values are seen in the last weeks of pregnancy, regardless of the methodology used (direct measurement, dye-dilution, or semiquantitative sonographic methods). Furthermore, animal and human data suggest a physiologic decline in amniotic fluid volume in the few days before the spontaneous onset of labor. A group of normal pregnant women (N = 646) underwent ultrasound evaluation at 39⁰/₇ to 39²/₇ weeks' gestation. Women who entered spontaneous labor within 7 days of the ultrasound were more likely to have a lower maximum vertical pocket measurement than those who delivered later.[13]

These findings point out the lack of sophistication in our current interpretation of the physiology and pathophysiology of amniotic fluid dynamics. The failure of sonographic estimates of amniotic fluid volume to consistently correlate with outcome is probably the result of applying a crude tool to a complex biologic system. Amniotic fluid estimates are only one component in the evaluation of fetal status. Thus, particularly in the otherwise normal

Table 8–2. Perinatal Outcomes of High-Risk Women with and without Oligohydramnios

Outcome Measure (%)	AFI ≤ 5 cm (N = 79)	AFI > 5 cm (N = 79)	OR (95% CI)
Thick meconium	6.3	12.6	0.47 (0.15–1.43)
Severe variable decelerations	5.1	10.1	0.47 (0.14–1.64)
Late decelerations	10.1	7.6	1.37 (0.45–4.15)
Cesarean for fetal distress	8.8	7.6	1.18 (0.38–3.69)
NICU admission	7.6	10.1	0.73 (0.24–2.21)

AFI, amniotic fluid index; CI, confidence interval; NICU, neonatal intensive care unit; OR, odds ratio.

Data from Magann EF, Kinsella MJ, Chauhan SP, et al: Does amniotic fluid index of < 5 cm necessitate delivery in high-risk pregnancies? A case-control study. Am J Obstet Gynecol 1999;180:1354–1359.

pregnancy at term, an "abnormal" value for amniotic fluid volume should be interpreted with wisdom. Current evidence suggests that such a finding is not a mandate for intervention.[14]

Editor's Note

The optimal management of isolated amniotic fluid abnormalities at or near term continues to be problematic. With the increasing utilization of ultrasound, more gravida are found to have either oligohydramnios or "decreased" fluid (less than average but not meeting diagnostic criteria for oligohydramnios). At many hospitals, labor induction for "abnormal fluid volume" is a common reason for admission to the labor ward. It is my impression that many clinicians are becoming increasingly aggressive in their management of isolated decreased fluid and oligohydramnios. Some will even deliver preterm gestations for isolated decreased fluid because they are concerned about potential fetal compromise.

As physicians, we are taught to not intervene unless the potential benefits outweigh the potential risks. In cases of isolated oligohydramnios or decreased fluid, the risks of fetal compromise and demise must be weighed against the risks and costs of labor induction, as well as potential fetal morbidity in preterm gestations. Unfortunately, there are insufficient data to clearly support an optimal course of management; a large prospective clinical trial is needed. Until then, the studies presented in this chapter should give us pause to carefully review our management of these cases, especially when there is isolated decreased amniotic fluid.

References

1. Crowley P, O'Herlihy C, Boylan P: The value of ultrasound measurement of amniotic fluid volume in the management of prolonged pregnancies. Br J Obstet Gynaecol 1984;91:444–448.
2. Tongsong T, Srisomboon J: Amniotic fluid volume as a predictor of fetal distress in intrauterine growth retardation. Int J Gynaecol Obstet 1993;40:131–134.
3. Fischer RL, McDonnell M, Bianculli KW, et al: Amniotic fluid volume estimation in the postdate pregnancy: A comparison of techniques. Obstet Gynecol 1993;81:698–704.
4. O'Brien JM, Mercer BM, Friedman SA, Sibai BM: Amniotic fluid index in hospitalized hypertensive patients managed expectantly. Obstet Gynecol 1993;82:247–250.
5. Kjos SL, Leung A, Henry OA, et al: Antepartum surveillance in diabetic pregnancies: Predictors of fetal distress in labor. Am J Obstet Gynecol 1995;173:1532–1539.
6. Conway DL, Adkins WB, Schroeder B, Langer O: Isolated oligohydramnios in the term pregnancy: Is it a clinical entity? J Matern Fetal Med 1998;7:197–200.
7. Magann EF, Chauhan SP, Kinsella MJ, et al: Antenatal testing among 1001 patients at high risk: The role of ultrasonographic estimate of amniotic fluid volume. Am J Obstet Gynecol 1999;180:1330–1336.
8. Magann EF, Kinsella MJ, Chauhan SP, et al: Does amniotic fluid index of < 5 cm necessitate delivery in high-risk pregnancies? A case-control study. Am J Obstet Gynecol 1999;180:1354–1359.
9. Kilpatrick SJ, Safford K: Maternal hydration increases amniotic fluid index in women with normal amniotic fluid. Obstet Gynecol 1993;81:49–52.
10. Flack NJ, Sepulveda W, Bower S, Fisk NM: Acute maternal hydration in third-trimester oligohydramnios: Effects on amniotic fluid volume, uteroplacental perfusion, and fetal blood flow and urine output. Am J Obstet Gynecol 1996;173:1186–1191.
11. Lagrew DC, Pircon RA, Nageotte M, et al: How frequently should the amniotic fluid index be repeated? Am J Obstet Gynecol 1992;167:1129–1133.
12. Garmel SH, Chelmow D, Sha SJ, et al: Oligohydramnios and the appropriately grown fetus. Am J Perinatol 1997;14:359–363.
13. Farina A, Rizzo N, Di Luzio L, et al: Amniotic fluid volume and onset of labor in physiological pregnancy. Am J Perinatol 1999;16:217–221.
14. American College of Obstetricians and Gynecologists: Antepartum fetal surveillance (ACOG Practice Bulletin No. 9). Washington, DC, American College of Obstetricians and Gynecologists, 1999.

CHAPTER

NINE

Severe Prematurity: Implications and Counseling

Seetha Shankaran

The survival of extremely-low-birth-weight (ELBW) infants (500 to 1000 g) has increased dramatically during the 1990s. Current information regarding survival of ELBW infants is now available from large prospectively collected multicenter programs and should be used when counseling families. In the National Institute of Child Health and Human Development (NICHD) Neonatal Research Network registry, the survival rate of 501 to 750 g infants increased from 41% in the early 1990s to 54% in 1996; among those with birth weights from 751 to 1000 g, survival increased from 81% to 86%.[1] Two other large prospective registries have also demonstrated similar improvements in survival. In the Vermont Oxford Network,[2] the survival rate of neonates with a birth weight of 501 to 750 g born in 1994 to 1996 is currently 59%, whereas those with a birth weight ranging from 750 to 1000 g is 89%. A reduction in mortality has been noted in the California linked birth/death cohort files from 1987 to 1993 for 500 to 749 g birth-weight infants from 72% to 58% and for the 750 to 999 g birth-weight category from 37% to 20%.[3] The survival rate of 401 to 500 g neonates is only 11% to 15%. See Table 9–1 for neonatal survival according to gestational age (based on the best obstetric estimate) and birth weight. The survival rate is influenced by gender and gestational age; at 25 weeks, a 700-g neonate has a predicted mortality of 61% if male, but only a 35% predicted mortality if female.[1]

The improvement in survival rate of the ELBW infant is associated with changes in perinatal and neonatal practices. These include willingness to perform cesarean delivery, administration of antenatal corticosteroids and antibiotics, delivery room resuscitation, and use of surfactant.[1, 2] The

Table 9–1. Neonatal Survival as a Function of Birth Weight and Gestational Age

GA (wk)	Survival (%)	Birth Weight (g)	Survival (%)
21–23	25	501–600	25
24	50	601–700	65
25	75	701–800	72
26	80	801–900	85
27	90	901–1000	90
28	92		

GA, gestational age in weeks by best obstetric estimate.

majority of women delivering neonates of 501 to 750 g birth weight received corticosteroids (63%) and antibiotics (62%), and 44% were delivered by cesarean section. Among women delivering 751- to 1000-g infants, 76% received corticosteroids, 65% received antibiotics, and 60% were delivered by cesarean section. The willingness to perform cesarean section was associated with an increased likelihood of both survival and intact survival above 26 weeks' gestation.[4]

Prospective data collected from birth registries demonstrate that respiratory distress syndrome continues to be the most frequent pulmonary disease among infants weighing less than 750 g as well as those between 750 and 1000 g.[1] Surfactant use reflects severity of disease, with nearly 70% of infants in the ELBW category receiving surfactant. Late septicemia is seen in approximately half of the infants weighing 501 to 750 g at birth and in a third of the 750- to 1000-g infants. Chronic lung disease (defined as oxygen dependency at 36 weeks' postconceptional age) continues to be seen in a very high percentage of these infants (52% in the 501- to 750-g and 34% in the 751- to 1000-g neonates). Necrotizing enterocolitis (NEC) requiring surgery occurs in 14% and 9% in these two weight categories. The incidence of grade III and grade IV intracranial hemorrhage (ICH) combined is 26% in the 501- to 750-g and 12% in the 751- to 1000-g infants. Periventricular leukomalacia (PVL) remains low in both weight groups (7%).[1]

In spite of early attempts at nutrition with parenteral and oral feeding, growth failure occurs in all ELBW infants. Most infants born between 21 and 29 weeks' gestation do not achieve the median birth weight of referenced fetuses at the same postconceptional age; almost all are below the 10th percentile for weight when they reach 36 weeks' postconceptional age. ELBW infants do not achieve the catch-up growth seen in larger preterm infants. At 18 months' corrected age, 46% of infants had a weight below the 10th percentile, 43% had a length below the 10th percentile, and 43% had a head circumference below the 10th percentile. Patterns of growth of ELBW infants reflect underlying disease processes. Appropriate-for-gestational-age infants who survived to hospital discharge without developing serious morbidities (chronic lung disease, severe ICH, NEC, or late-onset sepsis) gained weight faster than comparable infants with these morbidities.[5] Other factors negatively related to growth include small for gestational age at birth, decreasing birth weight, Caucasian ethnicity, and PVL. However, maternal educational levels are not associated with poor growth.[6]

The majority of deaths (56%) among ELBW neonates occur within the first 3 days of birth, with most other deaths occurring within the first 28 days. The length of hospital stay in survivors with a birth weight of 501 to 750 g is 116 days, and it is 86 days among those surviving in the 751- to 1000-g category. The length of stay of 501- to 750-g infants who die is 16 days, and in the 751- to 1000-g birth-weight group, it is 24 days.[1] The chance of survival in ELBW infants improves markedly with increases in postnatal age.[7] For example, 24- to 25-week-gestation infants have a survival of 35% at birth. This survival rate increases to 50% at 12 hours, 66% at 7 days, 78% at the end of 4 weeks.

Information regarding survival must be assessed in relationship to morbidity when counseling families. Survival to neonatal intensive care unit (NICU) discharge without major morbidity (grades III to IV ICH, NEC > stage 2, or chronic lung disease) is seen in 37% of 501- to 750-g and 58% of 751- to 1000-g infants.[1] Chronic lung disease is the most common morbidity in survivors (35% in 501- to 750-g and 26% in the 750- to 1000-g infants). Grade III ICH occurs in 6% and 5% of survivors in the two weight categories. When morbidity to NICU discharge was examined among infants weighing less than 1000 g in the early 1990s compared with the late 1990s in the NICUs participating in the NICHD Network, the rates of ICH and NEC remained stable. However, survivors with chronic lung disease increased from 17% to 23%, with the largest increase in infants weighing 501 to 750 g, from 41% in the early 1990s to 56% in 1996. It should be noted that the overall survival rate of ELBW infants continues to increase; therefore the number of infants surviving with each of these morbidities is actually increasing.

Data concerning short-term outcome after maternal-fetal and neonatal intensive care in the 1990s are now emerging. There is a close association between neurologic deficits and decreasing birth weight. Cerebral palsy (CP) occurs in 29% of infants weighing less than 500 g, 17% among infants weighing 501 to 600 g, and 21% among infants weighing 601 to 750 g. Blindness is also related to birth weight and gestational age (14% in <500-g infants and 18% in the 23- to 25-weeks' gestation infants, with a dramatic drop in risk in all other birth-weight ranges). Hearing impairment does not appear to be influenced by gestational age; 7% to 11% across all weight groups with a birth weight below 1000 g.[8, 9]

Cognitive outcome evaluated at an early age (18 months corrected age) appears to be related to gestational age and birth weight. The Bayley II Mental Developmental Index (MDI) was administered at 18 months to surviving ELBW infants weighing less than 1000 g in a large, prospectively followed cohort. Thirty-seven percent had a score of 2 standard deviations below the mean (<70).[9] Another study also evaluating ELBW infants demonstrated developmental delay (a score of <70) among 39% of 24- to 26-week survivors, 30% of 26-week survivors, and 11% of longer-than-26-week survivors.[10] Neuromotor scores appear to be better among ELBW infants; 29% of infants weighing less than 1000 g scored less than 70 on the Psychomotor Developmental Index (PDI).[9] Among all survivors with a birth weight of 401 to 1000 g, 51% were completely normal, whereas one or more major neurodevelopmental abnormalities (cerebral palsy, blindness, deafness, MDI <70, or PDI < 70) was identified in 49% of infants. Factors associated with an increasing neurodevelopmental morbidity included chronic lung disease, grades III to IV ICH, PVL, and male gender. Increasing birth weight, female gender, higher maternal education, and Caucasian ethnicity were associated with lower morbidity at 18 months after term.[9] When the rates of disability are compared among survivors receiving intensive care in the late 1990s with the 1990 to 1994 infants in the same health care system, mild neuromotor disabilities and blindness appear to increase along with an increase in survival rate.[8]

The survival rate of the ELBW infant continues to rise owing to changes in obstetric and neonatal care. Along with the increase in survival rate, there are more survivors with morbidity associated with neonatal intensive care (ICH and chronic lung disease). Lack of adequate weight gain is present in more than one third of infants with birth weight less than 1000 g. Only 50% of survivors are completely free of any neurologic and developmental deficits in infancy. Currently, only short-term outcome has been assessed in ELBW infants surviving in the early 1990s. The long-term outcome of these very-high-risk infants needs to assessed. The prevention of prematurity and its associated morbidity continues to be a challenge to the obstetrician and the neonatologist.

References

1. Lemons JA, Bauer CR, Oh W, et al: Very low birth weight outcomes of the National Institute of Child Health and Human Development neonatal research network, January 1995 through December 1996. NICHD Neonatal Research Network. Pediatrics 2001;107E1.
2. Finer NN, Horbar JD, Carpenter JH, for the Vermont Oxford Network: Cardiopulmonary resuscitation in the very low birth weight infant: The Vermont Oxford Network experience. Pediatrics 1999;104:428–434.
3. Gould JB, Benitz WE, Liu H: Mortality and time to death in very low birth weight infants: California, 1987 and 1993. Pediatrics 2000;105:E37.
4. Bottoms SF, Paul RH, Iams JD, et al: Obstetric determinants of neonatal survival: Influence of willingness to perform cesarean delivery on survival of extremely low-birth-weight infants. Am J Obstet Gynecol 1997;176:960–966.
5. Ehrenkranz RA, Younes N, Lemons JA, et al: Longitudinal growth of hospitalized very low birth weight infants. Pediatrics 1999; 104:280–289.
6. Dusick A, Vohr BR, Steichen JJ, et al: The NICHD Neonatal Research Network Follow-up Study. Factors affecting growth outcome at 18 months in extremely low birthweight (ELBW) infants. Pediatr Res 1998;43:213A.

7. Cartlidge PHT, Stewart JH: Survival of very low birthweight and very preterm infants in a geographically defined population. Acta Paediatr 1997;86:105–110.

8. Emsley HCA, Wardle SP, Sims DG, et al: Increased survival and deteriorating developmental outcome in 23 to 25 week old gestation infants, 1990–4 compared with 1984–9. Arch Dis Child Fetal Neonatal Ed 1998;78:F99–F104.

9. Vohr BR, Wright LL, Dusick AM, et al: Neurodevelopmental and functional outcomes of extremely low birth weight infants in the National Institute of Child Health and Human Development Neonatal Research Network, 1993–1994. Pediatrics 2000;105:1216–1226.

10. Piecuch RE, Leonard CH, Cooper SA, et al: Outcome of infants at 24–26 weeks gestation: Neurodevelopmental outcome. Obstet Gynecol 1997;90:809–814.

Management of Preeclampsia

Kristine Y. Lain and James M. Roberts

Preeclampsia is a pregnancy-specific disorder diagnosed by the new appearance of hypertension and proteinuria, usually in late pregnancy. It is a leading cause of maternal mortality and increases perinatal mortality fivefold. The mainstay of therapy, delivery, has not changed over the last 100 years, and thus part of the perinatal morbidity is due to iatrogenic prematurity. It is estimated that preeclampsia occurs in 6% to 8% of pregnancies, and that 15% of preterm births are secondary to delivery for preeclampsia.

Although increased blood pressure is the cornerstone of diagnosis, the syndrome is far more than simply pregnancy-induced hypertension. Although the precise etiology remains unclear, the emerging view is that preeclampsia is secondary to the interactions of reduced placental perfusion with diverse maternal factors to alter endothelial function.[1] The pathophysiologic changes of preeclampsia support the concept of reduced maternal systemic organ perfusion, in part secondary to profound vasoconstriction.

CLASSIFICATION OF THE HYPERTENSIVE DISORDERS OF PREGNANCY

Hypertensive disorders of pregnancy are usually classified according to those disorders that antedate and those specific to pregnancy. The term *pregnancy-induced hypertension* is nonspecific, and its use is not recommended.

Gestational Hypertension

Gestational hypertension is defined as gestational blood pressure elevation only, without proteinuria. The term *gestational hypertension* will therefore include three types of patients. The first is the patient with new-onset gestational blood pressure elevation that resolves by 12 weeks postpartum. This is termed *transient hypertension,* and the diagnosis can be made only retrospectively. The second is the patient who goes on to develop proteinuria and thus satisfy diagnostic criteria for preeclampsia. The third is the patient whose elevated blood pressures persist postpartum, indicating chronic hypertension.[2]

Minimally elevated blood pressures or gestational blood pressure elevation without proteinuria is not a reliable indicator of maternal or fetal morbidity or mortality and primarily mandates close attention to mother and fetus.[3] In certain patients, the elevation in blood pressure without proteinuria may be accompanied by other signs of the syndrome that influence the degree of follow-up, further testing, and management.

Preeclampsia

Preeclampsia is a pregnancy-specific hypertensive disorder that usually occurs after 20 weeks of gestation, but can occur earlier with fetal hydrops or hydatidiform mole. Preeclampsia, unlike gestational hypertension, increases maternal and perinatal morbidity and mortality. *Preeclampsia* is defined as gestational blood pressure elevation with proteinuria.[2] The nonspecific diagnostic criteria of edema has been abandoned. *Eclampsia* is the occurrence of seizures that cannot be otherwise explained in a woman with preeclampsia.

Chronic Hypertension

Chronic hypertension is the presence of increased blood pressure before pregnancy or before 20 weeks' gestational age or if there is unknown persistent hypertension 12 weeks postpartum. Chronic hypertension with superimposed preeclampsia is indicated by the presence of exacerbated blood pressures, a change in baseline proteinuria, or evidence of end-organ dysfunction.

DIAGNOSTIC CRITERIA

Gestational Blood Pressure Elevation

Gestational blood pressure elevation is 140 mm Hg systolic or 90 mm Hg diastolic in a woman normotensive before 20 weeks. For many years, an alternative definition, an incremental increase of 30 mm Hg systolic or 15 mm Hg diastolic, has been used. The lack of specificity of this finding (about 25% of pregnant women) and the absence of evidence that this degree of blood pressure elevation without achieving a pressure of 140 or 90 is associated with excess fetal or maternal mortality or morbidity has led to the removal of these criteria from the definition of preeclampsia.[2] Nonetheless, the young woman who increases her usually low pressure by this amount without achieving absolute diagnostic levels requires close attention.

Blood pressures should be taken with the patient seated with her arm at the level of the heart. If the patient is in bed, the semi-Fowler position is most accurate. It is important to remember that blood pressure measured in an artery only indicates central blood pressure if the cuff is at the level of the heart. If the cuff is higher than the heart, blood pressure will be falsely low. The obstetric tradition of measuring blood pressure in the upper arm of a woman lying on her side is inappropriate and should be abandoned. It is also recommended that gestational blood pressure elevation be defined on the basis of at least two determinations. The repeat blood pressure should be performed in a manner to reduce the likelihood of artifact and/or patient anxiety.[2]

Proteinuria

Proteinuria is defined as the urinary excretion of 300 mg or more of protein in a 24-hour period. In theory, this should correlate with 30 mg/dL or 1+ on a dipstick.[2] Random urine dipstick measurements have been shown to vary substantially from 24-hour collections and cannot be relied on to either detect or exclude the presence of proteinuria in the preeclamptic patient.[4, 5] A more effective screening test is the protein/creatinine (P/C) ratio, which has been used extensively in obstetrics.[6, 7] When a value of 0.2 is used as the upper limit of normal, significant proteinuria can essentially be ruled out. Although the P/C ratio is a better screening test than a dipstick measurement, it is recommended that the diagnosis of proteinuria be based, if at all possible, on the "gold standard," a timed urine collection.

CLINICAL PRESENTATIONS AND MANIFESTATIONS OF PREECLAMPSIA

Preeclampsia manifests a spectrum of clinical findings that ranges from mild to more severe disease with signs and symptoms of end-organ involvement (Table 10–1). "Severe-range" blood pressures are 160 systolic or higher or 110 diastolic or higher, and "severe-range" proteinuria is 2 g/24 hr or higher.[2] Although patients most likely progress through the continuum over time, their rate of progression differs. Maternal and neonatal morbidity and

Table 10–1. Clinical Spectrum of Preeclampsia

Preeclampsia
Preeclampsia with severe-range blood pressures
Preeclampsia with evidence of end-organ involvement
HELLP syndrome (hemolysis, elevated liver enzymes, low platelets)
Eclampsia

Table 10–2. Evidence of End-Organ Involvement

Renal
Oliguria ($\leq$500 mL/24 hr)
Creatinine > 1.2 mg/dL
Neurologic
Cerebral disturbances
Visual disturbances
Persistent headache
Hepatic
Epigastric or RUQ pain
Elevated liver enzymes ($\geq$2 times normal)
Pulmonary
Pulmonary edema
Hematologic
Platelets < 100,000/mm^3
Microangiopathic hemolysis (increased LDH or bilirubin)
Placental
IUGR
Oligohydramnios
Abnormal Doppler studies

IUGR, intrauterine growth retardation; LDH, lactate dehydrogenase; RUQ, right upper quadrant.

mortality depend on multiple factors, including the gestational age at delivery and the severity of the disease.

The woman with overt preeclampsia is vasoconstricted, with evidence of activation of the coagulation cascade, and may have multiple organ dysfunction secondary to reduced perfusion. End-organ dysfunction may manifest in renal, neurologic, hepatic, pulmonary, hematologic, or placental abnormalities (Table 10–2).[2] The presence of evident end-organ involvement increases the certainty of the diagnosis.

There is ample evidence that preeclampsia may occur in women already hypertensive (chronic hypertension with superimposed preeclampsia), and the prognosis for mother and fetus is much worse than with either condition alone. The differentiation of superimposed preeclampsia from worsening chronic hypertension is often difficult, and for clinical management, overdiagnosis is appropriate.

MANAGEMENT OF PREECLAMPSIA

Several concepts are critical to the understanding of the treatment of preeclampsia. First, delivery, although always appropriate for the mother, may not be so for the fetus. Successful treatment other than delivery must reduce perinatal morbidity and mortality without increasing maternal morbidity. A decision as to whether the fetus is more likely to survive without significant neonatal complications in utero or in the nursery is the cornerstone of management. Second, the signs and symptoms of preeclampsia are not of pathogenic importance. Finally, the pathogenic changes of preeclampsia are present long before clinical diagnostic criteria are manifest.[8]

ANTEPARTUM MANAGEMENT

Initial Assessment

Once the diagnosis of preeclampsia has been established, the subsequent management includes thorough maternal and fetal assessment.[2] For maternal assessment, the extent of disease should be determined by laboratory studies (Table 10–3) and symptom evaluation for end-organ involvement. Fetal evaluation includes a nonstress test and, if delivery is not immediately planned, a detailed ultrasound including biometrics, amniotic fluid volume, and a biophysical profile. All of these fetal variables should be interpreted in light of gestational age.

Management Options

Following diagnosis and assessment, there are two management options. The first, delivery, should be considered for patients at term, patients preterm with severe end-organ involvement especially with evidence of rapid progression, and patients with non-reassuring fetal status.

The second option is expectant management. This ranges from short-term delivery delay to obtain steroid benefit or, less commonly, longer-term delivery delay for the extremely premature fetus. There is ample evidence that expectant management of preeclampsia in selected patients can prolong gestation sufficiently to improve perinatal survival.[9] However, this approach is always accompanied by the possibility of unavoidable maternal and fetal

Table 10–3. Laboratory Assessment

Laboratory Test	Rationale
Routine	
Hemoglobin	Decrease suggests hemolysis; elevation suggests hemoconcentration
Platelet count	Thrombocytopenia suggests more severe disease and may warrant further testing or specific management
Serum creatinine level	To guide magnesium therapy
Serum transaminase levels	Elevated transaminase suggests more severe disease and may warrant further testing or specific management
Optional	
LDH	In presence of thrombocytopenia and elevated transaminases to diagnose HELLP
Bilirubin	In presence of thrombocytopenia and elevated transaminases to diagnose HELLP
Peripheral blood smear	In presence of thrombocytopenia and elevated transaminases to diagnose HELLP
Coagulation profile	Occasionally helpful in severe disease; rarely abnormal without attendant thrombocytopenia

HELLP, hemolysis, elevated liver enzymes, low platelets; LDH, lactate dehydrogenase.

morbidity. Again, the gestational age at presentation, the maternal and fetal well-being, and the availability of supportive care for either the mother or the fetus weighs heavily on the decision. Unfortunately, there are too numerous variations to apply a strict formula for management schemes.

Long-Term Expectant Management

Expectant management, short or long term, may be reasonable in preterm patients with mild disease, very preterm patients with severe-range blood pressures controlled without evidence of end-organ dysfunction, or even the extremely preterm patient with some evidence of end-organ involvement. Expectant management schemes for early disease with severe hypertension have been proposed by several investigators.[9]

Observational Period

Any patient considered a candidate for expectant management should be observed for a sufficient period of time after the initial assessment to ensure that the disorder is not rapidly progressing. In selected patients without severe-range hypertension, severe-range proteinuria, or end-organ dysfunction, this observation may be as an outpatient with home blood pressure measurements and follow-up within 24 hours. For all other patients, this observation should be in the hospital. During this observational period, the degree of intervention should be guided by the severity of maternal disease.

Outpatient Management

If initial observation indicates mild maternal involvement with no evidence of progression and stable fetal condition, selected patients may be managed as outpatients.[10] Weekly to semiweekly fetal nonstress test and/or biophysical profile should be performed in addition to daily kick counts. The maternal condition should be monitored with daily symptom assessment, home blood pressure measurements, weight, and urine dip for protein with weekly to semiweekly physician evaluations and platelet studies. Patients should be hospitalized for disease progression or poor compliance. Delivery should be considered at term or with progression depending on the severity.

Hospital Management

Hospital management is indicated for the preterm patient with severe-range blood pressures, severe-range proteinuria, or evidence of end-organ dysfunction, or the patient with mild disease who has failed home management. The decision to continue expectant management will be made daily. Maternal assessment includes daily symptom assessment, blood pressure measurements, weight, and urine dip for protein. Which laboratory studies to obtain other than frequent platelet counts depend on the individual patient's disease, and their frequency is guided by disease progression and severity. Fetal assessment should include daily kick counts, daily nonstress test or biophysical profile, and biometrics every 2 to 3 weeks.[2]

Delivery is indicated at any gestational age with nonreassuring fetal assessment, labor, premature preterm rupture of the membranes, severe maternal symptoms, hemodynamic instability despite antihypertensives, or rapid disease progression.[2] An especially important maternal indication for delivery is the presence of hepatic subcapsular hematoma with risk of hepatic rupture. This is suggested by increased liver size (on physical examination or ultrasound) associated with tenderness and elevated liver enzymes. Once fetal lung maturity is reached, delivery should always be considered in preeclampsia with severe-range blood pressures, end-organ involvement, or intrauterine growth retardation. Finally, delivery at term for any woman with preeclampsia is always appropriate.

INTRAPARTUM MANAGEMENT OF PREECLAMPSIA

Delivery Mode

The optimal route of delivery for the preeclamptic patient is vaginal because it avoids the additional stress of surgery. With the availability of cervical ripening agents, even the patient with an unfavorable cervix can be given a trial of labor. Although delivery cures preeclampsia, this cure is not immediate and time saved by cesarean section must be weighed against the increased maternal risk. A carefully constructed plan of management including clear end points for delivery should be established based on maternal and fetal condition. Labor induction should be aggressive, and cesarean section should be considered if a vaginal delivery cannot be achieved within the time determined in the original plan or for usual obstetric indications.[2] Additionally, evidence of impending hepatic rupture, as described previously, mandates immediate cesarean delivery for maternal indications.

Seizure Prophylaxis

There is general agreement for the use of seizure prophylaxis in the eclamptic patient and the patient with more severe disease.[2] However, the routine use of anticonvulsants with mild disease or with gestational hypertension is controversial. There are currently no reliable predictors of seizures, and no one sign or symptom predicts more than 83% of seizures.[11] In order to prevent the maximum number of seizures, all women with hypertension would need to be treated. However, as the indications for prophylaxis

are expanded, many more women at no risk for seizures will be treated.

The drug of choice is parenteral magnesium sulfate.[12] Magnesium sulfate is renally excreted and has a half-life of 4 hours in a patient with normal renal function. The usual dose is a 4-g IV load followed by a 2-g/hr maintenance dose by mechanically controlled infusion. Monitoring should consist of frequent deep tendon reflex assessment and close monitoring of urine output. Serum levels can be checked when toxicity is in question. Magnesium should not be administered to patients with myasthenia gravis. Doses need to be adjusted in women with compromised renal function. In these women, the initial dose is similar because the initial volume of distribution is not influenced by renal function. However, subsequent magnesium infusions should be at 1 g/hr with hourly serum magnesium determination until a steady state is reached with dosage guided by these findings. In addition, phenytoin is metabolized independent of renal excretion and can be considered as an alternative.

Antihypertensives

Diastolic blood pressures persistently greater than 105 to 110 mm Hg should be treated with antihypertensive agents. The ideal drug should have a fairly rapid onset of action and reduce pressures in a controlled fashion without lowering cardiac output (Table 10–4). Pharmacologic treatment should have no adverse maternal or fetal effects.[2]

Corticosteroids

Depending on the severity of the disease and the gestational age of onset, many infants may benefit from delivery delay for the purpose of receiving antenatal corticosteroids. There has also been experimental use of corticosteroids for the stabilization of the patient with laboratory evidence of end-organ involvement, but this is not currently in routine use.[13, 14]

Fluid Management

The patient with preeclampsia should be given isotonic crystalloid during labor with a maintenance rate of 100 to 125 mL/hr. Oliguria, urine output of 20 to 30 mL/hr for 2 hours, should be treated with isotonic crystalloid bolus of no more than 1000 mL over 1 hour. Central monitoring should be considered if further fluid management other than maintenance is chosen. Alternatively, the patient may be continued on reduced fluid input with the recognition that the problem will almost certainly resolve postpartum.

POSTPARTUM MANAGEMENT
Follow-up

Women with preeclampsia require close follow-up in the postpartum period. An oral antihypertensive should be

Table 10–4. Antihypertensive Agents

Agent	Mechanism of Action	Onset of Action	Duration of Action	Initial Dose	Repeat Dose (until BP controlled)	Maximum Dose	Side Effects
Hydralazine	Arteriolar dilatation	10–20 min	3–8 hr	5 mg IV	5–10 mg every 20 min	25 mg	Tachycardia, headache, epigastric pain
Labetalol	α- and β-adrenergic blockers	1–2 min	6–16 hr	20 mg IV	40 mg after 10 min; 80 mg after 10 min	220 mg	Avoid in asthma, CHF, DM
Nifedipine	Calcium channel blocker	5–10 min	4–8 hr	10 mg PO	10 mg every 20 min	30 mg	Tachycardia, headache, interaction with $MgSO_4$
Sodium nitroprusside	Arteriole and venous dilatation	½–2 min	3–5 min	0.5 μg/kg/min IV drip	Titrate for effect	5 μg/kg/min	Fetal cyanide toxicity

BP, blood pressure; DM, diabetes mellitus; CHF, congestive heart failure.

considered in a woman previously normotensive who has persistent hypertension (>160/100) in the days after delivery. These women should have blood pressure monitoring twice-weekly secondary to the normalization of blood pressures by 6 weeks postpartum. Women with persistent hypertension 12 weeks postpartum will most likely require long-term treatment. Any abnormal laboratory studies that do not normalize in the immediate postpartum period should also be re-evaluated at 6 weeks postpartum.[2]

Counseling

Women with preeclampsia complicating their pregnancies should be counseled regarding their risk of hypertension complications in future pregnancies. Risk is related to gestational age at onset, race, paternity, parity, and other medical complications.

Women with early onset preeclampsia should also be counseled regarding the association with thrombophilias. Testing strategies include antiphospholipid antibodies, homocysteine, factor V Leiden mutation, protein S, and protein C.[15, 16]

Recommended Reading

National High Blood Pressure Education Program: Working Group report on high blood pressure in pregnancy. Am J Obstet Gynecol 2000;183:S1–S22.

Roberts JM: Pregnancy-related hypertension. In Creasy RK, Resnik R (eds): Maternal-Fetal Medicine, 4th ed. Philadelphia, WB Saunders, 1999, pp 833–873.

Schiff E, Friedman SA, Sibai BM: Conservative management of severe preeclampsia remote from term. Obstet Gynecol 1994;84:626–630.

References

1. Roberts JM, Taylor RN, Musci TJ, et al: Preeclampsia: An endothelial cell disorder. Am J Obstet Gynecol 1989;161:1200–1204.
2. National High Blood Pressure Education Program (NHBPEP): Working Group report on high blood pressure in pregnancy. Am J Obstet Gynecol 2000;183:S1–S22.
3. Brown MA, Wang M-X, Buddle ML, et al: Albumin excretory rate in normal and hypertensive pregnancy. Clin Sci 1994;86:251–255.
4. Meyer NL, Mercer BM, Friedman SA, Sibai BM: Urinary dipstick protein: A poor predictor of absent or severe proteinuria. Am J Obstet Gynecol 1994;170:137–141.
5. Kuo VS, Koumantakis G, Gallery ED: Proteinuria and its assessment in normal and hypertensive pregnancy. Am J Obstet Gynecol 1992;167:723–728.
6. Young RA, Buchanan RJ, Kinch R: Use of the protein/creatinine ratio of a single voided urine specimen in the evaluation of suspected pregnancy-induced hypertension. J Fam Pract 1996;42:385–389.
7. Robert M, Sepandj F, Liston RM, Dooley KC: Random protein-creatinine ratio for the quantitation of proteinuria in pregnancy. Obstet Gynecol 1997;90:893–895.
8. Roberts JM: Pregnancy-related hypertension. In Creasy RK, Resnik R (eds): Maternal-Fetal Medicine, 4th ed. Philadelphia, WB Saunders, 1999, pp 833–873.
9. Schiff E, Friedman SA, Sibai BM: Conservative management of severe preeclampsia remote from term. Obstet Gynecol 1994;84:626–630.
10. Helewa M, Heaman M, Robinson MA, Thompson L: Community-based home-care program for the management of pre-eclampsia: An alternative. CMAJ 1993;149:829–834.
11. Sibai BM, Lipshitz J, Anderson GD, Dilts PV Jr: Reassessment of intravenous $MgSO_4$ therapy in preeclampsia-eclampsia. Obstet Gynecol 1981;57:199–202.
12. Witlin AG, Sibai BM: Magnesium sulfate therapy in preeclampsia and eclampsia. Obstet Gynecol 1998;92:883–889.
13. Magann EF, Bass D, Chauhan SP, et al: Antepartum corticosteroids: Disease stabilization in patients with the syndrome of hemolysis, elevated liver enzymes, and low platelets (HELLP). Am J Obstet Gynecol 1994;171:1148–1153.
14. Magann EF, Perry KG Jr, Meydrech EF, et al: Postpartum corticosteroids: Accelerated recovery from the syndrome of hemolysis, elevated liver enzymes, and low platelets (HELLP). Am J Obstet Gynecol 1994;171:1154–1158.
15. Dekker GA, de Vries JI, Doelitzsch PM, et al: Underlying disorders associated with severe early-onset preeclampsia. Am J Obstet Gynecol 1995;173:1042–1048.
16. Kupferminc MJ, Eldor A, Steinman N, et al: Increased frequency of genetic thrombophilia in women with complications of pregnancy. N Engl J Med 1999;340:9–13.

Shoulder Dystocia

Richard Bronsteen and Bernard Gonik

Shoulder dystocia is a true obstetric emergency that can lead to significant adverse neonatal consequences. Owing to its low frequency and often unexpected and unpredicted occurrence, obstetricians need to be prepared for it. In this chapter, we briefly review this topic, including risk factors for its occurrence, maneuvers to treat it, and evaluate the possibility of altering obstetric management to avoid it.

Shoulder dystocia results when the normal descent of the fetal shoulders into the maternal pelvis is arrested, resulting in a delay in the fetal delivery. Shoulder dystocias can first be suspected when the fetal vertex is noted to retract toward the perineum on delivery; a finding some have called the *turtle sign*. In other cases, the shoulder dystocia is found when downward traction on the fetal vertex fails to produce significant progress toward delivery. This can result from an impaction of the anterior shoulder at the pubis symphysis and/or the posterior shoulder at the sacral promontory.

Subjectively, shoulder dystocia can be defined as a difficult delivery. There is currently no uniformly accepted and clinically utilized objective definition. This has, at least in part, contributed to the variable incidence at which shoulder dystocia is reported. The incidence can vary widely from 0.15% to 11% of all deliveries. One definition of shoulder dystocia is any delivery in which ancillary maneuvers are needed. Sponge and associates[1] observed vaginal deliveries to better quantitate the delivery process. Ancillary maneuvers were needed in 11% of the deliveries, only half of which were reported as shoulder dystocia. A mean delivery time of 24 seconds was noted in normal deliveries, as opposed to 79 seconds when shoulder dystocia was diagnosed. The authors proposed a head-to-body delivery time cutoff of 60 seconds or the use of ancillary maneuvers to define shoulder dystocia.

RISK FACTORS

Several gestational factors have been found to be associated with the occurrence of shoulder dystocia, and these can be classified as maternal, fetal, and intrapartum. Maternal factors include diabetes, postdate gestation, obesity, increased weight gain, multiparity, and prior history of shoulder dystocia. Fetal factors include macrosomia; intrapartum factors include protraction and arrest disorders of the first and second stages of labor, precipitous labor, and the use of an operative vaginal delivery.

The most common association generally placed with shoulder dystocia is the presence of a large baby. Increasing birth weight does result in an increase in the incidence of shoulder dystocia, with reported incidences up to 10% seen with birth weights of 4 to 4.5 kg, and up to 30% with birth weights above 4.5 kg. Although commonly linked together in physician's minds, birth weight is not a sensitive marker for shoulder dystocia in the general population. Approximately half of identified cases of shoulder dystocia are seen with birth weights of less than 4 kg. Diabetes has been found to be an independent risk factor for shoulder dystocia and, as is detailed later in this section, is also additive to the risk factor of birth weight. Infants of diabetic mothers, besides having an increased risk of larger birth weights, also have asymmetrical growth, resulting in a larger torso size for their body weight than babies from nondiabetic pregnancies. Patients with a prior history of shoulder dystocia have been found to have a similar result in up to 14% of subsequent pregnancies.[2, 3]

Controlling for birth weight in a macrosomic diabetic population (birth weight > 4 kg), Nesbitt and colleagues[4] found vacuum extraction was associated with an approximately 35% to 50% increase in shoulder dystocia versus spontaneous vaginal deliveries. Labor abnormalities with either protraction or arrest disorders have been inconsistently seen in association with shoulder dystocia. Paradoxically precipitous labor has also been seen in association with shoulder dystocia, possibly due to insufficient time to allow for the appropriate alignment of the fetal shoulders in the usual oblique orientation as they begin to descend into the maternal pelvis.

Increasing the number of risk factors present will have an additive effect, increasing the risk for shoulder dystocia. Several studies have evaluated the dual risks of diabetes and macrosomia. Typical of these is Langer and coworkers review[5] of nearly 76,000 deliveries. The results here showed a threefold increase in shoulder dystocia when diabetes was present in babies with a birth weight greater than 4 kg (15% vs. 5% in the normal population), and a fourfold increase when the birth weight was greater than 4.5 kg (42% vs. 10%). The data also showed that both the accuracy of prediction and the risk of shoulder dystocia are increased in diabetes. Although Langer and coworkers found a sensitivity of only 30% in predicting shoulder dystocia in the general population using a cutoff of 4250 g, in diabetics a similar cutoff increased the sensitivity to 80%. Acker and associates[6] also found improved accuracy in diabetics with macrosomic babies, with a 31% incidence of shoulder dystocia when the birth weight was above 4 kg, and a sensitivity of 73%.

OUTCOME

The primary concern when shoulder dystocia is encountered is the possibility of permanent neonatal damage. The neonatal mortality has been reported to range from 21 to 290 per 1000 cases, with approximately 20% to 25% of cases showing immediate morbidity.[7, 8] Neurologic damage can result from trauma to the brachial plexus. Damage to the upper brachial plexus (C5 and C6 roots) will result in an Erb palsy, whereas damage to the lower brachial plexus (C7 and C8 roots) results in a Klumpke palsy. Brachial plexus damage has been reported in 17% of shoulder dystocia cases.[8] Although the majority of these cases resolve by 1 year of age, in 5% to 10% of cases the damage persists, giving a low overall incidence of permanent nerve damage.[7, 9] It should be noted that not all fetal injuries are due to birth trauma, because in utero injuries similar to those seen with shoulder dystocia have been reported.

Neonatal depression as defined by need for resuscitation and low Apgar scores has been associated with deliveries complicated by shoulder dystocia. These outcome measures, however, can be confounded by a variety of clinical factors. Orthopedic damage with fractured clavicles and humeruses can also result from shoulder dystocia.

Maternal morbidity can also arise from damage to pelvic tissues. Increases reported in postpartum hemorrhage may be due, at least in part, to large babies and prolonged labor, rather than from the dystocia itself.

ANTEPARTUM PREDICTION AND PREVENTION

Given the presence of identifiable risk factors, and the possibility of permanent neonatal sequelae, it would be quite helpful to the clinician if shoulder dystocia could be accurately predicted before its occurrence. This would give the physician an opportunity to alter management to avoid the shoulder dystocia. The areas of both prediction and alteration of clinical management have been evaluated with, unfortunately, limited success.

Individual risk factors taken alone lack sufficient accuracy to be of clinical use. Birth weight, probably the best single predictor of shoulder dystocia, is limited by the finding that approximately half of the shoulder dystocia cases are encountered with birth weights less than 4 kg. Many of the cases of shoulder dystocia are notable for the absence of any of the previously described risk factors.

Combining risk factors also has not been a useful practice for predicting cases of shoulder dystocia. Although increasing the number of risk factors present does increase the risk, such combinations show a poor sensitivity for the diagnosis. Using multivariable analysis, both Gross and colleagues[10] and Perlow and coworkers[11] were unable to

accurately predict the occurrence of shoulder dystocia. In the former study, only 16% of the cases of shoulder dystocia could be predicted, whereas 19% were predicted by the analysis in the latter study.

For the general population, risk factors for shoulder dystocia appear to be at best weak predictors, and thus our ability as clinicians to identify these cases prospectively appears to be limited. Thus, although appropriate risk factors are known, they lack reasonable accuracy in predicting shoulder dystocia. Increasing the number of risk factors present will increase the risk of shoulder dystocia, although the potential usefulness of multiple risk factors is limited. In diabetics, the accuracy of predictions somewhat improved compared with the general population, as shown previously. However, adding to the problem of antenatal prediction is that the best single predictor, birth weight, cannot be reliably detected by ultrasound before delivery.[12]

Studies have been done with alterations of clinical management in an attempt to decrease shoulder dystocia. Gonen and associates[12] randomized 273 term nondiabetic gravidas with estimated fetal weights between 4 and 4.5 kg (ultrasonic estimate) to either elective induction or expectant management. No differences were noted in outcome in regard to incidence of shoulder dystocia or cesarean birthrates in the two groups; however, the mean time till delivery in the expectant management group was only 3.2 days, and all patients in this group were delivered within 6 days. In a retrospective review of a similar group of term large-for-gestational-age (LGA) fetuses (by ultrasound), Combs and colleagues[13] found elective induction associated with an increase in cesarean sections, but no decrease in shoulder dystocia when compared with expectant management. Here again, the interval to delivery in the expectant management was small, with the average time to delivery being 1.5 days.

Thus, the physician must be aware not only of the potential lack of success of avoiding shoulder dystocia for term LGA fetuses but also of the potential of increasing the chances of a cesarean birth. Weeks and coworkers[14] evaluated the route of delivery for babies that were LGA at birth. In those pregnancies in which the large size was diagnosed prenatally, there was a higher cesarean section rate than in those pregnancies in which the large fetal size was not diagnosed before delivery. Similarly, Levine and associates[15] evaluated the delivery outcome for appropriate-for-gestational age (AGA) fetuses incorrectly labeled as LGA on ultrasound in comparison to correctly diagnosed AGA fetuses. The inappropriately labeled LGA group had a higher incidence of diagnosed labor abnormalities and cesarean sections compared with the similar in weight but appropriately labeled group.

A study using a decision analytic model was also not encouraging on the use of elective cesareans for macrosomia.[16] Estimates were taken from the literature for multiple factors including the accuracy of antenatal prediction of macrosomia and shoulder dystocia rates. Three clinical management protocols were modeled: no intervention; ultrasound estimated fetal weight (EFW) with elective cesarean section for EFW greater than 4 kg; and ultrasound with cesarean section for EFW greater than 4.5 kg. Using a cutoff of an EFW of 4500 g, it was predicted that 3695 cesarean deliveries would have to be done in the normal population to prevent 1 case of permanent brachial plexus palsy. In the diabetic population, the number of cesarean sections was reduced to 443 to prevent 1 permanent palsy, although for just preventing shoulder dystocia in this group, 7 cesarean sections are needed for each shoulder dystocia prevented.

Given the increased incidence of shoulder dystocia in the diabetic population, one would predict that this group might be more amenable to prenatal diagnosis and prevention. Conway and Langer[17] scanned all diabetics between 37 and 38 weeks in a protocol calling for elective cesarean section when the EFW was above 4250 g and elective induction for an EFW below this cutoff but above the 90th percentile. Their data showed that 80% of shoulder dystocias in diabetics occurred in babies above this birth weight (as opposed to only 30% in their nondiabetic population). Using this approach compared with recent historical controls whose delivery management was not dictated by fetal size, they were able to decrease the incidence of shoulder dystocia in the diabetic vaginal deliveries from 18.8% to 7.4%, with an increase in diabetic cesarean sections from 21.7 to 25.1%. From their data, 10 cesarean sections were performed for each case of shoulder dystocia avoided. Another study in diabetics (classes A2 and B) showed no significant difference in outcome between induced and expectantly managed pregnancies.[18] Although randomized, this study included only fetuses found to be AGA at randomization at 38 weeks. The lack of success in avoiding shoulder dystocia may be due to the use of only those babies predicted to be of normal size, a low risk group for shoulder dystocia.

Other ultrasonic parameters, including chest-to-head difference, shoulder-to-head difference, abdominal circumference, and abdominal-to-head differences, have been suggested as alternatives to EFW as predictors of shoulder dystocia. These parameters have yet to be fully evaluated. It is not clear whether they will be clinically superior to EFW in predicting birth weight and shoulder dystocia.

Thus, currently, our overall ability to predict and prevent neonatal damage from shoulder dystocia is quite limited. In the general population, risk factors are at best limited and weak predictors for shoulder dystocia. A significant percentage of these cases do not have any risk factors, and the positive predictive value of individual risk factors is poor. In the diabetic population, in which birth weight is the most widely studied risk factor, the numbers look more promising for prepartum diagnosis and prevention. Here, though, our efforts are hampered by our limited accuracy in predicting birth weight. Prenatal ultrasound has not yet reached the level at which the use of the scale in the delivery room becomes redundant. At this time, for the general population, the routine use of either elective induction or elective cesarean section is not predicted to be helpful in improving neonatal outcome. In the diabetic population, given the increase in neonatal size and delivery complications, the numbers are somewhat more favorable, but active intervention should be done cautiously. Single factors lack sufficient accuracy to be clinically helpful; however, the clinician should be wary in situations in which multiple risk factors are present. Although the presence of multiple risk factors lacks sensitivity for general usefulness in preventing shoulder dystocia, the factors are additive for increasing predictive value.

MANAGEMENT

Once shoulder dystocia is suspected or diagnosed, the physician should take necessary steps to maximize a safe delivery. Appropriate assistants should be obtained from the obstetric, pediatric, and anesthetic fields. The patient should also be quickly informed of the situation, especially when an epidural has not been placed, because a cooperative patient will help facilitate delivery more than an uncontrolled one. Although a large episiotomy is recommended by some, the clinician must remember that this is usually a bony dystocia, and an episiotomy may only add potential maternal morbidity without assisting in fetal delivery. A large episiotomy may be helpful in certain situations, such as when the posterior shoulder is being held up in its descent by the posterior vaginal wall and when extra room is needed vaginally for fetal manipulation. Thus, its use should be individualized rather than routine. Throughout the delivery process, the physician must avoid placing excessive traction on the fetal head to minimize damage to the brachial plexus.

The McRoberts maneuver is recommended as the initial step for relieving the shoulder dystocia. Initially described by Gonik and coworkers,[19] this maneuver is easily and quickly performed. With this maneuver, the patient flexes and abducts her thighs on her abdomen. Although the diameters of the maternal pelvis are not increased by this maneuver, it does change the pelvic angle by flattening the sacrum in relation to the maternal spine and elevating the symphysis. This maneuver has been associated with a decrease in force needed to deliver the fetal shoulders and a decrease in force applied to the brachial plexus; with this change in pelvic orientation, the fetal shoulders can now hopefully continue with the descent into the maternal pelvis. Along with this maneuver, suprapubic pressure can be given in an attempt to dislodge the fetal shoulders from their impacted anteroposterior alignment, so that they can obliquely enter the pelvis. The McRoberts maneuver, alone or with suprapubic pressure, will be successful in relieving up to 90% of shoulder dystocias. Fundal pressure is not recommended with this or any other of the maneuvers because it may only worsen the shoulder impaction at the pelvic inlet.

If the maneuvers described previously are unsuccessful, variations of the Woods screw maneuver should be tried. This maneuver was initially described as a one-person operation combining fundal pressure with rotating pressure on the fetal shoulder. It is now recommended that torsion is placed on either the anterior (Woods maneuver) or the posterior (Rubin maneuver) surfaces of the posterior shoulder in an attempt to rotate the fetus 180 degrees. This can also be done in conjunction with suprapubic pressure. Here again, one is trying to dislodge the fetal shoulders off their impacted anteroposterior alignment, to promote entry into the pelvic inlet and descent. If this too is unsuccessful, the physician's hand can be placed into the vagina in an attempt to deliver the posterior arm out along the fetal abdomen. This is accomplished by inserting a hand into the uterus to the posterior fetal elbow, flexing the lower arm at the elbow, and then sweeping the arm out along the fetal abdomen and chest. Once the arm is delivered, the impaction has been broken. The baby can then be rotated 180 degrees, with the new posterior shoulder descending into the pelvis. In severe cases, the physician may need to attempt these maneuvers several times before being successful with delivery.

These maneuvers should be successful in relieving the majority of shoulder dystocias. If still unsuccessful, several choices remain. Choosing among these can be difficult, because in the majority of cases, the physician will have no experience in performing the maneuver. Intentional clavicular fracture has been suggested to decrease the bisacromial diameter. This can be attempted either manually or with scissors. Owing to the difficulty in performing this maneuver and the potential for fetal morbidity this maneuver currently is reserved mostly for shoulder dystocias with intrauterine fetal death. The Zavanelli maneuver has gained notoriety in the decade and a half since it was first described. Here the fetal vertex is manually rotated back to the direct occiput anterior position, flexed, and pushed back into the vagina. In a recent literature review of 92 cases, this maneuver was successful 85% of the time on the initial attempt and, overall, had a 94% success rate when repeat attempts with anesthesia are included. Once this is successfully performed, the fetus is then delivered by cesarean section. Of the 8 cases not relieved by the Zavanelli maneuver, 6 were delivered with a symphysiotomy and 2 were delivered with the aid of fetal manipulation through a laparotomy.[20] Not unexpectedly, neonatal and maternal morbidity was seen in association with these deliveries, including 15 cases of Erb palsy, 10 with abnormal neurologic outcome, 7 neonatal deaths, and 7 uterine ruptures. These outcomes should not be attributed solely to the performance of the Zavanelli maneuver, because the presence of the severe dystocia along with the prior maneuvers certainly played a role in the outcomes. Another final resort–type of maneuver is a pubic symphysiotomy. Here a scalpel is used to separate the fibrous connecting tissues between the pubic symphysis. Care must be taken not to damage the underlying urethra.

An alternative maneuver from the midwifery field is the "all-fours" maneuver described by Gaskin.[21] This maneuver was brought into her practice in 1976 after she observed its use by midwives in the Guatemalan Highlands. The patient is turned to her hands and knees, placing equal weight on each extremity, delivering the baby from this position. Its successful use in 82 cases has subsequently been reported.[22] It is currently unclear where in the protocol described previously this maneuver may best be utilized.

At the present time, there does not appear to be a good solution to eliminating the problem of shoulder dystocia. Thus, physicians should be familiar with the steps to take once a shoulder dystocia is encountered and be able to institute them promptly. Periodic review of the maneuvers to be used can be quite helpful, because this situation is often encountered without warning.

References

1. Sponge CY, Beall M, Rodrigues D, et al: An objective definition of shoulder dystocia: Prolonged head-to-body intervals and/or the use of ancillary obstetric maneuvers. Obstet Gynecol 1995;86:433–436.
2. Smith RB, Lane C, Pearson JF: Shoulder dystocia: What happens at the next delivery? Br J Obstet Gynecol 1994;101:713–715.
3. Lewis DF, Raymond RC, Perkins MD, et al: Recurrence rate of shoulder dystocia. Am J Obstet Gynecol 1995;172:1369–1371.
4. Nesbitt TS, Gilbert WM, Herrchen B: Shoulder dystocia and associated risk factors with macrosomic infants born in California. Am J Obstet Gynecol 1998;179:476–480.
5. Langer O, Berkus MD, Huff RW, et al: Shoulder dystocia: Should the fetus weighing > 4000 grams be delivered by cesarean section? Am J Obstet Gynecol 1991;165:831.
6. Acker DB, Sachs BP, Friedman EA: Risk factors for shoulder dystocia in the average-weight infant. Obstet Gynecol 1986;67:614–618.
7. Gherman RB, Ouzounian JG, Goodwin TM: Obstetric maneuvers for shoulder dystocia and associated fetal morbidity. Am J Obstet Gynecol 1998;178:1126.
8. Benedetti TJ, Gabbe SG: Shoulder dystocia: A complication of fetal macrosomia and prolonged second stage of labor with midpelvic delivery. Obstet Gynecol 1978;52:526.
9. Gordon M, Rich H, Deutschberger J, et al: The immediate and long-term outcome of obstetric birth trauma. Am J Obstet Gynecol 1973;117:51.
10. Gross TL, Sokol RJ, Williams T, Thompson K: Shoulder dystocia: A fetal-physician risk. Am J Obstet Gynecol 1987;156:1408.
11. Perlow JK, Wigton T, Hart J: Birth trauma—a 5-year review of incidence and associated perinatal factors. J Reprod Med 1996;41:754.
12. Gonen O, Rosen D, Zipora D, et al: Induction of labor versus expectant management in macrosomia: A randomized study. Obstet Gynecol 1997;89:913.
13. Combs CA, Singh NB, Khoury JC: Elective induction versus spontaneous labor after sonographic diagnosis of fetal macrosomia. Obstet Gynecol 1993;81:492–496.
14. Weeks JW, Pitman T, Spinnato JA: Fetal macrosomia: Does antenatal prediction affect delivery route and birth outcome? Am J Obstet Gynecol 1995;173:1215.
15. Levine AR, Lockwood CJ, Brown B, et al: Sonographic diagnosis of the large-for-gestational age fetus at term: Does it make a difference? Obstet Gynecol 1992;79:55.
16. Rouse DJ, Owen J, Goldenberg RL, Cliver SP: The effectiveness and costs of elective cesarean delivery for fetal macrosomia diagnosed by ultrasound. JAMA 1996;276:1480–1486.
17. Conway DL, Langer O: Elective delivery of infants with macrosomia in diabetic women: Reduced shoulder dystocia versus increased cesarean deliveries. Am J Obstet Gynecol 1998;178:922.
18. Kjos SL, Henry OA, Montoro M, et al: Insulin-requiring diabetes in pregnancy: A randomized trial of active induction of labor and expectant management. Am J Obstet Gynecol 1993;169:611.
19. Gonik B, Stringer CA, Held B: An alternate maneuver for management of shoulder dystocia. Am J Obstet Gynecol 1983;145:882.
20. Sandberg EC: The Zavanelli maneuver: 12 years of recorded experience. Obstet Gynecol 1999;93:312–317.
21. Gaskin IM: Shoulder dystocia: Controversies in management. Birth Gazette 1988;5:14.
22. Bruner JP, Drummond SB, Meenan AL, Gaskin IM: All-fours maneuver for reducing shoulder dystocia during labor. J Reprod Med 1998;43:439.

Recently Described Hereditary Thrombophilias and Obstetric Outcome

Donna Dizon-Townson

As a result of the human genome project and the major advances in gene identification, the exciting area of the study of pregnancy and thrombophilia has emerged. Several recent letters to the editor in the *New England Journal of Medicine* have referred to this area of investigation as novel and challenging to clinicians and scientists.[1,2] Several common genetic predispositions to thrombophilia, including factor V Leiden, prothrombin G20210A, and the 5,10-methylenetetrahydrofolate reductase (5,10-MTHFR) mutations, have been described recently. The discovery of these common genetic predispositions has facilitated investigations into the effects of thrombophilic predispositions on pregnancy outcome for mother, fetus, and neonate. This review presents a discussion of the most recently identified thrombophilias and their reported associations with adverse pregnancy outcomes.

FACTOR V LEIDEN, PROTHROMBIN G20210A, AND 5,10-METHYLENETETRAHYDROFOLATE REDUCTASE

Factor V Leiden

Resistance to activated protein C (APC), most commonly due to a mutation of the factor V gene known as the Leiden mutation, is by far the most common identified genetic predisposition to thrombosis.[3–5] Normally, the protein C system provides anticoagulant properties critical for limiting thrombosis. Stimulation of the protein C system is dependent on the binding of thrombin to thrombomodulin on the endothelial cell surface. Protein C is activated by the thrombin-thrombomodulin complex. In the presence of protein S, APC selectively degrades the coagulation factors Va and VIIIa. Inactivation of factor V normally occurs in a three-step process, beginning with cleavage of the protein at Arg 506. In turn, this allows exposure and cleavage of the protein at Arg 306. The factor V Leiden mutation is a missense mutation in the factor V gene (1691 G-A), which produces an amino acid substitution of glutamine for arginine at position 506. Factor V protein encoded by the Leiden mutation is resistant to degradation by APC, thus conferring resistance to APC.[6]

Resistance to APC is assessed by determining the ratio of the activated partial thromboplastin time (aPTT) measured in the presence and the absence of APC. Normally, individuals will show a prolongation (>2.0) of the APC ratio. However, individuals with resistance to APC demonstrate a decrease in the APC ratio (<2.0). Resistance to APC, as determined by the functional assay, has been shown to increase during the second and third trimesters of normal pregnancy secondary to alterations in other coagulation proteins. Therefore, most experts currently recommend that the DNA test for factor V Leiden be used for screening for APC resistance during pregnancy. The DNA test is unaffected by either pregnancy or anticoagulant drugs.

Ninety percent to 100% of individuals with laboratory-confirmed APC resistance are either heterozygous or homozygous for the factor V Leiden mutation. Heterozygous carriers have a sevenfold increased risk for venous thrombosis, whereas homozygous carriers have an 80-fold increased risk. Carrier rates for factor V Leiden are 6% to 8% in northern Europeans and 4% to 5% in American whites. Ridker and colleagues[7] evaluated carrier frequencies for the mutation in over 4000 Americans of different ethnic origins and reported the following frequencies: whites, 5.27% (95% confidence interval 4.42 to 6.22), Hispanic Americans, 2.21% (1.01 to 4.16), African Americans, 1.23% (0.53 to 1.63), Asian Americans, 0.45% (0.05 to 1.63), Native Americans, 1.25% (0.03 to 6.77), and an overall carrier rate of 3.71% (3.14 to 4.33). Given the incidence of this condition, it is not surprising that APC resistance also has emerged as the single most common predisposition to thrombosis in pregnancy. In one study of deep venous thrombosis (DVT) in pregnancy, nearly 80% of cases had APC resistance.[8]

Prothrombin G20210A

A mutation in the prothrombin gene, prothrombin G20210A, is associated with an increased risk of venous thrombosis. Similar to factor V Leiden, this is another missense mutation, a G–A translation in nucleotide 20210 in the 3′ untranslated region of the prothrombin gene. This mutation is associated with elevated prothrombin levels

(>155%) and a 2.1-fold increased risk for thrombosis. Heterozygous carriers of the 20210A allele have a 2.8-fold increased risk for thrombosis, both DVT and cerebral vein thrombosis. The prevalence of the mutation in the white population is about 2%. The prevalence is 6% among unselected patients with thrombosis and about 18% in families with unexplained thrombophilia.

5,10-Methylenetetrahydrofolate Reductase

Epidemiologic evidence strongly implicates hyperhomocysteinemia as an independent risk factor for vascular disease in the coronary, cerebral, and peripheral vasculature.[9] Homocysteine, a sulfur-containing amino acid formed during the metabolism of methionine, is metabolized by one of two pathways: remethylation and trans-sulfuration. N^5,N^{10}-Methylenetetrahydrofolate reductase functions as a catalyst in the remethylation process. Kang and coworkers[10] reported a thermolabile variant caused by a missense mutation (C677T) in the coding region for the N^5,N^{10}-methylenetetrahydrofolate reductase binding site, resulting in the substitution of valine for alanine. This mutation correlates with elevated plasma homocysteine concentrations. Other data support an increased risk of thrombosis with hyperhomocysteinemia. It is therefore plausible that this mutation, which results in increased levels of homocysteine, may confer an increased risk for venous thrombosis.

OBSTETRIC OUTCOMES ASSOCIATED WITH HEREDITARY THROMBOPHILIA
Thromboembolism

Some 50% of thrombotic episodes in individuals with inherited thrombophilia occur in relation to another thrombogenic circumstance, such as with the use of oral contraceptives or in association with pregnancy or surgery. Thromboembolism, albeit an uncommon event, remains the number one cause of maternal mortality in both black and white populations in the United States.

The rate of thrombosis during pregnancy in asymptomatic women with APC resistance is uncertain. In a retrospective analysis of unselected obstetric patients, 14 of 403 (3.4%) individuals were found to carry the Leiden mutation.[11] Of these 14, 4 (28%) experienced a DVT during the pregnancy or postpartum period. In another study, 78% of women who experienced a DVT during pregnancy carried the factor V Leiden mutation.[8] Most recently, Gerhardt and associates[12] studied 119 women with a history of venous thromboembolism during pregnancy and the puerperium, compared with 233 age-matched normal women. They tested for the thrombotic mutations described. Among the women with a history of thromboembolism, the prevalence of factor V Leiden was 43.7%, compared with 7.7% among the normal women (relative risk of venous thrombo-

embolism, 9.3; 95% confidence interval 5.1 to 16.9). The prevalence of the prothrombin gene mutation was 16.9%, compared with 1.3% (relative risk, 15.2; 95% confidence interval, 4.2 to 52.6). The prevalence of both factor V Leiden and the G20210A prothrombin gene mutation was 9.3%, compared with 0 (estimated odds ratio 107).

Compared with patients who were heterozygous for factor V alone, the risk of spontaneous recurrent DVT has been shown to be increased in individuals who carry both factor V Leiden and the G20210A prothrombin mutation (relative risk 3.7; 95% confidence interval 1.7 to 7.7; $P <$ .001).[13] Carriers of both these mutations have an increased risk of recurrent DVT after a first episode and are candidates for lifelong anticoagulation. These worrying figures highlight the need for prospective observational studies to determine the actual risks of thrombosis in these patients. If the risk is confirmed to be medically substantial, trials of heparin prophylaxis may be justified.

Preeclampsia, Intrauterine Growth Restriction, and Fetal Loss

An expanding body of evidence suggests that thrombophilias, either inherited or acquired, are associated with preeclampsia, intrauterine growth restriction (IUGR), and pregnancy loss. The working hypothesis is that thrombotic predispositions interfere with establishment and maintenance of normal uteroplacental circulation. Thrombophilias may interfere with initial formation of spiral artery-intervillous circulation, eventually leading to limited placental (and hence fetal) perfusion. Thrombophilias also may result in the formation of thrombi in the low-pressure intervillous system and thereby lead to infarction and poor perfusion. In either event, the condition commonly known as uteroplacental insufficiency results.

Placentas from pregnancies exhibiting clinical features of uteroplacental insufficiency, even in the absence of known thrombophilias, often are characterized by intervillous fibrin deposition and infarction. One group found the factor V Leiden mutation in nearly 50% of 379 placentas with greater than 10% placental infarction.[14] Although it is unknown whether treatment with antiplatelet agents or anticoagulants has a beneficial effect on these common obstetric conditions, one might hypothesize that pregnancies at risk for these complications might benefit from anticoagulation during pregnancy. Readers should recognize, however, that properly designed trials to test this hypothesis are not yet available.

Preeclampsia

Four groups have shown that the frequency of APC resistance or the factor V Leiden mutation is significantly elevated among women with preeclampsia.[15–18] Dekker and colleagues[16] reported a 16% carrier rate of resistance to APC in women with severe early-onset preeclampsia. In comparison, by using well-defined criteria for severe pre-eclampsia, another group found a twofold increase in the carrier rate for the Leiden mutation in women with severe preeclampsia, compared with normotensive controls.[15] The higher rate of resistance to APC (16%) reported by Dekker and associates may be due to population differences, as they studied a Dutch population and used a broader definition of pregnancy-induced hypertension (39% had chronic hypertension and 53% had hemolysis, elevated liver enzymes, and low platelets—the HELLP syndrome).

The most comprehensive study of thrombophilias and pregnancy outcome to date is by Kupferminc and colleagues.[18] They studied the frequency of both hereditary and acquired thrombophilias in 110 women with the obstetric complications of preeclampsia, abruptio placentae, fetal growth retardation, and stillbirth compared with 110 women with normal pregnancies. They assessed for factor V Leiden, prothrombin G20210A, and 5,10-MTHFR mutations. In addition, patients were tested for deficiencies of protein S, protein C, and antithrombin III, and the presence of anticardiolipin antibodies. Women with obstetric complications delivered their babies at an earlier gestational age (32.1 ± 4.7 weeks) compared with women with normal pregnancies (39.5 ± 1.7 weeks [$P < .001$]) and had smaller neonates (1375 ± 693 g versus 3406 ± 402 g [$P < .001$]). Seventy-one of 110 (65%) of women with obstetric complications tested positive for one or more of the thrombophilias, compared with 20 of 110 (18%) of women with normal pregnancies ($P < .001$). The odds ratio was 8.2 (4.4 to 15.3). The prevalence of inherited thrombophilias in women with specific obstetric complications was as follows: severe preeclampsia, 5.4 (2.3 to 12.4); abruptio placentae, 7.2 (2.6 to 20.0); fetal growth retardation, 4.8 (2.2 to 10.3); and stillbirth, 3.4 (1.0 to 11.9).

Intrauterine Growth Restriction

Thrombosis and infarction of both the maternal and the fetal interfaces of the uteroplacental circulation are hypothesized to be the cause of uteroplacental insufficiency and subsequent IUGR. Correlation among placental histology, obstetric outcome, and IUGR has been reported by a number of investigators. An elegant description of placental thrombi and other vascular lesions in association with the maternal thrombophilias of protein C and protein S deficiency and antiphospholipid antibodies was reported by Rayne and colleagues.[19] Three of eight pregnancies in women with a thrombophilia were complicated with IUGR. Five of eight pregnancies suffered an intrauterine fetal demise. In another study reporting an adverse pregnancy outcome in association with resistance to APC, seven individuals had resistance to APC, defined as an APC ratio of less than 1.7, and six of the seven were heterozygous for the factor V Leiden mutation. Five of the seven pregnancies had IUGR and three of the seven suffered severe preeclampsia.[20]

Recurrent Fetal Loss

Recurrent miscarriage has been associated with certain hypercoagulable states. Antiphospholipid syndrome, which is characterized by recurrent fetal loss or venous or arterial thrombosis or both, has proved a valuable model for study. Based on the histologic findings of extensive infarction and necrosis in the placentas from pregnancies complicated by antiphospholipid syndrome, researchers have postulated that uteroplacental thrombosis may lead to placental infarction and eventual fetal death.

Inherited thrombophilias also have been shown to be associated with pregnancy loss; however, there is controversy regarding whether this association holds for first trimester (preembryonic or embryonic) loss, second trimester (fetal) loss and stillbirth, or both. Some investigators have found APC resistance associated with first trimester loss, whereas others have not.[21, 22] However, the association between APC resistance and second or third trimester fetal death is more secure. Rai and coworkers[23] found that 20% of women with second trimester fetal loss had resistance to APC as detected by the functional assay, compared with 4.3% of parous controls. In the European Prospective Cohort on Thrombophilia (EPCOT), investigators noted that the odds ratio for stillbirth in women with inherited thrombophilias was significant (3.6; 95% confidence interval 1.4 to 9.4).[23a] And for women with combined inherited thrombophilias, the odds ratio for stillbirth was quite high at 14.3 (95% confidence interval 2.4 to 8.6).

CEREBRAL PALSY

Several lines of evidence now support an association between thrombophilia and cerebral palsy. A proposed mechanism for the association of thrombophilia and cerebral palsy stems from the observation of thrombotic lesions in the placenta, leading to subsequent alterations in the uteroplacental blood flow that may result in either diffuse global fetal cerebral hypoperfusion or focal embolic events with resultant neurologic sequelae. It is important to realize that the fetal cerebral circulation is essentially unprotected in utero. Owing to the patency of the foramen ovale, the fetal circulation from umbilical vein to the brain is in direct communication and essentially bypasses the pulmonary circulation. Kraus and associates[24] observed thrombi in vessels from placentas of 11 of 15 children with cerebral palsy. An alternative basis for the injury was identified in the four placentas without thrombi. Moreover, in one infant who died at 1 month, autopsy confirmed the presence of cerebral thrombi and infarcts. The investigators concluded that thrombotic events may explain the pathogenesis of a proportion of cases of cerebral palsy. The association of placental thrombotic lesions and neurologic impairment and cerebral palsy has been confirmed by others.[25]

Following the discovery of factor V Leiden, Thorarensen and colleagues[26] reported three cases of neonatal cerebrovascular disorders, including ischemic infarction and hemiplegic stroke in babies who were heterozygous for the factor V Leiden. In addition, homozygosity has been proposed as a genetic cause of perinatal thrombosis and cerebral palsy.[27] Nelson and coworkers[28] reported 8 of 31 children (26%) with cerebral palsy, in contrast to 1 of 65 control children (1%) who were positive for factor V Leiden. They used a novel technique of recycling immunoaffinity chromatography, coupled with laser-enhanced fluorescence and chemiluminescence detection. We[29] have recently confirmed the findings of Nelson and coworkers by using the standard DNA techniques of allele-specific amplification. The carrier rate for factor V Leiden in children attending a mutidisciplinary cerebral palsy clinic was 6 of 28 (21%), compared with 3% in individuals without cerebral palsy ($P = .00001$).

SUMMARY

The discovery of these common thrombophilic mutations has enabled investigators to study the impact of thrombophilia on obstetric outcome. The findings to date have several important implications. First, these thrombophilic mutations may serve as disease markers. If large, prospective, observational studies support the association of thrombophilia and obstetric complications, then increased surveillance for these individuals may be warranted. Second, these thrombotic predispositions may be amenable to medical anticoagulant therapy. Prospective randomized trials of anticoagulation appear justified in certain high-risk groups. Third, these genetic traits may be identified in related asymptomatic family members prior to a thromboembolic event. Appropriate counseling and possible thromboprophylaxis may then be offered in a directed fashion.

References

1. Sibai BM: Thrombophilias and adverse outcomes of pregnancy—what should a clinician do? N Engl J Med 1999;340:50–52.
2. Greer IA: The challenge of thrombophilia in maternal-fetal medicine. N Engl J Med 2000;342:424–425.
3. Dahlback B: Inherited resistance to activated protein C, a major cause of venous thrombosis, is due to a mutation in the factor V gene. Haemostasis 1994;24:139–151.
4. Zoller B, Dahlback BD: Linkage between inherited resistance to activated protein C and factor V gene mutation in venous thrombosis. Lancet 1994;343:1536–1538.
5. Bertina RM, Koeleman BPC, Koster T, et al: Mutation in blood coagulation factor V associated with resistance to activated protein C. Nature 1994;369:64–67.
6. Kalafatis M, Rand MD, Mann KG: The mechanism of inactivation of human factor V and human factor Va by activated protein C. J Biol Chem 1994;269:31869–31880.
7. Ridker PM, Miletich JP, Hennekens CH, Buring JE: Ethnic distribution of factor V Leiden in 4047 men and women. JAMA 1997;297:1094–1099.
8. Hallak M, Denderowicz J, Cassel A, et al: Activated protein C resistance (factor V Leiden) associated with thrombosis in pregnancy. Am J Obstet Gynecol 1997;176:889–893.
9. Kang SS, Wong PW, Malinow MR: Hyperhomocyst(e)inemia as a risk factor for occlusive vascular disease. Annu Rev Nutr 1992;12:279–298.
10. Kang SS, Zhou J, Wong PWK, et al: Intermediate homocysteinemia: A thermolabile variant of methylenetetrahydrofolate reductase. Am J Hum Genet 1988;43:414–421.
11. Dizon-Townson D, Nelson L, Jang H, et al: The incidence of the factor V Leiden mutation in obstetrical population and its relation to deep vein thrombosis. Am J Obstet Gynecol 1997;176:883–886.
12. Gerhardt A, Scharf RE, Beckmann MW, et al: Prothrombin and factor V mutations in women with a history of thrombosis during pregnancy and the puerperium. N Engl J Med 2000;342:374–380.
13. De Stefano V, Martinelli I, Mannucci PM, et al: The risk of recurrent deep venous thrombosis among heterozygous carriers of both factor V Leiden and the G20210A prothrombin mutation. N Engl J Med 2000;341:801–806.
14. Dizon-Townson D, Meline L, Nelson L, et al: Fetal carriers of the factor V Leiden mutation are prone to miscarriage and placental infarction. Am J Obstet Gynecol 1997;177:401–405.
15. Dizon-Townson D, Nelson L, Easton K, Ward K: The factor V Leiden mutation may predispose women to severe preeclampsia. Am J Obstet Gynecol 1996;175:902–905.
16. Dekker GA, de Vries JIP, Doelitzsch PM, et al: Underlying disorders associated with severe early-onset preeclampsia. Am J Obstet Gynecol 1995;173:1042–1048.
17. Lindoff C, Ingemarsson I, Martinsson G, et al: Preeclampsia is associated with a reduced response to activated protein C. Am J Obstet Gynecol 1997;176:457–460.
18. Kupferminc MJ, Eldor A, Steinman N, et al: Increased frequency of genetic thrombophilia in women with complications of pregnancy. N Engl J Med 1999;340:9–13.
19. Rayne SC, Kraus FT: Placental thrombi and other vascular lesions: Classification, morphology, and clinical correlations. Pathol Res Pract 1993;189:2–17.
20. Rotmensch S, Liberati M, Mittelmann M, Ben-Rafael Z: Activated protein C resistance and adverse pregnancy outcome. Am J Obstet Gynecol 1997;177:170–173.
21. Dizon-Townson D, Kinney S, Branch DW, Ward K: The factor V Leiden mutation is not a common cause of recurrent miscarriage. J Reprod Immunol 1997;34:217–223.
22. Metz J, Kloss M, O'Malley CJ, et al: Prevalence of factor V Leiden is not increased in women with recurrent miscarriage. Clin Appl Thromb Hemostas 1996;3:137–140.
23. Rai R, Regan L, Hadley E, et al: Second-trimester pregnancy loss is associated with activated protein C resistance. Br J Haematol 1996;92:489–490.
23a. Preston FE, Rosendaal FR, Walker ID, et al: Increased fetal loss in women with heritable thrombophilia. Lancet 1996;348:913–916.
24. Kraus FT: Cerebral palsy and thrombi in placental vessels of the fetus: Insights from litigation. Hum Pathol 1997;28:246–248.
25. Redline RW, Wilson-Costello D, Borawski E, et al: Placental lesions associated with neurologic impairment and cerebral palsy in very low-birth-weight infants. Arch Pathol Lab Med 1998;122:1091–1098.
26. Thorarensen O, Ryan S, Hunter J, Younkin DP: Factor V Leiden mutation: An unrecognized cause of hemiplegic cerebral palsy, neonatal stroke, and placental thrombosis. Ann Neurol 1997;42:372–375.
27. Harum KH, Hoon AH, Kato GJ, et al: Homozygous factor V Leiden mutation as a genetic cause of perinatal thrombosis and cerebral palsy. Dev Med Child Neurol 1999;41:777–780.
28. Nelson KB, Dambrosia JM, Grether JK, Phillips TM: Neonatal cytokines and coagulation factors in children with cerebral palsy. Ann Neurol 1998;44:665–675.
29. Dizon-Townson D, Nelson L, Baksh L, et al: Factor V Leiden may predispose fetuses to cerebral palsy. Am J Obstet Gynecol 2000;182:S64.

THIRTEEN

Vaccines in Pregnancy

Theodore B. Jones

The U.S. Centers for Disease Control and Prevention (CDC) has cited 10 great public achievements in the United States during the previous century. The success of vaccination programs was at the top of their list; most vaccine-preventable diseases are now not common in the United States. Significant strides have been made in childhood immunization rates throughout the United States. In fact, rates are at an all-time high, resulting in most of the critical childhood vaccines achieving a utilization rate of almost 90%. However, immunization rates among adults are not as successful. It is estimated that 45,000 adults die each year of infections related to influenza, pneumoccocal disease, and hepatitis B; this is despite the availability of safe and effective vaccines to prevent these diseases and their complications.

Unfortunately, specific problems related to vaccine-preventable diseases persist. Much of the remaining morbidity and mortality related to vaccine-preventable diseases occurs among older adolescents and adults. These individuals escaped natural infection or were not vaccinated against diphtheria, tetanus, measles, mumps, rubella, and poliomyelitis and remain at risk of these infections and their complications. Lack of awareness of the safety of vaccines and the risks of vaccine-preventable diseases, concerns about adverse reactions related to vaccine administration, and missed opportunities by health providers to vaccinate adults in ambulatory settings adds to the existing difficulties with adult immunizations. Recognition of this problem led to the formation of the National Coalition for Adult Immunizations in 1988. It comprises voluntary, private, professional, and public organizations that share the goal of improving vaccine use among adults through the education of health care providers and patients.

The timeliness of this information for health care workers is important. Obstetricians-gynecologists are being asked to provide primary and preventive care for their patients during their reproductive years and thereafter. In most offices, there are dozens of daily opportunities to assess the vaccination status of women and to offer indicated protection before they depart the office. Unfortunately, many practicing obstetrician-gynecologists have a low awareness of the need to protect against vaccine-preventable diseases. A key factor that impedes a practitioner's use of vaccines in the office is the absence of skills and information by the physician and the office staff concerning the proper administration of vaccines and documentation of their use.

An important group is pregnant women. In many cases, prenatal care represents an opportunity for women to obtain insurance coverage that allows them access to health care. Perinatal care providers are well aware of the need to avoid all unnecessary medications or interventions that might injure the mother or her fetus during pregnancy (Table 13–1). However, the risks associated with vaccination are largely theoretical, and generally, the advantages outweigh the potential risks for adverse reactions. This is ever more important when exposure to infection is probable, if the infection poses particular danger to the mother or fetus, and if harm from the vaccine is unlikely. Additionally, information continues to accrue that confirms the safety of vaccines given inadvertently during pregnancy.

GENERAL CONSIDERATIONS

Immunobiologics have undergone significant change during the last 50 years. Modern immunobiologics are effective and extremely safe; however, adverse events have been associated with their administration. The spectrum of adverse events ranges from minor local reactions, which occur with some frequency, to severe systemic illnesses, such as paralysis associated with the live oral poliovirus.

Table 13–1. Vaccine Safety during Pregnancy

Vaccines Contraindicated during Pregnancy

Measles
Mumps
Rubella
Polio (OPV and IPV)*
Varicella
Japanese encephalitis
Vaccinia
Yellow fever*

Vaccines That May Be Used If Otherwise Indicated

Tetanus/diphtheria
Hepatitis B
Influenza
Pneumococcal
Hepatitis A
Cholera
Meningococcal
Plaque
Rabies
Typhoid (parenteral and Ty21a)

*Exception with travel to high-risk endemic area.
IPV, inactivated polio vaccine; OPV, oral polio vaccine.

The National Childhood Vaccine Injury Act of 1986 requires careful investigation of these events. Frequently, a cause-and-effect relationship cannot be established: temporal association alone does not always indicate causation. Temporally associated events severe enough to require medical attention by the recipient should be evaluated and reported in detail to the Vaccine Adverse Event Reporting System in order to foster better knowledge about adverse reactions.

Immunobiologics fall into three major categories: vaccines, toxoids, and immune globulins. Vaccines are further divided into two categories: live attenuated and inactivated. No problems in the developing fetus have been recognized in the administration of inactivated vaccines to pregnant women. However, there is a theoretical risk to the fetus posed by the administration of live virus vaccines. When a vaccine or toxoid is indicated during pregnancy, immunization after the end of the first trimester is reasonable, despite the absence of proven risks with earlier immunizations. Avoidance of live virus vaccines is necessary unless specifically indicated. Four requirements are expected of vaccines in order to be indicated during pregnancy:

1. The benefits of the vaccination are greater than the risk.
2. There is a high risk of exposure to the infectious agent.
3. The vaccine is effective and safe.
4. There is a risk for infection to the mother and/or the fetus.

There are particular benefits for the fetus and neonate when immunization occurs later in pregnancy. Although the maternal humoral response to immunization does not differ in the pregnant state, transplacental transfer of antibodies is known to be delayed. Additionally, although immunoglobulin G (IgG) antibody transfer starts at 16 weeks, the majority of IgG transfer does not occur until 32 weeks' gestation. This is a result of the increase in capacity for active transport of antibody as the placenta matures. For this reason, the benefits of maternal immunization are greater for the infants carried to term. Women of childbearing age are best served by possessing immunity to tetanus, diphtheria, measles, mumps, rubella, poliomyelitis, and varicella-zoster before conception. An important key to assessment for the need for vaccination is the review of history of previous illnesses and immunizations. Unfortunately, most adults have no records or unreliable records. Current perinatal guidelines recommend assessing all pregnant patients for evidence of immunity to rubella and hepatitis B.

SPECIFIC INDICATIONS IN PREGNANCY

Table 13–2 is an overview of vaccines in pregnancy and represents the most recent recommendations.[1, 2] The remainder of this section discusses selected indications of importance to the clinician.

Tetanus and Diphtheria

Tetanus occurs rarely in the United States, with most of the cases appearing to be a result of incomplete primary immunization series in elderly persons. Tetanus has been documented to occur among neonates born in conditions of poor hygiene to inadequately immunized mothers. Unfortunately, many adults are not protected from tetanus; several surveys performed since 1997 indicate that 11% of adults between the ages of 18 and 39 years are either inadequately immunized or not immunized. Vaccination for diphtheria, another disease that rarely occurs in the United States, is coupled with tetanus and pertussis as a normal part of childhood immunization series.

It is not unusual for obstetricians to encounter adolescents and adults with uncertain histories. Such cases should receive primary immunization utilizing the three-dose series. In individuals who have not received all of their series, the series should be completed with the necessary doses. Tetanus diphtheria toxoid booster doses should be given every 10 years beginning at the age of 11 or 12 years. Booster doses may be given during pregnancy. Additional booster doses are often given when a wound is believed to be significant and to be at risk of contamination. In general, a booster is appropriate if none has been given within the preceding 5 years. An incentive to the administration of tetanus toxoid in pregnancy is its effectiveness in the production of specific antibody that readily crosses the placenta, providing protection of the newborn against tetanus neonatorum, and also protecting the woman against puerperal tetanus. Adverse effects are rare.

Influenza Vaccination

Morbidity in the mother and the neonate from maternal influenza infection has been noted along with the possibility of teratogenicity. In addition, the theoretical neonatal protection supplied by transplacental transfer of preternal IgG influenza antigen-specific antibody after influenza vaccination has been suggested. The season for influenza infections lasts from the beginning of November through the month of March. The incubation period is approximately 1 to 4 days. The clinical diagnosis of influenza infection includes the recognition of symptoms such as fever, malaise, myalgias, and headache. The severity of influenza infection during pregnancy has varied during the 20th century, with maternal mortality reaching a zenith of 50% during the 1918 epidemic. Although no recent outbreaks of the disease have resulted in such high morbidity and mortality, reports of isolated fatalities continue. The explanations commonly cited for the predisposition of pregnant women to more severe morbidity include: pulmonary changes resulting in decreased residual lung capacity, hormonal changes causing smooth muscle relaxation and ineffective cough reflex, and an attenuated immune response.

Hepatitis B Vaccine

Hepatitis B remains an infectious disease with worldwide importance. The statistics are impressive: over 200,000 persons are infected with hepatitis B in the United

Table 13–2. Overview of Vaccines

Immunobiologic Generic Name	Primary Schedule and Booster(s)	Indications	Major Precautions and Contraindications	Special Considerations
Tetanus/diphtheria (Td) toxoid, adsorbed (for adult use)	Two doses IM 4 wk apart; third dose 6–12 mo after second dose; booster every 10 yr	All adults	Except in the first trimester, pregnancy is not a contraindication; history of a neurologic reaction or immediate hypersensitivity reaction after a previous dose; history of severe local (Arthus-type) reaction after previous dose, such individuals should not be given further routine or emergency doses of Td for 10 yr	Tetanus prophylaxis in wound management
Live Virus Vaccines				
Measles vaccine, live	One dose SC; second dose at least 1 mo later, at entry into college or post–high school education, beginning medical facility employment, or before traveling; susceptible travelers should receive one dose	All adults born after 1956 without documentation of live vaccine on or after first birthday, physician-diagnosed measles, or laboratory evidence of immunity; persons born before 1957 are generally considered immune	Pregnancy; immunocompromised persons; history of anaphylactic reactions after egg ingestion or receipt of neomycin	MMR is the vaccine of choice if recipients are likely to be susceptible to rubella and/or mumps as well as to measles; persons vaccinated between 1963 and 1967 with a killed measles vaccine alone, killed vaccine followed by live vaccine, or a vaccine of unknown type should be revaccinated with live measles virus vaccine
Mumps vaccine, live	One dose SC; no booster	All adults believed to be susceptible can be vaccinated; adults born before 1957 can be considered immune	Pregnancy; immunocompromised persons; history of anaphylactic reaction following egg ingestion	MMR is the vaccine of choice if recipients are likely to be susceptible to measles and rubella as well as to mumps
Rubella vaccine, live	One dose SC; no booster	Indicated for adults, both male and female, lacking documentation of live vaccine on or after first birthday or laboratory evidence of immunity, particularly young adults who work or congregate in places such as hospitals, colleges, and military facilities, as well as susceptible travelers	Pregnancy; immunocompromised persons; history of anaphylactic reaction following receipt of neomycin	Women pregnant when vaccinated or who become pregnant within 3 mo of vaccination should be counseled on the theoretical risks to the fetus; the risk of rubella vaccine–associated malformations in these women is so small as to be negligible; MMR is the vaccine of choice if recipients are likely to be susceptible to measles or mumps as well as to rubella
Live Virus and Inactivated Virus Vaccines				
Polio vaccines: enhanced-potency inactivated polio virus vaccine (eIPV); oral poliovirus vaccine, live (OPV)	eIPV preferred for primary vaccination; two doses SC 4 wk apart; a third dose 6–12 mo after second; for adults with a completed primary series and for whom a booster is indicated, either OPV or eIPV can be administered; if immediate protection is needed, OPV is recommended	Persons traveling to areas where wild poliovirus is epidemic or endemic; certain health care personnel	Although there is no convincing evidence documenting adverse effects of either OPV or eIPV on the pregnant woman or developing fetus, it is prudent on theoretical grounds to avoid vaccinating pregnant women; however, if immediate protection against polio is needed, OPV is recommended; OPV should not be given to immunocompromised individuals or to persons with known or possibly immunocompromised family members; eIPV is recommended in such situations	Although a protective immune response to eIPV in the immunocompromised person cannot be assured, the vaccine is safe, and some protection may result from its administration

Table continued on following page

Table 13–2. Overview of Vaccines *Continued*

Immunobiologic Generic Name	Primary Schedule and Booster(s)	Indications	Major Precautions and Contraindications	Special Considerations
Inactivated Virus Vaccines				
Hepatitis B (HB) inactivated virus vaccine	Two doses IM 4 wk apart; third dose 5 mo after second; booster doses not necessary within 7 yr of primary series Alternate schedule for one vaccine: three doses IM 4 wk apart; fourth dose 10 mo after the third	Adults at increased risk of occupational, environmental, social, or family exposure	Data are not available on the safety of the vaccine for the developing fetus; because the vaccine contains only noninfectious HBsAg particles, the risk should be negligible; pregnancy should not be considered a vaccine contraindication if the woman is otherwise eligible	The vaccine produces neither therapeutic nor adverse effects on HBV-infected persons; prevaccination serologic screening for susceptibility before vaccination may or may not be cost effective depending on costs of vaccination and testing and on the prevalence of immune persons in the group
Influenza vaccine (inactivated whole virus and split virus) vaccine	Annual vaccination with current vaccine; either whole or split virus vaccine may be used	Adults with high-risk conditions, residents of nursing homes or other chronic care facilities, medical care personnel, or healthy persons ≥ 65 yr	History of anaphylactic hypersensitivity to egg ingestion	No evidence exists of maternal or fetal risk when vaccine is administered in pregnancy because of an underlying high-risk condition in a pregnant woman; however, it is reasonable to wait until the second or third trimester, if possible, before vaccination
Pneumococcal polysaccharide vaccine (23 valent)	One dose; revaccination recommended for those at highest risk ≥ 6 yr after the first dose	Adults who are at increased risk of pneumococcal disease and its complications because of underlying health conditions; older adults, especially those ≥ 65 yr of age who are healthy	The safety of vaccine for pregnant women has not been evaluated; it should not be given during pregnancy unless the risk of infection is high; previous recipients of any type of pneumococcal polysaccharide vaccine who are at highest risk of fatal infection or antibody loss may be revaccinated ≥ 6 yr after the first dose	
Immune globulin (IG)	Hepatitis A prophylaxis Preexposure: one IM dose of 0.02 mL/kg for anticipated risk of 2–3 mo; IM dose of 0.06 mL/kg for anticipated risk of 5 mo; repeat appropriate dose at above intervals if exposure continues	Nonimmune persons traveling to developing countries		For travelers, IG is not an alternative to continued careful selection of foods and water; frequent travelers should be tested for hepatitis A antibody. IG is not indicated for persons with antibody to hepatitis A
	Postexposure: one IM dose of 0.02 mL/kg administered within 2 wk of exposure	Household and sexual contacts of persons with hepatitis A; staff, attendees, and parents of diapered attendees in day care center outbreaks		
	Measles prophylaxis 0.25 mL/kg IM (maximum 15 mL) administered within 6 day after exposure	Exposed susceptible contacts of measles cases	IG should not be used to control measles	IG administered within 6 days after exposure can prevent or modify measles; recipients of IG for measles prophylaxis should receive live measles vaccine 3 mo later
Hepatitis B immune globulin (HBIG)	0.06 mL/kg IM as soon as possible after exposure (with HB vaccine started at a different site); a second dose of HBIG should be administered 1 mo later (percutaneous/mucous membrane exposure) or 3 mo later (sexual exposure) if the HB vaccine series has not been started	After percutaneous or mucous membrane exposure to blood known to be HBsAg positive (within 7 days); after sexual exposure to a person with acute HBV or an HBV carrier (within 14 days)		

Table 13–2. Overview of Vaccines *Continued*

Immunobiologic Generic Name	Primary Schedule and Booster(s)	Indications	Major Precautions and Contraindications	Special Considerations
Tetanus immune globulin (TIG)	250 U IM	Part of management of nonclean, nonminor wound in a person with unknown tetanus toxoid status, with less than two previous doses or with two previous doses and a wound more than 24 hr old		
Rabies immune globulin, human (HRIG)	20 IU/kg, up to half infiltrated around wound; remainder IM	Part of management of rabies exposure in persons lacking a history of recommended preexposure or postexposure prophylaxis with HDCV	Although preferable to administer with the first dose of vaccine, can be administered up to the eighth day after the first dose of vaccine	
Varicella-zoster immune globulin (VZIG)	Persons < 50 kg: 125 U/ 10 kg IM Persons > 50 kg: 625 U	Immunocompromised patients known or likely to be susceptible with close and prolonged exposure to a household contact case or to an infectious hospital staff member or hospital roommate		

HBsAg, hepatitis B surface antigen; HBV, hepatitis B virus; HDCV, human diploid cell (rabies) vaccine; MMR, measles-mumps-rubella (vaccine).
Adapted from Update on Adult Immunization Recommendations of the Immunization Practices Advisory Committee (ACIP). MMWR 1991;40(RR12):1–52.

States each year. Of these, 11,000 will require hospitalization and 20,000 will develop chronic disease. There are 1.25 million Americans with chronic infection, with nearly 6000 dying annually from related hepatic diseases, such as cirrhosis and hepatocellular carcinoma.

The risk of vertical transmission ranges from 10% to 85%. Neonates infected with hepatitis B have a greater than 90% chance of developing a chronic infection, with a 25% risk of mortality related to chronic liver disease as adults. Over 90% of vertical infections can be prevented by vaccination and passive immunization with hepatitis B immune globulin at birth. Women who have household or sexual contact with carriers, intravenous drug users, recipients of blood products, health care workers, women with a recent episode of sexually transmitted disease or multiple male sex partners, or travelers to certain countries with high rates of endemic infection should be vaccinated. To increase the population-wide coverage, there is an aggressive effort to immunize all neonates as well as all adolescents younger than 20 years. Vaccine administration consists of a three-dose regimen over a 6-month period that induces immunity in 90% of healthy persons.

VACCINES IN THE NEAR FUTURE

Vaccine research is targeted at other causes of infectious morbidity and mortality in our communities. Efforts are coupled with the exploration of new strategies for safe and effective use. Maternal immunization can improve the passive immunity of infants to infectious agents that produce life-threatening illnesses in the first few months of life. The key to this protective effort is the generation of persistently high antibody titers when administered to adolescents and women of childbearing age. Similar to tetanus toxoid and influenza vaccine, additional vaccines have been suggested for maternal immunization as generators of persistently high antibody titers if given to adolescents and women of childbearing age (Table 13–3). These vaccines are being studied for safety and immunogenicity during pregnancy with an attempt toward devising an approach for women who present for antenatal care without prior evidence of adequate immunization.[3]

Table 13–3. Investigational Vaccines (in Development)

Vaccine	Status
Group B *Streptococcus* conjugate	Tested in women of childbearing age
Purified fusion protein for respiratory syncytial virus	Tested in postpartum women
Pneumococcal conjugate	Tested in women of childbearing age; preliminary tests
Meningococcal conjugate	Adult testing
Influenza, attenuated	Adult trial pending
Pertussis, acellular	Adult trial pending

Haemophilus influenzae Type b Vaccine

In parts of the world where *Haemophilus influenzae* type b occurs during the first few months of life, maternal immunization with *Haemophilus influenzae* type b vaccines could be very important. As a conjugate vaccine, it has been well tolerated and generates significantly higher levels of antibody in pregnant women than purified polysaccharide vaccines. The desired effect would be to produce higher levels of maternal antibodies for transmission to the fetus.

Pneumococcal Vaccine

Pneumococcal infection is a common cause of acute otitis media, meningitis, and pneumonia. Throughout the world, over 1 million children younger than 5 years of age die annually of pneumococcal pneumonia. Because infections occurring early in infancy pose the greatest risk for permanent sequelae or death, much consideration has been given to augmentation of the infants' passive immunity by boosting maternal titers. Active consideration is being given to using a conjugate vaccine in place of the current polysaccharide vaccine. The advantage to this modification would be to induce a greater protective immune response, although it would provide for protection against fewer antigen serotypes.

Group B Streptococcus

The most common cause of neonatal bacteremia and meningitis in the United States is group B streptococcus infection. It is common for pregnant women to have genitourinary colonization with group B streptococcus, and 25% of women receive antibiotics during labor to reduce the risk of neonatal infection (see Chapter 32, Prevention of Group B Streptococcal Disease). Maternal illness related to group B streptococcus is primarily chorioamnionitis or urinary tract infection. Polysaccharide vaccines have been studied in the past with limited success. Several conjugate vaccines are being evaluated clinically for promoting active maternal and passive fetal and neonatal immunity.

Respiratory Syncytial Virus

Respiratory syncytial virus (RSV) is a significant cause of respiratory disease during the first several months of life. Efforts to create an effective vaccine have been unsuccessful thus far. However, clinical trials are under way to evaluate a respiratory syncytial virus vaccine that has been shown to reduce the morbidity of a respiratory infection in children with cystic fibrosis as well as being safe and immunogenic in women of childbearing age.

Because information on vaccine recommendation changes are not always prominently displayed in the obstetric literature, periodic updating using web-based resources can be helpful. Sites associated with the CDC (www.cdc.gov/nip) contain new recommendations as they become available. In addition, organizations such as the Immunization Action Coalition (www.immunize.org) provide a wealth of information for clinicians.

References

1. American College of Physicians Task Force on Adult Immunization: Guide for Adult Immunization, 3rd ed. Philadelphia, American College of Physicians, 1994.
2. Update on Adult Immunization Recommendations of the Immunization Practices Advisory Committee (ACIP). MMWR 1991;40(RR12):1–52.
3. Glezen WP, Alpers M: Maternal immunization. Clin Infect Dis 1999;28:219–224.

FOURTEEN

Vaginal Birth after Cesarean: A Re-evaluation

Alan M. Peaceman

Prior to 1970, the primary cesarean delivery rate in the United States was below 4%. With the infrequency of this procedure, a policy of routine repeat cesarean birth had little impact on overall cesarean rates. However, with the rise in utilization of cesarean delivery in the 1970s, the contribution of repeat cesarean section to the overall cesarean rate became considerable. Traditional teaching was that a trial of labor carried unacceptable risk for the mother with a scarred uterus, but this concern originated from a time when cesarean scars were predominantly vertical in nature. There were few data regarding the experience with trials of labor in this setting until case series began to appear in the 1980s. As a consequence of this early experience, plus the efforts to lower overall cesarean rates, increasing numbers of women with low transverse uterine incisions have undergone a subsequent trial of labor. Vaginal birth after cesarean section (VBAC) rates, defined as the number of vaginal deliveries per 100 live births of women after a previous cesarean delivery, rose from 3% in 1980 to 28.3% in 1996.

With the rise in the number of women with a uterine scar undergoing a trial of labor has come the recognition of potential complications. Reports of rising numbers of adverse outcomes plus fear of litigation have tempered the enthusiasm of some patients and physicians for attempts at VBAC. As a result, a small downturn was seen in the VBAC rate in 1997, the first such downturn in the previous two decades. This chapter considers the risks and benefits of VBAC to assist the practitioner to arrive at a strategy for managing the patient with a prior cesarean delivery, and it discusses issues of patient management and counseling.

VBAC SUCCESS RATES

Literally hundreds of articles have been published regarding the issue of VBAC, with virtually all reporting vaginal delivery rates greater than 50% in the patients. Most studies report a vaginal delivery rate of between 60% and 80%. It is not surprising that a range this wide is seen, given the underlying variation in cesarean section rates. Clearly, success rates will vary with the patient population, the clinical setting, and the practice style of the physician.

A number of studies have examined whether circumstances of the first cesarean section influence VBAC success rates. Factors that have been associated with a higher likelihood of successful VBAC include a more dilated cervix at the time of admission, smaller birth weight, spontaneous labor, a prior vaginal delivery (either before the cesarean section or after), and prior cesarean for an indication other than dystocia (Table 14–1). Although these factors may convey an advantage to a patient, patients without them still have a likelihood of a successful trial of labor. Indeed, it should be remembered that as many as two thirds of women with an initial cesarean delivery for dystocia will have a subsequent VBAC, even if the subsequent birth weight is larger. Most studies did not find a significant difference in VBAC success rates based on the maximum cervical dilatation achieved before the previous cesarean. This would argue that arrest of labor is often due to factors other than cephalopelvic disproportion and that these factors often do not recur in the next labor.

Two risk-scoring systems have been published in an effort to describe a patient's chances of a successful VBAC based on the identified risk factors.[1, 2] These systems take into account indication for prior cesarean birth, cervical dilatation and effacement at admission, prior vaginal delivery, labor induction, and maternal age. In both studies, patients with the highest scores had VBAC success rates of over 90%. Even with the lowest scores, however, approximately 50% of patients had a successful VBAC.

It is important to remember that there are benefits to vaginal delivery in a patient with a prior cesarean section. Recovery time is often shortened for the mother who re-

Table 14–1. Reported VBAC Success Rates with Various Clinical Factors

Factor	VBAC Success (%)
Cervix at admission	
0–3 cm	61
4–6 cm	89
7–10 cm	90
Birth weight	
<4000 g	81
≥4000 g	67
Prior vaginal delivery	
Yes	87
No	73
Prior cesarean indication	
Dystocia	67
Other	80
Induced labor	53

turns home to care for multiple children. Repeat cesarean is associated with increased risks of anesthesia, infection, and blood loss, and patients encounter longer lengths of stay and increased costs. Further, repeat cesarean section places the patient at higher risk for placenta accreta in future pregnancies, with its attendant morbidity.

VBAC COMPLICATIONS

Although the high rate of successful vaginal delivery in patients attempting labor with prior cesarean birth has been seen consistently in most VBAC studies, significant complications for both the mother and the baby are also noted. The most feared complication is disruption of the uterine incision. This can result in extrusion of the fetus into the abdomen, a prolonged fetal heart rate deceleration, fetal demise, or extension of the incision into the broad ligament, necessitating hysterectomy. There are differences in terminology used by different investigators, but *uterine dehiscence* is defined by a scar separation that is asymptomatic, whereas *uterine rupture* is used when operative intervention is needed. In the largest prospective study to date involving over 7000 patients,[3] complications were relatively infrequent. Specifically, the incidence of uterine rupture was 0.8%, the incidence of 5-minute Apgar scores of less than 7 was 1.5%, and the incidence of hysterectomy was 0.06%. This series showed no maternal or perinatal deaths related to uterine rupture. In another series of more than 2000 patients with a trial of labor with prior cesarean delivery,[4] the dehiscence or rupture rate was 1.2%, with 1 neonatal death and 2 cases of apparent hypoxic ischemic encephalopathy. Therefore, it is appropriate to counsel patients that the risk of a symptomatic uterine disruption is likely in the 0.5% to 1.0% range, and that risk of perinatal death or significant neurologic injury is approximately 1 to 2 per 1000 trials of labor. The newborn risk is likely dependent on the ability to move quickly to operative intervention, because neonatal complications appear to be less frequent when the delivery can be accomplished within 20 minutes of the onset of abnormalities in the fetal heart rate tracing.

The diagnosis of uterine rupture during a trial of labor is based entirely on clinical signs. Originally, it was thought that a sudden increase in abdominal pain was the best predictor, and women were at times denied epidural analgesia for fear of masking this sign. Intrauterine pressure catheters were then encouraged, in the belief that a uterus with a defect would show a loss of the normal contraction pattern as the pressure would be transmitted into the abdominal cavity. Subsequently, it has been recognized that the best predictor of a uterine rupture is the development of a non-reassuring fetal heart rate tracing—variable decelerations, late decelerations, or a prolonged deceleration. Other signs that may support the suspicion of a rupture are uterine or abdominal pain, loss of station of the presenting part, vaginal bleeding, and maternal hypotension.

SPECIAL CASES

The experience just described relates primarily to those patients with one prior low transverse cesarean incision who are undergoing a subsequent trial of labor with a singleton vertex infant at term. There is considerably less experience with other obstetric circumstances, and therefore success rates and complication rates are less well defined. The risk of uterine dehiscence appears to increase in patients with more than one prior uterine incision, but it is still in the acceptable range to some motivated patients. A rate of rupture of approximately 1% has been observed in a cohort of patients with a prior low vertical uterine incision. Increased rates of complications have not been seen in studies involving VBAC in patients with twin gestation, breech presentation, fetal macrosomia, and unknown prior uterine scar. Although the experience is limited, motivated patients with these factors can be supported in their decision to attempt vaginal delivery.

CLINICAL RECOMMENDATIONS

During an initial prenatal visit, a history of prior uterine surgery should be elicited, along with its circumstances and any complications. Most patients with a single prior cesarean delivery can be encouraged to undergo a trial of labor. Patients should be apprised of the risks of VBAC, including the possibilities of uterine rupture, hemorrhage, neonatal injury or death, and the need for hysterectomy but also told that the neonatal risks are not significantly different from those seen in patients with unscarred uteruses. Further, they should also be informed of the benefits of VBAC, including the decreased disability, length of stay, cost, and maternal morbidity. No specific alterations in antenatal care are indicated. When admitted for labor, patients with prior cesarean birth should have continuous fetal monitoring and observation for clinical signs of scar disruption. Facilities to expedite delivery should be available as in other obstetric emergencies. Epidural analgesia can be offered to patients, and labor can be augmented with oxytocin as needed. Intrauterine pressure catheters do not seem to play an important role in the diagnosis of scar dehiscence. After delivery, some physicians routinely explore the uterus and examine the prior scar for signs of dehiscence—if one is identified, that may justify recommending against another trial of labor in future pregnancies.

References

1. Troyer LR, Parisi VM: Obstetric parameters affecting success in a trial of labor: Designation of a scoring system. Am J Obstet Gynecol 1992;167:1099–1104.
2. Flamm BL, Geiger AM: Vaginal birth after cesarean delivery: An admission scoring system. Obstet Gynecol 1997;90:907–910.
3. Flamm BL, Goings JR, Liu Y, Wolde-Tsadik G: Elective repeat cesarean delivery versus trial of labor: A prospective multicenter study. Obstet Gynecol 1994;83:927–932.
4. Socol ML, Peaceman AM: Vaginal birth after cesarean: An appraisal of fetal risk. Obstet Gynecol 1999;93:674–679.

Updates in Red Cell Isoimmunization

Mark E. Redman and Stanley M. Berry

Red blood cell isoimmunization remains a significant clinical problem.[1] The management of this condition continues to be a source of controversy despite the triumphs achieved in the prevention, detection, and treatment of hemolytic disease of the fetus and newborn. Increasing use of anti-D immune globulin prophylaxis and refinements in the diagnosis and treatment of fetal hemolytic anemia represent continued improvements in one of medicine's finest examples of the evolution of disease prevention and therapy. In the past, isoimmunization caused hemolytic disease in 9 to 10 in 1000 pregnancies, and was one of the major causes of perinatal morbidity and mortality.[2] Rh isoimmunization remains a significant obstetric complication but now occurs considerably less often. Pregnancy complications resulting from incompatibility of Rh antigens between fetus and mother occur in approximately 1 in 1000 pregnancies.[1] Whereas the most common cause of isoimmunization remains the immune response to the D antigen of the erythrocyte, minor antigens cause an increasing proportion of fetal and neonatal hemolytic disease as more potential cases of anti-D antigen isoimmunization are prevented.

This chapter reviews the pathophysiology that causes isoimmunization and can result in hemolytic and/or anemia resulting from the suppression of erythropoietic tissue, hydrops fetalis, and perinatal death. Attention is focused on recent advances in the prevention, screening, diagnosis, and treatment of Rh isoimmunization in pregnancy, as well as emerging techniques in these areas. Some investigators have assessed the cost effectiveness of Rh screening and immune prophylaxis. Others have examined extending the utility of amniocentesis in the diagnosis of Rh incompatibility and hemolytic disease. Research continues to refine the feasibility of noninvasive, as well as invasive and minimally invasive, diagnostic tests of Rh incompatibility and fetal anemia. Future techniques that appear promising include sonographic prediction of fetal anemia and assessment of fetal erythrocyte antigen status, by using both fetal cell retrieval from maternal blood and polymerase chain reaction (PCR)–based DNA analysis.

ISOIMMUNIZATION PATHOPHYSIOLOGY

Rh System

Among blood group systems, such as ABO and Rh, the Rh system is the primary source of isoimmunization in pregnancy. For this reason, we use the Rh system as our primary example when describing pathophysiology and clinical management. The reader must realize, however, that some antigen-antibody systems may have a different pathophysiology and, therefore, may require different management. The Rh system consists of a set of erythrocyte membrane-bound antigens. The Rh antigen subtypes, according to the nomenclatures of Fisher and Race, are C, c, D, E, and e.[2a] No alternate allele to D has been identified. Thus, "d" is merely a symbol that denotes the absence of D. In this chapter, *Rh-positive* and *Rh-negative* refer to the presence or absence, respectively, of the D antigen of the Rh system. Other nomenclatures are used to describe this group of erythrocyte antigens,[3, 4] but that of Fisher and Race[2a] is most commonly used in obstetrics.

Sensitization

When a patient who is naïve to one or more Rh antigens is exposed to an erythrocyte antigen of that type, a predominantly immunoglobulin M (IgM) antibody response may be mounted over 6 to 12 weeks. In the midst of the IgM response, an IgG response begins and persists for months to years after the initial stimulus is no longer present. After such a response to exposure, the patient has been "sensitized." Subsequent exposure to the sensitizing antigen in a sensitized patient provokes a rapid and prolific IgG response, facilitated by the presence of memory T cells from the initial exposure. A minority of maternal-fetal pairs with Rh incompatibility who cannot receive anti-D immune globulin develop sensitization. Rh-negative mothers of Rh-positive fetuses who do not receive prophylaxis have a 17% rate of sensitization during a single Rh-incompatible, ABO-compatible pregnancy.[5]

Variability in sensitization among maternal-fetal pairs at risk appears to be due to the requirement of sufficient fetal-maternal red cell passage to expose the maternal immune system to the novel antigen and to individual differences in immune response to antigens of the Rh system. It is now understood that fetal to maternal red cell passage occurs in nearly 100% of pregnancies.[6] The likelihood of increasing volumes of fetal-maternal red cell passage increases as pregnancy progresses. The incidence of maternal-fetal hemorrhage detectable by Kleihauer-Betke testing is approximately 3% in the first trimester, 12% in the second, and 45% in the third.[7] The average volume of fetal-maternal hemorrhage is 0.03 ml in the first and 0.1 ml in the second trimester. One recent study proposes that some variability in the maternal immune response to fetal

D antigen may be determined by fetal sex.[8] This retrospective review of 104 patients describes a significantly higher requirement for intrauterine transfusions (IUTs), lower gestational age at initial IUT, and lower cord blood hemoglobin and hematocrit for male fetuses than for female fetuses. The adjusted odds ratio (OR) for development of hydrops by male versus female fetuses was 13.1 (confidence interval [CI], 2.69 to 63.6). These investigators postulated that "rejection" of red blood cells of male fetuses might be augmented by a maternal immune response to a fetal intracellular antigen specific to males owing to location of the encoding gene on the Y chromosome.[8] One attempt to replicate the results of this investigation did not confirm the difference in disease severity based on sex.[9] Similar proportions of male and female fetuses were found in 207 pregnancies that were severely affected by anti-D antigen isoimmunization. There was no difference in prevalence of males versus females among fetuses that required transfusion, developed hydrops, or suffered perinatal death.[9]

ABO incompatibility reduces the chance of sensitization to 1.5% to 2% of susceptible maternal-fetal pairs.[7] In ABO-incompatible pregnancies, antibodies to ABO antigens may facilitate the clearing of fetal erythrocytes from maternal blood before sensitization to the Rh antigen occurs.[7]

Furthermore, maternal sensitization to a fetal erythrocyte antigen does not necessarily result in fetal hemolytic disease. At least 75% of patients have evidence of fetal-maternal hemorrhage after delivery, yet only 50% of sensitized patients develop fetal hemolytic disease. The development of hemolytic disease in an Rh-incompatible pregnancy depends on the volume of fetal blood exposure and on individual differences in maternal immune response.[7]

Immune Hydrops

In a sensitized gravida, maternal IgG antibodies may cross the placenta and bind to their target antigen on fetal red blood cell membranes. Fetal erythrocytes bound to maternal antibodies may interact with the Fc receptor of cells of the reticuloendothelial system. This interaction damages the erythrocyte membrane and leads to lysis of the erythrocyte. By this process, hemolysis may cause fetal anemia and accumulation of heme breakdown products, such as bilirubin. The resulting hypoxia promotes erythropoiesis. In the fetus, extramedullary erythropoiesis can result in hepatosplenomegaly and congestion of the portal circulation. The concomitant decrease in hepatic protein synthesis yields decreased intravascular oncotic pressure. Fetal ascites, skin edema, as well as pericardial and pleural effusions may result. In addition, the heme breakdown products circulating in the fetal intravascular space are believed to act as an osmotic diuretic that causes an increase in fetal urination, which leads to polyhydramnios. The accumulation of fluid in any two of the previously mentioned fetal compartments is known as fetal hydrops.

Circulating fetal bilirubin reaches the amniotic fluid by two pathways. Fetal urination, referred to earlier, is one of these pathways and tracheal efflux is the other. The amniotic fluid bilirubin serves as one clinically identifiable sign of disease severity, especially in isoimmunization related to the D antigen.

Differences in Pathophysiology with Minor Antigens

A somewhat different pathophysiology may give rise to the development of fetal hydrops when erythrocyte antigen incompatibilities other than those involving the D antigen are present. Although hemolysis is the cause of anemia in anti-D antigen isoimmunization, it appears less important in isoimmunization owing to atypical erythrocyte antigens such as Kell. Although maternal anti-Kell antibodies bind fetal erythrocytes, the principal pathology in Kell isoimmunization appears to be suppression of hematopoiesis.[10] Because fetal anemia due to Kell isoimmunization results from a process other than hemolysis, the fetus may be severely anemic without significant accumulation of heme breakdown products, such as bilirubin. This elucidates the poor correlation that has been observed between severity of hemolytic disease and levels of amniotic fluid bilirubin in patients with isoimmunization related to the Kell antigen.[11, 12] A review comparing Kell and RhD isoimmunization described significantly lower maternal antibody titers and poor correlation between fetal condition and amniotic fluid ΔOD_{450} for patients with Kell isoimmunization.[13] This difference in the pathophysiology of Kell isoimmunization may require deviations in the diagnostic strategy from that used in RhD isoimmunization. Reliance on amniotic fluid indicators of hemolysis will risk failing to predict anemia in pregnancies complicated by Kell isoimmunization.

SCREENING AND PROPHYLAXIS

Regimen

Pregnant women should be screened universally for Rh-negative status as well as the presence of antierythrocyte antibodies. Women who are Rh negative, who do not have antibodies to Rh antigens, and who have no history of sensitization are candidates for anti-D immune globulin prophylaxis. Patients found to have the Du antigen do not require administration of the anti-D immune globulin. The Du antigen is an erythrocyte surface marker that is a portion of the D antigen. Although some case reports describe the development of sensitization to D antigen in Du-positive patients, most evidence suggests that D-positive and Du-positive women are equivalent for purposes of prophylaxis.[6]

The timing and dose of anti-D antigen administered to eligible patients varies geographically. In the United States, and in some other countries, prophylaxis is administered antenatally as well as postnatally. Typically 300 μg of anti-D immune globulin is administered to Rh-negative unsensitized patients at approximately 28 weeks' gestation. A second dose is administered postpartum to parturients delivered of Rh-positive offspring. Prophylactic doses are also administered after clinical events that may be complicated by fetal-maternal hemorrhage, such as invasive diagnostic procedures, antepartum bleeding, abdominal trauma, and therapeutic or spontaneous abortion. In the United Kingdom, clinicians commonly administer 100 μg of anti-D immune globulin to Rh-negative unsensitized patients soon after delivery, and, increasingly, antenatal prophylaxis in the dose of 100 μg is administered at 28 and 34 weeks.

Antenatal prophylaxis of eligible patients became standard practice in the United States after publication of the findings of the McMaster Conference.[14] These results showed convincingly that a significant decrease in sensitization could be achieved by administering anti-D immune globulin universally at 28 weeks to nonsensitized Rh-negative women.[14] This policy has been resisted in the United Kingdom owing to uncertainty regarding the cost effectiveness of the practice. Postnatal prophylactic administration of anti-D immune globulin has been demonstrated to reduce the incidence of isoimmunization in susceptible patients from 17% to 1.5% to 2%. Some have questioned the added value of additional prophylaxis administered antenatally, especially in light of concerns that anti-D immune globulin may become scarce. The cost effectiveness of universal screening and prophylaxis of selected patients and the degree to which screening and prophylaxis recommendations are followed have been evaluated.

Administration of Anti-D Immune Globulin

In 1999, MacKenzie and coworkers[15] described the frequency with which prophylaxis recommendations are followed for Rh-negative primigravidas as well as both retrospective and prospective data that compared a cohort of patients who received antenatal prophylaxis with those who had not. This investigation revealed that antenatal prophylaxis significantly reduced the incidence of isoimmunization in second pregnancies when compared with both historical (OR, 0.28; CI, 0.14 to 0.53) and contemporary (OR, 0.43; CI, 0.22 to 0.86) control cohorts. The effectiveness of prophylaxis was limited, however, by poor adherence to guidelines for its use. Only 89% of eligible patients received at least one antepartum dose of anti-D immune globulin. Only 74% of eligible patients received two doses of anti-D immune globulin, which was the recommendation in the location where the study was conducted. This report documented that only 29% received anti-D immune globulin at the correct gestational ages (28 and 34 weeks). These investigators then estimated the cost savings of antenatal prophylaxis and the costs of routine antenatal prophylaxis for all Rh-negative gravidas. They

concluded that the costs of universal antenatal prophylaxis of all Rh-negative patients would exceed the savings.[15]

Cost Effectiveness

Other efforts have been undertaken to clarify the cost effectiveness of screening for patients at risk of isoimmunization and providing antenatal and postnatal prophylaxis. At the Consensus Conference on Anti-D Immune Globulin Prophylaxis held in Edinburgh, the literature pertaining to the economics of antenatal prophylaxis was summarized.[16] The review included eight studies that assessed the costs and benefits of antenatal prophylaxis for all Rh-negative patients or for only Rh-negative primigravidas.

Two studies were reviewed that compared antenatal prophylaxis for all with antenatal prophylaxis for only primigravidas. The studies yielded conflicting results, and comparisons between them are complicated by variation in their design and the economic details provided. Most of the studies used information from fee schedules rather than actual costs. The assessment of the actual costs of production of anti-D immune globulin is complicated because the anti-D immune globulin–related costs are joined with the costs of simultaneous production of other blood products. Whereas some studies demonstrate cost savings from antenatal prophylaxis of all Rh-negative gravidas, others do not, although they show cost savings from antenatal prophylaxis of only primigravidas.

Studies comparing the cost effectiveness of different antenatal prophylaxis strategies find that antenatal prophylaxis of only primigravidas is more cost effective than prophylaxis of all Rh-negative patients. This is presumably because primigravid patients are more likely to have subsequent pregnancies, which, of course, is requisite for the subsequent development of isoimmunization that could cause fetal hemolytic disease.[16] Thus, the cost effectiveness of antenatal prophylaxis of all Rh-negative patients remains unproved. Nevertheless, the supply of anti-D immune globulin is currently adequate, and the effectiveness, although not necessarily the cost effectiveness, of antenatal prophylaxis for all patients at risk is well documented. Accordingly, the American College of Obstetricians and Gynecologists continues to recommend routine antenatal prophylaxis for all Rh-negative patients, as outlined in its May 1999 Practice Bulletin.[17] Similarly, the Consensus Conference in the United Kingdom also concluded in its 1998 Consensus Statement[18] that the recommendation for prophylaxis in the United Kingdom should be changed to include antenatal prophylaxis for all Rh-negative patients.

Monoclonal Anti-D Antigen

Additional controversy regarding anti-D antigen centers on the source of the product. Because anti-D antigen is derived from donated blood, the potential of contamination exists. Prior to the use of screening tests for the hepatitis

C virus (HCV), a batch of anti-D antigen was contaminated with HCV from an infected donor. A 1999 report describes the outcome of 376 of the 390 patients who were exposed by receiving the anti-D antigen in Ireland between 1977 and 1978 and who were subsequently found to have HCV infection. Inflammation was found in 98% of the 363 study patients who underwent liver biopsy, with evidence of fibrosis in 186 (51%), and 2% had probable or definite cirrhosis.[19] Uncertainty regarding the continued availability of anti-D immune globulin also raises concerns about the source of the product.

Monoclonal anti-D immune globulin could offer a source of immune prophylaxis that is less susceptible to contamination and theoretically limitless in supply. Transformed human B cell lines producing Rh antibody have been shown to serve as reliable sources of anti-D immune globulin.[20] The safety and efficacy of this type of anti-D immune globulin have been assessed in a limited fashion; a large-scale clinical trial should be conducted to validate more confidently the clinical effectiveness of this form of anti-D immune globulin.

DIAGNOSIS

Titers

Maternal sensitization to the D antigen may occur despite proper anti-D immune globulin administration. Because pregnancies in different sensitized patients carry different risks for fetal hemolytic disease,[5] some assessment of the risk to a given pregnancy is required. The maternal anti-D antibody titer serves as an indicator of the presence and, in some cases, an initial approximation of the degree of maternal immune response to RhD antigen. Although titer values vary widely between laboratories and within an individual laboratory,[21] the titer is used to identify pregnancies that require further investigation. Owing to the variation in titers, as well as limited data to correlate titer values with severity of fetal anemia, no consensus exists regarding the titer level that marks a "critical titer" of anti-D antibodies in pregnancy. Nevertheless, many identify 1:16 as the titer value that prompts additional investigation because fetal hemolytic disease can occur when anti-D antibody titers are at least 1:16 or 1:32 and is rare when titers are below 1:16. Decisions to undertake further investigation after a given titer result will also depend on other factors specific to the patient, such as past obstetric history.

Amniocentesis

Amniocentesis has been utilized as a traditional means of diagnosing fetal hemolysis and estimating the severity of fetal anemia in pregnancies complicated by isoimmunization. The pioneering work of Liley[22] produced a chart correlating the severity of rhesus disease with the amniotic fluid bilirubin content, as reflected by the spectrophotometric change in optical density at 450 nm. This chart has facilitated use of amniotic fluid specimens to predict the severity and guide the management of hemolytic disease in fetuses between 27 and 40 weeks' gestation. Work by Queenan and associates[23] yielded a chart of ΔOD_{450} values between 14 and 40 weeks, thus extending the gestational age range in which clinicians might use amniocentesis results to guide management of hemolytic disease. One previous limitation of the Queenan chart was that it lacked clinical validation. A more recent study sought to assess the clinical usefulness of the Queenan chart compared with the Liley chart.[24] This investigation measured anti-D antibody titers and amniotic fluid ΔOD_{450} levels before intrauterine transfusion and found that the Queenan chart predicted the severely affected pregnancies before 27 weeks with a sensitivity of 100% and specificity of 79.4%. The moderately affected fetuses before 27 weeks were predicted with a sensitivity of 83.3% and specificity of 94.4%. The authors[24] concluded that the Queenan chart served as an acceptable substitute for the Liley chart before 27 weeks' gestation. Another evaluation of amniotic fluid ΔOD_{450} before 27 weeks found that single assessments via amniocentesis yielded a high rate of false-positive and false-negative results.[25] The authors[25] recommended, therefore, that diagnosis of fetal anemia before 27 weeks be made either by cordocentesis or by serial, rather than single, amniocentesis.

Amniocentesis can also be used to perform antenatal genotyping to determine fetal blood type and the potential for hemolytic disease. Assays utilizing the PCR to amplify fetal DNA from amniocytes obtained via amniocentesis or DNA from chorionic villi offer potential promise for identifying pregnancies in which further invasive procedures are unnecessary.[26]

Cordocentesis

The only method for directly quantitating the fetal hemoglobin remains fetal blood sampling, and cordocentesis is the most common method used to obtain fetal blood. Other procedures that can be used to obtain fetal blood include hepatocentesis and cardiocentesis. Intravascular transfusion via the umbilical vein remains the preferred method for fetal transfusion. Cordocentesis also is the primary method for fetal red cell antigen typing. The overall 1% to 2% risk of fetal death from cordocentesis and the paucity of centers that perform enough procedures to maintain high skill levels have inspired attempts to develop noninvasive techniques for predicting the severity of fetal anemia due to isoimmunization.

Noninvasive Assessment of Fetal Hemoglobin Levels

Ultrasound evaluation of the pregnancy complicated by isoimmunization provides the primary noninvasive means of assessment. Traditionally, however, the sonographic findings that have been recognized as signs of fetal anemia often represent severe disease after fetal decompensation has progressed. Findings such as ascites, pleural and pericardial effusions, and subcutaneous edema may be readily identified, but are not sensitive enough to predict severe anemia *before* it occurs and thus direct the timing of intrauterine transfusion.

Investigation into the use of biometry has revealed potential for predicting fetal anemia. Investigators who hypothesized that splenomegaly would predict the presence of hemolytic disease resulting in anemia obtained measurements of splenic circumference before cordocentesis in 21 singleton pregnancies and compared the values with measurements from 121 normal controls.[27] The investigators found that splenic circumference expressed in multiples of the median was significantly correlated with fetal anemia in cases with no prior transfusion. This method has not been shown to be an accurate predictor of anemia in large-scale clinical trials.

Doppler interrogation of fetal vessels provides another potential application of ultrasound in the assessment of anemia due to isoimmunization. Mari et al[28] have associated the peak systolic velocity of the middle cerebral artery with hemoglobin level. They assessed the potential utility of Doppler ultrasonography of the middle cerebral artery for predicting fetal anemia. In a study of 111 fetuses with isoimmunization, increased peak systolic velocity (PSV) in the middle cerebral artery (MCA) predicted moderate or severe anemia with 100% sensitivity and a false-positive rate of 12%.[28] The ability to anticipate the severity of anemia using sonographic evaluation could improve outcome by decreasing the number of invasive procedures required for diagnosing or treating hemolytic disease. This has not yet been assessed. The utility of MCA PSV for the prediction of anemia was not confirmed when other investigators attempted to replicate the results. In 223 measurements of MCA PSV in 61 pregnancies, elevated MCA PSV had a 56% sensitivity and 85% specificity for predicting fetal anemia.[29] These investigators noted improvement in prediction of anemia later in the study, suggesting the utility of the test improved with operator experience. Still, the sensitivity for anemia improved to only 75%.[29] Further investigation will be required before Doppler assessment of the MCA can be proposed to be the primary modality for predicting anemia in the management of isoimmunization.

Analysis of Maternal Blood

The emerging technology for identification of fetal cells in maternal plasma, along with the cloning of the RhD gene, offers significant promise of a practical and accurate method of identifying fetal Rh status without risk to the fetus. Geifman-Holtzman and colleagues[30] and Zheng and coworkers[31] have reported promising results with diagnos-

ing fetal RhD type by assessment of fetal genetic material in maternal blood. In light of concerns regarding the expense, technical difficulty, and reliability of identification of fetal Rh status from maternal blood samples, Lo and associates[32] sought to assess the feasibility of the technique by analyzing the fetal Rh status of 57 pregnancies from 10-ml maternal blood samples. After fluorogenic PCR analysis for fetal RhD DNA, the investigators correctly identified 78% of Rh-positive fetuses in the first trimester and 100% in the second and third trimesters.[32] These results suggest that assessment for fetal DNA in maternal blood may eventually provide a reliable method that poses no risk to the fetus and identifies pregnancies of Rh-negative patients that are at risk for fetal hemolytic disease.

CONCLUSION

Preventing isoimmunization by use of universal screening of maternal blood type and routine antenatal and postnatal immune prophylaxis for Rh-negative patients has been demonstrated to be cost effective in the primigravid patient and is recommended for all patients. The pathophysiology of Kell isoimmunization requires use of modalities other than amniocentesis for prediction of anemia. Although evidence is accumulating to validate the use of the Queenan chart to guide management of pregnancies with Rh isoimmunization by assessment of amniocentesis specimens beginning early in the second trimester, a large clinical experience with this methodology is still lacking. Techniques that do not involve invasion of the amniotic cavity to identify which pregnant women with red cell isoimmunization are at risk for fetal hemolytic disease and significant fetal anemia appear promising. Doppler insonation of the fetal middle cerebral artery for the determination of fetal anemia is a promising noninvasive technique. However, this modality needs independent validation by several centers before it can replace invasive techniques. Cordocentesis remains the only diagnostic modality that permits direct quantitation of fetal hemoglobin and assessment of fetal red blood cell antigens. In addition, it is the preferred method for treating fetal anemia due to isoimmunization.

References
1. Van Den Veyver IB, Subramanian SB, Hudson KM, et al: Prenatal diagnosis of the RhD fetal blood type on amniotic fluid by polymerase chain reaction. Obstet Gynecol 1996;87:419–422.
2. Joseph KS, Kramer MS: The decline in Rh hemolytic disease: Should Rh prophylaxis get all the credit? Am J Public Health 1998;88:209–215.
2a. Race RR: The Rh genotype and Fisher's theory. Blood 1948;3:27.
3. Wiener AS, Wexler IB: Heredity of the Blood Groups. New York, Grune & Stratton, 1958.
4. Rosenfield RE, Allan FH, Swisher SN, Kochwa S: A review of Rh serology and presentation of a new terminology. Transfusion 1962;2:287.
5. Bowman JM: Controversies in Rh prophylaxis. Who needs Rh immune globulin and when should it be given? Am J Obstet Gynecol 1985;151:289–294.

6. Berry SM: Red cell isoimmunization and fetal hemolytic disease. In Gleicher N, Buttino L Jr, Elkayam U, et al (eds). Principles and Practice of Medical Therapy in Pregnancy, 3rd. ed. Norwalk, Conn, Appleton & Lange, 1998, pp. 213–222.

7. Bowman JM: Maternal alloimmunization and fetal hemolytic disease. In Reece EA, Hobbins JC (eds): Medicine of the Fetus and Mother 2nd ed. Philadelphia, Lippincott-Raven; 1999, pp. 1241–1269.

8. Ulm B, Svolba MR, Ulm G, et al: Male fetuses are particularly affected by maternal alloimmunization to D antigen. Transfusion 1999;39:169–173.

9. Colombo DF, Knight PL, Buchholz V, O'Shaughnessy RW: Lack of a fetal sex predilection in a severe Rh-immunization in pregnancy. J Soc Gynecol Investig 2000;7:243A.

10. Vaughn JI, Manning M, Warwick R, et al: Inhibition of erythroid progenitor cells by anti-Kell antibodies in fetal alloimmune anemia. N Engl J Med 1998;338:798–803.

11. Vaughn JI, Warwick R, Letsky E, et al: Erythropoietic suppression in fetal anemia because of Kell alloimmunization. Am J Obstet Gynecol 1994;171:247–152.

12. Weiner CP, Widness JA: Decreased fetal erythropoiesis and hemolysis in Kell hemolytic anemia. Am J Obstet Gynecol 1996;174:547–151.

13. Babinszki A, Lapinski R, Berkowitz RL: Prognostic factors and management in pregnancies complicated with severe Kell alloimmunization: Experiences of the last 13 years. Am J Perinatol 1998;15:695–701.

14. McMaster conference on prevention of Rh Immunization. Sept. 28–30, 1977. Vox Sang 1979;36:50–64.

15. MacKenzie IZ, Bowell P, Gregory H, et al: Routine antenatal Rhesus D immunoglobin prophylaxis: The results of a prospective 10 year study. Br J Obstet Gynaecol 1999;106:492–497.

16. Cairns JA: Economics of antenatal prophylaxis. Br J Obstet Gynaecol 1998;105:19–22.

17. American College of Obstetricians and Gynecologists: Prevention of Rh D alloimmunization. ACOG Practice Bulletin, Clinical Management Guidelines for Obstetrician-Gynecologists 1999:4.

18. Urbaniak SJ, Farquhar MAF, Lowe GDO: Br J Obstet Gynaecol 1998;105:1–2.

19. Kenny-Walsh E: Clinical outcomes after hepatitis C infection from contaminated anti-D immune globulin. N Engl J Med 1999;340:1228–1233.

20. Hughes-Jones NC, Dash CH, Robson SC: Monoclonal anti-D issues. Br J Obstet Gynaecol 1998;105:29–30.

21. Goldsmith KLG, Mourant AE, Bangham DR: The international standard for anti-Rho (Anti-D) incomplete blood-typing serum. Bull World Health Organ 1967;36:435.

22. Liley AW: Liquor amnii analysis in the management of pregnancy complicated by rhesus sensitization. Am J Obstet Gynecol 1961;86:485–494.

23. Queenan JT, Tomai TP, Ural SH, King JC: Deviation in amniotic fluid optical density at a wavelength of 450 nm in Rh-immunized pregnancies from 14–40 weeks' gestation: A proposal for clinical management. Am J Obstet Gynecol 1993;168:1370–1376.

24. Scott F, Chan FY: Assessment of the clinical usefulness of the "Queenan" chart versus the "Liley" chart in predicting severity of Rhesus iso-immunization. Prenat Diagn 1998;18:1143–1148.

25. Rahman F, Detti L, Ozcan T, et al: Can a single measurement of amniotic fluid delta optical density be safely used in the clinical management of Rhesus-alloimmunized pregnancies before 27 weeks' gestation? Acta Obstet Gynecol Scand 1998;77:804–807.

26. Dildy GA, Jackson GM, Ward K: Determination of fetal RhD status from uncultured amniocytes. Obstet Gynecol 1996;88:207–210.

27. Bahado-Singh R, Oz U, Mari G, et al: Fetal splenic size in anemia due to Rh-alloimmunization. Obstet Gynecol 1998;92:828–832.

28. Mari G, Deter RL, Carpenter RL, et al: Noninvasive diagnosis by Doppler ultrasonography of fetal anemia due to maternal red-cell alloimmunization. N Engl J Med 2000;342:9–14.

29. Nesler S, Yankowitz J, Rijhsinghani A, et al: Value of middle cerebral artery peak velocity in evaluation of possible fetal anemia. J Soc Gynecol Investig 2000;7:118A.

30. Geifman-Holtzman O, Bernstein IM, Berry SM, et al: Fetal RhD genotyping from fetal cells flow sorted from maternal blood. Am J Obstet Gynecol 1996;174:818–822.

31. Zheng YL, Zhen DK, DeMaria MA, et al: Search for the optimal fetal cell antibody: Results of immunophenotyping studies using flow cytometry. Human Genet 1997;100:35–42.

32. Lo YMD, Hjelm M, Fidler C, et al: Prenatal diagnosis of fetal RhD status by molecular analysis of maternal plasma. N Engl J Med 1998;339:1734–1738.

Pregnancy and Medical Complications of Diabetes

Barak M. Rosenn and Menachem Miodovnik

Diabetes is one of the most common medical disorders of this era, affecting approximately 10.5 million people in the United States, or 4% of the population. The majority, approximately 90%, have type 2 diabetes (formerly known as maturity-onset, or non–insulin-dependent diabetes, NIDDM), and only 10% have type 1 diabetes (formerly termed juvenile diabetes, or insulin-dependent diabetes, IDDM). In the 18- to 44-year-old age group, the prevalence of diabetes is much lower, affecting approximately 1.5% of the population, but the representation of people with type 1 diabetes is disproportionately larger in this group because of the overall tendency of this form of the disease to occur at an earlier age. Thus, 1 to 2 of every 100 pregnant women may have preexisting diabetes, and many, if not most, of these have type 1 disease.

Diabetes is a chronic disease that is associated with the development of microvascular and macrovascular complications, manifested by retinopathy, nephropathy, neuropathy, coronary artery disease, peripheral vascular disease, and hypertension. These complications do not develop in every patient with diabetes, and the rate of progression varies from patient to patient. Some of the risk factors for developing these complications appear to be genetically determined. Others, such as glycemic control and hypertension, may be modified to alter the natural course of the disease, but adding pregnancy into this equation creates a significant dilemma for the patient and her health care provider. Thus, for the woman with diabetes who is pregnant, or who is planning to conceive, two main questions need to be addressed: (1) How will maternal diabetes affect the pregnancy and the health of her unborn child, particularly in the presence of microvascular or macrovascular disease? (2) How will pregnancy affect maternal diabetes and, specifically, the development and progression of microvascular and macrovascular disease?

MATERNAL EVALUATION

Preconceptional or prenatal care should include an evaluation of maternal status with respect to her diabetes and any existing complications. Some patients are highly self-conscious, visit their physician according to schedule, use their glucose meters on a regular and frequent basis, maintain good glycemic control, adhere to a prescribed diet, and exercise regularly. Unfortunately, most patients do not fall into this category. Many have very poor control of their diabetes and may be unaware of end-organ complications. Furthermore, a significant proportion of the population may actually have undiagnosed glucose intolerance and even overt type 2 diabetes for several years before being diagnosed and treated appropriately. Therefore, evaluation of the patient's status and risk in terms of diabetic complications should include the following components:

1. Evaluation of glycemic control, including hemoglobin A_{1c} concentration and review of daily self-monitoring of blood glucose concentrations obtained at least 5 to 7 times a day and recorded with a memory glucose meter.
2. Evaluation of blood pressure, including assessment of postural hypotension.
3. Evaluation of renal status: 24-hour urine collection for determination of creatinine clearance and total protein excretion (the possibility of a urinary tract infection should be excluded if proteinuria is present), and a renal panel to determine creatinine serum and BUN concentrations.
4. Evaluation of retinal status, preferably by an ophthalmologist who specializes in retinal disease. Documentation is best accomplished by a written description of findings accompanied by color photographs of the fundi for comparison with later examinations.
5. An ECG should be obtained on all women 35 years of age or older, those with hypertension, nephropathy, or peripheral vascular disease, those who are obese or have hypercholesterolemia, and those who have had diabetes for more than 20 years. Suspicious findings on ECG or suspicious symptomatology should be followed by a stress test.
6. Clinical evaluation of peripheral and autonomic neuropathy.
7. Clinical evaluation of hypoglycemic symptoms, their frequency, severity, and typical manifestations.
8. Clinical evaluation of peripheral vascular disease.

After evaluation of the patient's disease status, some insight into the expected course of pregnancy and the expected maternal and fetal outcome can be made, and this can be discussed with the patient and her family. The following sections summarize current concepts regarding pregnancy and medical complications of pregnancy and suggest some management recommendations. Be aware, however, that there are currently many gaps in our knowledge in this area, and that much of our clinical practice is guided by subjective experience rather than by objective data.

DIABETIC NEPHROPATHY
General Considerations

Diabetic nephropathy is a progressive disease that affects 30% to 40% of patients with diabetes. It is the most common cause of end-stage renal disease in the United States: in 1994, the rate of new cases of end-stage renal disease was 107 per million population, over three times more than in 1984. Clinically, diabetic nephropathy progresses through four distinct phases. Initially, there is a phase of glomerular hyperfiltration manifested by an increased glomerular filtration rate that is believed to result in renal structural damage. Within a few years, minute amounts of protein appear in the urine. This is the phase of microalbuminuria, defined variably as 30 to 300 mg of albumin excretion per 24 hours, or 20 to 200 μg per minute.

Within a few years, overt nephropathy develops (> 300 mg of albumin excretion per 24 hours or 200 μg per minute) characterized by excretion of progressively larger amounts of protein. Ultimately, progressive renal insufficiency and end-stage renal disease occur, manifest as decreasing creatinine clearance, increasing serum creatinine, and uremia. Diabetic nephropathy rarely manifests within the first 10 years of diabetes, but by 30 years, most of the 30% to 40% of those destined to develop nephropathy will already have done so. In the recent past, progression of nephropathy generally proceeded to end-stage renal disease, with creatinine clearance declining at a rate of approximately 10 mL/min every year, so that by the end of 10 years, most patients had reached the stage of renal failure requiring dialysis or renal transplant.

During the 1990s, however, it became clear that the development and progression of nephropathy can be modified by maintaining strict glycemic control and by meticulous control of blood pressure, and it is now recommended to maintain blood pressure values under 135/80. Furthermore, it became clear that antihypertensive treatment of patients with nephropathy using angiotensin-converting enzyme (ACE) inhibitors has a beneficial effect on nephropathy, even in the absence of hypertension.

Why Should Pregnancy Affect Nephropathy?

At least three factors that are associated with pregnancy could, hypothetically, increase the risk of nephropathy:

1. During normal pregnancy, there is a 40% to 60% increase in glomerular filtration rate. Because it is generally accepted that the primary insult leading to diabetic nephropathy is glomerular hyperfiltration, this could accelerate the development and progression of nephropathy.
2. Pregnancy-induced hypertension and preeclampsia affect 15% to 20% of all women with diabetes and an even greater proportion of those with nephropathy. Because systemic hypertension plays an important role in the progression of nephropathy, hypertensive disorders of pregnancy might be expected to exert a detrimental effect in this context.
3. Because diets with high protein content can result in

increased glomerular filtration rates, increased dietary protein intake, such as is recommended during pregnancy, may exacerbate glomerular hyperfiltration and accelerate the course of diabetic nephropathy.

Conversely, the strict glycemic control that is commonly recommended and instituted during pregnancy actually may have a beneficial effect on nephropathy, so it is difficult to predict the overall effect of pregnancy on the course of diabetic renal disease. To date, only a few studies, involving relatively few pregnant women have examined the short-term and long-term effects of pregnancy on renal function, and most have no nonpregnant controls.

How Does Pregnancy Affect the Course of Diabetic Nephropathy?

Pregnancy in women with microalbuminuria or overt nephropathy is often associated with a marked increase in proteinuria. This, however, is generally an acute and transient phenomenon. In most cases, even when massive proteinuria develops during pregnancy, it usually subsides after delivery and returns to prepregnancy levels. Of more concern to the patient is an issue that is much more difficult to determine, namely, the ultimate long-term effects of pregnancy on the course of diabetic nephropathy.

Several uncontrolled studies have attempted to address this issue.[1, 2, 3] Because of their design, none of these studies can account for all the possible confounding factors that might affect the outcome, and most studies include a relatively small number of subjects, explaining some of the conflicting conclusions. Taken together, most of these studies suggest that pregnancy is not associated with development of nephropathy or with accelerated progression of preexisting nephropathy. Some data, however, suggest that in patients with moderate or advanced renal disease (serum creatinine concentrations > 1.4 mg/dL or creatinine clearance < 75 mL/min) pregnancy may have a detrimental effect on progression to end-stage renal disease.[4] This fact should be taken into account when counseling this selective group of high-risk patients.

How Does Diabetic Nephropathy Affect Pregnancy Outcome?

The presence of diabetic nephropathy significantly affects the outcome of pregnancy, primarily for three reasons:

1. Pregnant women with diabetic nephropathy have an increased risk of developing hypertensive complications. Many of these women have preexisting chronic hypertension, and even in those who do not, preeclampsia is a common complication of pregnancy. Although the diagnosis of preeclampsia and superimposed preeclampsia in women who have preexisting proteinuria or hypertension sometimes may be difficult, it appears

that preeclampsia develops in up to 50% of women with nephropathy.

2. Women with nephropathy have an increased risk of fetal prematurity, caused by deteriorating maternal status or compromised fetal well-being. Approximately 25% to 30% of these pregnancies need to be delivered before 34 weeks' gestation, and approximately 50% are delivered before 37 weeks.

3. The fetuses of women with diabetic nephropathy are at an increased risk of fetal distress and fetal growth restriction, which occurs in approximately 20% of pregnancies. In these patients, chronic hypertension, decreased creatinine clearance, worsening nephropathy, and superimposed preeclampsia are all associated with an increased risk of fetal distress and fetal growth restriction.

In general, the worst perinatal outcomes occur in women who have measurable impaired renal function, with decreased creatinine clearance and increased serum creatinine concentrations. Aggressive control of maternal hypertension is of utmost importance to optimize pregnancy outcome, but the choice of antihypertensive medications is somewhat limited. The use of ACE inhibitors during pregnancy is contraindicated owing to their potential adverse effects on the fetus. The most widely used medications are methyldopa, nifedipine, and alpha-adrenergic blockers, for a targeted blood pressure in the range of 135/80.

Perinatal survival of infants born to mothers with diabetic nephropathy has been consistently close to 100% since about 1980. However, the increased rate of prematurity in this population is associated with an increased risk of long-term infant morbidity. Thus, although women with diabetic nephropathy may usually expect to deliver a viable fetus and take home a reasonably healthy infant, this group of patients is the one most likely to have a complicated course of pregnancy, requiring expert care and intensive management.

Guidelines for Management of Pregnant Women with Diabetic Nephropathy

Based on the observations reviewed in the previous sections, the following general guidelines may serve as a basis for the management of pregnant women with diabetic nephropathy or microalbuminuria:

1. Initial evaluation of the patient should be performed as outlined in the previous section on evaluation. If the serum creatinine concentration is 1.5 mg/dL or above, or if the creatinine clearance is 75 mL/min or less, the patient and her family should be advised that the risk of maternal and fetal complications is high, and that it is possible that pregnancy will accelerate progression of nephropathy toward end-stage renal disease. The physician should make every effort to ensure that the patient fully comprehends the significance of these risks.

2. Patients with hypertension should be managed aggressively to maintain blood pressure values under 135/80. Patients treated with ACE inhibitors should be switched to an alternative medication as soon as the pregnancy test becomes positive. Methyldopa can be used at doses of up to 3 g/day, and nifedipine or alpha-adrenergic blockers can be used when control of blood pressure cannot be achieved with methyldopa.

3. Insulin therapy should be adjusted to maintain near normoglycemia. This usually involves 3 to 4 injections of insulin a day, with frequent self-monitoring of capillary blood glucose concentrations. The goals of glycemic control should be less than 95 mg/dL before meals and less than 120 mg/dL 2 hours after meals. Hemoglobin A_{1c} levels should be obtained at the first prenatal visit and once each trimester.

4. A 24-hour collection of urine should be obtained at the first prenatal visit and at least once each trimester for determination of total protein content and creatinine clearance. A urine culture should be obtained simultaneously to rule out the coexistence of a urinary tract infection. Proteinuria may often increase during pregnancy to nephrotic ranges but will usually subside after delivery and is not, in itself, an indication for delivery. In the presence of massive proteinuria, serum albumin levels should be monitored, and peripheral edema often becomes a severe problem that requires supportive management.

5. Serial sonographic assessments of fetal growth should be obtained on a regular basis, at least every 4 weeks from 20 weeks' gestation onward. Antenatal fetal testing should start at 28 to 32 weeks, depending on the severity of the underlying disease and on fetal status as determined by sonography. Maternal bed rest is often prescribed to optimize the function of the fetoplacental unit, particularly in the presence of maternal hypertension or evidence of fetal growth restriction.

6. Timing of delivery should be guided by the usual obstetric indications, taking into account maternal and fetal status.

DIABETIC RETINOPATHY
General Considerations

Diabetic retinopathy is the leading cause of blindness in the United States, and it ultimately affects the majority of patients with diabetes. The etiology of diabetic retinopathy is not well understood, but the process involves progression from nonproliferative retinopathy, with development of capillary microaneurysms, excessive vascular permeability, and the formation of vascular occlusions, to the phase of proliferative retinopathy, with blood vessel proliferation and formation of fibrous tissue, contraction of fibrous tissue and vitreous, and the onset of hemorrhage leading ultimately to blindness. After 20 years of diabetes, practically 100% of patients who had onset of diabetes before age 30 years develop diabetic retinopathy, and approximately 50% of them have proliferative retinopathy. Thus, most pregnant women with type 1 diabetes have some degree of diabetic retinopathy and many have proliferative retinopathy.

The risk of progression from nonproliferative to proliferative diabetic retinopathy is directly related to the current degree of retinopathy. Patients who have only mild nonproliferative disease have approximately a 15% risk of progressing to high-risk proliferative disease within 5 years, whereas patients with severe nonproliferative disease have a 50% to 60% risk of progression. Regular periodic fundal examinations are extremely important in patients with diabetes, because laser photocoagulation is an effective therapy for proliferative retinopathy that can often prevent further progression of the disease. This, in combination with other treatment modalities such as vitrectomy, has greatly improved the prognosis for patients with diabetic retinopathy.

Why Should Pregnancy Affect Retinopathy?

Several recent large, prospective, randomized clinical trials have demonstrated that intensified glycemic control of diabetes is associated with significantly slower development and progression of retinopathy in patients with type 1 and type 2 diabetes.[5] Because the current consensus is to institute strict glycemic control in pregnant women with diabetes, this is expected to have a beneficial effect on retinopathy. At the same time, other studies have shown that rapid normalization of high blood glucose levels can cause acute progression of retinopathy, so that acute institution of strict glycemic control during pregnancy actually may be associated with deterioration of retinopathy.[6] Nevertheless, recent evidence indicates that over a longer period of follow-up of up to 4 years, patients who have been managed with intensive insulin therapy have slower progression of retinopathy compared with patients managed less intensively despite rapid initial progression.

In addition to institution of strict glycemic control, other changes occurring during pregnancy may affect retinopathy. Circulating and local factors such as growth hormone, insulin-like growth factor 1, and other angiogenic factors may have a role in development of retinopathy. These and similar factors are produced by the placenta in abundance and may, theoretically, affect the progression of retinopathy. Hypertension has also been consistently linked to the severity of retinopathy. The relation of hypertension to retinopathy may be particularly important during pregnancy because 10% to 20% of women with diabetes develop pregnancy-induced hypertension. Indeed, the development of pregnancy-induced hypertension, or preeclampsia, is associated with an increased risk for progression of retinopathy during pregnancy. Another theoretical concern related to pregnancy is that the abrupt increases in blood pressure that occur with maternal expulsive efforts during delivery may cause acute retinal hemorrhages in mothers with preproliferative changes. This concern, however, has not been substantiated by the limited available data addressing this issue.

How Does Pregnancy Affect Retinopathy?

Several studies have addressed this question and have reached varying conclusions. Some of this variance may be attributed to differences in study design and limited follow-up, but, taken together, the following conclusions may be drawn:

1. It appears that progression of retinopathy is related to the severity of preexisting disease: women with no background retinopathy, or with mild retinopathy, are less likely to have progression than those with more advanced retinopathy. Nevertheless, approximately 5% to 10% of patients with no retinal disease or with background retinopathy before pregnancy may develop proliferative retinopathy during pregnancy, requiring photocoagulation. It is impossible to determine whether such progression reflects the natural course of their disease and would have occurred even without pregnancy.
2. In many patients, regression of retinal changes occurs during the postpartum period, suggesting that short-term observations related to pregnancy may not predict the overall long-term effects of pregnancy on diabetic retinopathy.
3. The quality of glycemic control at conception, and the degree of change in glycemic control during pregnancy, reflected in the drop of hemoglobin A_{1c} concentration, are directly associated with progression of retinopathy. Obviously, these two factors are closely associated, and it is impossible to determine the independent effect of each on the progression of retinopathy. Consequently, it is possible that good glycemic control before pregnancy may offer the best opportunity to avoid progression of retinopathy during pregnancy.
4. Progression of retinopathy is more likely to occur in patients with hypertensive disorders. Approximately 50% to 60% of women with chronic hypertension or pregnancy-induced hypertension had progression of retinopathy during pregnancy.

Unlike nephropathy, the presence of retinopathy per se does not seem to have an adverse effect on pregnancy outcome. Some women have coexisting retinopathy and nephropathy, but it appears that in these patients the increased risk of adverse pregnancy outcome is related to the presence of nephropathy and not retinopathy.

Guidelines for Management of Pregnant Women with Diabetic Retinopathy

1. Whenever possible, women with diabetes should be encouraged to obtain preconception counseling and un-

dergo evaluation before pregnancy, as outlined previously. This will also allow gradual institution of strict glycemic control before pregnancy that may decrease the risk of progression related to abrupt glycemic control.

2. Women with diabetes should undergo funduscopic examinations once each trimester and approximately 6 to 12 weeks postpartum. This should preferably be done by an ophthalmologist specializing in retinal disease and documented with colored photographs.

3. Women with proliferative retinopathy should undergo phototherapy and other treatment before pregnancy, and they should not conceive before the proliferative process has been completely stabilized.

4. Any complaints related to changes in vision should be addressed immediately by referring the patient to an ophthalmologist.

5. Management of labor and delivery should be determined according to usual obstetric guidelines, regardless of retinopathy.

CORONARY ARTERY DISEASE

General Considerations

Women with diabetes have a threefold risk of atherosclerosis and fatal myocardial infarction (MI). In women who have preexisting coronary artery disease, the cardiovascular changes associated with pregnancy and delivery can result in inadequate myocardial oxygenation, leading to MI and heart failure. Increased cardiac output, decreased systemic vascular resistance with shunting of blood away from the coronary arteries, increased oxygen consumption during physical activity, increased vascular return during uterine contractions, and acute blood loss at delivery may all contribute to an absolute or relative decrease in the ability of the coronary blood flow to meet the demands of the myocardium. Additionally, these women are extremely vulnerable to myocardial damage and pulmonary edema in the immediate postpartum period. After a vaginal delivery, there is an immediate 60% to 80% increase in cardiac output due to release of venacaval obstruction, autotransfusion of uteroplacental blood, and rapid mobilization of extravascular fluid, resulting in increased venous return and stroke volume. These fluid shifts are less pronounced after cesarean delivery using controlled analgesia.

Of particular concern in these patients are the consequences of hypoglycemia. Institution of strict glycemic control in pregnant women with type 1 diabetes is associated with a significant risk of hypoglycemia, primarily during the first half of pregnancy. Activation of the counterregulatory responses to hypoglycemia will cause release of catecholamines, resulting in tachycardia, possible arrhythmia, and increased demands on the myocardium. These changes are particularly hazardous in a patient with underlying coronary artery disease and may result in an acute myocardial infarction.

Diabetic Coronary Artery Disease and Outcome of Pregnancy

The information in the medical literature concerning pregnancy in women with diabetes and coronary heart disease is limited and is composed primarily of case reports. To our knowledge, 20 cases have been reported in the literature between 1953 and 1998, of mothers with diabetes who suffered an MI or ischemic cardiac event before, during, or shortly after pregnancy.[9] Among the 13 women whose event occurred during pregnancy or in the puerperium, 7 mothers and 7 infants died. Among the 7 women whose myocardial event occurred before pregnancy, all the mothers and infants survived. The difference in outcome between women who had an MI before pregnancy and those who had an MI during pregnancy or the puerperium may reflect the grave consequences of having an MI during pregnancy but might also reflect a selection bias, in that this group of women with prior MI may have had minimal or no residual cardiac dysfunction after an MI and might represent the group that was less emphatically discouraged from conceiving or from carrying on with a pregnancy. It is also noteworthy that before 1980, the overall maternal mortality rate was 70% (7 of 10 women), whereas among cases reported after 1980, the mortality rate has dropped to 0 (0 of 10). This may reflect improved care, heightened awareness of the risks associated with these pregnancies, better counseling for women with diabetic coronary artery disease, or reporting bias of unexpectedly successful outcomes despite preexisting coronary artery disease.

Guidelines for Management of Pregnant Women with Diabetic Coronary Artery Disease

Despite the more recently published encouraging results of pregnancy outcome in women with diabetic coronary artery disease, these pregnancies continue to be extremely hazardous. Management should include the following elements:

1. Whenever possible, preconception consultation should be obtained. This should include a thorough evaluation by a cardiologist to determine the extent of coronary artery disease and myocardial function.

2. After the initial evaluation, either preconceptionally or as early in pregnancy as possible, the patient should be made aware of the serious maternal risks associated with pregnancy. The risk of maternal death should be explicitly discussed with the patient and her family. It is impossible to quantify this risk, but it is most likely related to the degree of cardiac dysfunction. It may also be prudent to obtain a psychological consultation to evaluate the patient's decision making and aid her in that process.

3. The option of termination of pregnancy should be discussed with the patient and her partner.
4. In the patient who decides to continue her pregnancy, a concerted effort should be made by the patient, the perinatologist, and the cardiologist to follow maternal and fetal status carefully and on a frequent basis. Maternal physical activity should be limited to the bare minimum, and follow-up visits with the perinatologist and the cardiologist should be scheduled every week from the second trimester onward. Antenatal fetal testing should begin at 28 gestational weeks, and serial sonograms should be performed to monitor fetal growth.
5. Every effort should be made to attain adequate glycemic control without risking hypoglycemia. Targets of glycemic control should be adjusted in those patients who have a history of frequent hypoglycemia or who experience hypoglycemic episodes during pregnancy.
6. The patient should deliver at a tertiary care center. Anesthesia during labor and delivery should be planned well in advance in consultation with an experienced anesthesiologist. Maternal hemodynamic status should be monitored closely during labor and delivery with the aid of invasive measures, if necessary. Maternal effort should be kept to a minimum, and delivery should be assisted electively.
7. A method for permanent sterilization should be discussed with the patient well in advance, so that the procedure might be performed after delivery.
8. The patient should be monitored extremely closely and carefully during the first 48 hours after delivery, owing to the increased risk of hemodynamic decompensation. Even after a vaginal delivery, the patient should be kept in the hospital at least 3 to 4 days before being discharged. This should be followed by an extended period of close postpartum follow-up.

DIABETIC NEUROPATHY

Little, if any, is known about the effects of diabetic neuropathy on pregnancy and the possible effects of pregnancy on neuropathy. Some studies suggest that a short-term increase in the incidence of polyneuropathy may occur in association with pregnancy, but that in the long-term, pregnancy is not associated with an increase in the prevalence of this complication.[10]

The presence of autonomic neuropathy with gastroparesis is particularly relevant to pregnancy in that, with the hyperemesis of pregnancy, it results in exacerbation of nausea and vomiting. This may result in irregular absorption of nutrients, inadequate nutrition, and aberrant glucose control. Exacerbation of autonomic neuropathy during pregnancy has been reported by some investigators, whereas others have noticed transient improvement in symptoms during pregnancy.[11] Overall, it seems that pregnancy does not alter the natural course of diabetic autonomic neuropathy, a complication associated with severe morbidity and mortality. From the few reported cases of pregnancy in women with autonomic neuropathy, it may be concluded that, although a successful outcome of the pregnancy is possible, there is a significant risk of maternal morbidity.

SUMMARY

Many women with diabetes develop complications of their chronic disease that may have a tremendous impact on their quality of life and their ultimate prognosis. Because type 1 diabetes often begins at a very early age, it is quite common for women in their childbearing age to be affected by these complications. As described in this chapter, diabetic complications and pregnancy may significantly affect each other, but it is not always easy to predict the course of either and to counsel these patients accordingly. Nevertheless, it appears that only in rare occasions should women with diabetes be advised against pregnancy, and that in most situations, with careful and knowledgeable management, a favorable outcome of pregnancy can be expected for both the mother and her infant.

Bibliography

1. Klein BEK, Moss SE, Klein R: Effect of pregnancy on progression of diabetic retinopathy. Diabetes Care 1990;13:34–40.
2. Gordon M, Landon MB, Samuels P, et al: Perinatal outcome and long-term follow-up associated with modern management of diabetic nephropathy. Obstet Gynecol 1996;87:401–409.
3. Miodovnik M, Rosenn BM, Khoury JC, et al: Does pregnancy increase the risk for development and progression of diabetic nephropathy? Am J Obstet Gynecol 1996;174:1180–1191.
4. Purdy LP, Hantsch CE, Molitch ME, et al: Effect of pregnancy on renal function in patients with moderate-to-severe renal insufficiency. Diabetes Care 1996;19:1067–1074.
5. The Diabetes Control and Complications Trial Research Group. The effect of intensive treatment of diabetes on the development and progression of long-term complications in insulin-dependent diabetes mellitus. N Engl J Med 1993;329:977–986
6. Dahl-Jorgesnsen K, Brinchmann-Hansten O, Hanssen KF, et al: Rapid tightening of blood glucose leads to transient deterioration of retinopathy in insulin-dependent diabetes mellitus: The Oslo study. Br Med J 1985;290:811–815.
7. Rosenn B, Miodovnik M, Kranias G, et al: Progression of diabetic retinopathy in pregnancy: Association with hypertension in pregnancy. Am J Obstet Gynecol 1992;166:1214–1218.
8. Chew EY, Mills JL, Metzger BE, et aL: Metabolic control and progression of retinopathy. National Institute of Child Health and Human Development Diabetes in Early Pregnancy Study. Diabetes Care 1995;18:631–637.
9. Gordon MC, Landon MB, Boyle J, et al: Coronary artery disease in insulin-dependent diabetes mellitus of pregnancy (class H): A review of the literature. Obstet Gynecol Surv 1996;51:437–444.
10. Hemachandra A, Ellis D, Lloyd CE, et al: The influence of pregnancy on IDDM complications. Diabetes Care 1995;18:950–954.
11. Scott AR, Tattersall RB, McPherson M. Improvement of postural hypotension and severe diabetic neuropathy during pregnancy. Diabetes Care 1988;11:369.

SEVENTEEN

Operative Vaginal Delivery

David E. Seubert and Mitchell P. Dombrowski

The use of instruments to assist a vaginal birth remains an art that the skilled practitioner can employ to minimize morbidity and mortality. Although instrumental deliveries have been performed for centuries, controversy has increased in recent decades about their safety for the fetus and mother. In addition, there has been increasing concern about the training and experience of graduating residents in regard to performing operative deliveries.

HISTORY

Hippocrates wrote about the problem of difficult labor in 400 BC describing extraction of a dead fetus.[1] Clearly, the earliest described forceps functioned to mutilate and extract a dead or live fetus. Avicenna, a Persian physician, was probably the first to write about a forceps used to save a fetus, around AD 1000.[1] During the 17th century, the Chamberlain family of physicians, who practiced in England, is credited with developing a pair of forceps for the delivery of a live infant. For centuries, the Chamberlain family kept the identity of their instruments a secret and enjoyed fame throughout Europe for their instrumental deliveries.[1] The first reference to a vacuum type of extractor appeared in 1706 in a paper by James Yonge describing a device with an air pump.[1]

Modern-day forceps are derived from either Simpson or Elliott forceps. In 1848, James Simpson of Edinburgh described both long and short forceps that consisted of fenestrated blades with parallel but separated shanks. Simpson is also credited with developing a flexible cuplike vacuum extractor in 1849.[1] About a decade later, Elliott of New York developed forceps that consisted of fenestrated blades with overlying shanks as a means to regulate lateral pressure.[1]

Further variations have evolved from both the Simpson and the Elliott models. Luikart forceps are Elliott-like forceps with pseudofenestrated blades; Tucker-McLane forceps have solid blades. Kielland forceps, which are used for midpelvic rotations, have a wide cephalic curve and minimal pelvic curve. Piper forceps, consisting of a cephalic and a pelvic curve, were introduced to keep the aftercoming head of a breech presentation in a flexed position. Barton forceps, introduced to the New York Obstetrical Society in 1925, are designed for deep transverse arrest and consist of an anteriorly hinged blade and a 50-degree angulation of the shanks and blades.[1]

Malmstrom, whose original instrument consisted of a rubber cover over a metal rim cup, accomplished further development of the vacuum.[1] The vacuum extractors of today typically are molded of synthetic materials and do not contain metal components.

PREPARATION

The art of instrumental delivery is knowing both when and when not to attempt to use a forceps for vacuum-assisted delivery. A number of conditions must be met before attempting an operative delivery:

- The cervix must be fully dilated.
- The vertex should be engaged.
- The membranes are ruptured.
- The position of the vertex is known with certainty (ultrasound may be helpful).
- The pelvis should be assessed for adequacy.
- The patient should receive adequate anesthesia.
- The bladder should be empty.
- The obstetrician should have requisite skill.
- There is a willingness to abandon the procedure if delivery does not proceed readily.

Ideally, before the procedure, the obstetrician has written a preoperative note documenting the indications for operative delivery, and the patient has given her consent.

Maternal indications for instrumental delivery include poor propulsive efforts from maternal exhaustion or regional anesthesia and conditions in which maternal Valsalva maneuvers are contraindicated, as in certain intracranial and cardiac conditions. Fetal indications include nonreassuring fetal status as indicated by fetal heart tones. The American College of Obstetricians and Gynecologists (ACOG) has classified operative deliveries according to station and rotation (Table 17–1). Such criteria can also be used for vacuum deliveries.

Vacuum Extractions

Proper application of the vacuum extractors requires knowledge of fetal presentation, position, and station. After ensuring that the maternal bladder is empty, the surgeon grasps the vacuum cup in one hand and compresses it together to place into the vagina. The cup is then placed over the occiput to ensure that the head remains flexed. According to ACOG Technical Bulletin 196,[2] when the vertex is in the occipitoanterior position, the center of the cup should be over the sagittal suture, about 3 cm in front of the posterior fontanel. The surgeon must ensure that maternal vaginal and cervical tissue is not underlying the

Table 17–1. Criteria of Forceps Deliveries according to Station and Rotation

Type of Procedure	Criteria
Outlet forceps	Scalp visible at the introitus without separating labia
	Fetal skull has reached pelvic floor
	Sagittal suture is in anteroposterior diameter or right or left occiput anterior or posterior position
	Fetal head is at or on perineum
	Rotation does not exceed 45°
Low forceps	Leading point of fetal skull is at station ≥ +2 cm and not on the pelvic floor
	Rotation 45° or less (left or right occiput anterior to occiput anterior, or left or right occiput posterior to occiput posterior)
	Rotation greater than 45°
Midforceps	Station above +2 cm but head engaged
High	Not included in classification

From American College of Obstetricians and Gynecologists: Operative Vaginal Delivery (ACOG Practice Bulletin: Clinical Management Guidelines for Obstetrician-Gynecologists. Number 17). Washington, DC, American College of Obstetricians and Gynecologists, 2000.

cup in order to avoid lacerations. Once the cup is placed, a vacuum of 400 to 600 mm Hg can be created by either wall suction or handheld pump. Propulsive efforts should be coordinated with maternal pushing efforts.

It is unclear what the threshold is for both timing and number of pull-offs before the vacuum technique is abandoned and another mode of delivery used. Whether the suction should be discontinued while the patient is resting between contractions is controversial. It has been speculated that the amount of time that the vacuum cup is in contact with the fetal scalp and the degree of asynclitism at the time of application are related to the risk of cephalohematoma.

The safety of the vacuum extractor remains controversial. In 1999, Towner and associates[3] reported a study of 583,340 live-born singleton infants born to nulliparous women between 1992 and 1994 weighing between 2500 and 4000 g. Neonates were delivered spontaneously, by vacuum extraction, by forceps, or by cesarean section before labor, or during labor. Intracranial hemorrhage was significantly higher among neonates delivered by vacuum extraction (1 in 860) compared with those delivered either spontaneously (1 in 1900) or by cesarean section before labor (1 in 2750). However, the rate of intracranial hemorrhage was similar to that of neonates delivered by cesarean section during labor (1 in 907). Vintzileos and colleagues[4] found that, when used electively, vacuum extraction was associated with lower pH in both umbilical cord artery and vein, lower venous base excess, and higher venous carbon dioxide tension, compared with normal spontaneous vaginal delivery. However, these cord blood gases resulted in no differences in perinatal morbidity and mortality or in the number of neonates born with acidemia.

ACOG issued a Committee Opinion in 1998[5] regarding the report entitled "Need for Caution When Using Vac-

uum-Assisted Delivery Devices" issued by the U.S. Food and Drug Administration (FDA) Public Health Advisory. The FDA based its report on 12 deaths and 9 serious injuries occurring over 4 years among infants delivered by vacuum extraction. This proportion of affected neonates represents 1 per 45,455 vacuum extractions. The Committee on Obstetric Practice stated that "as with any other obstetric procedure, obstetric care clinicians using vacuum-assisted delivery devices to effect operative vaginal deliveries should be properly trained and familiar with the indications and contraindications for the use of the device, as well as with its proper application and traction procedure." The opinion concluded with the statement that "the Committee on Obstetric Practice strongly recommends the continued use of vacuum-assisted delivery devices in appropriate clinical settings."

Forceps

The choice of forceps is a matter of clinical presentation as well as personal preference. Compared with Tucker-McLane forceps, Simpson forceps have a longer cephalic curve and are more suited for a molded fetal head. The open blades of the Simpson forceps facilitate traction but are more prone to injure maternal soft tissue. Solid blades such as in the Tucker-McLane forceps are less likely to cause maternal soft tissue injury with rotations but may increase the risk of slippage on the fetal head. The selected forceps should glide onto the fetal head with ease and should not be forced, which might injure both mother and fetus.

According to ACOG Technical Bulletin 196,[2] the left blade is usually applied first; however, if the position is not directly occiput anterior, the posterior blade should be applied first to prevent rotation toward the occiput transverse as the anterior blade is adjusted into place. The sagittal suture should lie perpendicular to the plane of the shanks, and the posterior fontanel should be palpable 1 fingerbreadth above this plane.

Traction should be applied in the direction of the birth canal, which may be facilitated by use of a Bill axis traction device. Traction in the plane of the pelvis can also be applied by the operator grasping the handles with both hands, thumbs beneath the handles, with the thumbs pointing toward the operator. The direction of traction changes progressively with descent, depending on the station at application; it begins well below the horizontal and rises to 45 degrees above the horizontal with extension and delivery of the head.[2] Excessive compression on the handles transmits compression to the fetal head. Care must be taken to provide perineal support, both with and without the performance of an episiotomy during the delivery process, to minimize lacerations.

Rotation of a nonocciput anterior vertex can be accomplished either by manual rotation or by using Kielland forceps, which can be applied by either the direct, the inversion, or the wandering technique. The rotation is performed to change the position of the engaged fetal head from either occiput transverse or occiput posterior to a more favorable diameter, such as occiput anterior. Rotation may need to be accomplished by "disengaging" the engaged fetal head in some instances. After rotation to occiput anterior position, the operator may remove the blades and allow the patient to continue with propulsive efforts or assist delivery with low forceps or vacuum.

SAFETY

Two randomized and prospective trials comparing spontaneous vaginal deliveries and elective forceps deliveries exist. Carmona and coworkers[6] randomized 50 patients and found that in the spontaneous delivery group the elapsed time from randomization to delivery was significantly longer (18 vs. 10.2 minutes), and the mean cord arterial pH was significantly lower (7.23 vs. 7.27), than in the forceps delivery group. They concluded that elective low forceps delivery might be used to shorten the second stage of labor without immediate adverse maternal or neonatal effects. Yancey and associates[7] found no significant differences in Apgar scores or umbilical arterial pH values between fetuses of patients randomized to spontaneous vaginal delivery or to outlet forceps delivery. It is interesting that they found that 17 infants in the forceps groups and 16 in the control group had cephalohematomas, facial bruising, subconjunctival hemorrhage, or scalp abrasions, a difference that was not significant. However, in contrast to Carmona and coworkers,[6] these investigators found that the use of outlet forceps did not significantly shorten the second stage of labor and was associated with an increased incidence of maternal perineal trauma.

Gilstrap and group[8] analyzed 704 women undergoing either elective, indicated low, or indicated midforceps deliveries. They found no significant difference between indicated low or midforceps deliveries, for either fetal distress or arrest of descent with regard to fetal acidosis, Apgar scores, fetal trauma, or neurologic deficit at discharge. However, they found a significant difference between midforceps versus low forceps regarding pre- and postdelivery hematocrits and vaginal lacerations.

The previously discussed large study by Towner and associates[3] also analyzed morbidity associated with forceps delivery. Similar to the results of vacuum-assisted deliveries, Towner and associates reported the rate of intracranial hemorrhage among forceps deliveries (1 in 664) to be similar among neonates delivered by cesarean section after labor (1 in 907), but significantly higher than those delivered spontaneously (1 in 1900), or delivered by cesarean section before the onset of labor (1 in 2750). The most important finding of this study is that vaginal delivery with vacuum extraction or forceps appears not to carry excess risk of neonatal intracranial hemorrhage, compared with cesarean section during labor. Their data suggest that the common risk factor for intracranial hemorrhage is abnormal labor per se rather than the application of a forceps or vacuum extractor. It should be noted that the combination of both vacuum extraction and forceps significantly increased the risk of intracranial hemorrhage.

Hankins and Rowe,[9] writing in 1996 about "Operative vaginal delivery—year 2000," concluded after reviewing published data that outlet and low forceps deliveries with less than 45 degrees of rotation are effective and safe for both mother and baby. They believe that the greatest risk to mother or fetus occurs with operations performed at the 0 or +1 station or those involving operations greater than 45 degrees. They suggested that operation deliveries involving greater than 45 degrees of rotation will be abandoned in the future.

CONCLUSION

The best data suggest that the skillful application of operative vaginal delivery does not significantly increase the incidence of serious fetal morbidity. Without question, an operative vaginal delivery is associated with less maternal morbidity than cesarean delivery. It therefore seems appropriate that obstetrics residents should continue to be trained in the judicious use of vacuum extraction and forceps deliveries. However, with the declining utilization of these procedures, especially of forceps, it is unclear whether many residents in training will achieve the minimum number of procedures to ensure competence in the performance of forceps deliveries. Physicians must make the judgment call in the delivery room regarding whether or not to use forceps or vacuum extractors and must additionally make the judgment when to abandon the procedure.

References

1. Lauffe LE, Berkus MD: Assisted Vaginal Delivery. New York, McGraw-Hill, 1992.
2. American College of Obstetricians and Gynecologists: Operative Vaginal Delivery (ACOG Technical Bulletin 196). Washington, DC, American College of Obstetricians and Gynecologists, 1994.
3. Towner D, Castro M, Eby-Wilkens E, Gilbert W: Effect of mode of delivery in nulliparous women on neonatal intracranial injury. N Engl J Med 1999;341:1709–1714.
4. Vintzileos AM, Nochimson DJ, Antsaklis A, et al: Effect of vacuum extraction on umbilical cord blood acid-base measurements. J Matern-Fetal Med 1996;5:11–17.
5. American College of Obstetricians and Gynecologists: Delivery by Vacuum Extraction (ACOG Committee Opinion 208). Washington, DC, American College of Obstetricians and Gynecologists, 1998.
6. Carmona F, Martinez-Roman S, Manau D, et al: Immediate maternal and neonatal effects of low-forceps delivery according to the new criteria of The American College of Obstetricians and Gynecologists compared with spontaneous vaginal delivery in term pregnancies. Am J Obstet Gynecol 1995;173:55–59.
7. Yancey MK, Herpolsheimer A, Jordan GD, et al: Maternal and neonatal effects of outlet forceps delivery compared with spontaneous vaginal delivery in term pregnancies. Obstet Gynecol 1991;78:646–650.
8. Gilstrap LC, Hauth JC, Schiano S, Connor KD: Neonatal acidosis and method of delivery. Obstet Gynecol 1984;681–685.
9. Hankins GDV, Rowe TF: Operative vaginal delivery—year 2000. Am J Obstet Gynecol 1996;175:275–272.

Issues in Cervical Ripening/Labor Induction

Lawrence D. Devoe and Steven H. Golde

According to the most recent national statistics, one in six pregnancies in the United States is induced for medical or obstetric indications. It is estimated that in many settings an almost equal number of patients require augmentation of labor or prelabor ripening of the uterine cervix. Given the frequency of these interventions, it is important that obstetric care providers are very familiar with not only the array of available cervical ripening/induction agents but also the indications and contraindications for their use in the best-practice scenarios.

INDICATIONS AND CONTRAINDICATIONS FOR CERVICAL RIPENING/INDUCTION OF LABOR

Cervical ripening is a process involving many biochemical and biophysical alterations. These are mediated by the local actions of cytokines and prostaglandins, which lead to the breakdown of cross-linked collagen fibers within the cervical stroma and increase the content of proteoglycans that draw and hold water within the intercellular space. Combined, these changes result in cervical softening and provide decreased resistance to stretch. A variety of pharmacologic and mechanical agents are available to initiate or augment these natural processes. However, each agent has inherent risks that must be weighed against the benefits.

A 1995 educational bulletin published by the American College of Obstetrics and Gynecology (ACOG)[1] presents a summary of principal indications and contraindications for labor induction (Table 18–1). Although these criteria are not all-inclusive, they account for the majority of cases in which labor induction must be weighed against the maternal or fetal risks of continued pregnancy. In the absence of urgent obstetric or medical problems, fetal maturity should be established before the induction of labor. Maturity may be established either by biochemical analysis of the amniotic fluid or by other clinical criteria (see Chapter 23, Fetal Lung Maturity Testing).

Because both maternal and fetal risks are associated with the cervical ripening and induction of labor, these interventions should follow careful explanation to and the receipt of consent from patients. They must be conducted in a setting in which close observation of mother and fetus is possible on a continuous basis. Because uterine hyperstimulation is the most common adverse effect associated with the agents described later, resuscitative measures, such as oxygen and tocolytics, should be readily available.

Prior to initiation of either cervical ripening or induction of labor, a careful assessment of fetal well-being, estimation of fetal weight and maternal pelvic capacity, establishment of vertex presentation, knowledge of placental implantation, and status of the amniotic membranes are necessary.

AGENTS/METHODS FOR CERVICAL RIPENING/INDUCTION OF LABOR

An induction of labor with an unfavorable cervix is associated with prolonged use of oxytocin at higher infusion rates, longer duration of labor, increased rates of cesarean delivery, as well as increased maternal and fetal morbidity. Consequently, patients with an unripe cervix (generally defined as a Bishop score < 6) who satisfy the criteria for safe induction of labor (as outlined earlier) will be candidates for cervical ripening.[2]

A number of methods for cervical ripening have been used in past obstetric practice (Table 18–2). In general, they may be categorized as mechanical (balloon-tipped catheters, natural/synthetic laminaria, maternal breast stimulation) or hormonal (oxytocin, prostaglandins). Additional methods for induction of labor include membrane stripping and amniotomy. Other approaches have been studied but remain experimental, such as the use of porcine relaxin and local application of estrogen.

In general, mechanical methods of cervical ripening are associated with increased risk of infection and inadvertent premature rupture of membranes. Conversely, when properly placed, their application nearly always results in some mechanical dilatation and effacement of the cervix. Breast stimulation has been studied as a method for reducing the need for induction of labor, especially in pregnancies beyond due dates. However, it carries an unknown but potentially serious risk for uncontrollable uterine hyperstimulation. Hormonal methods other than oxytocin are discussed in the following section. Low-dose oxytocin has been used as a gradual cervical ripener with widely varying rates of success. However, its lack of consistent response and need for constant monitoring make it less practical in some obstetric units.

Oxytocin remains the standard pharmacologic agent for labor induction. Many protocols exist for its administration, ranging from low-dose (1 to 2 mIU incremental increases every 30 to 40 minutes) to high-dose "active management" schedules that may involve much larger and more frequent

Table 18–1. Principal Indications and Contraindications for Labor Induction

Indications	Contraindications	Special Considerations
Pregnancy-induced hypertension	Placenta previa	Multifetal
Premature rupture of membranes	Vasa previa	Hydramnios
Chorioamnionitis	Transverse lie	Maternal cardiac disease
Suspected fetal jeopardy	Umbilical cord prolapse	Abnormal fetal heart rate patterns not requiring
e.g., severe fetal growth retardation,	Prior classic cesarean section	emergency delivery
isoimmunization	Myomectomy with invasion of endometrial	Grand multiparity
Maternal medical problems	cavity	Severe hypertension
e.g., diabetes mellitus, renal disease, chronic	Active genital herpes infection	Breech presentation
pulmonary disease		Unengaged presenting part
Fetal demise		
Logistic factors		
e.g., risk of rapid labor, distance from		
hospital, psychosocial indications		
Postdate pregnancy		

Modified from Committee on Obstetrics, American College of Obstetricians and Gynecologists: Induction of Labor (Practice Bulletin No. 10). Washington, DC, American College of Obstetricians and Gynecologists, November 1999.

increases in infusion rate. Pulsatile oxytocin delivery systems have been used experimentally but are not currently approved for clinical applications in the United States. The principal hazard associated with maternal oxytocin infusion is uterine hyperstimulation that may occur with any infusion schedule but is seen more frequently in patients entered into the active management of labor protocols.

CERVICAL RIPENING/INDUCTION WITH PROSTAGLANDINS

Since the 1980s, cervical ripening has been revolutionized by the introduction of low-dose intravaginal prostaglandin E_2 analogues (dinoprostone) derived from prepackaged suppositories. Original protocols used fractionated suppositories with estimated dosage ranging from 2 to 5 mg. Subsequently, many hospital pharmacies have dissolved the suppositories in a gel to obtain a more uniform dosage.

A significant breakthrough occurred with the introduction of intracervical dinoprostone (Prepidil) (0.5 mg/dose) as the first premeasured and U.S. Food and Drug Administration–approved agent for cervical ripening. Prepidil was reported to result in improved Bishop scores, shorten induction to delivery intervals, and lower oxytocin usage. However, its limitations included the need for frequent redosing and the requirement to delay administration of oxytocin for several hours after the last administration.

Table 18–2. Methods of Cervical Ripening

Method	Dose	Advantages	Disadvantages
Mechanical			
Balloon-tipped catheter	30-mL catheter placed into cervix	Usually well tolerated, success rates in the range reported for prostaglandin gels	Invasive, somewhat uncomfortable for patient, potential of infection
Laminaria tents	Multiple sterile tents placed in cervix	Usually well tolerated	Invasive, somewhat less effective than prostaglandin gels
Breast stimulation	Patient self-stimulation of areola	Patient initiated, low cost	Less effective than other means, risk of nonmonitored hyperstimulation, uncomfortable for patients
Pharmacologic			
Oxytocin	Oxytocin drip by infusion pump (1.0-to 22 mIU/min in 1.0 mIU/min increments q30min)	Can be titrated	Not particularly effective for cervical ripening, risk of hyperstimulation, water intoxication at high dose
Dinoprostone intracervical (Prepidil)	0.5-mg gel placed intracervically q6H (maximum cumulative dose: 1.5 mg/24 hr)	FDA approval for cervical ripening, low risk of hyperstimulation	Expensive, lack of easy removal method, requirement to wait 6–12 hr after last dose before augmentation with oxytocin
Dinoprostone vaginal insert (Cervidil)	10-mg insert placed in posterior vaginal fornix	FDA approval for cervical ripening, low risk of hyperstimulation, ease of removal	Expensive, oxytocin may be used on removal of insert
Misoprostol (Cytotec)	25–50 μg placed in posterior vaginal fornix	Inexpensive, low risk of hyperstimulation in 25 μg dose intravaginally, as effective as other prostaglandin preparations in comparative trials	Not approved by FDA, no means of easy removal

FDA, U.S. Food and Drug Administration.

Most importantly, as was the case with the local hospital dinoprostone compounds, Prepidil was an "all-or-none" approach; once administered, it depended on local absorption for its effectiveness and could be neither titrated nor discontinued should adverse reactions occur. More recently, vaginal dinoprostone (Cervidil), an intravaginal insert consisting of a polymeric base containing 10 mg of dinoprostone, has been approved for cervical ripening.[3] Unlike its predecessors, Cervidil relies on slow timed-release (at 0.3 mg/hr) of dinoprostone over 12 hours, following which conventional induction of labor may be started with an oxytocin infusion. Should hyperstimulation occur, the design of the insert allows it to be removed immediately from the vagina.

Studies comparing all these dinoprostone analogue preparations have shown similar trends in shortening the interval from admission to vaginal delivery, decreased needs for oxytocin administration, and shorter durations of active labor. A comparison of Cervidil and Prepidil by Chyu and Strassner[4] showed somewhat better efficacy of the former in achieving the aforementioned end-points.

Sanchez-Ramos and associates[5] summarized a number of clinical trials of the prostaglandin E_1 analogue misoprostol (Cytotec). Various dosage regimens have been studied, ranging from 25 to 100 μg repeated every 2 to 6 hours. Although shorter lengths of labor, induction, and time to delivery and lower oxytocin requirements have been uniformly reported compared with either placebo or dinoprostone, these differences diminish greatly as dosage is reduced. A significant concern registered in the early misoprostol trials was the consistent report of relatively high rates of uterine hyperstimulation and meconium passage. The incidence of these undesirable outcomes declined with decreased dosage schedules. Currently, Cytotec is not approved for this clinical indication and carries a special product warning on use in pregnancy. Use of this agent in any dosage schedule should be conducted under protocol.

CURRENT CONTROVERSIES IN CERVICAL RIPENING/INDUCTION

There can be little doubt that the advent of hormonal cervical ripeners, principally the prostaglandin analogues, has revolutionized our approach to the conduct of labor induction. The ability to overcome an unfavorable cervix and, consequently, decrease the length of labor, is appreciated not only by patients and hospital staff but also by those concerned with controlling the costs of health care. As these agents have seen greater use, some serious caveats have emerged. Two areas of greatest concern center on patients with premature rupture of membranes[6] and with prior uterine scar.[7] With premature rupture of the membranes, the hours of delay from insertion of cervical ripening agents to induction of labor must be weighed against the increasing risks of infection should these methods fail

and the risks of failed induction. Unfortunately, the evidence to support the use of cervical ripening agents in this context is still limited.

There is more reason to be concerned about the use of cervical ripeners for patients with prior cesarean scars. Several recent series have reported increased risks of catastrophic uterine rupture with dinoprostone and misoprostol among patients identified as good candidates for vaginal birth after cesarean delivery.[8, 9] Other contraindications to the use of cervical ripeners may emerge in the future, but prior uterine scar appears to present a significantly higher risk category for their use.

Selection of patients for entry into cervical ripening/induction protocols must continue to improve so that only the most appropriate candidates are included. At present, efforts to develop screening protocols for successful induction of labor (e.g., fetopelvic indices and modified Bishop scoring) have been limited. Given the frustration and excessive expense associated with induction of labor that fails to yield a normal vaginal delivery, efforts to solve this difficult problem must continue.

SUMMARY

Induction of labor is a frequently required obstetric intervention, with well-accepted indications and contraindications. In the case of patients with unfavorable cervices, induction of labor presents additional challenges that must be met with the use of a variety of adjunctive agents, including mechanical and hormonal cervical ripeners. Current practice favors the use of prostaglandin analogues. The benefits of inducing labor once cervical ripening has been achieved are well established and include shorter labors with lowered requirements for oxytocin administration. However, clinicians who use these potent agents must be well aware of their potential hazards (including the consequences of time delays before entry into active labor) and the best criteria for appropriate patient selection.

References

1. Committee on Obstetrics, American College of Obstetricians and Gynecologists: Induction of Labor (ACOG Technical Bulletin 217). Washington, DC, ACOG, December 1995.
2. Bishop EH: Pelvic scoring for elective induction. Obstet Gynecol 1964;24:266–268.
3. Witter FR, Rocco LE, Johnson TR: A randomized trial of prostaglandin E_2 in a controlled release pessary for cervical ripening at term. Am J Obstet Gynecol 1992;166:830–834.
4. Chyu JK, Stassner HT: Prostaglandin E_2 for cervical ripening: A randomized comparison of Cervidil versus Prepidil. Am J Obstet Gynecol 1997;177:606–611.
5. Sanchez-Ramos L, Kaunitz AM, Wears RL, et al: Misoprostol for cervical ripening and labor induction: A meta-analysis. Obstet Gynecol 1997;89:633–642.
6. Duff P: Premature ruptures of membranes at term. N Engl J Med 1996;334:1053–1054.
7. Flamm BL, Anton D, Goings JR, Newman BA: Prostaglandin E_2 for cervical ripening: A multicenter study of patients with prior cesarean delivery. Am J Perinatol 1997;14:157–160.

8. Plaut MM, Schwartz ML, Lubarsky SL: Uterine rupture associated with misoprostol in the gravid patient with a previous cesarean section. Am J Obstet Gynecol 1999;180:1535–1542.
9. Blanchette HA, Nayak S, Erasmus S: Comparison of the safety and efficacy of intravaginal misoprostol (prostaglandin E_1) with those of dinoprostone (prostaglandin E_2) for cervical ripening and induction of labor in a community hospital. Am J Obstet Gynecol 1999:180:1551–1559.

NINETEEN

Exercise in Pregnancy

James M. Pivarnik and Juanita Maria Rivera

Today's woman of childbearing age is much more involved in leisure time physical activities than her predecessors. Comprehensive high school athletic programs for girls have only been established since about the 1970s. In 1971, only 1 in 27 high school girls participated in athletics. Today, that number is approximately 1 in 3. In 1998, total participation was more than 2.6 million, an increase of more than 3% over the previous year. Although many of these girls do not continue organized team sports after high school, many maintain active lifestyles by participating in more individual endeavors, such as aerobics, running, cycling, and swimming.

From a public health perspective, it has become common knowledge that physical activity plays a major role in chronic disease prevention. The 1996 Surgeon General's Report on Physical Activity and Health[1] indicated that women should exercise at least moderately on most days of the week to help reduce their risk for heart disease, osteoporosis, cancer, and other chronic maladies. In addition, conditions that are risk factors for chronic disease, such as being overweight, are clearly related to childbearing. However, there is evidence that women who are physically active during pregnancy and the postpartum period are more likely than sedentary women to lose the weight gained during pregnancy. It makes sense that health professionals would want physically fit women to continue exercising throughout pregnancy if they are able, and encourage women who are primarily sedentary to begin a moderate physical activity program. With such emphasis on exercise and physical activity in women's lives, physicians must provide as much accurate information as possible so each pregnant woman can determine the best strategy for her particular needs.

RECENT HISTORY

In 1985, the American College of Obstetricians and Gynecologists (ACOG) published a six-page technical bulletin entitled "Exercise During Pregnancy and the Postnatal Period."[2] This document included a number of guidelines, as well as relative and absolute contraindications to physical activity. The Guidelines' "six commandments" for exercise during pregnancy included the following:

1. Maternal heart rate should not exceed 140 beats/min.
2. Strenuous activities should not exceed 15 minutes in duration.
3. No exercise should be performed in the supine position after the four month of gestation is completed.
4. Exercises that employ the Valsalva maneuver should be avoided.
5. Caloric intake should be adequate to meet the extra energy needs not only of pregnancy but also of the exercise performed.
6. Maternal core temperature should not exceed 38°C.

These original ACOG guidelines were conservative and based on the limited research information that was available at the time. In effect, the guidelines focused on the low end of the range of exercise levels recommended by the American College of Sports Medicine for individuals wishing to maintain or improve their cardiovascular fitness. However, the authors of the 1985 ACOG Guidelines noted that their basic recommendations were not appropriate for all women who wished to exercise during pregnancy.

It should be noted that recommendations designed for a general cross-section of the population may not be appropriate for a particular patient. A physically fit pregnant patient may tolerate a more strenuous program, whereas an unfit, overweight individual with a sedentary lifestyle should restrict activities to those that are less vigorous.

Since the 1985 ACOG Guidelines were written, dozens of research studies have been designed to examine the safety and efficacy of exercise during pregnancy. A brief summary of some of the basic physiologic responses to exercise is provided in the following section.

MATERNAL PHYSIOLOGIC RESPONSES

A number of physiologic changes occur in a woman during pregnancy that may affect her responses to exercise. These include, but are not limited to, changes in energy expenditure, cardiac output, respiratory mechanics, and gas exchange.

Resting energy expenditure increases as pregnancy progresses, but only when expressed in absolute terms (i.e., kcal/min). When indexed by body weight (kcal/min/kg), most research indicates little change in resting energy expenditure. During physical activity, absolute energy cost for an activity increases, but less so when energy expenditure is indexed by weight. Regardless of how energy utilization is computed, the result is that as pregnancy progresses, a given physical activity task becomes a greater percentage of a woman's exercise capacity. Thus, she will either have to (1) decrease her activity to remain at the same relative intensity as before pregnancy or (2) work at a greater percentage of her exercise capacity to perform the same task as during the prepartum period (e.g., continue to run at the same speed).

Resting cardiac output (or cardiac index) also increases during pregnancy. Although some researchers argue over the relative contribution and timing of changes in heart rate (HR) and stroke volume (SV), suffice it to say that increases in both components contribute to the enhanced delivery of blood to metabolically active tissues. It is possible that the enhanced blood volume, which increases some 40% to 60% during pregnancy, is partially responsible for the change in cardiac output. However, increases in HR and SV are found very early in pregnancy, long before a woman's blood volume increases substantially. Thus, most experts feel that the initiation of enhanced cardiac output is hormonally controlled. During a given bout of exercise, both HR and SV are usually shown to be greater than in nonpregnant conditions. However, the relative contribution of each is somewhat dependent on type of exercise performed.

Respiratory mechanics have also been shown to be affected by pregnancy. An increased tidal volume leads to a mild gestational respiratory alkalosis. During exercise, minute ventilation increases due to increases in both depth and rate of breathing. However, alveolar ventilation is largely unchanged as pregnancy progresses.

FETAL RESPONSES AND BIRTH OUTCOMES

Most studies show an increase in fetal HR in response to maternal exercise. This is a normal physiologic response, facilitating placental perfusion in the face of redistribution of maternal cardiac output to the exercising muscles. Although a few studies document instances of transient fetal bradycardia in response to maternal exercise,[3] none have reported adverse outcome. Although many studies have shown no effect of exercise behavior on birth outcome, some research indicates that women who remain physically active throughout pregnancy have shorter labors and fewer complications compared with women who discontinue their activities.[4] The issue of whether chronic physical activity results in lighter or heavier babies remains controversial because research findings are equivocal. This may be due in part to inadequate study design and difficulty in measuring physical activity accurately during pregnancy.

EFFECT OF CHRONIC EXERCISE

Compared with sedentary women, physically active women have enhanced responses to exercise during pregnancy. At a given HR, SV is greater in the exercise-trained woman, resulting in a greater cardiac output. This may be due in part to the higher blood volumes achieved by exercise-trained women during pregnancy, compared with their sedentary counterparts. Some researchers have shown enhanced left ventricular ejection fraction in physically active women.[3]

When compared with controls, the higher cardiac output seen in exercise trained women is accomplished by a larger drop in systemic vascular resistance. Mean arterial pressure response is approximately the same in both groups.

Respiration also differs between sedentary and active women. Active women show greater respiratory response at a given HR level. This additional ventilation is primarily due to increased depth of breathing, leading to greater alveolar ventilation in the active compared with the sedentary women.

Issues of maternal and fetal safety must continue to be addressed scientifically in the future. However, in most cases, research has shown that exercise is not harmful and most likely beneficial to the mother and fetus.[5]

CURRENT EXERCISE GUIDELINES

As a result of numerous research reports on exercise and pregnancy published in the mid-1980s and early 1990s, the ACOG Guidelines were revised in 1994.[6] Basic recommendations from the 1994 ACOG Guidelines are listed in the following section. Although they are more proactive and less precautionary than the 1985 version, they are still not very individualized. Some additional detail is provided with each basic tenet.

There Is Benefit from Mild to Moderate Exercise, and at Least 3 Days per Week Is Preferable

The 1994 ACOG Guidelines are largely in sync with U.S. Centers for Disease Control and Prevention recommendations and the Surgeon General's report regarding physical activity and exercise for healthy adults.[1] It is apparent that when it comes to maternal exercise behaviors, an uncomplicated pregnancy should be viewed as a healthy experience.

What is not discussed in great detail in the 1994 Guidelines is the issue of exercise intensity. For example, what is meant by mild to moderate, and can physically active women exercise at a greater intensity than sedentary women? Traditionally, the best way to gauge exercise intensity is by monitoring HR. This is because of the linear relationship that exists between HR response and energy expenditure during aerobic activities. Authors of the 1985 ACOG Guidelines believed that 140 beats/min should be the upper limit of maternal HR during exercise in pregnancy. After much research on this topic, the 1994 ACOG Guidelines *do not* include this caveat. As a matter of fact, the term *heart rate* does not even appear in the 1994 ACOG Guidelines. Rather, the authors refer the reader to a 1992 ACOG technical bulletin entitled "Women and

Exercise"[7] for specific details on exercise programs and intensity. This publication includes the use of a target HR "zone" during exercise. The authors believe that women should typically exercise between 60% and 80% of their maximum HR (HR_{max}). There is no way to accurately predict a woman's true HR_{max} without actually measuring it during an all-out effort. However, the usual method used to estimate HR_{max} is to subtract a woman's age from 220. Following this approach, the HR zone formula works out to:

$$[(220-age) \times 0.60] \text{ through } [(220-age) \times 0.80]$$
$$= \text{ target HR zone}$$

Thus, a 20-year-old woman would use an HR zone of 120 to 160 beats/min, a 30-year-old would use 114 to 152 beats/min, and so on. Whereas researchers might debate the actual HR zone numbers, health care providers should emphasize that a *range* of HR values is appropriate, rather than focusing on a single number. That is, most untrained women should exercise at the lower end of the zone when starting a mild-to-moderate exercise program, whereas women with a history of activity may exercise at the high end of the zone with no difficulty. Unfortunately, we have found that many clinicians do not take the time (or perhaps are not aware of this HR zone concept) to discuss this issue with their patients who seek advice on exercise intensity throughout pregnancy.

Avoid Supine Exercise after the First Trimester

Overwhelming evidence indicates that aerobic exercise, particularly when performed in moderation, is acceptable for most healthy mothers-to-be.[5, 6] Less is known about resistance training exercises that may involve more strenuous "weight-lifting" efforts that emphasize small muscle groups. Although this area is understudied, that does not mean that it is not important. Many women would like to begin or continue resistance training throughout pregnancy because they can do so with little bouncing and pounding, compared with weight-bearing activities such as jogging. The caveat regarding resistance training is that it may result in elevated maternal blood pressure, which could possibly lead to decreased venous return, and subsequent blunting of uterine blood flow. Resistance exercises performed in the supine position (e.g., bench press) are of greatest concern. From what we know at this time, it appears fetal heart rate decelerations are few, if any, when (1) the emphasis of a weight-training session is on repetition rather than absolute resistance and (2) the woman avoids the supine position, particularly late in pregnancy.

Modify Exercise Intensity According to Maternal Symptoms

Of all the recommendations, this one makes the most intuitive sense. However, women should understand that the absolute amount of exercise they perform will likely decrease as pregnancy progresses. Also, because HR response to exercise may differ greatly from woman to woman, it is best to include subjective feelings of perception of effort involved with each exercise session. Based on published[5] and unpublished observations, we recommend that women who are not regularly physically active keep their exercise routines in the moderate range. That is, they should perform exercises that are coincident with a perception that the overall exertion level required is moderate. For women who are chronic exercisers, a more vigorous upper limit can usually be maintained throughout much of an uncomplicated pregnancy. However, women must keep in mind that a given subjective rating will result in decreased exercise intensity (e.g., running changing to fast walking) toward the end of gestation.

Loss of Balance May Be a Concern, Particularly in the Third Trimester

This is of particular concern for women who either are not regular exercisers and/or are changing their activities to those that require unstable positioning, such as step aerobics. This may not be the best exercise late in pregnancy for someone either who is not used to aerobics in general or someone who has participated in aerobics classes in which stepping activities were limited to the floor. Other exercises that challenge a woman's balance late in pregnancy should also be viewed with caution.

Avoid Exercise When Blunt Trauma Is Possible

Some activities may increase a pregnant woman's risk of experiencing blunt trauma, even though a skilled participant may not always consider this possibility. Examples include downhill snow skiing, speed skating, surfing, and water skiing. Although the fetus is protected to a great extent in the womb, it is prudent to avoid activities in which circumstances beyond the control of even the most experienced participant can lead to high-impact falls while moving at high rates of speed. Cross-country skiing or ski simulators are reasonable alternatives during pregnancy.

Be Careful to Ensure an Adequate Diet to Replace Calories Burned during Exercise

Pregnant women involved in a physical activity program should appreciate the effect of their activity level on caloric balance. In a time when weight gains of 10 to 15 kg should be commonplace, energy balance requires even greater consideration. This is particularly relevant in highly active women with low prepregnancy body mass indexes (<20 kg/m²). On a few occasions, we have witnessed the maternal mind set that "if I can't continue to exercise at a high level, at least I can keep my weight down." However, it is recommended that women with a low body mass index gain even more weight than their more "normal" weight counterparts during pregnancy. Thus, careful consideration must be given to ensuring that caloric intake is adequate to meet the energy needs of pregnancy. This may require daily energy intake-versus-expenditure calculations, stressing that a positive caloric balance is expected during pregnancy. In some cases, it is prudent for women to seek counsel from a registered dietitian for specifics. Above all, women should be reassured that postpartum weight loss will occur when more vigorous activities can be resumed.

Ensure Adequate Heat Dissipation via Hydration, Clothing, Environment

Animal studies have demonstrated a teratogenic effect from high maternal temperatures due to febrile conditions.[5] Thus, thermoregulation remains a concern for physicians, because maternal core temperature rises linearly with exercise intensity. Also, neural tube defects occur in the first trimester, which may be before a woman even knows she is pregnant (particularly a woman who exercises regularly). In spite of this sensible concern, there is no evidence that maternal heat production during exercise leads to any detrimental effects on the human fetus. This is partially due to the fact that a woman is more readily able to divert heat from the fetus due to increased tissue conduction and enhanced radiation, convection, and evaporation to the environment. Still, a woman should take caution when exercising in hot environments. She should wear appropriate lightweight, loose-fitting clothing to aid heat removal and maintain adequate fluid replacement during and after exercise. Occasionally, this is a difficult "sell" for a woman who makes frequent trips to the bathroom as her pregnancy progresses! For women working out indoors, where convection may be reduced due to stationary exercise equipment, using an electric fan will enhance the cooling process.

Swimming has been recommended as the exercise of choice for many women who have the necessary skill and available facilities. Heat removal is rarely an issue, and the non–weight-bearing nature of swimming makes it ideal during pregnancy. In late gestation, some women switch to swimming on their backs, due to ease of breathing. Because gravity is not an issue, the "supine" nature of swimming on the back should not result in a significant reduction of blood flow to the uterus.

Another environmental concern is exercise at high (e.g., altitude) or low (e.g., scuba diving) ambient pressures. Hypoxia, resulting from low barometric pressure, is a concern for pregnant exercisers at altitude. Also, acute mountain sickness may be more pronounced during pregnancy, because a woman's acid-base status is altered owing to pregnancy-induced respiratory changes. Unless a woman is native to such conditions, exercise at elevations of much greater than a mile should be avoided if at all possible.

Likewise, scuba diving may cause problems because of increased nitrogen and oxygen pressures associated with breathing under water. Although little evidence is available to support a lower limit for depth, most physicians do not recommend diving deeper than to the bottom of the local swimming pool.

Resume Prepregnancy Routines Gradually Based on Capabilities

"When can I start exercising again?" may be the most frequently asked question regarding physical activity during pregnancy and the postpartum period. Unfortunately, there is no standard answer that fits all women. When to resume exercise depends largely on maternal (and fetal) outcomes related to the birthing process, motivation, and postpartum pain and symptoms. Many physicians suggest waiting at least 6 weeks after delivery. Whereas this seems reasonable, it is much like all suggestions about exercise during pregnancy. Some women may be able to return to activities such as light jogging in less than half that time with no problems. Others may take much longer than 6 weeks before they can return to even mild exercise programs. This is particularly true after cesarean section delivery when return to activity should not be hurried. Pain is usually the best guide, assuming there are no other medical concerns, such as bleeding or breast pain. Basically, if the exercise hurts, a woman should back off on the intensity.

It is worth noting that we have found aerobic fitness levels of physically active women are virtually unchanged (compared with early in pregnancy), even if they do not return to vigorous training some 12 weeks' postpartum. Hopefully, this is of some comfort to those women who believe that they must rush into returning to competition before they are ready.

The role of breastfeeding on postpartum exercise, as well as the role of postpartum exercise on breastfeeding, is of concern to most women. Good data are available indicating that, in general, exercise does not affect the volume or nutrient composition of breast milk.[8, 9] Some evidence indicates that lactic acid concentration in the breast milk increases with exercise.[8, 9] This is associated primarily with maximal exercise performed immediately before breastfeeding. In some cases, breast milk acceptance may be affected if feeding occurs soon after cessation of intense exercise. An obvious solution to this is to change workout times if a woman desires to train at high intensity levels. Modern conveniences such as breast pumps facilitate this strategy. The pump will allow the postpartum woman greater flexibility in the workout/feeding schedule and should result in a more comfortable exercise experience if her breasts are not full.

EXERCISE PRECAUTIONS

The following are the contraindications to exercise as stated in the 1994 ACOG Guidelines.[6]

- Pregnancy-induced hypertension
- Preterm premature rupture of membranes (pPROM)
- Preterm labor during the prior or the current pregnancy or both
- Incompetent cervix/cerclage
- Persistent second or third trimester bleeding
- Intrauterine growth restriction

In addition to the contraindications indicated previously, other maternal chronic conditions (e.g., chronic hypertension, diabetes) must be considered carefully when advising a woman on physical activity during pregnancy. Previously, in the 1985 ACOG Guidelines,[2] diagnosis of multiple gestation was considered an absolute contraindication for exercise. In twin pregnancies, the concern is an increased risk of pPROM, as well as the potential for insufficient oxygen and nutrients required by both fetuses. Whereas these concerns appear justified, there is no evidence available that performing physical activity exacerbates cases of pPROM or fetal hypoxia/malnutrition. However, in cases in which it appears that growth restriction may be occurring, or pPROM may be imminent, the obvious course of action is to cease physical activity. In any event, twin pregnancies should be monitored more closely than singleton births, particularly in a physically active woman. This requires even more thorough communication than is ordinarily required between patient and health care provider. In cases of more than two fetuses, the special monitoring and care required usually mean extensive physical activity is contraindicated.

SUMMARY

It is important for physicians to realize that pregnant women have different needs and abilities in the area of exercise and physical activity. It is not sufficient to simply say "go out and exercise, but not too strenuously." The women want, and deserve, more specific information related to their own individual circumstances. Whereas it is impossible to have a written "cookbook" answer for every maternal situation, the health care provider should present women with as much up-to-date, thorough, and relevant information as possible.

References

1. U.S. Department of Health and Human Services: Physical Activity and Health: A Report of the Surgeon General. Atlanta, U.S. Department of Health and Human Services, Centers for Disease Control and Prevention, National Center for Chronic Disease Prevention and Health Promotion, 1996.
2. American College of Obstetricians and Gynecologists: Exercise during Pregnancy and the Postnatal Period. Washington, DC, ACOG, 1985.
3. Veille JC: Maternal and fetal cardiovascular response to exercise during pregnancy. Semin Perinatol 1996;20:250–262.
4. Pivarnik JM: Potential effects of maternal physical activity on birth weight: Brief review. Med Sci Sports Exerc 1998;30:400–406.
5. McMurray RG, Mottola MF, Wolfe LA, et al: Recent advances in understanding maternal and fetal responses to exercise. Med Sci Sports Exerc 1993;25:1305–1321.
6. American College of Obstetricians and Gynecologists: Exercise during Pregnancy and the Postpartum Period (Technical Bulletin No. 189.) Washington, DC, ACOG, 1994.
7. American College of Obstetricians and Gynecologists: Women and Exercise (Technical Bulletin No. 173.) Washington, DC, ACOG, 1992.
8. Clapp JF III: Exercise Through Your Pregnancy. Champaign, IL, Human Kinetics. 1998.
9. Artal R, Wiswell R, Drinkwater B: Exercise in Pregnancy, 2nd ed. Baltimore, Williams & Wilkins, 1991.

TWENTY

Thrombocytopenia

Philip Samuels

Platelets are blood components that are anucleated, rich in phospholipids, and an integral part of the homeostasis of coagulation. With a prevalence of up to 7%, thrombocytopenia is the most frequent reason for consulting a hematologist during pregnancy.[1] Most pregnant patients with thrombocytopenia are asymptomatic. With improvements in automated blood cell counters in the 1980s, laboratories started reporting platelet counts as a standard part of the CBC. This advance in clinical pathology resulted in an "epidemic" of thrombocytopenia in pregnant women. Indeed, obstetricians obtaining a routine CBC as part of their routine prenatal battery are identifying completely asymptomatic women with depressed platelet counts.[2]

EVALUATION OF THE PATIENT WITH THROMBOCYTOPENIA DURING GESTATION

It is not always easy to determine the etiology of thrombocytopenia during pregnancy, but accurate diagnosis is essential to formulating a treatment plan. An accurate medical history is time consuming but paramount in arriving at a diagnosis. It is essential to know whether the patient has a past history of a depressed platelet count or a history of symptoms suggestive of thrombocytopenia.[3] It is important to know whether there is a history of easy bruising, petechiae, unexplained bleeding, epistaxis, and other signs and symptoms. Do cuts stop bleeding easily? Is there a history of conjunctival petechiae? Also, it is important to know whether the patient has taken any medications that can cause thrombocytopenia. Many medications have this possibility, with unfractionated heparin being the most notorious.

The patient must also be questioned about signs and symptoms suggestive of preeclampsia, because this is a common cause of thrombocytopenia. An obstetric history should focus on excessive bleeding from prior episiotomies or deliveries, from cesarean delivery incision sites, or from a neonate's circumcision. It is also important to determine whether the patient ever needed blood component therapy owing to bleeding. Because HIV infection can cause thrombocytopenia, patients must be asked about risk factors for this disorder. On examination, look for scleral hemorrhages, petechiae, and bruises. More than likely, the history and physical examination will be benign.

The following discussion elucidates the different causes of thrombocytopenia that coexist and/or complicate pregnancy and considers how to assess and treat (or ignore) these problems. The causes of thrombocytopenia complicating pregnancy are delineated in Table 20–1.

GESTATIONAL THROMBOCYTOPENIA

Gestational thrombocytopenia complicates 4% to 7% of pregnancies.[4] Its existence was first suggested by Hart and colleagues in 1986.[5] Burrows and Kelton[4] showed that a significant percentage of pregnant women with no medical or obstetric problems had a mildly depressed platelet count and delivered without maternal or neonatal complications. Samuels and associates[3] further defined gestational thrombocytopenia as a distinct entity. They also showed that there is no test for this disorder and that it cannot be distinguished from immune thrombocytopenia purpura (ITP) by the presence of platelet antibodies. Gestational thrombocytopenia is usually mild and progressive. The thrombocytopenia is usually mild (100,000 to 150,000/mm³) or moderate (50,000 to 100,000/mm³). In our referral practice, which covers a large geographic area, we have even encountered a few patients with gestational thrombocytopenia whose platelet counts could be classified as se-

---

Table 20–1. Causes of Pregnancy-Associated Thrombocytopenia

Common Causes

Gestational thrombocytopenia
Severe preeclampsia
HELLP syndrome
DIC from abruptio placentae
DIC from severe maternal hemorrhage

Infrequent Causes

DIC from retained dead fetus
DIC from maternal sepsis
Immune thrombocytopenia purpura
HIV infection

Rare Causes

Lupus anticoagulant and antiphospholipid syndrome
Systemic lupus erythematosus
Thrombotic thrombocytopenic purpura
Hemolytic-uremic syndrome
Folic acid deficiency
Congenital thrombocytopenia
Type IIB von Willebrand's disease

DIC, diffuse intravascular coagulation; HELLP, hemolysis, elevated liver enzymes, low platelets.

vere ($<50,000/mm^3$). At one time, it was thought that this disorder was just dilutional secondary to the increase in plasma volume during pregnancy. However, it has been demonstrated that there is increased platelet destruction and turnover in patients with gestational thrombocytopenia.

Gestational thrombocytopenia is rarely a cause of maternal or neonatal complications; it is more of an annoyance than a risk. The main risk to the patient is that she may be subjected to a prolonged, unnecessary evaluation for ITP, which may even include a bone marrow aspiration and biopsy. Also, if the patient's platelet count is less than $100,000/mm^3$ (occurring in $< 1\%$ of *all* pregnancies), many anesthesiologists will not perform a conduction anesthetic owing to the possibility of an epidural hematoma. This can cause frustration and disappointment for the patient.

The treatment for gestational thrombocytopenia is observation and delivery at term. If you decide to obtain a hematologic consultation, make certain that the hematologist knows that this entity exists. Glucocorticoids may possibly increase the platelet count in these patients. We have inadvertently given glucocorticoids to three patients with gestational thrombocytopenia because we mistakenly thought they had ITP. All three had rises in their platelet counts to greater than $100,000/mm^3$ within 2 weeks using moderate doses of steroids. We certainly do not advocate using glucocorticoids in patients with gestational thrombocytopenia, but we do want to mention this because it brings forth the possibility that this disorder may have an immune etiology.

The differential diagnosis of benign gestational thrombocytopenia must include an in vitro clumping phenomenon, which causes a factitious thrombocytopenia. This is found in approximately 3 per 1000 individuals. In this phenomenon, platelets clump when collected in ethylenediaminetetraacetic acid (EDTA), the diluent used in lavender-topped tubes in which CBCs and platelet counts are collected. When this is suspected, blood should simultaneously be collected in lavender-topped tubes (containing EDTA) and blue-topped tubes (containing citrate). A platelet count should be performed simultaneously on both tubes. The platelet count will be significantly higher in the citrate-containing tube if there is an in vitro clumping disorder. Also, a finger-stick platelet count can be manually counted, and the technician will notice clumping if there is a clumping disorder. The finger-stick count is the most labor-intensive but best test to diagnose clumping disorder.

SEVERE PREECLAMPSIA

This subject is covered in Chapter 10, Management of Preeclampsia. A platelet count below $100,000/mm^3$ is a criterion for diagnosing *severe* preeclampsia. The decreased platelet count in preeclampsia is probably due to increased platelet destruction and not to decreased production.[6] Potentially, endothelial cell damage from intense vasospasm causes increased platelet aggregation, which leads to depo-sition of platelets on the damaged vessel wall or increased clearance by the reticuloendothelial system, which results in a diminution of circulating platelets. The decrease in platelet count in preeclampsia can be gradual or sudden. A platelet count below $100,000/mm^3$ is usually an indication for delivery in a severely preeclamptic patient. This, however, is an overgeneralization because preeclampsia is a complex disease process and the decision making is dependent on many variables.

Many surgeons routinely transfuse patients with platelets at time of cesarean delivery if their count is below $50,000/mm^3$. This is certainly within the standard of care. In contrast, we have platelets in the operating room at the time of cesarean delivery, but do not transfuse unless the patient has abnormal bleeding at delivery. Untransfused packs of platelets usually upset the blood bank pathologist, but I really believe that platelet transfusion should be reserved for those who unequivocally need them. Platelet packs are occasionally from multiple donors, which increases the risk of transfusion-borne complications. In addition, the life span of transfused platelets in an individual who is actively destroying platelets is very short, and serves only as a stopgap measure. Platelet transfusion is helpful if the patient is actively bleeding, but of little use if the case is progressing normally and hemostasis is adequate. Meticulous surgical technique and hemostasis are essential in these patients. In the event of vaginal delivery, platelets should be available on the labor floor if the maternal platelet count is approaching $30,000/mm^3$. Platelet transfusion should be reserved for those who demonstrate increased bleeding.

The platelet count may remain depressed for some time after delivery of the patient with preeclampsia. An upward trend, however, usually begins by 48 hours after delivery. Unless the patient is exhibiting abnormal bleeding, do not check platelet counts too frequently, because this causes unnecessary discomfort, is expensive, and is unnecessary.

IMMUNE THROMBOCYTOPENIA PURPURA

ITP, which affects 3 per 1000 pregnant women, is the most publicized cause of thrombocytopenia complicating pregnancy. This is due to a misunderstanding of thrombocytopenia. Prior to 1990, gestational thrombocytopenia (which complicates 4% to 7% of pregnancies) was not recognized as a distinct entity. Almost every non-preeclamptic thrombocytopenic patient was diagnosed as having ITP, which resulted in a great overdiagnosis of the condition. In ITP, the patient synthesizes autoantibodies directed against her own platelets, leading to coating of the platelets with immune complexes resulting in their destruction by the reticuloendothelial system. Over 90% of individuals with ITP will have platelet-associated antibodies (positive direct test).[7] This means that by testing, we can detect immunoglobulins actually attached to the platelet surface. Over 50% of patients with ITP will have serum (free) antiplatelet antibodies (positive indirect test).[7] This means that there are free-floating, unattached immunoglobulins in the plasma and/or serum that are capable of attaching to platelets, leading to their ultimate destruction.

Platelet antibody testing has evolved since it was first introduced in 1979. The initial tests were radioimmunoassays (RIAs). They progressed to enzyme-linked immunosorbent assays (ELISAs). Now, many tests utilize flow cytometry. This progress is both fortunate and difficult for the practitioner. It is fortunate because tests are readily and more rapidly available from a variety of laboratories. It is difficult and confusing because different laboratories utilize different techniques that have different sensitivities and specificities, and there is no uniform way of reporting the results. Therefore, for the obstetrician who sees only a few patients with ITP annually, this can be frustrating and confusing. Remember that the diagnosis of ITP during pregnancy is based on history. Platelet antibody testing cannot distinguish between ITP and gestational thrombocytopenia.[3] There is no need to test platelet antibodies if a patient presents in the second or third trimester of pregnancy with a benign history and physical examination and mild-to-moderate thrombocytopenia.

ITP has been a source of interest and controversy for obstetricians because it has both maternal and fetal and neonatal implications. The free (unattached) immunoglobulin G (IgG) antiplatelet antibodies can cross the placenta and attach to fetal platelets, leading to their destruction and thus transient neonatal thrombocytopenia. Occasionally, this neonatal thrombocytopenia can be profound.[3] The true incidence of this phenomenon is controversial, but the reason for this confusion is easy to explain. As I mentioned in the beginning of this section, the existence of gestational thrombocytopenia (a common, benign entity) was not recognized until about 1990. Most studies conducted prior to that time included patients with gestational thrombocytopenia in their studies of ITP. Including a condition (gestational thrombocytopenia) with a prevalence of 4% to 7% in the study of a condition (ITP) with a prevalence of 0.3% greatly dilutes the study of the rarer event. In early studies, the majority of the patients actually had gestational thrombocytopenia and not ITP. This fictitiously reduced the true incidence of neonatal thrombocytopenia. The true incidence of profound neonatal thrombocytopenia (platelet count $< 50,000/mm^3$) in pregnancies complicated by ITP with indirect IgG antiplatelet antibodies is in the range of 15%, with a wide confidence interval.

The obstetric management of thrombocytopenia remains controversial. No large prospective studies have adequately evaluated the optimal mode of delivery. In a 1991 analysis of 474 pregnancies complicated by ITP that were reported in the literature,[8] 10% of the neonates had moderate thrombocytopenia and 15% had severe thrombocytopenia. The overall rate of intracranial hemorrhage was 3% and was not significantly related to mode of delivery.[8] In another study of 55 pregnancies complicated by ITP,[9] four infants had severe thrombocytopenia and the only neonate with intracranial hemorrhage was delivered by cesarean section.

In both of these studies, the authors concluded that intracranial hemorrhage is not related to the mode of delivery.

I believe that the default is to deliver these patients vaginally. However, although there are no data, I believe that a fetus known to be, or at risk to be, profoundly thrombocytopenic should not be delivered by vacuum extraction. I would be judicious in my use of scalp electrodes and obstetric forceps. Furthermore, I would not permit a prolonged second stage of labor in these patients. In addition, I would not circumcise a male infant born to a mother with ITP without knowing his platelet count. Other than these caveats, I would not alter routine obstetric care.

There are three methods of estimating the fetal platelet count before delivery. Each is cumbersome, and one has risks to the fetus. The utility of determining the fetal platelet count is controversial and should not be undertaken unless it will make a difference in the management of the pregnancy or delivery of the patient. A fetal scalp platelet count can be accomplished much like a scalp pH: the cervix must be dilated, the membranes ruptured, and the vertex at an accessible station. Scalp blood is drawn up into a pediatric counting chamber or into a capillary tube and then placed into a pediatric tube.[10] Fetal scalp blood can also be feathered onto a glass slide that can be stained with Wright stain after it dries. This can then be evaluated microscopically to see whether platelets are present in most high-power fields. This is circumstantial evidence that there are adequate platelets. Cordocentesis involves ultrasound-guided puncture of the umbilical cord and obtaining a platelet count. There are potential bleeding complications and fetal distress with this procedure, but in experienced hands, the complication rate is very low.[11] Again, fetal platelet determination should be undertaken only if it will affect the patient's treatment.

Not every pregnant woman with ITP warrants therapy. In general, our hematology colleagues do not routinely treat asymptomatic patients until their platelet counts are in the range of 20,000 to 30,000/mm³. Symptomatic patients with platelet counts below 50,000/mm³ should be treated. The initial therapy should be with a glucocorticoid. Patients with a bleeding complication should be treated with intravenous methylprednisolone. The usual dose is 1.0 to 1.5 mg/kg (total body weight) in two or three doses per day. It may take 2 or 3 days to see an initial response, and up to 2 weeks to see a maximal response. If oral therapy is initiated, the usual drug is prednisone, and the usual dose is 1 mg/kg/day. This is rapidly weaned after a response is seen, and the maintenance dose should keep the platelet counts at approximately 100,000/mm³.

Glucocorticoids are associated with diminished glucose tolerance, so women chronically on these medications should have early diabetes screening. Gastrointestinal ulceration with gastrointestinal bleeding is a potential side effect of corticosteroid therapy. These medications may also cause hirsutism, moniliasis, acne, and hypertension (owing to the mineralocorticoid component). Osteopenia is also a concern to patients chronically taking glucocorticoids. The patient should be counseled about these as well as potential fetal side effects before initiating therapy. Only about 10% of an ingested dose of prednisone actually crosses the placenta and reaches the fetus. After ingestion, prednisone is metabolized to its active form, prednisolone. In the placenta, the active prednisolone is metabolized by 11β-ol dehydrogenase to an inactive ketometabolite.

Although there are potential side effects, glucocorticoid therapy is generally the safest option for the mother and fetus, and is 70% effective in the patient with true ITP. In the 30% of patients who do not adequately respond, intravenous immunoglobulin (IVIG) or splenectomy may be indicated. Splenectomy is best accomplished in the second trimester because there is less chance of inciting preterm labor, organogenesis is completed, and the uterus is not large enough to make the procedure technically more difficult. Tocolysis is occasionally necessary after the procedure. The platelet count usually dramatically rises immediately after clamping the splenic vessels. My colleagues and I have, on three occasions, been able to temporize until term with patients poorly responsive to other therapies. During cesarean section, we consulted a general surgeon to perform a splenectomy through a midline skin incision. It is important to note that the spleen is not the only source of reticuloendothelial cells, so not every patient responds to splenectomy.

IVIGs are very expensive, but they are effective in raising the platelet count for varying amounts of time. Theoretically, immunoglobulins nonspecifically bind to receptors on reticuloendothelial cells. If receptors are saturated, there is no place for platelets to bind; hence, they are not destroyed. The usual dose is 0.4 to 1.0 g/kg/day in a continuous intravenous infusion. The infusions usually take about 8 to 12 hours to complete. This regimen is continued for 2 to 5 days. A response is usually seen in 2 to 3 days after initiating therapy, and it peaks in about 5 days. The length of response is highly variable. Some patients need to have the treatment repeated several times during the pregnancy. With modern IVIG therapy, there is minimal chance of viral infection because of the preparation precautions that are taken.[12]

Platelet transfusion should be saved for emergencies. ITP is a disease of platelet destruction. Transfused platelets, like endogenous platelets, will be rapidly destroyed. It is better to attack the problem by suppressing the reticuloendothelial system as the previous discussions have noted. In ITP, platelet transfusions are indicated when there is profound thrombocytopenia and the patient is actively and seriously bleeding. Simultaneously, other therapies should be instituted, even emergency splenectomy if necessary.

THROMBOTIC THROMBOCYTOPENIC PURPURA AND HEMOLYTIC-UREMIC SYNDROME

Thrombotic thrombocytopenic purpura (TTP) and hemolytic-uremic syndrome (HUS) are characterized by profound thrombocytopenia and microangiopathic hemolytic

Table 20–2. Pentad of Findings in Thrombotic Thrombocytopenic Purpura

Common Findings in 74% of Patients
Microangiopathic hemolytic anemia
Thrombocytopenia
Neurologic abnormalities
  Confusion
  Headache
  Paresis
  Visual hallucinations
  Seizures
Less Common Findings
Fever
Renal dysfunction

anemia; both disorders carry a high maternal mortality rate. Both conditions are extremely rare and may never be encountered during the course of a career in obstetrics and gynecology. Nonetheless, both should be considered in the differential diagnosis when pregnant women with acute thrombocytopenia are encountered. TTP is characterized by a pentad of findings cited in Table 20–2, but one must realize that only 40% of patients with this disorder have the complete pentad. TTP usually occurs in the late second or early third trimester. In contrast, HUS usually occurs in the third trimester and postpartum period, and usually in younger patients. Furthermore, it is rare for the platelet count to be below 100,000/mm³ in patients with HUS, whereas the platelet count is often below 50,000/mm³ in patients with TTP. Cytotoxic drugs and oral contraceptives predispose an individual to HUS, which often follows an infection with an enteric bacteria. Up to 25% of patients with HUS develop chronic renal insufficiency. Those who survive TTP usually do not have permanent renal impairment.

Plasma exchange has made a dramatic difference in the survival rate of those patients with TTP.[13] Even though plasma exchange has been used for treating TTP in pregnancy since 1984, the disease is rare enough that we are unable to quote a true success rate for this treatment during gestation. HUS does not respond as well to plasma exchange as TTP. Supportive therapy and dialysis, when necessary, remain the mainstays of treatment for HUS.

NEONATAL ALLOIMMUNE THROMBOCYTOPENIA

Although neonatal alloimmune thrombocytopenia (NAT) does not affect the maternal platelet count, no discussion of thrombocytopenia in pregnancy would be complete without mentioning NAT. NAT is analogous to red blood cell isoimmunization, but it involves platelets. It usually involves maternal antibodies directed against fetal PLA-1 antigens, but may also involve PLA-2, Bak-a, Bak-b, or other antigens. As in red blood cell isoimmunization, the course of NAT is worse with successive pregnancies.

The neonatal thrombocytopenia is usually profound, and intracranial hemorrhage in the newborn is common.

Therapy includes administration of IVIG to the mother.[14] Some protocols also include glucocorticoids. The optimal therapy has not been delineated. Cordocentesis to determine the fetal platelet count is common. Often, intrauterine intravascular fetal platelet transfusion is performed, using the mother's platelets as donors, because they do not carry the antigen that elicits the antibody response. Another alternative is for the mother to undergo artifical insemination with sperm from a donor lacking the antigen triggering this dramatic antibody response. There are several excellent reference laboratories throughout the United States where this antigen-antibody testing can be performed.[15, 16]

In summary, thrombocytopenia complicates about 4% of all pregnancies. The vast majority of complications are secondary to gestational thrombocytopenia, a benign disorder that requires no extensive evaluation and no therapy. Severe preeclampsia is also a common cause and is usually treated by delivery. With a careful history and physical examination, as well as with the judicious use of laboratory tests, a proper diagnosis can usually be obtained in an expeditious manner. Only after an accurate diagnosis is made can the obstetrician decide whether therapy is warranted and which therapy is most appropriate for the individual patient.

References

1. McRae KR, Samuels P, Schreiber AD: Pregnancy-associated thrombocytopenia: Pathogenesis and management. Blood 1992;80:2697.
2. Aster RH: Gestational thrombocytopenia. A plea for conservative management. N Engl J Med 1990;323:264.
3. Samuels P, Bussel JB, Braitman LE, et al: Estimation of the risk of thrombocytopenia in the offspring of pregnant women with presumed immune thrombocytopenic purpura. N Engl J Med 1990;323:229.
4. Burrows RF, Kelton JG: Fetal thrombocytopenia and its relation to maternal thrombocytopenia. N Engl J Med 1993;329:1463.
5. Hart D, Dunetz C, Nardi M, et al: An epidemic of maternal thrombocytopenia associated with elevated antiplatelet antibody in 116 consecutive pregnancies: Relationship to neonatal platelet count. Am J Obstet Gynecol 1986;154:878.
6. Samuels P, Main EK, Tomaski A, et al: Abnormalities in platelet antiglobulin tests in preeclamptic mothers and their neonates. Am J Obstet Gynecol 1987;107:109.
7. Cines DB, Schreiber AD: Immune thrombocytopenia: Use of a Coombs antiglobulin test to detect IgG and C3 on platelets. N Engl J Med 1979;300:106.
8. Cook RL, Miller RC, Katz VL, Cefalo RC: Immune thrombocytopenia purpura in pregnancy: A reappraisal of management. Obstet Gynecol 1991;78:578–583.
9. Payne SD, Resnik R, Moore TR, et al: Maternal characteristics and risk of severe neonatal thrombocytopenia and intracranial hemorrhage in pregnancies complicated by autoimmune thrombocytopenia. Am J Obstet Gynecol 1997;177:149–155.
10. Scott JR, Cruikshank DR, Kochenour NK, et al: Fetal platelet counts in the obstetric management of immunologic thrombocytopenic purpura. Am J Obstet Gynecol 1980;136:495.
11. Ghidini A, Sepulveda W, Lockwood CJ, Romero R: Complications of cord blood sampling. Am J Obstet Gynecol 1993;168:1339.
12. Roussel RH, Budinger MD, Pirofsky B, Schiff RI: Prospective study on the hepatitis safety of intravenous immunoglobulin, pH 4.25. Vox Sang 1991;60:65.
13. Weiner CP: Thrombotic microangiopathy in pregnancy and the postpartum period. Semin Hematol 1987;24:119.
14. Bussel JB, McFarland JG, Berkowitz R: Antenatal treatment of fetal alloimmune thrombocytopenias. Blut 1989;59:136.
15. Colorado Coagulation Consultants. www.colorado-coag.com
16. Blood Center of Southeastern Wisconsin. www.bloodctrwise.org

TWENTY-ONE

Management of Asthma in Pregnancy

Mitchell P. Dombrowski

Asthma may be the most common potentially serious medical complication of pregnancy. Approximately 4% of women of childbearing age have a history of asthma, but up to 10% of the population appears to have nonspecific airway hyperresponsiveness.[1] In general, the prevalence, morbidity, and mortality from asthma are increasing. Insight into the pathogenesis of asthma has changed with the recognition that airway inflammation is present in nearly all cases. The effects of pregnancy on asthma are controversial because previous studies have had conflicting results, but pregnancy may be associated with a worsening of more severe asthma. Asthma has been associated with considerable maternal morbidity, with 32.1% of patients having at least one exacerbation and 8.9% requiring hospitalization during pregnancy.[2]

Ethnicity may be a particularly important confounding factor in assessing the relationship between asthma and pregnancy outcomes, because African Americans (ages 15 to 44 years) are five times more likely to die from asthma and are twice as likely to be hospitalized from asthma compared with whites. A summary of possible maternal, fetal, and neonatal complications related to asthma and asthma therapy is presented in Table 21–1.

Studies have shown that patients with more severe asthma may have the greatest risk for complications during pregnancy.[3, 4] Quantifying this risk is problematic, because most studies have not categorized the severity of the asthma of their subjects. In 1993, the National Asthma Education Program (NAEP) Working Group[1] defined mild, moderate, and severe asthma according to symptomatic exacerbations (wheezing, cough, and/or dyspnea) and objective tests of pulmonary function. The most commonly used parameters are the peak expiratory flow rate (PEFR) and the forced expiratory volume in 1 second (FEV_1). The 1993 guidelines did not list the need for regular medication to be a factor for classifying asthma severity during pregnancy.

In a recent prospective observational study of pregnant women with asthma, patients with mild asthma but who required regular medications (β-agonist, theophylline, or inhaled corticosteroids) were similar to subjects with moderate asthma in respect to asthma exacerbations.[2] Pregnant patients requiring regular systemic corticosteroids to control asthma symptoms were similar to severe asthmatics in respect to exacerbations. See Table 21–2 for modified NAEP asthma severity criteria.

ASTHMA MANAGEMENT

The ultimate goal of asthma therapy is maintaining adequate oxygenation of the fetus by prevention of hypoxic episodes in the mother. The effective management of asthma during pregnancy relies on four integral components: (1) objective measures for assessment and monitoring, (2) avoiding or controlling asthma triggers, (3) patient education, and (4) pharmacologic therapy.

Assessment and Monitoring

Subjective measures of lung function by the patient and physician provide an insensitive and inaccurate assessment of airway hyperresponsiveness, airway inflammation, and asthma severity. The FEV_1 after a maximal inspiration is the single best measure of pulmonary function. However, measurement of FEV_1 requires a spirometer. The PEFR correlates well with the FEV_1 and has the advantage that it can be measured reliably with inexpensive, disposable, portable peak flow meters. Patient self-monitoring of PEFR provides valuable insight into the course of asthma throughout the day, assesses circadian variation in pulmonary function, and helps detect early signs of deterioration so that timely therapy can be instituted.

Asthma Triggers

Limiting adverse environmental exposures during pregnancy is important for controlling asthma. Irritants and allergens that provoke acute symptoms also increase airway inflammation and hyperresponsiveness. Avoiding or controlling such triggers can reduce asthma symptoms, airway hyporesponsiveness, and the need for medical therapy. Association of asthma with allergies is common: 75% to 85%

Table 21–1. Reported Effects of Asthma and Asthma Treatment Regimens

Increased Maternal Effects

Preeclampsia
Cesarean delivery
Asthma exacerbations
Preterm rupture of membranes

Increased Perinatal Effects

Mortality
Prematurity
Low birth weight
Hypoxia/asphyxia
Hypoadrenalism
Theophylline toxicity

Table 21–2. Modified NAEP Asthma Severity Classifications

Mild Asthma

Brief (<1 hr) symptomatic exacerbations ≤ twice/wk
PEFR ≥ 80% of personal best
FEV_1 ≥ 80% of predicted when asymptomatic

Moderate Asthma

Symptomatic exacerbations > twice/wk
Exacerbations affect activity levels
Exacerbations may last for days
PEFR, FEV_1 range from 60%–80% of predicted
Regular medications necessary to control symptoms

Severe Asthma

Continuous symptoms/frequent exacerbations limit activity levels
PEFR, FEV_1 < 60% of expected and are highly variable
Regular oral corticosteroids necessary to control symptoms

FEV_1, forced expiratory volume in 1 sec; NAEP, National Asthma Education Program; PEFR, peak expiratory flow rate.
From National Asthma Education Program: Management of Asthma During Pregnancy; Report of the Working Group on Asthma and Pregnancy (NIH Publication 93-3279). Washington, DC, National Institutes of Health, September, 1993.

of patients with asthma have positive skin tests to common allergens like animal dander, house dust mites, cockroach antigens, pollens, and molds. Other common nonimmunologic triggers include tobacco smoke, strong odors, air pollutants, food additives such as sulfites, and certain drugs, including aspirin and β-blockers. Another trigger can be strenuous physical activity. For some patients, exercise-induced asthma can be avoided with inhalation of $β_2$-agonist 5 to 60 minutes before exercise. Specific measures for avoiding asthma triggers are listed in Table 21–3.

Patient Education

Patients should be made aware that controlling asthma during pregnancy is especially important for the well-being of the fetus. Inform patients that they can reduce asthma triggers. The patient should have a basic understanding of the medical management during pregnancy, including self-monitoring of PEFRs and the correct use of inhalers.

Asthma Pharmacotherapy

Although animal studies have indicated an association of corticosteroids with increased risk of cleft palate and

Table 21–3. Limiting Exposure to Asthma Triggers

Use plastic mattress and pillow covers
Weekly washing of bedding in hot water
Animal dander control
  Weekly bathing of the pet
  Keep pets out of the bedroom
  Remove the pet from the home
Cockroach control
Avoid tobacco smoke
Inhibit mite and mold growth by reducing humidity
Do not be present when home is vacuumed

Table 21–4. Typical Dosages of Common Asthma Medications

Cromolyn sodium	2 inhalations qid
Beclomethasone	2–5 inhalations bid to qid
Triamcinolone	2 inhalations tid or qid or 4 inhalations bid
Budesonide	2–4 inhalations bid
Fluticasone	88–220 µg bid
Flunisolide	2–4 inhalations bid
Theophylline	Maintain serum levels of 8–12 µg/mL; decrease dosage by half if treated with erythromycin or cimetidine
Prednisone	1-wk 40 mg/day burst for active symptoms followed by 1-wk taper
Albuterol	2 inhalations q3–4h

decreased fetal survival, human studies have failed to suggest any increase in facial clefts or other birth defects. However, the use of oral corticosteroids has been associated with low birth weight. Potential adverse effects of oral or high-dose inhaled corticosteroids include adrenal suppression, weight gain, impaired fetal growth, hypertension, diabetes, cataracts, and osteoporosis.

In the United States, three classes of inhaled anti-inflammatory asthma medications are available at the present time: inhaled corticosteroids, nedocromil sodium, and cromolyn sodium. In controlled studies of nongravid subjects, use of inhaled corticosteroids or cromolyn sodium led to improvement in asthma symptoms, pulmonary function, nonspecific bronchial hyperactivity, emergency room relapses, and hospitalizations. Typical dosages of commonly used asthma medications are listed in Table 21–4.

Inhaled Corticosteroids

The use of inhaled corticosteroids among nonpregnant asthmatic patients has been associated with a marked reduction in fatal and near-fatal asthma.[5] In addition to their anti-inflammatory effect, corticosteroids increase the effectiveness of β-adrenergic drugs by inducing formation of new β-receptors. Inhaled corticosteroids produce clinically important improvements in bronchial hyperresponsiveness, which appear dose-related, can occur as early as a few weeks but take months to attain maximal effect, and include prevention of increased bronchial hyperresponsiveness after allergen. Inhaled corticosteroids are also more effective than β-agonists, theophylline, nedocromil sodium, and cromolyn sodium in reducing airway hyperresponsiveness during maintenance. In a prospective observational study of 504 pregnant subjects with asthma, 177 patients were not initially treated with either inhaled budesonide or inhaled beclomethasone.[6] This cohort had a 17% acute exacerbation rate compared with only a 4% rate among those treated with inhaled corticosteroids from the start of pregnancy.

A number of studies have found that inhaled corticosteroids can cause adrenal suppression and changes in bone metabolism in nonpregnant patients. Their potential effects on fetal adrenal function and fetal bone development are unknown. Inhaled corticosteroids can cause thrush and hoarseness, problems that may be mitigated by the use of metered-dose inhalers with spacers. Only about 10% to 20% of the inhaled dose of corticosteroid reaches the lungs; approximately 50% is deposited in the oropharynx. The use of spacers can increase delivery to the lungs, and mouth rinsing after inhalation will decrease oral absorption.

In 1993, the NAEP Working Group[1] recommended inhaled beclomethasone during pregnancy because most clinical studies had been conducted with beclomethasone. Since then, limited data during pregnancy and data from nonpregnant subjects suggest that the other inhaled corticosteroids may have therapeutic advantages compared with beclomethasone. Therefore, it seems reasonable to recommend beclomethasone as the preferred agent when commencing inhaled corticosteroids during pregnancy but to continue either triamcinolone acetonide, budesonide, fluticasone propionate, or flunisolide during pregnancy in a patient who is well controlled by that inhaled corticosteroid before pregnancy. All of the inhaled corticosteroids mentioned are currently labeled U.S. Food and Drug Administration pregnancy class C.

Beclomethasone Dipropionate

Inhaled beclomethasone has not been associated with increased rates of fetal malformations.[7-9] In a case analysis of 12,301 nonpregnant asthmatics, Ernst and associates[5] reported that use of beclomethasone for at least 1 year resulted in a significantly lower risk of fatal and near-fatal asthma compared with therapies not including inhaled corticosteroids. Inhaled beclomethasone has been associated with a reduced re-admission rate for asthma exacerbations in a randomized study of 84 pregnant patients.[9] Beclomethasone is identical to betamethasone except for having a chlorine instead of a fluorine at the 9-alpha position. This is significant because betamethasone is known to effectively cross to the fetus. Inhaled beclomethasone has been reported to impair growth in children as measured by height or lower leg growth.

Triamcinolone Acetonide

Data on inhaled triamcinolone use during pregnancy are limited to a single retrospective study,[10] which found a significantly lower incidence of hospital admissions for asthma exacerbations among 15 gravidas receiving inhaled triamcinolone (33%) compared with 14 patients treated with inhaled beclomethasone (79%; $P < .05$). This result may have been due to confounding factors and needs to be confirmed. Triamcinolone has been shown to have minimal systemic absorption after oral administration via metered dose inhalers with spacers.

Budesonide

To study possible teratogenic risks, the Swedish Medical Birth Registry was utilized in 2014 infants whose mothers had used inhaled budesonide in early pregnancy. A 3.8% (95% confidence interval, 2.9–4.6) frequency of congenital malformations was observed, which was similar to the general population rate of 3.5%.[11] Budesonide and theophylline may have synergistic effects. In a double-blind, placebo-controlled trial of nongravid subjects with moderate asthma, high-dose budesonide (800 µg) was compared with low-dose budesonide (400 µg), and with theophylline at serum concentrations below the recommended therapeutic range.[12] Compared with high-dose budesonide, the low-dose budesonide with theophylline regimen resulted in significantly improved FEV_1. Serum cortisol concentrations were significantly reduced in the group treated with high-dose budesonide but not the low-dose theophylline group.

Fluticasone Propionate and Flunisolide

Both fluticasone propionate and flunisolide are potent anti-inflammatory corticosteroids. There are no published studies of their use during human pregnancy. However, in contrast to inhaled beclomethasone that has been associated with growth decelerations in adolescent children, inhaled fluticasone propionate therapy was not found to be associated with a decrease in growth velocity in children.[13] In a randomized double-blind study of nonpregnant adults and adolescents, inhaled fluticasone propionate was found to be significantly more effective than theophylline in the treatment of mild to moderate asthma.

Cromolyn Sodium and Nedocromil Sodium

Given the potential for systemic effects of inhaled corticosteroids, even at low doses, it is important to identify nonsteroidal anti-inflammatory medications. At the present time, cromolyn sodium and nedocromil sodium are the only approved medications that fit into this category. Nedocromil sodium, a pyranoquinalone, exerts a number of anti-inflammatory effects in vivo and in vitro. Cromolyn sodium, which is virtually devoid of significant side effects, blocks both the early- and the late-phase pulmonary response to allergen challenge as well as prevents the development of airway hyperresponsiveness. Cromolyn sodium does not have any intrinsic bronchodilator or antihistaminic activity. Compared with inhaled corticosteroids, the time to maximal clinical benefit is longer for cromolyn sodium, 4 weeks versus 2 weeks. Nedocromil sodium and cromolyn sodium appear to be less effective than inhaled corticosteroids in reducing objective and subjective manifestations of asthma.

Bronchodilators

In some respects, these medications are now viewed as supplementary to nonbronchodilator antiasthma medications. An increased frequency of bronchodilator use could be an indicator of the need for additional anti-inflammatory therapy.

Theophylline

Theophylline has been used for over 50 years, and no increased risk of developmental problems has been identified. Theophylline serum concentrations should be maintained at 8 to 12 μg/mL during pregnancy.[1] Subjective symptoms of adverse theophylline effects, including insomnia, heartburn, palpitations, and nausea, may be difficult to differentiate from typical pregnancy symptoms. Theophylline can have significant interactions with other drugs, causing decreased clearance and resultant toxicity. Two commonly used drugs are cimetidine, which can cause a 70% increase, and erythromycin, which causes a 35% increase in theophylline serum levels.

The main advantage of theophylline is the long duration of action, 10 to 12 hours with the use of sustained-release preparations, which is especially useful in the management of nocturnal asthma. Theophylline should be used as an additional therapy when β-agonists and inhaled anti-inflammatory agents do not adequately control symptoms. Theophylline is indicated only for chronic therapy and is not effective for the treatment of acute exacerbations during pregnancy.[9] Theophylline has anti-inflammatory actions that may be mediated from inhibition of leukotriene production and its capacity to stimulate prostaglandin (PG) E_2 production.

Inhaled β-Agonists

β-Agonists are currently recommended for use with all degrees of asthma during pregnancy.[14] This group of medications has evolved from those that are relatively short acting (epinephrine, isoproterenol) to those of longer duration of action (albuterol, terbutaline, pirbuterol) but still lasting only 4 to 6 hours. Their greatest advantage is a rapid onset of effect in the relief of acute bronchospasm via smooth muscle relaxation. They are also excellent bronchoprotective agents for pretreatment before exercise. Before allergen exposure, β-agonists effectively block the pulmonary response but are of insufficient duration of action to prevent the late-phase pulmonary response unless administered in high doses.

Although $β_2$-agonists are associated with tremor, tachycardia, and palpitations, recent studies have found more serious complications, including an association with an increased risk of death with chronic use. They do not block the development of airway hyperresponsiveness.[15] Indeed, a comparison of an inhaled glucocorticoid, budesonide, with the inhaled $β_2$-agonist terbutaline, raised the question whether routine use of this medication could result in increased airway hyperresponsiveness.

Leukotriene Pathway Moderators

Leukotrienes are arachidonic acid metabolites that have been implicated in transducing bronchospasm, mucus secretion, and increased vascular permeability.[16] Bronchoconstriction associated with aspirin ingestion can be blocked by leukotriene receptor antagonists.[17] Treatment with the leukotriene receptor antagonist montelukast has been shown to improve pulmonary function significantly, as measured by FEV_1. The leukotriene receptor antagonists zafirlukast (Accolate) and montelukast (Singulair) are both rated pregnancy category B. The 5-lipoxygenase inhibitor zileuton (Zyflo) is rated pregnancy category C because of reduced weight and skeletal variations among rats at 18 times the recommended maximum human dosage. It should be noted that there are no data regarding the efficacy or safety of these agents during human pregnancy.

Step Therapy

The step-care therapeutic approach increases the number and frequency of medications with increasing asthma severity (Table 21–5). A burst of oral corticosteroids is indicated for exacerbations not responding to initial β-agonist therapy regardless of asthma severity. Additionally, patients who require increasing inhaled $β_2$-agonist therapy (>12 puffs per day) to control their symptoms may benefit from oral corticosteroids. In such cases, a short course of oral prednisone, 40 to 60 mg per day for 1 week, followed by 7 to 14 days of tapering, may be effective.

ANTENATAL MANAGEMENT

Patients with moderate and severe asthma should be considered to have high-risk pregnancies. Underestimation of asthma severity and undertreatment of asthma exacerbations can increase adverse outcomes. The first prenatal visit should include a detailed medical history, with attention to

---

Table 21–5. Step Therapy in Medical Management of Asthma

Mild
Inhaled $β_2$-agonist as needed*

Moderate
Inhaled $β_2$-agonist as needed*
Inhaled corticosteroids (or cromolyn)
Theophylline for nocturnal asthma or increased symptoms

Severe
Inhaled $β_2$-agonist as needed*
Inhaled corticosteroids (or cromolyn)
Theophylline for nocturnal asthma or increased symptoms
Oral systemic corticosteroids

---

*PEFR or FEV_1 < 80%, asthma exacerbations, or exposure to exercise or allergens (oral corticosteroid burst if inadequate response to $β_2$-agonist regardless of asthma severity).

FEV_1, forced expiratory volume in 1 sec; PEFR, peak expiratory flow rate.

Table 21–6. Individualized Peak Expiratory Flow Rate Zones

Establish personal best PEFR, then calculate:
1. Green zone > 80% of personal best PEFR
2. Yellow zone 50%–80% of personal best PEFR
3. Red zone < 50% of personal best PEFR

PEFR, peak expiratory flow rate. (Typical PEFR = 380–550 L/min.)

medical conditions that could complicate the management of asthma, including diabetes mellitus, hypertension, cardiac disease, adrenal disease, hyperthyroidism, HIV infection, hemoglobinopathies, hepatic disease, and active pulmonary disease (cystic fibrosis, bronchiectasis, tuberculosis, sarcoidosis, recurrent sinopulmonary infections, bronchitis). The patient should be questioned about the presence and severity of symptoms, episodes of nocturnal asthma, the number of days of work missed due to asthma exacerbations, history of acute asthma emergency care visits, and smoking history. The type and amount of asthma medications, including the number of puffs of β_2-agonists used each day, should be recorded. Asthma severity should be determined (see Table 21–2).

Gravidas with mild, well-controlled asthma may receive routine prenatal care. Moderate and severe asthmatic patients should have scheduling of prenatal visits based on clinical judgment; most will need prenatal visits at least every 2 weeks, then weekly at 36 weeks' gestation. In addition to routine care, antenatal visits should include an evaluation of asthma severity and symptom frequency, nocturnal asthma, FEV_1 or PEFR, medications (assess compliance and dosage), and emergency visits and hospital admissions for asthma exacerbations. Patients should be instructed on proper dosing and administration of their asthma medications.

Instruct patients on proper peak flowmeter technique; PEFR should be determined with peak flowmeters before medications, in the morning and after dinner. The patient should make the measurement while standing, after a maximum inspiration. Personal best PEFR should be determined, and personalized green, yellow, and red zones should be established and explained (Table 21–6). Those with moderate to severe asthma should be instructed to maintain an asthma diary containing daily assessment of asthma symptoms, including morning and evening peak flow measurements, symptoms and activity limitations, indication of any medical contacts initiated, and a record of regular and as-needed medications taken.

As previously discussed, avoidance and control of asthma triggers (see Table 21–3) are particularly important in pregnancy because pharmacologic control of asthma potentially has adverse fetal effects. Specific recommendations should be made for appropriate environmental controls, based on the patient's history of exposure and, when available, demonstrated skin test reactivity.

Moderate and severe asthmatic patients should have additional fetal surveillance in the form of ultrasound examinations and antenatal fetal testing. Because asthma has been associated with intrauterine growth restriction and preterm birth, it is critical to establish pregnancy dating accurately. Repeat ultrasound examinations are recommended for patients with suboptimally controlled asthma and after asthma exacerbations, to evaluate fetal activity, growth, and amniotic fluid volume. The intensity of antenatal fetal surveillance is based on the severity of the asthma. Instruct all patients to be attentive to fetal activity and keep a record of fetal kick counts. In most cases, moderate and severe asthmatic patients should have fetal testing starting by 32 weeks' gestation.

Home Management of Asthma Exacerbations

An asthma exacerbation that causes minimal problems for the mother may have severe sequelae for the fetus. Indeed, abnormal fetal heart rate tracing may be the initial manifestation of an asthmatic exacerbation. A maternal Po_2 of less than 60 or a hemoglobin saturation less than 90% may be associated with profound fetal hypoxia. Therefore, asthma exacerbations in pregnancy must be aggressively managed. Patients should be given an individualized guide for decision making and rescue management.

Patients should be educated to recognize signs and symptoms of early asthma exacerbations, such as coughing, chest tightness, dyspnea, or wheezing, or by a 20% decrease in their PEFR. This is important so that prompt home rescue treatment may be instituted to avoid maternal and fetal hypoxia. In general, patients should use inhaled albuterol, 2 to 4 puffs every 20 minutes, up to 1 hour. A good response is considered to be if symptoms are resolved or become subjectively mild, if normal activities can be resumed, and if the PEFR is greater than 70% of personal best. The patient should seek further medical attention if the response is incomplete or if fetal activity is decreased (Table 21–7).

Table 21–7. Home Management of Acute Asthma Exacerbations

Use inhaled albuterol, 2–4 puffs, and check PEFR in 20 min
If PEFR < 50% predicted or symptoms are severe, obtain emergency care
If PEFR is 50%–70% predicted:
  Repeat albuterol treatment, check PEFR in 20 min
  If PEFR is still 50%–70% predicted:
    Contact caregiver or go for emergency care
If PEFR > 70% predicted:
  Continue inhaled albuterol (2–4 puffs q3–4hr for 6–12 hr as needed)
If decreased fetal movement:
  Contact caregiver or go for emergency care

PEFR, peak expiratory flow rate.

Table 21–8. Emergency Assessment and Management of Asthma Exacerbations

1. **Initial evaluation:**
   History, examination, PEFR, oximetry
   Fetal monitoring if potentially viable
2. **Initial treatment:**
   Inhaled β_2-agonist × three doses over 60–90 min
   O_2 to maintain saturation ≥ 95%
   If no wheezing and PEFR or FEV_1 > 70% baseline, discharge with follow-up
3. **If oximetry < 90%, FEV_1 < 1.0 L, or PEFR < 100 L/min on presentation:**
   Continue nebulized albuterol
   Start IV corticosteroids
   Consider IV aminophylline
   Obtain arterial blood gases
   Admit to intensive care unit
   Possible intubation
4. **If PEFR or FEV_1 > 40% but < 70% baseline after β_2-agonist:**
   Obtain arterial blood gases
   Continue inhaled β_2-agonist every 1–4 hr
   Start IV corticosteroids in most cases
   Consider IV aminophylline
   Hospital admission in most cases

FEV_1, forced expiratory volume in 1 sec; IV, intravenous; PEFR, peak expiratory flow rate.

Hospital and Clinic Management

The principal goal is the prevention of hypoxia. Continuous electronic fetal monitoring is initiated if gestation has advanced to the point of potential fetal viability. Albuterol is delivered by nebulizer (2.5 mg = 0.5 mL albuterol in 2.5 mL normal saline) driven with oxygen; treatments are given every 20 minutes. Occasionally, nebulized treatment is not effective because the patient is moving air poorly. In such cases, terbutaline, 0.25 mg, can be administered subcutaneously every 15 minutes for 3 doses. The patient is assessed for general level of activity, color, pulse rate, use of accessory muscles, and airflow obstruction determined by auscultation, and FEV_1 or PEFR or both before and after each bronchodilator treatment. Measurement of oxygenation via pulse oximeter or arterial blood gases is essential. Arterial blood gases are obtained if oxygen saturation remains below 95%; chest radiographs are not commonly needed. Guidelines for the management of asthma exacerbations are presented in Table 21–8.

LABOR AND DELIVERY MANAGEMENT

Asthma medications should not be discontinued during labor and delivery. Although asthma is usually quiescent during labor, consideration should be given to assessing PEFRs on admission and at 12-hour intervals. The patient is kept hydrated and is given adequate analgesia to decrease the risk of bronchospasm. If systemic corticosteroids have been used in the previous 4 weeks, then hydrocortisone (100 mg q8h IV) is administered during labor and for the 24-hour period after delivery to prevent adrenal crisis.[1]

It is rarely necessary to deliver a fetus via cesarean for an acute asthma exacerbation. Usually, maternal and fetal distress can be managed by aggressive medical management. Occasionally, delivery may improve the respiratory status of a patient with unstable asthma who has a mature fetus. PGE_2 or E_1 can be used for cervical ripening, the management of spontaneous or induced abortions, or postpartum hemorrhage; 15-methyl PGF_2-alpha and methylergonovine can cause bronchospasm. There are no reports of the use of calcium channel blockers for tocolysis among patients with asthma. Magnesium sulfate is a bronchodilator, but indomethacin can induce bronchospasm in the aspirin-sensitive patient.

Lumbar anesthesia has the benefit of reducing oxygen consumption and minute ventilation during labor. Fentanyl may be a better analgesic than meperidine, which causes histamine release, but meperidine is rarely associated with the onset of bronchospasm during labor. Ketamine is useful for induction of general anesthesia because it can prevent bronchospasm. Communication between the obstetric, the anesthetic, and the pediatric caregivers is important for optimal care.

BREAST FEEDING

In general, only small amounts of asthma medications enter breast milk. Prednisone, theophylline, antihistamines, beclomethasone, β-agonists, and cromolyn are not considered to be contraindications for breast feeding.[1] However, among sensitive individuals theophylline may cause toxic effects in the neonate, including vomiting, feeding difficulties, jitteriness, and cardiac arrhythmias.

References

1. National Asthma Education Program: Management of Asthma During Pregnancy; Report of the Working Group on Asthma and Pregnancy (NIH Publication 93-3279). Washington, DC, National Institutes of Health, September 1993.
2. Dombrowski MP: Should the definitions of asthma severity be modified during pregnancy? Poster #541. Am J Obstet Gynecol 2000;182:S167.
3. Greenberger PA, Patterson R: The outcome of pregnancy complicated by severe asthma. Allergy Proc 1988;5:539–543.
4. Perlow JH, Montgomery D, Morgan MA, et al: Severity of asthma and perinatal outcome. Am J Obstet Gynecol 1992;167:963–967.
5. Ernst P, Spetzer WO, Suissa S, et al: Risk of fatal and near-fatal asthma in relation to inhaled corticosteroid use. JAMA 1992;268:3462–3464.
6. Stenius-Aarniala BSM, Hedman J, Teramo KA: Acute asthma during pregnancy: Thorax 1996;51:411–414.
7. Greenberger PA, Patterson R: Beclomethasone diproprionate for severe asthma during pregnancy. Ann Intern Med 1983;98:478–480.
8. Fitzsimons R, Greenberger PA, Patterson R: Outcome of pregnancy in women requiring corticosteroids for severe asthma. J Allergy Clin Immunol 1986;78:349–353.
9. Wendel PJ, Ramin SM, Barnett-Hamm C, et al: Asthma treatment in pregnancy: A randomized controlled study. Am J Obstet Gynecol 1996;175:150–154.
10. Dombrowski MP, Brown CL, Berry SM: Preliminary experience with triamcinolone acetonide during pregnancy. J Matern Fetal Med 1996;5:310–313.

11. Kallen B, Fydhstroem H, Aberg A: Congenital malformations after use of inhaled budesonide in early pregnancy. Obstet Gynecol 1999;93:392–395.
12. Evans DJ, Taylor DA, Zetterstrom O, et al: A comparison of low-dose inhaled budesonide plus theophylline and high-dose inhaled budesonide for moderate asthma. N Engl J Med 1997;337:1412–1418.
13. Allen DB, Bronsky EA, Laforce CF, et al: Growth in asthmatic children treated with fluticasone propionate. Fluticasone Propionate Asthma Study Group. J Pediatr 1998;132:472–477.
14. Schatz M, Zeiger RS, Harden KM, et al: The safety of inhaled β-agonist bronchodilators during pregnancy. J Allergy Clin Immunol 1988;82:686–695.
15. Haahtela T, Jarvinen M, Kava T, et al: Comparison of β_2-agonist, terbutalline, with an inhaled corticosteriod, budesonide, in newly detected asthma. N Engl J Med 1991;325:338–392.
16. Knorr B, Matz J, Bernstein JA, et al: Montelukast for chronic asthma in 6- to 14-year-old children: A randomized, double-blind trial. JAMA 1998;279:1181–1186.
17. Wenzel SE: New approaches to anti-inflammatory therapy for asthma. Am J Med 1998;104:287–300.

Thyroid Disease in Pregnancy

Mark E. Redman

The importance of thyroid hormone function in pregnancy has long been recognized. The association of "cretinism" with hypothyroidism was described over one hundred years ago. Recent investigations regarding thyroid disease in pregnancy have enhanced the understanding of the mechanisms that link thyroid hormone levels to maternal and fetal physiology as well as the significance of these processes for pregnancy outcomes. The pathways that modulate maternal and fetal thyroxine (T_4) levels in pregnancy have been clarified by recent studies. The association between maternal hypothyroidism and neurologic development has been further illuminated. Investigations recently have examined the diagnosis and management of pregnancies complicated by maternal and fetal thyroid disorders, as well as the role of thyroid hormones in hyperemesis gravidarum and preeclampsia. This chapter reviews the physiology of thyroid disease in pregnancy with focus on the most recent developments.

THYROID HORMONE LEVELS IN PREGNANCY

Laboratory assessment of thyroid function during pregnancy provides the primary means for quantifying thyroid disease but also can yield results of undetermined significance. Controversy exists regarding the distinction between alterations in laboratory values due to thyroid disease versus alterations due to pregnancy. Total levels of T_4 and triiodothyronine (T_3) are elevated in pregnancy, along with the estrogen-stimulated increase in thyroid-binding globulin (TBG). Levels of thyroid-stimulating hormone (TSH) vary as pregnancy progresses. It is commonly stated that, although free T_4 and free T_3 levels change throughout pregnancy, they remain within the limits of normal established for nonpregnant patients.[1] A 1999 investigation, however, questions this convention. McElduff[2] described the experience of one institution with measuring TSH and free T_4 levels. Testing of 119 patients with apparently uncomplicated pregnancies, with no history or signs of thyroid dysfunction, revealed that free T_4 levels were significantly below the lower limit of normal for nonpregnant patients and fell as pregnancy progressed. Additionally, 16% of the study population (and 24% of those at less than 20 weeks' gestation) had TSH levels below the lower limit of normal for nonpregnant patients. The majority of the low TSH values were associated with normal or low T_4 values.[2] Such a rate of abnormal values in normal pregnant

patients suggests that further study should evaluate whether the usual reference ranges for TSH and free T_4 need to be redefined for pregnant patients.

The mechanisms by which fetal thyroid levels are maintained also have been investigated recently. Conventional conceptions once held that fetal thyroid function was independent of maternal thyroid status, except with respect to iodine intake or administration of pharmacologic agents known to cross the placenta. The independence of maternal and fetal thyroid function has been attributed to the impermeability of the placenta to factors related to thyroid function. More insight has been gained regarding the influence of maternal thyroid function on fetal development, as well as the role played by the placenta. The pharmacokinetics of maternal-fetal transfer of thyrotropin-releasing hormone (TRH) were assessed in a prospective cross-sectional study of women undergoing fetal blood sampling for clinical indications.[3] Patients in the study group received an intravenous bolus of TRH immediately prior to fetal blood sampling and were compared with the control group. The peak fetal TRH levels were 1000-fold lower than the peak maternal levels after administration of the bolus. The investigators believed this to serve as an in vivo confirmation of prior in vitro data demonstrating the poor transfer of TRH across the placenta. This information supports the notion that high fetal TRH levels arise from a mechanism independent of maternal TRH, such as decreased clearance of TRH of fetal origin. These findings may also have significance for proposals that have been made to administer TRH in conjunction with corticosteroids to enhance fetal lung maturity.[3]

Evidence has been accumulating to support the notion that the placenta functions not only passively as a barrier but also actively to maintain fetal thyroid homeostasis. An Italian group[4] studied serum levels of T_3, reverse T_3 (rT3), and T_3 sulfate in fetuses delivered at a range of gestational ages and compared specimens of umbilical cord blood at the time of delivery versus neonatal specimens obtained on the fifth postnatal day. The authors presented evidence that iodothyronine deiodinases within the placenta actively maintain the fetal T_3 and rT_3 levels throughout gestation, not only by limiting passage of maternal T_4 to the fetus but also by metabolizing hormone of fetal origin.[4]

Comprehension of the role of iodine in determining maternal and fetal thyroid levels in pregnancy has been enhanced by the finding that iodine supplementation in pregnancy can induce opposite changes in maternal and neonatal thyroid function. It has been well known that one setting in which thyroid disease causes adverse outcome in pregnancy is when severe iodine deficiency causes fetal, as well as maternal, hypothyroidism. Whereas it has been clear that the extremes of iodine intake affect fetal thyroid function, little data existed regarding the effects of mild to moderate iodine deficiency on thyroid levels in pregnancy. In 2000, Nohr and Laurberg[5] assessed thyroid hormone levels in maternal serum and cord blood at delivery in subjects receiving iodine supplementation during pregnancy compared with controls in an area characterized by mild to moderate iodine deficiency. Subjects receiving iodine supplementation had significantly lower TSH and significantly higher free T_4 in maternal serum samples than those without supplementation. In cord blood samples, however, TSH was significantly higher and free T_4 was significantly lower in the group receiving supplemental iodine. The differential response of mother and fetus in the setting of mild to moderate iodine deficiency suggests that the fetal thyroid may be more susceptible to suppression by iodine than the adult thyroid during pregnancy.[5] Iodine supplementation in the setting of mild deficiency may not benefit the fetus. Furthermore, the finding of elevated TSH in neonatal screening may not necessarily indicate antepartum iodine deficiency.

THYROID FUNCTION AND NEURODEVELOPMENT

Although the association between iodine deficiency and cognitive impairment of offspring has been long recognized, further study continues to enhance the understanding of the role of maternal and fetal thyroid function in neurodevelopment as well as the mechanisms by which perturbations in thyroid homeostasis affect the developing central nervous system. The potential influence of maternal hypothyroidism, independent of fetal hypothyroidism due to severe iodine deficiency, on fetal neurologic development has prompted further investigation. In 1999, Pop and colleagues[6] published evidence that low maternal free T_4 may be an important predictor of neurologic impairment among offspring of apparently uncomplicated pregnancies in a region with iodine sufficiency.

The investigators studied 220 patients without neonatal or overt maternal hypothyroidism in the Netherlands, with assessment of the offspring using the Bayley Psychomotor Development Index (PDI) at 10 months of age. Patients in this cohort with free T_4 levels below the 5th and the 10th percentiles at 12 weeks' gestation had children with significantly lower PDI scores.[6] Further evidence linking maternal thyroid status and neurologic development was provided by a study reported by Haddow and coworkers in 1999.[7] This investigation retrospectively identified 62 patients with laboratory evidence of hypothyroidism, discovered on analysis of stored samples, and 124 matched controls. Notably, a significant proportion of the study population had not been diagnosed with hypothyroidism during the pregnancy studied. None of the offspring of the

62 pregnancies complicated by hypothyroidism had been diagnosed with congenital hypothyroidism. Neuropsychological testing of the offspring performed at 7 to 9 years of age revealed significantly lower performance by the group with maternal hypothyroidism on 2 of 15 neuropsychological tests and a trend toward lower performance on all 13 of the remaining tests, although these differences were not significant. Larger differences in performance were noted in the children of patients whose hypothyroidism was not treated during pregnancy. The authors concluded that maternal hypothyroidism during pregnancy, in the absence of congenital hypothyroidism in the neonate, impaired neurologic development in the offspring, even for a cohort in which many of the subjects had only mild or subclinical hypothyroidism.[7] Study of a small series of patients in Toronto that assessed infant cognitive abilities found not only decreased attention and speed of information processing in infants of hypothyroid subjects but also an atypical behavior profile suggestive of hypervigilance among infants of hyperthyroid subjects treated with antithyroid agents.[8]

Investigation has provided further evidence of the mechanisms by which thyroid function may modulate neurodevelopment. In 1999, a Spanish study[9] mapped and quantified the expression of type 2 iodothyronine deiodinase (D_2) in different regions of the rat brain. The investigation demonstrated regional changes in D_2 expression in rat neonates subjected to hypothyroidism during development. The pattern of D_2 expression revealed that the strongest effect of hypothyroidism on the concentration of D_2 messenger RNA (mRNA) occurred in the primary sensory pathways, specifically the trigeminal and auditory pathways. Significant changes in D_2 expression were also demonstrated in the lateral geniculate nucleus of the thalamus, the lateral vestibular nucleus, and several nuclei related to the activating ascending reticular pathway. These changes were distinct from those produced by mere developmental delay. Since local D_2 expression holds great importance for thyroid effects in the brain, the investigators concluded that the regional pattern and quantity of D_2 expression in response to hypothyroidism revealed specific regions of developing brain that are susceptible to perturbations of thyroid hormone levels.[9] Similarly, Dowling and associates[10] described acute changes in the expression of thyroid hormone–responsive genes in specific regions of the brains of fetal rats exposed to maternal hypothyroidism. Thus, pathways by which fetal neurologic development may be altered by maternal thyroid status have been revealed. As evidence mounts that maternal thyroid levels serve as an independent risk factor for impaired neurologic development, further study should evaluate whether this problem is amenable to population-based screening and intervention.

DIAGNOSIS AND TREATMENT OF THYROID DISEASE IN PREGNANCY

Increased attention to the influence of maternal thyroid disease on fetal neurologic development underscores the importance of continuing to gather evidence regarding the incidence, pathophysiology, and treatment of thyroid disease in pregnant patients. One recent study evaluated the association between congenital hypothyroidism and maternal thyroid disease.[11] Maternal serum TSH and autoantibody levels were assessed in 259 patients who delivered infants with congenital hypothyroidism and in 1773 controls in Quebec. The investigation revealed a high incidence of transient congenital hypothyroidism as well as a significant association between congenital hypothyroidism and retrospectively diagnosed maternal autoimmune thyroid disease.[11]

When maternal hyperthyroidism is diagnosed during pregnancy, the most common form of treatment is the administration of antithyroid agents. Traditionally, propylthiouracil (PTU) has been favored over methimazole owing to the impression that there is less exposure of the drug to the fetus with use of PTU, as well as an association between methimazole and a rare scalp defect. A model examining a perfused human placenta, however, found similar levels of transfer of both antithyroid drugs across the placenta, adding to controversy regarding the putative advantage of PTU over methimazole.[12] Further evidence has been gathered regarding the treatment of fetal thyroid disease as well. A recent case report documented transplacental passage of antithyroid antibodies and observed a correlation between maternal and fetal levels of the antibodies in a pregnancy complicated by Hashimoto's thyroiditis. The authors suggested that the maternal levels of autoantibodies hold potential to guide therapy for fetal disease without invasive fetal testing, such as with cordocentesis.[13] Such an approach, however, has not been clinically validated. Whereas authors have previously described treatment of fetal hypothyroidism in utero, guided by direct assessment of fetal levels via cordocentesis, investigators have continued to find success with treating additional forms of fetal thyroid disease. For example, Asteria and colleagues in 1999[14] reported treating fetal thyroid hormone resistance by using cordocentesis to guide the dosing of triiodothyroacetic acid (TRIAC).

THYROID FUNCTION AND OBSTETRIC COMPLICATIONS

Significant controversy has existed regarding the use of antithyroid agents in patients with hyperemesis gravidarum because studies have revealed that as many as 60% have biochemical evidence of hyperthyroidism, but only a small proportion have other clinical evidence of hyperthyroidism. A Turkish group in 1999[15] investigated the relationship between immunologic factors and elevated levels of human chorionic gonadotropin (hCG) in hyperemesis and hyperthyroxinemia. The investigators found significantly higher hCG, free T_4, and TSH levels in patients with hyperemesis as well as in hyperthyroxinemia. hCG was found to correlate negatively with TSH and positively with free T_4, lymphocyte count, and complement levels in patients with hyperemesis.[15] In addition to the suggestion that the link between hyperemesis and hyperthyroidism in pregnancy may be related to immune function, the data presented appear to support an association between the level of hCG and the level of thyroid stimulation in pregnancy. Another report implicates sensitivity to hCG, rather than levels of hCG, in a familial predisposition to development of hyperthyroidism in pregnancy. Rodien and coworkers[16] identified a mutation of the TSH receptor gene that appeared to confer increased sensitivity to hCG in a mother and daughter who both suffered from transient gestational hyperthyroidism associated with hyperemesis gravidarum. Elevated hCG levels in the first trimester spontaneously decline as gestation progresses. Thus, one approach to management of transient abnormalities of thyroid function tests without other evidence of thyroid disease may be expectant management. Yet, some argue that antithyroid agents yield clinical improvement of hyperemesis gravidarum in patients with concomitant hyperthyroidism. The utility of antithyroid agents in this setting should be evaluated by therapeutic trials.

The association between hypothyroidism in pregnancy and increased risk of developing preeclampsia has also been a source of controversy. Further evidence of an association was found in a study that correlated decreased thyroid hormones and elevated TSH in pregnancy with high levels of endothelin and increased severity of preeclampsia and eclampsia.[17] This finding may provide a mechanism by which the proposed link between hypothyroidism and preeclampsia occurs.

CONCLUSION

Recent investigation regarding thyroid disease in pregnancy has illuminated the basic mechanisms by which thyroid levels change in pregnancy and affect fetal development as well as their relationship to other aspects of maternal hormonal and immune system function. The clinical outcomes of alterations of thyroid function in pregnancy have been further described as well. The additional insight gained by these developments should guide continued investigation into the mechanisms by which thyroid economy affects and is affected by pregnancy, as well as clinical questions regarding the diagnosis and treatment of thyroid disease in pregnancy. Some authors have promoted the potential advantage of screening for maternal hypothyroidism in early pregnancy, for example, but the degree to which such a strategy would improve outcomes should be evaluated before such a screen becomes standard practice in routine prenatal care.

References
1. Inzucchi SE, Burrow GN: Endocrine disorders in pregnancy. In Reece EA, Hobbins JC (eds): Medicine of the Fetus and Mother, 2nd ed. Philadelphia, Lippincott-Raven, 1999, pp 1107–1115.

2. McElduff A: Measurement of free thyroxine (T$_4$) levels in pregnancy. Aust N Z J Obstet Gynaecol 1999;39:158–161.

3. Bajoria R, Peek MJ, Fisk NM: Maternal-to-fetal transfer of thyrotropin-releasing hormone in vivo. Am J Obstet Gynecol 1998;178:264–269.

4. Santini F, Chiovato L, Ghirri P, et al: Serum iodothyronines in the human fetus and the newborn: Evidence for an important role of placenta in fetal thyroid hormone homeostasis. J Clin Endocrinol Metab 1999;84:493–498.

5. Nohr SB, Laurberg P: Opposite variations in maternal and neonatal thyroid function induced by iodine supplementation during pregnancy. J Clin Endocrinol Metab 2000;85:623–627.

6. Pop VJ, Kuijpens JL, van Baar AL, et al: Low maternal free thyroxine concentrations during early pregnancy are associated with impaired psychomotor development in infancy. Clin Endocrinol (Oxf) 1999;50:149–155.

7. Haddow JE, Palomaki GE, Allan WC, J et al: Maternal thyroid deficiency during pregnancy and subsequent neuropsychological development of the child. N Engl J Med 1999;341:549–555.

8. Mirabella G, Feig D, Astzalos E, et al: The effect of abnormal intrauterine thyroid hormone economies on infant cognitive abilities. J Pediatr Endocrinol Metab 2000;13:191–194.

9. Guadano-Ferraz A, Escamez MJ, Rausell E, Bernal J: Expression of type 2 iodothyronine deiodinase in hypothyroid rat brain indicates an important role of thyroid hormone in the development of specific primary sensory systems. J Neurosci 1999;19:3430–3439.

10. Dowling ALS, Martz GU, Leonard JL, Zoeller RT: Acute changes in maternal thyroid hormone induce rapid and transient changes in gene expression in fetal rat brain. J Neurosci 2000;20:2255–2265.

11. Dussault JH, Fisher DA: Thyroid function in mothers of hypothyroid newborns. Obstet Gynecol 1999;93:15–20.

12. Mortimer RH, Cannell GR, Addison RS, et al: Methimazole and propylthiouracil equally cross the perfused human term placenta lobule. J Clin Endocrinol Metab 1997;82:3099–3102.

13. Radetti G, Persani L, Moroder W, et al: Transplacental passage of anti-thyroid auto-antibodies in a pregnant woman with auto-immune thyroid disease. Prenat Diagn 1999;19:468–471.

14. Asteria C, Rajanayagam O, Collingwood TN, et al: Prenatal diagnosis of thyroid hormone resistance. J Clin Endocrinol Metab 1999;84:405–410.

15. Leylek OA, Toyaksi M, Erselcan T, Dokmetas S: Immunologic and biochemical factors in hyperemesis gravidarum with or without hyperthyroxinemia. Gynecol Obstet Invest 1999;47:229–234.

16. Rodien P, Bremont C, Sanson ML, et al: Familial gestational hyperthyroidism caused by a mutant thyrotropin receptor hypersensitive to human chorionic gonadotropin. N Engl J Med 1998;339:1823–1826.

17. Basbug M, Aygen E, Tayyar M, et al: Correlation between maternal thyroid function test and endothelin in preeclampsia-eclampsia. Obstet Gynecol 1999;94:551–555.

TWENTY-THREE

Fetal Lung Maturity Testing

Michele R. Lauria

BACKGROUND

The fetal pulmonary system is normally one of the last organ systems to mature. However, fetal lung maturation is an inducible event that may occur as early as 25 weeks' gestation; therefore, lung maturity per se may not reflect overall preparation for extrauterine life in fetuses remote from term. Before the introduction of the lecithin to sphingomyelin (L/S) ratio in 1971 by Gluck and colleagues,[1] fetal lung maturity tests (i.e., staining patterns of amniotic fluid cells and amniotic fluid creatinine and osmolality) were actually measures of gestational age rather than lung maturation. The L/S ratio was the first test that predicated lung maturation independently of gestational age. Since the advent of the L/S ratio, numerous other easier and less expensive tests have been developed. However, the L/S ratio remains the standard against which these newer tests are compared.

INDICATIONS

Amniotic fluid assessment of fetal lung maturity should be performed before delivery at less than 39 weeks' gestation, when the potential for fetal or maternal compromise is not great enough to justify the risk of iatrogenic prematurity. Some examples include repeat cesarean section, stable placenta previa, or growth-restricted fetuses with reassuring antenatal testing.

In order to decrease the incidence of iatrogenic prematurity, the American College of Obstetricians and Gynecologists[2] suggested the following criteria for clinical confirmation of fetal maturity. If these criteria do not confirm menstrual dating of 39 weeks or greater in a patient with regular menstrual cycles and no recent oral contraceptive use, testing of amniotic fluid for maturity should be performed as clinically indicated.

- Fetal heart tones have been documented for 20 weeks by nonelectronic fetoscope or for 30 weeks by Doppler fetoscope.
- It has been 36 weeks since a serum or urine human chorionic gonadotropin pregnancy test was found to be positive by a reliable laboratory.
- Ultrasound measurement of the crown-rump length at 6 to 11 weeks' gestation supports a gestation age equal to or greater than 39 weeks.
- Ultrasound measurement at 12 to 20 weeks' gestation supports a clinically determined gestation age of 39 weeks or greater.

INTERPRETATION

In general, tests for lung maturity are highly specific at the expense of sensitivity. Consequently, when testing yields a mature result, there is very little chance that the delivered neonate will develop hyaline membrane disease (HMD). Conversely, even with immature results, the majority of neonates will have functional lung maturity. This is an important fact to consider when deciding to use amniotic fluid testing in the management of patients with serious prenatal complications. At gestational ages beyond 35 weeks, delivery without amniotic fluid testing is often the best choice because immature test results are poorly predictive of HMD. Despite the advances in lung maturity testing, one must remember that gestational age is still the best predictor of neonatal outcome.[3] Lung maturity testing is most useful for patients with uncertain dating, or with clinical scenarios where the indication for delivery does not justify any risk of HMD.[3]

The high specificity of fetal lung maturity tests makes them ideal for cascade testing protocols. Technically easy and inexpensive tests are used first; more complex tests, such as L/S and phosphatidyl glycerol (PG), are utilized if initial tests yield immature results. If any of the tests performed is mature, then functional lung maturity is assured.[4]

DIABETES

Diabetes is associated with a delay in PG production and other histologic and anatomic differences that predispose the neonate to HMD and transient tachypnea of the newborn. It appears that this is related to glycemic control, making the evaluation of maturity tests in diabetes a difficult research issue. In nondiabetic pregnancies, the mean gestational age for pulmonary maturity is 34 to 35 weeks, with more than 99% of fetuses having lung maturity at 37 weeks. With diabetic pregnancies, the risk of respiratory distress is significant until 38.5 weeks. Therefore, pregnancies complicated by diabetes should not undergo delivery before 39 weeks without documentation of lung maturity, unless there are clear maternal or fetal indications that justify the risk of respiratory complications. PG appears to be the most specific lung maturity test in diabetes, probably because it is one of the last surfactants to appear. Most other tests have not been adequately evaluated in diabetic populations that have poor glycemic control.[5]

TWINS

Testing in diamniotic twins raises questions about the need to test both fetuses. Clinicians often perform amniocentesis on the larger twin, assuming that it is less stressed and less likely to be mature. In a recent study[6] of 58 diamniotic twin pairs, a high correlation was found when testing was performed at 32 weeks or greater and was unaffected by fetal size. Disparity was most likely at less than 32 weeks when one twin was found to have an L/S ratio that was advanced for gestational age. Therefore, it seems reasonable to perform amniocentesis on only one fetal twin when close to term and to choose the technically easier twin.

EVALUATION OF TEST PERFORMANCE

Evaluation of various tests for fetal lung maturity can be difficult because of the variety of statistical analyses used, as well as the outcome measure being analyzed, for example, respiratory distress syndrome (RDS) versus lung maturity. Most tests have low specificity (30% to 50%) for predicting RDS but high specificity for predicting lung maturity (95% to 100%). Listed in the following section are the most commonly used tests for fetal lung maturity. *Sensitivity* and *specificity* refer to the ability of the test to predict lung maturity.

SPECIFIC FETAL MATURITY TESTS

L/S Ratio

Biochemical basis: The L/S ratio determines the ratio of saturated phosphatidyl choline (lecithin) to sphingomyelin. Lecithin is the principle surface-active component of surfactant. Sphingomyelin is a general membrane lipid found in all cells. It is used to adjust for variations in amniotic fluid volume.

Interpretation: The value that indicates lung maturity depends on the use of acetone precipitation, which lowers the L/S ratio. If acetone precipitation is used, then an L/S ratio of 2.0 or higher is mature, ratios below 1.0 confer a high risk of RDS. If acetone precipitation is not used, then mature ratios are 3.5 or higher.

Sensitivity: Low, 55% to 65%.

Specificity: High, 95% to 100%.

Diabetes: L/S ratio may be less reliable.

Effects of contamination: Blood contains sphingomyelin and lowers the L/S ratio. Meconium lacks sphingomyelin; however, it has a substance that migrates with these moieties, having a variable effect on the ratio. In a study

looking at the effects of specimen source and clarity on the ability of the L/S ratio to predict functional lung maturity, blood and meconium had minimal effects.[3]

Cost: $$$$.

Turnaround time: 2 to 3 hours.

Special considerations: Centrifugation causes lamellar bodies and lipid aggregates to separate out and falsely lowers results. Temperature changes and small variations in technique can significantly affect results, so the technique must be continuously validated. In addition, it requires highly trained laboratory personnel.

Phosphatidyl Glycerol (PG)

Biochemical basis: PG accounts for 10% of surfactant by weight, and appears only at the end of gestation in functionally mature lungs.

Interpretation: Values of greater than 1% are considered mature.

Sensitivity: Extremely low.

Specificity: High.

Diabetes: Reliable.

Effects of contamination: Some bacteria produce PG that may cause false-positive results, especially in heavily contaminated vaginal pool specimens. PG is not affected by contamination with blood or meconium.

Cost: $$$$.

Turnaround time: 2 to 3 hours.

Special considerations: Technically difficult to perform, requires skilled laboratory personnel.

Foam Stability Index (FSI)

Biochemical basis: Serial dilutions of amniotic fluid are mixed with ethanol. The highest dilution at which there is still stable foam is reported.

Interpretation: Mature is 47 or greater.

Sensitivity: Low.

Specificity: High.

Effects of contamination: Unreliable with blood, meconium, and vaginal secretion contamination.

Cost: $$.

Turnaround time: 30 minutes.

Special considerations: Suggested as a first test in cascade protocols.

Fluorescence Polarization (Abbott TDx/FLM)

Biochemical basis: Fluorescent probe that changes activity when it interacts with surfactant. The change in fluorescence is measured relative to the albumin content in the amniotic fluid.

Interpretation: Mature is 55 mg surfactant/g of albumin or greater.

Sensitivity: Low.

Specificity: High.

Diabetes: Preliminary studies suggest reliability in gestational diabetes; however, the degree of glycemic control for the study group was not reported.[7]

Effects of contamination: Both blood and meconium may affect interpretation by making immature fluids seem mature and mature fluids seem immature.

Cost: $.

Turnaround time: 30 minutes.

Special considerations: Requires minimal training.

Lamellar Body Count (LBC)

Biochemical basis: The LBC counts the number of lamellar bodies using the platelet channel of a hematology analyzer.

Interpretation: A variety of thresholds have been reported. For unspun fluid, an LBC of 8000 or less is 100% specific for biochemical immaturity based on L/S and PG testing. An LBC greater than 32,000 is 98% specific for biochemical maturity based on L/S and PG. For a review of recent articles discussing LBC, see Lewis and associates.[8]

Sensitivity: See above.

Specificity: See above.

Effects of contamination: Preliminary reports suggest minimal effects; however, this has not been adequately studied.

Cost: $.

Turnaround time: 30 minutes.

Special considerations: Centrifugation and the type of hematology analyzer used may significantly affect LBC. Centrifugation decreases the LBC by 10% to 40%. LBC has been proposed as an initial test in a cascade protocol.

Dipalmitoylphosphatidylcholine (DPPC)

Biochemical basis: Saturated DPPC is the major surface-active component of surfactant. This test measures the concentration of DPPC using enzyme hydrolysis and high-performance, thin-layer chromatography.

Interpretation: Mature is 12 μg/mL or greater.

Sensitivity: High.

Specificity: High.

Valid in diabetics: Unknown.

Effects of contamination: Negligible.

Cost: $$$.

Turnaround time: 2 hours.

Special considerations: This is a technically demanding test. The high sensitivity and specificity reports come from a single center,[9] and have yet to be validated at other institutions.

Optical Density (OD) at 650 nm

Biochemical basis: Lamellar bodies increase with gestational age and lung maturity. This test measures the amount of light absorbed by lamellar bodies at 650 nm.

Interpretation: Mature is greater than 0.15.

Sensitivity: Very low.

Specificity: High.

Effects of contamination: Both blood and meconium will interfere with light absorbance.

Cost: $.

Turnaround time: 2 hours.

Special considerations: OD can be performed on very small amounts of amniotic fluid. Centrifugation will cause lamellar bodies to be removed from the amniotic fluid sample.

References

1. Gluck L, Kulovich MV, Borer JC Jr, et al: Diagnosis of the respiratory distress syndrome by amniocentesis. Am J Obstet Gynecol 1971;109:440–445.
2. American College of Obstetricians and Gynecologists: Assessment of fetal lung maturity (Education and Technical Bulletins No. 230). Washington, DC, American College of Obstetricians and Gynecologists, 1996.
3. Lauria M, Dombrowski M, Delaney-Black V, Bottoms S: Lung maturity tests. Relation to source, clarity, gestational age and neonatal outcome. J Reprod Med 1996;41:685–691.
4. Bonebrake R, Towers C, Rumney P, Reimbold P: Is fluorescence polarization reliable and cost efficient in a fetal lung maturity cascade? Am J Obstet Gynecol 1997;177:835–841.
5. Jobe AH: Fetal lung development, tests for maturation, induction of maturation and treatment. In Creasy RK, Resnik R (eds): Maternal-Fetal Medicine. Philadelphia, WB Saunders, 1999.
6. Whitworth N, Magann E, Morrison JC: Evaluation of fetal lung maturity in diamniotic twins. Am J Obstet Gynecol 1999;180:1438–1441.
7. Livingston EG, Herbert WN, Hage ML, et al: Use of the TDx-FLM assay in evaluating fetal lung maturity in an insulin-dependent diabetic population. The Diabetes and Fetal Maturity Study Group. Obstet Gynecol 1995;86:826–829.
8. Lewis P, Lauria M, Dzieczkowski J, et al: Amniotic fluid lamellar body count: Cost-effective screening for fetal lung maturity. Obstet Gynecol 1999;93:387–391.
9. Alvarez JG, Slomovic B, Ludmir J: Analysis of dipalmitoyl phosphatidylcholine in amniotic fluid by high-performance liquid chromatography. J Chromatogr B 1997; 690:338–342.

Antenatal Magnesium Sulfate Exposure and the Risk of Cerebral Palsy in Preterm Neonates: An Update

Sean C. Blackwell and Yoram Sorokin

Despite intensive research and clinical efforts toward prevention and treatment for preterm delivery, the incidence of preterm birth in the United States since about 1980 has essentially remained unchanged. However, dramatic improvements in survival have occurred. The decreased mortality has been due to a combination of the antenatal administration of corticosteroids, technical advancements in neonatal intensive care medicine, and the postnatal use of surfactant.[1] These significant improvements in mortality have also resulted in a profound increase in the incidence of neurologic impairments in surviving neonates.[2] For instance, at 24 weeks' gestation, survival now approaches 47%, whereas 20% of these neonates will later develop cerebral palsy (CP). There has been little progress in our ability to decrease the rate of neurologic morbidity in these preterm neonates; approximately 28% of cases of disabling CP are in infants born weighing less than 1500 g.[3]

In 1995 to 1996, data from three observational studies[4-6] suggested a possible neuroprotective effect of magnesium sulfate (MgSO₄) exposure in utero. These findings have inspired much interest and hope and have contributed to initiation of three large, randomized clinical trials. The purpose of this review is to summarize the currently available literature and ongoing trials on the use of MgSO₄ as a fetal neuroprotective agent.

CLINICAL REPORTS OF ANTENATAL MAGNESIUM SULFATE EXPOSURE AND NEUROLOGIC OUTCOMES

In 1995, Nelson and Grether[4] reported data from a study that evaluated a cohort of very-low-birth-weight (VLBW; birth weight < 1500 g) infants delivered in a four-county area of California from 1983 to 1985. In a case-control study design, these authors compared antenatal and obstetric factors between infants who developed moderate or severe congenital CP with those of survivors without neurologic complications. After controlling for confounding factors such as indication for MgSO₄ (preterm labor to-

colysis or preeclampsia [pregnancy-induced hypertension {PIH}] seizure prophylaxis) and the use of antenatal corticosteroids, MgSO₄ exposure was associated with a decreased incidence of CP (odds ratio [OR] 0.18, 95% confidence interval [CI] 0.05 to 0.74). In that same year, Hauth and coworkers[5] reported developmental outcomes at 1 year of life or older for infants ($N = 389$) who weighed 500 to 1000 g at birth who delivered from 1979 to 1991. Regression analysis to adjust for multiple confounding factors indicated a reduced rate of CP with maternal antenatal MgSO₄ therapy (OR 0.35, CI 0.16 to 0.99). Of the 212 (55%) patients with MgSO₄ exposure, 7.6% of surviving infants developed CP compared with 19% of infants without exposure ($P = .001$). This reduction in the rate of CP was most pronounced at 24 to 25 weeks.

These studies were followed by the work of Schendel and associates,[6] who described developmental outcomes of VLBW infants delivered from 1986 to 1988 in 29 Georgia counties. These authors examined a cohort of VLBW infants at 1 year of age and again at 3 to 5 years and found that antenatal MgSO₄ was inversely associated with the risk of CP (crude OR 0.11, CI 0.02 to 0.81) and possibly mental retardation (crude OR 0.03, CI 0.07 to 1.29). The reductions in CP were not accounted for by a higher mortality rate for MgSO₄-exposed neonates. For the entire cohort of 1097 VLBW neonates, there was no association between MgSO₄ and infant mortality (adjusted OR 1.02, CI 0.83 to 1.25). It implied that MgSO₄ did not improve neurologic outcomes by means of increasing the mortality rate of the most "fragile" neonates.[7]

Owing to the observational nature of these positive studies, the authors concluded that placebo-controlled, randomized clinical trials (RCTs) would be necessary to determine whether antenatal MgSO₄ had neuroprotective effects. To date, there have been 15 clinical reports that have measured the effects of MgSO₄ on different neurologic outcomes (mortality, CP, mental retardation, intraventricular hemorrhage, and periventricular leukomalacia). These studies are summarized in Table 24–1. In all, 9 reported improvement in outcomes, 5 reported no difference, and 1 detailed a detrimental effect.

Table 24–1. Summary of Clinical Trials That Describe the Effects of Magnesium Sulfate on Neonatal Mortality and Neurologic Morbidity

Study	Population	Results
Nelson, 1995[4]	BW < 1500 g	Decreased CP at age 3 yr
Hauth et al, 1995[5]	BW 500–1000 g	Decreased CP at ≥ 1 yr of age
Schendel et al, 1996[6]	BW < 1500 g	Decreased CP at age 3 to 5 yr
Wisewell et al, 1996[8]	GA < 33 wk	Decreased IVH, PVL, CP
Lemons et al, 1996[9]	BW 401–1500 g	Decreased neonatal deaths; no difference in IVH
Kumar et al, 1996[10]	GA 23–32 wk	No difference in IVH
Paneth et al, 1997[11]	BW ≤ 2000 g	No difference in CP or IVH but decreased disabling CP in neonates with late-onset white matter lesions
FineSmith et al, 1997[12]	BW < 1750 g	Decreased PVL
Leviton et al, 1997[13]	BW 500–1500 g	No difference in IVH, white matter damage
Abbassi et al, 1997[14]	BW < 1000 g	No difference in IVH
Perlman et al, 1997[15]	BW < 1500 g	Decreased PV-IVH
Mittendorf et al, 1997[16]	GA < 34 wk	Increased risk of pediatric (fetal, neonatal, postnatal) deaths
Kimberlin et al, 1998[17]	BW ≤ 1000 g	No difference in IVH, PVL, ROP, seizures, death
Grether et al, 1998[18]	BW < 1500 g	Decreased neonatal deaths
Canterino et al, 1999[19]	BW 500–1750 g	No difference in IVH or PVL

BW, birth weight; CP, cerebral palsy; GA, gestational age; IVH, intraventricular hemorrhage; PV-IVH, periventricular-intraventricular hemorrhage; PVL, periventricular leukomalacia; ROP, retinopathy of prematurity.

There is no universal agreement as to whether the possible beneficial effects attributed to $MgSO_4$ are due to $MgSO_4$ exposure or to selection biases related to treatment.[20] Patients who develop premature labor (PTL) or preterm premature rupture of the membranes (pPROM) may present to the hospital with advanced labor and not receive $MgSO_4$. These pregnancies may be at a higher risk for CP owing to a higher rate of intrauterine infection, which has been associated with CP in preterm pregnancies.[21] Therefore, the apparent beneficial effect of $MgSO_4$ may be due to a greater risk for CP in the "control" group rather than a true neuroprotective effect. Furthermore, the risk for CP may be due to the indication for treatment, for example, an increased risk in pregnancies complicated by PTL and pPROM compared with those complicated by preterm PIH.

It has also been argued that the presence of PIH rather than $MgSO_4$ may be neuroprotective for the fetus.[22–25] In a study of neonates delivered at less than 32 weeks, Murphy and colleagues[24] showed that PIH was associated with a decreased risk of CP (OR 0.4, CI 0.2 to 0.9) independent of $MgSO_4$. In Western Australia, where $MgSO_4$ seizure prophylaxis is not used, Palmer and coworkers[25] found that PIH was associated with a decreased rate of CP in VLBW (<1500 g) neonates. Several other studies also reported that PIH was associated with decreased rates of intraventricular hemorrhage, germinal matrix hemorrhage, and other non-neurologic outcomes in preterm neonates (Table 24–2).

RANDOMIZED CLINICAL TRIALS INVESTIGATING ANTEPARTUM MAGNESIUM SULFATE THERAPY AND THE RISK OF CEREBRAL PALSY

In 1996, Rouse and associates[30] described the feasibility of an RCT to test whether antenatal $MgSO_4$ would decrease the rate of CP in surviving preterm neonates. They stated that such an effort would be difficult owing to the requirements for both a large study sample size and long-term neonatal follow-up. They also stated that a population with a high preterm delivery rate for which aggressive obstetric and pediatric efforts for extremely-low-birth-weight neonates are conducted would be necessary. Preterm pregnancies complicated by pPROM rather than PTL or PIH would most likely be the majority of eligible candidates. An RCT BEAM (Randomized Clinical Trial of the Beneficial Effects of Antenatal Magnesium) is currently being conducted by the National Institute of Child Health and Human Development Maternal Fetal Medicine Units Network (NICHHD-MFMU) and the National Institute of Neurologic Disorders and Stroke.[31] The BEAM study, with a planned sample size of 2200 patients, begun in 1997, is designed to determine whether $MgSO_4$, when given to patients between 24 and 32 weeks' gestation, decreases the

Table 24–2. Summary of Clinical Trials That Report a Beneficial Effect of Maternal Preeclampsia on Neonatal Neurologic Outcomes in Preterm Pregnancies

Study	Population	Results
Kuban et al, 1992[26]	BW < 1500 g	Decreased risk GMH-IVH
Murphy et al, 1995[24]	GA < 32 wk	Decreased CP
Perlman et al, 1997[15]	BW < 1500 g	Decreased IVH
Leviton et al, 1988[27]	BW ≤ 1500 g	Decreased GMH
van de Bor et al, 1987[28]	BW < 1500 g or GA < 32 wk	Decreased IVH
Spinillo et al, 1998[29]	GA < 33 wk	Decreased CP
Leviton et al, 1997[13]	BW 500–1500 g	Decreased IVH

BW, birth weight; CP, cerebral palsy; GA, gestational age; GMH, germinal matrix hemorrhage; IVH, intraventricular hemorrhage.

incidence of death or moderate to severe CP in surviving infants. The MgSO$_4$ protocol includes a 6-g loading dose followed by continuous infusion at 2 g/hr for at least 12 hours. Two other RCTs are in progress: the Australian Collaborative Trial of Magnesium Sulfate (ACTOMgSO$_4$) and the Pre-Mag French Multicentre Collaborative Trial.[32, 33]

CONTROVERSIAL RESULTS OF THE MAGNESIUM AND NEUROLOGIC ENDPOINTS TRIAL

In 1997, Mittendorf and colleagues[16] reported, as a research letter to the *Lancet,* the results of the Magnesium and Neurologic Endpoints Trial (MAGnet trial). The MAGnet trial was conducted at the University of Chicago and funded by the United Cerebral Palsy Research and Education Fund. It consisted of two mutually exclusive components: a tocolytic study and a preventive study. The preventive study sought to determine whether antenatal MgSO$_4$ decreases the frequency of CP among very preterm neonates. PTL patients of less than 34 weeks' gestation who presented with advanced cervical dilatation and not eligible for tocolysis were candidates for the preventive study. In the tocolytic component of the study, the use of MgSO$_4$ was compared with other tocolytics; in the preventive component, MgSO$_4$ was compared with placebo. The dosing for tocolytic MgSO$_4$ involved a 4-g bolus followed by a 2- to 3-g/hr continuous infusion; the preventive MgSO$_4$ dose was a single 4-g bolus.

After 1 year, the study was stopped owing to concerns over an excess of "total pediatric deaths" in the patients exposed to MgSO$_4$. The authors defined this outcome as a sum of fetal, neonatal, and postneonatal deaths. There were 10 pediatric deaths (5 singletons, 3 twin pairs with 1 death, and 1 twin pair with death of both twins) in the 65 patients (10 twin gestations) who received MgSO$_4$ and 1 pediatric death (1 singleton) in the 69 patients (6 twin gestations) who received other tocolytics or saline solution. This difference was statistically significant (risk difference 10.7%, 95% CI 2.9 to 18.5%; $P = .02$). This was the first clinical report suggesting a significantly adverse effect of maternal MgSO$_4$ treatment on the fetus. In the associated commentary discussing the results and the implications of the MAGnet trial, it was suggested that MgSO$_4$ should be used in preterm pregnancies for seizure prophylaxis but not for tocolysis. These same investigators later elaborated the possible clinical significance of the MAGnet Trial in a commentary to *Obstetrics and Gynecology.*[34] In this commentary, the authors summarized mortality data from previous studies and speculated on the potential impact of MgSO$_4$ therapy on infant mortality in the United States.

After the initial report in the *Lancet,* a series of "letters to the editor" were published that questioned several aspects of the MAGnet Trial and its accompanying commentary. Authors challenged whether it was appropriate to

consider MgSO$_4$ as a causative factor in deaths related to congenital anomalies, twin-twin transfusion syndrome with severe prematurity, or deaths well beyond the neonatal period. Also challenged was a possible imbalance of multiple gestations in the study group as well as a very low incidence of mortality in the control population. Another important issue raised was that neither the authors of the MAGnet Trial nor the accompanying commentary made reference to the fact that several large RCTs investigating MgSO$_4$ as both a tocolytic and an anticonvulsant have found no association between MgSO$_4$ treatment and mortality. Finally, investigators for two of the three on-going RCTs (Premag[33] and ACTOMgSO$_4$[32]) indicated that in planned blinded interim analyses, there was no evidence of excess mortality in the MgSO$_4$ treatment groups. Mittendorf and coworkers[16, 34] replied that the dosing of MgSO$_4$ in the MAGnet trial (median total dose of 50 g) was significantly higher than that of the ACTOMgSO$_4$ and BEAM studies (total dose 28 to 30 g), and thus the question of whether there is a dose-response relationship between MgSO$_4$ and death may not be answered by these trials.

CONCLUSION

The potential use of antenatal MgSO$_4$ as a neuroprotective agent is based on promising epidemiologic data as well as experimental evidence that provides biologic plausibility for such an effect. The magnesium ion is an integral factor in many biologic processes; its potential mechanisms for neuroprotection are numerous. Whether its neuroprotective effect would be central, for example, in the fetal brain, or peripheral and whether it would be due to a single mechanism or a combination remains unclear. MgSO$_4$ is an ideal agent because it is easy to dose and administer, has a low side effect profile, is safe to the mother, and is relatively inexpensive. It has also been used since about 1980 in obstetrics, and its properties are familiar to most clinicians.

The results of the RCTs that will provide data on the safety and neuroprotective properties of MgSO$_4$ are expected in the next few years. Based on the sum of all available evidence, antenatal MgSO$_4$ should not be administered to preterm pregnancies for the prevention of CP until the results of these RCTs are available; however, its use as a tocolytic agent should not be considered deleterious to the fetus.

References

1. Kuban KC, Leviton A: Cerebral palsy. N Engl J Med 1994;330:188–195.
2. Bhushan V, Paneth N, Kiely JL: Impact of improved survival of very low birth weight infants on recent secular trends in the prevalence of cerebral palsy. Pediatrics 1993;91:1094–1100.
3. Cummins SK, Nelson KB, Grether JK, Velie EM: Cerebral palsy in four northern California counties, births 1983 through 1985. J Pediatr 1993;123:230–237.
4. Nelson KB, Grether JK: Can magnesium sulfate reduce the risk of

cerebral palsy in very low birth weight infants? Pediatrics 1995;95:263–267.

5. Hauth JC, Goldenberg RL, Nelson KG, et al: Reduction of cerebral palsy with maternal magnesium sulfate treatment in newborns weighing 500–1000 g. Am J Obstet Gynecol 1995;172:419.

6. Schendel DE, Berg CJ, Yeargin-Allsopp M, et al: Prenatal magnesium sulfate exposure and the risk for cerebral palsy or mental retardation among very low-birth-weight children aged 3 to 5 years. JAMA 1996;276:1805–1810.

7. Nelson KB: Magnesium sulfate and risk of cerebral palsy in very low-birth-weight infants. JAMA 1996;276:1843–1844.

8. Wisewell TE, Graziani LJ, Caddell JL, et al: Maternally administered magnesium sulfate ($MgSO_4$) protects against early brain injury and long term adverse neurodevelopmental outcomes in preterm infants: A prospective study. Pediatr Res 1996;39:253A.

9. Lemons J, Stevenson D, Verter J, et al: In utero magnesium exposure: Risk of death and of intraventricular hemorrhage (IVH) in very low birth weight (VLBW) infants. Pediatr Res 1996;39:225A.

10. Kumar V, Holman M, Rosenkrantz T: Is magnesium protective to the fetus? Pediatr Res 1996;39:223A.

11. Paneth N, Jetton J, Pinto-Martin J, Susser M: Magnesium sulfate in labor and risk of neonatal brain lesions and cerebral palsy in low birth weight infants. The Neonatal Brain Hemorrhage Study Analysis Group. Pediatrics 1997;99:E1.

12. FineSmith RB, Roche K, Yellin PB, et al: Effect of magnesium sulfate on the development of cystic periventricular leukomalacia in preterm infants. Am J Perinatol 1997;14:303–307.

13. Leviton A, Paneth N, Susser M, et al: Maternal receipt of magnesium sulfate does not seem to reduce the risk of neonatal white matter damage. Pediatrics 1997;99:E2.

14. Abbasi S, Tolosa J, Grous MK, et al: Effect of antenatal magnesium exposure on neonatal mortality and morbidity. Pediatr Res 1997;41:134A.

15. Perlman JM, Risser RC, Gee JB: Pregnancy-induced hypertension and reduced intraventricular hemorrhage in preterm infants. Pediatr Neurol 1997;17:29–33.

16. Mittendorf R, Covert R, Boman J, et al: Is tocolytic magnesium sulphate associated with increased total paediatric mortality? Lancet 1997;350:1517–1518.

17. Kimberlin DF, Hauth JC, Goldenberg RL, et al: The effect of maternal magnesium sulfate treatment on neonatal morbidity in ≤ 1000–gram infants. Am J Perinatol 1998;15:635–641.

18. Grether JK, Hoogstrate J, Selvin S, Nelson KB: Magnesium sulfate tocolysis and risk of neonatal death. Am J Obstet Gynecol 1998;178:1–6.

19. Canterino JC, Verma UL, Visintainer PF, et al: Maternal magnesium sulfate and the development of neonatal periventricular leukomalacia and intraventricular hemorrhage. Obstet Gynecol 1999;93:396–402.

20. Allred EN, Dammann O, Kuban KKC, et al: Prenatal magnesium exposure and the risk of cerebral palsy. JAMA 1997;277:1033–1034.

21. Murphy DJ, Johnson A: Placental infection and risk of cerebral palsy in very low birth weight infants. J Pediatr 1996;129:776–778.

22. Collins M, Paneth N: Preeclampsia and cerebral palsy: Are they related? Dev Med Child Neurol 1998;40:207–211.

23. Blair E, Palmer L, Stanley F: Cerebral palsy in very low birth weight infants, pre-eclampsia and magnesium sulfate. Pediatrics 1996;97:780–782.

24. Murphy DJ, Sellers S, MacKenzie IZ, et al: Case-control study of antenatal and intrapartum risk factors for cerebral palsy in very preterm singleton babies. Lancet 1995;346:1449–1454.

25. Palmer L, Blair E, Petterson B, Burton P: Antenatal antecedents of moderate and severe cerebral palsy. Paediatr Perinatal Epidemiol 1995;9:171–184.

26. Kuban KC, Leviton A, Pagano M, et al: Maternal toxemia is associated with reduced incidence of germinal matrix hemorrhage in premature babies. J Child Neurol 1992;7:70–76.

27. Leviton A, Kuban KC, Pagano M, et al: Maternal toxemia and neonatal germinal matrix hemorrhage in intubated infants less than 1751 g. Obstet Gynecol 1988;72:571–576.

28. van de Bor M, Verloove-Vanhorick SP, Brand R, et al: Incidence and prediction of periventricular-intraventricular hemorrhage in very preterm infants. J Perinat Med 1987;15:333–339.

29. Spinillo A, Capuzzo E, Cavallini AN, et al: Preeclampsia, preterm delivery and infant cerebral palsy. Eur J Obstet Gynecol Reprod Biol 1998;77:151–155.

30. Rouse DJ, Hauth JC, Nelson KG, Goldenberg RL: The feasibility of a randomized clinical perinatal trial: Maternal magnesium sulfate for the prevention of cerebral palsy. Am J Obstet Gynecol 1996;175:701–705.

31. Phelan JP, Mittendorf RL, Morales WJ, Rouse D: Does magnesium help or harm the preterm fetus? OBG Management. September 1999, pp. 56–78.

32. Crowther C, Hiller J, Doyle L, et al: Tocolytic magnesium sulphate and paediatric mortality. Lancet 1998;351:291.

33. Benichou J, Zupan V, Fernandez H, et al: Tocolytic magnesium sulphate and paediatric mortality. Lancet 1998;351:290–291.

34. Mittendorf R, Pryde P, Khoshnood B, Lee KS: If tocolytic magnesium sulfate is associated with excess total pediatric mortality, what is its impact? Obstet Gynecol 1998;92:308–311.

Management of Epilepsy

William C. Mabie

This discussion is divided into two sections: management of epilepsy in general and, more specifically, management during pregnancy. One percent of the population has epilepsy; 0.3% to 0.5% of pregnancies are complicated by epilepsy.

As shown in Table 25–1, seizures may be divided into two types: partial and generalized. Partial seizures are also known as focal seizures and raise the possibility of a brain tumor or focal injury to the brain. In contrast, generalized seizures involve diffuse regions of the brain simultaneously and bilaterally. Generalized seizures may result from cellular, biochemical, or structural abnormalities that have a more widespread distribution.

Simple-partial seizures cause motor, sensory, autonomic, or psychic symptoms, with consciousness being fully preserved. For example, a partial seizure arising from the right motor cortex in the vicinity controlling hand movement would result in involuntary movement of the contralateral left hand. Two additional features deserve comment. If the abnormal movement begins in a restricted region, such as the fingers, and gradually progresses to involve a larger portion of the extremity, the phenomenon is known as a *jacksonian march.* Second, patients may experience localized paresis (Todd's paralysis) lasting from minutes to hours in the involved region after the seizure. *Complex-partial seizures* are focal seizures associated with loss of consciousness. Automatisms associated with complex-partial seizures may include lip smacking, chewing, swallowing, or "picking" movements of the hands. Partial seizures may also spread to involve both cerebral hemispheres and produce a generalized seizure. A partial seizure with secondary generalization is difficult to distinguish from a primarily generalized tonic-clonic seizure, because bystanders may overlook the more subtle focal symptoms present at the onset. Often, the focal onset can be established only through electroencephalographic analysis during a seizure. If a careful history identifies a stereotypic aura or warning preceding a tonic-clonic seizure, this probably represents a simple-partial seizure with secondary generalization.

Generalized seizures arise from both hemispheres simultaneously and are divided into *tonic-clonic* (grand mal), *absence* (petit mal), and myoclonic (brief muscle jerks).

Causes of seizures include idiopathic (60%), trauma, brain tumor, arteriovenous malformation, drug withdrawal (alcohol, cocaine, amphetamines), infection, metabolic disorders (uremia, hepatic failure, electrolytes, hypoglycemia), stroke, and cardiac arrest.

Evaluation of the seizure patient includes history of the event, past medical history, physical examination, and laboratory data (Tables 25–2 and 25–3).

Goals of therapy are to eliminate the cause of epilepsy, to suppress the seizures, and to deal with the psychosocial consequences. The last problem is the greatest. Many patients with epilepsy underestimate their potential and feel as if they are subnormal. They may have difficulty obtaining a driver's license, maintaining employment, or finding a mate.

Antiepileptic drug therapy does not have to start with the first seizure. The decision must be made with the patient's informed participation. Social variables, such as loss of driving privileges and the situational embarrassment of recurrent seizures, will influence the decision to treat a patient with an isolated seizure. More than 50% of patients who have a recurrence will do so in the first 6 months

Table 25–1. Seizure Types

Partial	Generalized
Simple-partial	Tonic-clonic
Complex-partial	Absence
Secondary generalized	Myoclonic

Table 25–2. Evaluation of Seizures

History of the Event

Preceding activities
Prodromal symptoms (aura)
Description of seizures
   Interact with environment
   Motor function
Postictal behavior
   Focal/lateralizing signs
   Time to recovery

Medical History

Family history of seizures
Febrile convulsions
Head injury
Cerebrovascular or cardiovascular disease
Progressive cognitive dysfunction (Alzheimer's)
Infection
Substance abuse
Cancer (metastases)

Complete Physical Examination

Table 25–3. Laboratory Evaluation

Routine laboratory studies
  Complete blood count, urinalysis, glucose, calcium, magnesium, hepatic and renal function, drug screen of blood and urine
  Lumbar puncture if any suspicion of meningitis or encephalitis or if patient is infected with HIV
Electroencephalogram
Neuroimaging (MRI preferred)
Split-screen video-EEG monitoring

EEG, electroencephalographic; MRI, magnetic resonance imaging.

after the initial seizure. The recurrence rate after a first unprovoked seizure varies from 36% to 77%. Risk factors associated with recurrent seizures are the following: (1) abnormal neurologic examination, (2) seizures presenting as status epilepticus, (3) postictal Todd's paralysis, (4) a strong family history of seizures, or (5) an abnormal electroencephalogram. The risk of recurrence after two seizures approaches 80% to 90%. Such patients should be treated with anticonvulsants.

Treatment with antiepileptic drugs (AEDs) is based on the type of seizures. Monotherapy is preferred. First-line therapy for partial seizures in adults is phenytoin or carbamazepine. Primidone, phenobarbital, and valproate are only slightly less effective. Monotherapy with one of the first-line drugs provides adequate control of approximately 70% of adults with partial epilepsy. Another 15% to 20% can be controlled with combination drug therapy including one or two additional drugs. Unsatisfactory control remains in about 15% of patients, who then become candidates for surgery or experimental drug therapy. New AEDs for adjunctive care include lamotrigine, gabapentin, felbamate, tiagabine, and topiramate.[1]

First-line initial monotherapy for generalized seizures is valproate. Phenytoin, carbamazepine, phenobarbital, or primidone can be used if valproate is ineffective or poorly tolerated. The new AEDs have not been extensively studied for the treatment of generalized epilepsies. Lamotrigine, topiramate, and felbamate show promise as adjunctive or alternative therapy. Ethosuximide or valproate are best for petit mal epilepsy. Myoclonic seizures may be treated with primidone, valproate, or clonazepam.[1]

Advantages of monotherapy are the following: (1) enhanced patient compliance, (2) lower drug costs, (3) fewer side effects, and (4) no risk of AED-AED interactions. Side effects and pharmacokinetic profiles of the commonly used drugs are shown in Tables 25–4 and 25–5.

EPILEPSY AND PREGNANCY

One of the main concerns of pregnant women with epilepsy is the teratogenic potential of AEDs. Minor malformations in children of epileptic mothers were described before the first anticonvulsant drug was marketed. Trimethadione is thought to be a teratogen and should not be used in pregnancy. It is rarely used in the nonpregnant patient. The four standard AEDs have all been associated with syndromes of anomalies. For example, phenytoin syndrome consists of a broad nasal bridge, short upturned nose, low-set ears, epicanthal folds, hypertelorism, wide mouth, ptosis or strabismus, distal digital hypoplasia, nail hypoplasia, intrauterine growth retardation, and mental deficiency. However, there is much overlap between all of these syndromes, and current thinking is that a specific syndrome referable to one drug is less likely than previously suggested. There is evidence that the risk of neural tube defects is greatest for infants of epileptic women taking valproate (1% to 2%) and carbamazepine (0.5% to 1%).

Because all AEDs are considered about equally teratogenic, the medication that is most efficacious for the woman's seizure type should be selected. If a woman presents for prenatal care taking a single drug that is effective, a medication change should not be attempted. Malformations occur from drug exposure early in pregnancy. The risk of teratogenesis is increased by exposure to a second agent. There is also a risk of poorer seizure control during the medication change.

Except for topiramate, which is associated with limb agenesis in rodents, none of the newer AEDs has been teratogenic in animals. Human experience with the newer AEDs is limited but growing. On the basis of available information, the newer AEDs should be considered with the standard AEDs as appropriate first-line treatment in pregnancy.[2]

Table 25–4. Commonly Used Anticonvulsant Drugs, Dosages, and Side Effects

Generic Name	Trade Name	Dosage	Side Effects
Phenytoin	Dilantin	300–400 mg/day	Gum hyperplasia, coarsening of facial features, hirsutism, lymphadenopathy, cerebellar toxicity
Carbamazepine	Tegretol	600–1800 mg/dL	GI upset, bone marrow suppression, liver toxicity
Valproate	Depakene/Depakote	750–2000 mg/dL	GI upset, hair loss, weight gain, bone marrow suppression, liver toxicity
Phenobarbital	Luminol	60–180 mg/day	Sedation, dulling of intellect
Ethosuximide	Zarontin	750–1250 mg/day	GI upset, drowsiness, agranulocytosis
Gabapentin	Neurontin	900–2400 mg/day	Sedation, dizziness
Felbamate	Felbatol	1800–4800 mg/day	Aplastic anemia (1/2000), liver failure (1/5000)
Lamotrigine	Lamictal	150–500 mg/day	Sedation, dizziness, rash

GI, gastrointestinal.

Table 25–5. Pharmacokinetic Profile

Generic Name	Plasma Protein Binding (%)	Half-life (hr)	Time to Steady State (day)	Therapeutic Serum Level (μg/mL)
Phenytoin	90	15–30	5–15	10–20
Carbamazepine	70–80	11–17	3–10	4–12
Valproate	60–95	6–18	2–4	50–150
Phenobarbital	40–60	30–50	16–21	10–50
Ethosuximide	0	40–50	6–12	40–100

The risk of major malformations in pregnancy is 2% to 3%. In epilepsy, the risk of malformation is increased two- to threefold to 4% to 9%. Still, greater than 90% of epileptic women will have an infant without malformations. The increase in malformations may be multifactorial. Polytherapy and higher drug dosages increase teratogenic risk. The increased risk of epilepsy in the offspring is not increased compared with that of the general population risk of 0.7% to 1%.[3]

Discontinuation of AED can be considered in the patient who has been seizure free for 2 to 5 years and has a single type of seizure, a normal neurologic examination, and a normal electroencephalogram. The drug should be tapered slowly over 2 to 3 months and withdrawal completed 6 months before planned conception.[3]

Contraception

Phenytoin, carbamazepine, phenobarbital, and primidone are inducers of the hepatic cytochrome P-450 system of mixed function oxidases. This results in reduction of exogenous estrogen and progesterone levels. Breakthrough bleeding and pregnancy may occur in women taking oral contraceptives. Formulations containing at least 50 μg of estradiol or mestranol are more protective. Valproate, which inhibits the hepatic microsomal enzyme system, and the new AEDs (gabapentin and lamotrigine) have no significant effect on hormone levels.

Levonorgestrel implants do not appear to be a good alternative for contraception in women using the enzyme-inducing AEDs. Intramuscular medroxyprogesterone acetate delivers higher dosages of progestin, but its effectiveness has not been well evaluated in women with epilepsy.[4]

Pregnancy

There is a rare entity known as gestational epilepsy in which the patient has seizures only during pregnancy. This may not recur in the next pregnancy. When one considers the effect of pregnancy on epilepsy, seizure frequency has been reported to have no change (50%), to increase (40%), and to decrease (10%). Noncompliance with medications occurs during pregnancy because of a fear of teratogenicity and because of hyperemesis. Sleep deprivation may increase seizure frequency. Plasma levels of AEDs may be lowered by malabsorption, by increased renal and hepatic clearance, and by plasma volume increases; however, the fall in serum albumin decreases protein binding and may increase the free or active component of the drug.

Eclampsia is not increased in epileptic women. Slight increases in preeclampsia, abruptio placenta, preterm labor, stillbirth, microcephaly, mental retardation, and childhood seizures have been reported, but the literature is inconsistent. Fetal bradycardia and hypoxia may occur during maternal seizures. Serum folate, vitamin D, and vitamin K levels are decreased in pregnancy. Because of delayed gastric emptying and reduced esophageal sphincter pressure in pregnancy, aspiration pneumonia is more likely during a seizure.

The best possible seizure control should be achieved before conception. A woman requiring high-dose AED therapy can be changed to lower individual doses administered more frequently to minimize fetal exposure. Total or free plasma AED levels should be monitored before conception to establish a baseline and then every 3 months throughout pregnancy. If seizure control is maintained during pregnancy regardless of plasma concentration, an argument could be made not to implement dosage increases.[4]

Prenatal Testing

Prenatal testing consists of a serum α-fetoprotein or a triple screen at 15 to 20 weeks' gestation and an anomaly ultrasound at 18 to 20 weeks' gestation. If the patient received valproate or carbamazepine, detailed ultrasound examination should be performed to rule out a neural tube defect.

Folic Acid

Low serum and red blood cell folate levels have been associated with spontaneous abortion and fetal malformations in animal models and in humans. Treatment with phenytoin, carbamazepine, and barbiturates can impair folate absorption. There is a substantial scientific basis for recommending prepregnancy and early pregnancy supplementation with folic acid at 0.4 mg/day. Higher doses (4 mg/day) have been recommended for women who have previously delivered an infant with a neural tube defect. This guideline applies to all women—not just those taking

AEDs. Women receiving valproate or carbamazepine also may benefit from the 4-mg/day dose because these drugs are associated with neural tube defects.[4]

Vitamin K Supplementation

There are conflicting data in the medical literature about the effects of vitamin K supplementation on the frequency of neonatal hemorrhage. Infants of women who take enzyme-inducing AEDs have higher levels of PIVKA (protein induced by vitamin K absence), which is considered a marker for coagulopathy related to vitamin K deficiency. Vitamin K supplementation has been associated with normalization of PIVKA levels. The problems are that vitamin K crosses the placenta poorly, all newborns are routinely given 1 mg of vitamin K intramuscularly at birth, and outcome studies have not been conducted to confirm the usefulness of prenatal vitamin K supplementation.[5]

Breastfeeding

Women with epilepsy should be encouraged to breastfeed their infants because of the immunologic and nutritional benefits. Nevertheless, breastfed infants receiving AEDs should be watched for somnolence, poor feeding, and poor weight gain.

Postpartum AED Adjustment

For many women, AED dosage increases will be necessary during pregnancy. Monitoring serum AED levels should continue post partum. With reversal of the physiologic changes of pregnancy, AED dosages usually may be reduced to prepregnancy levels by 8 weeks' postpartum.

References

1. Mattson RH: Medical management of epilepsy in adults. Neurology 1998;51(Suppl 4):S15–S20.
2. Morrell MJ: Guidelines for the care of women with epilepsy. Neurology 1998;51(Suppl 4):S21–S27.
3. American Academy of Neurology: Practice parameter: Management issues for women with epilepsy (summary statement). Report of the Quality Standards Subcommittee of the American Academy of Neurology. Neurology 1998;51:944–948.
4. American Academy of Neurology: Consensus statements: Medical management of epilepsy. Neurology 1998;51(Suppl 4):S39–S43.
5. Zahn CA, Morrell MJ, Collins SD, et al: Management issues for women with epilepsy: A review of the literature. Neurology 1998;51:949–956.

TWENTY-SIX

Herpes Infections in Pregnancy

Debora F. Kimberlin and William W. Andrews

Herpes simplex virus (HSV) infection is the most common cause of genital ulcerative disease in the United States and other developed countries. Approximately 5% of women of reproductive age have a history of genital herpes,[1] and up to 30% have serologic evidence of HSV-2 infection.[2] Since about 1975, the prevalence of HSV infection has increased dramatically.[3] The most serious consequence of HSV infection during pregnancy is transmission of infection to the fetus or neonate. Neonatal herpes is a devastating disease; despite antiviral therapy, more than 40% of affected neonates die or suffer significant neurologic sequelae.[3] Current clinical management guidelines have been developed in an effort to reduce the frequency of maternal-fetal transmission.

THE HERPES SIMPLEX VIRUS

Genital herpes is a sexually transmitted disease caused by HSV types 1 and 2 of the Herpesviridae family. Both HSV-1 and HSV-2 are double-stranded DNA viruses that are surrounded by a glycoprotein envelope. Although homology between the two viruses is extensive, they may be differentiated by minor immunologic and biochemical differences.

Transmission of HSV occurs when the mucous membranes or abraded skin of a susceptible person comes in contact with virus from an infected host who is actively shedding infectious viral particles. This most often occurs during close, intimate contact. Although both HSV-1 and HSV-2 can cause genital and nongenital infections, HSV-1 most commonly infects the oropharynx and nongenital mucosae. Initial infection with HSV-1 typically occurs in childhood and is usually asymptomatic.[4] In the United States, the majority (85%) of genital HSV infections are caused by HSV-2.[5]

Diagnosis

The "gold standard" for diagnosis of HSV infection is isolation of virus by tissue culture. Most cultures will be positive within 48 to 72 hours. However, most laboratories will not report a culture as negative until it has been held for 7 days. Viral culture has a sensitivity of 90% to 95% if specimens are obtained early in the vesicular or ulcerative stage; sensitivity decreases to less than 50% once lesions begin to re-epithelialize.[6] Cytologic methods such as the Tzanck preparation and the Papanicolaou smear have low sensitivities and high false-negative rates that limit their clinical utility. Amniocentesis is not effective in diagnosing fetal infection.

DNA polymerase chain reaction is a powerful new technique that provides a more sensitive means of detecting HSV DNA.[7] At present, this technology is available only through selected research laboratories. Serologic assays for HSV-1 and HSV-2 are available from many commercial laboratories. Despite claims of specificity, these assays cannot reliably differentiate between the two viral serotypes. Western blot and glycoprotein immunoassays are type-specific for HSV serology, but these tests are available only in selected research laboratories. The limited availability of reliable type-specific serologic assays makes definitive disease classification impractical for most HSV-infected patients.

Clinical Spectrum of Disease

Genital herpes infections are classified into one of three categories based on serologic antibody status (Table 26–1). First-episode *primary infection* results when an individual who lacks preexisting antibody is exposed to HSV-1 or HSV-2. Viral reactivation after the establishment of latency results in *recurrent infection*, and *first-episode, nonprimary infection* occurs when a person with preexisting antibody to one type of HSV experiences a first infection with the heterologous virus type. Patients with any one of these types of infection may be either symptomatic (prodromal symptoms and clinically evident lesions) or asymptomatic (viral shedding occurs in the absence of symptoms or clinically evident lesions).

Table 26–1. Clinical Designation of Herpes Simplex Virus Infection

Primary genital HSV: antibodies to both HSV-1 and HSV-2 are absent at the time the patient acquires genital HSV caused by HSV-1 or HSV-2

Nonprimary first-episode genital HSV: acquisition of genital HSV (due to HSV-1) with preexisting antibodies to HSV-2 or acquisition of genital HSV (due to HSV-2) with preexisting antibodies to HSV-1

Recurrent genital HSV: reactivation of genital HSV in which the HSV type recovered from the lesion is the same type as the antibody in the sera

HSV, herpes simplex virus.
From Riley LE: Herpes simplex virus. Semin Perinatol 1998;22:284–292.

Table 26–2. First-Episode and Recurrent Genital Herpes Outbreaks

	First Episode		Recurrent Symptomatic
	Primary	*Nonprimary*	
Incubation period (days)	3–6		
Viral shedding (days)	12	7	4
Lesions present (days)	20	15	9

From Corey L, Adams H, Brown A, Hommes K: Genital herpes simplex virus infections: Clinical manifestations, course, and complications. Ann Intern Med 1983; 98:958–972; and Cook CR, Gall SA: Herpes in pregnancy. Infect Dis Obstet Gynecol 1994;1:298–304.

The clinical diagnosis of genital herpes is based on recognition of a viral prodrome and subsequent development of vesicular or ulcerative lesions. Lesions typically are found on the vulva or perineum; however, they may also be found in the vagina and cervix or perianal region. The classic description of a primary infection includes multiple, bilateral genital lesions; lymphadenopathy; fever; and systemic symptoms (malaise, fatigue, lethargy). With recurrent outbreaks, systemic symptoms typically are absent, lesions are fewer in number and resolve more quickly, and viral shedding occurs for a shorter period of time. First-episode, nonprimary infections are generally less symptomatic than primary infections; the heterologous HSV antibody is believed to afford partial protection, resulting in blunting of clinical symptoms. The duration of viral shedding and of the presence of lesions varies among primary, first episode nonprimary, and recurrent infections (Table 26–2).

Clinical evaluation must be correlated with culture and type-specific serologic assay results to classify genital herpes infections correctly. In a prospective trial, Hensleigh and associates[8] found that only 1 of 23 pregnant women with clinical signs and symptoms of primary HSV actually had a primary outbreak; 18 had recurrent HSV and 4 had first-episode nonprimary infections. Thus, at least in pregnant women, usual clinical indices of infection may not be adequate to classify the infection accurately. Furthermore, based on the report by Hensleigh and associates,[8] most infections in pregnant women that clinically appear to be primary are, in fact, recurrent.

Impact of Infection during Pregnancy

Although several studies have reported that first-episode genital HSV infection acquired during pregnancy is associated with spontaneous abortion, intrauterine growth restriction, and preterm delivery,[9–11] the number of reported patients is small. A more recent study did not confirm an increased risk of spontaneous abortion.[12] Recurrent HSV infections are not associated with an increased risk of preterm labor, spontaneous pregnancy loss, or intrauterine growth restriction, and there are no reports of a herpes-associated embryopathy.

Impact of Infection on the Neonate

The most serious consequence of maternal HSV infection is that of vertical transmission of infection to the fetus or neonate. Intrapartum contact of the fetus with an infected maternal genital tract is the most common source of neonatal HSV infection, accounting for 85% of all cases. Postnatal transmission of HSV is responsible for approximately 10% of cases, and the remaining 5% of neonatal infections result from intrauterine acquisition of infection. Vertical transmission rates vary depending on the type of maternal disease. With primary infection, higher concentrations of virus are shed in the genital tract, viral excretion occurs for up to 21 days, and concomitant cervical shedding frequently (85%) occurs.[5, 13]

In contrast, lower concentrations of virus are recovered, shedding occurs for an average of only 2 to 5 days, and cervical involvement is much less common with recurrent outbreaks. If a patient has an active primary HSV outbreak at the time of vaginal delivery, the risk of neonatal transmission is 50%.[9, 14, 15] The risk for transmission is approximately 33% with asymptomatic first-episode disease.[15, 16] With exposure to a recurrent lesion, the risk of neonatal infection falls to 3% to 4%.[9, 15]

Clinical Management and Controversies

To reduce the risk of vertical transmission of infection, cesarean delivery is recommended for women who have active genital lesions or prodromal symptoms at the time of labor or membrane rupture at term. Prior to the late 1980s, weekly HSV cultures were recommended in women with a history of genital herpes in order to detect asymptomatic shedding. Cesarean delivery was performed in women who had positive HSV cultures near term or active lesions in labor. The American College of Obstetricians and Gynecologists recommended that this practice be abandoned after Arvin and colleagues[17] demonstrated that antepartum cultures did not predict which patients would have viral shedding at delivery.

Although the current management guidelines represent an improvement over previous protocols, several concerns remain. (1) Cesarean delivery is not entirely protective against neonatal transmission. In fact, approximately 20% to 30% of HSV-infected infants are born by cesarean section,[18] and 8% of neonatal infections occur despite cesarean delivery with intact membranes.[19] (2) In addition, the majority (60% to 80%) of HSV-infected infants are born to women who have neither active genital lesions nor a history of HSV infection.[18, 20, 21] (3) Lastly, the practice of cesarean delivery for women with active recurrent lesions remains controversial. The majority of women with active recurrent lesions do not have evidence of viral shedding, and the risk of neonatal transmission is low.

Randolph and coworkers[22] estimated that $2.5 million are spent and 1580 cesarean sections performed in order to prevent one case of neonatal herpes. Despite these legitimate concerns, it seems unlikely that the long-established practice of cesarean section for active recurrent genital HSV lesions will change.

Women who have recurrent distal (e.g., buttocks, thigh) lesions at the time of labor are believed to be at very low risk for neonatal transmission and may be delivered vaginally.[23] The lesions should be covered by an occlusive dressing during labor and delivery.

Preterm Premature Rupture of the Membranes

In managing a patient who has preterm premature rupture of the membranes (pPROM) and active HSV lesions, one must weigh the risks of ascending HSV infection, with potential transmission of infection to the fetus, against the risks of neonatal morbidity incurred as a result of preterm birth. No randomized data exist, but numerous case reports or series suggest that expectant management is reasonable in very preterm (<32 weeks) gestations.[23–25] In addition, the American College of Obstetricians and Gynecologists recommends that glucocorticoids be administered and that antiviral therapy be given to these women.[23] Despite this recommendation, no data currently confirm that antiviral therapy is efficacious in preventing ascending HSV infection in women with pPROM who are being expectantly managed. Clinical management must be individualized in this setting, and the patient should be informed fully of these difficult management issues.

Suppressive Antiviral Therapy

Acyclovir is an antiviral agent that has been shown to reduce both the frequency and the duration of genital HSV recurrences in nonpregnant patients. Although it has not been approved by the U.S. Food and Drug Administration for use in pregnancy, acyclovir has been used in hundreds of gravid women without apparent adverse fetal effects.[26] Suppressive acyclovir therapy during late pregnancy has been proposed as a strategy to reduce both the frequency of HSV recurrence in labor and the need for cesarean delivery. In a small, randomized prospective trial, Scott and associates[27] found that suppressive acyclovir therapy (400 mg, three times daily) reduces the need for cesarean delivery in women with first-episode HSV in pregnancy. None of the women treated with acyclovir required a cesarean section for HSV, whereas 9 of 25 patients (36%) receiving placebo did.

Another randomized trial of suppressive acyclovir therapy in women with recurrent HSV[28] demonstrated a reduction in the number of recurrences during treatment among acyclovir recipients. Although there was a trend toward a reduction in cesarean section for HSV in the acyclovir group, this was not statistically significant. The investigators concluded that there was "little evidence to suggest acyclovir should be used outside randomized controlled trials for the suppression of recurrent genital herpes infection during pregnancy."

Valacyclovir (Valtrex), a prodrug of acyclovir, is absorbed in the gastrointestinal tract more effectively and has enhanced bioavailability compared with its parent drug. A small pharmacokinetic trial was performed in pregnant women,[29] and additional clinical trials of suppressive valacyclovir therapy in pregnancy are ongoing. Additional data are needed before any definitive conclusions can be reached regarding the effectiveness of suppressive antiviral therapy in pregnancy.

The American College of Obstetricians and Gynecologists recently recommended that acyclovir be given to women during an acute primary HSV outbreak in pregnancy. Continued suppressive therapy was also recommended to be considered in these women.[23] Nevertheless, currently no objective data are available indicating a benefit to this use.

Breastfeeding and Infant Contact

Women may be allowed to breastfeed unless active lesions are present on the breast. Oropharyngeal or cutaneous lesions are potential sources for neonatal infection. Mothers who have cutaneous lesions should practice meticulous handwashing technique and avoid contact of the neonate with the lesion.

SUMMARY

Genital HSV infection continues to be a common clinical problem in the United States. The most serious sequelae of this infection in pregnant women is vertical transmission, with substantial risk of neonatal morbidity and mortality. Although devastating, neonatal HSV infection is fortunately rare despite the fact that exposure to active viral particles during the birth process is almost certainly a common event. Current guidelines for pregnancy management have changed little during the 1990s. The effectiveness of current guidelines to reduce vertical transmission remains uncertain, but clearly these guidelines are responsible for increased maternal operative morbidity and substantial financial expenditure. Additional research is of paramount importance before new clinical management recommendations can be issued.

Suggestions for Future Reading

American College of Obstetricians and Gynecologists: Management of herpes in pregnancy (Practice Bulletin No. 8). Washington, DC, ACOG, October 1999.

Cook CR, Gall SA: Herpes in pregnancy. Infect Dis Obstet Gynecol 1994;1:298–304.

References

1. Prober C, Corey L, Brown Z, et al: The management of pregnancies complicated by genital infections with herpes simplex virus. Clin Infect Dis 1992;15:1031–1038.
2. Fleming D, McQuillan G, Johnson R, et al: Herpes simplex virus type 2 in the United States, 1976 to 1994. N Engl J Med 1997;337:1105–1111.
3. Whitley R, Arvin A, Prober C: Predictors of morbidity and mortality in neonates with herpes simplex infections. N Engl J Med 1991;324:450–454.
4. Cesario T, Poland J, Wulff H, Chin T, Wennder H: Six years experiences with herpes simplex virus in a children's home. Am J Epidemiol 1969;90:416.
5. Corey L, Adams H, Brown A, Hommes K: Genital herpes simplex virus infections: Clinical manifestations, course and complications. Ann Intern Med 1983;98:958–972.
6. Moseley R, Corey L, Benjamin D, et al: Comparison of viral isolation direct immunofluorescence, and indirect immunoperoxidase techniques for detection of genital herpes simplex virus infection. J Clin Microbiol 1981;13:913–918.
7. Cone R, Hobson A, Brown Z, et al: Frequent detection of genital herpes simplex virus DNA by polymerase chain reaction among pregnant women. JAMA 1994;272:792–796.
8. Hensleigh P, Andrews W, Brown Z, et al: Genital herpes during pregnancy: Inability to distinguish primary and recurrent infections clinically. Obstet Gynecol 1997;89:891–895.
9. Nahamias A, Josey W, Naib Z, et al: Perinatal risk associated with maternal genital herpes simplex virus infection. Am J Obstet Gynecol 1971;110:825–837.
10. Brown Z, Vontver L, Benedetti J: Effects on infants of a first episode of genital herpes during pregnancy. N Engl J Med 1987;313:1246–1251.
11. Brown Z, Benedetti J, Selke S: Asymptomatic maternal shedding of herpes simplex virus at the onset of labor. Relationship to preterm labor. Obstet Gynecol 1996;87:483–488.
12. Brown Z, Selke S, Zeh J, et al: The acquisition of herpes simplex virus during pregnancy. N Engl J Med 1997;337:509–515.
13. Whitley R: Herpes simplex virus infections. In Remington JS, Klein JO (eds): Infectious Diseases of the Fetus and Newborn Infant, 3rd ed. Philadelphia, WB Saunders, 1990, pp 282–305.
14. Nahamias A, Roizman B: Infection with herpes simplex viruses 1 and 2. N Engl J Med 1973;289:781–789.
15. Brown Z, Benedetti J, Ashley R: Neonatal herpes simplex virus infections in relation to asymptomatic maternal infections at the time of labor. N Engl J Med 1991;324:1247–1252.
16. Prober C, Hensleigh P, Boucher F, et al: Use of routine viral cultures at delivery to identify neonates exposed to herpes simplex virus. N Engl J Med 1988;318:887–891.
17. Arvin A, Hensleigh P, Prober C: Failure of antepartum maternal cultures to predict the infant's risk of exposure to herpes simplex virus at delivery. N Engl J Med 1986;315:796–800.
18. Whitley R, Corey L, Arvin A, et al: Changing presentation of herpes simplex virus infection in neonates. J Infect Dis 1988;158:109–116.
19. Stone K, Brooks C, Guinan M, Alexander E: National surveillance of neonatal herpes simplex virus infections. Sex Transm Dis 1989;16:152–156.
20. Whitley R, Nahmias A, Visitine A, et al: The natural history of herpes simplex virus infection of mother and newborn. Pediatrics 1980;66:489–494.
21. Yeager A, Arvin A: Reasons for the absence of a history of recurrent genital infections in mothers of neonates infected with herpes simplex virus. Pediatrics 1984;73:188–193.
22. Randolph A, Washington E, Prober C: Cesarean delivery for women presenting with genital herpes lesions. JAMA 1993;270:77–82.
23. American College of Obstetricians and Gynecologists: Management of herpes in pregnancy (Practice Bulletin No. 8). Washington, DC, ACOG, October 1999.
24. Ray D, Evans A, Elliott J: Maternal herpes infection complicated by prolonged premature rupture of membranes. Am J Perinatol 1985;2:96–100.
25. Utley K, Bronberger P, Wagner L: Management of primary herpes in pregnancy complicated by ruptured membranes and extreme prematurity: Case report. Obstet Gynecol 1987;69:471–473.
26. Andrews E, Yankaskas B, Cordero J, et al: Acyclovir in pregnancy registry: Six years' experience. Obstet Gynecol 1992;79:7–13.
27. Scott L, Sanchez P, Jackson G, et al: Acyclovir suppression to prevent cesarean delivery after first-episode genital herpes. Obstet Gynecol 1996;87:69–73.
28. Brocklehurst P, Kinghorn G, Carney O, et al: A randomised placebo controlled trial of suppressive acyclovir in late pregnancy in women with recurrent genital herpes infection. Br J Obstet Gynaecol 1998;105:275–280.
29. Kimberlin D, Weller S, Whitley R, et al: Pharmacokinetics of oral valacyclovir and acyclovir in late pregnancy. Am J Obstet Gynecol 1998;179:846–851.

TWENTY-SEVEN

Maintenance Therapy following Successful Arrest of Preterm Labor

Debra A. Guinn and Marsha Wheeler

OVERVIEW

Approximately 9% to 10% of births in the United States occur before 37 weeks' gestation. These preterm births are responsible for 70% to 85% of all the neonatal morbidity and mortality in nonanomalous fetuses in the United States. The majority of serious complications occur in neonates born at less than 32 weeks' gestational age. These complications include respiratory distress syndrome, intraventricular hemorrhage, necrotizing enterocolitis, and sepsis. It is not surprising that at least 50% of all long-range neurologic handicaps in children are associated with extreme prematurity. It has been estimated that 5% of the entire nation's health care expenditure goes to caring for premature infants.

Currently, the only potentially preventable cause of preterm birth is idiopathic preterm labor or premature rupture of the membranes. Approximately 50% of all preterm births are caused by idiopathic preterm labor. Tocolytic agents, such as the beta-mimetics (ritodrine and terbutaline) and magnesium sulfate (MgSO$_4$), are commonly used to treat preterm labor and have been proved to delay preterm birth for 48 hours.[1] If preterm labor is arrested, the patient remains at high risk for a recurrent episode of preterm labor and preterm birth.[1] Maintenance tocolytic therapy may decrease chances for delivery in some cases. Several agents, including the beta-mimetics (ritodrine and terbutaline), MgSO$_4$, prostaglandin synthetase inhibitors, and calcium channel blockers, have been tested in randomized trials.

BETA-MIMETICS

Efficacy of Oral Tocolysis

We have been able to identify eight randomized placebo-controlled trials of oral beta-mimetic maintenance therapy to prevent recurrent preterm labor and preterm delivery. In 1980, Creasy and colleagues[2] randomized 55 patients whose preterm labor had been arrested with intramuscular ritodrine for 24 hours to receive either oral ritodrine or oral placebo. Therapy was continued until 38 weeks' gestation. The number of days gained after initiation of oral therapy was similar in both groups (oral ritodrine, 34 days, and oral placebo, 36 days). Patients who received ritodrine had significantly fewer recurrent episodes of "preterm labor"

requiring treatment. However, recurrent preterm labor was never defined and thus its use as an end point for the study is suspect.

In 1981, Brown and Tejani[3] reported on 51 patients who were randomized to oral terbutaline therapy or oral placebo after successful tocolytic therapy with ethanol. Participants were alternatively assigned to receive terbutaline or placebo. Preterm labor was defined solely as the presence of uterine contractions before 36 weeks' gestation. Patients who received terbutaline had fewer episodes of recurrent preterm labor and significantly longer time gained in utero (42.5 days vs. 29.4 days). This study's usefulness is limited by its lack of statistical power, its failure of proper randomization, and the use of a subjective definition of preterm labor.

In 1983, Smit[4] randomized 44 patients to oral ritodrine or oral placebo after successful tocolysis with intravenous ritodrine. There was no significant difference in the rates of preterm delivery between the groups. In 1991, Ricci and associates[5] randomized 75 patients who had been treated with MgSO$_4$ to one of three groups: oral ritodrine, oral magnesium, or oral placebo. No difference was found among the groups with respect to time gained in utero or the number of fetuses completing 36 weeks' gestation. In 1993, Parilla and associates[6] randomized 54 women to oral terbutaline or no therapy. Unlike the case in previous trials, preterm labor was prospectively defined as the presence of uterine contractions with progressive cervical change of at least 1 cm dilation and 1 cm of effacement. This more conservative definition of preterm labor is more likely to identify women who are really in labor who might benefit from therapy. There were no differences between groups in the mean days to delivery, or in the percent of patients who delivered at less than 34 and less than 37 weeks' gestation.

In 1995, How and coworkers[7] randomized 184 patients into four groups: (1) patients with a Bishop score of 5 or greater who received terbutaline ($n = 50$), (2) those with a Bishop score of 7 or greater who received no treatment ($n = 53$), (3) those with a Bishop score of less than 5 who received terbutaline ($n = 41$), and (4) those patients with a Bishop score of less than 5 who received no therapy ($n = 40$). Even when stratifying patients by cervical examination, the investigators did not detect any significant differences in the number of readmissions, the number of unscheduled hospital visits, and the neonatal outcomes among the four groups. Holleboom and colleagues[8] randomized 95 women to receive oral sustained-release ritodrine therapy or a similarly administered placebo. Women were treated for 1 week. There was a decrease in the number of women with recurrent preterm labor (ritodrine, 2%, vs. placebo, 24.4%, P = .06) but no difference in the rate of preterm delivery (ritodrine, 32%, vs. placebo, 28.9%, odds ratio 1.16 and 95% confidence interval, 0.48 to 2.78).

Two other larger trials were reported in 1996. Lewis and associates[9] randomized women between 24 0/7 and 34 6/7 weeks of pregnancy to receive either terbutaline (4 mg orally every 4 hours) or a similarly administered placebo until 37 weeks' gestation. No differences in the proportion of patients delivered 1 week after randomization, the median latency interval, the mean gestational age at delivery, the incidence of recurrent preterm labor, or neonatal morbidity were reported. However, they did note on post hoc analysis of the 96 women randomized at less than 32 weeks that there was a significant prolongation of pregnancy (P < .01) in the terbutaline group. Rust and coworkers[10] randomized 248 women to receive either placebo (n = 68), terbutaline (n = 72), or magnesium (n = 65). As in the previous trials, there was no difference among the groups in the length of gestation or preterm delivery rates. The terbutaline group had significantly more side effects from treatment.

A total of 915 patients was randomized in these eight trials. In six of the eight trials, there was no decrease in the preterm delivery rate or a prolongation of pregnancy with maintenance tocolytic therapy when compared with controls receiving no treatment. Seven of the eight trials reported on the number of women treated for recurrent preterm labor. Overall, for women receiving a beta-mimetic, the rate of recurrent preterm labor was 32.5% (range, 2% to 59%) and for patients receiving placebo or no therapy, 28.3% (range, 12.9% to 63%). Despite obvious differences in the trials, Sanchez-Ramos and associates[11] combined these data using meta-analysis. When the analysis was restricted to trials comparing beta-mimetics to placebo or no therapy, there was no benefit of treatment for prevention of preterm birth (odds ratio 1.08) (95% confidence interval, 0.82 to 1.43) or risk of recurrent preterm labor (0.90) (95% confidence interval, 0.63 to 1.28).

Meta-analysis is a powerful tool when used under ideal circumstances. Unfortunately, it is problematic when it is used to combine heterogeneous trials comparing different drugs and dosing regimens. In addition, there is no consistency among the trials in inclusion criteria and definitions of preterm labor and recurrent preterm labor. Nevertheless, whether the trials are evaluated individually, cumulatively as a review, or using meta-analysis, there appears to be no benefit from oral beta-mimetic tocolysis.

Several potential explanations of why oral beta-mimetic therapy appears to be ineffective are possible. Oral administration of terbutaline results in inconstant drug levels, characterized by peaks and troughs. The need to take the drug every 2 to 4 hours throughout the day, including waking at regular intervals throughout the night, may decrease compliance. Finally, long-term exposure to beta-mimetic agents results in desensitization of the beta-adrenergic receptors in the myometrium. Development of tolerance is related to both the duration of therapy and the total dose of the beta-mimetics.[12]

Efficacy of Continuous Subcutaneous Administration of Terbutaline

Researchers have developed a continuous portable subcutaneous pump (MiniMed model 404-S, Sylmar, Calif), similar to the insulin pump, for administration of terbutaline for maintenance therapy. Its theoretical advantages in oral maintenance therapy are the continuous low maintenance drug levels elicited and the ability to administer a drug bolus if uterine contractions develop, thus preventing or decreasing the development of tolerance of the β-receptors to the β-agonist terbutaline.

A number of descriptive studies of terbutaline pump therapy for prevention of preterm birth have been published in peer review journals. Results of the first series of patients undergoing terbutaline pump therapy were published by Lam and coworkers in 1988.[13] They "selected" nine patients who had persistent uterine contractions on oral terbutaline after successful parenteral tocolysis with $MgSO_4$ to receive pump therapy. During the course of hospitalization, pump dosing was adjusted according to the patient's contraction pattern. Patients were educated in management of the pump and were discharged once they demonstrated proficiency with pump therapy. In addition to the pump therapy, patients underwent home uterine activity monitoring. Patients were placed on the monitors a minimum of 8 hours per day. Patients adjusted their terbutaline dose and activity according to their contraction pattern.

The mean gestational age at initiation of therapy was 29.6 weeks, and pregnancy was prolonged an average of 9.2 ± 4.3 weeks. The minimum gestational age at delivery was 37.3 weeks. Unfortunately, it is not clear from this small series whether pump therapy, home uterine activity monitoring, or anything contributed to the prolongation of these gestations. In addition, patients treated in this series demonstrated only minimal cervical dilatation (mean, 1.2 cm) at entry. It is likely and certainly possible that these "selected" patients, despite the presence of uterine contractions, were not in preterm labor and not at risk for delivering preterm.

Next, Lam and associates[13a] published in a nonpeer review journal the results of a randomized trial of terbutaline pump therapy and oral terbutaline. Without giving any details regarding study design or execution, they reported that the terbutaline pump was more efficacious than oral terbutaline in achieving delivery after 36 weeks of gestation (93% vs. 34%). Subsequently, a number of investigators described their clinical experience with pump therapy. In

1997, Wenstrom and coworkers[14] published the first randomized, placebo-controlled trial of the terbutaline pump. These researchers assigned women in preterm labor to receive either terbutaline pump therapy ($n = 15$), placebo pump therapy ($n = 12$), or oral terbutaline ($n = 15$). If women developed recurrent preterm labor, the blind was broken and women receiving placebo were switched to terbutaline. Although conclusions were limited by the small number of patients in each group and the crossover design, no differences were reported in the mean delay to delivery or in neonatal morbidity.

In 1998, we reported our randomized double-blind trial of terbutaline pump therapy.[15] Preterm labor was defined prospectively as the presence of uterine contractions and 1 cm or greater cervical dilatation, 80% or greater effacement, and/or cervical change. All gravidas were treated with $MgSO_4$ until contractions were arrested for a minimum of 24 hours. Indomethacin was added as a second-line agent if the patient's labor was progressing on $MgSO_4$. Women with singleton gestations and intact membranes at between 22 and 33⁶/₇ weeks' gestation were eligible. Consenting women were randomized to receive terbutaline pump ($n = 24$) or placebo pump therapy ($n = 28$). Pump therapy was initiated by the research nurse using a standard protocol. The protocol was similar to the one Lam and associates[13a] recommended in their review of pump therapy.

In addition to their programmed infusion, patients were allowed to administer up to two additional boluses (either 0.25 mg terbutaline or 0.25 ml saline, depending on the treatment group) for uterine contractions. All women were educated in the signs and symptoms of preterm labor. Twenty-four-hour nursing support was available. A sample size of 48 women was required to detect a 2-week intergroup difference in mean time to delivery. At randomization, the groups were well balanced with respect to parity, prior preterm delivery, gestational age, and cervical examination. Overall, there was a 1-day difference in mean time to delivery between the groups (terbutaline, 29 days, and placebo, 28 days, $P = .78$). There were no differences in the rates of preterm delivery at less than 34 and less than 37 weeks' gestation or rates of neonatal morbidity. There were no differences in rates of recurrent preterm labor (terbutaline, 38%, and placebo, 37%, $P = .89$). A substantial number of patients discontinued therapy prematurely for various reasons.

We compared the outcomes of women who continued terbutaline pump therapy ($n = 13$) and those who continued placebo therapy ($n = 19$). There were no significant differences in any of the outcome measures. There was only a 2-day difference in mean time to delivery in the women who continued terbutaline therapy compared with the women who continued pump therapy (23 days vs. 25 days).

Despite very limited information regarding terbutaline pump therapy, its use has been widely promoted by several home health care corporations that target the majority of their services to the obstetric patient. Terbutaline pump therapy, whether used alone or in conjunction with home uterine activity monitoring programs, is extremely expensive, averaging over $200 per day, when compared with oral therapy or no therapy.[16] As its use has increased, so have reports of complications related to therapy. As a result, the U.S. Food and Drug Administration recently issued an alert regarding the potential dangers associated with terbutaline pump therapy and the lack of data supporting the efficacy of this treatment.[17] Nevertheless, its widespread use continues.

Risks Associated with Oral or Subcutaneous Beta-mimetic Therapy

Frequent unwanted effects of beta-mimetic therapy include palpitations, tremor, nausea, vomiting, headache, thirst, nervousness, and restlessness.[18] Complications of the oral beta-mimetics and the subcutaneous administration of terbutaline include sudden death,[19] pulmonary edema, cardiac arrhythmias, hepatitis, glucose intolerance, and gestational diabetes.[20] One case of neonatal myocardial necrosis in a woman receiving high doses of subcutaneous terbutaline has been reported.[21]

SUMMARY OF BETA-MIMETICS FOR MAINTENANCE THERAPY

The beta-mimetics, administered orally or via the pump, are widely used for women who have an episode of preterm labor requiring intervention. No compelling evidence from the randomized controlled trials supports the use of beta-mimetics for maintenance therapy. Given the potential risks associated with the beta-mimetics, there is no justification for their continued use as a chronically administered therapy.

However, evidence suggests that acute therapy with terbutaline reduces uterine activity. Intermittent treatment may result in symptomatic relief from annoying or painful contractions. Terbutaline may also provide emotional benefits for women at risk for preterm delivery. Many women in our experience want to feel that they are "doing something" to reduce their risk of preterm delivery. Self-administration of terbutaline gives some women a sense of control and reduces their anxiety. The efficacy and safety of this approach needs to be further evaluated.

OTHER MAINTENANCE TOCOLYTIC AGENTS

Compared with the beta-mimetics, relatively few trials exploring other options for maintenance therapy exist. $MgSO_4$ has been administered on a chronic basis intravenously and orally. Long-term magnesium exposure can result in significant maternal and neonatal osteopenia, especially when magnesium is used in conjunction with multiple doses of corticosteroids and bed rest. In the two randomized trials that compare oral magnesium with placebo, no apparent benefits were noted in time to delivery or neonatal outcomes.[5, 10]

Long-term tocolysis with the prostaglandin synthetase inhibitors is contraindicated. The fetal risk is far in excess of any potential benefits. It is possible that more selective cyclooxygenase-2 (COX-2) inhibitors will be useful for maintenance therapy. The calcium channel blockers appear to be gaining popularity for reducing recurrent preterm labor. Nifedipine has been compared with the beta-sympathomimetic agents.[22, 23] These investigations showed that calcium channel blockers and nifedipine were equivalent or superior to the beta-mimetics for prolonging pregnancy, with fewer maternal side effects. Carr and colleagues[24] published in 1999 the only randomized trial of nifedipine compared with no therapy. They randomized 74 women to receive oral nifedipine (20 mg every 4 to 6 hours) or no treatment. The groups were well balanced at randomization for potential confounders. There were no differences in the time gained from initiation of therapy until delivery in the two groups (37 days for the nifedipine group and 32 days for the no-therapy group) or in gestational age at delivery (35.4 weeks, nifepine group, and 35.3 weeks, no-therapy group). Oral nifedipine after successful tocolysis with MgSO₄ did not improve pregnancy outcome. Although this study did not report any significant complications of therapy, there has been a report of a myocardial infarction after treatment with nifedipine for maintenance tocolysis.[25]

Summary

At this time there is no evidence that any of the available maintenance tocolytic agents are effective in prolonging gestation, reducing preterm births, or improving neonatal outcome. Each of the therapies has been associated with significant complications. Therefore, we cannot recommend that any of these agents be used outside of properly designed randomized trials.

Our approach to women whose preterm labor has been successfully arrested with tocolytic agents is to observe them in the hospital for 2 to 3 days. If the patient has advanced cervical dilatation or is significantly premature, we watch them longer. During the hospitalization, we attempt to determine what the patient's normal contraction pattern is without intervening, unless there is cervical change. For example, many women contract in the evening. If a woman experiences six contractions an hour every evening without progressing into labor, she is instructed to return to the hospital if she is contracting greater than six times an hour. In addition, she is to return immediately if the character of her contractions changes or other new symptoms suggestive of preterm labor are present. In the first couple of weeks of outpatient management, it is not uncommon for us to see the women urgently in the office or the hospital on several occasions. We check the cervix, and as long as a woman is not continuing to dilate, we continue outpatient management. If the woman has progressive dilatation, she is admitted to the hospital for observation and potential re-treatment with indomethacin or MgSO₄.

This management scheme has not been formally tested. However, we believe it is reasonable, given the lack of evidence to support the efficacy or safety of drug therapy in this setting. Obviously, this strategy will not work for all patients, and some may require prolonged observation in the hospital or other interventions.

References

1. Gyetvai K, Hannah ME, Hodnett ED, Ohlsson A: Tocolytics for preterm labor: A systematic review. Obstet Gynecol 1999;94:869–877.
2. Creasy R, Golbus M, Laros R, et al: Oral ritodrine maintenance in the treatment of preterm labor. Am J Obstet Gynecol 1980;137:212–216.
3. Brown S, Tejani N: Terbutaline sulfate in the prevention of recurrence of premature labor. Obstet Gynecol 1981;57:22–25.
4. Smit D: Efficacy of Orally Administered Ritodrine after Initial Intravenous Therapy [thesis]. Limburg, Netherlands, University of Limburg, 1983.
5. Ricci J, Hariharan S, Helfgott A, et al: Oral tocolysis with magnesium chloride: A randomized controlled prospective clinical trial. Am J Obstet Gynecol 1991;165:603–610.
6. Parilla B, Dooley S, Minogue J, Socol M: The efficacy of oral terbutaline after intravenous tocolysis. Am J Obstet Gynecol 1993;169:965–969.
7. How H, Hughes S, Vogel R, et al: Oral terbutaline in the outpatient management of preterm labor. Am J Obstet Gynecol 1995;173:1518–1522.
8. Holleboom C, Merkus M, Elferen LV, Kerise M: Double-blind evaluation of ritodrine sustained release for oral maintenance of tocolysis after active preterm labour. Br J Obstet Gynaecol 1996;103:702–705.
9. Lewis R, Mercer B, Salama M, et al: Oral terbutaline after parenteral tocolysis: A randomized, double-blind, placebo-controlled trial. Am J Obstet Gynecol 1996;175:84–87.
10. Rust O, Bofill J, Arriola R, et al: The clinical efficacy of oral tocolytic therapy. Am J Obstet Gynecol 1996;175:838–842.
11. Sanchez-Ramos L, Kaunitz A, Gaudier F, Delke I: Efficacy of maintenance therapy after acute tocolysis: A meta-analysis. Am J Obstet Gynecol 1999;181:484–490.
12. Ryden G, Andersson R, Berg G: Is the relaxing effect of beta-adrenergic agonists on the human myometrium only transitory? Acta Obstet Gynecol Scand Suppl 1982;108:47–51.
13. Lam F, Gill P, Smith M, et al: Use of the subcutaneous terbutaline pump for long-term tocolysis. Obstet Gynecol 1988;72:810–813.
13a. Lam F, Elliott J, Jones S, et al: Clinical issues surrounding the use of terbutaline-sulfate for preterm labor. Obstet Gynecol Surv 1998;53(11 Suppl):S85–S95.
14. Wenstrom K, Weiner C, Merrill D, Niebyl J: A placebo-controlled randomized trial of the terbutaline pump for prevention of preterm delivery. Am J Perinatol 1997;14:87–91.
15. Guinn D, Goepfert A, Owen J, et al: Terbutaline pump maintenance therapy for prevention of preterm delivery: A double-blind trial. Am J Obstet Gynecol 1998;179:874–878.
16. Adkins R: Reply: Terbutaline pump treatment of premature labor. South Med J 1993;86:1076.
17. U.S. Food and Drug Administration: Warning on the use of terbutaline-sulfate for premature labor. JAMA 1998;297:1.
18. King JF, Grant A, Keirse MJ, Chalmers I: Beta-mimetics in preterm labour: An overview of the randomized controlled trials. Br J Obstet Gynaecol 1988;95:211–222.
19. Hudgens DR, Conradi SE: Sudden death associated with terbutaline sulfate administration. Am J Obstet Gynecol 1993;169:120–121.
20. Bessinger RE: A systematic review of adverse events documented in

the use of currently available treatment of preterm labor. Res Clin Forums 1994;16:89–126.

21. Fletcher S, Fyfe D, Case C, et al: Myocardial necrosis in a newborn after long-term supression of preterm labor. Am J Obstet Gynecol 1991;165:140–144.

22. Meyer W, Randall H, Graves W: Nifedipine versus ritodrine for suppressing preterm labor. J Reprod Med 1990;35:649–654.

23. Lockwood CJ: Calcium-channel blockers in the management of preterm labour. Lancet 1997;350:1339–1340.

24. Carr D, Clark A, Kernek K, Spinnato J: Maintenance oral nifedipine for preterm labor: A randomized clinical trial. Am J Obstet Gynecol 1999;181:822–827.

25. Oei SG, Oei SK, Brolmann HA: Myocardial infarction during nifedipine therapy for preterm labor. N Engl J Med 1999;340:154.

TWENTY-EIGHT

Trauma in Pregnancy

Jennifer Gunter

Trauma is the leading cause of death for women of reproductive age and is the most common nonobstetric cause of death in pregnancy. Trauma in pregnancy is not only a major cause of maternal morbidity and mortality but also a significant cause of adverse perinatal outcome. Because trauma complicates approximately 7% of pregnancies, it is essential that any practitioner providing health care to the gravid patient have an understanding of both the maternal and the fetal effects of trauma and of the complex management issues surrounding care of the pregnant trauma victim.[1] Maternal anatomy and physiology are altered with advancing gestational age, potentially contributing to diagnostic delays. The trauma team must also consider possible adverse fetal effects of radiologic procedures, medications, and surgery. Special attention is warranted once fetal viability is suspected, because delivery may be indicated in situations with fetal distress. These many issues are best managed by a multidisciplinary team approach, including the obstetrician, emergency medicine specialists, trauma surgeons, and other specialists as required.

EPIDEMIOLOGY

Trauma encompasses accidents, homicides, and adverse effects, such as assaults or falls. In industrialized countries, the leading cause of trauma in pregnancy is motor vehicle accidents, accounting for approximately 60% of cases. The majority of the remaining causes of trauma in pregnancy are almost evenly divided between assaults and falls.[2, 3]

According to the National Center for Health Statistics,[4] motor vehicle accidents were the eighth leading cause of death in the United States in 1997, but the leading cause of death for women ages 15 to 24 years and the second leading cause of death for women ages 25 to 44 years. The use of restraints dramatically reduces the rate of both maternal and fetal complications from motor vehicle accidents; however, pregnant women may be less likely to employ restraints than nonpregnant women. In studies of pregnant trauma victims, seat belt use ranged from 7% to 75%.[5–8] The appropriate use of seat belts should be reviewed at the first prenatal visit and reinforced throughout the pregnancy. For proper seat belt use in pregnancy, as described by Pearlman in 1997,[9] the lap belt should be placed low, beneath the uterus, and the shoulder belt should run down the midportion of the clavicle, between the breasts and beside the uterus. Although air bags have proved to be beneficial for the adult population in general, few data exist regarding air bag use and pregnancy.[9]

Domestic violence and assaults are significant causes of both adverse maternal and fetal sequelae. As reported by Gazmararian and colleagues in 1996,[10] the incidence of domestic violence may be higher in pregnancy, with rates ranging from 4% to 20%, and so the importance of screening for domestic violence in all pregnant patients cannot be overemphasized. Not only is intimate partner violence a significant cause of maternal morbidity and mortality, but also direct blows to the pregnant abdomen are common during these violent encounters. Pregnant victims of domestic violence have a greater risk of perinatal complications compared with other trauma victims.[7] Pregnant victims of intimate partner violence are also at increased risk for subsequent assaults during their pregnancy.[11] All pregnant women should be routinely screened for intimate partner abuse using the intimate partner violence screen or other appropriate tool. Women ideally should be screened at least once a trimester because the incidence of domestic violence increases with advancing gestational age.[12] Documentation of injuries and referral to appropriate services should be made available to all women who screen positive.

MATERNAL CONSIDERATIONS

Maternal outcome after a traumatic event is not altered by the pregnancy itself; however, physiologic changes of pregnancy may contribute to diagnostic delays or change the patterns of injury. Changes of pregnancy must be considered in the physical examination of the gravid trauma victim. Care must be exercised in positioning the pregnant patient for both examination and resuscitation purposes. The pregnant uterus, especially after 20 weeks' gestation, will occlude the vena cava in the dorsal position, reducing venous return and consequently decreasing cardiac output. Every effort should be made to place the pregnant trauma victim in the dorsal position, with a wedge under the right flank at all times to displace the gravid uterus from the vena cava.

The normal physiologic adaptations to pregnancy must also be considered in the evaluation of the pregnant trauma patient. The increase in resting heart rate and the decrease in both systolic and diastolic blood pressures in pregnancy may be misinterpreted as signs of impending hypovolemia. Similarly, the tachypnea of pregnancy, which increases with advancing gestational age, should not be confused with respiratory distress. Other normal adaptations of pregnancy include an increase in white blood cell count of up to 12,000 cells/mm, a dilutional anemia, and an elevation in the serum alkaline phosphatase.

The abdominal examination may be more difficult in the pregnant patient with advancing gestational age. Intra-abdominal contents will be displaced into the upper abdomen by the enlarged uterus, and peritoneal signs, such as rebound tenderness and guarding, may be more difficult to elicit during pregnancy.

The two most common causes of maternal death after trauma in pregnancy are neurologic injury and hemorrhage.[5, 8] There is no evidence to suggest that the risk of death from serious trauma is greater for the gravida; however, patterns of injury after abdominal trauma may vary in the pregnant patient as a result of the anatomic changes associated with advancing gestational age. In later gestations, the enlarging uterus may actually protect the patient from injuries caused by direct abdominal trauma, especially penetrating wounds. Not only can the uterus itself act as a shield, but it also displaces the bowel upward, out of the lower abdomen and pelvis. In advancing gestations with most of the bowel displaced cephalad, injuries to the upper abdomen may produce more extensive bowel injuries than suspected. Splenic rupture and retroperitoneal hemorrhage may also be more common after abdominal trauma in pregnancy.[1, 5, 8] Another consideration for the pregnant patient is the increased risk of bladder injury with abdominal trauma, due to the upward displacement of the bladder into the abdomen after approximately 12 weeks' gestation.

Direct uterine injury must also be considered because this may also result in catastrophic maternal and fetal consequences. Uterine blood flow approaches 600 mL/min at term; therefore, injury to the uterus can result in significant maternal blood loss in a very short time. Uterine rupture is a rare complication of trauma during pregnancy, and it is usually associated with severe concurrent maternal injuries. Although uniformly fatal for the fetus, uterine rupture is associated with a maternal mortality of less than 10%, with most maternal deaths resulting from other injuries.[5]

Fetal Considerations

Maternal trauma during pregnancy significantly increases the risk of adverse perinatal outcome. A point that cannot be overemphasized is the inability to calculate the risk of adverse fetal sequelae based on the degree of maternal injury. Although severe maternal injuries are more likely to result in fetal compromise, there is a definite risk of adverse perinatal outcome with minor trauma, which is extremely important because minor trauma occurs with greater frequency in pregnancy than severe trauma.[5, 8]

The most common cause of adverse fetal sequelae after trauma during pregnancy is abruptio placentae. Placental detachment is more common after severe trauma, complicating approximately 20% to 50% of cases of severe maternal trauma and 6% of cases of minor trauma.[5, 6, 8] Direct abdominal trauma and decelerative forces cause a shearing force that may result in placental separation, but these traumatic events also cause an increase in intra-amniotic pressure that contributes to placental shearing from the decidua.[5] Separation of the placenta interrupts fetal gas exchange, causing hypoxemia, accumulation of carbon dioxide and resulting acidosis, and even fetal death. In addition, blood is a potent uterine irritant, and uterine contractions may begin shortly after placental separation that is associated with a traumatic event.

In a prospective cohort study in 1990, Pearlman and colleagues[8] identified frequent uterine contractions (more than 8/hr) as a sensitive, but not specific, predictor of patients who are at increased risk for adverse perinatal outcome from abruptio placentae. Once the lower limits of fetal viability have been reached, cardiotocographic monitoring for a minimum of 4 hours should be used as a screening tool to identify patients at risk for placental separation.[2] Physical findings, including uterine tenderness, and ultrasound are not predictors of placental separation.

Abruptio placentae and the subsequent uterine activity place the pregnant trauma victim and the fetus at risk for premature delivery and therefore the sequelae of prematurity. Tocolysis, however, is generally not recommended in the face of suspected placental separation.[5] Trauma in pregnancy may also produce direct fetal injury, although this is a less common sequelae. Skull fractures and intracranial hemorrhages are most commonly reported.[5, 13] Fetal injury may also result from penetrating abdominal trauma and uterine rupture.

It is equally important to consider fetal sequelae that may result from diagnostic procedures and interventions. Almost all trauma patients, except perhaps those with the most minor of injuries, will require some form of radiographic imaging. At any gestational age few concerns exist with exposures of 5 rads or less.[14] In the first trimester, the threshold for developmental sequelae from radiation is approximately 15 to 20 rads; however, in the late second and the third trimester, much higher doses of radiation are required to produce adverse neurologic outcome.[15, 16] With adequate lead shielding, the radiation dose to the fetus from most procedures, with the exception of a computed tomography scan of the pelvis, is well below 5 rads. With good communication between the trauma team, the obstetrician, and the radiologist, the radiation dose to the fetus from abdominopelvic computed tomography usually can be reduced to less than 5 to 10 rads by limiting the number and thickness of slices. Diagnostic procedures that do not rely on ionizing radiation, such as ultrasound or magnetic resonance imaging, may in some instances be acceptable alternatives.

Management

The initial management of any trauma victim, including the pregnant patient, should be based on the "ABCs," as defined by the Advanced Trauma Life Support guidelines:

A: airway; B: breathing; C: circulation; D: disability or neurologic deficit; E: exposure and environmental control.[17] In assessing the pregnant trauma victim, especially patients who are hypotensive, it is essential that the uterus be reflected off the inferior vena cava in order to maintain adequate venous return. This may be accomplished with a wedge under the patient's right flank, or, if the patient is on a backboard, a wedge can be placed under the backboard. Another option is to have an individual assigned to deflect the uterus manually to the left, off the vena cava and aorta.[18]

The importance of airway protection in the pregnant patient cannot be overemphasized, because pregnancy is associated with a reduction in resting tone of the lower esophageal sphincter and a delay in gastric emptying, thus increasing the risk of pulmonary aspiration of gastric contents. Every attempt should be made to keep oxygen saturation above 90%; therefore, patients should be on continuous pulse oximetry.[18] Supplemental oxygen may be required, by either nasal cannula, mask, or endotracheal intubation. If intubation is required, either for oxygenation or for airway protection, rapid-sequence induction with cricoid pressure is recommended. Failed intubation is more common in the pregnant patient.

After airway protection and oxygenation have been secured, an assessment of the circulatory status should ensue, with appropriate fluid resuscitation. Intravenous access should be secured; patients with visible evidence of trauma should have two large-bore intravenous lines established. Crystalloid should be used as initial fluid resuscitation either lactated Ringer's solution or normal saline solution, in a 3:1 ratio to replace estimated blood loss. Estimation of maternal blood loss is often difficult in the pregnant patient. Although blood pressures are generally lower in pregnancy, the expanded maternal blood volume often delays manifestations of hypovolemia until there has been a significant amount of blood loss.

Military antishock trousers (MAST) increases systemic vascular resistance and preload and is an invaluable tool in the stabilization and transport of the hypovolemic trauma patient. Inflating the abdominal compartment could compress the uterus on the vena cava with adverse affects on preload; however, no data exist concerning its use in pregnancy. MAST may be considered for transportation of the pregnant trauma patient in extremis.[5]

Diagnostic peritoneal lavage may be performed during pregnancy, although open lavage is preferred to blind needle insertion to reduce the risk of injury to the uterus or other viscus.[2] With advancing gestational age, the incision should be made above the umbilicus to avoid the uterus. The indications for diagnostic peritoneal lavage are unchanged in pregnancy and include some of the following: signs or symptoms suggestive of intraperitoneal bleeding, altered sensorium, unexplained shock, major thoracic injuries, and multiple orthopedic injuries.[2]

Maintaining maternal blood pressure is essential not only for maternal reasons but also for fetal oxygenation. If hypovolemia ensues, blood flow to the uterine artery will be reduced and oxygen delivery to the placenta impaired. For this reason, vasopressors should be avoided, if possible, because they may reduce uterine blood flow. Volume replacement should be the first step in managing the gravid accident victim with hypovolemia. If vasopressors are required for the patient refractory to volume replacement, ephedrine or mephentermine is preferred, because each will increase both maternal and uterine blood flow.

If abruptio placentae is suspected, the following laboratory tests are indicated: blood type, crossmatch, complete blood count, international normalized ratio, partial thromboplastin time, fibrinogen, and an evaluation for products of fibrin degradation, because a placental separation may result in disseminated intravascular coagulation. Laboratory testing for fetal-maternal hemorrhage, such as the Kleihauer-Betke test, is controversial. The use of this testing has been proposed to identify the fetus at risk for the sequelae of hemorrhage and also to identify those Rh-negative women who may need more than 1 ampule (300 μg) of Rh immune globulin to prevent sensitization. Severe fetal hemorrhage with resulting anemia should be identified by fetal heart rate abnormalities, and clinical management of the pregnant trauma victim is usually decided before these results are available. Over 90% of fetal-maternal hemorrhages associated with maternal trauma are less than 30 mL; therefore administration of 1 ampule (300 μg) would be sufficient for most patients.[2] One ampule of Rh immune globulin should be administered to all D-negative pregnant trauma victims to prevent Rh sensitization, and the decision to perform a Kleihauer-Betke test should be individualized.[9]

In fetuses at or approaching viability, cardiotocographic monitoring should be initiated as soon as the maternal condition allows. A minimum of 4 hours of fetal heart rate and uterine activity monitoring is recommended.[8] Patients with less than one contraction every 10 minutes are unlikely to have abruptio placentae; however, almost 20% of women with a contraction frequency greater than one every 10 minutes will have a separation and so fetal heart rate monitoring should be extended for these patients.[2] Monitoring should also be extended past 4 hours for the following conditions: fetal heart rate abnormalities, vaginal bleeding, significant uterine tenderness, serious maternal injury, and ruptured membranes. The use of tocolytics for uterine contractions after maternal trauma is generally not recommended.[5]

Special concerns exist for the pregnant woman who suffers a cardiac arrest. To achieve maximum benefit from cardiopulmonary resuscitation, the patient should be placed in the dorsal position. To maximize cardiac return, the pregnant uterus must not compress the inferior vena cava, and so one member of the team should be assigned to push the uterus to the left during cardiopulmonary resuscitation.[5] There are few data concerning the indications for perimortem cesarean section; however, after cardiopulmonary arrest if initial resuscitation efforts are unsuccessful, cesarean delivery may improve maternal venous return and help the resuscitative effort. Although resuscitation efforts generally extend well past 30 minutes in young, healthy women, fetal survival is doubtful after 15 to 20 minutes without maternal vital signs. Cesarean section, therefore, should be considered for both maternal and fetal indications after 4 minutes of unsuccessful cardiopulmonary resuscitation.[2, 19]

Suggestions for Future Reading

American College of Obstetricians and Gynecologists: Obstetric Aspects of Trauma Management (Technical Bulletin 251). Washington, DC, ACOG, 1998.

American College of Obstetricians and Gynecologists: Domestic Violence (Technical Bulletin 257). Washington, DC, ACOG, 1999.

Pearlman MD, Tintinalli JE, Lorenz RP: Blunt trauma during pregnancy. N Engl J Med 1990;323:1609–1613.

References

1. Stone IK: Trauma in the obstetric patient. Obstet Gynecol Clin North Am 1999;26:459–467.
2. American College of Obstetricians and Gynecologists: Obstetric Aspects of Trauma Management (Technical Bulletin No. 251). Washington, DC, ACOG, 1998.
3. Connolly A, Katz VL, Bash KL, et al: Trauma and pregnancy. Am J Perinatol 1997;14:331–336.
4. National Center for Health Statistics: Deaths: Final data for 1997. Morbid Mortal Wkly Rep 1997;47:99–1120.
5. Pearlman MD, Tintinalli JE, Lorenz RP: Blunt trauma during pregnancy. N Engl J Med 1990;323:1609–1613.
6. Reis PM, Sander CM, Pearlman MD: Abruptio placentae after auto accidents: A case-control study. J Reprod Med 2000;45:6–10.
7. Goodwin TM, Breen MT: Pregnancy outcome and fetomaternal hemorrhage after noncatastrophic trauma. Am J Obstet Gynecol 1990;162:665–671.
8. Pearlman MD, Tintinalli JE, Lorenz RP: A prospective controlled study of outcome after trauma during pregnancy. Am J Obstet Gynecol 1990;162:1502–1510.
9. Pearlman MD: Motor vehicle crashes, pregnancy loss and preterm labor. Int J Gynecol Obstet 1997;57:127–132.
10. Gazmararian JA, Lazorick S, Spitz AM, et al: Prevalence of violence against pregnant women. JAMA 1996;275:1915–1920.
11. Pak LL, Reece EA, Chan L: Is adverse pregnancy outcome predictable after blunt abdominal trauma? Am J Obstet Gynecol 1998;179:1140–1144.
12. American College of Obstetricians and Gynecologists: Domestic Violence (Technical Bulletin No. 257). Washington, DC, ACOG, 1999.
13. Sherer DM, Anyaegbunam A, Onyeije R: Antepartum fetal intracranial hemorrhage, predisposing factors and prenatal sonography: A review. Am J Perinatol 1998;15:431–441.
14. American College of Obstetricians and Gynecologists: Teratology (Educational Bulletin No. 236). Washington, DC, ACOG, 1997.
15. American College of Obstetricians and Gynecologists: Guidelines for Diagnostic Imaging During Pregnancy (Committee Opinion No. 158). Washington, DC, ACOG, 1995.
16. Brent RL: The effect of embryonic and fetal exposure to x-rays, microwaves, and ultrasound: Counseling the pregnant and nonpregnant patients about these risks. Semin Oncol 1989;16:347–369.
17. American College of Surgeons Committee on Trauma: Advanced Trauma Life Support for Doctors. 1997, Chapter 1, pp 21–86.
18. American College of Surgeons Committee on Trauma: Advanced Trauma Life Support for Doctors. 1997, Chapter 11, pp 315–323.
19. Katz VL, Dotters DJ, Droegmueller W: Perimortem cesarean delivery. Obstet Gynecol 1986;68:571–576.

TWENTY-NINE

Peripartum Pulmonary Edema

Brian A. Mason

BACKGROUND

Pulmonary edema is one of the most common problems leading to severe respiratory compromise in pregnant women. Whereas it affects only about 0.05% of normal pregnancies, 3% to 5% of pregnancies with preeclampsia or preterm labor are complicated by pulmonary edema. The fact that up to 1 in 20 women with complicated pregnancies develop this condition may seem impressive; what is more remarkable is that clinical pulmonary edema is so uncommon, given a few basic realities of physiology. First is the fact that the lung is a wet organ. If the blood is removed from a human lung, 400 mg of its 500-mg weight is water, and yet the separation of the wet and dry compartments of the lung (in which 80% of its weight is water) is absolutely critical to maintaining ventilation. Furthermore, up to 80% of all pregnancies are associated with some form of clinical edema. The lung's ability to maintain wet and dry separation and to avoid clinical pulmonary edema is a credit to its tightly regulated homeostatic apparatus.

PATHOPHYSIOLOGIC BASICS

To understand pulmonary edema, it is important to have some familiarity with the forces that govern normal lung fluid homeostasis. The normal lung is in a state of constant dynamic equilibrium in which fluid filters back and forth from the wet to the dry spaces. Fluid continually leaks across the capillary membrane into the interstitial space and into the alveolus and filters back, from the alveolus and interstitial space, into the capillary. Although the fluid passes in both directions, on average a larger percentage of the fluid is within the capillary at any given time. In hemodynamic terminology, the net fluid flux is inward toward the capillary. Minor local variations in this process may cause a small amount of fluid to build up within the alveolus. In these instances, the excess fluid within the alveolus is taken up by the lymphatics, which serve as the body's back-up "sump drain."

The interplay of these factors is described by the mathematical equation known as Starling's formula ($Q = K(P_c - P_{is}) - K(COP_c - COP_{is})$; Fig. 29–1). Although daunting at first viewing, closer examination reveals its elegant simplicity. Q is the net flow (the amount and direction of fluid flux). P represents hydrostatic pressure, with P_c indicating the hydrostatic pressure outward from the capillary and P_{is} representing the hydrostatic pressure inward

toward the capillary from the interstitial space. COP represents colloid osmotic pressure: the tendency of a fluid to flow toward osmotically active substances. (COP_c is the COP within the capillary that pulls fluid toward itself, and COP_{is} is the COP within the interstitial space that pulls fluid out of the capillary.) K is the permeability constant, which reflects how easily fluid passes through the wall of a given vessel. In a normal, healthy lung, the sum of the forces pulling and pushing inward (COP_c and P_{is}) is greater than the sum of the forces pulling and pushing outward (COP_{is} and P_c). A change in one or more of these factors or in K can lead to a disruption of the normal homeostasis, a net flux of fluid out of the capillary and into the interstitial

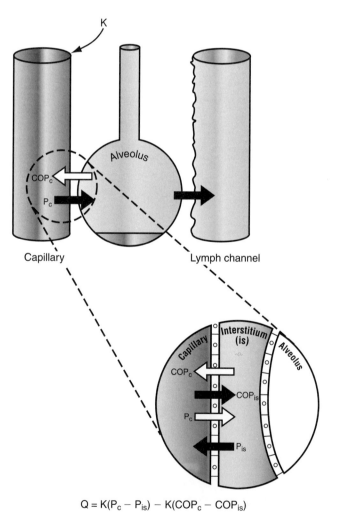

$$Q = K(P_c - P_{is}) - K(COP_c - COP_{is})$$

Figure 29–1. Starling's formula. See text for explanation.

and alveoli spaces, in a condition we clinically refer to as *pulmonary edema.*

DIAGNOSIS

Overall mortality and recovery times are greatly reduced if pulmonary edema is diagnosed early and corrected quickly. In practice, however, this may be more difficult than it might seem. The diagnosis of pulmonary edema is classically made in the acutely hypoxic patient who has audible fine crackles or rales on auscultation bilaterally (particularly in the lower lung fields), with no other apparent cause for the hypoxemia. Often, patients will display signs of tachypnea and air hunger, and a chest radiograph (Fig. 29–2) generally will reveal bilateral symmetrical fine infiltrates in the lower lung fields. Additional radiographic findings may be consistent with volume overload, including mild cardiac silhouette enlargement and cephalization of vascular markings. Unfortunately, by the time such oxygenation and chest film changes are apparent, lung fluid volume may increase up to 30%. It is, therefore, critically important that action be taken quickly once the clinical manifestations of pulmonary edema are apparent.[1]

Traditionally, pulmonary edema has been divided into two categories, cardiogenic and noncardiogenic. Unfortunately, this simple classification fails to account for important differences in various types of pulmonary edema. Accurately distinguishing between the various subtypes of pulmonary edema is important, because treatment and prognosis may be different depending on which subtypes are responsible for the patient's symptoms. Currently, a more physiologically precise classification is used to define three principal subtypes of pulmonary edema: disturbance of normal Starling's forces, lymphatic insufficiency, and increased capillary permeability (Table 29–1). The disturbance of the normal Starling force category is further divided into two subtypes: increased capillary hydrostatic pressure and osmotic derangement.

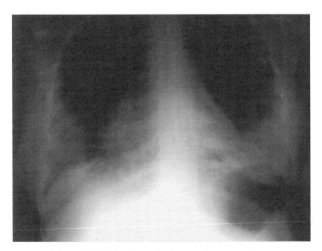

Figure 29–2. Radiograph shows pulmonary edema.

DISTURBED STARLING'S FORCES PULMONARY EDEMA

Increased Capillary Hydrostatic Pressure

This subtype of the disruption of normal Starling's forces pulmonary edema has classically been referred to as *cardiogenic pulmonary edema.* It can be due to an abnormality in the heart rate, contractility, preload, or afterload of the cardiovascular system. Underlying causes may be volume overload, heart disease, or hypertension. Hemodynamically, it is associated with an increased pressure within the pulmonary capillaries as measured by an elevated pulmonary capillary wedge pressure (PCWP). In some instances, an increase in mean arterial pressure can create sufficient afterload and increased resistance to left ventricular outflow that hydrostatic pressure builds up, back into the pulmonary vasculature, precipitating hydrostatic pulmonary edema.

Osmotic Derangement Pulmonary Edema

This subtype of disturbed Starling's forces pulmonary edema is caused by an abnormally low COP intravascularly. The reduction in this force pulling water into the intravascular space can allow a net flow of fluid out of the vessels and accumulation in the extravascular space. Any number of factors common in pregnancy may adversely affect COP: nutritional deficits, hepatic impairment, and tocolytics (particularly magnesium sulfate and beta mimetics). COP may also be affected by severe conditions, such as sepsis or preeclampsia, or seemingly benign conditions, such as intravenous (IV) hydration or the postpartum state.[2]

In addition, these effects can be additive. For example, if a patient's COP in pregnancy is 22 mm Hg, she may experience a 4 mm Hg drop immediately after delivery simply by virtue of this normal postpartum effect on COP. If she also has preeclampsia, she may experience an additional 4 mm Hg drop and may now have a COP of 14 mm Hg.[3] A continuous exposure to magnesium sulfate infusion for as little as 36 hours can cause an additional drop in COP. It is therefore easy to see how such a patient could be at extreme risk for developing disturbed Starling's forces pulmonary edema of the osmotic derangement subtype.

Lymphatic Insufficiency Pulmonary Edema

The lung has a back-up system for clearing excess fluid from the alveolus. The lymphatic system serves as this overflow drain; however, if it is occluded or damaged, fluid could build up in the alveolus with resulting pulmonary edema. This can occur even when the Starling forces are otherwise normal.[4] Lymphatic insufficiency pulmonary

Table 29–1. Potential Etiologies of Pulmonary Edema by Subtype

Hydrostatic	Osmotic Derangement	Increased Permeability	Uncertain Etiology
Congenital heart disease	Preeclampsia	Sepsis/infection	Acute fatty liver of pregnancy
Patent ductus arteriosus	Routine fluids	Chorioamnionitis/subclinical uterine infection	Pulmonary embolism
Ischemic heart disease	Magnesium sulfate tocolysis	Amniotic fluid embolism	Asthma
Beta mimetics	IV crystalloid use	Abruptio placentae	Pulmonary hypertension
Peripartum cardiomyopathy	Preload boluses for conduction anesthesia	Smoke	Hyperthyroidism
Twins/increased physiologic volume expansion	Beta mimetics (decreased COP, decreased urine output, retained sodium and water)	Beta mimetics	Steroids
Acquired valvular lesions		Appendicitis	Airway obstruction
Mitral stenosis		Pneumonia	Foreign body
Myocardial infarction		Aspiration pneumonitis	Pneumothorax
Electrolyte disturbance		Intrauterine fetal demise	Amnioinfusion
Dysrhythmias		Chemical	Pulmonary venous dysfunction
Ventricular septal defect		IV nitroglycerin for tocolysis	Edema
Mitral regurgitation		Pyelonephritis	Failed intubation/laryngospasm
Transient cardiac dysfunction		Blood transfusion reaction	Tumor
Myocarditis		Disseminated intravascular coagulation	Neurogenic
Volume overload (intravascular)		Inhalation injury	
		Inhaled drug use (especially heroin)	

COP, Colloid osmotic pressure.

edema is extremely rare in pregnancy because the factors that can precipitate it include such things as lymphatic carcinoma and silicosis, which are extraordinarily uncommon in pregnancy. It should, however, be kept in a differential diagnosis if the patient has a smoking history, environmental exposure, or crush injuries to the chest.

Increased Capillary Permeability Pulmonary Edema

A very common cause of pulmonary edema in pregnancy is increased capillary permeability. This is also referred to as the capillary leak syndrome or noncardiogenic pulmonary edema (under the older nomenclature). If the capillary leak is severe or unchecked, the interstitial space can become so overloaded with fluid and protein that there is spillover into the alveolar compartment and damage to the alveolar epithelium as well. A number of pregnancy-related factors may precipitate increased capillary permeability pulmonary edema, including tocolytics, infections, acute blood loss, aspiration, and amniotic fluid embolism.[5] Capillary leak pulmonary edema is the most ominous of the types of pulmonary edema and can be associated with the worst prognosis because, in severe instances, it may give rise to the acute respiratory distress syndrome if the precipitating event is extreme.

Treatment
General Measures

A number of initial maneuvers are performed as soon as the diagnosis of pulmonary edema is made, regardless of its underlying etiology. First, administer oxygen to the patient. Usually, a 50% Ventimask is sufficient to correct hypoxemia while minimizing any oxygen toxicity. However, this may be increased as needed in the acute setting. Next, if possible, place the patient in a seated upright position. This allows optimization of the pulmonary physiology by allowing an appropriate distribution of ventilation and perfusion. Place a pulse oximeter on the patient in order to continuously monitor the percentage of oxygen saturation. Minimize all fluid input, especially IV infusions. Most IV infusion pumps will allow a 10 to 20 mL/hr "keep vein open" rate, and this should not be exceeded for the main IV access. If other infusions are necessary in the acute setting, consider double-concentrating them to minimize the amount of fluid vehicle instilled.

Perform a quick initial survey to look for precipitating insults, such as magnesium sulfate infusions and beta mimetic therapies. Arterial blood gas should then be measured, because this will give information not only about oxygenation but also about ventilation and acid-base status. Do not hold oxygen therapy simply to obtain a "room air blood gas" measurement. Calculations such as the arterial-alveolar gradient can be made as long as the fraction of inspired oxygen (FIO_2) is defined, and there is thus no reason to subject the patient to the risk of hypoxemia while arterial blood gas data are being obtained.

Once these initial measures have been undertaken, consider forced diuresis. As an initial therapy, 20 mg of furosemide may be given as an IV injection. Most patients will demonstrate a brisk diuresis within 15 to 30 minutes of administration of the drug.

Immediate delivery of the fetus is rarely necessary in cases of acute pulmonary edema. In most instances, the fetus will stabilize as soon as the maternal oxygenation status has been improved. If pregnancy is thought to be a precipitator of the pulmonary edema, as in the case of preeclampsia, then strong consideration should be given to delivery, but only after the maternal condition has been stabilized.

Advanced Diagnosis and Treatment

Once the initial measures have been completed, a more thorough evaluation of the patient is undertaken. The detailed physical examination and history should pay special attention to preexisting conditions such as cardiac or hypertensive disease. Signs and symptoms of preeclampsia, infection, chemical exposure, seizures, murmurs, peripheral edema, or any other historical or physical clues that might illuminate the specific cause for the pulmonary edema should be carefully investigated. At the very least, a shielded chest radiograph with both posteroanterior and lateral views should be performed to confirm the radiographic features of pulmonary edema and rule out other confounding diagnoses, such as pneumonia. If an underlying cause for the edema is not immediately apparent, an echocardiogram should be ordered; this will help investigate possible systolic or diastolic dysfunction and will help quantify this dysfunction. If the patient is slow to respond to therapy and multiple arterial blood gas analyses are anticipated, an indwelling arterial catheter might be helpful. The arterial catheter also gives the added advantage of continuous, accurate real-time evaluation of mean arterial pressure, which reflects afterload.

In complicated cases of severe pulmonary edema, particularly if cardiac dysfunction is present, a pulmonary artery (Swan-Ganz) catheter can be extremely helpful if there is significant capillary leak or uncertainty over the volume status of the patient.[6] Using this device, an accurate evaluation of central volume status can be easily determined. As a result, hydrostatic pressures can be minimized without unwittingly compromising cardiac performance. It is important to note that the central venous pressure catheter is not a suitable substitute for the indwelling pulmonary artery catheter. The central venous pressure catheter is extremely prone to inaccuracy in pregnancy and pregnancy-related conditions, such as preeclampsia due to intrapulmonic shunting. At best, it gives a representation of right-sided preload to the heart, which is less useful information than the left-sided heart preload value that is given with greater precision by the PCWP obtained from the Swan-Ganz catheter. Furthermore, the Swan-Ganz catheter allows for the continuous monitoring of cardiac performance and, most importantly, oxygen delivery to the patient's tissues and fetus (Fig. 29–3).

If the PCWP obtained from the Swan-Ganz catheter is used in concert with a measurement of COP obtained from a laboratory analysis of the patient's plasma, a COP-to-PCWP difference can be determined when the value for a

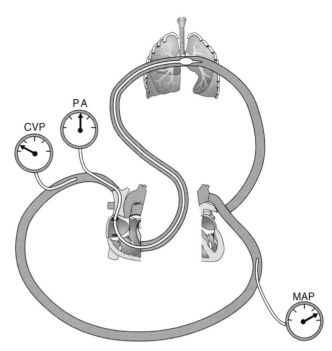

Figure 29–3. Diagram of the use of the Swan-Ganz catheter. CVP, central venous pressure; MAP, mean arterial pressure; PA, pulmonary artery.

PCWP in millimeters of mercury is subtracted from the COP in millimeters of mercury. The difference should be greater than 4 mm Hg; if it is not, then the Starling forces are such that they favor ongoing or increasing pulmonary edema.

Subtype-Specific Therapies

If the pulmonary edema appears to be principally hydrostatic in nature after careful evaluation, then preload must be reduced. This is best accomplished through aggressive diuresis, generally through the use of furosemide or other potent diuretic agents, as well as by limiting fluid intake. Attention is given to afterload reduction, especially if left ventricular dysfunction is present.[7] Afterload reduction is accomplished through blood pressure control with afterload reducing agents such as hydralazine or (if the patient is no longer pregnant) angiotensin-converting enzyme inhibitors such as enalapril.

If the clinical setting, presentation, or measurement of COP suggests that the primary lesion leading to pulmonary edema is an osmotic derangement, then a careful search for factors that reduce the COP should be undertaken and those conditions eliminated. PCWP should be lowered to an optimally low level, preferably a COP minus PCWP difference of 4 or greater. Although appealing in theory, increasing COP with exogenously administered colloids like albumin has not proved to be useful and may exacerbate the long-term recovery of patients, especially if an undiagnosed capillary leak is present. These colloids tend to extravasate into the extravascular space and pull fluid toward themselves, further exacerbating the pulmonary edema. As a result, colloid administration is almost never indicated in these patients. If evaluation reveals that capillary permeability is the most likely etiology, then an aggressive search for precipitating causes such as infection is undertaken.

Broad-spectrum antibiotic coverage is started early and later targeted to the organisms cultured. In these cases, strong consideration should be given to invasive monitoring with a pulmonary artery catheter owing to the difficulty in managing these patients and the extreme morbidity that can be associated with this condition. Because we have little direct control over the capillary permeability, Starling's forces must be made best use of to minimize further exacerbation of the pulmonary edema in these patients.

CONCLUSION

By the time physical manifestations of pulmonary edema are present, the pathophysiologic conditions leading to it are well established. Consequently, prevention is the best cure in these cases if possible. However, once the clinical symptoms are present, basic measures should be begun promptly. Then an effort is made to characterize the subtype responsible and to treat it appropriately, employing advanced techniques as needed.

Suggestions for Future Reading

1. Mabie WC, Hackman BB, Sibai BM: Pulmonary edema associated with pregnancy: Echocardiographic insights and implications for treatment. Obstet Gynecol 1993;81:227–234.
2. Yeast JD, Halberstadt C, Meyer BA, et al: The risk of pulmonary edema and colloid osmotic pressure changes during magnesium sulfate infusion. Am J Obstet Gynecol 1993;169:1566–1571.
3. Benedetti TJ, Carlson RW: Studies of colloid osmotic pressure in pregnancy-induced hypertension. Am J Obstet Gynecol 1979; 135:308–311.
4. Taylor AE: Capillary fluid filtration: Starling forces and lymph flow. Circ Res 1981;49:557–575.
5. Le Jemtel TH, Demopoulos L, Tavel ME: A problem of pulmonary edema developing postpartum. Chest 1995;108:1478–1479.
6. Keefer JR, Strauss RG, Civetta JM, et al: Non-cardiogenic pulmonary edema and invasive cardiovascular monitoring. Obstet Gynecol 1981;58:46–51.
7. Sibai BM, Mabie WC, Harvey CJ, et al: Pulmonary edema in severe preeclampsia-eclampsia: Analysis of 37 consecutive cases. Am J Obstet Gynecol 1987;156:1174–1179.
8. Jones MM, Longmire S, Cotton DB, et al: Influence of crystalloid versus colloid infusion on peripartum colloid osmotic pressure changes. Obstet Gynecol 1986;68:659–661.

Medication Use during Pregnancy

John T. Repke

Since antiquity, pregnant women have been advised to avoid certain foods and medications during pregnancy lest harm come to the fetus. Early admonitions to avoid alcohol use date back to biblical times. Indeed, although the in utero environment is privileged, it is not immune to exposure from exogenous substances. The interest in medication use in pregnancy stems from several sources of concern. The overriding concern is the potential effects of medication on the developing fetus, so-called teratogenesis. Beyond classic teratogenesis, mutagenesis is also a concern, as is the medical legal risk of medication exposure during pregnancy, from the physician's perspective.

TERATOGENESIS

A *teratogen* is defined as a drug or other agent that causes abnormal development. The word derives from the Greek words *teras,* meaning monster, and *genesis,* meaning origin. *Teratogenesis* has been defined as the origin or mode of production of a monster or a disturbed growth process involved in the production of a monster. Whereas this may be a rare effect of a drug during pregnancy, certainly examples exist of severe developmental abnormalities that have been caused by in utero exposure to medications.

Teratogenesis can be classified as morphologic, which would be classic teratogenesis, functional teratogenesis, and even behavioral teratogenesis. In the human being, the classic teratogenic period is from approximately day 17 to

day 54 postconception. The clinician should remember, in counseling a patient, that only 2% to 3% of teratogenic events can be explained by drug exposure, with approximately 70% of teratogenesis causes being unknown. The remaining cases may be part of genetic syndromes or other exposures. Teratogenic effects may depend on the total dose of medication to which the fetus is exposed, the timing or duration of the exposure, host susceptibility, and interactions between the environment and genetically predisposed individuals.

DRUG CLASSIFICATIONS

In an effort to better understand risk, the U.S. Food and Drug Administration (FDA) had incorporated a categorization of medications to guide the use of such medications in pregnancy (Table 30–1). More recently, however, it has been recognized that this classification system is not very functional. With the release of hundreds of new medications each year, it is impossible for adequate studies in pregnancy to be accomplished to ensure their safe use in the pregnant patient. Therefore, more recent opinion has favored elimination of this classification system, since most new drugs end up in category C anyway, substituting a system of reporting of malformations with specific agents or classes of agents as they occur, provided that preliminary testing or precedence suggests a reasonable probability of their being safely used. In general, older drugs with an established record of safety can be used for most disorders

Table 29–1. U.S. Food and Drug Administration*

Category A	Category B	Category C	Category D	Category X
L-Thyroxine	Hydrochlorothiazide	Theophylline Nifedipine	Cytoxan	Aminopterin Oral Contraceptives
Essentially safe, based on controlled studies in pregnancy	Safe in animals, or, if adverse effect demonstrated, not confirmed in human studies Controlled studies in women either are not available or do not confirm adverse effects	Animal studies reveal adverse effects on the fetus (embryocidal, teratogenic, other), no controlled studies in women, or Studies in women and animals not available Use only if potential benefit justifies risk to fetus	Positive evidence of human fetal risk Benefits may be acceptable despite risk Drug may be necessary in life-threatening situations	Contraindicated in women who are or may become pregnant

*Drugs listed are examples of each category.

Table 30–2. Selected Drugs in Pregnancy

I. Drugs with Human Teratogenic Potential

Thalidomide
Isotretinoin
Warfarin (Coumadin)
Methotrexate
Aminopterin
Phenytoin
Carbamazepine
Valproic acid
Lithium
Angiotensin-converting enzyme inhibitors
Angiotensin receptor blockers*
Alcohol

II. Other Drugs to Avoid during Pregnancy

Drug	Comment
Methimazole	Aplasia cutis, fetal goiter; propylthiouracil preferred agent
Tetracycline	Bone and tooth enamel effects if used in latter two trimesters
Aminoglycosides	High levels may affect fetal vestibular and auditory systems
Quinolone antibiotics	Skeletal abnormalities in rats; should be used only if no alternative
Immunosuppressives	Fetal toxicities similar to maternal

III. Drugs without Conclusive Adverse Effects

Acetaminophen
Penicillin derivatives
Cephalosporins
Macrolides (erythromycin)
Metronidazole
Hydrochlorothiazide
Calcium channel blockers
Beta-blockers
Acyclovir
Zidovudine (AZT)

of pregnancy, and newer medications should be avoided except when benefit clearly outweighs risk. A summary of the potential fetal effects of selected drugs is presented in Table 30–2.

PRECONCEPTION COUNSELING

As obstetricians, perhaps the most important function we can serve is to provide for adequate preconception counseling of patients who are at risk for particular disorders or whose medical disorders require continued medication use during the conception and periconception periods. Such preconception counseling allows for a truly informed patient to undertake pregnancy knowing what the risks to her unborn child will be from her underlying illness or the medication that she is required to take. Of course, other preconception issues may also be addressed at this time.

Folic Acid

One of the best examples of preconception counseling is preconception intake of folate, or folic acid. Folate, a necessary component for proper hematopoiesis, when

deficient, has been demonstrated to be associated with an increased risk of neural tube defects. Although the recommended daily intake of folate is 0.4 mg/day, populations at high risk for having a child with a neural tube defect—specifically, those individuals who have had a previous affected infant or who have a first-degree relative with a neural tube defect—have been recommended to increase their folic acid intake to 4.0 mg/day[1] starting at least 30 days before conception and continuing at least until complete closure of the neural tube at approximately day 24 postconception. This strategy has been estimated to result in a 72% reduction in the occurrence of neural tube defects in these high-risk populations.

Other Vitamins and Nutrients

Most prenatal care providers would suggest proper nutrition with vitamin supplementation when needed, yet it is essential that patients recognize that more is not necessarily better. Two specific examples relative to vitamins: vitamin B_6 (pyridoxine) has been demonstrated to be safe for use in pregnancy and may also be an effective antiemetic,[2] but, despite being a water-soluble vitamin, it may cause signs of neurotoxicity at doses exceeding 200 mg/day.[3] Additionally, vitamin A, an essential vitamin (recommended daily allowance, 800 μg/day) may be teratogenic at doses exceeding 8000 μg/day.[4] Reported anomalies have been primarily cranial-facial, although liver toxicity may also occur.

With the increase in popularity of complementary alternative medicine, it is essential that providers of prenatal care caution their patients about using over-the-counter preparations. Many of these preparations are safe, but quality control issues, specifically relating to the actual dose delivered by any given tablet or quantity of liquid, do raise concerns with respect to potential fetal toxicity. Information about specific alternative medicine remedies should be sought from either a qualified health care provider or a pharmacist, or through contacting the FDA.[5]

THERAPEUTIC MEDICATIONS

As the subspecialties of perinatology and neonatology have advanced, many more patients with medical illnesses are now able to become pregnant and carry their pregnancy successfully to viability. This success has resulted in an increased cohort of pregnant women who require that medications be continued throughout normal pregnancy. Some of the more common medications used during pregnancy, as well as their potential risks, are reviewed here.

Anticoagulants

Patients requiring anticoagulation therapy include those with histories of thromboembolic disease or who are at high risk for thromboembolic disease, such as those carrying the factor 5 Leiden mutation.

Heparin, a parenterally administered anticoagulant, has a high molecular weight and charge, and, therefore, does not cross the placenta and is not teratogenic. No fetal risks are directly attributable to heparin use, although maternal risks, especially with prolonged use, include osteopenia or osteoporosis. Heparin is also safe for use during lactation.

Warfarin (Coumadin), however, is teratogenic. The warfarin embryopathy was first reported in 1966.[6] It is a constellation of abnormalities that includes nasal hypoplasia, optic atrophy, scoliosis, epiphyseal stippling, mental retardation, and microcephaly. In general, for the warfarin embryopathy to occur, exposure must have taken place before the seventh week of gestation. For this reason, some practitioners, most notably those in Europe, have utilized heparin in the first trimester of pregnancy and converted these patients to the orally efficacious agent warfarin for use in the second and third trimesters, then reconverted these patients back to heparin as term approached so as to minimize the anticoagulation effects of the transplacentally passed drug warfarin on the fetus. This technique has not achieved great popularity in the United States.

Anticonvulsants

Epilepsy is one of the more common medical complications of pregnancy.[7] Nearly 40 years ago, data from the Collaborative Perinatal Project suggested that epilepsy itself was associated with an increased risk of congenital anomalies, whether treated or untreated. Phenytoin (Dilantin) is among the more widely prescribed anticonvulsant medications. A fetal hydantoin syndrome has been described, consisting of microcephaly, mental retardation, small-for-gestational-age, developmental delays, cranial-facial dysmorphism, and nail and distal phalangeal hypoplasia. It has been estimated that this syndrome will occur in approximately 5% to 10% of exposed fetuses. It has been suggested that there may be a fetal genetic predisposition to this syndrome, possibly the result of a single gene recessive allele with a resultant deficiency in epoxide hydrolase, an enzyme necessary for inactivation of one of the reactive intermediates of phenytoin.[8]

Because of these findings with phenytoin, it was hoped that an alternative anticonvulsant could be found without the associated risks. Unfortunately, although initial studies on carbamazepine (Tegretol) were promising, with increasing experience it was noted that a syndrome similar to the fetal hydantoin syndrome also occurred with carbamazepine.[8] In addition, a slightly increased risk of neural tube defect was associated with the use of this drug. Another anticonvulsant agent, valproic acid, is also associated with an approximate risk of neural tube defect approaching 1%.

With respect to epilepsy, with or without treatment epilepsy is associated with an increased rate of fetal anomalies. Ideally, women contemplating pregnancy should be seen preconceptionally, and, if they have been seizure-free for greater than 2 years, an attempt should be made to withdraw their anticonvulsant medication before conception. All anticonvulsant medications potentially can cause some degree of bone marrow suppression, and the practitioner should be aware of this. The benefit of third trimester administration of vitamin K to patients receiving anticonvulsant medications has not been conclusively established.

Thyroid Medications

Thyroid disorders may complicate up to 2.5% of all pregnancies.[9] It is known that thyroid hormone is essential for proper fetal development. Management of hypothyroidism is generally accomplished with the administration of L-thyroxine. L-Thyroxine is a category A drug and is extremely safe for use in pregnancy. Hyperthyroidism is managed with the administration of antithyroid medications, the most common of which is propylthiouracil. Propylthiouracil is preferable over methimazole because the latter drug has been associated with certain dermatologic abnormalities. Excessive administration of antithyroid medications can result in an increased risk of fetal goiter, congenital hypothyroidism, and mental retardation. The requirements for antithyroid medications decrease throughout pregnancy, and frequently these medications may be discontinued entirely in the third trimester. A general principle is to minimize fetal exposure to propylthiouracil by using the lowest dose necessary to maintain free thyroxine (T_4) levels in the upper range of normal.

Cardiovascular Medications

The most commonly used cardiovascular medications in pregnancy are the antihypertensives. Alpha-methyldopa is used most in pregnancy, in large part because of its safety record and classification as a category B drug. Other medications, such as the calcium channel blockers and β-blockers, are perhaps more effective but have been relegated to second-line agents because of their designation as category C drugs. Any of these drugs are suitable for use in pregnancy once a proper diagnosis of hypertension has been established. Angiotensin-converting enzyme inhibitors and angiotensin receptor blockers are the exception, however, and should not be used during pregnancy, particularly in the second or third trimester, because they have been associated with certain congenital anomalies and neonatal renal failure.[10]

Antibiotics

Almost all antibiotics are safe for use in pregnancy. A recommendation to proceed with caution when using sulfa drugs in the third trimester persists, although the likelihood of clinically significant neonatal hyperbilirubinemia secondary to proper use of maternally administered sulfa drugs in the third trimester is extremely small. Quinolone antibiotics should be avoided during pregnancy. As stated earlier, older, more established antibiotics are preferred over newer, less established drugs for the treatment of minor bacterial infections during pregnancy. Metronidazole, a treatment for trichomoniasis as well as bacterial vaginosis, may be used safely during pregnancy regardless of trimester.

Antineoplastics/Immunosuppressants

These agents will not be commonly used during pregnancy; when they are, most likely it will be in the setting of a pregnancy complicated by lupus or neoplastic disease. In general, the decision to use these drugs is based on the estimated risk versus the estimated benefits. Utilization of these medications during pregnancy should be undertaken only after careful consultation with a maternal-fetal medicine specialist.

Nonprescription Drugs

Prescription medications may represent a potential risk to the developing fetus, but a greater risk is probably the injudicious use of readily available nonprescription or so-called over-the-counter preparations.

Analgesics

The use of nonsteroidal anti-inflammatory drugs (NSAIDs) such as aspirin has long been discouraged during pregnancy. NSAIDs have not been demonstrated to be teratogenic, although, in general, they nonreversibly bind platelets, which may increase bleeding tendencies. Since the early 1990s, an increased use of low-dose (80 mg) aspirin for the management or prevention of certain medical conditions has changed this previous pattern of avoidance. Alternative analgesic medications are available, and the most commonly recommended is acetaminophen, which also has been demonstrated to be nonteratogenic. NSAIDs should be avoided, especially during the third trimester, unless specifically recommended, because they cause oligohydramnios and premature closure of the fetal ductus arteriosus. Again, older, more established medications are preferable over newly released drugs with a less established safety record.

Antihistamines

Most antihistamines are safe for use in pregnancy. Chlorpheniramine, diphenhydramine, and meclizine are all safe. Some of the newer antihistamines, such as astemizole (Hismanal) and loratadine (Claritin), have a less well-established record for safe use in pregnancy. Although no adverse effects have been reported, they offer no clear advantage over some of the more established older medications.

RECREATIONAL MEDICATIONS

The four most commonly used "recreational" medications are alcohol, caffeine, marijuana, and cocaine. Nicotine is not discussed.

Alcohol

It has long been known that alcohol use, especially when heavy, may result in adverse fetal effects. In fact, the potential for adverse fetal effects has led to the conclusion that no absolute safe level of alcohol consumption in pregnancy has been established.[11, 12] The major concern of excessive alcohol use during pregnancy is fetal alcohol syndrome. This syndrome requires one characteristic from each of the following categories: growth restriction (pre- or postnatal), facial anomalies, and central nervous system dysfunction. It is unclear whether other confounders associated with alcohol use or certain nutritional deficiencies may alter the risk of developing the complete fetal alcohol syndrome.

Marijuana

Marijuana has not been established to be a teratogen. Its use in pregnancy may be a marker for other substance use, including alcohol and tobacco. Carbon monoxide exposure after smoking marijuana is similar to that seen after smoking tobacco. Some studies have reported a slightly increased risk of preterm delivery and small-for-gestational-age infants among marijuana users, although it is recognized that other confounding variables may exist that could account for these findings.

Cocaine

Cocaine use during pregnancy has been associated with lack of prenatal care and may be a marker for polysubstance abuse. Congenital anomalies have been reported after cocaine use and are thought to be possibly secondary to intense vasoconstriction and thrombosis. Fatal cardiac arrhythmias, abruptio placentae, hypertension, and seizures have all been associated with cocaine use. Reported anomalies in the fetus include limb reduction defects, necrotizing enterocolitis, and porencephalic cysts. In addition, long-term behavioral effects on the child have been reported after cocaine exposure in utero, including but not limited to attention deficit disorders.

Caffeine

Caffeine is not teratogenic. As a mild stimulant, it has not been found to have adverse effects on pregnancy up to a level of 300 mg/day. Excessive caffeine was thought to have an impact on such things as gestational age at delivery and fetal weight, but these studies were confounded by tobacco use, alcohol use, and weight gain during pregnancy. The FDA's recommendation with respect to caffeine is that it may be used safely during pregnancy in moderation.

ANTIVIRAL THERAPY

In the era of retroviral illness, antiviral therapy has become more commonplace during pregnancy. Initially, in response to the herpes epidemic of the 1970s and early 1980s, practitioners began using medications like acyclovir to reduce the number of herpes outbreaks and the need for cesarean section at term. Acyclovir, although listed as a category C medication, has no reported apparent teratogenicity associated with it. Its use should be in situations when recurrent outbreaks are incapacitating or should be avoided for other reasons.

Antiretroviral therapy such as zidovudine (AZT) has been effective in reducing the vertical transmission of HIV.[13] In addition, multiagent antiretroviral therapy most recently has been associated with reducing viral load and potentially further reducing the risk of vertical transmission. Although the long-term effects of certain substances like protease inhibitors remain unknown, nearly a decade of use of AZT suggests that it may be safely used in pregnancy and that the benefits of its use in the setting of HIV disease outweighs the risks.

SUMMARY

Medication use in pregnancy creates a challenge for the health care provider as well as the patient. Judging benefits and risks can be objective but in many instances is largely subjective. Excellent communication between health care providers and recipients is essential to optimize pregnancy outcome under these circumstances. More importantly, the contribution of effective preconception counseling to improving pregnancy outcome cannot be overstated.

Suggestions for Future Reading

Briggs GG, Freeman RK, Yaffe SJ (eds): Drugs in Pregnancy and Lactation. Baltimore, Williams & Wilkins, 1990.
Gazaway PJ, Niebyl JR, Repke JT, et al: Antibiotics, analgesics, arthritis drugs in pregnancy. Patient Care 1993;27:71–82.
Gazaway PJ, Niebyl JR, Repke JT, et al: Drugs in pregnancy: Epilepsy, cancer and more. Patient Care 1993;27:79–89.
Gazaway PJ, Niebyl JR, Repke JT, et al: Cardiac and respiratory drugs in pregnancy. Patient Care 1993;27:53–66.
Koren G, Pastuszak A, Ito S: Drugs in pregnancy. N Engl J Med 1998;338:1128–1137.
Niebyl JR (ed): Drug Use in Pregnancy, 2nd ed. Philadelphia, Lea & Febiger, 1988.

References

1. Rothenberg SP: Increasing the dietary intake of folate: Pros and cons. Semin Hematol 1999;36:65–74.
2. Sahakian V, Rouse D, Sipes S, et al: Vitamin B_6 is effective therapy for nausea and vomiting of pregnancy: A randomized, double-blind placebo-controlled study. Obstet Gynecol 1991;78:33–36.
3. Bender DA: Non-nutritional uses of vitamin B_6. Br J Nutr 1999;81:7–20.
4. Wiegand UW, Hartmann S, Hummler H: Safety of vitamin A: Recent results. Int J Vitam Nutr Res 1998;68:411–416.
5. Houston RF, Valentine WA: Complementary and alternative therapies in perinatal populations: A selected review of the current literature. J Perinat Neonatal Nurs 1998;12(3):1–15.
6. Ginsberg JS, Hirsh J: Use of antithrombotic agents during pregnancy. Chest 1998;114(5 Suppl):524S–530S.
7. Crawford P, Lee P: Gender difference in management of epilepsy—what women are hearing. Seizure 1999;8:135–139.
8. Gelineau van Waes J, Bennett GD, Finnell RH: Phenytoin-induced alterations in craniofacial gene expression. Teratology 1999;59:23–34.
9. Utiger RD: Maternal hypothyroidism and fetal development. N Engl J Med 1999;341:601–602.
10. Kumar D, Moss G, Primhak R, Coombs R: Congenital renal tubular dysplasia and skull ossification defects similar to teratogenic effects of angiotensin-converting enzyme (ACE) inhibitors. J Med Genet 1997;34:541–545.
11. Bagheri MM, Burd L, Martsolf JT, Klug MG: Fetal alcohol syndrome: Maternal and neonatal characteristics. J Perinat Med 1998;26:263–269.
12. Hankin JR, Sokol RJ: Identification and care of problems associated with alcohol ingestion in pregnancy. Semin Perinatol 1995;19:286–292.
13. Hanson IC, Antonelli TA, Sperling RS, et al: Lack of tumors in infants with perinatal HIV-1 exposure and fetal neonatal exposure to zidovudine. J Acquir Immune Defic Syndr Hum Retrovirol 1999;20:463–467.

THIRTY-ONE

Anticoagulation

Renee A. Bobrowski and

Jeffery S. Dzieczkowski

Obstetricians encounter patients requiring anticoagulation for a variety of reasons: acute thromboembolism, prior thrombosis, antiphospholipid antibody syndrome, or mechanical heart valve. The goals of anticoagulation include prevention or treatment of deep vein thrombosis (DVT), pulmonary embolism (PE), postphlebitic syndrome, and systemic emboli in patients with a mechanical heart valve. This chapter addresses practical aspects of anticoagulation in the pregnant patient.

INDICATIONS FOR ANTICOAGULATION DURING PREGNANCY

Thromboembolism in the Current Pregnancy

Several diagnostic algorithms are available for evaluation of suspected DVT or PE. Imaging studies may be performed before anticoagulation in a patient with symptoms of DVT. A pulmonary embolus, however, is life threatening. Anticoagulation should be started immediately when PE is suspected, unless the patient is at high risk for bleeding. Anticoagulation can then be discontinued once PE is excluded.

Therapeutic anticoagulation within the first 24 hours after diagnosis is important to decrease recurrence risk. Three dosing regimens for intravenous (IV) unfractionated heparin (UFH) have been recommended for nonpregnant patients. They are commonly employed but have not been rigorously tested in pregnant patients. The first regimen is a weight-based nomogram. An IV bolus of 80 U/kg is administered followed by 18 U/kg/hr continuous IV infusion. Adjustments in hourly dose are based on the activated partial thromboplastin time (APTT) result and patient weight (Table 31–1). The second option is a 5000 U IV bolus followed by 30,720 U/day (1280 U/hr). Finally, 40,000 U/day (1667 U/hr) or 30,000 U/day (1250 U/hr) can be empirically administered to patients without and with risks for bleeding, respectively. IV therapy using UFH is recommended for the initial 5 to 10 days after the diagnosis of DVT or PE.

Low-molecular-weight heparin (LMWH) is increasingly being used as an alternative to UFH. Several manufacturers produce LMWH, and the dosage varies with the preparation. Enoxaparin (Lovenox) is the most commonly used preparation. The therapeutic dosage is 1 mg/kg subcutaneously (SQ) twice daily.

Long-term heparin therapy during pregnancy is possible by SQ injection. Once the dosage of IV UFH necessary to achieve therapeutic APTTs is stable, the total units of IV heparin required in 24 hours are divided into SQ twice-daily (bid) dosing. Alternatively, 250 U/kg SQ bid can be used to calculate the initial dose. The heparin dose is thereafter adjusted to maintain a therapeutic 6-hour postinjection APTT or heparin level. Twice-daily injections can be problematic for some patients because the APTT may be subtherapeutic for many hours. The frequency of administration (i.e., bid or three times daily [tid]) must therefore be individualized. Long-term therapy with enoxaparin is continued at 1 mg/kg SQ bid. Monitoring LMWH therapy is unnecessary in nonpregnant patients but should be strongly considered during pregnancy to ensure adequate dosage. Monitoring guidelines have not been established, but a heparin level measured every 4 to 6 weeks in a stable patient is reasonable.

Several issues must be considered when an anticoagulated patient enters labor. Prophylactic UFH may be continued during labor or withheld until 4 to 6 hours after delivery. Therapeutic UFH can be continued during labor and stopped 4 hours before anticipated delivery. A continuous IV infusion offers better control over the SQ route. Full-dose UFH is resumed after delivery for patients requiring continued therapeutic anticoagulation. A waiting period of 4 to 6 hours after vaginal delivery or 6 to 12 hours after cesarean section is recommended. Patients requiring therapeutic anticoagulation may also be changed to prophylactic UFH during labor. Patients taking prophylactic or therapeutic LMWH present an intrapartum management dilemma. The risk of epidural hematoma appears increased when regional anesthesia is administered to patients receiving LMWH. One option is to discontinue LMWH at 36 to 37 weeks' gestation and substitute UFH for the remainder of the pregnancy. Alternatively, LMWH may be administered during labor, but spinal or epidural anesthesia is not an option.

Women experiencing DVT or PE during pregnancy require therapeutic anticoagulation for the duration of the pregnancy and 6 weeks postpartum. At least 3 months of treatment is required. A woman suffering a thrombotic event 12 or more weeks before delivery, for example, requires therapeutic anticoagulation for the remainder of the pregnancy and 6 weeks postpartum. If the event occurs less than 12 weeks before delivery, the duration of postpartum anticoagulation will exceed the usual 6-week period to complete 3 months of therapy. A recent study[1] suggested

Table 31–1. Body Weight–Based Dosing of Intravenous Heparin

Loading Dose: 80 IU/kg Maintenance Dose: 18 IU/kg/hr APPTs	Dose Change (U/kg/hr)	Additional Action	Next APTT (hr)
<35 (1.2 × mean normal)	+4	Rebolus with 80 IU/kg	6
35–45 (1.2–1.5 × mean normal)	+2	Rebolus with 40 IU/kg	6
46–70 (1.5–2.3 × mean normal)	0	0	6*
71–90 (2.3–3.0 × mean normal)	−2	0	6
>90 (>3 × mean normal)	−3	Stop infusion 1 hr	6

Heparin, 25,000 IU in 250 μL D₅W. Infuse at rate dictated by body weight through an infusion apparatus calibrated for flow rates. The therapeutic range in seconds should correspond to a plasma heparin level of 0.2–0.4 IU/mL by protamine sulfate, or 0.3–0.6 IU/mL by amidolytic assay. When APTT is checked at 6 hr or longer, steady-rate kinetics can be assumed.

*During the first 24 hr, repeat APTT every 6 hr. Thereafter, monitor APTT once every morning unless it is outside the therapeutic range.

APTT, activated partial thromboplastin time.

Modified from Hyers TM, Agnelli G, Hull RD, et al: Antithrombotic therapy for venous thrombotic disease. Chest 1998;114(5 Suppl):561S–578S.

that more than 3 months' treatment may be necessary to prevent recurrence, but the optimal time period has not been determined. However, patients with recurrent thrombosis or a predisposition to thrombosis (i.e., antiphospholipid antibodies [APLAs], homozygous factor V Leiden mutation, deficiency of antithrombin, protein C or S, malignancy) require indefinite anticoagulation. Postpartum treatment options include subcutaneous UFH or LMWH, or warfarin. Warfarin is compatible with breastfeeding because the metabolite excreted into breast milk is not an anticoagulant.

Thrombolytic agents and vena caval interruption are adjunctive treatments. Thrombolytics have been administered to the rare pregnant patient suffering a life-threatening PE. Inferior vena caval interruption is considered when a patient has contraindications to or complications of anticoagulation, or recurrent pulmonary emboli despite adequate anticoagulation.

History of Thromboembolism before Pregnancy

Ideally, women with a prior thrombotic event have been evaluated for a hypercoagulable state before their next pregnancy. However, laboratory studies should not be performed during the acute thrombosis because some anticoagulant protein levels are altered. Candidates for evaluation include those with (1) a prior DVT or PE during pregnancy; (2) a family history of thrombotic events or known thrombophilia, (3) a thrombotic event in a nonpregnant patient younger than 45 years, and (4) a thrombus in an atypical site. Testing should include (1) activated protein C resistance (APCR)/factor V Leiden assay, (2) protein C activity, (3) protein S activity, (4) antithrombin activity, (5) APLAs, (6) prothrombin gene mutation, and (7) lupus anticoagulant. Several additional inherited procoagulant states are known, but their incidence and prevalence are yet to be determined. The APCR assay, protein C and antithrombin activity, APLAs, and lupus anticoagulant should not be

altered by normal pregnancy and can be obtained for women without a prior evaluation.

Pregnant women with a history of thrombosis but a negative thrombophilia evaluation should be treated with prophylactic heparin. The dosage of UFH has traditionally been 5000 U SQ bid. However, this regimen may not provide adequate prophylaxis as gestation advances. Second and third trimester dosages of 7500 U SQ bid and 10,000 U SQ bid or higher may be required. The dosage of prophylactic UFH is best adjusted to maintain a heparin level (also known as anti-Xa activity) of 0.1 to 0.2 U/mL. When enoxaparin is administered for prophylaxis, 30 mg bid is recommended. Women who have not undergone a thrombophilia evaluation are managed as detailed earlier. A family history of thromboembolic events or known thrombophilia should be considered when a treatment regimen is developed.

Women with a thrombophilia who have had a thrombosis are frequently committed to lifelong warfarin anticoagulation. They require continued therapeutic anticoagulation during pregnancy. The majority of these women are anticoagulated with warfarin when not pregnant. Women who seek preconception care can be converted from warfarin to heparin anticoagulation as detailed in the section on warfarin therapy.

Thrombophilia Carrier

Asymptomatic thrombophilia carriers are typically discovered after a family member suffers a thrombotic event and is diagnosed with a clotting disorder. The asymptomatic carrier is at increased risk for thrombosis, particularly during pregnancy and surgery. The lifetime incidence of a thrombotic event in a carrier varies with the coagulant protein mutation. Heterozygous and homozygous factor V Leiden carriers have a 10- and a 100-fold higher risk, respectively, whereas antithrombin-deficient patients have a 50-fold higher risk of thrombosis than the general population. The frequency of DVT during pregnancy in a small group of untreated women with the factor V Leiden mutation (13 heterozygotes, 1 homozygote) was 28% (see Chapter 12, Recently Described Hereditary Thrombophilias and Obstetric Outcome).

Antiphospholipid Antibody Syndrome

APLAs are associated with an increased risk for thrombosis, preeclampsia, intrauterine growth restriction, and fetal loss. Women with APLAs and no history of thrombosis or pregnancy loss may be managed with close clinical surveillance for DVT or heparin prophylaxis throughout pregnancy and the postpartum period. Women with APLAs and a prior thrombosis require therapeutic UFH or LMWH for the duration of pregnancy and postpartum. These women require indefinite anticoagulation and can be converted to warfarin after delivery. Women with APLAs and a prior pregnancy loss should be treated with low-dose aspirin and prophylactic heparin.

Mechanical Heart Valve

Women with a mechanical valve require lifelong anticoagulation with warfarin. During pregnancy, therapeutic UFH is typically administered with twice-daily SQ dosing. An increased risk of embolism has been reported with heparin therapy, but it is unclear whether those patients received sufficient heparin. It is extremely important to ensure that patients with a valve receive adequate heparin dosage and frequent laboratory monitoring. The APTT is obtained 6 hours postinjection, and the recommended target is twice the baseline value. Heparin levels may also be used to monitor the adequacy of therapy. LMWH is an option for gravidas with a mechanical valve, but experience is limited. Low-dose aspirin may be given in addition to heparin for patients at high risk for embolism.

THERAPEUTIC OPTIONS AND COMPLICATIONS OF ANTICOAGULATION

Heparins

UFH has been used for many years, but LMWHs are becoming increasingly popular. Both UFH and LMWH accelerate antithrombin's inhibition of thrombin and activated factor X (Xa). UFH has equal activity against thrombin and factor Xa, but LMWHs have greater activity against Xa. LMWHs' advantages include better bioavailability, a longer half-life, and a lower incidence of heparin-induced thrombocytopenia. LMWH is a safe and effective alternative to UFH for pregnant patients.

Laboratory monitoring of heparin therapy depends on whether UFH or LMWH is being administered. UFH is monitored with either the APTT or heparin level/factor Xa

activity. A therapeutic APTT is one and a half to two times the patient's baseline APTT. A therapeutic heparin level is 0.4 to 0.6 U/mL, but this range may vary among laboratories. LMWH must be monitored with a heparin level; the APTT cannot be used. Monitoring LMWH is not required in the general population because of the excellent bioavailability and predictable response. The pharmacokinetics of LMWH are not well established in pregnant patients, and increasing dosages may be required with advancing gestation. Therefore, monitoring of the Xa activity should be considered in gravidas receiving therapeutic LMWH.

Bleeding is the most common complication of heparin therapy. If the APTT is excessively prolonged and the patient is not bleeding, brief discontinuation (30 to 60 minutes) of the IV infusion or withholding the next SQ injection is sufficient. The heparin dosage is adjusted and then resumed with continued monitoring of the APTT (see Table 31–1). If the patient suffers life-threatening bleeding, protamine sulfate may be administered. The half-life of heparin (60 minutes) and the total amount of circulating heparin are used to calculate the amount of protamine required. One milligram of IV protamine neutralizes approximately 100 U of UFH. The dosage should never exceed 50 mg, as a large dose may potentiate the coagulopathy. IV protamine must be infused slowly over 10 minutes to avoid hypotension. Patients previously exposed to protamine (including NPH insulin) have a 1% risk of anaphylaxis with re-exposure.

Two forms of thrombocytopenia occur with UFH administration. A nonimmune heparin-induced thrombocytopenia (HIT) occurs in 3% of patients receiving therapeutic UFH and 0.5% to 1% of those receiving prophylaxis. It can occur within 24 hours of therapy if the patient has previously been exposed to heparin. Patients with no prior heparin exposure can develop HIT within 5 to 10 days of initiating therapy. The second type of HIT is immune mediated and associated with thrombosis (HITTS). Thirty percent to 60% of patients who develop HIT will suffer from HITTS, with 25% to 37% mortality.

The diagnosis of HIT is primarily clinical and based on the development of thrombocytopenia. Monitoring a daily platelet count is recommended for nonpregnant patients receiving UFH. This is impractical during pregnancy because patients receive heparin for many months. Given the natural history of HIT, a daily platelet count during the initial week of UFH therapy, weekly for the next 3 weeks, and then monthly is a reasonable approach. However, this guideline is not clearly established. A sudden, unexplained 30% to 50% decrease in platelets from preheparin baseline is highly suggestive of HIT. Because HIT/HITTS can occur despite a platelet count of greater than $100,000/mm^3$, no absolute threshold can be used in the diagnosis. No laboratory test can predict HIT or HITTS, and none of the currently available assays is 100% sensitive for the diagnosis.

Heparin administration should be immediately discontinued when thrombocytopenia is detected. Continued anticoagulation, however, is required and should be in concert with a hematologist. Danaparoid and recombinant hirudin are approved for treatment of HIT/HITTS. Warfarin increases the risk for thrombosis in acute HIT/HITTS and is contraindicated. LMWH cannot be substituted for UFH in patients with acute or prior HIT/HITTS because there is strong cross-reactivity between LMWH and UFH.

Prolonged heparin exposure has been associated with osteoporosis. It occurs in less than 5% of patients on long-term therapy. Symptomatic vertebral fractures have been reported in 2% of women receiving heparin during pregnancy. The risk is correlated with the duration and dosage of heparin therapy. Bone density studies have been recommended if a patient receives UFH for more than 6 months at less than 20,000 U/day or for more than 3 months with more than 20,000 U/day. Adequate calcium supplementation should be encouraged.

Warfarin

Warfarin exposure during the first trimester of pregnancy is associated with embryopathy. The true incidence of fetal malformations is uncertain, but the risk with exposure during the 6th to 12th week of pregnancy is approximately 30% (95% confidence interval, 15% to 45%). Warfarin exposure during any trimester of pregnancy is associated with fetal central nervous system malformations and hemorrhage. A recent small study[2] of warfarin exposure during pregnancy suggested that the risk of adverse fetal outcome is strongly correlated with the warfarin dose. Women requiring less than 5 mg/day of warfarin during pregnancy appeared to have fewer fetal complications than those requiring more than 5 mg/day.

Women receiving long-term anticoagulation with warfarin have three options when considering pregnancy. The first is frequent pregnancy testing. Warfarin is discontinued and heparin initiated immediately when the test is positive. The risk of fetal malformations is minimal, provided that warfarin is discontinued before the sixth week of pregnancy. The second approach is discontinuation of warfarin and administration of heparin before conception; heparin is then continued throughout pregnancy. This has the disadvantage of prolonged heparin exposure if conception does not occur quickly. A third option is discontinuation of warfarin by 6 weeks' gestation with initiation of therapeutic heparin. Warfarin is resumed between 12 and 36 weeks' gestation, after which time heparin is restarted until delivery. Although this approach is employed in Europe, American obstetricians are reluctant to use warfarin antenatally owing to the small but real risk to the fetus. Regardless of the approach chosen, women must be counseled on the risks of warfarin exposure during pregnancy and the importance of early pregnancy detection.

Warfarin has limited indications during pregnancy but the indications include patients with mechanical valves who have suffered emboli despite therapeutic heparinization and patients with HIT/HITTS. Patients with severe antithrombin deficiency are frequently heparin resistant and require either antithrombin concentrates or warfarin to prevent thrombosis.

Patients who require postpartum, indefinite, or lifelong anticoagulation can be converted from heparin to warfarin after delivery. Therapeutic heparinization is extremely important before administering the first warfarin dose. Patients with subtherapeutic heparin levels are at increased risk for thrombosis if warfarin is started. A loading dose of 5 mg/day of warfarin achieves a therapeutic, steady state by day 5 of therapy in most patients. A higher loading dose may result in a transient hypercoagulable state and increased thrombosis risk. Therapeutic heparin should be continued for 2 additional days once the target International Normalized Ratio (INR) is reached.

The adequacy of warfarin dosage is monitored with the INR. It is obtained daily until therapeutic for 2 days, then 2 to 3 times per week for 1 to 2 weeks and less often thereafter. The target INR in patients being treated for DVT or PE is 2.5 (range 2.0 to 3.0) and 3.0 (range 2.5 to 3.5) for APLAs or a mechanical heart valve. Long-term care of the patient receiving warfarin is best achieved by an internist, hematologist, or anticoagulation clinic.

Aspirin

Aspirin is a class C medication that irreversibly inhibits platelet function. Studies using aspirin during pregnancy have concentrated on attempts to reduce the incidence of preeclampsia on low- and high-risk gravidas and improve outcomes for patients with APLAs. The safety of aspirin in pregnancy has been examined in several large studies. A small but statistically significant increased risk of abruptio placentae for low-risk nulliparous women was noted in one trial.[3] The relationship between aspirin and congenital anomalies has not been clearly established. Aspirin ingestion does increase the risk of postpartum hemorrhage. Full-dose aspirin (doses $\geq$ 325 mg) during the week before delivery may affect the neonate's hemostatic mechanism. Low-dose aspirin is beneficial for select women, including those with APLAs and prior adverse pregnancy outcome, a mechanical heart valve and high risk of embolization, systemic lupus erythematosus and prior arterial emboli, and platelet hyperactivity.

Suggestions for Future Reading

Bick RL, Frenkel EP: Clinical aspects of heparin-induced thrombocytopenia and thrombosis and other side effects of heparin therapy. Clin Appl Thromb/Hemost 1999;5(Suppl 1):S7–S15.

Cruickshank MK, Levine MN, Hirsh J, et al: A standard nomogram for the management of heparin therapy. Arch Intern Med 1991;151:333–337.

Ginsberg JS, Hirsh J: Use of antithrombotic agents in pregnancy. Chest 1998;114:524S–530S.

Hirsh J, Warkentin TE, Raschke R, et al: Heparin and low-molecular-weight heparin: Mechanism of action, pharmacokinetics, dosing considerations, monitoring, efficacy and safety. Chest 1998;114:489S–510S.

Lodwick A: Warfarin therapy: A review of the literature since the Fifth American College of Chest Physicians' Consensus Conference on Antithrombotic Therapy. Clin Appl Thromb/Hemost 1999;5:208–215.

References

1. Kearon C, Gent M, Hirsh J, et al: A comparison of three months of anticoagulation with extended anticoagulation for a first episode of idiopathic venous thromboembolism. N Engl J Med 1999;340:901–907.
2. Vitale N, De Feo M, De Santo LS, et al: Dose-dependent fetal complications of warfarin in pregnant women with mechanical heart valves. J Am Coll Cardiol 1999;33:1637–1641.
3. Sibai BM, Caritis SN, Thom E, et al: Prevention of preeclampsia with low-dose aspirin in healthy, nulliparous pregnant women. The National Institute of Child Health and Human Development Network of Maternal-Fetal Medicine Units. N Engl J Med 1993;329:1213–1218.

THIRTY-TWO

Prevention of Group B Streptococcus Disease

Brian Thomas Pierce, Byron C. Calhoun,

and Roderick F. Hume, Jr.

BACKGROUND

Lancefield group B streptococcus (GBS), or *Streptococcus agalactiae,* is a gram-positive coccus that causes invasive disease in newborns, pregnant women, and adults with underlying medical conditions, such as diabetes, liver disease, and cancer. GBS is of particular concern to obstetricians and pediatricians in that GBS infections are the leading cause of bacterial disease and bacterial death among newborns in the United States.[1] GBS disease in infants is classified as early-onset if the disease occurs at younger than 7 days of age or late-onset if the disease occurs at 7 days of age or later. To date, prenatal surveillance and intrapartum chemoprophylaxis have not decreased the incidence of late-onset GBS disease, but have been shown to substantially decrease the incidence of early-onset GBS disease.[2, 3] GBS infections resulted in an estimated 7600 serious illnesses and 310 deaths among United States infants aged 90 days or younger yearly, with 80% of these illnesses occurring as early-onset disease.[4] The rate of late-onset GBS disease appears constant since the early 1990s, but, with the more widespread use of intrapartum chemoprophylaxis, the incidence of early-onset GBS disease is declining.[2]

The probable human reservoir for GBS is the gastrointestinal tract, with secondary spread to the genitourinary tract being common. Colonization rates are similar among pregnant and nonpregnant women, although they differ among ethnic groups, geographic locales, and age groups.[5] Overall, approximately 10% to 30% of pregnant women are estimated to be colonized with GBS in the vaginal or rectal area.[4]

NEONATAL COMPLICATIONS

The neonatal manifestations of GBS invasive disease include signs and symptoms of sepsis, pneumonia, and meningitis, with 90% of neonates being symptomatic within 12 hours of birth.[1, 5] The overall mortality rate from early-onset GBS disease ranges from 5% to 20%, with the rate decreasing since about 1980. Long-term sequelae occur in 15% to 30% of survivors, primarily in the form of neurologic impairment, including psychomotor delay or spastic disorders.[4, 5]

MATERNAL/PREGNANCY COMPLICATIONS

Several maternal complications have been attributed to GBS colonization, including cystitis and, rarely, pyelonephritis, chorioamnionitis, endometritis, and wound infection.[6] Conflicting reports link GBS to premature labor and delivery.

PREGNANCY RISK FACTORS

Specific clinical findings have been associated with increased rate of early-onset GBS disease (Table 32–1).

In addition, neonates delivered from African American women and women younger than 20 years of age are at increased risk for early-onset GBS sepsis.[5, 7] Women with multiple gestations are also more likely to develop GBS sepsis, which is apparently due to preterm delivery and low birth weight.[5] Preterm delivery is associated with increases in both GBS attack rate and fatality rate, with approximately 25% of cases occurring in premature infants.[5] Possible explanations include decreased placental antibody transport in early gestation and the increased incidence of preterm premature rupture of membranes (pPROM) associated with early delivery.[2] Lower-birth-weight infants are also at a significantly increased risk for both invasive GBS disease and disease-related fatality.

As expected, the incidence of early-onset GBS disease is higher in women colonized with GBS who have risk factors, followed by those colonized who do not have risk factors (Fig. 32–1). The risk factor of colonization alone has a higher rate for early-onset disease than the other risk factors combined. In addition, early-onset disease does occur in noncolonized women who do not have risk factors, indicating that not all cases of this disease may be prevented with a risk factor or screening approach.[5]

PREVENTION

Early-onset GBS disease prevention has focused on antepartum, intrapartum, and postpartum intervention strate-

Table 32–1. Risk Factors for Early-Onset Group B Streptococcus Disease

Maternal GBS colonization
Rupture of membranes > 18 hr
Premature delivery
Intrapartum fever
GBS bacteriuria
Prior infant with GBS disease

GBS, group B streptococcus.
Data from references 4, 5, 7.

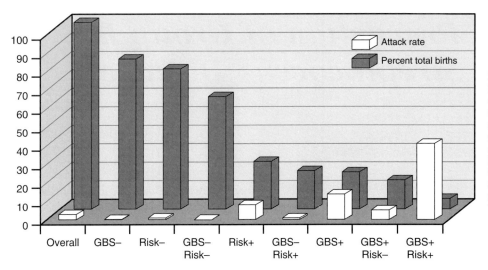

Figure 32–1. Attack rate per 1000 births for early-onset group B streptococcal (GBS) disease by colonization status and risk factors. Risk factors are defined as temperature $> 37.5°C$; membrane rupture > 12 hours; delivery at < 37 weeks' gestation. (From Prevention of perinatal group B streptococcal disease: A public health perspective. Centers for Disease Control and Prevention. MMWR Morb Mortal Wkly Rep 1996;45[RR-7]:1–24.)

gies, with intrapartum intervention clearly having the greatest impact on GBS disease incidence.

Antepartum Chemoprophylaxis

Antepartum antibiotic treatment in an attempt to reduce GBS colonization at delivery intuitively makes sense. However, most studies have shown that antepartum therapy of asymptomatic women does not eradicate GBS, and no substantial difference in delivery colonization has been observed between the treated and the untreated groups. Antepartum treatment should not be withheld for women with GBS bacteriuria or other symptoms related to maternal or fetal GBS disease.

Intrapartum Chemoprophylaxis

Many studies have addressed the efficacy of intrapartum chemoprophylaxis on reducing the incidence of neonatal colonization and early-onset GBS disease. These studies differ in the method of intervention used, but overall they show a significant reduction in colonization and GBS disease. One meta-analysis estimated a 30-fold reduction in early-onset GBS disease with the use of intrapartum chemoprophylaxis.[3]

In unusual circumstances in which antibiotics may be unavailable or contraindicated, vaginal lavage with chlorhexidine has been shown to be effective in reducing GBS load and neonatal intensive care unit admissions.

Postpartum (Neonatal) Chemoprophylaxis

Several studies have addressed the issue of postpartum chemoprophylaxis to newborns.[2, 4, 5, 10] No significant differences were found in the incidence of early-onset or late-onset GBS disease or mortality. Furthermore, there may

be increased neonatal mortality from penicillin-resistant pathogens in prophylactically treated infants.

GROUP B STREPTOCOCCUS CARRIER DETECTION

The majority of studies addressing the reduction of early-onset GBS disease incidence have specifically studied the population of GBS-colonized women. In addition, the vast majority of infants affected by early-onset GBS disease are born to colonized mothers. Because of this, an accurate method for detecting carrier status at time of delivery is crucial.

One important finding of carrier detection studies is that the later in pregnancy GBS cultures are obtained, the higher the positive and negative predictive values for GBS disease carrier status at delivery.[2, 4, 5, 8] A substantial number of patients with a negative culture obtained in the late second trimester will have positive cultures at term. Yancey and coworkers[8] demonstrated that the critical time for screening patients for GBS colonization is within 5 weeks of delivery. The sensitivity, specificity, positive predictive value, and negative predictive value of culture obtained within 5 weeks of delivery are significantly higher than cultures obtained more than 5 weeks after delivery (sensitivity, 87% vs. 43%; specificity 96% vs. 85%; positive predictive value, 87% vs. 50%; negative predictive value, 96% vs. 81%).

CULTURE METHODS

Bacterial culture on selective broth media, such as Lim broth or Todd-Hewitt broth, remains the "gold standard" for diagnosing GBS disease, with culture swabs obtained from the lower vagina and rectum.

A significant increase in GBS detection is found (97.4% vs. 64.1%) when culture swabs are inoculated onto selective broth culture medium compared with swabs inoculated onto nonselective sheep blood agar plates.[9] Also, GBS-colonized women have the highest rate of positive cultures from anorectal swabs, followed by vaginal swabs, with much decreased detection from cervical swabs. Therefore, maximum detection is obtained with swabs collected in the lower third of the vagina and the anorectum.[9]

Women can also be instructed on self-collection without a decrease in culture yield. In addition, immediate inoculation onto culture medium is not necessary and GBS carrier detection is not decreased by delayed inoculation while transporting the culture to the laboratory.

Following incubation onto selective broth for 18 to 24 hours, the broth is subcultured to sheep blood agar plates and inspected for organisms suggestive of GBS. Various tests may then be utilized for specific GBS identification.

Rapid detection tests for detecting GBS colonization have been developed and are reliable in detecting GBS in heavily colonized women. These rapid tests currently do not have the sensitivity for reliably detecting GBS in lightly colonized women.

PREVENTION GUIDELINES

Centers for Disease Control and Prevention

In 1996, the Centers for Disease Control and Prevention (CDC) published two alternative guidelines for decreasing early-onset GBS disease. The first is based on prenatal screening for patients who have not had a previous infant with invasive GBS disease or GBS bacteriuria during the current pregnancy and who are 37 weeks' gestation or later. A rectal and vaginal swab for GBS culture is performed at

35 to 37 weeks' gestation, and, for those patients who are positive, intrapartum chemoprophylaxis is offered. Patients who have not had the culture performed, or in whom the results of which are incomplete or unknown, are offered treatment for intrapartum temperature 100.4°F (38.0°C) or higher or membrane rupture of 18 hours or longer. Otherwise, no intrapartum prophylaxis is needed (Fig. 32–2).

The second guideline bases treatment on risk factors alone. Should a patient have any of the following risk factors, GBS disease prophylaxis is offered: Previous infant with invasive GBS disease, GBS bacteriuria during this pregnancy, delivery at less than 37 weeks' gestation, duration of ruptured membranes 18 hours or longer, or intrapartum temperature of 100.4°F (38.0°C) or higher (Fig. 32–3).

The CDC also states that routine use of prophylactic antibiotics for infants born to mothers who receive intrapartum GBS disease prophylaxis is not recommended and that individual circumstances or institutional preferences may be appropriate. Two potential treatment algorithms are provided in their policy statement.

American College of Obstetricians and Gynecologists

The American College of Obstetricians and Gynecologists (ACOG) endorses the CDC guidelines, in a change from their prior policy of only treating women based on risk factors alone.[4] For patients with pPROM, ACOG and the CDC recommend obtaining culture of GBS in all women. After culture, providers may initiate treatment until culture results return negative or withhold treatment until culture results return positive or the patient begins labor.

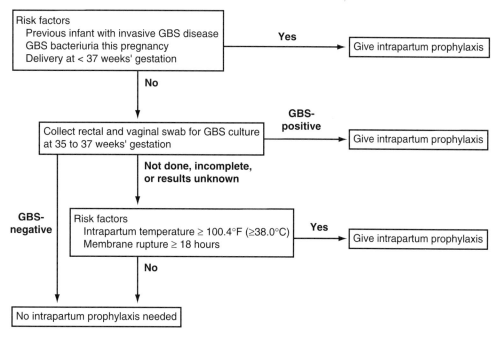

Figure 32–2. Algorithm for prevention of early-onset GBS disease in neonates: screening approach. (From Prevention of perinatal group B streptococcal disease: A public health perspective. Centers for Disease Control and Prevention. MMWR Morb Mortal Wkly Rep 1996;45[RR-7]:1–24.)

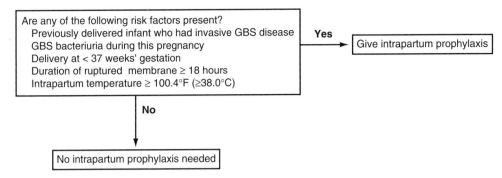

Figure 32–3. Algorithm for prevention of early-onset GBS disease in neonates: risk factor approach. (From Prevention of perinatal group B streptococcal disease: A public health perspective. Centers for Disease Control and Prevention. MMWR Morb Mortal Wkly Rep 1996;45[RR-7]:1–24.)

An adequate length of treatment for GBS-positive women and pPROM is not yet known.[4]

American Academy of Pediatrics

In March 1997, the American Academy of Pediatrics (AAP) published revised guidelines for the prevention of early-onset GBS infection, which also endorse the CDC recommendations and base treatment either on the results of GBS cultures obtained at 35 to 37 weeks' gestation or on the presence of risk factors.[10] These new guidelines are a change from the 1992 guidelines, which had recommended GBS screening at 28 weeks' gestation followed by intrapartum chemoprophylaxis for GBS-positive women who had certain risk factors including multiple gestation and pPROM after 12 hours. Criticism for the previous recommendations were based on the poorer predictive value of 28-week cultures of GBS positivity at term and the fact that many obstetricians felt obliged to treat the GBS-positive women antenatally with antibiotics, which has little or no effect in irradicating the organism.

In addition, the AAP also discusses guidelines for managing neonates in regards to decreasing GBS disease.

STRATEGY COMPARISON

Different treatment strategies in reducing early-onset GBS disease and antibiotic administration in a hypothetical population were compared in the CDC guidelines. Prenatal culture at 35 to 37 weeks' gestation with intrapartum prophylaxis for preterm deliveries and all GBS carriers would result in an 86% rate of prevention of early-onset GBS disease with 26.7% of deliveries receiving antibiotics, whereas a prevention guideline employing no prenatal cultures and utilizing prophylaxis for only women with risk factors would result in a 68.8% reduction in early-onset GBS disease with 18.3% of deliveries receiving antibiotics.[5]

To date, no clinical trials comparing the different strategies have been performed with sufficient numbers to detect a difference. Power analysis reveals the necessity for 100,000 pregnant women in each arm of a randomized

prospective clinical trial for a difference in mortality to be detected.[11]

COST COMPARISON

Several studies[5, 12] have concluded that a protocol based on treatment for risk factors will be less expensive and require fewer personnel than a protocol based on prenatal cultures. This may hold true for obstetric costs; however, few of these studies address the overall costs, which include increased newborn septic workups. Russell and colleagues[12] found a significant obstetric cost reduction following a hospital protocol change from a culture method to a risk-factor method; however, total costs increased substantially.

ANTIBIOTICS

GBS remains universally susceptible to penicillin G, which is the first-line prophylactic medication in the CDC guidelines (Table 32–2).[5] Many of the prior studies evaluating the efficacy of intrapartum prophylaxis were based on ampicillin administration.

The pharmacokinetics of penicillin G and ampicillin are similar in that both medications cross the placenta and achieve bactericidal levels in fetal tissue. Owing to decreased protein binding when compared with that of peni-

Table 32–2. Recommended Antibiotics for Group B Streptococcus Prophylaxis

Primary	Penicillin G	5 million units IV load followed by 2.5 million units q4h until delivery
Alternative	Ampicillin	2 g IV load followed by 1 g IV q4h until delivery
Penicillin-allergic primary	Clindamycin	900 mg IV q8h until delivery
Penicillin-allergic alternative	Erythromycin	500 mg IV q6h until delivery

Data from Prevention of perinatal group B streptococcal disease: A public health perspective. Centers for Disease Control and Prevention. MMWR Morb Mortal Wkly Rep 1996;45(RR-7):1–24.

cillin, ampicillin does achieve a higher fetal-maternal concentration ratio, although the concentration of penicillin remains above the minimum inhibiting concentration of 0.02 mg/mL for GBS.

One potential drawback of ampicillin is that, although it covers GBS adequately, antimicrobial resistant microorganisms may emerge. Indeed, there are now several reports of adverse perinatal outcomes by ampicillin-resistant bacteria after treatment with ampicillin for pPROM or GBS-positive cultures.[2, 5, 13]

There also appears to be a critical time period for treatment before delivery. The incidence of neonatal GBS surface colonization is significantly reduced with maternal antibiotic treatment for at least 2 to 4 hours before delivery. By inference, GBS invasive disease should also be reduced with longer duration of treatment.

The CDC guidelines also recommend clindamycin or erythromycin for GBS prophylaxis in patients allergic to penicillins. The efficacy of these medications for reducing early-onset GBS disease has not been evaluated in clinical trials. In addition, clinically isolated GBS has shown resistance to both clindamycin and erythromycin. Nevertheless, although these agents are not ideal, they remain the best practical alternatives for patients with contraindications to the penicillins and cephalosporins.

The prevention strategies recommend treatment for intrapartum temperature higher than 100.4°F; in this circumstance, it may be prudent to change to a broader-spectrum antibiotic.

One more important issue concerning antibiotic administration is the 1:50,000 to 100,000 risk for fatal anaphylaxis, which has been estimated to result in 4 to 12 maternal deaths per year.[5] With more widespread use of intrapartum chemoprophylaxis, the true impact of this is yet to be realized.

VACCINATIONS

Conjugated vaccines against the major serotypes of GBS have been produced and offer potential nonantibiotic therapy for reducing the incidence of early-onset GBS disease. Because infants with early-onset GBS disease are more likely to have low levels of antibody to GBS capsular polysaccharide, maternal vaccination has been hypothesized to increase these antibody levels. Several drawbacks to vaccination include maternal apprehension of vaccination in pregnancy and a shift in serotypes of GBS strains causing disease. Even so, vaccination may prove to reduce early-onset GBS disease, and clinical trials are in progress to determine their impact.[2, 5]

SUMMARY

Although declining in incidence, early-onset GBS disease remains the most important infectious newborn complication, with substantial morbidity, mortality, and cost. The CDC, ACOG, and AAP give evidence-based prevention recommendations, and it is imperative that obstetric and newborn providers adopt one of these strategies to reduce the incidence of this devastating disease.

Suggestions for Future Reading

American College of Obstetricians and Gynecologists: Prevention of early-onset group B streptococcal disease in newborns (ACOG Committee Opinion No. 173). Washington, DC, ACOG, June 1996.

Prevention of perinatal group B streptococcal disease: A public health perspective. Centers for Disease Control and Prevention. MMWR Morb Mortal Wkly Rep 1996;45(RR-7):1–24.

Revised guidelines for prevention of early-onset group B streptococcal (GBS) infection. American Academy of Pediatrics, Committee on Infectious Diseases and Committee on Fetus and Newborn. Pediatrics 1997;99:489–496.

Schuchat A: Group B streptococcus. Lancet 1999;353:51–56.

References

1. Decreasing incidence of perinatal group B streptococcal disease–United States, 1993–1995. MMWR Morb Mortal Wkly Rep 1997;46:473–477.
2. Schuchat A: Group B streptococcus. Lancet 1999;353:51–56.
3. Allen UD, Navas L, King SM: Effectiveness of intrapartum penicillin prophylaxis in preventing early-onset group B streptococcal infection: Results of a meta-analysis. Can Med Assoc J 1993;149:1659–1665.
4. American College of Obstetricians and Gynecologists: Prevention of early-onset group B streptococcal disease in newborns (ACOG Committee Opinion No. 173). Washington, DC, ACOG, June 1996.
5. Prevention of perinatal group B streptococcal disease: A public health perspective. Centers for Disease Control and Prevention. MMWR Morb Mortal Wkly Rep 1996;45(RR-7):1–24.
6. Yancey M, Duff P, Clark P, et al: Peripartum infection associated with vaginal group B streptococcal colonization. Obstet Gynecol 1994;85:816–819.
7. Schuchat A, Deaver-Robinson K, Plikaytis BD, et al: Multistate case-control study of maternal risk factors for neonatal group B streptococcal disease. The Active Surveillance Group. Pediatr Infect Dis J 1994;13:623–629.
8. Yancey M, Schuchat A, Brown L, et al: The accuracy of late antenatal screening cultures in predicting genital group B streptococcal colonization at delivery. Obstet Gynecol 1996;88:811–815.
9. Philipson E, Palermino D, Robinson A: Enhanced antenatal detection of group B streptococcus colonization. Obstet Gynecol 1995;85:437–439.
10. Revised guidelines for prevention of early-onset group B streptococcal (GBS) infection. American Academy of Pediatrics Committee on Infectious Diseases and Committee on Fetus and Newborn. Pediatrics 1997;99:489–496.
11. Landon MB, Harger J, McNellis D, et al: Prevention of neonatal group B streptococcal infection. Obstet Gynecol 1994;84:460.
12. Russell CS, Griffin D, Hume R, et al: Cost consequences of elimination of the routine group B streptococcus culture at a teaching hospital. J Matern Fetal Med 2000;9:1–5.
13. McDuffie R, McGregor J, Gibbs R: Adverse perinatal outcome and resistant enterobacteriaceae after antibiotic usage for premature rupture of the membranes and group b streptococcus carriage. Obstet Gynecol 1993;82:487–489.

THIRTY-THREE

Adolescent Pregnancy: Improving Outcomes through Focused Multidisciplinary Obstetric Care

Elizabeth Golladay Hancock,

Byron C. Calhoun, and Roderick F. Hume, Jr.

Adolescent pregnancies have been associated with poor perinatal outcome. Historically, women 19 years of age and younger have double the maternal mortality, double the risk of low-birth-weight infants, and triple the neonatal death rate of the general population. Numerous studies have consistently demonstrated that young age in and of itself does not provide for the increased risk of adverse pregnancy outcome. Since the 1970s, we have known that removal of the psychosocial and socioeconomic barriers to prenatal care reduces the risk of adverse outcome in teenage pregnancy to that of the general population. Adolescent pregnancy is a social problem with medical implications. Development of a multidisciplinary approach to care of the pregnant adolescent is essential in providing optimal outcomes.

STATISTICS

The 1997 Youth Risk Behavior Survey revealed that 48.4% of high school students report sexual intercourse, 16% reported four or more long-term partners and only half used condoms.[1] According to the most recent complete estimate (1995), the *pregnancy rate,* defined as the sum of live births, spontaneous abortions, and elective terminations, for adolescents aged 15 to 19 years was 101.1/1000, and that for adolescents younger than 15 years of age was 2.91/1000. Abortions in the two groups were 34.5% and 47%, respectively. Because unintended pregnancies account for the majority of adolescent conceptions, abortion is a commonly chosen option among this age group (Fig. 33–1).[2]

Only 8% of those adolescent mothers choosing to continue pregnancy gave the infant up for adoption.[3] The United States birthrate among adolescents is 4 to 8 times higher than that of Western European countries and 18 times that of Japan (Fig. 33–2).[4]

Risk factors for early intercourse are early pubertal development, a history of sexual abuse, cultural and family patterns of early sexual experience, parents on welfare, poor school performance, nonwhite race, and living in rural areas, especially the South.[3, 4] Peer pressure also plays an important role in teenage pregnancy. Teenagers with poor self-esteem or who fail scholastically or athletically are especially susceptible. Giving birth to a baby is seen as an accomplishment, and the attention that it attracts is reinforcing. This encouragement may play a role in the high rate of repeat pregnancy among teens. Approximately 25% of teenage births are second and higher-order births. Children of teenage parents have an increased risk of developmental delay, academic difficulties, behavioral disorders, substance abuse, and becoming adolescent parents themselves.[5]

LOW BIRTH WEIGHT

Low birth weight (<2500 g) is one of the most significant factors in predicting infant perinatal morbidity and mortality. This includes those infants born appropriate for gestational age but preterm and those born small for gestational age. Intrauterine growth restriction can result from a variety of conditions that interfere with the delivery of nutrients or oxygen to the fetus. Smoking, low caloric intake, and poor weight gain are well-established risk factors for intrauterine growth restriction. Every day, it is estimated that 3000 adolescents start to smoke. According to the National Center for Health Statistics, the overall rate of smoking during pregnancy dropped from 20% to 13.2% between 1990 and 1997. However, for pregnant women aged 15 to 19 years, the smoking rate actually increased to 17.2%.[6] Data from the Camden Study, an ongoing study of the effects of maternal nutrition and growth during pregnancy, reveals that prepregnancy weight and maternal weight gain are important determinants of infant birth weight. Diets chosen by adolescents are variable, and ingestion of vitamin supplements is erratic. The importance of adequate prenatal care in this population cannot be overemphasized. Women who get insufficient prenatal care (either inadequate in frequency or initiated late in pregnancy) are about twice as likely as those who receive

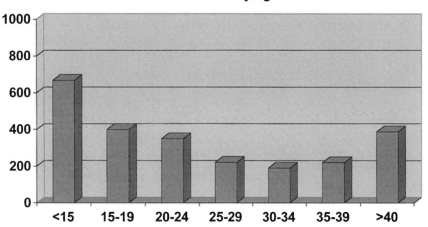

Figure 33–1. Abortion ratio (number of abortions per 1000 live births) by age group of women who obtained a legal abortion, United States, 1995. (From Koonin LM, Smith JC, Ramick M, Strauss LT: Abortion surveillance—United States, 1995. CDC Surveill Summ. MMWR Morb Mortal Wkly Rep 1998;47[SS-2]:31–40.)

sufficient care to have a low-birth-weight infant. Teens typically present late for prenatal care. Only 66.7% present for care in the first trimester (compared with 76% in 20- to 24-year-olds and 88% in 30- to 34-year-olds) (Fig. 33–3).

Although a large proportion of preterm births remains unexplained, psychological stress has been hypothesized to influence pregnancy outcomes. Whether this occurs directly by influencing neurologic, endocrine, and immunologic systems or indirectly by influencing behaviors such as smoking, drug use, and sexual promiscuity is unknown. Adolescent pregnancies are associated with poverty, inadequate nutrition, poor preconceptual health, genital tract infection, smoking, and alcohol and drug abuse. An impoverished living environment has a negative impact on birth weight. Additionally, adolescents suffer an increased incidence of physical and sexual abuse.

SEXUAL ABUSE

Pregnancy in a young adolescent is an established sign of potential sexual abuse. Younger teens are especially vulnerable to coercive and nonconsensual sex. Involuntary sexual activity has been reported in 74% of sexually active girls younger than 14 years and 60% of those younger than 15 years.[5] Women who are abused during pregnancy have ambivalent feelings toward the pregnancy, enter prenatal care late, and have violence toward them escalate during the pregnancy. Almost two thirds of adolescent mothers have partners older than 20 years of age. Medical professionals are obligated under law to report suspected sexual abuse of minors. Ask patients at their initial prenatal visit whether they have ever been or are currently being physically or sexually abused. Prenatal care in a multidiscipli-

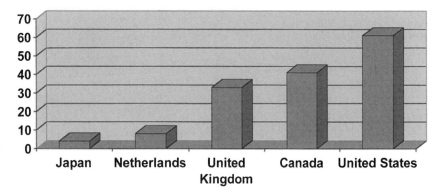

Figure 33–2. Birth rates (1992 data) for selected developed countries for females 15 to 19 years old. (Adapted from American Academy of Pediatrics, Committee on Adolescence: Adolescent pregnancy—current trends and issues: 1998. Pediatrics 1999;103:516–520.)

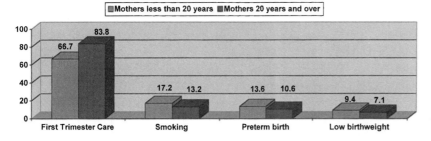

Figure 33–3. Selected characteristics for teenage mothers and mothers aged 20 years and older: United States, 1996. (From Ventura SJ, Matthews TJ, Curtin SC: Declines in teenage birth rates, 1991–1997: National and state patterns. National Center for Health Statistics. Natl Vital Stat Rep 1998;47[12]:5.)

nary clinic provides a unique opportunity to teach adolescent females how to protect themselves and their future children from abuse.

THE VERY YOUNG ADOLESCENT

Several studies that stratify outcomes into two separate age groups have identified middle-school-age adolescents as particularly high risk for low-birth-weight infants.[7–9] In Satin and colleagues study[7] of an indigent population, the 11- to 15-year-old study group, which was disproportionately black and obtained less prenatal care, had double the rate of very-low-birth-weight infants. This age group is typically unmarried, living at home, and still in school. There is particular concern that girls 15 years old and younger may experience pregnancy complications owing to their physiologic immaturity. Scholl and coworkers[8] demonstrated that despite adequate weight gain during pregnancy, younger adolescents did not mobilize the fat reserves late in pregnancy that typically enhances fetal growth. They hypothesized that the adolescent preferentially utilizes this fat reserve for their own continued development. The Rochester Study of Adolescent Pregnancy did not support this theory of competition for nutrients in a population that was well nourished in the prepregnant state. In the Rochester study, Stevens-Simon and associates[9] found that very young parturients actually transferred more of their gestational weight gain to the fetus than did older adolescents.

Fraser and colleagues[10] studied an entirely white population in Utah and confirmed earlier findings that sociodemographic factors, particularly inadequate prenatal care, resulted in a marked increase in premature birth. However, when the analysis was limited to nonsmoking, teenage mothers who were married, had age-appropriate educational levels, and received adequate prenatal care, the youngest mothers (aged ≤ 17 years) still had the highest relative risk of low-birth-weight, premature delivery, and small-for-gestational-age infants. No data were provided on maternal weight gain in this population. These studies suggest that when sociodemographic variables are controlled for, a small but statistically significant portion of the hazards

associated with adolescent pregnancy may be due to physiologic immaturity. Middle-school-aged mothers, especially if underweight, should be a special target for pregnancy intervention.

PREGNANCY MANAGEMENT

The adolescent pregnancy clinic should provide quality medical care and attend to the broad range of psychosocial, educational, and economic problems that surround teenage childbearing. Emphasis must be placed on the need for early and regular prenatal care, adequate nutrition, education, and reduction of risk factors, such as sexually transmitted diseases, smoking, and drug use. A multidisciplinary team approach has proved to be the most successful in achieving these goals.[5, 11, 12] This team consists, minimally, of the health care provider, nurse educator, social worker, and nutritionist.

A single health care provider is optimal (whether physician, nurse midwife, nurse practitioner, or physician's assistant) because continuity of care facilitates compliance. The nurse educator conducts an "exit interview" with the teen after each visit to ensure understanding of its contents and that patient-specific problems and needs are not overlooked. Additionally, an educational curriculum that covers specific learning objectives ensures that important topics are addressed at appropriate gestational ages throughout pregnancy. Educational groups such as parenting classes, childbirth classes, and tours of the labor and delivery area are quite useful. Significant others (fathers-to-be, grandparents-to-be) should be encouraged to actively participate in these groups.

The nutritionist's evaluation must have priority because of the high frequency of anemia and nutritional problems among adolescents. The only *biologic* factors that have been associated consistently with negative pregnancy results are low prepregnancy weight, parity, and poor pregnancy weight gain. Although total weight gain is important to successful pregnancy outcome, the pattern of weight gain also appears to play a significant role. According to Hediger and coworkers,[13] both early and late weight gain in pregnancy have independent effects on pregnancy outcome.

Inadequate gains early in pregnancy (<24 wk) result in increased risk of having a growth-restricted infant, even if weight appears to improve late in the second or third trimester. Failing weight gain from 24 weeks to delivery (<400 g/wk) is strongly associated with preterm birth. The social worker helps to identify and remove obstacles to care, such as transportation to clinic visits, access to school services, referral to the Special Supplemental Food Program for Women, Infants, and Children (WIC), and adequate housing.

Many successful programs utilize a community outreach worker to visit the home of the adolescent and serve as an advocate, friend, and role model. Early postpartum discharge is contraindicated to ensure that the mother is capable of caring for her child and has resources available for assistance.

PREVENTION OF RECURRENT PREGNANCY

It is not uncommon for adolescents to become pregnant again. Repeat pregnancies may be as prevalent as 30% to 50% by the second postpartum year. Oral contraceptives, depo medroxyprogesterone acetate, and the subdermal implant system have all been studied extensively and found to be safe for teenagers. Compliance is the main issue with the adolescent. Continuation rates for oral contraceptives are very low. Better continuation rates are achieved with Depo-Provera (56% at 2 years) and Norplant (95% at 15 months).

SUMMARY

During the 1990s, teenage pregnancy rates have declined substantially. The overall teenage birth rate dropped by 20% between 1991 and 1999, from 62.1 to 49.6 live births per 1000 teenagers, respectively.[14] The abortion rate among this population has also declined by a similar rate. Compared with the 1980s, teenagers are more likely to use contraceptives at first intercourse, especially condoms. In addition, the use of injectable and implantable contraception has increased among adolescents. The most significant decline in teenage births was in the rate of second births to teenagers. This rate declined from 25% in 1991 to 22% in 1997, representing a 21% decrease.[5] Numerous health care dollars have been spent in the effort to reduce the incidence of teen pregnancy. Optimism surrounds the latest reports that suggest educational programs are effective in preventing unintended pregnancy. The crisis of a teen pregnancy offers a ''teachable moment'' that should not be squandered. Prenatal care should be tailored to the medical, social, nutritional, and educational needs of the adolescents

and should include child care training and contraceptive counseling. Care for the pregnant adolescent in a multidisciplinary clinic approach reduces the risk of low birth weight, maternal mortality, and neonatal death to that of the general population. It is important to provide this care in an environment in which adolescents feel comfortable and valued as individuals.[12]

Suggestions for Future Reading

American Academy of Pediatrics, Committee on Adolescence. Adolescent pregnancy—Current trends and issues: 1998. Pediatrics 1999; 103:516–520.

American College of Obstetricians and Gynecologists: Adolescent Pregnancy Facts. Washington, DC, ACOG, 1999.

Foster HW, Bond T, Ivery DG, et al: Teen pregnancy—problems and approaches: Panel presentations. Am J Obstet Gynecol 1999;181:32S–36S.

Rogers MM, Peoples-Sheps MD, Suchindran C: Impact of a social support program on teenage prenatal care use and pregnancy outcomes. J Adolesc Health 1996;19:132–140.

References

1. Centers for Disease Control and Prevention: Trends in sexual risk behaviors among high school students—United States, 1991–1997. MMWR Morb Mortal Wkly Rep 1998;47:749–752.
2. Koonin LM, Smith JC, Ramick M, Strauss LT: Abortion surveillance—United States, 1995. CDC Surveill Summ. MMWR Morb Mortal Wkly Rep 1998;47(SS-2):31–40.
3. American College of Obstetricians and Gynecologists: Adolescent Pregnancy Facts. Washington, DC, ACOG, 1999.
4. American Academy of Pediatrics, Committee on Adolescence: Adolescent pregnancy—current trends and issues: 1998. Pediatrics 1999;103:516–520.
5. Foster HW, Bond T, Ivery DG, et al: Teen pregnancy—problems and approaches: Panel presentations. Am J Obstet Gynecol 1999;181:32S–36S.
6. Ventura SJ, Matthews TJ, Curtin SC: Declines in teenage birth rates, 1991–1997: National and state patterns. National Center for Health Statistics. Natl Vital Stat Rep 1998;47(12):5.
7. Satin AJ, Leveno KJ, Sherman ML, et al: Maternal youth and pregnancy outcomes: Middle school versus high school age groups compared with women beyond the teen years. Am J Obstet Gynecol 1994;171:184–187.
8. Scholl TO, Hediger ML, Schall JI, et al: Maternal growth during pregnancy and the competition for nutrients. Am J Clin Nutr 1994;60:183–188.
9. Stevens-Simon C, McAnarney E, Roghmann KJ: Adolescent gestational weight gain and birth weight. Pediatrics 1993;92:805–809.
10. Fraser AM, Brockert JE, Ward RH: Association of young maternal age with adverse reproductive outcomes. N Engl J Med 1995;332:1113–1117.
11. Perez R, Patience T, Pulous E, et al: Use of a focussed teen prenatal clinic at a military teaching hospital: Model for improved outcomes of unmarried mothers. Aust N Z J Obstet Gynaecol 1998;38:280–283.
12. Rogers MM, Peoples-Sheps MD, Suchindran C: Impact of a social support program on teenage prenatal care use and pregnancy outcomes. J Adolesc Health 1996;19:132–140.
13. Hediger ML, Scholl TO, Belsky DH, et al: Patterns of weight gain in adolescent pregnancy: Effects on birth weight and preterm delivery. Obstet Gynecol 1989;74:6–12.
14. Curtin SC, Martin JA: Births: Preliminary data for 1999. National Center for Health Statistics. Natl Vital Stat Rep 2000;48(14):1.

THIRTY-FOUR

Unintended Pregnancy

Diane M. Flynn, Jeffrey B. Clark, and

Roderick F. Hume, Jr.

Approximately 2.65 million unintended pregnancies are conceived annually in the United States. This represents one of the highest rates of unintended pregnancies among developed countries and accounts for nearly half (49%) of all pregnancies in the United States.[1] The Institute of Medicine advocates the adoption of a national consensus that all pregnancies should be intended.[2] The U.S. Department of Health and Human Services established as a priority the prevention of unintended pregnancy in its *Healthy People 2010* objectives.[3]

People are inclined to seek health care when they feel most susceptible to an undesired condition. Therefore, clinicians who provide primary and reproductive care to women often have the opportunity to counsel women when they are most receptive to contraceptive advice. The adolescent who is considering becoming sexually active and presents for a routine examination is unlikely to contemplate counseling that encourages abstinence as an option. The woman who presents to rule out an unintended pregnancy is likely to consider recommendations for contraception. This access to "teachable moments" can empower clinicians to positively influence contraceptive behavior.

CONSEQUENCES OF UNINTENDED PREGNANCY

Unintended pregnancy is associated with considerable costs to women, men, children, and society. Women who carry unintended pregnancies are less likely to seek early prenatal care than women with intended pregnancies.[2] They are more likely to be the victims of violence. A woman who carries an unintended pregnancy is more likely to expose the fetus to harmful substances, such as alcohol and tobacco, although these behaviors may be attributable to associated demographic factors rather than intention status.[2]

Most descriptive studies of pregnancy intendedness and birth weight report a higher risk of low birth weight in infants born as a result of an unintended pregnancy,[2] although this association was not observed in all studies. Infants born as a result of unintended pregnancies are less likely to be breastfed. They are more likely to live in poverty and to live in single-parent households.[2] Many studies suggest that these children are at greater risk of physical abuse and neglect.[2] They are more likely to die in the first year of life, particularly when the pregnancy was unwanted rather than mistimed.[2]

Induced abortion, elected by 54% of women with unin-tended pregnancies, is an important consequence of unintended pregnancy. In 1995, over 1.2 million induced abortions were reported to the Centers for Disease Control and Prevention. This represents a 15% decrease since 1990. The abortion-to-live-birth ratio was 311 abortions per 1000 live births in 1995, the lowest reported since 1975. These decreases may be due to a decrease in unintended pregnancies, a decrease in access to abortion services, or a change in attitudes about abortion.

Legal elective abortion is medically safe, but it often poses important moral and ethical dilemmas to the women and couples who consider it, as well as to the providers who perform it. Several studies have attempted to determine whether women who have induced abortions experience long-term psychological sequelae. Despite methodologic limitations, most studies consistently find rare instances of long-term negative psychological responses after elective termination and report decreased psychological distress after abortion compared with before abortion.[2]

Although the medical and psychological consequences of abortion appear to be minor for most women, elective abortion is a politically and socially divisive issue in the United States. Clearly, prevention of unintended pregnancy is the common goal that unites those who support and those who oppose legalized abortion.

DEMOGRAPHY OF UNINTENDED PREGNANCY

Contrary to the popular perception that unintended pregnancy is a problem primarily of adolescent, poor, unmarried, or minority women, it is experienced by women of all reproductive ages regardless of race, ethnicity, income, marital status, or educational level. The most comprehensive data on unintended pregnancy in the United States are compiled from the National Survey of Family Growth (NSFG), a federally funded survey representative of United States women aged 15 to 44 years, conducted by the National Center for Health Statistics. The NSFG has been completed every 3 to 6 years since 1973. The most recent survey, completed in 1995, includes interviews of 10,847 women and provides information on pregnancy intendedness, contraceptive use, and pregnancy outcomes between 1990 and 1995.[4]

According to the NSFG, pregnancies are defined as *intended* or *unintended* at conception. A pregnancy is considered *intended* if the woman did not practice contracep-

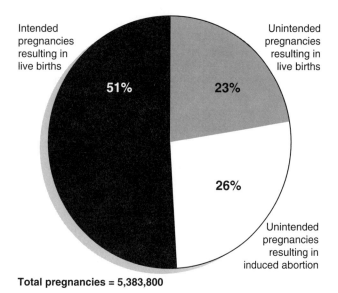

Total pregnancies = 5,383,800

Figure 34–1. Pregnancy intendedness in the United States, 1994, excluding spontaneous abortions. (Redrawn from Henshaw SK: Unintended pregnancy in the United States. Fam Plann Perspect 1998;30:24–29.)

tion at the time of conception and if she wanted to become pregnant at the time of conception or sooner. Pregnancies experienced by women who did not use contraception at the time of conception and were indifferent to becoming pregnant are also considered *intended*. A pregnancy is considered *unintended* if the woman practiced contraception at the time of conception or if she did not want to become pregnant at the time of conception. Among unintended pregnancies, a distinction is made between *mistimed* and *unwanted* pregnancies. A *mistimed* conception is one that is wanted by the woman, but occurred sooner than desired. An *unwanted* pregnancy is one that is conceived by a woman who did not want a(nother) baby ever.[4]

According to the 1995 NSFG, after spontaneous abortions are excluded, 49% of pregnancies and 31% of births[4] in the United States are unintended at the time of conception (Fig. 34–1). About 26% of pregnancies and 54% of unintended pregnancies end in induced abortion. The remaining unintended pregnancies lead to live births.[1]

Age is an important predictor of unintended pregnancy risk; the highest unintended pregnancy rates are observed

in women at both extremes of the reproductive years. The highest proportion of unintended pregnancies is observed in teenagers younger than 18 years, in whom 82% of pregnancies are unintended. The proportion of unintended pregnancies decreases with increasing age until the 30- to 34-year-old age group, in which one third of pregnancies are unintended. In age groups older than 35 years, the proportion increases, with slightly over one half of pregnancies among women over age 40 years unintended (Fig. 34–2).[1]

The proportion of unintended pregnancies is 31% among married women, 63% among formerly married women, and 78% among never-married women. Pregnancies among married women are much less likely to end in induced abortion (11%) than those among formerly married (41%) and never-married women (46%). Poverty is strongly associated with unintended pregnancy. Sixty-one percent of pregnancies in women living in poverty are unintended, compared with 53% of pregnancies in women living between 100% and 199% of the poverty level, and 41% of pregnancies in women living at 200% of the poverty level or above. Race and ethnicity are also strongly associated with pregnancy intendedness and correlate with economic trends. Seventy-two percent of pregnancies among African American women are unintended, compared with 43% among white women. The percentage of unintended pregnancies that end in induced abortion is also higher in African American women (60%) than in white women (50%). The percentage of pregnancies that are unintended is about the same in Hispanic women (48.6%) compared with non-Hispanic women (49.3%).[1]

Some decrease has been observed in unintended pregnancy trends in the United States in recent years. Between 1988 and 1995, the unintended pregnancy rate decreased from 54 per 1000 to 45 per 1000, and the percentage of pregnancies that were unintended decreased from 55% to 49%. Much of this improvement is attributable to a higher prevalence of contraceptive use and the use of more effective methods.[1]

CONTRACEPTION USE

According to the NSFG,[4] the proportion of women in the United States aged 15 to 44 years who use contracep-

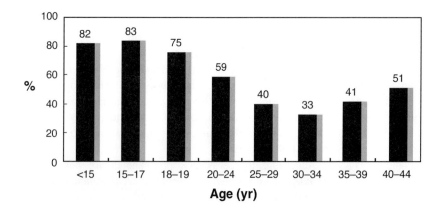

Figure 34–2. Percentage of pregnancies that are unintended by age in the United States, 1994. (Redrawn from Henshaw SK: Unintended pregnancy in the United States. Fam Plann Perspect 1998;30:24–29.)

tion increased from 56% in 1982 to 64% in 1995. This increase was observed in all age, ethnic and racial groups.[5] The 36% of contraception nonusers were composed of 5% of women who were infertile; 9% who were pregnant, postpartum, or trying to conceive at the time of the interview; 11% who had never had intercourse; 6% who were sexually experienced, but who had not had intercourse in the previous 3 months; and 5% who had had intercourse within the previous 3 months.[5] This last group, comprising the 5% of women of childbearing age who were sexually active but not using contraception, experienced nearly half (47%) of all unintended pregnancies. Women who used contraception at any time during the month of conception experienced the remaining 53% of unintended pregnancies.[1]

Determinants of Contraceptive Use

Whether or not a couple uses contraception is determined by social, cognitive, and psychological factors. These factors are incorporated into the basic tenets of behavioral theories such as the Health Belief Model, the Theory of Reasoned Action, and the Social Learning Theory. All three models consider two sets of factors: (1) *exogenous factors,* consisting of individual demographic characteristics and aggregate group characteristics, and (2) *proximal factors,* consisting of knowledge, beliefs, attitudes, and perceptions.[6]

The exogenous factors associated with contraceptive nonuse and misuse are young age, racial and ethnic minority, low socioeconomic status, strong religious commitment, low educational background, and unmarried status. Exogenous factors include the least modifiable risk factors, describe the most disadvantaged in our society, and are rarely the focus of prevention programs.[6]

Proximal determinants are the targets of most prevention programs because they are the predisposing, enabling, and reinforcing factors[7] most likely to be influenced by appropriate intervention. The main reasons some women do not use birth control include naiveté regarding pregnancy risk, limited knowledge about birth control methods, and negative attitudes about contraceptive use. Studies of adolescents and college students show that women and men often have incorrect information about the female reproductive cycle, the probability of conception, and the health risks and side effects of birth control.

Self efficacy is as important as knowledge, attitudes, and perceptions in determining contraceptive behavior. Women who believe they have the skills to control their own behavior and believe they should and can be responsible for their sexual activity are much less likely to experience an unintended pregnancy than are women without these beliefs.[6]

An important determinant of how well a reversible contraceptive works is the ability and motivation of the user and partner to use the method properly and consistently.

Available methods vary not only in effectiveness but also in ease of use. Methods that have high inherent effectiveness and require little patient skill, such as implants and injectables, have low failure rates. User motivation can affect highly efficacious methods like the pill, which requires daily use for contraceptive success. Methods that require user skill and motivation proximal to the time of intercourse, such as barrier methods, withdrawal, and periodic abstinence, have the highest failure rates.

Access to contraceptive services has been defined as the "degree of fit" between the patient and the health care system. Degree of fit has five dimensions: (1) *availability* is a measure of the number and types of providers and services available to meet the patient's needs; (2) *accessibility* is a measure of the convenience of location of services; (3) *accommodation* is a measure of the ease with which appointments that serve the patient can be made; (4) *affordability* is a measure of the patient's ability and/or willingness to pay for the service and whether the services are worth the cost; and (5) *acceptability* is a measure of whether or not the providers' personal and practice styles are suitable to the patient.

Note that even if contraception is free and available at an easily accessible clinic, other barriers, such as reluctance to undergo a medical examination, embarrassment about being sexually active, concerns regarding confidentiality, and dissatisfaction with available birth control methods, may prevent individuals from seeking contraceptive counseling.[6]

Choice of Contraceptive Method

Among women contraceptive users in 1995, the methods of contraception most widely used were female sterilization (28% of users), oral contraceptives (27% of users), and the male condom (20% of users). The next most commonly reported method was vasectomy, which 11% of women contraceptive users relied on to prevent unintended pregnancy. These methods were the most commonly reported in 1982 and 1988 as well. Ninety-one percent of contraceptive users reported use of a single method (Fig. 34–3).[5]

Overall, the distribution of contraceptive users by primary method changed little between 1988 and 1995. The most substantial change was an increase from 15% to 20% in the proportion of women contraceptive users who reported using the male condom. Fewer than 1% of women contraceptive users report using the female condom, which received U.S. Food and Drug Administration (FDA) approval in 1993. However, some reports suggest that use of the female condom has increased in some regions of the United States. Depot medroxyprogesterone acetate (DMPA) injectable contraceptives (Depo-Provera) and the levonorgestrel implant system (Norplant) were relatively new in 1995 and were reported by only 3% and 1% of all users, respectively. However, the proportions of contraceptive users younger than age 25 years who reported using

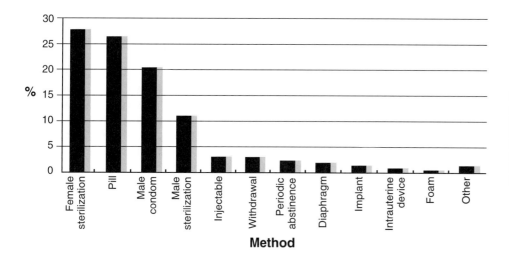

Figure 34–3. Distribution of contraceptive users aged 15 to 44 years in the United States by current method, 1995. (Redrawn from Piccinino LJ, Mosher WD: Trends in contraceptive use in the United States, 1982 to 1995. Fam Plann Perspect 1998; 30:4–10.)

injectable DMPA and the levonorgestrel implant were more than four times that of older women.[5]

Choice of contraceptive method is strongly influenced by demographic factors, including age, race, ethnicity, education, income, and marital status. Among contraceptive users, there was a substantial drop between 1988 and 1995 in oral contraceptive use by teenagers (from 59% to 44% of users) and women ages 20 to 24 years (from 68% to 52% of users). Use of the male condom increased in all age groups but most markedly among women in their 20s. Oral contraceptive use among never-married women declined from 59% to 44% of contraceptive users; this group showed a substantial increase in condom use, from 20% to 30% of users. Patterns of contraceptive use among currently married women changed little between 1988 and 1995; however, condom use among married women increased slightly from 14% to 17% of users, and diaphragm use declined from 6% to 2% of users. About 54% of contraceptive users with less than a high school education elect female sterilization for contraception, whereas women with higher educational experience are more likely to use reversible methods of contraception. Condom use increased in all educational groups between 1988 and 1995.[5]

Emergency Contraception

Emergency contraception prevents pregnancy after unprotected intercourse. The Yuzpe regimen of postcoital contraception, which includes two oral doses each of 100 μg ethinyl estradiol and 1 mg of DL-norgestrel within 72 hours of unprotected intercourse, was first described in 1977 by Yuzpe and colleagues.[8] Similar estrogen-progestin regimens have been used for postcoital contraception ever since, and in 1996, the American College of Obstetrics and Gynecology endorsed their use.[9] In February 1997, the FDA approved the use of combination oral contraceptive pills for this indication. The hormones studied in clinical trials of combination emergency contraceptive pills are found in several oral contraceptive brands available in the United States. Each dose of emergency combination pills contains 100 to 120 μg ethinyl estradoil and 0.5 to 0.6 mg of levonorgestrel.

Preven is the only brand of combination pills specifically formulated for use as emergency contraception in the United States.[10] However, the following contain the appropriate dosage for each dose (initial dose with repeat dose 12 hours later) of emergency contraception: Ovral (2 white pills), Nordette (4 orange pills), Levlen (4 orange pills), Levora (4 white pills), Lo/Ovral (4 white pills), Triphasil (4 yellow pills), Tri-Levlen (4 yellow pills), Trivora (4 pink pills), Levlite (5 pink pills), Alesse (5 pink pills), Low-Ogestrel (4 white pills), and Ogestrel (2 white pills). An antiemetic given 1 hour before each of the two doses will reduce nausea and vomiting.

Progestin-only pills (levonorgestrel 0.75 mg × 2 doses) are another safe and effective method of emergency contraception. A randomized clinical trial comparing combination emergency contraceptive pills with progestin-only pills found that the progestin-only regimen was more effective at preventing pregnancy and better tolerated.[11] Pregnancy risk is reduced by an estimated 74% with the estrogen-progestin regimen and by 85% with the progestin-only method. Regardless of which type of emergency contraceptive pill is selected, a first dose should be taken within 72 hours of unprotected intercourse and a second dose 12 hours later. The efficacy of both methods is highest the sooner after unprotected intercourse the first dose is taken. Plan B is the only progestin-only pill formulated for emergency contraception currently available in the United States,[12] but Ovrette 1.5 mg dose (20 pills of 0.075 mg norgestrel apiece) with a repeat 1.5-mg dose 12 hours later is an equivalent agent.

Less commonly used methods of postcoital contraception include high-dose estrogen (ethinyl estradiol 5 mg daily for 5 days); mifepristone (single 600-mg dose); danazol (400 to 800 mg every 12 hours for 2 doses or 400 mg every 12 hours for 3 doses); and the copper-T intrauterine device (IUD).

The precise mechanism of action of emergency contraceptive pills is unclear. Possible actions include inhibition of ovulation, inhibition of sperm transport through thickened cervical mucus, inhibition of tubal transport of sperm or egg, interference with fertilization, or prevention of implantation. A recent statistical analysis concluded that combination emergency contraceptive pills could not be as effective as they appear to be if their mechanism of action is limited to prevention or delay of ovulation.[13] Emergency contraception is not believed to be capable of interfering with pregnancy once implantation occurs, so by definition it is not an abortifacient. However, because some people oppose contraceptive methods that act after fertilization, health professionals are obliged to explain to patients the potential postfertilization mechanism of emergency contraceptive pills.

Although emergency contraceptive pills are typically prescribed within 72 hours of unprotected intercourse, they can also be prescribed in advance so that they are readily available should the need arise.[14] Since 1997, Washington State pharmacists who receive training in emergency contraception have been permitted to dispense emergency contraceptive pills without a prescription to women who fulfil eligibility criteria. Nearly 12,000 prescriptions were written by Washington State pharmacists during a 2-year pilot of this program. Several other states are investigating the feasibility of similar initiatives.[15]

A recent cross-sectional analysis of more than 1000 women in the United States and 307 obstetrician-gynecologists found that only 26% of women at risk for unintended pregnancy were aware of emergency contraceptive pills and knew that these could be taken up to 3 days after unprotected intercourse. The percentage was even lower among demographic groups at highest risk of unintended pregnancy. Although 83% of women at risk of unintended pregnancy stated that they relied on health professionals for information about contraception, only 7% of obstetrician-gynecologists reported that they usually discussed emergency contraception during routine contraceptive counseling.

Women who are prescribed emergency contraceptive pills in advance of need do not appear to take more chances with contraception than women who are not. Clinicians should inform patients at risk of unintended pregnancy about emergency contraception and either prescribe emergency contraceptive pills in advance of need or ensure that patients know how to obtain them should the need arise.

Cost-Effectiveness of Contraception

Contraception allows women of reproductive age to avoid the costs of induced abortions and unintended births. A recent cost-effectiveness analysis[16] compared the direct medical costs of 15 contraceptive methods: tubal ligation, vasectomy, oral contraceptives, progestin implant, injectable medroxyprogesterone acetate (DMPA), progesterone-T IUD, copper-T IUD, diaphragm, male condom, fe-

male condom, sponge, spermicides, cervical cap, withdrawal, and periodic abstinence. The analysis concluded that regardless of payment mechanism or contraceptive method, contraception saves money. For couples who desire no future children, surgical sterilization procedures are the most cost effective over time despite their higher initial costs. The most cost-effective reversible methods are the copper-T IUD, the progestin implant, and DMPA injectable contraceptives. Barrier methods could become significantly more cost effective if imperfect use was minimized. Emergency contraceptive pills are cost effective regardless of whether they are prescribed after the emergency arises or in advance of need. The IUD is not cost effective if used solely as emergency contraception, but becomes cost effective if its use continues for as few as 4 months.[14]

UNINTENDED PREGNANCY PREVENTION

Despite our understanding of the demography and consequences of unintended pregnancy in the United States, we have limited understanding of how to prevent it. Some of the difficulty in identifying effective strategies lies in the complexities involved in measuring outcomes of prevention programs. In a nationwide search to identify local programs designed to decrease unintended pregnancy, the Institute of Medicine Committee on Unintended Pregnancy identified more than 200 programs. Of those, only 23 fulfilled the committee's inclusion criteria of being well designed, systematically evaluated, completed since 1980, and reported in a peer-reviewed journal.

Analysis of the 23 programs reveals the following information.[2]

1. Because most programs were targeted at adolescents, little is known about prevention of unintended pregnancy in adults.
2. Evidence is insufficient to determine whether abstinence-only programs are effective in delaying age at first intercourse. However, programs that encouraged both abstinence and contraception use seem to succeed in both delaying onset of sexual intercourse and increasing use of contraception in adolescents.
3. Although most programs encouraged contraceptive use, few programs dispensed contraceptives or included specific instructions on how participants can obtain contraceptives.
4. About half of programs that attempted to decrease rapid repeat pregnancy were effective. The optimal time to intervene is in the second postpartum month, when sexual activity typically resumes.

There is a growing emphasis in health education on tailoring educational efforts to the readiness of the individual to change health behaviors. The Transtheoretical Model of Behavior Change proposed by Prochaska and DiClemente[17] and initially used to study smoking cessation has been used to study contraceptive behavior.[18] It asserts that individuals progress through defined stages of decision making before abandoning high-risk behaviors and/or adopting healthy behaviors. With regard to contraceptive behavior, the *precontemplative* stage describes a period in which the individual is not using contraception consistently and does not plan to do so within the following 6 months. *Contemplation* describes the period in which individuals are considering consistent contraception use within the next 6 months. *Preparation* is the period in which an individual plans to begin consistent contraception use within the next month. The *action* stage of change describes the first 6 months after an individual begins consistent use of contraception. The *maintenance* stage of change describes the period starting 6 months after an individual begins to use contraception consistently, and continues until contraception misuse or nonuse ceases to be a problem behavior for the individual. If decisions regarding contraceptive use are reached in a manner similar to that for other health behaviors, such as smoking cessation and weight loss, then unintended pregnancy prevention intervention efforts should be tailored to the behavioral stage of individuals at risk.

One Community-Based Unintended Pregnancy Prevention Program

The Unintended Pregnancy Prevention Program (UPPP) is an intervention designed to decrease unintended pregnancy in a military population (unpublished research protocol No. 97050, Madigan Army Medical Center, Tacoma, Wash). It includes a 3-hour interactive class and a program of enhanced access to contraceptive services. The program was developed after a descriptive study of U.S. Army women presenting for prenatal care found that 55% reported that their pregnancies were unintended and nearly two thirds of women with unintended pregnancies used no birth control during the month they conceived. Military women with unintended pregnancies share many of the same consequences as civilian women. In addition, unintended pregnancy poses substantial costs to military readiness.

The UPPP was implemented on a large military installation in 1997. One distinctive feature of the program is its inclusion of men in the educational program. The entire social and work groups of men and women learn from the same source and share the same health care resources. The UPPP class incorporates many of the principles of adult learning theory. Specifically, the program's design was based on a needs assessment of military women. The curriculum was designed to teach what is immediately useful to program participants and emphasizes respect for each participant's ability to reach the reproductive decisions that are best for him or her. Because adults learn well together in teams, the class incorporates small group activities to allow participants to explore what they have learned. The UPPP includes a measurement of the stage of behavioral change of participants. The program will require further study to determine its effectiveness. It may be adapted to civilian and adolescent populations with few modifications (unpublished research protocol No. 97050, Madigan Army Medical Center, Tacoma, Wash.).

SUMMARY

Unintended pregnancy is a major public health problem in the United States. Among the core goals of the Institute of Medicine Committee on Unintended Pregnancy are to improve knowledge about contraception, to increase access to contraceptive services, and to address the role of feelings and attitudes in contraceptive decisions. Clinicians, by virtue of their access to teachable moments and their opportunity to determine the readiness of individuals to change behavior, are in key positions to promote these goals in the examination room.

References

1. Henshaw SK: Unintended pregnancy in the United States. Fam Plann Perspect 1998;30:24–29.
2. Brown SS, Eisenbery L: The Best Intentions: Unintended Pregnancy and the Well-Being of Children and Families, Washington, DC, National Academy Press, 1995.
3. U.S. Department of Health and Human Services: Healthy People 2010, 2nd ed, 2 vols. Washington, DC, U.S. Government Printing Office, Nov 2000.
4. Abma JC, Chandra A, Mosher WD, et al: Fertility, family planning, and women's health: New data from the 1995 National Survey of Family Growth. National Center for Health Statistics. Vital Health Stat 23 1997;19:1–114.
5. Piccinino LJ, Mosher WD: Trends in contraceptive use in the United States: 1982–1995. Fam Plann Perspect 1998;30:4–10.
6. Tanfer K: Determinants of contraceptive use: A review. Paper prepared for the Committee on Unintended Pregnancy, Institute of Medicine. Washington, DC, 1994.
7. Green LN, Kreuter MW: Health Promotion Planning, an Educational and Ecological Approach, 3rd ed. Mountain View, CA, Mayfield, 1999, pp 152–182.
8. Yuzpe AA, Lancee WJ: Ethinylestradiol and DL-norgestrel as a postcoital contraceptive. Fertil Steril 1977;28:932–936.
9. American College of Obstetricians and Gynecologists: Emergency Oral Contraception (ACOG Practice Pattern No. 3). Washington DC, ACOG, Dec 1996.
10. FDA approves application for Preven emergency contraceptive kit, FDA talk paper T-98-49). Rockville, Md, U.S. Department of Health and Human Services, Food and Drug Administration, Sept 2, 1998.
11. von Hertzen H, Piaggio G, Van Look P, for the Task Force on Postovulatory Methods of Fertility Regulation: Randomised controlled trial of levonorgestrel versus the Yuzpe regimen of combined oral contraceptives for emergency contraception. Lancet 1998; 352:428–433.
12. Food and Drug Administration application 021045, approved July 28, 1999. FDA website: www.fda.gov/cder/da/da0799.htm
13. Trussell J, Raymond EG: Statistical evidence about the mechanism of action of the Yuzpe regimen of emergency contraception. Obstet Gynecol 1999;93:872–876.
14. Trussell J, Koenig J, Ellertson C, Stewart F: Preventing unintended pregnancy: The cost-effectiveness of three methods of emergency contraception. Am J Public Health 1997;87:932–937.
15. Emergency Contraception Collaborative Agreement Project: Expanding women's access to emergency contraceptive pills through

direct pharmacy provision. Program for Appropriate Technology in Health. www.path.org/resources/ec_better_access_to_ecps.htm

16. Trussell J, Leveque JA, Koenig JD, et al: The economic value of contraception: A comparison of 15 methods. Am J Public Health 1995;85:494–503.

17. Prochaska JO, DiClemente CC: Stages and processes of self-change of smoking: Toward an integrative model of change. J Consult Clin Psychol 1983;51:390–395.

18. Grimley DM, Riley GE, Bellis JM, Prochaska JO: Assessing the stages of change and decision-making for contraceptive use for the prevention of pregnancy, sexually transmitted diseases, and acquired immunodeficiency syndrome. Health Educ Q 1993;20:455–470.

Selective Arterial Embolization in the Management of Obstetric Hemorrhage

Vern L. Katz and Honor M. Wolfe

Arterial embolization (AE) is one of the most important advances for the control of obstetric hemorrhage since about 1985. Although not available in every hospital, AE is a technique more effective than hypogastric artery ligation and safer than exploratory laparotomy; it also allows preservation of fertility. As such, AE is changing the algorithm for the management of obstetric hemorrhage.

The technique of AE was first developed in the 1960s with the use of diagnostic angiography for localization of arterial vessels in cases of acute, active gastrointestinal bleeding. Angiography was a useful adjunct when surgical exploration failed to identify the focus of bleeding.[1] In the 1970s, the use of such methods shifted from primarily diagnostic to therapeutic. The use of percutaneous catheters to inject pharmacologic agents for vasoconstriction, balloon occlusion, and arterial embolization became an accepted technique, which is now becoming widespread in surgery, gynecology, and obstetrics.

Sequential surgical ligation of pelvic vessels for the control of pelvic bleeding in obstetrics was reported with success in the 1980s.[2, 3] Reports on the use of AE of these pelvic vessels for control of obstetric hemorrhage began to emerge in the late 1970s. Pais and colleagues in 1980[4] suggested that AE be attempted before surgery for the treatment of obstetric hemorrhage. Brown and coworkers[5] described AE as "an alternative approach" to surgical correction of hemorrhage.

Arterial embolization has several advantages in the control of obstetric hemorrhage:

1. Laparotomy, which can be extremely dangerous in an already hemodynamically unstable patient, often with an associated coagulopathy, is not required. This avoids anesthetic risks and surgical blood loss.
2. Identification of vessels involved in bleeding is definitive with the use of the diagnostic angiographic phase. Additionally, after embolization, hemostasis or the presence of ongoing bleeding can be verified.
3. Fertility is preserved.

POSTPARTUM HEMORRHAGE
Definition and "Traditional" Management

Postpartum hemorrhage (PPH) remains a major cause of morbidity and mortality in the United States and world-wide. It has been defined as either a 10% drop in hematocrit or the need for transfusion of red blood cells after delivery.[6] Conservative estimates suggest that PPH occurs in approximately 5% of deliveries, although PPH requiring surgical intervention occurs less commonly. A comprehensive review of PPH is beyond the scope of this chapter.

The two major etiologies of PPH are uterine atony and lacerated blood vessels, with uterine atony being by far the major cause. Women whose pregnancies are complicated by uterine overdistention, prolonged labor, infection, multiparity, or oxytocin use are all at increased risk for PPH. Initial management includes vigorous uterine massage, oxytocin, prostaglandins, and, in selected cases, methylergonovine (Methergine). If pharmacologic methods are unsuccessful in controlling PPH, experts traditionally have recommended dilatation and curettage (D&C), uterine packing, or laparotomy.

At laparotomy, there are several choices. Most investigators recommend that the initial attempt at surgical control of PPH consist of uterine artery ligation, followed, if necessary, by hypogastric artery ligation. In a retrospective study, O'Leary[7] found that uterine artery ligation was successful in 95% of cases. In view of its relative ease and low complication rate, it is a logical option after failure of conservative management. Ligation of the hypogastric artery involves careful dissection of the retroperitoneal space. This more technically difficult procedure is associated with higher complication rates, including inadvertent ligation of the external iliac artery, ureteral injury, laceration of the internal or external iliac veins, and formation of a retroperitoneal hematoma. In addition, the efficacy of this approach is less than that reported for uterine artery ligation and ranges from 20% to 60%. If either uterine or hypogastric vessel ligation is unsuccessful, then the next step in surgical intervention is hysterectomy.

Conservative pharmacologic therapy followed by sequential surgical intervention has been the cornerstone of management for PPH. AE represents an alternative to laparotomy, concurrent with maintenance of hemodynamic stability, in the patient with uncontrolled PPH. Uterine or vaginal packing may be used as a temporizing measure while preparing for angiographic diagnosis and intervention. Throughout any management schema, attention to hemodynamic stability is essential. Adequate crystalloid and blood replacement, as well as monitoring the coagulation profile, are all critical. With increasing blood and fluid infusions, dilutional coagulopathy will develop frequently, and the patient must be closely monitored for the development of fluid overload, pulmonary edema, or both.

ARTERIAL EMBOLIZATION

Technique

Angiographic AE is a well-established technique for control of bleeding in most areas of the body. The general principles for AE include (1) catheterization of the nearest accessible major vessel, (2) fluoroscopic manipulation of the catheter to the required site, (3) injection of radiopaque dye with confirmation of a distal "blush," (4) placement of the catheter tip into the distal vessel with inflation of a small balloon to prevent backwash of embologenic material, (5) injection of an embologenic material, (6) confirmation of hemostasis with reinjection of dye, and (7) deflation and removal of the catheter.

The pelvic structures are supplied by multiple collateral vessels, as well as an extensive primary circulation. The number of potential bleeding vessels involved in puerperal hemorrhage is a characteristic of PPH that favors embolization over surgery in its management. Many of these vessels are difficult to dissect, with potential for further bleeding and damage to surrounding nerves and vessels. In cases of PPH, the aorta and pelvic vessels are imaged, and an attempt is made to identify bleeding vessels. The catheter is advanced into the internal iliac artery under fluoroscopic guidance. Injection of dye allows identification of specific bleeding vessels, seen as sites where contrast medium pools or extravasates. Following occlusion of the vessel(s), hemostasis can be documented before removal of the catheter.

Although the anterior branch of the internal iliac artery (hypogastric) is usually embolized, bleeding from branches of the ovarian arteries, posterior branches of the internal iliac, lumbar and iliolumbar, and femoral-circumflex arteries have all been reported.[8] Superselective catheterization of specific bleeding vessels is possible but often requires more time than is available in cases of massive PPH. In addition, embolization of the hypogastric artery(ies) is generally effective and complications associated with catheterization of such a peripheral vessel are minimal, especially when compared with potential problems associated with delay in therapy.

Several substances have been used to achieve hemostasis through embolization. The materials can be either absorbable (autologous blood clot, Gelfoam, Oxycel, Avitene) or nonabsorbable (silicone microspheres, dextran microspheres, stainless steel coils, sclerosing agents, liquid polymers). Choice of the material depends on the size of the vessel to be occluded and whether temporary or permanent occlusion is desired. Pelage and associates,[9] in a series of 27 women, used polyvinyl alcohol in 4 patients without problems.

Most investigators have used dissolvable gelatin sponge (Gelfoam, Upjohn, Kalamazoo, Mich) cut into 1-mm slices. In cases of PPH, these pledgets have the advantage of being well tolerated, nonantigenic, easy to work with, and, most importantly, dissolvable within 2 to 3 weeks.[4, 5, 8, 10] Gelfoam powder is not used because of the potential for passage into more peripheral vessels and consequent ischemic damage.[8] After the catheter is placed, dye injected, balloon inflated, and pledgets injected, dye is reinjected to confirm hemostasis. It is important to evaluate other areas to confirm that no additional sources of bleeding are present.

Nearly all authorities have emphasized the importance of correcting any coagulopathies before embolization. Embolization has the advantage of occluding vessels distal to the main vessel embolized, markedly improving its success rate relative to surgical ligation. When consideration is given to AE, the operator should avoid surgical ligation of the internal iliac arteries, because this precludes the most common site of entry for embolization in cases of PPH.

Disadvantages and Complications

Although there are clear advantages to the use of embolotherapy, particularly its efficacy and the avoidance of surgical risks, this method is not suited for every patient experiencing a PPH. Beyond the need for practitioners experienced and skilled in this specialized technique, the greatest limitation of this method is the time required from a request for the procedure until the control of bleeding. This varies from institution to institution, and several estimates from experienced programs have been published.

Hansch and colleagues[11] in a recent review estimated that at their institution the time from notification of a PPH by the interventional radiology department to the beginning of actual embolization was between 45 and 60 minutes. Once the embolization procedure was begun, selective catheterization of the anterior division of the internal iliac arteries was usually achieved within 30 minutes. The investigators conclude that the availability of appropriate imaging equipment and radiolucent beds in a labor and delivery suite could shorten this period of time significantly. They further suggest that installation of this equipment in tertiary care centers be considered. Similarly, Vedantham and coworkers[12] reported that team assembly and patient preparation took 40 to 60 minutes. Although the full procedure time ranged from 1 to 3 hours, adequate hemostasis in major bleeding vessels was generally achieved in 30 to 60 minutes from the onset of the procedure.

Thus, when deciding on the use of embolotherapy for management of bleeding, particularly in the postpartum period, the physician should allow a minimum of 1.5 to 2 hours from "decision" to control of bleeding. It is important to assess the condition of the patient, the rate of blood loss, and the ability of the patient to wait that period of time for definitive intervention to control ongoing blood loss. As AE becomes widespread, we predict that before the patient begins to develop distress from continued blood loss, the practitioner will pack the uterus and call for embolization rather than proceeding down the current algorithm of chemotherapy, D&C, and then laparotomy. If medical management is unsuccessful, the next step will become (1) uterine packing for tamponade, (2) correction of any coagulopathy and anemia, and (3) AE.

Radiation exposure is a second concern in the use of AE, particularly when catheters are placed prophylactically before scheduled cesarean section. It is estimated that preoperative placement of catheters in the anterior divisions of the internal iliac artery can usually be accomplished in less than 5 to 8 minutes of actual fluoroscopy time.[11] During fluoroscopy, radiation exposure to the fetus and pelvic structures is estimated to be up to 2 rad/min. Prophylactic placement of catheters into the internal iliac vessels has been described for situations such as placenta accreta and has been achieved in under 1 minute of fluoroscopy time.[13] Fluoroscopy time is obviously less critical after delivery. The approach to the pelvis is generally obtained in nonprophylactic cases via the femoral arteries to the iliac vessels or aorta. However, before delivery of a viable pregnancy, researchers have used an approach through the axillary arteries to decrease radiation exposure.[11, 13, 14]

Other than radiation exposure and the time involved, specific complications are few. Many patients are already near fluid overload, anemia, and coagulopathy. AE does not affect the course of these conditions. Patients with pelvic hematomas often develop infection, and AE is not thought to affect the management of these infections.

A procedure-related complication is potential ischemia of embolized tissue. Because of the extensive collateral vascularization of the pelvis and the use of Gelfoam pledgets over Gelfoam powder, ischemia is very rare.[10] In close to 100 patients described in the literature, only 1 case of mild, self-limited buttock pain has been described as an ischemic complication.[8] Perforation of blood vessels with the guide wire is a potential complication, as is irritation at the arterial entry site.

Several investigators have reported transient temperature elevations and low-grade fever for 2 to 3 days after embolization.[11, 15, 17] Antibiotic therapy results in prompt resolution of fevers in patients with no evidence of large hematomas. It is difficult to identify the cause of the temperature elevations in most patients, but it is likely a function of devitalized tissues.

It is important to note that no deaths or permanent injuries have been reported with AE for obstetric hemorrhage. This is in contrast to women with gynecologic problems and malignancies, in whom ischemic damage and femoral artery thrombosis have not been reported.

EMBOLIZATION FOR POSTPARTUM HEMORRHAGE

Postpartum hemorrhage is caused in the great majority of cases by either uterine atony or lacerated vessels. If surgical treatment is chosen and bleeding continues, a combination of both etiologies may be involved. Brown and coworkers in 1979[5] reported on the use of AE for a large retroperitoneal hematoma that extended into the rectovaginal septum, occurring after a spontaneous vaginal delivery. The bleeding was managed initially with hypogastric artery ligation. After continued hemorrhaging, catheterization and embolization of the vaginal branch of the internal pudendal artery were successful in stopping the blood loss.

Yamashita and associates[13] described successful AE in six women. Five of the women had vaginal or cervical lacerations secondary to vacuum extraction, and one had a ruptured uterus. Four of the six had large retroperitoneal or paravaginal hematomas. In two of the six women, hysterectomy was performed first. In another, hypogastric artery ligation was attempted before AE. Hansch and colleagues[11] described six women treated with AE, three of whom had uterine atony. Gilbert and associates[17] reported on 10 other women, 3 with postcesarean section bleeding, 4 with vaginal side wall hematomas, and 1 with bleeding associated with a large myoma. Chin and colleagues[10] described a woman with hemorrhage and a large vulvovaginal hematoma secondary to a forceps delivery. In all these cases, arterial embolization was fast and successful in controlling the hemorrhage.

In one of the largest series to date, Pelage and associates[9] reported on 27 women with life-threatening PPH who were treated successfully with embolization. Notably, two patients required repeat embolization 1 day later. All women who retained their uteri had resumption of normal menses. Other case series and reports exist, but they are now much less commonly reported in the literature because the procedure is well accepted and familiar to so many physicians.

Overall, success rates for the use of AE in the control of PPH are above 95%, with a recent literature review quoting a 100% (49/49) success rate for those undergoing vaginal delivery and 89% (16/18) for those delivered by cesarean section.[12]

PROPHYLACTIC CATHETERIZATION

Because of the time involved in achieving hemostasis with embolotherapy and the rapid rate of blood loss associated with PPH, some investigators have described the preoperative placement of catheters with or without embolization. Although not all cases of PPH can be anticipated, careful evaluation by history and ultrasound examination can identify patients at particularly high risk for life-threatening hemorrhagic complications at the time of delivery.

The prophylactic placement of catheters for AE has been reported with great success in gynecologic patients believed to be at high risk for intraoperative blood loss. Mitty and coworkers[14] compared the use of emergency and prophylactic placement of arterial catheters for embolization in 18 patients. Control of bleeding was successful in all nine patients undergoing emergency embolotherapy. Of the nine patients in whom arterial catheters were placed prophylactically, two underwent preoperative embolization, and two intrapartum embolization; the five remaining patients obtained surgical hemostasis without need for embolization. The researchers caution that when embolotherapy is considered, surgical ligation of the hypogastric arteries should be avoided, because it "virtually ends access to the uterine arteries for transcatheter therapy." However, multiple reports have documented successful hemostasis with AE even after hypogastric artery ligation or hysterectomy.[8, 10, 13, 17] Our opinion is that hemostasis can be obtained temporarily with packing, and then embolization should be attempted as a safer alternative.

Dubois and colleagues[16] described two multiparous women with placenta percreta with bladder involvement, diagnosed sonographically. Prior to planned cesarean-hysterectomy, bilateral internal iliac catheters were placed via the axillary arteries, 5-French balloon occluding catheters were secured, and the patients moved to the operating room. The infants were delivered and the balloons inflated. Distal Gelfoam pledgets were injected before hysterectomy and bladder repair. Estimated blood loss was 2000 mL for one of the women, and 1800 mL for the other.[16] Hansch and colleagues[11] described two similar women in whom balloon catheters were placed before a cesarean delivery.

CERVICAL AND ABDOMINAL PREGNANCY

Cervical pregnancies are rare, comprising an estimated 0.15% of all ectopic pregnancies. This diagnosis is associated with major maternal morbidity and historically has been managed by surgical intervention, most commonly hysterectomy, to control hemorrhage. Intraoperative techniques such as bilateral internal iliac artery ligation have been successful in controlling hemorrhage prophylactically, prior to removal of a cervical pregnancy.

Lobel and associates[18] were among the first to report the use of preoperative AE in the management of cervical pregnancy. In two cases of cervical ectopic pregnancies, each at 7 weeks' gestation, AE of the uterine artery permitted pregnancy termination and evacuation without hysterectomy. In the same year, Martin and coworkers[19] reported successful management of intra-abdominal hemorrhage after laparotomy for an abdominal pregnancy, using angiographic transcatheter embolization of a large abnormal arterial branch of the left internal iliac artery.

Marston and associates[20] reported a patient with an 8-week cervical ectopic pregnancy, initially treated with methotrexate, in whom bleeding necessitated emergency embolization with Gelfoam of the anterior division of the right internal iliac artery and the left uterine artery. The patient became pregnant 4 months after this procedure and delivered a healthy infant at term.

Frates and colleagues[21] reported 12 consecutive patients with a sonographically diagnosed cervical ectopic pregnancy with an estimated gestational age of from 5.0 to 7.9 weeks. Embolization of the uterine artery followed by evacuation was successful in the four patients in whom it was attempted. However, the investigators concluded, based on their small series, that injection of potassium chloride was their treatment of choice in the clinically stable patient because it was rapid and less invasive than the combination of angiographic embolization and subsequent dilatation and evacuation.

HEPATIC RUPTURE

Spontaneous hepatic rupture is a rare and life-threatening complication of preeclampsia, with reported maternal mortality rates of up to 86%. Ten percent to 15% of preeclampsia-related maternal deaths result from hepatic rupture. Surgical intervention in such cases is accompanied by massive blood loss and frequently by associated coagulopathy. Surgical hemostasis is often difficult to achieve because of the diffuse nature of liver involvement.

Terasaki and coworkers[22] reported four patients with severe preeclampsia and associated spontaneous subcapsular hepatic hematomas. All four patients, one of whom had failed surgical intervention, had successful transcatheter embolization of the hepatic artery with Gelfoam particles.

In reporting on eight patients with spontaneous hepatic rupture, Stain and colleagues[23] concluded that hepatic arterial interruption is the preferred treatment for spontaneous hepatic rupture in pregnancy. In their series, three of eight patients died: one after operative hepatic artery interruption and two when arterial interruption was used after attempts at localized hemostasis failed. They advise operative interruption if the rupture is discovered at the time of cesarean section and percutaneous angiographic embolization if it is discovered in the postpartum period.

Commonly observed complications after embolization of the hepatic artery include fever, nausea, right upper quadrant pain, and transient elevations of liver enzymes. Unlike the case in embolization of pelvic vessels, more serious complications have been reported after embolization of the hepatic artery, including acute necrosis of the liver or gallbladder, cholecystitis, sepsis, and death.

LONG-TERM EFFECTS

There are questions regarding the impact of selective AE of pelvic vessels on women's menstrual and reproductive functions. Although the literature supports the immediate safety and efficacy of this procedure, its long-term effects have not been well established. However, possibly as an effect of the extensive system of collateral flow in the pelvis, no long-term adverse outcomes related to changes in blood flow have been demonstrated.

Stancato-Pasik and coworkers[15] reported on 17 women who were followed for 1 to 6 years after embolus therapy for obstetric-related hemorrhage. Five women subsequently underwent hysterectomy for indications unrelated to obstetric events or embolization; normal menses resumed in all but one patient whose amenorrhea was medication related, and three women delivered normal, full-term infants.[15]

As mentioned earlier, Marston and associates[20] reported on the successful delivery of a term infant after angiographic embolization for a cervical pregnancy. Greenwood and coworkers[8] in their series also described a patient who delivered a healthy term infant after embolization in a previous pregnancy. Pelage and associates[9] commented on several women who resumed normal menses, one of whom became pregnant by the time their series was in press. Yamashita and associates[13] reported four of four women who resumed menses after AE. Their menses were reported to be normal in regard to duration, timing, symptoms, and amount of blood loss, as well as basal body temperature. Gelfoam is absorbable, and, unlike the case in hypogastric artery ligation, uterine flow should return to normal after recanalization of embolized vessels. Even after hypogastric artery ligation, normal pregnancies may occur.

CONCLUSION

AE is an excellent procedure with much less risk and fewer long-term problems than laparotomy for obstetric hemorrhage. Its primary limitation is the time involved in setup. However, we expect that to change as invasive radiology becomes more common for multiple indications and the various embolizing techniques become widespread. The safety alone, compared with surgery, makes it a procedure that should be considered early in the management of bleeding and considered for prophylactic management in women with potential hemorrhage.

References

1. Baum S, Nusbaum M, Clearfield HR, et al: Angiography in the diagnosis of gastrointestinal bleeding. Arch Intern Med 1967;119:16–24.
2. O'Leary JL, O'Leary JA: Uterine artery ligation in the control of intractable postpartum hemorrhage. Am J Obstet Gynecol 1974;43:849–853.
3. Clark SL, Phelan JP, Yeh S-U, et al: Hypogastric artery ligation for obstetric hemorrhage. Obstet Gynecol 1985;66:353–356.
4. Pais SO, Glickman M, Schwartz P, et al: Embolization of pelvic arteries for control of postpartum hemorrhage. Obstet Gynecol 1980;55:754–758.
5. Brown BJ, Heaston DK, Poulson AM, et al: Uncontrollable postpartum bleeding: A new approach to hemostasis through angiographic arterial embolization. Obstet Gynecol 1979;54:361–365.
6. American College of Obstetrics and Gynecology: Postpartum hemorrhage. (Educational Bulletin No. 243). Washington, DC, ACOG, January 1998.
7. O'Leary JA: Stop of hemorrhage with uterine artery ligation. Contemp ObGyn 1986;28:13.
8. Greenwood LH, Glickman MG, Schwartz PE, et al: Obstetric and nonmalignant gynecologic bleeding: Treatment with angiographic embolization. Radiology 1987;164:155–159.
9. Pelage J-P, Dref OL, Mateo J, et al: Life-threatening primary postpartum hemorrhage: Treatment with emergency selective arterial embolization. Radiology 1998;208:359–362.
10. Chin HG, Scott DR, Resnik R, et al: Angiographic embolization of intractable puerperal hematomas. Am J Obstet Gynecol 1989;160:434–438.
11. Hansch E, Chitkara U, McAlpine J, et al: Pelvic arterial embolization for control of obstetric hemorrhage: A five-year experience. Am J Obstet Gynecol 1999;180:1454–1460.
12. Vedantham S, Goodwin SC, McLucas B, Mohr G: Uterine artery embolization: An underused method of controlling pelvic hemorrhage. Am J Obstet Gynecol 1997;176:938–948.
13. Yamashita Y, Takahashi M, Ito M, Okamura H: Transcatheter arterial embolization in the management of postpartum hemorrhage due to genital tract injury. Obstet Gynecol 1991;77:160–163.
14. Mitty HA, Sterling KM, Alvarez M, Gendler R: Obstetric hemorrhage: Prophylactic and emergency arterial catheterization and embolotherapy. Radiology 1993;188:183–187.
15. Stancato-Pasik A, Mitty HA, Richard HM III, Eshkar N: Obstetric embolotherapy: Effect on menses and pregnancy. Radiology 1997;204:791–793.
16. Dubois J, Garel L, Grignon A, et al: Placenta percreta: Balloon occlusion and embolization of the internal iliac arteries to reduce intraoperative blood losses. Am J Obstet Gynecol 1997;176:723–726.
17. Gilbert WM, Moore TR, Resnik R, et al: Angiographic embolization in the management of hemorrhagic complications of pregnancy. Am J Obstet Gynecol 1992;166:493–497.
18. Lobel SM, Meyerovitz MF, Benson CC, et al: Preoperative angiographic uterine artery embolization in the management of cervical pregnancy. Obstet Gynecol 1990;76:938–941.
19. Martin JN, Ridgway LE, Connors JJ, et al: Angiographic arterial embolization and computed tomography–directed drainage for the management of hemorrhage and infection with abdominal pregnancy. Obstet Gynecol 1990;76:941–943.
20. Marston LM, Dotters DJ, Katz VL: Methotrexate and angiographic embolization for conservative treatment of cervical pregnancy. South Med J 1996;89:246–248.
21. Frates MC, Benson CB, Doubilet PM, et al: Cervical ectopic pregnancy: Results of conservative treatment. Radiology 1994;191:773–775.
22. Terasaki KK, Quinn MF, Lundell CJ, et al: Spontaneous hepatic hemorrhage in preeclampsia: Treatment with hepatic arterial embolization. Radiology 1990;174:1039–1041.
23. Stain SC, Woodburn DA, Stephens AL, et al: Spontaneous hepatic hemorrhage associated with pregnancy: Treatment by hepatic arterial interruptions. Ann Surg 1996;224:72–78.

THIRTY-SIX

Diagnosis and Management of Premature Rupture of the Membranes

Laura A. Gorski and Brian M. Mercer

Preterm premature rupture of the membranes (pPROM) occurs in 2% to 4% of pregnancies. pPROM results in about one third of preterm deliveries, complicating over 120,000 pregnancies annually in the United States. Midtrimester premature rupture of the membranes (PROM), generally defined as occurring between 16 and 26 weeks, complicates 0.6% to 0.7% of pregnancies. pPROM is a cause of significant maternal morbidity as well as infant morbidity and mortality. The frequency and severity of these complications vary primarily with the gestational age at membrane rupture, but also with the underlying pathology and complications related to oligohydramnios and conservative management. In some cases, management will be dictated by the presence of overt intrauterine infection, advanced labor, or evident fetal compromise. However, when the mother is particularly remote from term, conservative management of pPROM may offer the potential for significant benefit to the neonate. In this chapter we address the etiology, diagnosis, and clinical course of pPROM, as well as the maternal and fetal risks associated with conservative and active management. We review the current data regarding adjunctive therapies to conservative management.

Etiology

A number of mechanisms have been proposed for PROM. Generally, these can be grouped into intrinsic membrane weakness, mechanical stress, or ascending intrauterine infection. Factors that could cause weakening of the fetal membranes and have been associated with PROM include poor maternal nutrition, maternal smoking, subchorionic hemorrhage, and collagen deficiency syndromes. Factors associated with mechanical stress or distention include polyhydramnios, twin gestation, and incompetent cervix. Trauma may also be associated with pPROM through an acute rise in intra-amniotic pressure or through the production of occult contractions. The lower genital tract is a potential reservoir for bacteria that may ascend the cervical canal and cause localized decidual inflammation. Membrane protein degradation and local prostaglandin production secondarily cause weakening of the chorioamnion and occult contractions. Intrauterine infection appears to play an important role in pPROM, especially at early gestational ages. Prior preterm delivery and prior preterm labor

in the current pregnancy have also been associated with pPROM. Midtrimester leakage has been specifically associated with amniocentesis, chorionic villus sampling, and cervical cerclage. However, in many cases, the cause of early membrane rupture is unknown.

Clinical Course

pPROM is generally followed by brief latency, with subsequent labor and delivery. At term, half of expectantly managed gravidas will deliver within 5 hours, and 95% will deliver within 28 hours of membrane rupture. After pPROM, half will deliver within 48 hours, and 80% will deliver within 1 week.[1] Regarding midtrimester PROM, half of gravidas will deliver within 1 week of membrane rupture.[2] Alternatively, up to 22% of women with midtrimester PROM will remain undelivered for at least 1 month. With expectant management, a small proportion of women suffering membrane rupture can anticipate cessation of fluid leakage (2.6% to 13%).[3, 4]

Maternal Complications

The incidence of chorioamnionitis after pPROM is approximately 15% to 20% overall. The risk of infection increases with the duration of membrane rupture. This risk of infection also increases with decreasing gestational age at membrane rupture and with digital vaginal examination.[4] After midtrimester PROM, 40% to 60% of histologic specimens demonstrate evident inflammation, and clinical endometritis will occur in 2% to 13% of women.[5] Abruptio placentae (4% to 12%) may lead to PROM, or it may occur secondarily.[6] Amniotic fluid leakage will cease in 2.6% to 11% of pPROM pregnancies and in 9.7% to 21% of pregnancies complicated by midtrimester PROM. (Mercer, 1997). Retained placenta and postpartum hemorrhage necessitating dilatation and curettage (12%), maternal sepsis (0.8%), and death (0.14%) are uncommon but serious complications after midtrimester PROM.[2]

Fetal/Neonatal Risks

Because latency after membrane rupture is generally brief, the most significant risks to the fetus after pPROM are complications of prematurity. For all gestations, respiratory distress syndrome (RDS) is the most common complication. Although some investigators have suggested that membrane rupture accelerates fetal pulmonary maturity, this finding remains controversial. Near term, other serious acute morbidities, including necrotizing enterocolitis, intraventricular hemorrhage (IVH), and sepsis, are relatively uncommon. Alternatively, with pPROM remote from term, there is significant risk of serious perinatal morbidity or death due to extreme prematurity and infection. Infants delivered after pPROM may be at particular risk for sepsis, including group B streptococcal sepsis, owing to the combined risks of prolonged membrane rupture, amnionitis, and low birth weight. In addition, there is a 1% to 2% risk of stillbirth due to umbilical cord compression after pPROM.

Midtrimester PROM is particularly associated with a high risk of perinatal mortality and long-term sequelae. Before the 1970s, delivery in the second trimester was generally associated with rapid neonatal death. However, the limit of potential viability has decreased progressively. Infant survival after delivery at 24 to 26 weeks' gestation is currently reported to be between 50% and 75%.[7] Survival rates after PROM are comparable but decrease in the presence of amnionitis or malformations.

Delivery before fetal viability will result in rapid perinatal death. With conservative management, a survival rate of 23% after PROM at or before 22 weeks' gestation has been reported. Alternatively, those fetuses delivered at 24 to 26 weeks' gestation will have morbidity and mortality appropriate to the gestational age at birth. The incidence of stillbirth subsequent to midtrimester PROM (15%) is higher than that seen with membrane rupture at later gestations.[2] This may be due to increased susceptibility of the umbilical cord to compression or of the fetus to hypoxia and intrauterine infection. Alternatively, this finding may reflect the lack of intervention for fetal distress before fetal viability.

The most significant risks to the fetus after pPROM are complications of prematurity, with RDS being the most common consequence. It is controversial whether or not membrane rupture accelerates fetal pulmonary maturity. Other serious consequences, including necrotizing enterocolitis, IVH, and sepsis, are uncommon near term. Lethal pulmonary hypoplasia and restriction deformities are complications specific to midtrimester PROM. The estimated risk of pulmonary hypoplasia after midtrimester PROM varies greatly, between 1% and 27%. Lethal pulmonary hypoplasia rarely occurs with membrane rupture subsequent to 24 to 26 weeks' gestation, presumably because alveolar growth adequate to support postnatal development has occurred.

The pattern of fetal restriction deformities occurring after prolonged intrauterine crowding is similar to that seen with Potter's syndrome. The nonpulmonary features include abnormal facies and limb-positioning abnormalities. The ears may be low set, and epicanthal folds may be present. The extremities may be flattened and malpositioned. Developmental delay, delayed motor development, cerebral palsy, chronic lung disease, hydrocephalus, and mental retardation are serious sequelae that have been reported to occur after midtrimester PROM.[2] Intact long-term survival after midtrimester PROM has been reported to be 56% to 69%. However, reports of the frequency of complications may be biased owing to the lack of complete long-term follow-up in several studies.

DIAGNOSIS

An accurate diagnosis is critical to the management of suspected rupture of membranes. Over 90% of cases can be diagnosed by means of history and careful physical examination. The majority of patients presenting with pPROM will provide an adequate clinical history, including a sudden gush of fluid from the vagina, followed by continued, uncontrollable vaginal fluid leakage. Occasionally, patients will present with an equivocal history of perineal dampness, intermittent leakage, or an isolated gush of fluid. In this setting, other possible causes of abnormal discharge, such as urinary leakage, excess vaginal discharge with advanced dilatation or membrane prolapse, cervicitis, bloody show, semen, and vaginal douches, should be considered.

The diagnosis of membrane rupture can be confirmed by seeing a pool of amniotic fluid in the posterior fornix or passing through the endocervical canal. Further information can be obtained by swabbing the posterior fornix (avoiding cervical mucus) with a sterile swab. The presence of "ferning" on a microscopic slide confirms the diagnosis. Nitrazine paper will turn blue when exposed to amniotic fluid, but false-positive results may occur with blood or semen contamination, or if bacterial vaginosis is present. Alternatively, false-negative results may occur with prolonged leakage and minimal residual fluid.

Examination should be performed in a manner that minimizes the risk of introducing infection, particularly if early delivery is not anticipated. Digital cervical examination should be avoided if the patient is not in labor, because it may increase the risk of intrauterine infection, and it adds little information to that available with speculum examination. Further, sterile speculum examination can provide the opportunity to inspect for cervicitis, occult umbilical cord, or fetal prolapse; visually inspect for cervical dilatation and effacement (correlation coefficient with digital examination: 0.74); and perform appropriate cultures (e.g., endocervical *Chlamydia trachomatis* and *Neisseria gonorrhoeae*, anovaginal *Streptococcus agalactiae*). Occasionally the diagnosis will remain in question after speculum examination. In this circumstance, amnioinfusion of indigo carmine dye (1 mL in 9 mL of sterile saline solution) can confirm or exclude the diagnosis. The standard for detecting an intra-amniotic infection is amniocentesis with Gram stain and culture. A number of investigators have confirmed the association between Gram stain and maternal temperature elevation, tachycardia, and leukocytosis.

MANAGEMENT

Despite much controversy regarding the management of PROM, there is a consensus in some areas. When the diagnosis of PROM is confirmed, the patient should be carefully evaluated for evidence of advanced labor, chorioamnionitis, abruptio placentae, or fetal distress. Those with advanced labor, evident intrauterine infection, significant vaginal bleeding, and fetal distress are best delivered expeditiously. In the presence of advanced dilatation and membrane rupture, extended latency is unlikely. Further, if fetal malpresentation coexists, there is an increased risk of umbilical cord prolapse. Other than in exceptional circumstances, women with advanced cervical dilatation should be delivered. Intrapartum prophylaxis against group B streptococcus (GBS) is recommended for gravidas delivering preterm and for those delivering at term with membrane rupture ≥18 hours, or with intrapartum fever, unless recent anovaginal GBS cultures are negative.[8]

Conservative management of the patient depends highly on the gestational age at presentation. Optimally, the gestational age will be apparent based on prior clinical examination or ultrasound. In the absence of prior obstetric care, ultrasound should be performed to estimate gestational age and to evaluate the fetus for presentation and malformations when appropriate. Subsequent management can be directed by these findings. If conservative management of pPROM is feasible, the patient should be admitted to a facility capable of emergency delivery and intensive neonatal resuscitation and care. If patient transfer is to be considered, it should be undertaken early in the course of management to avoid emergency transfer once labor or complications ensue.

PROM at Term

The ultimate goal of management after PROM at term is expeditious delivery while minimizing the risk of intrauterine infection and cesarean delivery. The gravida presenting in labor should be monitored for labor progress and fetal well-being, with oxytocin augmentation as required. The gravida presenting without contractions should be offered labor induction. Continuous low-dose oxytocin infusion is acceptable. Both oxytocin infusion and prostaglandin E_2 have been demonstrated as effective for gravidas with term PROM and unripe cervices.[9, 10] Digital cervical examinations should be kept to a minimum. Therapeutic antibiotic treatment may be given for suspected intrauterine infection.

pPROM

Labor induction should also be considered for the woman with PROM and documented fetal pulmonary maturity near term (after 32 to 34 weeks). Expectant management in this setting increases the potential for development of maternal amnionitis, umbilical cord compression, and prolonged hospitalization and increases the likelihood of neonatal evaluation and treatment for suspected infection, despite offering only brief potential increase in latency.[11] Given the risks of conservative management, some clinicians will elect to deliver all patients with PROM at ≥ 32 weeks, regardless of documented pulmonary maturity. Studies evaluating conservative management of PROM at 30 to 34 weeks and 32 to 36 weeks (without adjunctive antibiotics or corticosteroids) have found increased amnionitis and prolonged hospitalization, but no significant reduction in RDS, IVH, necrotizing enterocolitis, or death.

The stable gravida with pPROM remote from term is generally best served by conservative management in an attempt to reduce the risk of gestational age–dependent neonatal morbidity. The patient should be informed that the majority of patients would not have a prolonged latency, but that initial assessment cannot accurately differentiate those who will subsequently develop complications. Conservative management generally consists of modified bed rest, to potentially enhance amniotic fluid re-accumulation and complete pelvic rest to avoid infection. Patients should be assessed periodically for evidence of infection or labor. The presence of fever (temperature exceeding 38.0°C or 100.4°F), uterine tenderness, and/or maternal or fetal tachycardia may indicate intrauterine infection.

Leukocyte counts are nonspecific, especially if antenatal corticosteroids have been administered. If intrauterine infection is suspected and additional confirmation is required, amniocentesis may provide further suggestive information, including a glucose concentration of less than 20 mg/dL, a positive Gram stain, or a positive amniotic fluid culture. The presence of amniotic fluid leukocytes alone is not diagnostic in the setting of membrane rupture. Recent study has suggested that elevated amniotic fluid interleukin-6 levels are associated with an increased risk of intrauterine infection.[11]

During conservative management, the initial step is extended continuous fetal monitoring. Subsequent testing is performed at least daily. Smith and colleagues demonstrated a 32% incidence of variable decelerations after pPROM. Similarly, Moberg and associates demonstrated a 79.9% risk of fetal distress after pPROM, with 76% of patients showing evident cord compression.[12] Whereas the biophysical profile can identify a potentially compromised fetus, the nonstress test provides additional information regarding periodic heart rate changes, including variable and late decelerations, as well as subclinical uterine activity. An abnormal test should result in reassessment of the clinical picture and possibly lead to delivery. Because of the risk of fetal cord compression, women with PROM should undergo early fetal heart rate monitoring in labor.

Antibiotics

The efficacy of adjunctive antibiotics during conservative management of pPROM has been widely studied and summarized in two meta-analyses.[1, 13] It is clear that antibiotics in this setting are associated with an increased likelihood of prolonged latency. The two meta-analyses also suggested a potential reduction in IVH with antibiotic treatment during conservative management. The National Institutes of Child Health and Human Development, Maternal-Fetal Medicine Research Unit, evaluated a regimen of intravenous and oral antibiotics given for 1 week after PROM.[14] No corticosteroids or tocolytics were given. This trial found significant pregnancy prolongation of up to 3 weeks after initiation of therapy, as well as a reduction in the number of infants with serious outcomes, RDS, and necrotizing enterocolitis. Those who were negative for GBS suffered less neonatal sepsis and pneumonia with antenatal antibiotic administration.

Although a meta-analysis of five trials in which corticosteroids were administered found no reduction in neonatal morbidity or mortality with antibiotics, a recent prospective, double-blind trial of women with pPROM (before 32 weeks' gestation) found a reduction in composite morbidity (any instances of death, sepsis, or RDS) with the adjunctive antibiotics.[15] The optimal antibiotic regimen during conservative management of pPROM remote from term has not been established. The National Institutes of Child Health and Human Development trial demonstrated significant perinatal benefit with a combination of ampicillin and erythromycin given intravenously for the first 48 hours, followed by oral amoxicillin and erythromycin for an additional 5 days if delivery did not occur.[14] Two additional trials have found broad-spectrum ampicillin-sulbactam, or the combination of ampicillin-sulbactam and ampicillin-clavulanate, to be superior to ampicillin alone.[15, 16] Limited-duration therapy is generally recommended ($\leq$ 7 days). Regardless of adjunctive antibiotic therapy, the need for intrapartum GBS prophylaxis should be reassessed once delivery is anticipated.[8]

Corticosteroids

The use of corticosteroids after pPROM is controversial. Despite the demonstrated benefit in gravidas with intact membranes, it has been suggested that corticosteroids may not be effective after pPROM because many patients will deliver before accruing the benefit of corticosteroid administration, and membrane rupture itself might lead to accelerated fetal pulmonary maturation. Further, it has been suggested that corticosteroid administration after pPROM may lead to neonatal infectious complications.

Two meta-analyses evaluating the impact of corticosteroid use on RDS after pPROM produced conflicting results.[17, 18] Both studies found significant reduction in RDS with antenatal corticosteroids; one failed to show benefit when the study with the lowest quality score was subsequently removed. The other demonstrated additional benefits of antenatal corticosteroids, including reduced periventricular hemorrhage, necrotizing enterocolitis, and death. A

trial of corticosteroids in women given adjunctive antibiotics after pPROM found a significant reduction in RDS with corticosteroid administration (18 vs. 44%).[19]

A number of prospective trials have evaluated neonatal infection with corticosteroid administration after pPROM. These studies have yielded inconsistent results. Overall, there does not appear to be a significant neonatal risk of infection with corticosteroid use after pPROM (9.1% vs. 7.2%).

The National Institutes of Health Consensus Development Panel recommended corticosteroid use for women with pPROM before 30 to 32 weeks' gestation in the absence of intra-amniotic infection.[20] The available data indicate that the benefit of antenatal corticosteroids may outweigh the risk in these patients between 24 and 32 weeks of gestation. Currently, no data evaluate the potential benefits and risks of weekly corticosteroid administration in this population.

Tocolysis

Prophylactic tocolysis after pPROM has been shown to prolong latency briefly. However, a practice of therapeutic tocolysis only after the onset of contractions has not been shown to prolong latency. No study has demonstrated that tocolytics improve neonatal outcome, but none has evaluated tocolysis when corticosteroids and antibiotics are given concurrently. Possibly, short-term pregnancy prolongation with prophylactic tocolysis would enhance the potential for corticosteroid effect and allow time for antibiotics to act against subclinical decidual infection. In the absence of data, no recommendation regarding tocolytic administration during conservative management of pPROM can be given.

Antepartum Discharge

Generally, hospitalization for bed rest and pelvic rest is indicated after pPROM. With the recognition that latency is frequently brief, that intrauterine and fetal infection may occur, and that the fetus is at risk for umbilical cord compression, ongoing surveillance of both mother and fetus is necessary.

One clinical trial of discharged patients after pPROM has suggested that gravidas can be discharged before delivery to reduce health care costs.[21] Those with pPROM and no evidence of intrauterine infection, labor, or fetal compromise were evaluated in the hospital for 72 hours. Those with negative cervical cultures and no evident labor, intrauterine infection, or fetal compromise were then randomly assigned to either continued inpatient management or discharge. Only 18% of women were eligible for discharge at 72 hours. There were no identifiable differences in latency, nor in the incidences of intra-amniotic infection, variable decelerations, or cesarean delivery. Infant outcomes were also similar, but the trial lacked the necessary power to adequately evaluate the impact of discharge on these outcomes. Because of the potential risks of occult cord compression and abruption, further study is warranted before this practice becomes "routine."

Midtrimester PROM

Initial management of gravidas with midtrimester PROM should reflect the potential neonatal survival. Fetuses presenting at 24 to 26 weeks' gestation are generally considered potentially viable and should be treated conservatively to prolong latency where feasible. Clinical management is generally the same as that of women presenting with pPROM remote from term.

Women presenting with PROM before presumed fetal viability should be counseled regarding the impact of immediate delivery and the potential risks and benefits of conservative management. Counseling should include a realistic appraisal of neonatal outcomes, including the availability of obstetric monitoring and neonatal intensive care facilities. The patient electing conservative management after previable PROM should be counseled regarding the potential for delivery near viability and the risks of extreme prematurity should a brief delay in delivery occur.

There are currently no data on which to base initial management of the woman with previable PROM. The benefits of an initial period of inpatient observation may include strict bed and pelvic rest to enhance the opportunity for resealing and early identification of infection or abruption. Ultrasound should be performed to identify coexistent fetal anomalies. No consensus exists regarding the potential benefits of inpatient and outpatient management in this setting. A number of novel treatments, including amnioinfusion and fibrin sealing of the membranes, have been suggested. However, the clinical utility of these techniques remains to be confirmed.

SUMMARY

Management of PROM requires an accurate understanding of the risks and benefits of continued pregnancy versus early delivery. Knowledge of gestational age–dependent neonatal morbidity and mortality is important in determining the potential benefits of conservative management and risks of delivery. When possible, the treatment of pregnancies complicated by PROM remote from term should be directed toward pregnancy prolongation for reduction of perinatal morbidity due to prematurity. At or near term, pPROM usually is best managed by expeditious delivery with attention to risk factors for perinatal infection, particularly if fetal pulmonary maturity can be documented.

References

1. Mercer B, Arheart K: Antimicrobial therapy in expectant management of preterm premature rupture of the membranes. Lancet 1995; 346:1271–1279.
2. Schucker JL, Mercer BM: Midtrimester premature rupture of the membranes. Semin Perinatol 1996;20:389–400.
3. Johnson JWC, Egerman RS, Moorhead J: Cases with ruptured membranes that "reseal." Am J Obstet Gynecol 1990;163:1024–1032.
4. Schutte MF, Treffers PE, Kloosterman GJ, et al: Management of premature rupture of membranes: The risk of vaginal examination to the infant. Am J Obstet Gynecol 1983;146:395–400.
5. Garite TJ, Freeman RK: Chorioamnionitis in the preterm gestation. Obstet Gynecol 1982;59:539–545.
6. Vintzileos AM, Campbell WA, Nochimson DJ, Weinbaum PJ: Preterm premature rupture of the membranes: A risk factor for the development of abruptio placentae. Am J Obstet Gynecol 1987;156:1235–1238.
7. Stevenson DK, Wright LL, Lemons JA, et al: Very low birth weight outcomes of the National Institute of Child Health and Human Development Neonatal Research Network, January 1993 through December 1994. Am J Obstet Gynecol 1998;179:1632–1639.
8. American College of Obstetricians and Gynecologists, Committee on Obstetric Practice: Prevention of early-onset group B streptococcal disease in newborns (Committee Opinion No. 173). Washington, DC, ACOG, 1996.
9. Hannah ME, Ohlsson A, Farine D, et al: Induction of labor compared with expectant management for prelabor rupture of the membranes at term. N Engl J Med 1996;334:1005–1010.
10. Mercer BM, Crocker LG, Boe NM, Sibai BM: Induction versus expectant management in premature rupture of the membranes with mature amniotic fluid at 32 to 36 weeks: A randomized trial. Am J Obstet Gynecol 1993;169:775–782.
11. Romero R, Yoon BH, Mazor M, et al: A comparative study of the diagnostic performance of amniotic fluid glucose, white blood cell count, interleukin-6, and Gram stain in the detection of microbial invasion in patients with preterm premature rupture of membranes. Am J Obstet Gynecol 1993;169:839–851.
12. Moberg LJ, Garite TJ, Freeman RK: Fetal heart rate patterns and fetal distress in patients with preterm premature rupture of membranes. Obstet Gynecol 1984;64:60–64.
13. Egarter C, Leitich H, Karas H, et al: Antibiotic treatment in premature rupture of membranes and neonatal morbidity: A meta-analysis. Am J Obstet Gynecol 1996;174:589–597.
14. Mercer B, Miodovnik M, Thurnau G, et al: Antibiotic therapy for reduction of infant morbidity after preterm premature rupture of the membranes: A randomized controlled trial. JAMA 1997;278:989–995.
15. Lovett SM, Weiss JD, Diogo MJ, et al: A prospective, double-blind, randomized, controlled clinical trial of ampicillin-sulbactam for preterm premature rupture of membranes in women receiving antenatal corticosteroid therapy. Am J Obstet Gynecol 1997; 176:1030–1038.
16. Lewis DF, Fontenot MT, Brooks GG, et al: Latency period after preterm premature rupture of membranes: A comparison of ampicillin with and without sulbactam. Obstet Gynecol 1995;86:392–395.
17. Ohlsson A: Treatments of preterm premature rupture of the membranes: A meta-analysis. Am J Obstet Gynecol 1989;160:890–906.
18. Crowley P: Antenatal corticosteroid therapy: A meta-analysis of the randomized trials, 1972 to 1994. Am J Obstet Gynecol 1995; 173:322–335.
19. Lewis DF, Brody K, Edwards MS, et al: Preterm premature ruptured membranes: A randomized trial of steroids after treatment with antibiotics. Obstet Gynecol 1996;88:801–805.
20. National Institute of Health Consensus Development Conference Statement: Effect of corticosteroids for fetal maturation on perinatal outcomes, February 28–March 2, 1994. Am J Obstet Gynecol 1995; 173:246–252.
21. Carlan SJ, O'Brien WF, Parsons MD, Lense JJ: Preterm premature rupture of membranes: A randomized study of home versus hospital management. Obstet Gynecol 1993; 81:61–64.

THIRTY-SEVEN

Benefits and Perils of Computers in Medical Care

Mitchell P. Dombrowski, Michael
Dombrowski, and Scott B. Ransom

This chapter provides an overview of benefits and risks of the increasing use of computers in the practice of medicine. We make no attempt at being comprehensive; this would be far beyond the scope of the chapter. Rather, we present information that we think would be potentially useful to most physicians who use computers. We believe that in the next few decades, computerization will dramatically change the practice of medicine.

HARDWARE AND SYSTEMS ROBUSTNESS

It is critical that a computer and its network infrastructure support the demands of a working hospital environment; health care workers must have continuous and reliable access to computerized records and other services. A robust computer infrastructure must also address stringent security requirements. The hardware of a campus-computing environment has three sectors: servers, client computers, and the network that connects them. A failure in any of the components means that data and services cannot be accessed.

To ensure availability on the server level, several steps must be taken. One of the most important is redundancy of critical systems such as power supply. Electrical feeds must be redundant; a short in a junction box should not bring down the whole network. Uninterruptible power supply (UPS) battery backups provide constant power in the case of an electrical failure until power is restored. Redundant servers provide another level of security; if the primary computer fails, the "failover" server automatically takes over operations with no or minimal downtime. Optimally, there should be multiple paths for data to travel from server to client; in case a wire gets cut or a router fails, the network still functions. The client computer is an often-overlooked component of the system. An information technology (IT) department must have adequate spares and be able to replace broken computers in a timely fashion. A computer's software configuration must be sufficiently secure so that the users cannot accidentally change settings, thus disabling the computer.

Many of these precautions are not limited to large, expensive servers and can be used by the home user. UPS devices are inexpensive and prevent data loss in the case of a power failure. Recordable compact disks (CDs) and tape drives can provide essential backups for important files and operating systems. Redundant array of inexpensive disks (RAID) systems allow for uninterrupted functioning in the case of hard disk failure.

VIRUSES

Historically, computer viruses were spread by sharing infected programs or floppy disks. Modern computer viruses can be much more insidious. Viruses can surreptitiously infect the host computer and spread to other computers while waiting for a specific date or command to take further action. Some viruses log keystrokes and send them to a specified email address, thus stealing usernames and passwords.

Sending emails to everyone in the user's address book is also a very common viral practice to infect other computers. One of the most common vectors for viruses is Microsoft's Outlook family of email clients. The addition of multiple features can paradoxically create security holes that can be exploited by virus programmers. Virus writers exploit built-in scripting features that allow them to program Outlook to violate the host's security. An example is the Sircam virus, which randomly sends a user's documents via email to everyone listed in the email address book. The most common method of introducing a virus into a computer is via an email attachment. Attachments from unknown persons should never be opened, especially if they contain a ".bat", ".exe", or ".com" extension. Care must be taken even when opening email attachments from trusted colleagues; their computer may be sending unauthorized virus-containing emails without their knowledge.

Antivirus software such as Norton Antivirus and McAfee's VirusScan offer continuous protection against many viruses. Such software programs scan all incoming email and downloaded files, and periodically scan the computer's hard drives. Owing to the continual introduction of new viruses, a user must remember to have the antivirus scanner updated; most virus-scanning programs can be set to do this at automatic intervals.

HACKING SECURITY RISKS

Home computers are often very vulnerable to other types of attack. Hackers may exploit security holes in a software program running in the background that the user is not even aware is running. File sharing is sometimes enabled for a variety of reasons, and if not properly secured, the entire hard drive contents may be accessible to unauthorized persons. Malicious users can then read private documents and/or gain remote control of the computer. Personal web servers, especially if continuously connected to the Internet, are at risk from unauthorized entry. Web servers may be subjected to hundreds of break-in attempts per day from locations around the world by automated hacking programs.

A common form of hacking called *social engineering* requires no computer knowledge on the part of the perpetrator. A computer user will receive a call or email from a person claiming to be from the IT department asking for that user's password to check for "security leaks," or to make sure that "the email system is working." The IT department should make it clear to their clients that they will never ask for passwords and that any such requests must be immediately reported.

SECURITY LEVELS

In general, electronic medical records should be held to well-established standards of confidentiality and security that have been applied to written medical records. In most circumstances, the written medical record or chart is primarily protected by being stored in a secure place, such as a nursing station. Medical personnel are permitted access to charts by either visual recognition, display of a badge, or other identification. Electronic medical records security can be managed in an equivalent fashion. In high-volume units, such as a labor and delivery triage, an open system (computers without usernames and passwords) is a reasonable alternative. Such open systems must be in a restricted area, such as a nursing station, so that only authorized personnel have access. Personnel have access to view-only medical records that are limited to patients currently admitted to the unit. This is analogous to access to the written medical record. The benefits of a no–log-in open system allow immediate retrieval of prenatal examination records, laboratory data, and ultrasound and prenatal histories by busy medical personnel.[1] A no–log-in system was implemented and has successfully run for a decade without a single known case of inappropriate access.

In contrast, on-campus access to patients in other units or hospitals in a medical system should be secure because the potential for unauthorized access is increased. On-campus authority to order medications and medical or nursing care should be only by a system that identifies the user. Username and password is by far the most common form of authentification currently in place in hospitals. Newer, more robust technologies such as badge scanners, iris scans, and finger- or thumbprint recognition are viable alternatives. Face-recognition technology is a promising system that in our opinion has not yet achieved acceptable levels of reliability.

Off-campus review of patient electronic records introduces new levels of security concerns, especially if access is Internet based. It should be remembered that the security of a system is only as strong as its weakest link. The security of a superbly designed and protected system can be violated by a stolen username and password. The ramifications of inappropriate access to personal and confidential medical records cannot be overstated. Usernames and passwords can be stolen by people observing an individual logging-in, by stealing them from an individual's home computer (see earlier), or when they are "lent" to medical students, nursing staff, or other personnel.

Many administrators assume that a simple username and password is sufficient security to order medical therapy off-campus, typically through the Internet. Log-ins and encryption offer a level of security. The potential ramifications of a stolen password can be horrific. Not only could there be a breach of confidentiality, but there can also be intentionally inappropriate medical therapy ordered for scores of patients. The authors are not aware that this has ever occurred, but any off-campus system that supports medical ordering must be extremely secure.

Unfortunately, most electronic medical systems use a single level of security (username and password) for all levels of security risk. In case of an open no–log-in computer in a secure site limited to only data retrieval, this level of security is too robust and interferes with data access. In cases of off-campus ordering via the Internet, this level of security may be woefully inadequate. The important principle is that the security of an electronic medical system should be tailored to the level of risk.

COMPUTERIZED MEDICAL RECORDS
Decreasing Error Rates in Obstetric Practice

Computerization of obstetric medical records can significantly reduce the error rate. In a 1995 study, computerized admission forms were found to be significantly more accurate than handwritten forms in an obstetric triage unit. Computer-generated admission forms, which included medical history, medications, allergies, gestational dating, and ultrasound and laboratory results, had an average of 0.9 errors compared with matched written admit notes, which had an average of 8.3 errors.[1] Handwritten admission form errors, typically omissions, appeared to be secondary to incomplete assessment of prenatal records. This problem is exacerbated by the hectic and frequently "crisis" atmosphere of a busy obstetric triage center, which is not conducive to accurate and complete assessment of lengthy and complicated prenatal records. Because of its nature, that is, having generally well-defined and delineated problems, the discipline of obstetrics is ideally suited to computerization of the clinical record.

Computers should be designed to minimize the requirements for human functions that are known to be particularly fallible, such as vigilance (prolonged attention) and short-term memory.[2] Software should provide checklists, protocols, and computerized decision aids; physicians should not have to rely on memory to retrieve a laboratory test, and nurses should not have to remember the time a medication is due. Mundane tasks such as these are performed much more reliably by computers than by humans. A computerized medication system can prevent overdoses or administration of incompatible medication or one to which the patient has an allergy. Error reduction in medicine can be modeled after the aviation industry, which relies heavily on standardization and computerization.[2]

In addition to greater accuracy, computerized records have other advantages, including instantaneous access, which can be critical in obstetric emergencies. Another advantage is electronic transmission for review by doctors anywhere in the world. Computerization of the medical record also facilitates research, quality assurance, departmental reports, administrative reporting, and billing. The use of computerized medical records can help control care costs by reducing repeat baseline laboratory tests ordered because of unavailable written records at patient admission.

PEARLS AND PITFALLS

Carpal tunnel syndrome and other repetitive stress injuries are common afflictions for regular computer users. These types of injuries can be avoided or mitigated by maintaining proper posture and using ergonomically designed keyboards and trackball input devices rather than a standard mouse. Operating the mouse on occasion with the nondominant hand will also help. Surprisingly, most computer monitors have their refresh screen rates set at 60 Hz, which can cause eyestrain and headaches even when screen flicker is not apparent to the user. The refresh rate can be adjusted to a more appropriate rate of 70 Hz or greater rate for most monitors by clicking the "Start" button then "Settings," "Control Panel," "Display," "Settings," "Advanced," then "Monitor" on Windows-based computers.

A fundamental advantage of computers is that they are far superior to humans in regard to mundane tasks such as tracking routine events; coordinating events, time, dates, and data, and managing data. Poorly designed software can obviate all theoretical advantages of the computer, especially in cases when a rush is made to introduce computerized medical care. A case in point is a program to track and bill for nonstress testing (NST). This program relies on the person using the computer to confirm the correct date, time, and nursing shift of the NST, and makes no provision for correcting an inaccurately entered nursing shift. This program also relies on data entry that must alternate between keyboard and mouse. Poorly designed programs may decrease efficiency and increase the opportunity for error. Hospitals frequently purchase software systems by departments (e.g., billing, nursing, transcription, departmental) that are incompatible with each other. We have seen nursing stations with as many as five different and incompatible computers.

Physicians may be asked to remember multiple usernames and passwords and are sometimes requested to change them on a monthly basis. In effect, physicians may be asked to remember dozens of different usernames and passwords per year; yet hospital IT administrators may wonder why some physicians resist computerization. A slow log-in sequence is frequently a disincentive for harried physicians to use computers. Many physicians find it easier and faster to simply call the laboratory or radiology for results. Technologies such as biometric identification systems, smart cards, or magnetic-stripe cards can simplify and speed up the log-in process.

A very important advantage of computers is the documentation of events and patient information. Fetal monitoring archiving systems are especially useful. The entire purchase cost can be recouped by the retrieval of fetal monitor strips in a single malpractice case where the paper copies have been lost. Well-designed systems that allow secure and easy retrieval of patient lists, laboratory, ultrasound, radiographic reports, dictation and operative summaries, and consultations, among other data, are a tremendous help. Advanced systems can reduce the error rates of medication orders and can serve to prompt physicians to give care that is consistent with protocols and standards of care. Systems should also document all alterations in charting and ordering by time and personnel.

Computer users should also remember that any entries must be considered to be permanent and irretrievable. A common error is sending emails that in years hence would be damaging. Emails often cannot be deleted by erasing them or even formatting a hard drive; they probably reside on one or more servers. Emails are frequently subpoenaed in lawsuits—much to the dismay of sender and/or recipient.

INTERNET RESOURCES

Most people in North America have access to the Internet either at home, at school, or at work. The Internet provides instantaneous access to information that was previously difficult or impossible to obtain. Much of the information available on the web is accurate and even peer-reviewed, such as in Medline and government institutes. However, physicians and their patients must be aware that thousands of sites purporting to provide accurate information are in reality completely unreliable. Table 37–1 presents a sampling of Internet sites that may be useful to many obstetricians and gynecologists.

TELEMEDICINE

The use of telemedicine and teleconferencing has been increasing. The transmission of real-time ultrasound images (telesonography) has been shown to be reliable and acceptable to both patients and physicians.[3] A bandwidth of

Table 37–1. Selected Internet Resources*

www.nichd.nih.gov	National Institute of Child Health and Human Development
www.cdc.gov	Centers for Disease Control and Prevention
www.acog.org	American College of Obstetricians and Gynecologists
www.genetests.org	Resource for genetic diseases and reference laboratories
www.harrisonsonline.com	*Harrison's Principles of Internal Medicine*
www.ncbi.nlm.nih.gov	National Center for Biotechnology Information
www.ovid.com	Medline (subscription based)
www.google.com	Powerful general search engine
www.bsc.gwu.edu/mfmu	NICHD Maternal Fetal Medicine Units Network
www.ncbi.nlm.nih.gov/PubMed	National Library of Medicine PubMed
www.ncbi.nlm.nih.gov/entrez/query.fcgi	National Library of Medicine Medline
www.nlm.nih.gov/medlineplus/druginformation.html	Prescription and over-the-counter medications
www.rxlist.com	Prescription and over-the-counter medications
www.cochrane.org	Cochrane Library
www.ahrq.gov	Healthcare research and quality
www.hotmail.com	Email service
www.immunize.org	Immunization information
www.mc.vanderbilt.edu/prevmed/ps.htm	Statistical power and sample size software
www.cdc.gov/epiinfo	Epidemiology and statistical software
www.geneclinics.org	Information related to genetic testing
www.corhealth.com	References to multiple medically related sites (subscription-based)
www.colorado-coag.com	Specialized laboratory services including coagulation
www.bloodctrwise.org	Blood products and laboratory services
www.hcfa.gov	Information about Medicaid and Medicare Services
www.nim.nih.gov/nichsr.html	Information from the National Information Center on Health Services Research and Health Care Technology
www.acpe.org	American College of Physician Executives website
www.apha.org	American Public Health Association
www.hrsa.dhhs.gov	Department of Health and Human Services
www.himss.org	Healthcare Information and Management Systems Society
www.jcaho.org	Joint Commission on Accreditation of Healh Care Organizations
www.ncqa.org	National Committee for Quality Assurance
www.webmd.com	WebMD provides a resource for medical information and services

*Services are free unless indicated.

384 kbit/sec was found to provide adequate image quality. The increasing availability and decreasing costs of broadband will greatly increase the feasibility of modalities such as telesonography. Telemedicine has the potential to bring imaging and expert consulting to areas that were previously too small to support specialized services. At this time, the limitations to telemedicine are not technological, but rather are issues relating to cross-state medical licensure, malpractice, and insurance.

BUSINESS STRATEGY AND INFORMATION TECHNOLOGY

IT is a tool to potentially provide a strategic advantage in improving quality, reducing cost, and improving revenues. The purchase and utilization of IT tools should be considered from a strategic perspective. Many large and previously successful health care organizations and providers have purchased expensive information systems without an eye toward strategy. These organizations have often been disappointed and frequently develop a precarious financial situation owing to the purchase of these systems without a real consideration of expected outcomes. The implications on care processes, quality, cost, and revenue should be carefully entertained before making a decision

to purchase an IT product. That is, a purchaser should expect specific outcomes from its purchase, including:

1. Reduced cost of care owing to more efficient processes, reduced duplication of services, and improved throughput
2. Improved revenue collection or capture
3. Improved quality with reduced medical errors and clinical variation
4. Improved perception of quality by consumers by providing direct access to medical records, appointment scheduling, and health information resources

As mentioned previously, IT may provide a strategic advantage to reduce adverse clinical events. Bates[4] showed that the use of a computerized physician order entry system decreased the rate of nonintercepted serious medication errors by more than 50%. IT tools may provide an aid to reduce adverse clinical events, as shown in Table 37–2. In addition, physician order entry reduces the potential for transcription errors by clerks and pharmacists caused by a difficulty in reading a physician's writing.

Computers can provide alerts to the physician for specific issues, including the need to complete an α-fetoprotein test, streptococcal culture, and HIV assessment at an appropriate time for a pregnant patient. Ransom and coworkers[5] showed that 43.2% of medical malpractice cases on an

Table 37–2. Information Technology Tools to Reduce Adverse Clinical Events

Drug allergy alerts
Drug-drug interaction alerts
Drug laboratory alerts
Menu of medications from inpatient formulary
Default doses for each medication
Range of potential doses for each medication
Relevant laboratory results displayed online for a number of medications
Patient characteristic checking (adjusting doses based on age and condition)

obstetric service were related to not following a minimal standard of care for appropriate testing, documentation, and therapeutic intervention, which could be reduced by an effective IT reminder system. Similarly, we showed that 11.7% of all patients cared for on an obstetric service varied from the minimal standard of care owing to physicians and nurses forgetting to complete necessary tests or interventions. IT has a strong potential to improve the care process through automation (Table 37–3) and has great potential to improve clinical quality and reduce adverse clinical events. Nevertheless, before a specific implementation, the purchaser must have a clear idea of the ways the system will affect the care process.

Disease management software has the capacity to enhance clinical and service quality as well as the efficiency of care delivery. IT can assist the disease management process by providing on-line clinical pathways, ordering sets, assembling relevant data and outcome information, and engaging the provider to supply the most cost-effective care process. Disease management programs can facilitate physicians and nurses to become better care managers to improve quality, reduce cost, and enhance revenues. In addition, comprehensive disease management programs improve information access and process efficiency to caregivers, payors, patients, employers, and purchasers.

The health care system must be concerned with the three major aspects of quality: clinical, service, and financial. When implementing an information system, the impact on clinical quality must be considered for such things as adverse drug events, accurate diagnostic testing, and efficient therapeutic interventions. Similarly, service quality

Table 37–3. Process Automation with Information Technology

Bring all information about patient orders together in one location
Increase transmission speed of orders
Reduce or eliminate transcription errors
Eliminate paper orders
Improve legibility of orders
Facilitate JCAHO compliance by improving legibility of prescriber's signature
Optimize insurance contracting
Improve data access to understand care outcomes and quality

JCAHO, Joint Commission on Accreditation of Health Care Organizations.

must be considered in such areas as efficient and possibly patient-directed appointment scheduling, email access to providers by patients, access to medical records by patients with appropriate security and confidentiality provisions, and provision of health information to the population serviced. Last, financial concerns must be addressed as related to information system direct and variable cost, impact on revenue collections, cost reductions, and efficient contracting. Thus, all three areas of quality must be considered in order to develop an optimal health system or clinical practice. While physicians tend to focus on clinical quality, patients generally can understand only service quality, and if the financial situation is not adequate, the provider will go out of business, which will not support the overall quality mission.

A key strategic focus for IT is to reduce the cost of care in two areas:

1. Improved care efficiencies by selecting the most cost-effective diagnostic or therapeutic options
2. Reduced cost of business processes in areas such as contracting, accounting, human resource requirements, and data input

As cost-effectiveness analysis become available, the information system can provide this information to facilitate the care process. For example, cost-effectiveness analysis has been completed to better understand the use of CA 125 testing for an early diagnosis of ovarian cancer. Through direct and immediate access to these cost-effectiveness analyses, the IT tool can provide assistance to select testing only for patients with a net benefit. Similarly, IT tools can facilitate the care of an obstetric patient considering genetic testing. This technology can help the provider council the patient and family on genetic testing based on the patient's specific expectations and risk factors.

The critical success factors in selecting an information system for health care include substantial physician involvement, expertise in systems development, ease of use and speed of the system, well-thought-out implementation policies, and strong support from other administrative and clinical leadership. Further, the IT vendor must be considered for its quality and long-term viability for future product support. While many vendors have pre-alpha, alpha, and beta products with an intent to produce products for IT consumers, the purchaser must be aware of the pitfalls and realities of partnering with a technology company for these products. The IT development process is very time consuming and difficult, with an unknown outcome. Given reasonable expectations, these products may be appropriate; however, the purchaser must be aware of the realities of this option rather than going with an established and known product. Therefore, IT should be considered from a strategic perspective. Substantial and specific benefits should be understood before the purchase of an IT product to coincide with the health care organization's goals and desired outcomes.

References

1. Dombrowski MP, Tomlinson MW, Bottoms SF, et al: Computer generated admission forms have greater accuracy. Am J Obstet Gynecol 1995;173:847–848.
2. Leape LL: Error in medicine. JAMA 1994;272:1851–1857.
3. Landwehr JB Jr, Zador IE, Wolfe HM, et al: Telemedicine and fetal ultrasonography: Assessment of technical performance and clinical feasibility. Am J Obstet Gynecol 1997;177:846–848.
4. Bates D: Effect of computerized physician order entry and a team intervention on prevention of serious medication errors. JAMA 1998;280:15–19.
5. Ransom SB, Studdert DM, Dombrowski MP, et al: Reduced medical legal risk by optimal obstetrical clinical pathway implementation: A case control trial. (Submitted.)
6. Tan JT, Hanna J: Integrating health care with information technology: Knitting patient information through networking. Health Care Manage Rev 1994;19(2):72–80.

Postpartum Endometritis

CHAPTER

THIRTY-EIGHT

Sebastian Faro

Postpartum endometritis is an infection that commonly originates from the patient's own vaginal microflora. The incidence after vaginal delivery is 5% or lower, and after cesarean section is between 10% and 20%, with higher rates occurring in high-risk populations. This infection probably begins during labor. Bacteria advance, during labor, from the vagina through the cervix into the uterus and invade the myometrium. Infection is enhanced by factors, such as cesarean delivery, that decrease blood flow to the uterine tissue. This is seen with incision of the tissue and placement of suture, both of which decrease blood flow to the lower segment of the uterine myometrium.

The infection process begins with bacteria of the vagina ascending through the endocervix, gaining entrance to the decidua, and simultaneously colonizing the amniotic membranes. If the amniotic membranes are ruptured, the bacteria have direct access to the uterine cavity and its contents: amniotic fluid, amniotic membrane, and fetus. Pinell and colleagues[1] demonstrated that facultative bacteria, *Escherichia coli,* and gram-positive bacteria (e.g., *Streptococcus agalactiae*) can reproduce in amniotic fluid during labor. Bacterial colony counts, over a 12-hour period, increase from 10^2 to 10^6 or more bacteria/mL of amniotic fluid. Obligate anaerobic bacteria increase from 10^2 to 10^4 or more bacteria/mL of amniotic fluid. This number is of sufficient inoculum size to initiate bacterial infection.

The vaginal microflora plays a significant role in whether or not the patient is likely to develop postpartum endometritis. In a healthy vaginal ecosystem, the number of potential pathogenic bacteria is typically 10^2 or fewer bacteria/mL of vaginal fluid. This inoculum is insufficient to initiate infection even in the presence of a foreign body. Infection can begin de novo if the inoculum is 10^6 or more; however, in the presence of a foreign body, an inoculum as low as 10^3 bacteria/mL can initiate an infection. Cesarean delivery enhances the risk of postpartum infection because

1. The patient delivered by cesarean section typically has a prolonged labor.
2. The patient usually has ruptured amniotic membranes for a prolonged period of time.
3. Intrauterine pressure catheters and fetal scalp electrodes are used.
4. Numerous vaginal examinations have been performed.
5. The uterus is incised, thus compromising the blood supply to the myometrium in the area of trauma.
6. Use of suture to close the uterine defect can compromise the blood supply further.
7. Extension of the uterine incision during delivery often causes laceration of the uterine artery or its branches; this necessitates the use of additional suture material.

The process of bacterial ascent to the uterus during labor, leading to invasion of the myometrium, usually results in asymptomatic infection during the course of labor. These patients frequently develop chorioamnionitis, which can be asymptomatic as well. Patients who develop symptomatic chorioamnionitis typically experience fever, uterine tenderness, and possibly a dysfunctional labor.

Patients with asymptomatic intrapartum myometritis are likely to fail antibiotic prophylaxis. Additional risk factors for failure to respond satisfactorily to antibiotic prophylaxis are bacterial vaginosis, colonization by *S. agalactiae, E. coli,* or any bacterium that dominates the vaginal microflora, for example, *Lactobacillus.*[2] Typically, the patient with asymptomatic intrapartum myometritis will manifest signs and symptoms of infection within 12 to 24 hours of delivery.

The diagnosis of postpartum endometritis may be subtle or apparent. The diagnosis is suspected when a patient presents with the following:

1. An oral body temperature of 100.4°F or greater measured on two occasions and taken at least 6 hours apart, or a temperature 101°F or greater.
2. Presence of tachycardia that parallels the rise in temperature.
3. A white blood cell (WBC) count 14,000 or higher or greater than 10% in band forms.
4. Failure of the uterus to show signs of significant involution.
5. Cervix remains dilated.
6. Lochia can have an anaerobic odor.
7. Lochia can be purulent.
8. Uterus and parametria are tender to palpation.
9. Parametrium can be indurated.
10. Evidence of pelvic peritonitis may be present.
11. Patient may have evidence of an adynamic ileus.

The bacteria that are most likely to cause early postpartum endometritis, or infection occurring within the first 12 to 24 hours, are *S. agalactiae, E. coli, Gardnerella vaginalis,* and *Enterococcus faecalis.* Typically, early infection is unimicrobial but can involve anaerobic bacteria, for example, *Prevotella bivia* or *Peptostreptococcus.* Endometrial specimens for the culture of aerobic, facultative, and obligate anaerobic bacteria can be helpful, especially for the patient who fails to respond to initial empirical antibiotic therapy. It is not inappropriate to initiate treatment with a single antibiotic instead of using a combination (Table 38–1).

The range of activity of the new expanded-spectrum agents offers the opportunity to use single-agent therapy

181

Table 38–1. Intravenous Antibiotic Choices for the Treatment of Postpartum Endometritis

Piperacillin/tazobactam 3.375 g q6h
Ampicillin/sulbactam 3 g q6h
Ticarcillin/clavulanic acid 3.1 g q6h
Cefoxitin 2 g q6h
Ceftizoxime 2 g q8h
Cefotetan 2 g q12h
Clindamycin 900 mg q8h or metronidazole 500 mg q8h plus gentamicin 5 mg/kg body weight q24h (+ ampicillin 2 g q6h)
L-Ofloxacin 500 mg q24h (if the patient is not breastfeeding)
Clindamycin or metronidazole plus ofloxacin 400 mg q12h (if not breastfeeding)

and not sacrifice efficacy. The one potential complicating factor is that almost all patients delivered by cesarean section receive antibiotic prophylaxis. This is in contradistinction to the patients undergoing vaginal delivery, who do not receive antibiotic prophylaxis unless they have a heart condition necessitating the use of such therapy.

Typically, cephalosporins are almost universally chosen for prophylaxis. These agents do select for resistant bacteria, for example, *E. faecalis, E. coli,* and *Enterobacter cloacae.*[3, 4] This should be taken into consideration when initiating empirical antibiotic therapy for the treatment of postpartum endometritis. One should not specifically direct therapy against these bacteria, but appropriate choices can be made that will provide coverage against most of the bacteria.

Patients who develop postpartum endometritis typically respond to therapy within 48 to 72 hours of initiating antibiotic therapy. Those not demonstrating significant improvement within this time frame or with evidence of deterioration should be considered failures. Waiting longer for a positive response can result in the patient developing myometrial microabscesses and/or myonecrosis of the myometrium.[5] Thus, patients who have not demonstrated a positive response to antibiotic therapy within 48 hours should be thoroughly re-evaluated. A computed tomography scan of the pelvis can assist in determining if there is gas in the myometrium, necrosis of the myometrium, and/or pelvic vein thrombosis.

Patients with recurring high spiking temperatures and WBC counts of 20,000 or higher and a benign or unrewarding physical examination should be considered to have septic pelvic vein thrombosis. This patient should receive heparin 10,000 U as a loading dose intravenously and 1000 units/hr. The patient should also be maintained on antibiotic therapy until she is afebrile for 72 hours and the WBC count has returned to normal.

Individuals failing initial therapy still considered to have postpartum endometritis should have therapy expanded if they are being treated with a single agent. If they are receiving a cephalosporin, consider changing to a penicillin plus gentamicin. If they are receiving a combination of clindamycin or metronidazole plus gentamicin, add ampicillin. If they are receiving triple antibiotics, consider discontinuing gentamicin and adding amikacin until the bacteria causing the infection have been identified.

If the patient is receiving triple antibiotics and not responding, consider one of the following: myometrial abscesses, pelvic abscess, myonecrosis of the uterus, or septic pelvic vein thrombosis. Individual myometrial abscesses and/or myonecrosis of the uterus will not respond to antibiotic therapy because the underlying mechanism causing this is thrombosis of the uterine vasculature, thereby preventing sufficient blood flow to the myometrium, resulting in the failure to achieve adequate antibiotic levels in the myometrial tissue. These individuals will require hysterectomy to prevent sepsis, septic shock, and death.

Individuals considered to have septic pelvic vein thrombosis should receive heparin and antibiotic therapy. Heparin is administered as follows: 10,000 U intravenously as a loading dose followed by 1000 units/hr. Once the patient has become afebrile for 72 hours and there is no evidence of disseminated thrombi, the heparin and antibiotic therapy can be discontinued. In patients with evidence of disseminated thrombi—for example, deep vein thrombosis of an extremity, vena caval thrombosis, or pulmonary embolus—anticoagulation should be carried out for 6 months.

Patients with a WBC count of 13,000 or higher but 16,000 or lower and an unremarkable physical examination—that is, no localizing signs of infection, but may have general malaise and myalgias—should be considered to have a viral infection. These individuals do not need antibiotic therapy because it is ineffective against viral infection. These individuals usually have spiking temperatures, for example, 103°F or higher and experience spontaneous resolution of their disease within 48 to 72 hours.

Individuals with high spiking temperature or low-grade temperature and a negative physical examination should be considered to have drug fever. There is nothing pathognomonic concerning drug fever; however, approximately 50% of the patients can have an eosinophilia. Discontinuing all antibiotics and nonvital medications should result in resolution of the fever within 24 hours.

Postpartum endometritis is not an uncommon infection after delivery by cesarean section. Most women will respond, approximately 80% to 90%, to initial empirical therapy. However, this fact should not give the physician a false sense of confidence, and therefore, this infection should not be taken lightly. Women developing postpartum endometritis can manifest the disease soon after delivery, within 12 hours as seen with *S. agalactiae,* or late in the postpartum period. The disease can have a rapid course, and the patient can develop septic shock, adult respiratory distress syndrome, and death. Patients developing fever after delivery should be thoroughly evaluated, and antibiotic therapy should be instituted without delay if bacterial infection is suspected.

References

1. Pinell P, Faro S, Roberts S, et al: Intrauterine pressure catheter in labor: Associated microbiology. Infect Dis Obstet Gynecol 1993;1:60–64.
2. Faro S, Cox SM, Phillips LE, et al: Influence of antibiotic prophylaxis on vaginal microflora. J Obstet Gynaecol 1986;6(Suppl 1):4s–7s.
3. Faro S, Martens MG, Hammill HA, et al: Antibiotic prophylaxis: Is there a difference? Am J Obstet Gynecol 1990;162:900–907.
4. Martens MG, Faro S, Maccato M, et al: Susceptibility of female pelvic pathogens to oral antibiotic agents in patients who develop postpartum endometritis. Am J Obstet Gynecol 1991;164:1383–1386.
5. Gilstrap LC III, Faro S: Infections in Pregnancy, 2nd ed. New York, John Wiley & Sons, 1997.

THIRTY-NINE

Management of Antiphospholipid Syndrome

Robert M. Silver

Antiphospholipid antibodies (aPLs) are a heterogeneous group of autoantibodies that bind to epitopes expressed by negatively charged phospholipids, proteins, or a protein-phospholipid complex. Although several have been characterized, two aPLs, lupus anticoagulant (LA) and anticardiolipin antibodies (aCLs) are best characterized and generally accepted as having clinical relevance. Circulating levels of these antibodies are associated with several medical problems, including pregnancy loss, arterial and venous thrombosis, and autoimmune thrombocytopenia. In addition to fetal loss, several obstetric disorders have been associated with aPLs. Successful pregnancies are often complicated by preeclampsia, intrauterine growth retardation (IUGR), abnormal fetal heart rate tracings, and preterm delivery.

ANTIPHOSPHOLIPID SYNDROME

When characteristic clinical features occur in a patient with specified levels of aPLs, the patient is considered to have antiphospholipid syndrome (APS).

Clinical Criteria

1. *Vascular thrombosis*
   a. One or more episodes of arterial, venous, or small vessel thrombosis, in any tissue or organ, confirmed by imaging, Doppler studies, or histopathology
2. *Pregnancy morbidity*
   a. One or more unexplained fetal deaths of a morphologically normal fetus at or beyond the 10th week of gestation, with normal fetal morphology documented by ultrasound or direct examination of the fetus, or
   b. One or more premature births of a morphologically normal neonate at or before the 34th week of gestation because of severe preeclampsia or severe placental insufficiency, or
   c. Three or more unexplained consecutive spontaneous abortions before the 10th week of gestation with no evidence of maternal anatomic abnormalities, hormonal abnormalities, or parental balanced translocations.

Laboratory Criteria

1. *aCL* of immunoglobulin G (IgG) and/or IgM isotype in blood, present in medium or high titer, on two or more occasions, 8 weeks or more apart, and measured by a standardized enzyme-linked immunosorbent assay (ELISA) for β_2-glycoprotein-I (β_2-GP-I)–dependent aCLs, or
2. *LA* present in serum on two or more occasions 8 weeks or more apart and detected according to the guidelines of the Scientific and Standardization Committee (SSC) subcommittee on Lupus Anticoagulants/phospholipid dependent antibodies.

Connective tissue diseases, especially systemic lupus erythematosus (SLE), have also been associated with APS. Patients meeting criteria for APS who also have underlying autoimmune disease are considered to have "secondary" APS. "Primary" APS is diagnosed when individuals do not have another multisystem autoimmune disorder.

PREGNANCY LOSS AND ANTIPHOSPHOLIPID ANTIBODIES

A relationship between circulating aPLs and pregnancy loss has been recognized since the 1950s, and numerous studies have confirmed the association. Indeed, the rate of pregnancy loss in untreated patients with APS has been reported to be as high as 90%. A relatively large proportion of aPLs-related pregnancy losses are second or early third trimester fetal deaths. Fifty percent of pregnancy losses in a large cohort of women with APS at the University of Utah were fetal deaths and over 80% of women with APS suffered at least one fetal death.[1, 2] Thus, clinicians should be suspicious of APS in women with unexplained fetal death.

aPLs also account for some cases of recurrent spontaneous abortion. Positive tests for aPLs have been detected in up to 20% of women with recurrent pregnancy loss. However, many of these positive tests are for low levels of aPLs, or aPLs other than LA or aCLs. Low positive levels of aPLs and aPLs other than LA and aCLs (see later) are of questionable clinical relevance. At the University of Utah, APS is the cause in 4% to 5% of unselected couples with recurrent spontaneous abortion.

As opposed to recurrent pregnancy loss or fetal death, aPLs have not been associated with sporadic spontaneous abortions. This is not surprising, given the myriad causes of individual pregnancy loss and the infrequency of APS.

OBSTETRIC FEATURES OF ANTIPHOSPHOLIPID SYNDROME

Successful pregnancies in women with APS are often complicated by obstetric disorders associated with abnormal placentation. Very high rates of preeclampsia have been reported in women with well-characterized APS. At the University of Utah, half of the women with APS developed preeclampsia and a quarter had severe preeclampsia. APS is also an important cause of *very severe preeclampsia*. Several studies have noted aPLs in approximately 15% of women with early-onset (<34 weeks) severe preeclampsia.[1, 2] Testing for aPLs is recommended for women developing severe preeclampsia before 34 weeks' gestation but not for those with mild disease or preeclampsia at term.

IUGR is also common. IUGR has been reported in one third of APS pregnancies. However, aPLs have not been demonstrated to be a common cause of idiopathic growth impairment. Similarly, abnormal fetal heart rate tracings requiring delivery occur in half of pregnancies complicated by APS. As with IUGR, aPLs are rarely found in idiopathic cases of abnormal fetal heart rate tracings. Thus, idiopathic IUGR and "fetal distress" are not indications for testing for aPLs in the absence of other features of APS.

These obstetric disorders all dramatically increase the risk of preterm delivery in women with APS. Patients should be counseled that they have up to a 40% chance of delivering before 34 weeks' gestation if they are fortunate enough to achieve a live birth.

MEDICAL FEATURES OF ANTIPHOSPHOLIPID SYNDROME

One of the most worrisome complications of APS is thrombosis. A majority of thrombotic events (65% to 70%) are venous, but arterial thromboses and stroke are also common. The most common site of venous thrombosis is the lower extremity, and up to one third of patients will have at least one pulmonary embolus. However, thromboses in unusual locations have been reported in association with APS; hence, thrombosis in an unusual location should cause the clinician to contemplate this diagnosis. Unexplained venous thrombosis should be considered an indication for testing for aPLs, which are present in approximately 2% of cases.

Similarly, unexplained arterial thrombosis is also an indication for aPL testing. APS may explain up to 40% of cerebrovascular accidents in otherwise healthy individuals under age 50 years. Arterial thromboses can also occur in unusual locations, such as the retinal artery.

Both pregnancy and oral contraceptive use appear to increase the risk of thromboembolism in women with APS. In fact, the prospective risk of thrombosis has been reported as 5% to 12% during pregnancy and the puerperium. Thus, prophylactic anticoagulant therapy should be considered during pregnancy and the postpartum period (see later). In addition, women with APS should not be treated with estrogen-containing oral contraceptives.

Autoimmune thrombocytopenia is also strongly associated with aPL. Although APS-related thrombocytopenia is difficult to distinguish from idiopathic thrombocytopenic purpura, the two disorders are treated similarly. Numerous other medical disorders associated with APS include autoimmune hemolytic anemia, livedo reticularis, chorea gravidarum, pyoderma-like leg ulcers, and transverse myelitis.

LABORATORY TESTING FOR ANTIPHOSPHOLIPID ANTIBODIES

Laboratory testing for aPLs is a relatively new science that is still evolving. Problems have included nonstandardized assays, interlaboratory variation of assays, and confusion as to which aPLs to test for. Many of these issues are being resolved through international workshops, but the clinician is best served by utilizing a laboratory with a special interest and expertise in aPL testing.

The two aPLs that are best characterized and recommended for clinical use are LA and aCLs. The antibody causing a false-positive serologic test for syphilis is an aPL often present in individuals with LA and aCLs. However, it is not recommended for routine testing because the relationship between it and clinical disorders is less clear. Similarly, other aPLs such as antiphosphatidylserine antibodies (aPSs) are sometimes present in patients with APS. However, most individuals with aPSs also have LA or aCLs. Also, assays for aPLs other than LA and aCLs have not been subjected to any standardization. Thus, although assays for additional aPLs may prove useful, they cannot be recommended for routine clinical use at present.

"LA" is a classic misnomer and an unusual name for an autoantibody. Recall that many individuals with LA do not have SLE, and LA is associated with thrombosis, not anticoagulation. LA is detected in plasma using any of several phospholipid-dependent clotting assays. Examples include the activated partial thromboplastin time (APTT), dilute Russell viper venom time, and Kaolin clotting time. If LA is present, it will bind to phospholipid used in the assays, thus interfering with the assay and resulting in an apparent prolongation of the clotting time. This observation prompted the term *anticoagulant*. The sensitivity of these tests for LA is greatly affected by the reagents used and varies among laboratories.

Factors other than LA—for example, improperly processed specimens, clotting factor deficiencies, or anticoagulant medications—can also result in an apparent prolongation of clotting time. Thus, plasmas suspected of containing LA should undergo confirmatory testing. First, a mixing study is done wherein the patient's plasma is "mixed" with normal plasma. If an inhibitory antibody such as LA is present, the clotting test will remain abnormal. However, if the patient has a clotting factor deficiency, adding normal plasma will correct the clotting time. A second confirmatory test involves the addition or removal of phospholipid to the plasma. For example, if pretreatment with phospholipid normalizes the clotting time (by binding LA and removing it from the reaction), the patient is considered to have LA.

The clinician should order an LA screen, which will include some combination of phospholipid-dependent clotting assays and confirmatory tests. Regardless of the assay used, LA cannot be quantified and is reported as present or absent.

aCLs are detected by immunoassays. Interlaboratory variation in these assays prompted the development of standard sera, which can be obtained from the Antiphospholipid Standardization Laboratory in Atlanta, Georgia. Assays using standard sera are reliable and allow for the semiquantitation of antibody levels, reported as IgG binding units for IgG aCLs, IgM binding units for IgM aCLs, and IgA binding units for IgA aCLs. Results are reported as negative or low, medium, or high positive. Medium or high-positive IgG aCLs correlate well with clinical disorders and are considered to be laboratory criteria for APS. Low-positive results and isolated IgM or IgA antibodies are common, nonspecific, and of questionable clinical relevance. They should not be considered diagnostic of APS.

There is substantial overlap between LA and aCLs but the correlation is imperfect. Because both LA and aCLs independently correlate with clinical disorders, testing for both LA and aCLs is recommended.

Another controversial issue is whether or not individuals suspected of having APS should be tested for antibodies against β_2-GP-I (anti-β_2-GP-I). It appears that β_2-GP-I, an abundant circulating glycoprotein, may be the true epitope for aCLs. Also, aCLs that are associated with clinical features of APS require β_2-GP-I for binding. Fortunately, commercially available tests for aPLs all contain β_2-GP-I in the assay, and are β_2-GP-I dependent. Antibodies against β_2-GP-I can be directly measured and have been associated with the medical features of APS. However, the association between anti-β_2-GP-I and obstetric complications of APS is less clear. As with "other aPLs," testing for anti-β_2-GP-I in women with pregnancy loss or obstetric features of APS is not currently recommended.

Indications for Antiphospholipid Antibody Testing

1. Three or more first-trimester pregnancy losses
2. Unexplained second- or third-trimester fetal death
3. Severe preeclampsia less than 34 weeks' gestation
4. Unexplained arterial or venous thrombosis
5. Autoimmune thrombocytopenia
6. Stroke, transient ischemic attacks, or amaurosis fugax, especially in patients less than 50 years old
7. Autoimmune hemolytic anemia
8. SLE
9. False-positive serologic test for syphilis
10. Unexplained severe fetal growth impairment or uteroplacental insufficiency (testing of questionable benefit in the absence of other clinical features of APS)

Obstetric Management of Antiphospholipid Syndrome

Extremely high rates of pregnancy loss and obstetric complications prompted clinicians to seek treatments for use during pregnancy to improve fetal outcome. Although still unproved in optimally designed clinical trials, accumulating evidence indicates that fetal survival is dramatically improved in treated pregnancies.

Medical treatments are based on proposed mechanisms of fetal loss in women with APS. Strategies intended to suppress the immune system include administration of steroids and intravenous immune globulin (IVIG). Heparin and other anticoagulants are intended to prevent thrombosis in the uteroplacental circulation, and low-dose aspirin can increase the prostacyclin-to-thromboxane ratio by suppressing platelet production of thromboxane.

Considerable success has been reported after treatment with either high-dose prednisone (40 mg/day) and low-dose aspirin (81 mg/day) or prophylactic doses of heparin (e.g., 5000 to 10,000 U/day) and low-dose aspirin. At the University of Utah, both regimens have resulted in a 70% success rate in a cohort of women with only a 10% live-birth rate in previous pregnancies. In a small randomized trial by Cowchock and colleagues,[3] both prednisone and heparin were equally efficacious, but prednisone had more side effects. Because heparin has fewer side effects and may also provide prophylaxis against thrombosis, heparin and low-dose aspirin are recommended as primary therapy. Low-molecular-weight heparin has been used safely during pregnancy and may eventually replace unfractionated heparin.

Heparin use has several adverse effects, including bleeding, thrombocytopenia, and osteopenia, that can lead to vertebral compression fractures. Because the risks of osteoporosis and bleeding increase with increasing doses of heparin and "anticoagulant" doses of heparin are not superior to "prophylactic" doses with regard to fetal outcome, prophylactic doses should be used in the absence of acute thrombosis. Also, weight-bearing exercise and calcium and vitamin D supplementation should be encouraged to diminish the risk of osteoporosis. Heparin and high-dose prednisone should not be used simultaneously because they both predispose women to osteopenic fractures and combination therapy is no better than either drug alone.

Therapy should be initiated after confirmation of a viable embryo with cardiac activity. Any theoretical (and unproven) benefit of preconception treatment is offset by the side effects of prolonged therapy. Thromboprophylaxis should be continued during the postpartum period because of the risk of thromboembolism. Coumarin can be used postpartum to limit the risk of heparin-induced osteoporosis.

IVIG has been extremely promising in a small number of cases that were refractory to heparin or prednisone. However, it did not improve obstetric outcome beyond that achieved with heparin and low-dose aspirin in a recently completed pilot, randomized, controlled trial. Given that IVIG is extremely expensive, it cannot be recommended as primary therapy without further proof of efficacy.

Ideally, women with APS should receive preconceptional counseling regarding their risk for fetal loss, preterm birth, preeclampsia, fetal growth impairment, cesarean delivery, and thromboembolism. They should also have confirmation of relevant levels of aPLs. However, once the diagnosis of APS is made, serial antibody determinations are unnecessary. Intensive surveillance (weekly clinic visits and biweekly nonstress tests) for preeclampsia, fetal growth impairment, and uteroplacental insufficiency should be instituted at 30 to 32 weeks' gestation. Earlier (24 to 25 weeks' gestation) and more frequent ultrasounds and fetal testing are indicated in selected cases—for example, women with poor obstetric histories, fetal growth retardation, or preeclampsia. We and others have noted spontaneous decelerations in the second trimester in APS pregnancies. Intervention with preterm delivery may improve fetal outcome in severe cases. Finally, women with SLE, autoimmune thrombocytopenia, or other related diseases should receive specialized care as appropriate.

MEDICAL MANAGEMENT OF ANTIPHOSPHOLIPID SYNDROME

Women with APS are at substantial risk for the development of nonobstetric medical problems associated with aPLs. Individuals with previous thromboses and APS

should receive lifelong anticoagulation with coumarin to achieve an international normalized ratio of 2.5 to 3.0. Acute thromboses require anticoagulation with heparin to elevate the APTT to 1.5 to 2 times normal. Phospholipid-dependent clotting assays, such as the APTT, cannot be used to assess anticoagulation in women with LA. Anticoagulation is considered adequate when the thrombin time is elevated to 100 seconds or greater. It is unclear whether patients with APS and no previous thromboses require treatment. The issue is currently being studied. Meanwhile, these women should probably avoid estrogen-containing oral contraceptives and use thromboprophylaxis in high-risk circumstances, such as surgery and pregnancy.

Suggestions for Future Reading

Branch DW, Silver RM: Antiphospholipid Syndrome. American College of Obstetricians and Gynecologists Educational Bulletin No. 224, 1998.
Silver RM, Branch DW: Autoimmune disease in pregnancy. Clin Perinatol 1997;24:291–320.
Silver RM, Branch DW: Sporadic and recurrent pregnancy loss. In Reece EA, Hobbins JC (eds): Medicine of the Fetus and Mother, 2nd ed. Philadelphia, JB Lippincott, 1999a, pp. 195–216.
Silver RM, Branch DW: Immunologic disorders. In Creasy RK, Resnick R (eds): Maternal-Fetal Medicine: Principles and Practice, 4th ed. Philadelphia, WB Saunders, 1999b, pp. 465–483.

References

1. Branch DW, Silver RM, Blackwell JL, et al: Outcome of treated pregnancies in women with antiphospholipid syndrome: An update of the Utah experience. Obstet Gynecol 1992;80:614–620.
2. Branch DW, Andres R, Digre KB, et al: The association of antiphospholipid antibodies with severe preeclampsia. Obstet Gynecol 1989;73:541–545.
3. Cowchock FS, Reece EA, Balaban D, et al: Repeated fetal losses associated with antiphospholipid antibodies: A collaborative randomized trial comparing prednisone to low-dose heparin treatment. Am J Obstet Gynecol 1992;166:1318–1327.

CHAPTER FORTY

Induction of Ovulation

Kevin T. McGinnis and Kenneth A. Ginsburg

In the course of their reproductive life, about 15% of women will encounter the emotionally devastating problem of infertility. Whereas some of these women may go on to conceive on their own, a large number will seek help from their physician. Ovulation induction is an important tool for the gynecologist working with a patient trying to achieve pregnancy.

In this chapter we will provide an overview of the techniques of ovulation induction. A more detailed review is available in the classic texts of Speroff and associates and Seibel.[1–3]

In the normal menstrual cycle, a large number of ovarian follicles are recruited toward the end of the luteal phase of the previous menstrual cycle. Additional development of this cohort of recruited follicles is then further stimulated by endogenous follicle-stimulating hormone (FSH) released during the follicular phase of the current cycle until (usually) a single follicle is selected as the dominant follicle. With the selection of this dominant follicle, the remainder of the follicles in the cohort regress through a process of atresia. Luteinizing hormone (LH) is also required in this process to stimulate the production of androgens (particularly androstenedione) in the outer theca layer surrounding the follicle. This is then converted by the granulosa layer to estradiol (E_2). This production of E_2 provides key feedback to the hypothalamic-pituitary axis (in addition to the action of other ovarian factors, such as inhibin) both controlling the level of FSH in a negative feedback loop and triggering the gonadotropin surge at midcycle, which results in ovulation.

Ovulation induction is a process employing a variety of medications to hormonally produce a state of controlled ovarian hyperstimulation in order to induce the continued development of multiple ovarian follicles from the initially recruited cohort of follicles. Ovulation induction is generally used in conjunction with timed intercourse or intrauterine insemination, in order to optimize the chance of achieving pregnancy.

Three classes of medications are used for ovulation induction. (1) Estrogen antagonists such as clomiphene citrate (CC) act centrally on the hypothalamic-pituitary axis to block the negative feedback of E_2 on gonadotropin secretion. This results in an increase in the endogenous release of FSH.[2] (2) Gonadotropin-releasing hormone (GnRH) also acts centrally via direct stimulation of FSH/LH release from the pituitary gland, thus bypassing the hypothalamus.[3] (3) Gonadotropin preparations containing either FSH alone or FSH and LH in combination act directly on the ovary, bypassing the hypothalamic-pituitary axis. Each of these is discussed in turn. It is clear, however, that before beginning a therapeutic course of any of these medications, the etiology of a patient's infertility should be carefully investigated.

WHO ARE APPROPRIATE CANDIDATES FOR OVULATION INDUCTION?

The goal of controlled ovarian hyperstimulation is to cause the release of several oocytes concurrently, increasing the likelihood of pregnancy in a given cycle. Before beginning a therapeutic course that involves both financial and emotional expense as well as increased medical risks, it is only prudent to complete an initial evaluation for infertility. A careful history and physical examination should rule out obvious causes of infertility. Additional initial testing should also include a semen analysis, because about 40% of couples evaluated for infertility have a documented male factor contributing to their difficulty in achieving pregnancy. Common hormonal cause of anovulation or oligo-ovulation should be ruled out by checking prolactin and thyroid-stimulating hormone levels. In the absence of historical factors suggestive of a tubal or uterine factor, many physicians will begin an initial course of therapy with CC, because that is relatively low risk and inexpensive, before completing an anatomic evaluation that is both invasive and potentially more expensive. However, before proceeding with other therapy, such as gonadotropin controlled ovarian hyperstimulation, an evaluation of the uterine cavity and documentation of patent fallopian tubes as well as a more thorough infertility evaluation should be performed.

Patients who do not ovulate or ovulate only irregularly may be classified into one of three general categories:

- Hypothalamic-pituitary failure
These patients generally have a diagnosis of hypothalamic amenorrhea. This may be a result of stress, anorexia nervosa, Kallmann's syndrome, or one of the rare forms of gonadotropin deficiency. Medications may also contribute to failure of the hypothalamic-pituitary axis. On evaluation, these patients will be found to be *hypo*gonadotropic (low FSH) with consequent *hypo*gonadism (low E_2). As a result, these patients will fail to bleed in

189

response to a progestin challenge, although they will respond to an estrogen/progestin challenge.

- Hypothalamic-pituitary dysfunction
  These patients are generally anovulatory or oligo-ovulatory and may present with a variety of menstrual patterns from frequent bleeding to amenorrhea. E_2 and FSH levels in these patients are usually normal or near normal. LH levels may be elevated relative to the FSH level if the patient has polycystic ovarian syndrome (PCOS). Because E_2 levels are normal, these patients bleed in response to a progestin withdrawal challenge.
- Ovarian failure
  Patients with ovarian failure do not have a developing cohort of follicles. On evaluation, these patients are *hyper*gonadotropic (high FSH) and *hypo*gonadal (low E_2). As a result, these patients often do not respond to a progestin withdrawal challenge but do respond to an estrogen/progestin challenge.

The preceding classification is useful in evaluating candidates for ovulation induction and as a guide to the initial selection of therapy. The ideal candidate for ovulation induction is a patient who is anovulatory or oligo-ovulatory, with an otherwise normal evaluation. Patients who are anovulatory but with an intact (although possibly somewhat dysfunctional) hypothalamic-pituitary axis may respond to any of the previous therapies, but are often begun on CC. Patients with hypothalamic amenorrhea but with an intact pituitary-ovarian axis will respond to either GnRH therapy or gonadotropin therapy, but are not good candidates for CC. On the other hand, patients with ovarian failure will not respond to any form of ovulation induction.

Whereas patients with ovulatory dysfunction not related to ovarian failure are the optimal candidates for ovulation induction, patients with an otherwise normal workup (and thus fitting the category of unexplained infertility) often are begun on a therapeutic course of ovulation induction empirically, before advancing to in vitro fertilization.

USE OF CLOMIPHENE CITRATE

Pharmacology of Clomiphene Citrate

CC acts as an estrogen antagonist, with its primary effect occurring at the level of the hypothalamus. CC is distributed as a racemic mixture of the zu-stereoisomers and en-stereoisomers, with zu-clomiphene being the more active compound. Although the initial elimination of CC occurs with a half-life of about 6 days, significant levels of CC can be detected 4 to 6 weeks after administration.

The primary site of action of CC is at the level of the nuclear receptors in the hypothalamus, but other tissues are also affected. At the level of the ovary, CC acts as an agonist, enhancing FSH-induced buildup of LH receptors in granulosa cells. On the other hand, CC acts as an antagonist at the level of the endometrium, cervix, and vagina. When postcoital tests are performed in conjunction with CC, about 15% of patients will show unfavorable

mucus. Whether or not this is clinically significant continues to be debated.

Protocol for Administration

CC is usually administered for a total of 5 days, with a starting dosage of 50 mg daily beginning on days 3, 4, or 5 of the menstrual cycle in patients who menstruate. Patients with amenorrhea or oligomenorrhea can be withdrawn with progestin therapy (e.g., medroxyprogesterone acetate, 10 mg daily for 5 to 10 days) before starting CC. A course of an oral contraceptive agent may be used for the same purpose. Ovulation will occur 5 to 12 days after the last dose of CC, usually between 7 and 10 days after the last CC pill. Patients are usually advised to have intercourse every other day for 1 week beginning 5 days after the last dose of CC. Ovulation should be documented using either temperature charting, a urinary LH surge testing kit, or ultrasound documentation of one or more dominant follicles 5 days after the last dose of CC. If ovulation is not documented, the dosage of CC should be increased by 50 mg in the next cycle and in each subsequent anovulatory cycle in stepwise fashion. Although the maximum dosage of CC is 250 mg, most patients who achieve pregnancy will do so at a dosage of 150 mg or less. Once ovulation has been documented, there is usually no need to further increase the dosage.

If it is necessary to time ovulation more precisely, transvaginal ultrasound to determine the number and size of growing follicles can be performed starting 5 days after the last dose of CC. Patients are followed by serial ultrasound until the dominant follicle has reached a size of 18 to 20 mm, at which time 10,000 IU of human chorionic gonadotropin (hCG) is administered intramuscularly. Ovulation will usually occur approximately 36 hours later, and intrauterine insemination or intercourse is then timed to take place approximately 12 hours before ovulation.

Ovarian cysts occasionally occur as a result of therapy with CC. Most clinicians will therefore want to document the absence of ovarian cysts (which may be responsive to FSH/LH stimulation) before beginning another cycle of therapy. Cysts smaller than 2 cm are not usually clinically significant. When larger cysts are documented, medical therapy is withheld until they have resolved.

In anovulatory patients with a diagnosis of PCOS, some investigators are recommending the use of insulin-sensitizing drugs such as metformin in conjunction with CC. The hyperinsulinemic state associated with PCOS can contribute to infertility and anovulation. Indeed, some patients starting on metformin alone become spontaneously ovulatory and conceive without other intervention. The optimum protocol for metformin therapy has yet to be elucidated, but use of metformin appears promising in these select patients.

Ovulation and Pregnancy Rates

For appropriately selected patients (e.g., anovulatory patients with hypothalamic dysfunction), ovulation rates of

80% may be seen with CC. About 50% of these patients will achieve pregnancy. Once ovulation has been documented, CC is continued at that dosage for 3 to 6 months. Approximately 85% of pregnancies will occur within the first 3 months of CC therapy. If pregnancy has not been achieved after 3 to 6 months of CC therapy, a complete infertility evaluation should be performed and the patient considered for a more aggressive approach such as ovulation induction with gonadotropins or in vitro fertilization.

Adverse Effects

Before CC therapy is initiated, the patient should be counseled regarding expected side effects. The antagonistic effects of CC leads to a number of menopause-like side effects, including hot flushes, mood swings, and vaginal dryness. Other side effects include breast tenderness, nausea, and headaches. Visual changes such as blurred vision, scotomata, or changes in visual acuity are occasionally reported. These changes resolve with the discontinuation of CC. When visual changes do occur, further CC therapy is contraindicated.

Ovarian hyperstimulation syndrome (OHSS) occurs rarely with CC therapy. Nonetheless, providers supervising CC therapy should be familiar with the diagnosis and management of OHSS.

Therapy with CC is associated with a multiple birth rate of 5% to 10%. Although this is mostly dizygotic twinning, about 0.1% are triplets and higher-order multiples. The spontaneous abortion rate associated with CC is about 15%, which is comparable with the rate of spontaneous abortions in recognized natural conceptions. CC therapy is not associated with a higher than background risk of genetic or developmental defects in offspring. The risk of ectopic pregnancy with the use of CC therapy increases only minimally in patients whose sole risk factor for infertility is anovulation or oligo-ovulation.

Questions regarding the risk of epithelial ovarian cancer have been raised for the use of CC as well as other infertility medications. Infertility itself is a known risk factor for epithelial ovarian cancer. A number of retrospective studies[4, 5] of epithelial ovarian cancer and use of infertility drugs have suggested an increased risk for patients prescribed infertility drugs compared with the general population. However, these studies are poorly controlled and have the bias that most infertility patients have used infertility drugs at some time in their treatment. In the study by Rossing and coworkers,[4] analysis of patients using CC for longer than 12 months has shown a slight increase in risk of borderline ovarian tumors but not for malignant tumors. There was no increased risk for patients using CC for less than 12 months. Patients using CC for a prolonged period should be advised that although there may be a theoretical increased risk for ovarian epithelial cancer associated with CC, evidence for usage of less than 12 months is at best equivocal. Patients may also be advised that if they achieve pregnancy, it may offer some protection against epithelial ovarian cancer.

USE OF GONADOTROPINS
Pharmacology of the Gonadotropins

The gonadotropins FSH and LH are glycoproteins produced in the anterior pituitary under hypothalamic control via the pulsatile release of GnRH. Introduced commercially shortly after the introduction of CC in the 1960s, the first preparations were prepared from the urine of menopausal women. These human menopausal gonadotropins (hMGs) (Pergonal, Humegon) contain equal concentrations of FSH and LH. They are typically distributed as lyophilized powders for reconstitution in saline solution just before intramuscular injection. A typical vial of powder contains 75 IU each of FSH and LH. These preparations may contain other proteins in addition to FSH and LH, and this can sometimes result in a local reaction to the injections, especially if they are given subcutaneously. Following the introduction of hMGs into clinical practice, highly purified hMG (Repronex, Fertinex) was introduced. Also prepared from the urine of menopausal women, these preparations are further purified to remove most of the extraneous proteins as well as the LH. The highly purified hMG products can be given subcutaneously. Recently, recombinant preparations containing only human FSH produced in mammalian tissue cultures have become available (Follistim, Gonal-F). The primary differences between the preparations are the absence of LH (purified hMG and recombinant FSH), the source of the gonadotropins (human menopausal urine or recombinant tissue cultures), and the mode of administration (subcutaneous or intramuscular).

Recognition of the etiology of the patient's infertility is the key to selecting the appropriate gonadotropin preparation. Detailed discussion of these complex issues is beyond the scope of this chapter. For example, patients with hypothalamic hypogonadism have not only low FSH but low LH as well. Because low levels of LH are necessary for the production of ovarian androgens that will be aromatized to E_2, products containing only FSH may yield less satisfactory results in these patients. On the other hand, patients with hypothalamic-pituitary dysfunction, such as PCOS patients, will have circulating background levels of LH that may even be elevated relative to their FSH. In these patients, additional LH from hMG may increase the level of androgens in the follicular fluid to a level that is not beneficial to improving fertility.

The primary site of action of the gonadotropins is the ovary itself, where they participate in the process of follicular recruitment. The continued administration of exogenous gonadotropins as the lead follicle develops avoids the negative feedback of estrogen on the hypothalamic-pituitary axis, which would normally decrease endogenous gonadotropin production, thereby limiting follicular recruitment and subsequent stimulation. The administration of exogenous gonadotropins at this time in the cycle thus allows additional follicles to develop.

Protocol for Administration

Gonadotropin administration is associated with potentially lethal side effects. For this reason, these drugs should be administered only under the close supervision of a physician familiar with their use and experienced in the diagnosis and management of their potential complications. Supervision of gonadotropin administration requires access to pelvic ultrasonography and the availability of a rapid turnaround (<4-hour) serum estradiol assay, all on a 7-day-per-week basis. Also as previously mentioned, a complete evaluation for infertility should be performed before the initiation of gonadotropin therapy.

In a typical protocol, gonadotropins are administered beginning on day 2 or 3 of a natural cycle or after an induced withdrawal bleed. E_2 is measured before starting medication. If the E_2 level exceeds approximately 100 pg/ml, the medication is withheld until the following cycle. Likewise, if ovarian cysts larger than about 15 to 20 mm are seen, the cycle is likewise canceled and the patient is often placed on oral contraceptive pills for the remainder of the cycle. Larger cysts, particularly in the range of 18 to 24 mm, can prove problematic in monitoring the progress of stimulation, because this is the target range used to identify a mature follicle.

A starting dose of 1 to 2 ampules (75 to 150 IU FSH or FSH/LH) given in the evening is typical, although higher doses may be needed with older patients or patients who have previously failed to ovulate or achieve pregnancy with gonadotropin ovulation induction. Patients with PCOS may require lower doses and are sometimes started on ½ to 1 ampule (37.5 to 75 IU) daily. After 5 to 7 days of therapy, the patient returns for an E_2 measurement and possibly a pelvic ultrasound to measure the developing follicles. Ultrasound monitoring is not usually required until a rise in E_2 is noted. From that point, the dosage of gonadotropin is individually adjusted, carefully monitoring the growth of the follicles and the E_2 level. A follicle is designated as mature when it reaches an average diameter (measured in two dimensions) of 18 to 20 mm. The usual goal is to have one or two follicles reach this diameter. This generally requires 7 to 14 days of gonadotropins. When one or two mature follicles are identified, the patient is instructed to take 10,000 IU of hCG (Profasi, Pregnyl). The similarity of the α subunit of hCG with LH mimics the LH surge and triggers ovulation approximately 36 hours later. Gonadotropins are discontinued at the time of hCG administration. As with CC, intercourse or insemination is timed to occur about 12 hours before ovulation; it is timed to bracket ovulation.

Once hCG is administered, progesterone support is often added in the form of vaginal suppositories, cream, or intramuscular injections of progesterone in oil. An additional dosage of hCG is often given 6 to 7 days after the initial dose of hCG. This provides additional support to the corpus luteum. Adding progesterone support will lengthen the time to a spontaneous withdrawal bleed if pregnancy is not achieved. Patients started on progesterone support should be warned of this so as not to engender false hopes in this emotionally charged setting. Fourteen days after ovulation, patients should have a serum hCG performed and, if it is positive, followed with serial hCG and ultrasound measurements to track the progress of the pregnancy. If a patient achieves pregnancy, progesterone support if started is usually continued until about 10 to 12 weeks.

One of the problems with this protocol is that patients may respond to the high levels of E_2 with a premature endogenous LH surge, triggering ovulation of immature follicles and premature luteinization. To prevent this, a modified protocol is sometimes used for stimulation. In this modified protocol, a long-acting GnRH agonist such as leuprolide acetate (1.0 mg subcutaneously daily) is begun on day 21 of the previous cycle. Amenorrheic patients are started on oral contraceptive pills and then begun on leuprolide on day 21. After approximately 10 days of leuprolide therapy, a withdrawal bleed usually occurs. Gonadotropins are then started on day 2 or 3 of the new cycle. When gonadotropins are begun, the dose of GnRH agonist is halved. The tonic (as opposed to pulsatile) administration of a GnRH agonist results in a downregulation of the pituitary and helps to prevent a premature LH surge. However, it must be recognized that this complete suppression of endogenous pituitary gonadotropins may increase the dosage of gonadotropins required by the patient. The absence of endogenous tonic stimulation of the corpus luteum may also increase the need for post-hCG progesterone support.

A third, "flare," protocol is also in wide use. In this approach, the addition of a GnRH agonist is begun at the same time as initiation of gonadotropin therapy. The intent is to take advantage of the rise (flare) of endogenous FSH and LH that usually follows the initial dosing with GnRH agonist. This flare of endogenous FSH/LH augments the administered gonadotropins at the beginning of stimulation.

There are many variations on the protocols outlined previously. The key to successful ovulation induction with gonadotropins is a careful infertility evaluation followed by the closely supervised administration of a regimen of gonadotropins.

More recently, as is the case with CC, metformin use is being investigated for use with ovulation induction in patients with anovulation and PCOS.[6]

Ovulation and Pregnancy Rates

For properly selected patients (i.e., patients with hypothalamic anovulation), a cumulative pregnancy rate after 6 consecutive cycles may be as high as 90%. In general, about two thirds of women on gonadotropins will ovulate, with about 25% of them achieving pregnancy.

Three to six cycles of gonadotropin induction of ovulation should be sufficient to achieve pregnancy. If pregnancy has not occurred in this time frame, the infertility evaluation should again be reviewed and consideration given to proceeding to in vitro fertilization.

The rate of spontaneous abortion for clinically recognized pregnancies with gonadotropin induction is somewhat higher than that in the general population, about 25% compared with 15%. Some of this increase may be related to earlier diagnosis of pregnancy and consequent recognition of early miscarriage. There may also be a selection bias for this older, higher-risk patient population.

The multiple pregnancy rate is significantly higher than with natural cycles or CC cycles. With careful supervision, the multiple pregnancy rate can be limited to 15%. However, multiple pregnancy rates of 25% are often seen, and rates as high as 40% have been reported.[7] Most of these multiple pregnancies will be twins; however, 5% or more will be higher-order multiples. This represents a serious complication with high potential morbidity and mortality for both the mother and her offspring. Counseling about this complication, and the therapeutic options available for dealing with multiple gestation, should occur before initiating gonadotropin therapy.

Adverse Effects

In addition to the severe consequences of a multiple gestation, other potentially severe side effects are associated with gonadotropin administration. The most concerning of these is OHSS. Mild OHSS is common, whereas moderate to severe OHSS can occur in 1% to 2% of patients.

OHSS usually presents initially with a complaint of abdominal bloating and discomfort. In mild cases, the syndrome is associated with ovarian enlargement, abdominal distention, and weight gain. In the moderate to severe syndrome, the ovarian enlargement is more pronounced (with ovarian dimensions reaching 10 cm or greater). Release of vascular endothelial growth factor from the ovarian stroma appears to be a key factor in the pathophysiology of this process, resulting in markedly increased vascular permeability. This has predictable and dangerous consequences. Development of abdominal ascites, pleural effusion, hemoconcentration, oliguria, hypovolemia, hypercoagulability, and electrolyte imbalances are all features of the moderate to severe presentations of this syndrome. In the most severe cases, adult respiratory distress syndrome with its associated 50% mortality risk can occur.

Risk factors for development of moderate to severe OHSS include markedly elevated E_2 levels (>2000 pg/ml), multiple (>10 small or >5 intermediate sized) follicles, administration of hCG, and occurrence of pregnancy. When a patient is believed to be at significant risk for developing moderate to severe OHSS, hCG should be withheld, and she should be closely monitored for the development of symptoms.

Because of the greater number of follicles that develop with gonadotropin controlled ovarian hyperstimulation cycles, the ectopic pregnancy rate is higher than in the general population, approaching 3% to 5%. There is no evidence of an increase in congenital or developmental anomalies with the use of gonadotropins.

USE OF GnRH

Pharmacology of GnRH

GnRH is normally released from the hypothalamus in a pulsatile fashion, with a frequency of 1 pulse every 60 to 90 minutes in the follicular phase and 1 pulse every 100 to 200 minutes in the luteal phase. GnRH may be administered via a small portable pump that is worn continuously. It acts as a permissive hormone with regard to the release of FSH and LH, and so the pituitary-ovarian axis must be capable of functioning normally in order for pulsatile GnRH therapy to succeed. Thus, it is most appropriate for women with hypothalamic amenorrhea/anovulation. Also, women with hyperprolactinemia who cannot tolerate a dopamine antagonist, such as bromocriptine, may be good candidates for this treatment.

Protocol for Administration

GnRH is administered by an infusion pump. The portable pump can be programmed to administer pulses of GnRH either subcutaneously or intravenously at set intervals. For intravenous administration, heparin is added to the solution. Absorption through the intravenous route is more predictable, but this requires closer monitoring to avoid local reaction, infection, or other complications from intravenous access and indwelling catheter placement. For example, this route would not be appropriate for patients with a history that placed them at risk for development of bacterial endocarditis.

The pump must be worn 24 hours a day, which can be somewhat inconvenient. GnRH is administered as a 5-μg bolus (intravenous route) or a 20-μg bolus (subcutaneous route) every 90 minutes. The patient response can be evaluated by weekly measurement of E_2. If a patient fails to respond, the dose is increased in 5-μg increments. Once ovulation has occurred, the pump should be continued or replaced by using hCG to support the luteal phase.

Ovulation will typically occur around day 14 of the cycle, although it may occur anytime between day 10 and day 22. Ultrasound monitoring or an LH surge test kit may be used to facilitate the timing of intercourse or insemination.

Ovulation and Pregnancy Rates

For properly selected patients (i.e., hypothalamic anovulatory women), the pregnancy rate may be as high as 20% to 30% per cycle. This approaches the normal fertility rate. Cumulative pregnancy rates of 80% in six cycles have been reported. A spontaneous abortion rate of about 15% to 20% is associated with this approach. The ectopic pregnancy rate is similar to that in the general population (about 1%).[8]

Adverse Effects

Because this method of ovulation induction most closely mimics a natural cycle, the side effects are generally minimal. Mild to moderate OHSS occurs infrequently, and severe OHSS is very rare and usually associated with inappropriate dosing.

There is no evidence of increased risk of congenital malformations or developmental abnormalities associated with this method.[9] Other side effects include local reactions, and occasionally development of circulating antibodies to GnRH.

References

1. Speroff L, Glass RH, Kase NG (eds): Clinical and Gynecologic Endocrinology and Infertility, 6th ed. Baltimore, Lippincott Williams & Wilkins, 1999, pp 1097–1132.
2. Chamoun D, McClamrocki H, Adashi E: Ovulation initiation with clomiphene citrate. In Seibel M (ed): Infertility: A Comprehensive Text, 2nd ed. Stamford, CT, Appleton & Lange, 1997.
3. Lunenfeld B, Lunenfeld E: Ovulation induction with human memopausal gonadotropin. In Seibel M (ed): Infertility: A Comprehensive Text, 2nd ed. Stamford, CT, Appleton & Lange, 1997.
4. Rossing MA, Daling JR, Weiss NS, et al: Ovarian tumors in a cohort of infertile women. N Engl J Med 1994;331:771–776.
5. Whittemore AS, Harris R, Itnyre J: Characteristics relating to ovarian cancer risk: Collaborative analysis of 12 US case-control studies. IV. The pathogenesis of epithelial ovarian cancer. Collaborative Ovarian Cancer Group. Am J Epidemiol 1992;136:1212–1220.
6. Nestler JE, Jakubowicz DJ, Evans WS, Pasquali R: Effects of metformin on spontaneous and clomiphene-induced ovulation in the polycystic ovary syndrome. N Engl J Med 1998;338:1876–1880.
7. Guzick DS, Carson SA, Coutifaris C, et al: Efficacy of superovulation and intrauterine insemination in the treatment of infertility. National Cooperative Reproductive Medicine Network. N Engl J Med 1999;340:177–183.
8. Speroff L, Glass RH, Kase NG (eds): Clinical and Gynecologic Endocrinology and Infertility, 6th ed. Baltimore, Lippincott Williams & Wilkins, 1999, p 1114.
9. Shoham Z, Zosmer A, Insler V: Early miscarriage and fetal malformations after induction of ovulation (by clomiphene citrate and/or human menotropins), in vitro fertilization, and gamete intrafallopian transfer. Fertil Steril 1991;55:1–11.

Family Decision-Making in Prenatal Genetic Testing

Virginia L. Miller

Genetic testing has rapidly advanced since the 1970s. The Human Genome Project, with its aim of mapping and sequencing the entire human genome, will continue the explosion of information about the function of our genes.[1] Although this new knowledge will ultimately lead to the treatment, cure, and prevention of genetic disorders, the ability to diagnose disease is certain to outpace the development of effective treatment strategies.

As the Human Genome Project identifies more genes related to human disease, the range of conditions included in genetic testing is likely to expand. In the area of prenatal genetic testing, techniques such as chorionic villus sampling have been developed for prenatal diagnosis earlier in pregnancy than amniocentesis. Further, preimplantation diagnosis allows for prenatal genetic testing before the embryo is implanted in the uterus.

Couples who have entered into a pregnancy have already made reproductive decisions important to their future family. For example, decisions regarding the timing of the pregnancy are in the context of financial capabilities, work schedules and responsibilities, and commitments to other children and family members. For couples with a history of genetic disease, either among family members or through the previous diagnosis of an affected child, difficult personal decisions surround entering the pregnancy itself.

The discoveries made by the Human Genome Project will increase the number of decisions to be made by families. Since the 1980s, prenatal genetic screening and testing have become commonplace. Currently, the exchanges between health care providers and expectant parents regarding prenatal genetic testing occur very early in the pregnancy. The decisions surrounding screening and testing take place in the context of uncertainty because they carry with them the possibility of a sequence of multiple decisions that may affect the entire family. Much societal and ethical debate has developed about what is to be decided and who decides. Shiloh[2] has described the process of genetic testing as a series of decisions. The family must decide whether to even consider prenatal genetic testing. If they do, the first step is to receive genetic counseling. Second, after genetic counseling, if they reach the decision to have prenatal genetic testing, the next step is to choose which test to have. Finally, the most personally complex and challenging situation is the one in which a genetic disorder has been diagnosed in the fetus and the family must decide whether to continue or terminate the pregnancy. This chapter highlights literature relevant to decision making in each stage of prenatal genetic testing and emphasizes factors influencing families.

The first stage at which major reproductive decisions are made is actually embarking on the pregnancy. Once pregnancy has occurred, health care providers may discuss prenatal genetic testing with parents early in prenatal care. As McGee[3] has suggested, it raises the importance of family history. For example, what if the fetus develops late-onset Alzheimer's disease or breast cancer, like current relatives? In the future, testing may allow for gene therapy in the womb. At present, which tests should be offered to all expectant families? Questions such as these may call health care providers to develop protocols regarding which type of testing all expectant parents will be informed about and which should be recommended. Common indications for referral to prenatal genetic services include a family history of a genetic disorder, advanced maternal age, and abnormal screening test results.

The second stage of the decision-making process entails deciding about having genetic counseling. In a comprehensive review of the literature, Kessler[4] reports that much of the past research in the area examines the recall of information or the recognition of information presented. Whereas families may come to counseling to learn information and the information obtained is used to make reproductive decisions, it is unclear whether the information is used in decision making exactly as it is acquired. Kessler puts forth the idea that the information must be transformed into personally meaningful units for use in future problem solving. Lippman-Hand and Fraser in 1979[5] reported that genetic counseling information is transformed in a qualitative bipolar manner for decision making; the information is transformed into what is the better outcome and what is the worse outcome.

In a study of cystic fibrosis (CF) carriers, Denayer and associates[6] evaluated attitudes toward reproductive decision making in hypothetical situations. Study participants were asked how they would have reacted if they had been told before marriage that they had a one in four chance of having a child with CF in every pregnancy. None of the study participants would have considered the carrier status an obstacle to marriage. The majority reported that they would try to prevent having a child with CF, either by not having children or through prenatal diagnosis. In another study, Wertz and colleagues[7] assessed the reproductive plans of 836 women after genetic counseling. The following were found to be associated with uncertainty regarding reproductive decision making after genetic counseling: precounseling uncertainty along with uncertainty about the ideal family size; concerns about the effects of an affected child on social life; and problems caring for an affected child at home. Wertz and colleagues concluded that genetic counseling was not effective in facilitating reproductive decision making, but they noted that 78% came to counseling to learn information. After counseling, 65% of the women were still uncertain, but this dropped to 48% 6 months later. This suggests that the effects of genetic counseling may be part of an ongoing process contributing to reproductive decision making.[4]

In a study on the impact of predictive testing for Huntington's disease, Decruyenaere and coworkers[8] evaluated whether knowing one's carrier status reduces anxiety and uncertainty and whether reproductive decision making was clarified. The study suggests that test results had a definite influence on reproductive decision making. One year after testing, two thirds of the carriers with reproductive plans decided to refrain from having more children or to have prenatal diagnosis. In contrast, most of the noncarriers with reproductive plans had chosen to have a pregnancy. In a study regarding the reproductive decisions among adult males with different forms of muscular dystrophy, Eggers and Zatz[9] reported that high recurrence risks did not significantly reduce reproduction after genetic counseling. Further, high recurrence risks did not correlate with less prospective desire for children.

In a follow-up study of parents' counseling needs and experiences surrounding the diagnosis of a sex chromosome abnormality, one finding identified by Peirucelli and associates[10] was that about half of the interviewees had not had genetic counseling before receiving prenatal genetic testing. The authors suggest that without genetic counseling before prenatal genetic testing, families may not be making fully informed decisions. Marteau and Croyle[11] advocate for research to identify how much and what type of information and support should be provided to the growing number of people being offered genetic testing. They propose that further research is needed to learn the most practical and effective counseling strategies to achieve a thorough understanding of genetic testing.

In the third decision-making stage, after genetic counseling, families must decide whether to undergo prenatal genetic testing. Published research has examined several factors that have influenced decision making. Frets and colleagues[12] developed a model that correctly predicted reproductive decisions among 164 couples after genetic counseling in 91% of the cases. The model consists of eight factors divided into three groups: reproductive outcome before genetic counseling; desire to have more children; and interpretation of information gained from genetic counseling. In a 1992 study by Wertz and coworkers,[13] the psychosocial factors underlying decisions regarding prenatal diagnosis for CF were assessed among parents of affected children. Three factors that were identified as significantly related to plans to use prenatal diagnosis were willingness to abort for CF; siblings' approval of abortion for CF; and listing no accomplishments for the existing child with CF.

Some women and their families may find themselves in the situation in which they have not made a conscious decision regarding prenatal testing. For example, maternal serum α-fetoprotein (MS-AFP) has become commonplace and many prenatal care providers view it as a part of routine prenatal care. Health education and counseling efforts regarding this screening test may not adequately address its full implications. Women undergoing the test may not realize that if the screening test is abnormal, a repeat test will be performed. If that result is abnormal, then further testing with ultrasound and amniocentesis may be recommended. In a 1996 study by Browner and coworkers,[14] information retention regarding MS-AFP screening after a video was compared with that of using only an informational booklet. These authors concluded that the video drew attention to the decision the pregnant woman will be required to make regarding prenatal screening, and its value may be in the woman's ability to make thoughtful, more informed decisions regarding prenatal screening.

Once the decision to participate in prenatal genetic testing has been reached, the next step is to choose which test. Verp and Heckerling[15] examined women's decision making regarding the choice of chorionic villus sampling and amniocentesis. The authors propose that women with a personal or family history of genetic disease may have different preferences than those seeking testing owing to advanced maternal age. Their values regarding early diagnosis and first or second trimester termination may determine their decision regarding chorionic villus sampling or amniocentesis.

Several studies have examined parental decisions after prenatal diagnosis. In a 1990 study, Drugan and associates[16] identified determinants of parental decisions to abort for chromosome abnormalities among 80 families. The severity of the chromosome anomaly and, to a lesser extent, viewing the anomalies on ultrasound were the major determinants of the decision to terminate the pregnancy. Diagnosis in the first trimester was no more likely to lead to a termination of pregnancy than diagnosis in the second trimester. In a comprehensive review of the literature on the choices women make regarding acting on abnormal results, Pryde and colleagues[17] noted that for fetal aneuploidy, the specific karyotype and its prognosis are the major determinants of the decision to terminate the pregnancy.

In each stage of decision making, the decisions are reached within the broad context of uncertainty within a short time frame and with many intertwined factors. Examples of these factors include family and friends, ethnicity, culture, religion, educational background, existing children, and socioeconomic status. For example, the type and amount of information families obtain from health care professionals, family, friends, or their own research may influence decision making. Marteau and coworkers[18] described the process of developing a valid and reliable measure of women's knowledge of prenatal screening and diagnostic testing and examined the scores on a questionnaire before and after women had been given information about testing. In the development of the instrument, two aspects of knowledge were assessed: the familiarity with the test names; and the purpose of the test and to whom they are offered. Three groups of women were assessed: those attending their first prenatal appointment; those attending a family planning clinic who had never been pregnant; and those who were 2 days postpartum. Whereas the majority of women were familiar with the names of the tests, and knowledge was greater postpartum than prenatally, there were a number of women postpartum who were uncertain or incorrect about having undergone either amniocentesis (16 of 69) or MS-AFP screening (26 of 69). The authors concluded that the lack of knowledge may exist for several reasons: the information was never offered; the information was offered, but not understood; or the information was offered and understood, but not retained for cognitive or emotional reasons.

An additional factor influencing decision making is anxiety. Marteau and associates[19] studied the anxiety levels, attitudes toward the pregnancy and fetus, and health-related behaviors among women who had undergone prenatal screening and diagnosis. Women who had not had MS-AFP screening were significantly more anxious at 38 weeks' gestation than those women who had had the test. Similarly, whereas there were no significant first trimester differences in state or trait anxiety for women who had had an amniocentesis and those who had not, by 38 weeks' gestation, women who had not had amniocentesis were found to be significantly more anxious than those who had. In terms of attitude toward the pregnancy, women not having MS-AFP tended to be less positive in their attitude toward the pregnancy in the second trimester. Marteau and associates offered several possible explanations why not undergoing prenatal screening or diagnostic testing is associated with increased levels of anxiety in the third trimester. First, reassurance regarding one test may generalize to reassurance about other risks in the pregnancy. Second, there may be regret regarding not having the test, and as delivery approaches there may be concern about the normality of the infant. Third, it may reflect a coping style of avoiding concerns in the second trimester, which becomes increasingly difficult to do in the third trimester.

Given all the intertwined factors involved in decision making about prenatal genetic testing, and as it becomes increasingly widespread, the psychosocial impact on women, their families, and society as a whole needs to be systematically examined. Comprehensive longitudinal research is needed on the process leading from one decision to the next throughout all stages of prenatal genetic testing.

References

1. Andrews LB, Fullarton JE, Holtzman NA, Motulsky AG (eds): Assessing Genetic Risks: Implications for Health and Social Policy. Committee on Assessing Genetic Risks, Division of Health Sciences Policy, Institute of Medicine. Washington, DC, National Academy Press, 1994.
2. Shiloh S: Decision-making in the context of genetic risk. In Marteau TM, Richards M (eds): The Troubled Helix: Social and Psychological Implications of the New Human Genetics. Cambridge, Cambridge University Press, 1996.
3. McGee G: The Perfect Baby: A Pragmatic Approach to Genetics. Lanham, Md, Rowman & Littlefield, 1997.
4. Kessler S: Psychological aspects of genetic counseling: VI. A critical review of the literature dealing with education and reproduction. Am J Med Genet 1989;34:340–353.
5. Lippman-Hand A, Fraser FC: Genetic counseling—the postcounseling period: I. Parents' perceptions of uncertainty. Am J Med Genet 1979;4:51–71.
6. Denayer L, Welkenhuysen M, Evers-Kiebooms G, et al: Risk perception after CF carrier testing and impact of the test result on reproductive decision making. Am J Med Genet 1997;69:422–428.
7. Wertz DC, Sorenson JR, Heeren TC: Genetic counseling and reproductive uncertainty. Am J Med Genet 1984;18:79–88.
8. Decruyenaere M, Evers-Kiebooms G, Boogaerts A, et al: Prediction of psychological functioning one year after the predictive test for Huntington's disease and impact of the test results on reproductive decision making. J Med Genet 1996;33:737–743.
9. Eggers S, Zatz M: How the magnitude of clinical severity and recurrence risk affects reproductive decisions in adult males with different forms of progressive muscular dystrophy. J Med Genet 1998;35:189–195.
10. Peirucelli N, Walker M, Schurry E: Continuation of pregnancy following the diagnosis of a fetal sex chromosome abnormality: A study of parents' counseling needs and experiences. J Genet Couns 1998;7:401–415.
11. Marteau TM, Croyle RT: The new genetics: Psychological responses to genetic testing. BMJ 1998;316:693–696.
12. Frets PG, Duivenvoorden HJ, Verhage F, et al: Model identifying the reproductive decision after genetic counseling. Am J Med Genet 1990;35:503–509.
13. Wertz DC, Janes SR, Rosenfield JM, Erbe RW: Attitudes toward the prenatal diagnosis of cystic fibrosis: Factors in decision making among affected families. Am J Hum Genet 1992;50:1077–1085.
14. Browner CH, Preloran M, Press NA: The effects of ethnicity, education and an informational video on pregnant women's knowledge and decisions about a prenatal diagnostic screening test. Patient Education and Counseling 1996;27:135–146.
15. Verp MS, Heckerling PS: Use of decision analysis to evaluate patients' choices of diagnostic prenatal test. Am J Med Genet 1995;58:337–344.
16. Drugan A, Greb A, Johnson MP, et al: Determinants of parental decisions to abort for chromosome abnormalities. Prenat Diagn 1990;10:483–490.
17. Pryde PG, Drugan A, Johnson MP, et al: Prenatal diagnosis: Choices women make about pursuing testing and acting on abnormal results. Clin Obstet Gynecol 1993;36:496–509.
18. Marteau TM, Johnston M, Plencicar M, et al: Development of a self-administered questionnaire to measure women's knowledge of prenatal screening and diagnostic tests. J Psychosom Res 1988;32:403–408.
19. Marteau TM, Johnston M, Shaw RW, et al: The impact of prenatal screening and diagnostic testing upon the cognitions, emotions and behaviour of pregnant women. J Psychosom Res 1989;33:7–16.

FORTY-TWO

Ultrasound in Pregnancy: Routine or by Indication?

Huda B. Al-Kouatly, Stephen T. Chasen,

and Frank A. Chervenak

The question of whether or not every pregnant woman should have an ultrasound examination remains controversial.[1] All authorities agree that ultrasound plays a crucial role in obstetrics, and, to this end, the National Institutes of Health first developed an extensive list of indications for ultrasonography during pregnancy in 1984. This document was adapted later by the American College of Obstetricians and Gynecologists (ACOG).[2] Many clinicians feel strongly that the routine use of prenatal ultrasound can improve perinatal outcome by accurate dating of pregnancy, early diagnosis of multiple gestations, and diagnosis of fetal anomalies. For these reasons, they advocate ultrasound in all low-risk patients, at 18 to 20 weeks' gestation. Others believe that in the low-risk pregnancy, ultrasound is not warranted in the absence of a specific indication.[3] It should be noted that even when selective criteria are used, most patients exhibit at least one clinical indication for ultrasound at some point during pregnancy.

THE RADIUS STUDY

Since 1988, three large randomized studies have been published that address the issue of routine ultrasound in pregnancy. The Routine Antenatal Diagnostic Imaging Ultrasound (RADIUS) study intensified the level of debate over routine ultrasound in the United States.[4–6] The RADIUS trial was conducted from 1987 to 1991 at 28 sites in six states and included 15,530 pregnant women who were considered low risk by their physicians. Those women randomized to the study group had ultrasound examinations between 18 and 20 weeks and 31 and 33 weeks of gestation. Those in the control group received ultrasonography only as clinically indicated. This study, a randomized, prospective clinical trial, was designed to test the hypothesis that routine ultrasound screening in pregnancy would reduce perinatal morbidity and mortality. The researchers concluded that, compared with selective use of ultrasound, routine ultrasound did not contribute to a reduction in perinatal mortality or morbidity in low-risk pregnancies and thus resulted in excessive cost.

The conclusions of the RADIUS study have been widely disputed. The RADIUS trial assumed that routine ultrasound would be truly clinically important only if associated with a documented reduction in perinatal morbidity and mortality. Although perinatal morbidity and mortality are important measures, they do not represent the full array of possible clinical benefits. The researchers did not study other potential benefits of routine ultrasonography, including (1) increased detection of fetal anomalies, (2) earlier diagnosis of twin gestations, (3) decreased use of tocolytic therapy, and (4) fewer postdate inductions. Because routine management protocols were not utilized, it is also possible that potentially beneficial information provided by ultrasound did not result in improved perinatal outcomes.

The overall rate of 35% for detection of fetal anomalies in the RADIUS study and the detection rate of 16.6% in routine second trimester scans cannot be said to represent the capability of modern ultrasound in diagnosing fetal anomalies.[7] Despite this, significantly more anomalies were detected in the screened group than in the study control group, 16.6% versus 4.9%.[6]

OTHER STUDIES

The Helsinki Ultrasound Trial was a randomized, prospective, controlled study of 8662 gravidas in the greater Helsinki area from 1986 to 1988.[8] Ultrasound was routinely performed between 16 and 20 weeks in the study (screening) group. In the control group, 77% of women had an ultrasound examination at some point during their pregnancy. The first ultrasound examination was performed after 20 weeks in only 2.1% of the screening group, compared with 21.5% of those in the control group. In the screening group, there was a significantly decreased rate of postmaturity at the time of onset of labor compared with the control group, 5.5% versus 2.9%. Twin pregnancies were significantly more likely to be detected by 20 weeks' gestation in the screening group. The perinatal mortality rate was significantly lower in singletons and twins in the screening group compared with the control group. There was an increased rate of detection of congenital malformations in the screening group, leading to 11 cases of pregnancy termination. In contrast, there were no terminations due to malformations in the control group. The overall rate of perinatal mortality was 4.6 per 1000 in the screened group and 9.0 per 1000 in the control group. The increased rate of induced abortions due to congenital malformations in the screening group seemed to account for most of this difference.

Waldenström and colleagues[9] conducted a randomized controlled trial from 1985 to 1987 involving 4997 women in Sweden. Randomized subjects were less than 20 weeks' gestation and did not have any of 15 preset indications for ultrasound. Those randomized to the screening group had ultrasonography from 13 to 19 weeks' gestation; none in the control group had a scan before 19 weeks. Ultrasound after 19 weeks was performed at the discretion of the physicians in both groups. In this study, there was a decreased rate of induced labor for post-term pregnancy in the screening group, and twins were diagnosed earlier. There was no difference in perinatal mortality in singletons or twins between the two groups. The detection of fetal anomalies by ultrasound was not discussed in this study.

Several large series have been published recently that describe the sensitivity of routine ultrasound in detecting fetal anomalies. The Eurofetus study involved prospective data collected from ultrasound centers in 60 hospitals in 14 countries, most from the European union, with neonatal follow-up.[10] Obstetricians performed most ultrasound examinations. Of 3686 neonates with malformations, 2262 were diagnosed by ultrasound as abnormal (sensitivity, 61.4%). The sensitivity was 73.7% for major anomalies compared with a sensitivity of 45.7% for minor anomalies. Ultrasound detection was highest for anomalies of the central nervous system (88.3%) and urinary tract (84.4%) and lowest for the heart and great vessels (38.8%).

Papp and associates[11] conducted a prospective, nonrandomized study in Hungary to compare the effectiveness of ultrasound and maternal serum α-fetoprotein (MS-AFP) screening for detecting fetal anomalies. Ultrasound examinations were performed by nonphysicians, under the supervision of obstetricians. There were 496 major anomalies among 63,794 pregnancies; an 18- to 20-week ultrasound examination detected 317 (63.9%) of these. Ultrasound screening decreased the birth prevalence of severe congenital anomalies, compared with the midtrimester prevalence due to pregnancy terminations. The sensitivity of ultrasound was significantly higher than that of MS-AFP for every category of anomalies. Their data suggest that universal MS-AFP screening and scanning only those with elevated MS-AFP, although useful for detection of neural tube defects, would fail to detect most other types of congenital anomalies.

In 1998, Queisser-Luft and coworkers[12] published a retrospective case-control study assessing the detection rate of three-step ultrasound screening (at 9 to 12 weeks, 19 to 20 weeks, and 23 to 29 weeks) in Germany. Obstetricians performed a level 1 ultrasound examination. Data were reviewed on 20,248 livebirths, stillbirths, and abortions; 4525 (22%) of the pregnancies were categorized as high risk owing to at least one maternal or fetal risk factor. Ultrasound detected only 95 of 314 anomalies in 298 pregnancies, a sensitivity rate of 30.3%. The majority of these were not detected until the third trimester; two thirds were detected after 24 weeks of gestation. Fifty percent of these 298 pregnancies with anomalies belonged to the high-risk cohort. The investigators concluded that routine ultrasound screening was not very effective in detecting fetal anomalies in a low-risk population, but they did advo-

cate ultrasound screening for high-risk pregnancies. However, because of the low sensitivity rate, they proposed that ultrasound screening be accomplished by highly experienced personnel.

In reviewing these studies, it is apparent that there is a wide range of detection rates of fetal anomalies. In the RADIUS study, the sensitivity of second trimester ultrasound in university hospitals was 35%, compared with 13% in nontertiary (community and office-based) centers.[6] In the RADIUS study, ultrasound examinations were performed by 60 sonographers, 75 radiologists, and 13 maternal-fetal medicine specialists. In the Helsinki trial, the detection rate of fetal anomalies at the University Hospital was 76.9%, compared with only 36% at the City Hospital.[8] The ultrasound was performed mainly by trained nurses at both hospitals. The average ultrasound examination was 8 minutes longer when performed at the University Hospital.[13] From these data, it is obvious that operator experience is extremely important in diagnosing fetal anomalies and is a more important factor than whether or not the operator is an obstetrician.

COST ANALYSIS

The cost-effectiveness analysis of routine ultrasound is problematic for many reasons. Wide ranges of anomaly detection rates, as well as different rates of pregnancy termination in different populations, significantly alter any calculation. Ultrasound that is not of high quality can add costs owing to unnecessary interventions based on false diagnoses and can cause considerable parental anxiety. The lifelong care for infants surviving with anomalies poses very real problems for the individual, the family, and society. The continued physical, psychological, and financial requirements of a child with major anomalies are hard to define specifically and consequently difficult to quantify, a reason why most studies do not account for this factor in their analyses. A cost analysis based in countries with nationalized health care would not be applicable to the United States, which lacks uniformity in reimbursement. Finally, even the highest quality ultrasound cannot be effective in improving outcomes if the appropriate expertise in managing high-risk conditions diagnosed by ultrasound is not available.

The authors of the RADIUS study concluded that routine ultrasound in pregnancy would add considerable cost, with no improvement in perinatal outcome.[4] The cost analysis did not include the lifetime cost of caring for infants born with congenital anomalies. Because higher rates of anomaly detection in the second trimester will afford more women the choice of termination, those patients who undergo routine ultrasound are less likely to deliver an abnormal infant, resulting in considerable cost savings. DeVore[14] has shown that the cost per anomaly detected by screening ultrasound in the tertiary care centers of the RADIUS study was equivalent to the cost per anomaly detected using MS-

AFP screening in California, a standard for cost-effectiveness. Given the improved detection rate in tertiary centers, the cost per anomaly detected with quality ultrasound would actually be much less.[14] By this comparison alone, routine obstetric ultrasound is cost-effective.

The authors of a recent extensive cost analysis of the Helsinki trial[13] came to a different conclusion than did the authors of the RADIUS study. Their aim was to evaluate the cost-effectiveness of one second trimester ultrasound examination on perinatal mortality. Their exhaustive cost calculations are of clinical importance. For example, they took into account not only the direct cost of the ultrasound examination but also the indirect costs, such as complementary procedures induced by the screening program, lost working hours, and travel expenses for the patient. The cost of each avoided perinatal death was $21,938. However, combining all positive and negative costs, the net estimate showed a cost saving of $17,077 per each avoided perinatal death. They concluded that one second trimester ultrasound is cost-effective.

Roberts and coworkers[15] published a decision analysis in 1998 and compared 12 options for the use of routine ultrasound in pregnancy, based on combinations of one or more of the following: first trimester dating scan, first trimester anomaly scan, second trimester scan, and third trimester scan. Four target fetal anomalies were evaluated: cardiac, spina bifida, Down syndrome, and other lethal abnormalities. They determined the cost per anomaly detected in each screening option by using available data about anomaly detection rates and cost estimates based on data from the National Health Service in the United Kingdom. The researchers concluded that ultrasound screening was potentially within the range of cost-effectiveness of other accepted screening programs.

ETHICAL DIMENSIONS

In our view, ethics is an essential dimension of the routine obstetric ultrasound debate.[16] Providing patients with information about diagnostic and therapeutic alternatives is an essential component of respect for the patient's autonomy. Failure to provide the patients access to information deprives them of the opportunity to consider alternatives about the management of their pregnancy, some of which accord with the patient's values. Routinely offering obstetric ultrasound respects the autonomy of pregnant women; not routinely offering obstetric ultrasound systematically disrespects autonomy because their access to the diagnosis of serious anomalies and, therefore, access to abortion following possible serious fetal anomalies is restricted.[17] These matters are neither ethically nor clinically trivial.

The implication of respect for autonomy in clinical practice means that physicians should inform every pregnant patient of the availability of diagnostic ultrasound.[17] A practice of discussing ultrasound only when a woman initiates an inquiry lessens the patient's autonomy because many women are ignorant of this modality and of its ability to detect at least three times the background detection rate of fetal anomalies.[4, 17, 18] We believe that the clinical strategy of Prenatal Informed Consent for Sonogram (PICS) should be employed with every pregnant woman.[17]

PICS should be undertaken in several stages. Soon after the pregnancy has been diagnosed, the gravida should be provided with information about the actual and theoretical benefits and harms of obstetric ultrasound. She should then be given an opportunity to evaluate this information within the frame of her own values and should be asked to articulate her preference regarding the use of ultrasound in the management of her pregnancy. The physician should then provide his or her own recommendation, with a discussion of any disagreement that may emerge. On the basis of the foregoing, the patient makes her final decision that determines the use of ultrasound for that pregnancy. In essence, PICS establishes a patient-based indication for routine obstetric ultrasound.[17] We propose that obstetricians should be advocates of their patient's autonomy by offering access to routine obstetric ultrasound.

Treating a perceived lack of benefit of routine obstetric ultrasound as decisive implies that clinical considerations override autonomy-based considerations. Clinical judgment should not be based on the narrow end points of morbidity and mortality but should also include the prevention of significant harm in small but important subsets of patients. Prudent clinical judgment emphasizes the seriousness of the outcome rather than the low incidence of the outcome. For example, given the seriousness of the outcomes of undetected clinical complications, such as unexpected twins at the time of delivery, it is justifiably risk-averse to attempt to prevent those outcomes when in clinical judgment the risks of not performing the ultrasound outweigh the risks of performing it. In our view,[17] high-quality ultrasound that is required as a matter of professional integrity reduces the risk of harm from erroneous ultrasound and, therefore, tips the balance in favor of offering routine ultrasound.

An ethical analysis of routine ultrasound examination based on clinical judgment of the proper scope reaches two conclusions: (1) end points of overall perinatal morbidity and mortality are not the sole measures of clinical judgment but are only part of it and (2) prudent clinical judgment supports offering high-quality ultrasound. The significant benefit of PICS—namely, making an informed choice about pregnancy management—is central to the respect for autonomy. On balance, autonomy-based obligations should clearly be the physician's primary guide in response to objections based on lack of benefit.

Treating the cost of routine obstetric ultrasound as decisive asserts that justice-based considerations or fairness override autonomy-based considerations. A central justice-based consideration is cost-effectiveness, which concerns identifying the least expensive means to achieve an agreed-upon goal. An important goal of obstetric ultrasound is the detection of fetal anomalies. As previously discussed, DeVore[14] has shown that the cost per detected case of an anomaly in the RADIUS trial was not greatly different from the cost per detected anomaly in the California MS-AFP screening program. A second justice-based consideration is whether the current cost of an intervention saves a greater cost in the future. We interpret DeVore's analysis to suggest that routine ultrasound is cost-beneficial because the cost per anomaly detected with quality ultrasound is far below the neonatal and lifetime costs of those anomalies (assuming that, for many pregnancies in which serious anomalies are detected, women will seek a termination).

It is already well understood that respect for autonomy is very costly and that fact, by itself, does not override the importance of autonomy. Such matters as universal suffrage, protection of the rights of citizens accused or convicted of crimes, and the public accountability of government institutions to the electorate are very expensive. No credible argument based on excessive cost has been advanced to override such autonomy-based considerations. Therefore, no credible argument can be advanced against PICS, a far less costly form of respect for autonomy exercised around a central individual and social concern, namely human reproductive freedom.

At the very least, cost-based arguments must show that the cost per detected anomaly is so excessive as to establish conclusively that this excessive cost violates accepted theories of justice. Simply subordinating respect for autonomy to ill-defined considerations of cost falls far below this demanding intellectual standard and ill serves the specialty of obstetrics and gynecology and the women it serves. We are advocates for the best health care for women, and our respect for their autonomy is paramount.

CONCLUSION

Based on several studies, it is apparent that large cohorts can be routinely screened with obstetric ultrasound with high rates of anomaly detection. There is also the potential for lowering perinatal mortality by diagnosing multiple gestation early in pregnancy and by accurately assessing gestational age. For these benefits to be realized, however, those performing ultrasound examinations must have the appropriate training and expertise. In most studies, ultrasound examinations performed in tertiary care centers were significantly more likely to diagnose fetal anomalies than those performed elsewhere. Any cost analysis of routine examination is limited by many factors, but there are data to suggest that the costs of quality routine ultrasound are not prohibitive and may even result in a net cost savings. Ethical dimensions must be considered when evaluating whether all pregnant women should be offered an ultrasound examination.

Suggestions for Future Reading

Chervenak FA, McCullough LB, Chervenak JL: Prenatal informed consent for sonogram: An indication for obstetric ultrasonography. Am J Obstet Gynecol 1989;161:857–860.

Ecker JL, Frigoletto FD: Routine ultrasound screening in low-risk pregnancies: Imperatives for further studies. Obstet Gynecol 1999;93:607–610.

Grandjean H, Larroque D, Levi S, for the Eurofetus Team: Sensitivity of routine ultrasound screening of pregnancies in the Eurofetus database. Ann N Y Acad Sci 1998;847:118–124.

Leivo T, Tuominen R, Saari-Kemppainen A, et al: Cost-effectiveness of one-stage ultrasound screening in pregnancy: A report from the Helsinki Ultrasound Trial. Ultrasound Obstet Gynecol 1996;7:309–314.

Romero R: Routine obstetric ultrasound. Ultrasound Obstet Gynecol 1993;3:303–307.

References

1. Ecker JL, Frigoletto FD: Routine ultrasound screening in low-risk pregnancies: Imperatives for further studies. Obstet Gynecol 1999;93:607–610.
2. American College of Obstetricians and Gynecologists: Ultrasonography in pregnancy (Technical Bulletin No. 187). Washington, DC, ACOG, 1993.
3. Frigoletto FD: Commentary on routine OB ultrasound. ACOG Clin Rev 1996;1:4–5.
4. Ewigman BG, Crane JP, Frigoletto FD, et al, for the RADIUS Study Group: Effect of prenatal ultrasound screening on perinatal outcome. N Engl J Med 1993;329:821–827.
5. LeFevre ML, Bain RP, Ewigman BG, et al: A randomized trial of prenatal ultrasonographic screening: Impact on maternal management and outcome. Am J Obstet Gynecol 1993;169:483–489.
6. Crane JP, LeFevre ML, Winborn RC, et al, for the RADIUS Study Group: A randomized trial of prenatal ultrasonographic screening: Impact on the detection, management, and outcome of anomalous fetuses. Am J Obstet Gynecol 1994;171:392–399.
7. Romero R: Routine obstetric ultrasound. Ultrasound Obstet Gynecol 1993;3:303–307.
8. Saari-Kemppainen A, Karjalainen O, Ylöstalo P, Heinonen OP: Ultrasound screening and perinatal mortality: Controlled trial of systematic one-stage screening in pregnancy. The Helsinki Ultrasound Trial. Lancet 1990;336:387–391.
9. Waldenström U, Axelsson O, Nilsson S, et al: Effects of routine one-stage ultrasound screening in pregnancy: A randomised controlled trial. Lancet 1988;2:585–588.
10. Grandjean H, Larroque D, Levi S, for the Eurofetus Team: Sensitivity of routine ultrasound screening of pregnancies in the Eurofetus database. Ann N Y Acad Sci 1998;847:118–124.
11. Papp Z, Toth-Pal E, Papp CS, et al: Impact of prenatal mid-trimester screening on the prevalence of fetal structural anomalies: A prospective epidemiological study. Ultrasound Obstet Gynecol 1995;6:320–326.
12. Queisser-Luft A, Stopfkuchen H, Stolz G, et al: Prenatal diagnosis of major malformations: Quality control of routine ultrasound examinations based on a five-year study of 20,248 newborn fetuses and infants. Prenat Diagn 1998;18:567–576.
13. Leivo T, Tuominen R, Saari-Kemppainen A, et al: Cost-effectiveness of one-stage ultrasound screening in pregnancy: A report from the Helsinki Ultrasound Trial. Ultrasound Obstet Gynecol 1996;7:309–314.
14. DeVore GR: The Routine Antenatal Diagnostic Imaging with Ultrasound Study: Another perspective. Obstet Gynecol 1994;84:622–626.
15. Roberts T, Mugford M, Piercy J: Choosing options for ultrasound screening in pregnancy and comparing cost effectiveness: A decision analysis approach. Br J Obstet Gynaecol 1998;105:960–970.
16. McCullough LB, Chervenak FA: Ethics in Obstetrics and Gynecology. New York, Oxford University Press, 1994.
17. Chervenak FA, McCullough LB, Chervenak JL: Prenatal informed consent for sonogram: An indication for obstetric ultrasonography. Am J Obstet Gynecol 1989;161:857–860.
18. Ewigman BG, Le Fevre M, Bain RP, et al: Ethics and routine ultrasonography in pregnancy [letter]. Am J Obstet Gynecol 1990;163:256–257.

FORTY-THREE

Fetal Macrosomia: Antenatal Diagnosis and Management

Peter G. Pryde and Helen H. Kay

It is well known that excessive birth weight, designated *macrosomia,* is associated with increased risk of injury to both the fetus and the mother. However, a lack of consensus remains regarding several pertinent details relating to the disorder, including a clinically relevant definition, acceptable antepartum diagnostic methods, and the optimal management approach when the diagnosis is made. Notwithstanding these unsettled issues, clinicians must frequently make decisions about the management of pregnancies in which macrosomia is suspected. It is important to develop a rational approach to this common obstetric problem.

DEFINITION

Several definitions have been suggested for macrosomia. Most common are the *birth weight* criteria of either 4000 g or 4500 g, regardless of gestational age. The term *large for gestational age,* referring to infants having birth weights greater than the 90th percentile, has also been used. Because true birth weight can be known only after delivery, and the antenatal diagnosis of macrosomia remains imprecise, the American College of Obstetricians and Gynecologists has proposed that clinicians "consider any fetus with an estimated weight of more than 4500 g in utero to be macrosomic."[1]

PREVALENCE OF MACROSOMIA

The prevalence of macrosomia depends obviously on its definition, but it appears to be geographically variable as well (Table 43–1). In addition, there is evidence that the condition is increasing in recent decades. For example, a population survey indicated that the prevalences of babies

Table 43–1. Birth Prevalence of Macrosomia According to Definition and Population

Definition	National Health Statistics	Milwaukee, Wisconsin
>4000 g	8.9%	15.9%
>4500 g	1.5%	2.2%

Data from Sandmire HF: Whither ultrasound prediction of fetal macrosomia? Obstet Gynecol 1993;82:860–862.

with birth weights greater than 4 kg and those greater than 4.5 kg were 12.5% and 2.9%, respectively, in 1979 compared with 19.4% and 4.0% in 1992.[2] Nutritional factors undoubtedly explain much of the regional variation as well as the recently rising prevalence of macrosomia.

MECHANISMS OF MACROSOMIA

The mechanisms of fetal overgrowth are heterogeneous. This is clinically relevant because the mechanism, in a given case, determines its anatomic characteristics and the likelihood of attendant morbidity.[3] It is estimated that 50% to 60% of macrosomia is due to genetically programmed *intrinsic growth potential* in the upper 5th to 10th percentiles. These fetuses tend to be *symmetrically* large, with proportionate linear and circumferential growth. An additional 35% to 40% of macrosomia is attributed to nutritional phenomena including gestational and pregestational diabetes. Chronic maternal hyperglycemia leads to excessive transplacental glucose transfer with consequent hyperglycemia in the fetal compartment. This causes fetal overproduction of insulin and other insulin-like growth factors, leading to a metabolically driven form of macrosomia in which there is *disproportionate* circumferential growth (owing to increased muscle, fat, and solid organ mass particularly affecting the trunk and shoulders). It is this group of *asymmetrically* large fetuses that contributes predominantly to the morbidity, principally from birth trauma, associated with macrosomia.

MATERNAL MORBIDITY

Cesarean section rates, and their attendant morbidity, increase with macrosomic pregnancies. Although larger fetuses are more likely to be involved in true cephalopelvic disproportion, individual physician practice patterns also appear to influence the widely variable cesarean rates for this indication.[4] In fact, studies indicate that the antepartum suspicion of macrosomia, particularly following ultrasound diagnosis, increases cesarean rates independent of true birth weight. Thus, it is not only the macrosomic condition itself but also physician apprehension about *possible* macrosomia that contributes to the higher rates of cesareans performed for that indication. Other maternal risks in macrosomic pregnancy include postpartum hemorrhage and puerperal infection regardless of the route of delivery. Also, potential long-term consequences of pelvic floor injuries occur during a difficult second stage of labor, including urinary and fecal incontinence, pelvic pain, sexual dysfunction, and pelvic prolapse.

Fetal Morbidity

Macrosomic infants are at increased risk for birth trauma and asphyxial injury.[5] Whereas these injuries can occur with either vaginal or cesarean delivery, the incidence is greater among vaginally delivered infants. The fetal injury of greatest overall impact is Erb's palsy, a severe upper extremity paralysis caused by permanent damage to the brachial plexus. This injury most often results from shoulder dystocia occurring at the time of delivery, although cases of Erb's palsy have been reported subsequent to uncomplicated vaginal and cesarean deliveries.[6] The likelihood of shoulder dystocia increases with increasing fetal weight, but it is much more likely among infants of diabetic mothers at any birth weight exceeding 4000 g (Table 43–2). Among macrosomic infants experiencing a shoulder dystocia, approximately 15% to 30% will sustain a brachial plexus injury. Of these initial injuries, it is estimated that more than 80% resolve completely. Thus, not more than 1% to 5% of all shoulder dystocia events results in permanent injury. Another injury increased among macrosomic infants is fracture of the clavicle and, less commonly, the humerus. Fortunately, such fractures heal quickly and typically without sequelae. Severe asphyxia is rare, but even death can occur in difficult shoulder dystocia situations.

Risk Factors Associated with Fetal Overgrowth

Multiple risk factors have been identified in association with fetal macrosomia. Most patients having one or more of these factors, however, will deliver infants with normal birth weights. Already discussed is the strong association between macrosomia and maternal glucose intolerance. Additional important risk factors include postdatism, maternal obesity, excessive weight gain during pregnancy, and previous history of macrosomic delivery. Also associated with macrosomia, but independently less predictive, are multiparity, fetal male gender, and maternal birth weight more than 4000 g.

Prenatal Diagnosis of Fetal Macrosomia

Estimates of fetal weight by physical examination are inaccurate and worsen with increasing birth weight. Using clinical evaluation alone, more than half of fetuses with birth weights exceeding 4000 g are underestimated by 0.5 kg, and more than 80% are underestimated by that much if the actual birth weight exceeds 4500 g. Ultrasound estimates, although more widely accepted, are also poorly predictive.[4] Despite efforts using a variety of biometric formulas, no current method estimates birth weight with error less than 10% to 15% of the predicted value. For the purposes of predicting macrosomia, sensitivities in the 80% range and positive predictive values between 70% and 80% are reported when applied to diabetic populations. Applied to low-risk populations, however, sensitivities are in the 70% range and positive predictive values are closer to 60%. These test-performance characteristics translate into a failure to detect macrosomia (false-negative results) in 20% to 50% of affected cases, whereas erroneous predictions (false-positive results) occur in 20% to 40% of cases in which a macrosomia diagnosis has been made. Recently proposed novel imaging approaches may improve the accuracy of antenatal fetal macrosomia diagnosis and better predict dystocia risk. Using ultrasound, methods to evaluate increased soft tissue mass as an indicator of asymmetrical fetal overgrowth are being investigated. These include measurements of cheek-to-cheek diameter and humeral soft tissue thickness. Perhaps even more promising are efforts to simultaneously quantify fetal shoulder width and maternal pelvic dimensions using computed tomography or magnetic resonance imaging.

Clinical Predictors of Shoulder Dystocia

Antepartum risk factors for shoulder dystocia are essentially the same as those for macrosomia, with the addition of contracted maternal pelvis and prior history of shoulder dystocia. Intrapartum risk factors include a prolonged second stage of labor, midpelvic operative vaginal delivery, and a genuinely macrosomic fetus.[7] It would seem that by recognizing these well-delineated risk factors, the clinician should be able to predict most instances of shoulder dystocia. However, scrutiny of existing data reveals that the event is, in fact, generally unpredictable.[8] As shown in

Table 43–2. Shoulder Dystocia Related to Birth Weight and Diabetic Status*

Birth Weight (g)	Diabetics (Subset Incidence %) [Fraction of Total Dystocia Cases %]	Nondiabetics (Subset Incidence %) [Fraction of Total Dystocia Cases %]
<4000	8/1253 (0.63) [1.7]	168/68,548 (0.24) [37]
4000–4500	10/209 (4.8) [2.2]	159/4630 (3.4) [35]
>4500	32/77 (41) [7.0]	79/806 (9.8) [17]
Totals	50/1539 (3.2) [11.0]	406/73,984 (0.5) [89]

Data from Langer O, Berkus MD, Huff RW, Samueloff A: Shoulder dystocia: Should the fetus weighting greater than or equal to 4000 grams be delivered by cesarean section? Am J Obstet Gynecol 1991;165:831–837.

*The highest risk group for SD is the diabetic pregnancy subset with birth weight > 4500 g (41% risk). However, fewer than 10% of all SDs occur in this group. The subgroup having the highest contribution to overall SD prevalence is the nondiabetic group with birth weight < 4000 g (37% of all SD cases), whereas this is the group in which individuals carry the least risk (0.24%).

SD, shoulder dystocia.

Table 43–3. Financial and Maternal Cesarean "Costs" per Case of Permanent Brachial Plexus Injury Avoided by Policy of Cesarean for Ultrasound Estimates of Weight >4000 or 4500g*

Cost/Benefit (Policy)	Nondiabetics	Diabetics	BPI Avoided By Policy (%)
Cesareans/BPI avoided (4000 g)	2345	489	31
Cost/BPI avoided (4000 g)	$4.9 million	$880,000	
Cesareans/BPI avoided (4500 g)	3695	443	5
Cost/BPI avoided (4500 g)	$8.7 million	$930,000	

*Note that whether using EFW of 4000 or 4500 g, an enormous number of cesareans are required for a relatively small impact on the rare background occurrence rate of permanent BPI.

BPI, brachial plexus injury; EFW, estimated fetal weight.

Data from Rouse DJ, Owen J, Goldenberg RL, Cliver SP: The effectiveness and cost of elective cesarean delivery for fetal macrosomia diagnosed by ultrasound. JAMA 1996;276:1480–1486.

Table 43–2, infants having a birth weight greater than 4000 g account for only half of shoulder dystocia cases.[9] Moreover, among macrosomic infants, the relationship with shoulder dystocia is much stronger in the comparatively small group of *asymmetrically large* infants of diabetic mothers than in the much larger group of *proportionately large* infants born to women not having diabetes. Thus, whereas an individual diabetic pregnancy is more likely to be complicated with shoulder dystocia at any given birth weight, considerably more cases occur among the far larger population of nondiabetics. Finally, the majority of shoulder dystocias (more than two thirds) occur among patients having a normal labor pattern.

OBSTETRIC STRATEGIES FOR THE MANAGEMENT OF POTENTIAL MACROSOMIA

The obvious goal for the obstetrician relating to the problem of fetal macrosomia is to prevent maternal and fetal injury. The most desirable way to accomplish this is to prevent macrosomia altogether. Preventive strategies that have been investigated with variable degrees of success include the timely identification and treatment of gestational and pregestational diabetics and labor induction for anticipated "evolving" macrosomia. In cases in which a diagnosis of established macrosomia is suspected, three management strategies have been proposed: (1) elective cesarean section to avoid birth trauma, (2) induction of labor to avoid worsening of the condition, and (3) expectant management awaiting spontaneous labor. Regardless of the strategy selected, there is increasing consensus that when macrosomia is suspected, particularly with prolonged second stage, midpelvic operative vaginal delivery should be avoided.

PREVENTION OF MACROSOMIA

The prevalence of macrosomia in diabetic patients can be reduced by establishing euglycemia.[3] Also, a strategy of routine labor induction *in diabetic women* at 37 to 38 weeks (subsequent to maturity amniocentesis) for mac-

rosomia prevention has met with some success.[10] In contrast, studies evaluating induction of labor versus expectant management for macrosomia *in nondiabetic pregnancies* have failed to show a reduction in either utilization of cesarean section or prevalence of shoulder dystocia.[11]

CESAREAN SECTION TO PREVENT SHOULDER DYSTOCIA

Most controversial of all proposed management strategies for macrosomia is that of elective cesarean section for the prevention of birth trauma. Assumptions to justify this approach are (1) a high correlation between macrosomia and birth injury, (2) the clinical ability to reliably identify fetuses that are macrosomic, and (3) the consensus that overall fetal risks associated with macrosomia (principally permanent brachial plexus injury) exceed the overall maternal risks associated with the numerous extra cesarean sections resulting from such a strategy. These assumptions have been examined and debated in the literature. Several points deserve emphasis: As discussed previously, it is increasingly clear that (1) ultrasound biometry has limited accuracy in the prediction of macrosomia, (2) most cases

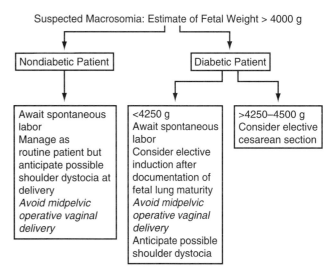

Figure 43–1. Suggested management protocol for suspected macrosomia: estimate of fetal weight > 4000 g.

of shoulder dystocia are not predictable by current identifiable risk factors, (3) most infants experiencing shoulder dystocia are not injured, and, among those who do sustain brachial plexus injury, the vast majority recover completely, and (4) nearly a third of brachial plexus injuries occur in cases in which there was not even clinical recognition of shoulder dystocia. Also, depending on the macrosomia cutoff weight estimate, large numbers of elective cesarean sections would need to be performed for comparatively small reductions in overall prevalence of shoulder dystocia (Table 43–3).[12] For this reason, the American College of Obstetricians and Gynecologists has published evidence-based guidelines[8] suggesting that "planned cesarean delivery on the basis of suspected macrosomia *in the general population* is not a reasonable strategy," but that such an approach "may be a reasonable strategy *for diabetic pregnant women* with estimated fetal weights exceeding 4250–4500 g" (Fig. 43–1).

References

1. American College of Obstetricians and Gynecologists: Fetal macrosomia (ACOG Technical Bulletin No. 159). Washington, DC, ACOG, 1991.
2. Geary M: Consideration of short term consequences of heavier babies is important. BMJ 1998;317:81–82.
3. Moore TR: Fetal growth in diabetic pregnancy. Clin Obstet Gynecol 1997;40:771–786.
4. Sandmire HF: Whither ultrasound prediction of fetal macrosomia? Obstet Gynecol 1993;82:860–862.
5. Baskett TF, Allen AC: Perinatal implications of shoulder dystocia. Obstet Gynecol 1995;86:14–17.
6. Gilbert WM, Nesbitt TS, Danielson B: Associated factors in 1611 cases of brachial plexus injury. Obstet Gynecol 1999;93:536–540.
7. Benedetti TJ, Gabbe SG: Shoulder dystocia: A complication of fetal macrosomia and prolonged second stage of labor with midpelvic delivery. Obstet Gynecol 1978;52:526–529.
8. American College of Obstetricians and Gynecologists: Shoulder dystocia (ACOG Practice Patterns No. 7). Washington, DC, ACOG, 1997.
9. Langer O, Berkus MD, Huff RW, Samueloff A: Shoulder dystocia: Should the fetus weighing greater than or equal to 4000 grams be delivered by cesarean section? Am J Obstet Gynecol 1991;165:831–837.
10. Kjos SL, Henry OA, Montoro M, et al: Insulin-requiring diabetes in pregnancy: A randomized trial of active induction of labor and expectant management. Am J Obstet Gynecol 1993;169:611–615.
11. Gonen O, Rosen OJ, Dolfin Z, et al: Induction of labor versus expectant management in macrosomia: A randomized study. Obstet Gynecol 1997;89:913–917.
12. Rouse DJ, Owen J, Goldenberg RL, Cliver SP: The effectiveness and cost of elective cesarean delivery for fetal macrosomia diagnosed by ultrasound. JAMA 1996;276:1480–1486.

FORTY-FOUR

Invasive Procedures for Prenatal Diagnosis

Arie Drugan and Mark I. Evans

Amniocentesis for prenatal diagnosis of fetal genetic disease has now been performed for more than three decades. Collaborative studies established the safety and accuracy of midtrimester amniocentesis,[1, 2] so that this technique became a routine part of prenatal care in patients at risk for chromosomal or biochemical disorders in the fetus. Amniocentesis is considered the "gold standard" against which other procedures for prenatal diagnosis are compared. However, despite its proven efficacy, a major disadvantage of amniocentesis is the availability of results late in the second trimester, generally after 20 weeks of gestation. The emotional and physical implications of termination of pregnancy at an advanced gestational age are obvious.

Technical developments in ultrasound machinery, increasing expertise in ultrasound-guided procedures, and increasing preference on the part of patients for early prenatal diagnosis[3] initiated attempts in the mid to late 1980s to perform prenatal diagnosis in the first trimester (chorionic villus sampling [CVS] and early amniocentesis). CVS results are usually available by the end of the first trimester. The accuracy and safety of CVS are comparable with those of amniocentesis.[4, 5] The early results, therefore, allow patients' privacy in reproductive decisions and, if so opted, an earlier and safer termination of pregnancy. A proposed alternative to CVS has been offered by early amniocentesis performed between 10 and 14 weeks of gestation.[6]

A change in the pattern of indications for prenatal diagnosis has also been observed over the years. Advanced maternal age (older than 35 years) is still the most common indication for genetic counseling and prenatal diagnosis, noted in more than 70% of cases. Other "classic" indications include a previous affected offspring or a balanced structural rearrangement of parental chromosomes, the latter being clinically evident as recurrent pregnancy loss (Table 44–1). Increased utilization of biochemical serum screening and ultrasound screening for fetal chromosome anomalies has caused more young patients, previously considered to be at low risk for fetal aneuploidy, to opt for invasive prenatal testing.[7] Using a risk cutoff for fetal Down syndrome equal to that of a 35-year-old, the combination of "triple" serum screening (α-fetoprotein [AFP], human chorionic gonadotropin, and unconjugated estriol) and maternal age will detect the need for invasive prenatal testing in about 65% of aneuploid conceptions. Five percent of pregnant patients will test positive and 1 in 50 amniocenteses performed for this indication will diagnose a chromosomal abnormal conception.[8] Sonographic markers for fetal chromosome anomalies (Table 44–2), observed in about 3% to 5% of pregnancies, are another emerging indication for evaluation of fetal karyotype. The most ominous of these findings are abnormalities of fetal neck. We believe that fetal chromosomes should be evaluated even in young patients with normal biochemical serum screening.[9] The results of biochemical and ultrasound screening may be also used to modulate the risk of aneuploidy in the population previously considered at risk (i.e., patients older

Table 44–1. Indications for Invasive Prenatal Diagnosis

Increased risk of chromosome anomalies
  Advanced maternal age
  Previous offspring with chromosome anomalies
  Parental balanced translocation or inversion
  Ultrasound diagnosis of fetal malformations or anomalies
  Abnormal biochemical screening in maternal serum

Previous offspring with neural tube defect

Parents carriers of a mendelian genetic trait
  Molecular DNA diagnosis (e.g., cystic fibrosis, sickle cell anemia, or fragile X)
  Enzymatic activity in villi or amniocytes (e.g., Tay-Sachs)
  Precursor levels in cell-free amniotic fluid (e.g., 17-OH progesterone)

Suspected fetal infection (e.g., cytomegalovirus, parvovirus B19, or toxoplasmosis)

Suspected fetal hematologic disorder (e.g., alloimmune thrombocytopenia)

Table 44–2. Relative Risk Associated with Sonographic Markers for Fetal Aneuploidy

Sonographic Marker	Prevalence (%)	Relative Risk*
Choroid plexus cysts	1.25	×9†
Nuchal edema or cysts	4–5	
>4 mm		×18
>5 mm		×28
>6 mm		×36
Left ventricular echogenic focus	5	×4
Hyperechoic bowel	0.6–0.8	×14–16
Pyelectasis	2	×3.3–3.9
Fetal biometry		
Short crown-rump length	7	×3
Short femur	4–5	×2.7
Short femur and humerus	2.4	×11.5

*Risk for trisomy 21 as calculated in relation to maternal age alone or in combination with biochemical screening.
†Risk is specific for trisomy 18; risk for trisomy 21 is negligible.

than 35 years). This may allow a reduction in the number of invasive diagnostic procedures in patients of advanced maternal age.[10, 11] On the other hand, "at-risk" patients previously tending to decline amniocentesis may be influenced to accept invasive prenatal diagnosis after a positive screen result.[11]

The need for rapid evaluation of fetal karyotype may arise when anomalies are suspected late, at a gestational age near the legal limit for termination of affected pregnancies. In those cases, the diagnostic options are "late" CVS[12] or cordocentesis and investigation of fetal blood karyotype. Other tests that may be performed on blood obtained by cordocentesis include hematologic disorders, acid-base balance, and immunologic status of the fetus.[13]

Genetic counseling should be a prerequisite to any invasive procedure for prenatal diagnosis.[14] Pedigree information obtained during the counseling session will allow the practitioner to ascertain genetic risks more accurately and to maximize the benefits of genetic evaluation of patients before CVS, amniocentesis, or cordocentesis.

PRENATAL DIAGNOSIS IN THE FIRST TRIMESTER

Chorionic Villus Sampling

CVS should be considered in almost every patient who needs prenatal diagnosis in the first trimester. The most common indication for CVS is advanced maternal age, which accounts for 70% to 80% of cases.[15] Other indications include a previous child with chromosome anomalies or a parent carrier of a balanced translocation or inversion. Biochemical genetic disorders can be diagnosed through enzyme levels or activity in fresh or cultured villi.[16] CVS is particularly suitable for prenatal diagnosis of classic genetic disorders with known mutations, using molecular analysis. The amount of DNA obtained from even a few villi is much larger than that contained in amniocytes from 40 mL of amniotic fluid.

Fetal viability and gestational age must always be confirmed before the procedure. CVS procedures are most commonly performed between 9 and 12 weeks of gestation, by either a transcervical or a transabdominal route. With the patient in the lithotomy position and a relatively full bladder, a catheter is inserted through the cervical canal and into the placenta, guided by transabdominal ultrasound. Instead of a catheter, some use a biopsy forceps for transcervical CVS.[17] With the sampling device in place, suction is applied using a 20-mL syringe, and some villi are separated from the placenta for analysis. Fetal heart activity should be verified before and after CVS.

The major determinant of the route of approach is placental location—transabdominal CVS is the procedure of choice for cases with anterior fundal placentas, whereas transcervical CVS should be performed when the placenta is posterior and low lying. Other factors may dictate the preferable approach to CVS in specific cases. Thus, trans-

cervical or transvaginal CVS should not be used in patients with active vaginal or cervical infection (e.g., genital herpes), whereas the transabdominal approach should be avoided in cases with interposed bowel or marked uterine retroversion and a posterior placenta.[18] In the latter situation, the procedure can be performed with a needle inserted through the vagina and the uterine walls, guided by transabdominal or transvaginal ultrasound.[19, 20]

After 13 weeks, the procedure usually is best done using a transabdominal approach,[18, 21] although a transcervical approach for late CVS using a thin biopsy forceps has also been employed successfully.[22] The use of variable approaches (e.g., transcervical versus transabdominal), real-time ultrasound guidance, and malleable catheters for villi aspiration have improved the yield and safety of CVS.[15, 23] Despite the preference of some American and European centers to use the transabdominal approach for CVS in most cases,[24, 25] in our experience, transabdominal sample size usually has been lower than that obtained transcervically.[26] Proficiency in both types of procedures is necessary, because tailoring the type of procedure to placental location is expected to reduce complication rates after CVS.[15, 27]

Safety of Chorionic Villus Sampling

The safety of CVS must be viewed from the perspective of the natural pregnancy loss rate in the first trimester. The likelihood of spontaneous abortion after documentation of a viable gestation in women at 8 to 11 weeks has been calculated by Simpson[28] as 3% to 5%, increasing with maternal age. Both the Canadian and the American collaborative studies documented an excess loss rate in the CVS group of 0.6% to 0.8%, which is not significantly different than the loss rate in the amniocentesis group.[3, 4] Fundal placental location, three catheter insertions, and obtaining small amounts of villi have been significantly associated with pregnancy loss after CVS. These factors may reflect technical difficulty during the procedure.[18]

In two small series, Firth and associates[29] and Burton and coworkers[30] claimed a 1% risk of limb reduction defects after CVS. Evaluation of over 135,000 cases from experienced centers worldwide reveals that the incidence of limb reduction defects or any other limb defects is identical to the background risk observed in the population.[31] Furthermore, closer assessment of cases of limb reduction defects reported after CVS has shown that several had not accounted for familial factors.[32] There may also be a slightly increased risk with CVS procedures done at 6 to 8 weeks of gestation or by inexperienced personnel, but available data suggest that the risk of limb deficiency after CVS at 10 weeks and beyond equals the background risk.[33]

Another concern regarding the safety of CVS is the potential for procedure related fetal-maternal transfusion. A transient rise in maternal serum AFP level after CVS has been reported.[34] The increase is correlated to sample size, but not to CVS technique, whether transabdominal or transcervical.[35] The calculated mean volume of transfused fetal blood was 5.4 mL. Others have reported the volume of fetal-maternal transfusion after CVS to reach 21% of fetal-placental blood volume.[36] Rh isoimmunization should be considered a relative contraindication to CVS, and Rh immunoprophylaxis (anti-D 300 μg) should be administered to Rh-negative patients.

Chromosomal Analysis

Simoni and Brambati and colleagues[37] developed laboratory techniques to obtain karyotypes adequate for interpretation from chorionic villi. They also reported the first diagnosis of trisomy 21 by direct analysis of villi, 5 hours after CVS was performed.[38] Over the years, the quality of chromosome preparation from CVS material has improved considerably, approaching the banding quality obtained from amniocytes or blood karyotypes.[39]

Two types of cells are observed in chorionic villi. The outer layer consists of cytotrophoblasts, which divide spontaneously, and is used for direct evaluation of metaphases. The inner mesenchymal core is used to initiate long-term cultures and is usually considered as more representative of fetal chromosomes. Karyotypes are obtained from either direct analysis or long-term culture or both in 99.6% of cases.[39] Results of direct analysis are equivocal in 1% to 2% of cases, the questions raised usually being resolved by long-term CVS or amniotic cell cultures.[18] Most commonly, an abnormal direct result that proves to be normal on long-term culture will not be confirmed in karyotypes obtained from amniocytes or fetal blood lymphocytes. The rare but more ominous situation is a normal direct result followed by an abnormal result in long-term culture. In half of these cases, the abnormality is confirmed in fetal tissue.[39] Studies suggest that the probability of a false-negative result after CVS is 10 times higher with the direct analysis as compared with culture results.[40, 41] However, when both direct analysis and culture are employed, the rate of false-negative results is about 1 in 3000 samples, similar to that observed in amniocentesis specimens.[41] Maternal cell contamination has been observed in 1.9% of long-term cultures, but that did not contribute to diagnostic errors in any case.[18] A simple polymerase chain reaction method to detect maternal cell contamination in prenatal diagnosis has been suggested.[42]

Chromosomal mosaicism in CVS material affects about 1.3% (range, 1.2% to 2.5%) of cases and is more common in direct preparations than in long-term cultures.[36] Mosaicism was restricted to extraembryonic tissue in 70% to 80% of cases. However, despite the fact that mosaicism was confined to the placenta, follow-up of these cases documented a significantly elevated fetal loss rate (7.5% to 16.7%), mostly in the second and third trimesters, suggesting that such placental mosaicism is not entirely benign.[43, 44] Intrauterine growth restriction also appears to be more common in this situation.[45] Mosaic trisomy 3 is one of the most common types of mosaicism observed in placental cells.[36] An adverse impact on pregnancy outcome seems to be most common in association with confined placental mosaicism of chromosomes 13, 16, and 22.[46] When further evaluation is needed, detailed ultrasound evaluation for fetal anomalies and amniocentesis or cordocentesis are adequate for follow-up.[44, 47] However, even if fetal blood karyotype is normal, there still will remain a small chance that mosaicism is confined to specific fetal tissues, as observed in trisomy 20 mosaicism.

"Early" Amniocentesis

"Early" amniocentesis (EA) refers to aspiration of amniotic fluid up to 14 weeks + 6 days from the last menstrual period. EA appeared to be an attractive alternative to CVS late in the first trimester because many obstetricians are familiar with the method of amniocentesis and gained increasing experience with ultrasound-guided invasive procedures. The technique of EA is relatively simple; using continuous ultrasound guidance and aseptic technique, a 22-gauge needle is inserted into a pocket of fluid, and about 1 mL of fluid per week of gestation is aspirated into a 20-mL syringe.

Complications of EA include bleeding (1.9%), uterine cramping (common), leakage of fluid (2.9%), and infection (1%). Tenting of membranes ahead of the needle is relatively common (about 5%), because membranes are not yet adhering to the uterine wall at this time in gestation. Rotating the needle or the use of a stylet longer than the needle allows the procedure to succeed in this situation.[6, 48] However, other complications associated with EA include an increased risk of musculoskeletal deformities (e.g., clubfoot)[49, 50] and increased respiratory morbidity in the offspring.[51] Findings from the collaborative Canadian study[49, 50] support an approximate 1% risk of clubfoot with procedures done up through 12 completed weeks. The American early amnio/transabdominal CVS trial, originally between 10 and 14 weeks, was scaled back to 13 to 14 weeks to reflect the consensus that early amniocenteses should not be done at less than 13 weeks except in exceptional circumstances.

These findings may be associated causally with reduction of amniotic fluid volume at a gestational age critical for lung and limb development. The total unintentional loss rate reported after EA (1.4% to 4.2%; mean, 2.7% ± 1%) probably includes losses not related causally to the early procedure.[52–55] However, increased loss rates have been observed in all series in association with amniocentesis performed *before 13 weeks* of gestation.[52, 56, 57]

A concern has also been raised about the risk of culture failure after EA. In our experience, the culture failure rate is 1 in 700 after midtrimester amniocentesis, but about 1% after early procedures, and nearly 5% in amniotic fluid samples obtained before 12 weeks' gestation.[26, 58] It should also be noted that failure of culture at amniocentesis has been reported more commonly in association with fetal chromosome anomalies.[59] The mean culture time may also be somewhat longer after EA than after midtrimester procedures.[60, 61] The use of a filter technique for EA may reduce the risk of culture failure to 0.2% and the time from sampling to harvest to 9 to 10 days.[62]

Analysis of early amniotic fluid specimens shows that AFP peaks at 12 to 13 weeks of gestation and then gradually declines, similar to fetal serum.[63] High amniotic fluid AFP levels have been observed with fetal neural tube defects or omphalocele even in these early samples,[64] and low amniotic fluid AFP values accompanied some conceptions diagnosed as aneuploid, but data are still questionable as to accuracy. Even more complex is the interpretation of acetylcholinesterase (AChE) in early amniotic fluid samples. AChE usually is analyzed on gel electrophoresis as a bimodal result, either positive or negative. In early amniotic fluid samples, a faint, inconclusive band is frequently observed. This finding seems, however, to be associated with fetal anomalies in only a minority of cases.[65] It appears that in early amniotic fluid samples, a negative AChE result may be reliable in the setting of elevated amniotic fluid AFP, but the interpretation of a positive AChE may necessitate quantitative evaluation of band density.[66] A normal sonogram in this situation is reassuring in regard to fetal neural or abdominal wall defects, but a higher rate of adverse outcome has been reported in these pregnancies.[67]

First Trimester Prenatal Diagnosis—Chorionic Villus Sampling or Early Amniocentesis?

Prenatal diagnosis in the first trimester enables us to reassure most patients with normal results 6 to 9 weeks earlier than would be possible with midtrimester amniocentesis. Patients undergoing CVS show a sharp drop in anxiety levels immediately after receiving results, whereas patients having amniocentesis at midtrimester remain anxious longer.[68] In cases that are diagnosed as abnormal, the mother can have a less traumatic and less risky termination of pregnancy.[69] However, which of the two procedures available for prenatal diagnosis in the first trimester is preferable?

Only a few prospective, randomized studies compare CVS and amniocentesis in the first trimester. Byrne and associates[70] suggest that the two techniques can be comparable in terms of accuracy and successful results. Nicolaides and coworkers[71] reported that the two procedures were similar in providing a sample for evaluation (CVS, 99.3%; EA, 100%) and in giving a nonmosaic cytogenetic result (CVS, 97.5%; EA, 97.9%). Spontaneous pregnancy loss after EA was, however, significantly higher than after CVS (4.9% vs. 2.1%, respectively). Nagel and colleagues[72] reported that the risk of unintentional loss and of mosaicism was actually higher after EA (6.2% and 5.4% respec-

tively) than after CVS. Moreover, the Canadian Early and Mid-Trimester Amniocentesis Trial (CEMAT) study showed that repeat amniocentesis was necessary in 2.2% of patients after EA.[61]

Thus, EA may be a viable alternative to CVS at 13 weeks. The possibility of analyzing amniotic fluid AFP and AChE also is tempting, especially for patients at high risk for neural tube defects per family history and for diabetics. It should be noted, however, that amniocentesis at 12 weeks or earlier is associated with significantly more culture failures and pregnancy loss than are observed at midtrimester. Furthermore, concerns have been raised that removal of amniotic fluid so early in gestation may affect fetal lung development and function.[51, 73] Thus, our opinion is that CVS is the procedure of choice before 12 weeks of gestation, for karyotyping as well as for DNA molecular analysis. In the first trimester, amniocentesis should be considered only in specific clinical situations (e.g., certain biochemical disorders or multiple pregnancy with fused placentas). In such conditions, amniocentesis should probably be performed at or after 13 weeks of gestation.

PRENATAL DIAGNOSIS IN THE SECOND AND THIRD TRIMESTERS

Midtrimester Amniocentesis

Midtrimester amniocentesis is the oldest, most commonly performed procedure for prenatal diagnosis. It also is considered the gold standard with which other procedures for prenatal diagnosis are compared. Indications for genetic amniocentesis include increased risk for chromosome anomalies or for structural anomalies that may be associated with elevated AFP. In addition, some metabolic genetic disorders may be diagnosed by measurement of precursor levels in cell-free fluid or by enzyme activity in cultured amniocytes.

Technical Aspects of Amniocentesis

An obstetrician trained and experienced in the procedure should perform amniocentesis. A detailed ultrasound examination is done to evaluate gestational age, placental location, and amount of amniotic fluid and to exclude fetal anomalies. After sterile preparation of the skin, a draped sterile ultrasound transducer is used to locate a suitable pocket of fluid. Using continuous ultrasound guidance, a 20- to 22-gauge, 3.5-inch-long spinal needle is inserted in a single smooth motion into the pocket of fluid. When the needle, which is visualized on ultrasound as a bright spot, is placed satisfactorily into the pocket of amniotic fluid, the stylet is removed, and a 5-mL syringe is used to aspirate the first 2 to 3 mL of fluid, which is then discarded. This is done to minimize the risk of contamination from maternal cells collected in the path of the needle. Twenty to 30 mL of amniotic fluid is then gently aspirated, transferred into sterile tubes, and transported at room temperature to the laboratory for processing.

The patient's blood type and antibody status should be known before amniocentesis. In Rh-negative women, the risk of Rh isosensitization from amniocentesis has been estimated to increase by 1% above the background risk.[74] Thus, transplacental passage of the needle should be avoided, if possible, in Rh-negative women,[75] and Rh immunoprophylaxis should be administered after the procedure.

In the cytogenetic lab, amniocytes are removed from the fluid by centrifugation and cultured in flasks or on cover glasses, to grow in monolayers. Colcimide is used to arrest dividing cells in metaphase, when chromosomes are maximally condensed. Cells are then harvested, placed in hypotonic saline solution, which causes intracellular swelling and better spreading of the chromosomes during slide preparation. After fixation, the chromosomes are stained with Giemsa or quinacrine for microscopic analysis. The use of triple gas incubators, specific growth media (e.g., Chang) that enhance cellular proliferation, and in situ culture on cover glass have considerably shortened the sampling-harvesting interval; in most laboratories, the results are available within 2 weeks. Additional improvement has been obtained by computerized cytoanalyzers that expedite recognition of metaphase spreads and obviate the need for darkroom and photography.

Safety and Complications

Amniocentesis is a relatively safe procedure when performed by trained personnel. In experienced hands, the procedure-related pregnancy loss rate has been quoted as between 0.2% and 0.5% over and above the spontaneous loss rate at 16 weeks of gestation, which has been estimated at 1% to 3%.[76] Pregnancy loss rates seem to be associated with the number of failed needle insertions at the same session and with vaginal bleeding after amniocentesis. Gestational age at the time of amniocentesis, volume of fluid removed, or repeat amniocentesis after a failed attempt at a different session does not seem to correlate with increased risk of pregnancy loss.[77] In experienced hands, transplacental amniocentesis does not appear to increase the rate of fetal loss.[78] Leakage of amniotic fluid is a relatively frequent complication, affecting approximately 1% to 2% of patients after amniocentesis, but it usually is of minor long-term consequence. In most cases, it resolves with bed rest for 48 to 72 hours.[79] Although it is rare, prolonged amniotic fluid leakage may lead to severe oligohydramnios, resulting in fetal pressure deformities and pulmonary hypoplasia.[80] Even patients with complete absence of fluid after amniocentesis, however, may accumulate amniotic fluid and go on to have normal outcomes.[81] Thus, as long as there is no evidence of infection, expectant management for several days seems prudent. The risk of severe amnionitis endangering maternal health appears to

be very low, around 0.1%.[82] Likewise, fetal injury by the needle should be very rare with ultrasound-guided amniocentesis.

Cytogenetic analysis of amniotic fluid cells accurately reflects fetal karyotype in over 99% of cases, although mosaicism sometimes may confuse the interpretation of results. Differentiation of cytogenetic abnormalities that truly reflect fetal chromosome aberrations from those that are the result of laboratory artifacts may be difficult. One or more hypermodal cells from one colony or one culture flask are identified in 2% to 3% of all amniocyte cultures and will be associated usually with a normal phenotype.[83] True fetal mosaicism should be considered when hypermodal cells are identified in separate colonies from the same culture flask or in different culture flasks, these being observed in 0.7% and 0.2% of amniotic cell cultures, respectively.[84, 85] Even in the latter situation, however, the abnormality in culture may not represent true fetal mosaicism, as reported by Gosden and associates.[47] In these cases, evaluation of fetal karyotype with blood sampling should help to avoid termination of pregnancy of some normal fetuses. In our experience, the frequency of results needing further investigation is similar in cultures from amniocentesis and from CVS.[86]

Late Chorionic Villus Sampling

The technique of transabdominal CVS as used in the first trimester has been applied successfully late in pregnancy for analysis of fetal karyotype from chorionic villi. Nicolaides and coworkers[87] first reported six successful placental biopsies at 14 to 37 weeks of gestation, and suggested that CVS should not be confined to the first trimester. Chieri and Aldini[88] performed transabdominal placental biopsy and amniocentesis in 220 patients at midtrimester; 210 of the procedures were indicated for advanced maternal age. A sample adequate for analysis (>2 mg of cleaned villi) was obtained in 90.9% of cases. The success rate was 94% with an anterior or fundal placenta, and 83.8% with a posterior placental location. In the latter situation, the approach to the placenta was through the amniotic cavity. Cytogenetic results were obtained in 95% of samples. No discrepancy could be found between cytogenetic results obtained in villi or in amniotic fluid. When fetal anomalies were observed on CVS, they were acted on without waiting for corroboration from the amniotic fluid culture.[88] Several other studies documented a sampling and diagnostic success of 98% to 99%, with a very low rate (0.3% to 1.8%) of late CVS-related pregnancy loss.[89–92]

The collaborative results of 2058 late CVS procedures performed at 24 centers were reported by Holzgreve and colleagues.[12] Fetal karyotype was available in 96% of procedures. The frequency of abnormal chromosome results was 21% when fetal anomalies were observed on ultrasound, and 6.2% with normal ultrasound findings. The pregnancy loss rate, excluding terminations, was 10.3% in the group with abnormal ultrasound findings, and 2.3% in the normal ultrasound group. Holzgreve and associates[93] further presented their own data on 301 CVS procedures in the second and third trimesters, 225 (74.7%) of which were performed for abnormal ultrasound scans. Karyotyping was successful in 99% of cases. The rate of chromosome anomalies was 20% in the group with abnormal ultrasound, and increased to 38% when the ultrasound findings included abnormalities of amniotic fluid volume.

It is apparent from these studies that despite the decrease in mitotic index with placental aging, direct results can be obtained even with small amounts of placental tissue. However, there was a trend for an increasing rate of failed direct preparation with gestational age.[92] The quality of karyotypes obtained from analysis of second and third trimester samples was similar to that in the first trimester.[89] The risk of maternal cell contamination in late CVS samples may actually be lower than that observed in the first trimester, because of less direct contact between villi and decidua at later gestational age.[94] Thus, placental biopsies in the second and third trimesters are technically feasible procedures for prenatal diagnosis, with results apparently as accurate as those of amniocentesis and probably associated with a smaller risk of pregnancy loss than percutaneous umbilical blood sampling. Late CVS also offers a distinct advantage over cordocentesis in cases complicated by oligohydramnios, when fetal karyotype is needed for decisions about pregnancy termination or management of labor. The decision how to manage intrapartum fetal distress, a common phenomenon in fetuses with chromosome anomalies, may be influenced significantly by identification of an abnormal fetal karyotype.

Cordocentesis (Percutaneous Umbilical Blood Sampling)

Daffos and coworkers[95] introduced cordocentesis in 1983 for the diagnosis of fetal infections. In experienced hands, the risk of fetal loss is relatively small, between 1% and 5.4%.[96–98] Other complications, usually associated with excessive needle manipulations, include hematoma of the umbilical cord and placental abruption,[8] chorioamnionitis (0.6%), and preterm delivery (9%).[98] Fetal exsanguination from the puncture site is a relatively rare complication that has been reported infrequently.[99] Maternal complications are negligible, although one case of life-threatening amnionitis has also been reported.[100] It appears that risks are higher when the mother is obese, the placenta is posterior, and the sampling is performed relatively early in gestation (i.e., before 19 weeks).[96]

Before cordocentesis, a detailed ultrasound examination should evaluate gestational age and placental location and exclude fetal anomalies. The most common site for cordocentesis is the placental insertion of the umbilical vein. When the placenta is anterior or lateral, the needle is introduced through the placenta into the umbilical cord. In cases with a posterior placenta, the needle is passed through the amniotic cavity and the cord is punctured close to its placental insertion or at the intra-abdominal section of the umbilical vein. Different guidance techniques (i.e., fixed needle guides vs. freehand), needles of lengths varying from 8 to 15 cm, gauges varying from 20 to 27 French, and patient preparation protocols are used by various centers. Nicolaides and colleagues[101] advocate an outpatient setting for the procedure, without maternal fasting or use of sedation, tocolytics, antibiotics, or fetal paralysis.

Molecular diagnoses now are available for many of the mutations resulting in thalassemia, sickle cell disease, and hemophilia A and B, enabling diagnosis in the first trimester by CVS, with blood sampling being performed only in cases that are noninformative or with ambiguous results. Cordocentesis is, however, necessary for the diagnosis and management of von Willebrand's disease and congenital alloimmune thrombocytopenia.[102] In alloimmune thrombocytopenia, cordocentesis allows the determination of fetal platelet phenotype and count. A low fetal platelet count in this situation can be treated by weekly infusion of platelets, until delivery.[103, 104]

In Rh isoimmunization, fetal blood sampling is performed for immediate confirmation of fetal antigenic status, obviating the need for further intervention in the Rh-negative fetus. If the fetus is Rh positive, cordocentesis enables a more accurate assessment of fetal anemia and an immediate correction of fetal erythrocyte count by intravascular transfusion. From case-control studies, it appears that intravascular correction of fetal anemia is more efficient and less risky to the mother and fetus than the intraperitoneal approach, at all gestational ages or levels of disease severity.[105] Moreover, the fetus suffering from Rh disease with high-output cardiac failure may be compromised by the volume overload needed to correct the severe anemia and may benefit from intravascular exchange transfusion.[106] It should be noted, however, that cordocentesis may enhance maternal sensitization more than does amniocentesis, especially if blood sampling is performed by a transplacental approach.[107] Thus, Rh immunoprophylaxis should be offered to all Rh-negative patients undergoing cordocentesis.

The diagnosis of fetal infection is based commonly on the demonstration of the agent-specific immunoglobulin M (IgM) in fetal blood, because the large molecule IgM does not cross the placenta. Fetal blood sampling should be scheduled to allow enough time from initial exposure for IgM to appear after immune competence develops in the fetus. For first trimester exposures, the best time for cordocentesis is probably after 22 weeks' gestation. In specific cases, in utero treatment also is available. Thus, after demonstration of IgM specific for toxoplasmosis in fetal blood, antibiotic treatment with spiramycin significantly reduced the risk of congenital toxoplasmosis as well as the risk of late sequelae.[108] Repeated blood transfusions in utero have been used in hydropic fetuses with hemolytic anemia caused by parvovirus B19 infection.[109]

In the evaluation of the small-for-dates fetus, cordocentesis allows for rapid fetal karyotyping, available within 48 to 72 hours. Other abnormalities observed in blood samples from fetuses with intrauterine growth restriction with normal chromosomes include hypoxemia, hypercapnia, lactic acidemia, leukopenia, thrombocytopenia, and disturbed carbohydrate, lipid, and protein metabolism.[107] Several studies have compared the prediction of fetal acidosis by Doppler or biophysical profile with cord blood gases. Weiner and associates[110] demonstrated a statistically significant correlation between an increased umbilical systolic-to-diastolic ratio (>3.5) and fetal hypoxia and acidemia in cord blood. This relationship was even more significant with absent or reversed diastolic flow. In another study, the biophysical profile significantly correlated with changes in cord pH including, to some extent, the degree of fetal acidemia.[111] In the situation of severe intrauterine growth restriction with equivocal biophysical score and umbilical blood flow studies, the availability of fetal Po_2 and pH may provide additional and crucial information in the balance between the risk of premature delivery and the risk of leaving the fetus to grow in a hostile intrauterine environment.

Summary

Invasive procedures for prenatal diagnosis have been performed at all gestational ages. Genetic counseling by a trained genetic counselor and evaluation of genetic risks should precede any invasive procedure. Patients should be informed about the risk of that pregnancy being affected by the conditions considered and the yield of information obtained through prenatal evaluation. The risk and potential complications of the procedure itself also should be discussed.

The most common indication for prenatal diagnosis is an increased risk for chromosome anomalies. The safest and most widely accepted procedures for prenatal diagnosis are CVS in the first trimester and amniocentesis in the second trimester of pregnancy. EA and cordocentesis with their higher inherent risk of pregnancy loss should probably be tailored to those specific situations in which no other options for prenatal diagnosis are available or that are associated with a relatively high risk of fetal anomalies.

References

1. Medical Research Council: Diagnosis of Genetic Disease by Amniocentesis during Second Trimester of Pregnancy. Ottawa, Ontario, Canada, Medical Research Council, 1977.
2. National Institute of Child Health and Human Development Amniocentesis Registry, 1978: The safety and accuracy of midtrimester amniocentesis (DHEW Publication No. [NIH] 78-190). Washington, DC, U.S. Department of Health, Education, and Welfare, 1978.
3. Evans MI, Drugan A, Koppitch FC, et al: Genetic diagnosis in the first trimester: The norm for the 1990s. Am J Obstet Gynecol 1989;160:1332.
4. Canadian Collaborative CVS—Amniocentesis Clinical Trial Group: Multicenter randomized clinical trial of chorionic villus sampling and amniocentesis. Lancet 1989;1:1.
5. Rhoads GG, Jackson LG, Schlesselman SE, et al: The safety and efficacy of chorionic villus sampling for early prenatal diagnosis of cytogenetic abnormalities. N Engl J Med 1989;320:609.
6. Hanson FW, Happ RL, Tennant FR, et al: Ultrasonography-guided early amniocentesis in singleton pregnancies. Am J Obstet Gynecol 1990;162:1376.
7. Olsen CL, Cross PK: Trends in the use of prenatal diagnosis in New York State and the impact of biochemical screening on the detection of Down syndrome: 1984–1993. Prenat Diagn 1997;17:1113.
8. Drugan A, Reichler A, Bronshtein M, et al: Abnormal biochemical serum screening versus second trimester ultrasound-detected minor anomalies as predictors of aneuploidy in low risk patients. Fetal Diagn Ther 1996;11:301.
9. Zimmer EZ, Drugan A, Ofir C, et al: Ultrasound anomalies of the fetal neck: Implications for the risk of aneuploidy and structural anomalies. Prenat Diagn 1997;17:1055.
10. Haddow JE, Palomaki GE, Knight GJ, et al: Reducing the need for amniocentesis in women 35 years of age or older with serum markers for screening. N Engl J Med 1994;330:1114.
11. Beekhuis JR, De Wolf BT, Mantingh A, Heringa MP: The influence of serum screening on the amniocentesis rate in women of advanced maternal age. Prenat Diagn 1994;14:199.
12. Holzgreve W, Miny P, Schloo R, et al: "Late CVS" International Registry: Complication of data from 24 centers. Prenat Diagn 1990;10:159.
13. Hoskins IA: Cordocentesis in isoimmunization and fetal physiologic measurement, infection and karyotyping. Curr Opin Obstet Gynecol 1991;3:266.
14. Cohn GM, Gould M, Miller RC, et al: The importance of genetic counseling before amniocentesis. J Perinatol 1996;16:352.
15. Copeland KL, Carpenter RJ, Penolio KR, et al: Integration of the transabdominal technique into an ongoing chorionic villus sampling program. Am J Obstet Gynecol 1989;161:1289.
16. Evans MI, Moore C, Kolodny F, et al: Lysosomal enzymes in chorionic villi, cultured amniocytes, and cultured skin fibroblasts. Clin Chim Acta 1986;157:109.
17. Borell A, Fortuny A, Lazaro L, et al: First trimester transcervical chorionic villus sampling by biopsy forceps versus midtrimester amniocentesis: A randomized controlled trial project. Prenat Diagn 1999;19:1138.
18. Simpson JL: Chorionic villus sampling. Semin Perinatol 1990;14:446.
19. Ghirardini G, Popp WL, Camurri L, et al: Vaginosonographic guided chorionic villi needle biopsy. Eur J Obstet Gynecol Reprod Biol 1986;23:315.
20. Sidransky E, Black SH, Soenksen DM, et al: Transvaginal chorionic villus sampling. Prenat Diagn 1990;10:583.
21. Podobnick M, Ciglar S, Singer Z, et al: Transabdominal chorionic villus sampling in the second and third trimesters of high-risk pregnancies. Prenat Diagn 1997;17:125.
22. Borrell A, Costa D, Delgado RD, et al: Transcervical chorionic villus sampling beyond 12 weeks of gestation. Ultrasound Obstet Gynecol 1996;7:416.
23. Jahoda MGJ, Pijpers I, Reuss A, et al: Transabdominal villus sampling in early second trimester: A safe sampling method for women of advanced age. Prenat Diagn 1990;10:307.
24. Brambati B, Oldrini A, Lanzani A: Transabdominal villus sampling: A free hand ultrasound guided technique. Am J Obstet Gynecol 1987;157:134.
25. Smidt-Jensen S, Hahnemann N: Transabdominal fine needle biopsy from chorionic villi in the first trimester. Prenat Diagn 1984;4:163.
26. Evans MI, Quigg MH, Koppitch FC, et al: First trimester prenatal diagnosis. In Evans MI, Fletcher JC, Dixler AO, et al (eds): Fetal Diagnosis and Therapy: Science, Ethics and the Law. Philadelphia, JB Lippincott, 1989, p. 17.
27. Brambati B, Lanzani A, Tului L: Transabdominal and transcervical chorionic villus sampling: Efficiency and risk evaluation of 2411 cases. Am J Med Genet 1990;35:160.
28. Simpson JL: Incidence and timing of pregnancy losses: Relevance to evaluating safety of early prenatal diagnosis. Am J Med Genet 1990;35:165.
29. Firth HV, Boyd PA, Chamberlain P, et al: Severe limb abnormalities after chorionic villus sampling at 56–66 days' gestation. Lancet 1991;337:762.
30. Burton BK, Schulz CJ, Burd LI: Limb anomalies associated with chorionic villus sampling. Obstet Gynecol 1992;79:726.
31. Kuliev A, Jackson L, Froster U, et al: Chorionic villus sampling

safety. Report of World Health Organization/EURO meeting. Am J Obstet Gynecol 1996;174:807.

32. Schloo R, Miny P, Holzgreve W, et al: Distal limb deficiency following chorionic villus sampling? Am J Med Genet 1992;42:404.

33. Firth H: Chorion villus sampling and limb deficiency—cause or coincidence? Prenat Diagn 1997;17:1313.

34. Blakemore KJ, Baumgarten A, Schonfeld Dimaio M, et al: Rise in maternal serum alpha-fetoprotein concentration after chorionic villus sampling and the possibility of isoimmunization. Am J Obstet Gynecol 1986;155:986.

35. Shulman LP, Meyers CM, Simpson JL, et al: Fetomaternal transfusion depends on amount of chorionic villi aspirated but not on method of chorionic villus sampling. Am J Obstet Gynecol 1990;162:1185.

36. McGowan KD, Blackemore KJ: Amniocentesis and chorionic villus sampling. Curr Opin Obstet Gynecol 1991;3:221.

37. Simoni G, Brambati B, Danesino C, et al: Efficient direct chromosome analyses and enzyme determinations from chorionic villi samples in the first trimester of pregnancy. Hum Genet 1983;63:349.

38. Brambati B, Simoni G: Letter to the editor. Lancet 1989;1:583.

39. Ledbetter DH, Martin AO, Verlinsky Y, et al: Cytogenetic results of chorionic villus sampling: High success rate and diagnostic accuracy in the United States Collaborative Study. Am J Obstet Gynecol 1990;162:495.

40. Qumsiyeh MB, Adhvaryu SG, Peters-Brown T, et al: Discrepancies in cytogenetic findings in chorionic villi. J Matern Fetal Med 1997;6:351.

41. Kennerknecht I, Barbi G, Djalali M, et al: False negative findings in chorionic villus sampling. An experimental approach and review of the literature. Prenat Diagn 1998;18:1276.

42. Batanian JR, Ledbetter DW, Fenwick RG: A simple VNTR-PCR method for detecting maternal cell contamination in prenatal diagnosis. Genet Test 1998;2:347.

43. Johnson A, Wapner RJ, Davis GH, et al: Mosaicism in chorionic villus sampling: An association with poor perinatal outcome. Obstet Gynecol 1990;75:573.

44. Sundberg K, Lundsteen C, Philip J: Early filtration amniocentesis for further investigation of mosaicism diagnosed by chorionic villus sampling. Prenat Diagn 1996;16:1121.

45. Kalousek DK, Dill FJ: Chromosomal mosaicism confined to the placenta in human conceptions. Science 1983;221:665.

46. Leschot NJ, Schuring Blum GH, Van Prooijen-Knegt AC, et al: The outcome of pregnancies with confined placental chromosome mosaicism in cytotrophoblast cells. Prenat Diagn 1996;16:705.

47. Gosden C, Rodeck CH, Nicolaides KH: Fetal blood sampling in the investigation of chromosome mosaicism in amniotic fluid cell culture. Lancet 1988;1:613.

48. Dombrowski MP, Isada NB, Johnson MP, Berry SM: Modified stylet technique for tenting of amniotic membranes. Obstet Gynecol 1996;87:455.

49. Farrell SA, Summers AM, Dallaire L, et al: Club foot, an adverse outcome of early amniocentesis: Disruption or deformation? CEMAT. Canadian Early and Mid-Trimester Amniocentesis Trial. J Med Genet 1999;36:843.

50. Delisle MF, Wilson RD: First trimester prenatal diagnosis: Amniocentesis. Semin Perinatol 1999;23:414.

51. Greenough A, Yuksel B, Naik S, et al: First trimester invasive procedures: Effects on symptom status and lung volume in very young children. Pediatr Pulmonol 1997;24:415.

52. Penso CA, Frigoletto FD: Early amniocentesis. Semin Perinatol 1990;14:465.

53. Brumfield CG, Lin S, Conner W, et al: Pregnancy outcome following genetic amniocentesis at 11–14 versus 16–19 weeks' gestation. Obstet Gynecol 1996;88:114.

54. Johnson JM, Wilson RD, Winsor EJ, et al: The early amniocentesis study: A randomized clinical trial of early amniocentesis versus midtrimester amniocentesis. Fetal Diagn Ther 1996;11:85.

55. Elejalde BR, de Elejalde MM, Acuna JM, et al: Prospective study of amniocentesis performed between weeks 9 and 16 of gestation: Its feasibility, risks, complications and use in early genetic amniocentesis. Am J Med Genet 1990;35:188.

56. Saltvedt S, Almstrom H: Fetal loss rate after second trimester amniocentesis at different gestational age. Acta Obstet Gynecol Scand 1999;78:10.

57. Johnson JM, Wilson RD, Singer J, et al: Technical factors in early amniocentesis predict adverse outcome. Results of the Canadian

58. Early (EA) versus Mid-trimester (MA) Amniocentesis Trial. Prenat Diagn 1999;19:732.

58. Rooney DE, MacLachlan N, Smith J, et al: Early amniocentesis: A cytogenetic evaluation. BMJ 1989;299:25.

59. Reid R, Sepuvelda W, Kyle PM, Davies G: Amniotic fluid culture failure: Clinical significance and association with aneuploidy. Obstet Gynecol 1996;87:588.

60. Diaz Vega M, De La Cueva P, Leal C, Aisa F: Early amniocentesis at 10–12 weeks' gestation. Prenat Diagn 1996;16:307.

61. Winsor EJ, Tomkins DJ, Kalousek D, et al: Cytogenetic aspects of the Canadian Early and Mid-trimester Amniotic fluid trial (CEMAT). Prenat Diagn 1999;16:620.

62. Sundberg K, Lundsteen P, Philip J: Comparison of cell cultures, chromosome quality and karyotypes obtained after chorionic villus sampling and early amniocentesis with filter technique. Prenat Diagn 1999;19:12.

63. Drugan A, Syner FN, Greb A, et al: Amniotic fluid alpha-fetoprotein and acetylcholinesterase in early genetic amniocentesis. Obstet Gynecol 1988;72:33.

64. Crandall BF, Chua C: Detecting neural tube defects by amniocentesis between 11 and 15 weeks' gestation. Prenat Diagn 1995;15:339.

65. Drugan A, Syner FN, Belsky RL, et al: Amniotic fluid acetylcholinesterase: Implications of an inconclusive result. Am J Obstet Gynecol 1988;159:469.

66. Burton BK, Nelson LH, Pettenati MJ: False positive acetylcholinesterase with early amniocentesis. Obstet Gynecol 1989;74:607.

67. Brown CL, Colden KA, Hume RF, et al: Faint and positive amniotic fluid acetylcholinesterase with a normal sonogram. Am J Obstet Gynecol 1996;175:1000.

68. Robinson GE, Garner DM, Olmsted MP, et al: Anxiety reduction after chorionic villus sampling and genetic amniocentesis. Am J Obstet Gynecol 1988;159:953.

69. Gosden CM: First trimester fetal karyotyping: CVS or early amniocentesis? (editorial). Ultrasound Obstet Gynecol 1991;1:233.

70. Byrne D, Marks K, Azar G, et al: Randomized study of early amniocentesis versus chorionic villus sampling: A technical and cytogenetic comparison of 650 patients. Ultrasound Obstet Gynecol 1991;1:235.

71. Nicolaides KH, Brizot ML, Patel F, Snijders R: Comparison of chorionic villus sampling and early amniocentesis for karyotyping in 1492 singleton pregnancies. Fetal Diagn Ther 1996;11:9.

72. Nagel HT, Vandenbussche FP, Keirse MJ, et al: Amniocentesis before 14 completed weeks as an alternative to transabdominal chorionic villus sampling: A controlled trial with infant follow-up. Prenat Diagn 1998;18:465.

73. Yuksel B, Greenough A, Naik S, et al: Perinatal lung function and invasive antenatal procedures. Thorax 1997;52:181.

74. Murray JC, Karp LE, Williamson RA, et al: Rh isoimmunization as related to amniocentesis. Am J Hum Genet 1983;16:527.

75. Golbus MS, Stephens JD, Cann HM, et al: Rh isoimmunization following genetic amniocentesis. Prenat Diagn 1982;2:149.

76. Reid KP, Gurrin LC, Dickinson JE, et al: Pregnancy loss rates following second trimester genetic amniocentesis. Aust N Z J Obstet Gynecol 1999;39:281.

77. Midtrimester amniocentesis for prenatal diagnosis: Safety and accuracy. JAMA 1976;236:1471.

78. Bombard AT, Power JF, Carter S, et al: Procedure related fetal losses in transplacental versus nontransplacental genetic amniocentesis. Am J Obstet Gynecol 1995;172:868.

79. Crane JP, Rohland BM: Clinical significance of amniotic fluid leakage after genetic amniocentesis. Prenat Diagn 1986;6:25.

80. Nimrod C, Varela-Gittings F, Machin G, et al: The effect of very prolonged membrane rupture on fetal development. Am J Obstet Gynecol 1984;148:540.

81. Gold R, Goyert G, Schwartz DB, et al: Conservative management of midtrimester post amniocentesis fluid leakage. Obstet Gynecol 1989;74:745.

82. Ayadi S, Carbillon L, Varlet C, et al: Fatal sepsis due to *Escherichia coli* after second trimester amniocentesis. Fetal Diagn Ther 1998;13:98.

83. Simpson JL: Amniocentesis: What it can tell you and what it can't. Contemp Obstet Gynecol 1988;31:33.

84. Hsu LYF, Kaffe S, Perlis ET: Trisomy 20 mosaicism in prenatal diagnosis: A review and update. Prenat Diagn 1987;7:581.

85. Worton RG, Stern RA: A Canadian collaborative study on mosaicism in amniotic fluid cell cultures. Prenat Diagn 1984;4:131.

86. Wright DJ, Brindley BA, Koppitch FC, et al: Interpretation of chorionic villus sampling laboratory results is just as reliable as amniocentesis. Obstet Gynecol 1989;74:739.

87. Nicolaides KH, Soothill PH, Rodeck CH, et al: Prenatal diagnosis: Why confine chorionic villus (placental) biopsy to the first trimester? Lancet 1986;1:543.

88. Chieri PR, Aldini AJR: Feasibility of placental biopsy in the second trimester for fetal diagnosis. Am J Obstet Gynecol 1989;160:581.

89. Smidt-Jensen S, Lundsteen C, Lind AM, et al: Transabdominal chorionic villus sampling in the second and third trimester of pregnancy: Chromosome quality, reporting time and feto-maternal bleeding. Prenat Diagn 1993;13:957.

90. Ko TM, Tseng LH, Hwa HL, et al: Prenatal diagnosis by transabdominal chorionic villus sampling in the second and third trimesters. Arch Gynecol Obstet 1995;256:193.

91. Podobnik M, Ciglar S, Singer Z, et al: Transabdominal chorionic villus sampling in the second and third trimesters of high-risk pregnancies. Prenat Diagn 1997;17:125.

92. Carroll SG, Davies T, Kyle PM, et al: Fetal karyotyping by chorionic villus sampling after the first trimester. Br J Obstet Gynaecol 1999;106:1035.

93. Holzgreve W, Miny P, Gerlach B, et al: Benefits of placental biopsies for rapid karyotyping in the second and third trimesters (late chorionic villus sampling) in high-risk pregnancies. Am J Obstet Gynecol 1990;162:1188.

94. Ganshirt-Ahlert D, Pohlschmidt M, Gal A, et al: Transabdominal placental biopsy in the second and third trimester of pregnancy: What is the risk of maternal contamination in DNA diagnosis? Obstet Gynecol 1990;75:320.

95. Daffos F, Cappella-Pavlovsky M, Forestier F: Fetal blood sampling via the umbilical cord using a needle guided by ultrasound: Report of 66 cases. Prenat Diagn 1983;3:271.

96. Nicolaides KH, Sniders RJM: Cordocentesis. In Evans MI (ed): Reproductive Risks and Prenatal Diagnosis. Norwalk, Conn, Appleton & Lange, 1992, p 201.

97. Buscaglia M, Ghisoni L, Bellotti M, et al: Percutaneous umbilical blood sampling: Indication changes and procedure loss rates in a nine years' experience. Fetal Diagn Ther 1996;11:106.

98. Bernaschek G, Yildiz A, Kolankaya A, et al: Complications of cordocentesis in high-risk pregnancies: Effects on fetal loss and premature deliveries. Prenat Diagn 1995;15:995.

99. Seligman SP, Young BK: Tachycardia as the sole fetal heart rate abnormality after funipuncture. Obstet Gynecol 1996;87:833.

100. Wilkins I, Mezrow G, Lynch L, et al: Amnionitis and life threatening respiratory distress after percutaneous umbilical blood sampling. Am J Obstet Gynecol 1989;160:427.

101. Nicolaides KH, Soothill PW, Rodeck CH, et al: Ultrasound guided sampling of umbilical cord and placental blood to access fetal well being. Lancet 1986;1:1065.

102. Bussel JB, Berkowitz RL, McFarland JG, et al: Antenatal treatment of neonatal thrombocytopenia. N Engl J Med 1988;319:1374.

103. Nicolini U, Rodeck CH, Kochenour NK, et al: In utero platelet transfusion for alloimmune thrombocytopenia. Lancet 1988;2:506.

104. Murphy MF, Pullon HWH, Metcalfe P, et al: Management of fetal allo-immune thrombocytopenia by weekly in utero platelet transfusions. Vox Sang 1990;58:45.

105. Harman CR, Bowman JM, Manning FA, et al: Intrauterine transfusion—intraperitoneal versus intravascular approach: A case-control comparison. Am J Obstet Gynecol 1990;162:1053.

106. Poissonier MH, Brossard Y, Demedeiros N, et al: Two hundred intrauterine exchange transfusions in severe blood incompatibilities. Am J Obstet Gynecol 1989;161:709.

107. Weiner CP, Grant S, Hudson J, et al: Effect of diagnostic and therapeutic cordocentesis on maternal serum alpha-fetoprotein concentration. Am J Obstet Gynecol 1989;161:706.

108. Daffos F, Forestier F, Capella-Pavlovsky M, et al: Prenatal management of 746 pregnancies at risk for congenital toxoplasmosis. N Engl J Med 1988;318:271.

109. Peters MT, Nicolaides KH: Cordocentesis for the diagnosis and treatment of human fetal parvovirus infection. Obstet Gynecol 1990;75:501.

110. Weiner CP: The relationship between the umbilical artery systolic/diastolic ratio and umbilical blood gas measurements in specimens obtained by cordocentesis. Am J Obstet Gynecol 1990;162:1198.

111. Ribbert LSM, Sniders RJM, Nicolaides KH, et al: Relationship of fetal biophysical profile and blood gas values at cordocentesis in severely growth retarded fetuses. Am J Obstet Gynecol 1990;163:569.

FORTY-FIVE

New Genetic Concepts

Ralph L. Kramer, Yuval Yaron,

Mark Paul Johnson, and Mark I. Evans

Half of what was taught in medical school genetics in 1990 is now known to be wrong. Although mendelian inheritance still constitutes the foundation of the science of genetics, not all heritable traits follow Mendel's laws. Exceptions include mitochondrial inheritance, genomic imprinting, uniparental disomy, mosaicism (somatic and germline), and trinucleotide repeat expansion. These modes of inheritance now explain previously unexplainable patterns of inheritance and recurrence.

MITOCHONDRIAL INHERITANCE

Each human cell contains thousands of mitochondria that are the major sites of ATP production. The mitochondrial genome is a circular DNA molecule with 16,569 nucleotides encoding 37 genes (Fig. 45–1). There are 2 to 10 copies of mitochondrial DNA per mitochondrion, encoding for 2 rRNAs, 22 tRNAs, and 13 polypeptide chains (complexes I to V), which are part of the oxidative phosphorylation system and the respiratory pathway.

Several features differentiate the mitochondrial genome from the nuclear genome. Nearly every nucleotide appears to be part of a coding sequence, either for a protein or for one of the RNAs. Hence, there are very few introns in the mitochondrial genome. Total noncoding DNA is just a little over 1 kb and is thought to be a control region containing both origins of replication for the H (heavy) strand of mtDNA and promoters for H strand and L (light) strand transcription. Both the H and the L strands contain coding sequences.

Comparison of mitochondrial gene sequences and the amino acid sequences of the corresponding proteins indicates that the genetic code in mtDNA is different from that which is used in the nuclear genome. Four of the 64 codons code for different amino acids in the mitochondrial genome. Whereas more than 30 tRNAs specify amino acids in the cytoplasm, mitochondrial protein synthesis requires only 22. Many of the tRNA molecules recognize any one of the four nucleotides in the third position that allows one tRNA to pair with any one of four codons, allowing protein synthesis with fewer tRNAs. In other words, the rules for codon-anticodon pairing appear to be "relaxed" in the mitochondrial genome.

Variability of phenotypic expression, which is characteristic of mitochondrial disease, is determined by the relative proportion of mutant and normal mtDNA in the affected tissue. Unlike nuclear DNA, which is evenly divided between daughter cells, the cytoplasm and therefore mtDNA are randomly distributed to daughter cells. The term *heteroplasmy* is used to refer to the presence of both normal and abnormal mitochondria, as opposed to homoplasmy, in which all the mitochondria are either normal or abnormal.

The ovum is the source of all mitochondria in the embryo, because sperm contain only a few mitochondria that are located in the tail region. Because only the nucleus of the sperm fuses with the ovum, the mitochondria from the sperm do not persist in the offspring. Hence, no known disease is thought to be inherited through the paternal mitochondrial genome, and mitochondrial inheritance is exclusively maternal.

Somatic mtDNA Mutations and Aging

Mitochondria carry out the majority of cellular oxidation and produce most of the cell's ATP. Free radicals are produced in the mitochondria during oxidative phosphory-

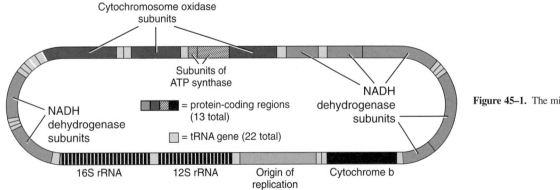

Figure 45–1. The mitochondrial genome.

lation and other reactions. Free radical production is increased by inhibition of the electron transport pathways and is thus a self-perpetuating process. Oxidative damage to mtDNA either directly or indirectly, by oxidative products such as lipids and proteins, can cause mtDNA mutations that further impair oxidative phosphorylation efficiency. mtDNA is more susceptible to damage by free radicals because of the close proximity of mtDNA to the site of free radical generation, the lack of protective histones, and the relatively poor repair mechanisms of the mitochondrial genome.

Mitochondrial Disease

Leber's Hereditary Optic Neuropathy (LHON). LHON is characterized by rapid loss of central vision during early adult life. Eyes may be affected simultaneously or sequentially. LHON patients and their maternal relatives have also been reported to manifest a variety of additional symptoms. Cardiac conduction defects have been noted in some families.

Myoclonus Epilepsy and Ragged-Red Fibers (MERRF) Syndrome. The term *ragged-red fibers* is derived from histologic characteristics observed with the modified Gomori trichome staining of fresh-frozen muscle in which accumulated mitochondria appear red, resulting from rearrangements of mtDNA or point mutations affecting tRNA genes. The syndrome consists of myopathy, myoclonus, generalized seizures, hearing loss, intellectual deterioration, and ataxia.

Mitochondrial Myopathy, Encephalopathy, Lactic Acidosis, and Strokelike Episodes (MELAS). This disorder is first manifest in childhood as stunted growth; recurrent strokelike episodes manifest as hemiparesis, hemianopsia, and cortical blindness. Focal or generalized seizures, myoclonic epilepsy, and hearing loss may also be seen, as well as episodic vomiting. Death often occurs before the age of 20 years. MELAS is associated with a point mutation in the tRNA for leucine.

Kearns-Sayre Syndrome and Chronic Progressive External Ophthalmoplegia (KSS/CPEO). This disease is characterized by ophthalmoplegia, atypical retinitis pigmentosa, and mitochondrial myopathy. Cardiac conduction defects may be present. The age of onset is usually before age 20 years. Other features may include ataxia, hearing loss, dementia, short stature, delayed secondary sexual characteristics, hypoparathyroidism, and hypothyroidism.

Neuropathy, Ataxia, and Retinitis Pigmentosa (NARP). As the name implies, this disorder is characterized by a variable combination of retinitis pigmentosa, ataxia, and sensory neuropathy. Other features include developmental delay, dementia, seizures, and proximal limb weakness.

Cytochrome C Oxidase Deficiency (Complex IV Deficiency). There are three established clinical syndromes of cytochrome C oxidase (COX) deficiency, two of which represent variant forms of infantile myopathy. One is benign, characterized by spontaneous recovery by the age of 2 to 3 years. The other form presents in the neonatal period and results in respiratory failure. The fatal form is also associated with a renal tubular defect. The fatal form is inherited as a recessive trait and is thought to represent a defect in a nuclear-encoded polypeptide in the respiratory chain. The third form of COX deficiency affects the central nervous system and is known as *Leigh's syndrome.* The typical presentation in the neonatal period is one of hypotonia, recurrent vomiting, and retinitis pigmentosa, leading to visual loss. Lactic acid levels are increased in blood and cerebrospinal fluid. Several heteroplasmic mtDNA mutations have been demonstrated in Leigh's syndrome.

Maternally Inherited Diabetes Mellitus. Several retrospective studies showed that patients with non–insulin-dependent diabetes mellitus (NIDDM) were much more likely to have a mother who was diagnosed with NIDDM than a father. This was also noted to be true for women with gestational diabetes. These studies may be subject to certain biases, however, because all of them used patient recollection to ascertain affected first-degree relatives.

Glucose intolerance, or NIDDM, has been reported in some subjects with mitochondrial myopathy. Up to 20% of patients with MELAS have been shown to be diabetic. Diabetes in this group of patients has been associated with nerve deafness and a point mutation in a mitochondrial gene for leucine tRNA. It therefore seems probable that mitochondrial mutations may be involved in the pathogenesis of a small but clinically significant proportion of cases of NIDDM.

GENOMIC IMPRINTING

Genomic imprinting refers to the process by which specific genes are differentially marked (imprinted) during parental gametogenesis. The result is differential expression of these genes depending on whether they are inherited either maternally or paternally. The existence of genomic imprinting was first suspected after experiments with pronuclear transplantation. If one of the pronuclei is removed and replaced with a pronucleus of the opposite parental origin, the result is lethal. However, depending on whether the pronuclei are of maternal or paternal origin, the consequences are very different. If both are of maternal origin (a gynogenetic embryo), the embryo initially develops normally, but development of the placenta and fetal membranes is deficient. If the pronuclei are both male (an androgenetic embryo), the membranes and placenta develop normally while the embryo develops poorly. This latter situation is seen in the case of the triploid conceptus with a partial molar pregnancy. These experiments and observations imply that both maternal and paternal genomes are necessary for normal growth and development. Therefore, their contributions cannot be equivalent.

Several theories have been proposed to explain the reason for the existence of genomic imprinting, including avoidance of genetic conflict, prevention of parthenogenesis, optimizing placental function while avoiding the development of gestational trophoblastic disease, dominance modification, and gene regulation. Genomic imprinting is also thought to be operative in X inactivation, which results in dosage compensation so that structural genes on the X chromosome are expressed at the same levels in males and females.

Genomic Imprinting in Human Disease

Prader-Willi and Angelman's Syndromes. Prader-Willi syndrome (PWS) is characterized by short stature, obesity, polyphagia, hypogonadism, and mental retardation. High-resolution chromosome banding studies revealed small interstitial deletions of the 15q11-q13 region in a large proportion of these patients.

An identical deletion was reported in 1987 by Magenis and colleagues[1] in patients with the much more uncommon Angelman's (or happy puppet) syndrome (AS), characterized by microcephaly, jerky movements, seizures, mental retardation, inappropriate laughter, a large mouth, and protruding tongue. In a rare subset of patients with PWS who did not have detectable cytogenetic deletion, Nicholls and associates[2] reported that both copies of chromosome 15 were maternal in origin. It was subsequently discovered in PWS that the deletion always involved the paternally derived chromosome 15, whereas the deletion was present on the maternal copy in AS. These findings strongly suggest a parent-of-origin effect or genomic imprinting in which PWS and AS are caused by two closely linked genes that are oppositely imprinted. Both PWS and AS have been documented to result from uniparental disomy, in which both copies of chromosome 15 are inherited from one parent (see later). In the case of PWS, both copies are maternal, whereas in AS both copies are paternal in origin.

Beckwith-Wiedemann Syndrome (BWS). This syndrome is characterized by general and regional overgrowth characterized by macrosomia, macroglossia, large kidneys with renal medullary dysplasia, and pancreatic hyperplasia, as well as cytomegaly within the fetal adrenal cortex. Omphalocele may also be present. Birth weight averages 4 kg, and excessive growth is noted in early childhood. There is a significant predisposition toward the development of certain malignancies, most commonly Wilms' tumor, but also adrenocortical carcinoma, hepatoblastoma, and rhabdomyosarcoma. The gene for BWS has been mapped to 11p15. Maternal genomic imprinting is operative. The proposed mechanism is failure of methylation to suppress the maternally derived gene insulin-like growth factor 2 (IGF-2).

UNIPARENTAL DISOMY

Uniparental disomy (UPD) refers to the inheritance of two copies of a chromosome (or part of a chromosome)

from the same parent. When a chromosome or gene is present in duplicate, it is called *isodisomy*. If both nonidentical homologues are present, it is designated as *heterodisomy*. UPD can involve both autosomes and sex chromosomes. Cystic fibrosis (CF) and growth deficiency have been diagnosed in a patient who had inherited two copies of the same mutation in the CF gene but had only one carrier parent with that mutation. The patient with CF had evidence of intrauterine growth restriction, which was thought to be secondary to the effects of UPD rather than of CF.

UPD has been discerned to cause both PWS and AS. UPD has been described for chromosomes 5, 6, 7, 9, 11, 13, 14, 15, 16, 21, 22, and the XY pair. Vidaud and coworkers[3] described a phenotypically normal boy with sex chromosome UPD that was detected because both the boy and his father had hemophilia. Maternal isodisomy for chromosome 16 is associated with pregnancy loss and severe intrauterine growth retardation but can be compatible with a viable pregnancy. The consequences of UPD depend on the existence of genomic imprinting for a given gene, the presence of recessive mutations in the case of isodisomy, and the extent of mosaicism that may be present in these individuals.

The most common cause of UPD is thought to be trisomy rescue, which occurs when a trisomic zygote loses the extra chromosome. If the loss happens randomly, two thirds of the cases will not exhibit uniparental disomy, and one third will. Isodisomy results when nondisjunction occurs during meiosis I, whereas heterodisomy results from nondisjunction in meiosis II. The existence of confined placental mosaicism, as evidenced on chorionic villus sampling, is thought to support the theory of trisomy rescue as the most common cause of UPD. Nondisjunction occurs far more commonly in female gametes than in male gametes, hence the significantly higher frequency of PWS compared with AS.

GERMLINE MOSAICISM

Germline mosaicism is defined as the presence of two or more genetically different populations of germline cells. These result from a somatic mutation in a germline precursor that subsequently persists in all the clonal descendants of that cell. Because only the germline cells are affected, the carrier of this mutation is phenotypically normal.

SOMATIC MOSAICISM

If a mutation within the primordial inner cell mass occurs before differentiation of somatic and germline cells, it will be present in both somatic and germline cells. If this mutation were present in progenitor cells from which the germline cells were derived, all subsequent germline cells would contain this mutation, which would be transmissible to all of the offspring, although the transmitting parent will be mosaic. If the mutation occurs only in the somatic cell line after separation of the somatic and germline cells, it will not be transmissible.

Chromosomal mosaicism may result from postzygotic nondisjunction. The significance of mosaicism is frequently difficult to determine. The effects of mosaicism will depend on the chromosome involved, the proportion of cells containing the abnormal chromosome complement, and the tissues containing this abnormality. The proportion of cells with the abnormal chromosome complement in one tissue may not reflect the proportions in another tissue.

One must consider the inherent ascertainment bias in attempting to predict the phenotypic effect of mosaicism, especially when diagnosed prenatally. People who are phenotypically normal are rarely karyotyped. Hence, people who are phenotypically normal but chromosomally mosaic would be unlikely to be ascertained.

TRINUCLEOTIDE REPEAT EXPANSION

About three fourths of the linear length of the genome consists of single-copy or unique DNA, with the remainder consisting of several classes of repetitive DNA. Tandem (head-to-tail) repeat sequences may be transcriptionally active or inactive. Tandem repeats in coding DNA can vary from short to very large repeat sequences that can include whole genes. Sequence exchange between the repeats can result in either a reduction or an increase (expansion) in the number of tandem repeats. Expansion of trinucleotide or triplet repeat sequences is now a recognized cause of human disease and provides an explanation of the phenomenon known as genetic anticipation.

Genetic anticipation is defined as the trend toward progressively earlier onset and increased severity of a disease with each subsequent generation. Anticipation was originally thought to reflect ascertainment bias—that is, the family was studied only when a severely affected individual was found. It is now known in at least 10 disorders that anticipation occurs as the result of instability of trinucleotide repeats. In certain disorders such as the fragile-X syndrome, the GC-rich triplet repeats can exist in a premutation state in which the number of repeats is greater than that found in alleles of the normal population, but insufficient to cause expression of the disease.

Fragile-X Syndrome. Fragile-X syndrome was the first disorder recognized to result from trinucleotide repeat expansion. It was originally diagnosed cytogenetically and identified by a fragile site—that is, a folate-dependent area in which the chromatin fails to condense during mitosis and consequently does not stain when cells are grown in folate-deficient media. On examination, the chromosome appears broken or distorted in this region. Fragile-X syndrome is now recognized to be the most common inherited form of moderate mental retardation and the second most common chromosomal cause of mental retardation. Current prevalence estimates suggest that 1 in 1200 males and 1 in 2500 females are affected with fragile-X syndrome. Approximately 1 in 700 females will carry a mutation in the gene for fragile-X syndrome *(FMR-1)*. Males affected with this disorder usually have mental retardation, coarse facial features, and macroorchidism. Affected females are less dysmorphic, but as many as one third will exhibit mild mental retardation.

The expression of the fragile-X mutation depends on the number of CGG repeats within the CpG island in the promoter region of the *FMR-1* gene. The *FMR-1* gene has one of the highest mutation rates of any gene in the human genome. The DNA diagnosis for the fragile-X syndrome is based on the size of the CGG expansion as well as the degree of methylation of the *FMR-1* gene.

In fragile-X syndrome, alleles of normal individuals have fewer than 50 copies of the CGG repeat. Small expansions known as premutations involve up to 200 repeats. Males and females carrying the premutation are said to be premutation carriers and are phenotypically normal. The disorder becomes clinically apparent when the triplet is expanded preferentially during maternal meiosis to greater than 200 repeats, and the gene is inactivated through methylation, with loss of the as-yet-unknown FMR-1 gene product.

Unaffected males who carry the premutation (normal transmitting males) may pass the mutation on to their daughters who will also be unaffected. However, their daughters may pass on the expanded allele to their offspring, who are then at risk for expansion to a full mutation and expression of the fragile-X syndrome.

Huntington's Disease (HD). HD is a progressive neurologic disorder characterized by chorea, dementia, rigidity, seizures, and, frequently, psychiatric symptoms. It has been observed that the offspring of affected males have a significantly younger age of onset than the offspring of affected females. This is thought to result from paternal genomic imprinting involving DNA methylation. Late-onset cases are much more likely to be inherited from an affected mother.

HD is inherited as an autosomal dominant trait. The gene is on the short arm of chromosome 4 and is now known as *huntingtin*. It contains an expanded, unstable CAG triplet repeat in HD patients. The risk of expansion is greater during spermatogenesis than in oogenesis. The normal range of CAG repeats is 11 to 34 copies; 30 to 37 copies define the premutation, and the disease is expressed when 38 to 86 copies are present.

Myotonic Dystrophy (DM). DM is characterized by myotonia and muscular dystrophy, as well as cataracts, hypogonadism, cardiac arrhythmias, and frontal balding. Symptoms usually appear in midlife, but the age of onset may be considerably earlier. Distal muscles of the extremities are initially affected, with later involvement of proximal muscles of the extremities and the extraocular and facial muscles.

The gene is located on chromosome 19 and codes for a protein kinase. The defect is an amplification of a CTG triplet repeat. Fewer than 30 copies of the repeat is considered normal; 30 to 50 copies is consistent with the premutation, whereas overt expression is seen with greater than 50 copies. The severity of the disease is directly correlated with the number of copies.

Spinocerebellar Ataxia Type I (SCA1). This neurodegenerative disease is characterized by ataxia, progressive dementia, and spasticity. Symptoms usually begin in the third or fourth decade of life.

The gene for SCA1 has been mapped to chromosome 6. The mutation consists of a CAG repeat expansion. Early-onset disease is associated with a larger number of repeats and paternal transmission. Twenty-five to thirty-six repeats is considered normal, 35 to 43 constitutes the premutation, and 42 to 81 copies coincides with expression of the disease.

Spinal and Bulbar Muscular Atrophy (Kennedy's Disease). Spinal and bulbar muscular atrophy was first described by Kennedy in nine males in two unrelated kindreds, in 1968.[4] Fasciculations followed by muscle weakness and wasting occurred at approximately 40 years of age. Pyramidal, sensory, and cerebellar signs were absent. The disorder is compatible with long life. The main feature of Kennedy's disease, distinguishing it from autosomal recessive and autosomal dominant forms of spinal muscular atrophy (SMA), is the presence of sensory abnormalities. Gynecomastia is frequently the first clinical sign suggesting androgen deficiency and estrogen excess.

The gene for SMA and bulbar muscular atrophy has been mapped to Xq11-q12 and is inherited as an X-linked autosomal disorder.

SUMMARY

Nontraditional inheritance is recognized with increasing frequency as the explanation for the inheritance of a diverse and increasing number of single-gene disorders. Such nonclassic modes of inheritance include mitochondrial inheritance, genomic imprinting, uniparental disomy, mosaicism, and trinucleotide repeat expansion. Examples of disorders associated with each of the these mechanisms will undoubtedly grow as the molecular basis of medical disorders continues to be elucidated, and gene defects linked to medical diseases emerge through the Human Genome Project.

Suggestions for Future Reading

Chatkupt S, Antonowicz M, Johnson WG: Parents do matter: Genomic imprinting and prenatal sex effects in neurological disorders. J Neurolog Sci 1995;130:1–10.

References

1. Magenis RE, Brown MG, Lacy DA, et al: Is Angelman syndrome an alternate result of lel(15)(q11q13)? Am J Med Genet 1987;28:829–838.
2. Nicholls RD, Knoll JH, Butler MG, et al: Genetic imprinting suggested by maternal heterodisomy in non-deletion Prader-Willi syndrome. Nature 1999;342:281–285.
3. Vidaud D, Vidaud M, Plassa F, et al: Father-to-son transmission of hemophilia A due to uniparental disomy. 1989; 40th Ann Meet Am Soc Hum Genet, Abstract 889.
4. Kennedy WR, Alter M, Sung JH: Progressive proximal spinal and bulbar muscular atrophy of late onset: a sex-linked recessive trait. Neurology 1968;18:671–680.

FORTY-SIX

Principles of Screening

Mark I. Evans, Erick L. Krivchenia,

and Frank A. Chervenak

In obstetrics and gynecology, there are two areas of nearly universally accepted established screening procedures: one for cervical cancer via the Papanicolau (Pap) smear, and the second for fetuses with neural tube defects and chromosome abnormalities, such as Down syndrome, via α-fetoprotein (AFP) and other biochemical markers.

PRINCIPLES OF SCREENING TESTS

One of the key elements of screening for any disease process is a fundamental understanding of the differences between diagnostic and screening tests. Diagnostic tests are intended to give a definitive answer to the question: Does the patient have this particular problem? They are generally complex tests and require sophisticated analysis and interpretation. They tend to be expensive, and they are usually performed only on patients believed to be at risk. Conversely, screening tests are administered to healthy patients and to the entire population. They should be cheap, easy to use, and interpretable by everyone; their function is to help define who, among the low-risk group, is, in fact, really at high risk (Table 46–1).

Screening test results are never pathognomonic for the disease. All they do is define who needs further testing. The concept of screening tests is certainly not new to obstetrics and gynecology, having been pioneered nearly 50 years ago with the development of the Pap smear for cervical cancer screening.

With regard to genetic diseases, asking the patient her age is nothing more than a cheap screening test. Using maternal age 35 years as a cutoff, 20% of chromosomal abnormalities, such as Down syndrome, can be detected because that is the percentage of women over that age who bear such a child. Invasive testing is offered on that basis.

Four key measures are used in the evaluation of diagnostic and screening tests: sensitivity, specificity, positive predictive value, and negative predictive value (Fig. 46–1). Sensitivity and specificity fundamentally look at the question from an epidemiologic viewpoint. For example, of all the people with the disease, what percentage were identified by the test? This is the *sensitivity*. Conversely, of all the people who do not have the disease process, what percentage of the patients tested negative? This is *specificity*. Physicians are generally more interested in different questions, because the patient first gets interested only after a positive test. Of all patients who have a positive test, what percentage of them actually have the disease? This is the *positive predictive value*. The *negative predictive value* is just the opposite: of all the people who have a negative test, what percentage of them are actually negative?

A key point to remember is that sensitivity and specificity do not vary as a function of prevalence, but positive and negative predictive values do. This has particular relevance, for example, to the mid-1980s when HIV testing first became a subject of public debate. One of the suggestions of the Reagan White House was to have mandatory testing of heterosexual couples about to marry. In a population in which the prevalence is very low, the proportion of positives that will be false-positive results will be much higher than in a population in which the prevalence is very high, in which case the great majority of positives will, in fact, be true-positive results. In both high- and low-prevalence areas, the sensitivity and specificity of the tests would be the same, but the positive and negative predictive values would be widely different.

Assume an example of HIV testing in a very high-risk population, for example, a sexually transmitted disease clinic in a large city known for its homosexual population. In this example of 1000 patients, we will say that there are 180 true positives, 20 false positives, 20 false negatives,

---

Table 46–1. Screening Tests Versus Diagnostic Tests

Screening Tests	Diagnostic Tests
Performed on healthy patients	Performed on "at-risk" population
Cheap	Commonly expensive
Easy	Commonly have risk
Reliable	Give definitive answer
Quick	
Define at-risk population	
Do not give definitive answer	

Sensitivity: $A/(A + C)$
Specificity: $D/(B + D)$

Positive predictive value: $A/(A + B)$
Negative predictive value: $D/(C + D)$

Figure 46–1. Four key measures used in evaluation of diagnostic and/or screening tests.

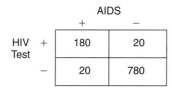

AIDS

	+	−
HIV + Test	180	20
−	20	780

Figure 46–2. HIV testing in a high-risk big-city sexually transmitted disease clinic.

Sensitivity: 180/200 = 90%
Specificity: 780/800 = 98%

Positive predictive value: 180/200 = 90%
Negative predictive value: 780/800 = 98%

AIDS

	+	−
HIV + Test	18	20
−	2	780

Figure 46–3. HIV testing in a low-risk population.

Sensitivity: 18/20 = 90%
Specificity: 780/800 = 98%

Positive predictive value: 18/38 = 47%
Negative predictive value: 780/782 = ~100%

Down Syndrome

	+	−
MS-AFP +	5	400
−	5	7590

Figure 46–4. Low maternal serum α-fetoprotein (MS-AFP) and Down syndrome.

Sensitivity: 5/10 = 50%
Specificity: 7590/7990 = 95%

Positive predictive value: 5/405 = 1.2%
Negative predictive value: 7590/7595 = ~100%

Down Syndrome

	+	−
Double/Triple +	6	300
−	4	7690

Figure 46–5. Double/triple screening and Down syndrome.

Sensitivity: 6/10 = 60%
Specificity: 7690/7990 = 96%

Positive predictive value: 6/306 = 2%
Negative predictive value: 7690/7694 = ~100%

and 780 true negatives (Fig. 46–2). Thus, the sensitivity is 180/(180 + 20), or 200, going vertically—that is, A/(A + C). This gives a sensitivity of 90%. The positive predictive value is likewise 180/200, but this time going horizontally, A/(A + B), which again gives a positive predictive value of 90%. Historically, a screening test is considered to be excellent if the sum of these two numbers equals at least 150. So, at 180, this would be considered a superb test.

If one moves the scenario to a very rural, conservative area, where, instead of the prevalence of HIV being put at 200 per 1000, it is going to be only 20 per 1000, then the implication can be quite different. In this example (Fig. 46–3) the sensitivity will now be 18/(18 + 2), or 18/20—again, vertically A/(A + C). The proportion stays the same because the fact that patients have false-negative results is a function of the disease, not of the laboratory test. However, the 20 false-positive results, which are a function of the laboratory test and not the disease, will still be there, so the positive predictive value is now 18/(18 + 20), or 18/38, or 47% going horizontally—that is, A/(A + B). Thus, from a clinical perspective, the true likelihood that a patient who has a positive test will in fact have HIV varies by a factor of 2, depending on whether the patient is rural low risk or inner-city high risk, in these examples. This is why national standards for certain tests can be very problematic.

In fact, both of these examples of population incidences for this screening test are far higher than those actually observed. This model can be used in AFP screening for Down syndrome, which is known to occur in approximately 1/800 births (Fig. 46–4). Thus, for an example in which there are 10 cases of Down syndrome, there will be a total of 8000 cases. AFP screening for Down syndrome, as described in Chapter 48, was known to identify approximately 50% of all the cases. Historically, for all patients who underwent an amniocentesis because of a "low maternal serum—α-fetoprotein (MS-AFP)," an abnormality was identified in approximately 1 in every 90 amnioceteses. Applying the earlier 2 × 2 grid for low MS-AFP, one would see 5 cases detected, 5 cases missed—that is, 5 false-negative results—and there were approximately 400 false-positive results, to find the 5 cases of Down syndrome, in a total of 7590 true-negative results. This gave a sensitivity of 50%, and a positive predictive value of approximately 1.2%. With the shift to double and triple screening, in which case approximately 60% of all cases were detected, there was a positive amniocentesis in approximately 1 of every 50 procedures performed. The table now shifts to 6 cases detected, 4 cases missed, for a sensitivity of 60%, and 6 positive Down syndrome cases found out of 300 amnioceteses performed, for a positive predictive value of approximately 2% (Fig. 46–5).

These examples illustrate the difficulties inherent in any screening program, and the need to understand the context to translate the implications of any positive test.

Suggestions for Future Reading

Hook EB: Rates of chromosomal abnormalities at indifferent maternal ages. Obstet Gynecol 1981;58:292.

Hook EB: Variability in predicted rates of Down syndrome associated with elevated maternal serum alpha-fetoprotein levels in older women. Am J Hum Genet 1988;43:160.

FORTY-SEVEN

First Trimester Screening

Terrence W. Hallahan, David A. Krantz,

and James N. Macri

Prenatal screening for Down syndrome and open neural tube defects has usually been performed in the second trimester of pregnancy, between 15 and 18 weeks' gestation. For those patients found to be at increased risk, amniocentesis may not be performed until 18 to 20 weeks, and the final laboratory result may not be available until 20 to 22 weeks of pregnancy. This is a time of great stress for couples, who are often left with very little time to face the necessary decisions brought about by an abnormal diagnosis.

Screening for Down syndrome can now be performed much earlier, from 11 to 14 weeks of pregnancy, using a combination of ultrasound and maternal serum markers. The prospect of prenatal screening in the first trimester of pregnancy, with subsequent diagnostic testing, offers distinct advantages over current second trimester screening protocols. Most patients will receive very early reassurance that they are not at increased risk for chromosomal abnormalities. Patients found to be at increased risk will have more time and more diagnostic options to choose from (chorionic villus sampling, early amniocentesis, or conventional amniocentesis). Moreover, a significantly greater percentage of Down syndrome cases can be detected with first trimester screening compared with second trimester screening. For those patients who choose not to proceed with an affected pregnancy, safer termination procedures are available during the first trimester before the patient is obviously pregnant.

First trimester screening combines the results of an ultrasound examination and a blood test performed between the 11th and the 14th week of pregnancy to determine the risk of Down syndrome and trisomy 18.

MATERNAL BLOOD MARKERS

Second trimester Down syndrome screening is conducted using two or more of the maternal blood markers α-fetoprotein (AFP), free β-human chorionic gonadotropin (β-hCG), intact hCG, and unconjugated estriol. Unfortunately, only free β-hCG is a useful biochemical marker in the first trimester as well. In addition to free β-hCG, pregnancy-associated plasma protein-A (PAPP-A) is a useful first trimester marker, which is not productive in the second trimester. To date, over 700 first trimester Down syndrome cases have been analyzed for free β-hCG and PAPP-A. Median levels in Down syndrome are 2.00 for free β-hCG and 0.47 for PAPP-A. Several studies, including 500 cases of Down syndrome, have shown that the combination of free β-hCG, PAPP-A, and maternal age can detect about

60% of Down syndrome cases in the first trimester (Table 47–1). This level of detection in the first trimester equals or exceeds that of most second trimester protocols.

Recently, dried blood spot collection and transport techniques have been used in the Down syndrome screening process. This technique offers significant advantages over the standard blood draw, including:

1. Simplification of the blood collection process
2. No syringe needles required
3. Reduced specimen degradation and hemolysis
4. Increased stability at extremes of temperature
5. Improved biohazard control for laboratory and transport personnel
6. No breakage, spillage, or aerosol hazards
7. Simple, low-cost shipping and storage
8. No centrifugation required
9. Potential for greater screening efficiency owing to reduced variance in biochemical analysis

ULTRASOUND EXAMINATION (NUCHAL TRANSLUCENCY)

Nuchal translucency (NT) is significantly increased in cases of Down syndrome and certain other fetal malformations, particularly major heart defects. The NT measurement can be taken between 11 weeks 1 day and 13 weeks 6 days of gestation. Although the procedure to measure NT is relatively simple, population-based prenatal screening programs depend on consistent determinations of normal marker distributions versus affected marker distributions. Therefore, it is essential that the sonographer undergo training to measure NT and that he or she participates regularly in quality control assessment. The Fetal Medicine Foundation in London provides such training and quality control assessment. Snidjers and associates[1] demonstrated that by following these training and quality control criteria, 77% of Down syndrome cases could be detected at a 5% false-positive rate. On the other hand, Haddow and colleagues[2] demonstrated that failure to follow training and quality control guidelines could result in poor performance.

PROSPECTIVE SCREENING WITH A COMBINED BLOOD AND ULTRASOUND TEST

Patient-specific Down syndrome risk may be calculated by combining NT, free β-hCG, and PAPP-A results with the patient's age-related a priori risk.

Table 47–1. First Trimester Down Syndrome Screening Studies Using Free β-hCG, PAPP-A, and Maternal Age

Study	Down Cases (N)	Gestational Wks	Detection Rate (%)
Krantz et al, 1996[1]	22	10–13	63
Wald et al, 1996[2]	77	8–14	62
Berry et al, 1997[3]	47	9–14	55
Orlandi et al, 1997[4]	11	9–14	61
Haddow et al, 1998[5]	48	9–15	60
Wheeler and Sinosich, 1998[6]	17	9–12	67
De Graaf et al, 1999[7]	37	10–14	55
Spencer et al, 1999[8]	210	10–14	67
Tsukerman, et al 1999[9]	31	8–13	69
Total	500	—	63

1. Krantz DA, Larsen JW, Buchanan PD, et al: First-trimester Down syndrome screening: Free beta human chorionic gonadotropin and pregnancy-associated plasma protein A. Am J Obstet Gynecol 1996;174:612–616.
2. Wald NJ, George L, Smith D, et al: On behalf of the International Prenatal Screening Research Group: Serum screening for Down's syndrome between 8 and 14 weeks of pregnancy. Br J Obstet Gynaecol 1996;104:407–412.
3. Berry E, Aitken DA, Crossley JA, et al: Screening for Down's syndrome: Changes in marker levels and detection rates between first and second trimester. Br J Obstet Gynaecol 1997;104:811–817.
4. Orlandi F, Damiani G, Hallahan TW, et al: First-trimester screening for aneuploidy: Biochemistry and nuchal translucency. Ultrasound Obstet Gynecol 1997;10:381–386.
5. Haddow JE, Palomaki GE, Knight GJ, et al: Screening of maternal serum for fetal Down's syndrome in the first trimester. N Engl J Med 1998;338:955–961.
6. Wheeler DM, Sinosich MJ: Prenatal screening in the first trimester of pregnancy. Prenat Diagn 1998;18:537–543.
7. De Graaf IM, Pajkrt E, Bilardo CM, et al: Early pregnancy screening for fetal aneuploidy with serum markers and nuchal translucency. Prenat Diagn 1999;19:458–462.
8. Spencer K, Souter V, Tul N, et al: A screening program for trisomy 21 at 10–14 weeks using fetal nuchal translucency, maternal serum free beta human chorionic gonadotropin, and pregnancy-associated plasma protein A. Ultrasound Obstet Gynecol 1999;13:231–237.
9. Tsukerman GL, Gusina NB, Cuckle HS. Maternal serum screening for Down syndrome in the first trimester; Experience from Belarus. Prenat Diagn 1999;19:499–504.
β-hCG, β-human chorionic gonadotropin; PAPP-A, pregnancy-associated plasma protein A.

In a prospective study, 10,251 patients between 9 weeks 0 days and 13 weeks 6 days underwent prospective first trimester biochemical screening.[3] Of the 10,251 patients, 5809 underwent ultrasound examination for NT. NT examination was performed only if the patient was between 10 weeks 4 days and 13 weeks 6 days and a sonographer trained by the Fetal Medicine Foundation was available.

Of 10,251 patients, 10,106 were unaffected, 50 carried Down syndrome fetuses, and 20 patients carried trisomy 18 fetuses. Using each patient's incidence rate based on maternal age and gestational age, the expected number of Down syndrome and trisomy 18 cases was 48.9 and 21.6, respectively. There were 75 additional cases with adverse

fetal outcomes, including 3 cases of trisomy 13, 5 cases of Turner's syndrome, and 4 cases of triploidy. Among the 5809 patients who had NT measurement, there were 33 Down syndrome cases and 13 cases of trisomy 18. In this subset, the expected number of Down syndrome and trisomy 18 cases was 31.7 and 13.6, respectively. In this subset were 45 of the additional cases with adverse fetal outcomes, including 3 cases of trisomy 13, 5 cases of Turner's syndrome, and 2 cases of triploidy.

Table 47–2 shows results of prospective screening, using the combined screening protocol for the 5809 patients who had both NT and biochemical analysis. In women under 35 years of age, the observed false-positive rate for Down

Table 47–2. Results of Prospective Screening with a Combined Biochemical and Ultrasound Protocol

Screening Result	Outcome				
	Unaffected N (%)	Down N (%)	Trisomy 18 N (%)	Other N (%)	Total N (%)
Patients Younger than 35 Yr of Age					
Within normative range	3552 (95.1)	1 (12.5)	0 (0.0)	10 (55.6)	3563 (94.6)
Increased risk for Down	168 (4.5)	7 (87.5)	0 (0.0)	8 (44.4)	183 (4.9)
Increased risk for trisomy 18	16 (0.4)	0 (0.0)	4 (100)	0 (0.0)	20 (0.5)
Total	3736 (100)	8 (100)	4 (100)	18 (100)	3766 (100)
Patients 35 Yr and Older					
Within normative range	1671 (84.3)	2 (8.0)	0 (0.0)	14 (51.9)	1687 (82.6)
Increased risk for Down	283 (14.3)	23 (92.0)	0 (0.0)	10 (37.0)	316 (15.5)
Increased risk for trisomy 18	28 (1.4)	0 (0.0)	9 (100)	3 (11.1)	40 (2.0)
Total	1982 (100)	25 (100)	9 (100)	27 (100)	2043 (100)

A cutoff equal to the age-related risk of a 35-yr-old patient was used for Down syndrome screening. A cutoff of 1 in 150 was used for trisomy 18.
Reprinted with permission from the American College of Obstetricians and Gynecologists (Obstetrics and Gynecology, 2000;96:207–213.)

Table 47–3. Screening Efficiency of First Trimester Down Syndrome Screening Protocols

Protocol	At a Fixed 5% False-positive Rate		At a Fixed 70% Detection Rate	
	Cutoff	Detection Rate (%)	Cutoff	False-positive Rate (%)
Free β-hCG	1/145	46	1/355	15.8
PAPP-A	1/105	38	1/395	19.0
Free β-hCG + PAPP-A	1/140	63	1/195	6.8
NT	1/195	74	1/90	3.4
Free β-hCG + NT	1/240	80	1/55	2.3
PAPP-A + NT	1/185	81	1/35	2.3
Free β-hCG + PAPP-A + NT	1/270	91	1/15	1.4

Note: All risks are in terms of first trimester risk. All protocols include maternal age. Data are modeled based on observed likelihood ratios and distribution of live births in the United States (ages 14–49 yr).

Free β-hCG, free β-human chorionic gonadotropin; NT, nuchal translucency; PAPP-A, pregnancy-associated plasma protein A.

Reprinted with permission from the American College of Obstetricians and Gynecologists (Obstetrics and Gynecology, 2000;96:207–213.)

syndrome screening was 4.5%, with a detection rate of 87.5%. The false-negative rate was 12.5%. In older patients, the observed false-positive rate was 14.3%, and the detection rate was 92%. For trisomy 18 in the younger age group, the observed false-positive rate was 0.4% and the observed detection rate was 100%. In the older age group, the observed false-positive rate was 1.4%, and the observed detection rate was 100%. The yield of either Down syndrome or trisomy 18 in the increased risk group was 11 of 195 (1 in 18) in younger patients and 32 of 343 (1 in 11) in older patients. Including other adverse outcomes, the yield would be 19 of 203 (1 in 11) in younger patients and 45 of 356 (1 in 8) in older patients. For results that were within normative range, the negative predictive value was 99.97% for younger patients and 99.88% after excluding other outcomes. Both cases of triploidy, all five cases of Turner's syndrome, and two of three cases of trisomy 13 were detected with combined screening.

Table 47–3 shows the detection efficiency of various combinations of markers at a fixed 5% false-positive rate, as well as false-positive rates at a fixed 70% detection efficiency, based on modeling for a general screening population. The data in this study are similar to those of other studies (Table 47–4).

FIRST TRIMESTER DOWN SYNDROME SCREENING PROTOCOL

Figure 47–1 illustrates the approximate timing of first trimester screening, starting with the patient's last menstrual period. It is noteworthy that first trimester screening will not detect open neural tube defects, and as a result a second trimester AFP test is needed to screen for this disorder. Because approximately 90% of Down syndrome cases can be detected with first trimester screening, additional Down syndrome screening in the second trimester

Table 47–4. Detection Rate at a 5% False-positive Rate in First Trimester Down Syndrome Screening Studies, Using Free β-hCG, PAPP-A, and Nuchal Translucency

Study	Down Cases (N)	Gestational Age (wk)	Detection Rate (%)
Brizot et al, 1994[1], 1995[2]	80	10–14	89
Orlandi et al, 1997[3]	11	9–14	87
De Graaf et al, 1999[4]	37	10–14	85
De Biasio et al, 1999*[5]	13	10–14	85
Spencer et al, 1999[6]	210	10–14	89
Krantz et al, 2000[7]	33	10–13	91
Total	384	—	89

* This study reported a false-positive rate of 3.3%.

1. Brizot ML, Snidjers RJM, Bersinger NA, et al: Maternal serum pregnancy-associated placental protein A and fetal nuchal translucency thickness for the prediction of fetal trisomies in early pregnancy. Obstet Gynecol 1994;84:918–922.

2. Brizot ML, Snidjers RJM, Butler J, et al: Maternal serum hCG and fetal nuchal translucency thickness for the prediction of fetal trisomies in the first trimester of pregnancy. Br J Obstet Gynaecol 1995;102:127–132.

3. Orlandi F, Damiani G, Hallahan TW, et al: First-trimester screening for aneuploidy: Biochemistry and nuchal translucency. Ultrasound Obstet Gynecol 1997;10:381–386.

4. De Graaf IM, Pajkrt E, Bilardo CM, et al: Early pregnancy screening for fetal aneuploidy with serum markers and nuchal translucency. Prenat Diagn 1999;19:458–462.

5. De Biasio P, Siccardi M, Volpe G, et al: First-trimester screening for Down's syndrome using nuchal translucency measurement with free beta hCG and PAPP-A between 10 and 13 weeks of pregnancy: The combined test. Prenat Diagn 1999;19:360–363.

6. Spencer K, Souter V, Tul N, et al: A screening program for trisomy 21 at 10–14 weeks using fetal nuchal translucency, maternal serum free beta human chorionic gonadotropin and pregnancy-associated plasma protein A. Ultrasound Obstet Gynecol 1999;13:231–237.

7. Krantz DA, Hallahan TW, Orlandi F, et al: First-trimester Down syndrome screening using dried blood biochemistry and nuchal translucency. Obstet Gynecol 2000;96:207–213.

β-hCG, Beta human chorionic gonadotropin; PAPP-A, pregnancy-associated plasma protein A.

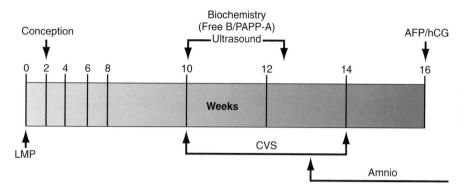

Figure 47–1. First trimester Down syndrome screening. AFP, α-fetoprotein; Amnio, amniocentesis; CVS, chorionic villus sampling; hCG, human chorionic gonadotropin; LMP, last menstrual period.

will likely lead to a significantly increased false-positive rate, with little additional detection capability.

Discussion

The data show that although biochemical screening alone (63% detection rate) or ultrasound screening alone (74% detection rate) each provide Down syndrome detection rates similar to or better than currently available second trimester methods, the combination of biochemical and sonographic screening protocols results in a significantly improved detection rate of 91%. In addition to increased detection, first trimester screening offers inherent advantages of early detection (Table 47–5). Most patients are found to be at low risk of chromosomal abnormalities and thus can be reassured substantially earlier in pregnancy. For patients found to be at increased risk, more time is available to decide on diagnostic options. The additional first trimester detection of affected cases destined to miscarry means that treatment may be offered in a medically controlled setting, and such diagnoses can alert patients to increased risks in future pregnancies. Finally, for patients who choose to terminate an affected pregnancy, safer and earlier procedures are available than those used at or around 20 weeks' gestation.

Table 47–5. Advantages of First Trimester Screening

Increased detection of Down syndrome and other chromosomal abnormalities
Earlier reassurance for low-risk patients
Additional time for decision making for high-risk patients
Greater privacy for those patients with affected fetuses
Safer termination procedures

Experience with second trimester screening indicates that significant maternal anxiety ensues after an increased risk result. It is essential, therefore, that diagnostic procedures be available and offered as quickly as possible after screening results have been reported. Chorionic villus sampling and early amniocentesis are the primary diagnostic procedures between 11 and 14 weeks' gestation.

First trimester screening using a combination of biochemistry and NT measurement is feasible, results in improved Down syndrome detection over currently employed second trimester protocols, and provides substantial advantages to clinicians and patients.

Suggestions for Future Reading

Krantz DA, Hallahan TW, Orlandi F, et al: First-trimester Down syndrome screening using dried blood biochemistry and nuchal translucency. Obstet Gynecol 2000;96:207–213.

Nicolaides KH, Sebire NJ, Snijders RJM (eds): The 11 to 14 Weeks' Scan; The Diagnosis of Fetal Abnormalities. London, Parthenon Publishing Group, 1999.

Orlandi F, Damiani G, Hallahan TW, et al: First-trimester screening for aneuploidy: Biochemistry and nuchal translucency. Ultrasound Obstet Gynecol 1997;10:381–386.

Snidjers RJM, Noble P, Sebire N, et al: UK multicentre project on assessment of risk of trisomy 21 by maternal age and fetal nuchal translucency thickness at 10–14 weeks' gestation. Lancet 1998; 352:343–346.

References

1. Snidjers RJM, Noble P, Sebire N, et al: UK multicentre project on assessment of risk of trisomy 21 by maternal age and fetal nuchal translucency thickness at 10–14 weeks' gestation. Lancet 1998;352:343–346.

2. Haddow JE, Palomaki GE, Knight GJ, et al: Screening of maternal serum for fetal Down's syndrome in the first trimester. N Engl J Med 1998;338:955–961.

3. Krantz DA, Hallahan TW, Orlandi F, et al: First-trimester Down syndrome screening using dried blood biochemistry and nuchal translucency. Obstet Gynecol 2000;96:207–213.

FORTY-EIGHT

Second-Trimester Screening

Mark I. Evans, Joseph E. O'Brien,

and Harry Harrison

NEURAL TUBE DEFECTS

It was in the early 1970s that Brock and Sutcliffe first described measuring α-fetoprotein (AFP) in amniotic fluid, and later in maternal serum, for the prenatal detection of neural tube defects. In the mid-1970s, routine prenatal screening was accepted in the United Kingdom, but it took until the mid-1980s to become "standard" in the United States. Evaluation of the impact of such screening has clearly shown that the birth rate of children with neural tube defects declined from 1.3 per 1000 births in 1970 to 0.6 per 1000 births in 1989.

It has long been appreciated that there are racial, geographic, and ethnic variations in the incidence of neural tube defects and that there are patients at increased risk based on other medical conditions. For example, diabetics are known to have an increased risk of neural tube defects, as are women taking antiepileptic drugs.

A very important question raised has been the association of folic acid deficiency and the incidence of neural tube defects. Experimental, clinical, and embryologic studies have investigated the role of vitamins as a causative factor. Special attention has focused on the essential B vitamin folic acid, which serves as a methyl donor involved in nucleic acid synthesis, purine-pyrimidine metabolism, and protein synthesis. Because of increased folic acid needs in pregnancy, pregnant women are particularly prone to develop relative deficiencies. Other possible influences include insufficient diet, physiologic hemodilution of pregnancy, increased plasma clearance, and genetic disorders that might affect production, transport, and metabolism.

Since the early 1990s, a number of studies have been made on supplementing folic acid in women at high risk for neural tube defects. These studies have generally shown a decrease in the recurrence risk for such supplemented women who have already had an affected child.

Wald and associates[1] have reported that women with a history of neural tube defects may have a different folate metabolism from controls, but that with supplementation at 4 mg daily, their levels of circulating folate can be greater than 160 μg/L, which is the lower limit of normal.

The use of multivitamins containing folic acid in the preconceptual period showed a statistically significant 60% reduction in the risk of neural tube defects among women who used daily vitamin supplements containing folic acid in the first month of pregnancy. After much debate, the U.S. Food and Drug Administration implemented, beginning in 1998, supplementation of breads and grains with folic acid.

It will be interesting to follow the epidemiologic data on the effects on both recurrence and primary incidence.

SCREENING FOR CHROMOSOME ABNORMALITIES

In 1984, Merkatz and coworkers[2] published a report on the association of low maternal serum α-fetoprotein (MS-AFP) with an increased risk of chromosome abnormalities, particularly Down syndrome.

The adoption of widescale screening with MS-AFP by the late 1980s effectively doubled the potential detection of chromosome abnormalities in the population. Only 20% of Down syndrome babies are born to women older than age 35 years. The addition of a well-coordinated MS-AFP screening program detected approximately 30% of the 80% of cases that are born to women younger than age 35 years (Fig. 48–1). The mechanics of biochemical screening—that is, with adjustments for gestational age, race, diabetic status, multiple gestation status, and maternal weight and adjustments via a different database or correction factors for maternal race—have been published previously and are not repeated here.

In 1988, Wald and colleagues[3] suggested that a combina-

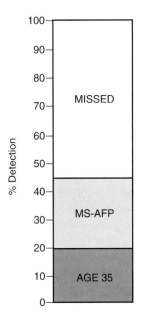

Figure 48–1. Detection of Down syndrome by maternal serum α-fetoprotein (MS-AFP).

tion of parameters, including AFP, β human chorionic gonadotropin (β-hCG), and unconjugated estriol (uE₃), could significantly increase the detection frequency of Down syndrome to approximately 60% of the total. There is essentially universal agreement that among the three parameters—AFP, β-hCG, and uE₃—if one could choose only one, β-hCG is by far the best. There is a virtual tie for second place in efficacy between AFP and uE₃. However, because AFP is already used in America and much of Western Europe for the detection of neural tube defects, the only real remaining question is whether adding uE₃ as a third parameter is cost beneficial.

The debate over the use of uE₃—that is, double screening versus triple screening—became very intense and very emotional, with staunch proponents on both sides, almost appearing to be a matter of "religion." We happen to belong to the "double religion" in believing that the studies as a whole suggest that there is no real effectiveness of adding the third marker. The literature is divided between several studies that say the third marker helps and others that say it does not. Furthermore, since 1991 when Crossley and group[4] first proposed that the β-hCG/AFP ratio be used as a marker, the question of how the data are interpreted has been added into the overall equation of sensitivity and specificity.

Several new markers have been investigated. The most important in the second trimester has been the use of free β-hCG as opposed to the intact β-hCG. Wald and associates[1] reported in 1993 that the use of free β-hCG compared with total β-hCG would increase the detection frequency by about 4% for a given false-positive rate used in conjunction with maternal age, AFP, and uE₃. Other studies have suggested that free β-hCG has both better sensitivity and specificity than the intact molecule, particularly at earlier gestational ages (e.g., 14 and 15 weeks), and in the first trimester.

Several other markers have been investigated. Cole and colleagues[5] have proposed "nicked" β-hCG, which is a structurally abnormal form. They have found increased effectiveness, but the molecule is relatively labile. In order for the research assay to be usable as a clinical screening test, stability has to be increased. The urea-resistant fraction of neutrophil alkaline phosphatase has also shown promising results. Its manual assay, first proposed by Tafas,[6] is too cumbersome for practical use, but automated methods have been developed that should make it practical.

More recently, dimeric inhibin A has been proposed as a 4th marker to create a "quadruple" test. Its proponents claim a 5% increase in sensitivity, along with an increase in specificity. Furthermore, the gestational age variation in normal values of inhibin is minimal, thereby removing one of the most common confounders of biochemical screening interpretation—gestational age inaccuracy.

Another promising marker has been the search for fetal cells in maternal circulation. Studies throughout the mid-1990s have suggested that isolation and analysis of fetal cells may, in fact, become practical and useful as a screen-

ing test. Data through the late 1990s have shown fetal cells to have a sensitivity no greater than that of other available markers, but a specificity that is much better. Laboratory methodologies for the isolation of fetal blood cells followed essentially two pathways: (1) fluorescent activated cell-sorting group, and (2) magnetic activated cell sorting. The most likely scenario for fetal cell use would be a two-stage process. Usually, most programs strive for a 5% screen positive rate that detects about 60% to 70% of abnormalities.

Instead, there would be a two-step process. First, using traditional means, about 10% would screen positive, for a sensitivity of 80%. Then fetal cell analysis would eliminate about two out of three of those, leaving 2% to 3% needing amniocentesis, but still almost all of the abnormal cases should be there (Fig. 48–2). Previous work by us has shown that reducing the number of amniocenteses needed by 1% (e.g., from 5% to 4%) would save the United States about $70 million per year in health care costs.[7]

The next several years will determine how successful fetal cell sorting is as a screening test. It was originally hoped that it could be a diagnostic test and replace the need for invasive testing. However, as of this writing, fetal karyotypes cannot be obtained from cells that are isolated, and therefore only fluorescent in situ hybridization (FISH)-related results are possible. While FISH is very good as a screening test for aneuploidy, our experiences show that approximately one third of abnormal karyotypes seen in prenatal diagnosis programs are, in fact, not ones that would be detected by the standard probes for chromosomes 13, 18, 21, X, and Y. Until and unless complete karyotypes can be obtained, fetal cells will not replace invasive testing, but they are a potentially important addition to the armamentarium of screening technologies.

Another area of potential applicability of fetal cells in maternal blood is for the isolation of the molecular diagnosis of mendelian disorders. Because the limitations of molecular diagnostic tests are irrelevant for mendelian disorders for which probes are available, fetal cells are more likely to succeed for mendelian disorders than aneuploidy. It further follows that as newborn screening becomes molecular, many of those screens could be done just as easily prenatally, giving couples reproductive choice, as well as the potential for fetal therapy.

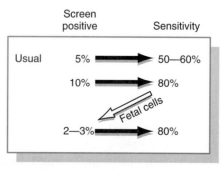

Figure 48–2. Two-step process.

TRISOMY 18

Although screening has generally focused on trisomy 21, our data, and those of others, have always shown a varied pattern of anomalies detected by screening. A different pattern of analyte levels has been observed in trisomy 18. The values of AFP, β-hCG, and uE$_3$ appear to be very low. This suggests a different pathophysiology than for Down syndrome. In Down syndrome, the low AFP and uE$_3$ and high β-hCG can be explained as reflecting immaturity of the fetus—that is, all values are consistent with a younger gestational age. In trisomy 18, therefore, that explanation does not work.

SECOND-TRIMESTER ULTRASOUND

Ultrasound can be either a diagnostic or a screening test. Anencephaly, gastroschisis, omphalocele, and limb reductions are all diagnoses unto themselves, but other findings such as cardiac anomalies are also commonly markers of underlying chromosome abnormalities.

Minor morphologic markers can be used to alter the a priori odds based on maternal age and maternal serum biochemical screening. Factors such as echogenic bowel, frontal thalamic distance, hypoplasia, clinodactyly of the middle phalanx of the fifth digit, simian crease, sandal gap, pyelectasis, foot-to-femur ratios, and choroid plexus cysts have all been used but are controversial to the extent that it is unclear when the documentation of such an anomaly requires the performance of a karyotype. Choroid plexus cysts have been a particular source of controversy, with series describing risks as much as 10% to considerably less than 1%. The current feeling is that an isolated small, nonprogressive choroid plexus cyst, in the absence of any other finding and good fetal growth, probably carries minimal risk.

In the second trimester, increased nuchal skin fold thickness, which is routinely seen in neonates with trisomy 21, has been identified as a marker in pregnancy. Detection rates have varied over the years as ultrasound has become more sophisticated.

As with biochemical screening, attempts have been made to create algorithms and combine multiple ultrasound markers to produce risk figures. These have predominantly been limited to relatively high-risk populations and have not been shown to be particularly usable in the general population screening.

SUMMARY

In sum, the past years have seen considerable progress in the area of biochemical screening. Increasing data have now clearly shown the advantages of multiple markers, particularly β-hCG, over AFP alone. Considerable controversy continues over the best mathematical algorithm and which markers are best (e.g., for β-hCG, uE$_3$). There appears to be a plateau of detection frequencies.

Suggestions for Future Reading

Evans MI, O'Brien JE, Dvorin E, et al: Biochemical screening. In Gleisher N, Buttino L Jr, Elkayam U, et al (eds): Principles and Practices of Medical Therapy in Pregnancy, 3rd ed. Norwalk, Conn, Appleton & Lange, 1998, pp 199–207.

Krantz DA, Hallahan TW, Orlandi F, et al: First-trimester Down syndrome screening using dried blood biochemistry and nuchal translucency. Obstet Gynecol 2000;96:207–213.

Nicolaides KH, Sebire NJ, Snijders RJM (eds): The 11 to 14 Weeks' Scan; The Diagnosis of Fetal Abnormalities. London, Parthenon Publishing Group, 1999.

Orlandi F, Damiani G, Hallahan TW, et al: First-trimester screening for aneuploidy: Biochemistry and nuchal translucency. Ultrasound Obstet Gynecol 1997;10:381–386.

Snijders RJM, Noble P, Sebire N, et al: UK multicentre project on assessment of risk of trisomy 21 by maternal age and fetal nuchal-translucency thickness at 10–14 weeks of gestation. Lancet 1998; 352:343–346.

References

1. Wald J, Schorah CJ, Sheldon TA, et al: Investigation of factors influencing folate status in women who have had a neural tube defect–affected infant. Br J Obstet Gynaecol 1993;100:546–549.
2. Merkatz IR, Nitowsky FM, Macri JN, et al: An association between low maternal serum alpha-fetoprotein and fetal chromosome abnormalities. Am J Obstet Gynecol 1984;148:886–894.
3. Wald NJ, Cuckle HS, Densem JW, et al: Maternal serum screening for Down syndrome in early pregnancy. BMJ 1988;297:883–887.
4. Crossley JA, Aitken DA, Connor JM: Prenatal screening for chromosome abnormalities using maternal serum chorionic gonadotrophin, alpha-fetoprotein, and age. Prenat Diagn 1991;11:83–101.
5. Cole LA, Kardana A, Park SY, Braunstein GD: The deactivation of hCG by nicking and dissociation. J Clin Endocrinol Metab 1993;76:704–710.
6. Tafas T, Cuckle HS, Nasr S, et al: An automated image analysis method for the measurement of neutrophil alkaline phosphatase in the prenatal screening of Down Syndrome. Fetal Diagn Ther 1996;11:254–259.
7. Evans MI, Chik L, O'Brien JE, et al: MOMs (multiples of the median) and DADs (discriminant aneuploidy detection): Improved specificity and cost-effectiveness of biochemical screening for aneuploidy with DADs. Am J Obstet Gynecol 1995;172:1138–1147.
8. Evans MI, Henry GP, Miller WA, et al: International collaborative assessment of 146,000 prenatal karyotypes: Expected limitations if only chromosome-specific probes and fluorescent in-situ hybridization are used. Hum Reprod 1999;14:1213–1216.

FORTY-NINE

Teratology

Christine M. Kovac, Byron C. Calhoun,

and Roderick F. Hume, Jr.

The perceived invulnerability of the fetus within the sanctity of the womb was lost with the recognition that rubella and radiation could cause birth defects. Indeed, it is not infrequent that the woman's primary care provider faces an anxious patient fearful of potential teratogen exposure. Recall the preschool teacher early in her first pregnancy concerned about the outbreak of fifth disease in her class. Much of prenatal care is aimed at the identification of risk factors and appropriate intervention to prevent subsequent problems (anemia, Rh status) or to recognize a problem in order to offer the optimal therapeutic choice (maternal analyte and ultrasound screening for fetal anomalies).

Screening ultrasound provides the opportunity to triage patients with abnormal findings.[1, 2] Referral to a center of excellence with the American Institute of Ultrasound in Medicine (AIUM) accreditation enhances care.[3] Teratology, classically defined as the study of abnormal formation of the developing embryo-fetus resulting in congenital anomalies, is now more commonly viewed as the study of extrinsic factors that cause birth defects. Teratogens include certain drugs, toxins, viral infections, and ionizing radiation.[4] However, teratogens as a whole make up a rather minor contribution to the total incidence of birth defects. The classification of congenital anomalies can be confusing in that the same birth defect may result from different underlying etiologies, each having a different prognosis and recurrence risk. Establishing future pregnancy (recurrence) risks within the family demands the precise diagnosis of the affected fetus-neonate, especially in cases of spontaneous or therapeutic abortion and stillbirth. The outcomes for an anomalous newborn are often directly related to the mode and place of delivery. Recognizing the fetal condition allows optimal delivery and immediate neonatal care.

Terminal fetal conditions may be candidates for perinatal hospice if pregnancy termination is not an option.[5] How do we offer such a system of care? Can we prevent the occurrence or recurrence of birth defects? The confirmation that simple preconception supplementation with folate reduces neural tube defects and that preconception control of diabetes in pregnancy reduces fetal anomalies is a monumental achievement attained during the 1990s. The goals of this chapter are to define and review recent developments in the study, treatment, and prevention of teratogenesis. More exhaustive treatment of this topic is available in recommended readings.[6–9]

DEFINITION OF TERMS

Congenital anomalies, or birth defects, are abnormalities of the structure and function recognized at birth. Dysmorphology is the study of human anomalies. Major structural anomalies, which occur in 2% to 3% of all live births, have medical or surgical consequences that must be repaired for normal function (cleft palate). Minor anomalies, which can be identified in 10% to 15% of newborns, do not directly contribute to mortality or morbidity (two-vessel umbilical cord). However, the careful search for minor anomalies is important because of the significantly increased association of multiple minor anomalies predicting underlying major birth defects. This association described in newborns is also true for fetal dysmorphology. It is also important to recognize that not all anomalies will be evident in utero, at birth, or within the first year of life. The constellation of physical features, family history (pedigree), and maternal history encompasses essential components of the differential diagnostic process for a birth defect. Teratogens are extrinsic, or environmental, factors that interfere with the normal development of the embryo and may cause morphologic abnormalities. Not surprisingly many teratogens interact adversely with the normal signal transduction molecules (morphogens) integral to the finely tuned developmental pathways. These molecular misadventures explain the diversity of possible etiologies for a given birth defect. For example, holoprosencephaly (HPE) may be due to an autosomal recessive disorder (familial HPE) involving the mutation of a signal molecule; a manifestation of trisomy 13, in which triplication of genes alters the proper balance of critical proteins; an expression of an inborn error of metabolism (Smith-Lemli-Opitz syndrome [SLOS]), in which a necessary ligand (cholesterol) for a signal molecule is lacking; or a consequence of teratogen exposure (fetal alcohol syndrome), in which the drug alters distribution within the molecular milieu. The timing of exposure is critical in determining causality for the specific anomaly. Teratogens must act during the critical period between conception and delivery. The first 8 weeks of gestation is the period of greatest vulnerability because it is the time of major organogenesis. For example, the severity of congenital rubella is directly correlated to the timing of the primary infection. Several distinct pathogenetic mechanisms are operative in humans, which provides a useful organizing conceptual framework for the evaluation of a patient or research hypothesis.

PATHOPHYSIOLOGIC MECHANISM

A congenital anomaly may be the result of one of three different teratogenic, or pathogenetic, processes: malformation, deformation, or disruption. *Malformation* involves an error during organogenesis, such that the structure was never formed normally. *Disruption* results from the destruction of a previously normally formed structure. *Deformation* involves the remodeling of a previously normal structure, generally by mechanical forces, resulting in a lasting birth defect. The concept of developmental fields can promote the understanding of embryologic mechanics and associated risks of the underlying etiology and pathogenetic mechanism. Hence, a midline facial defect should alert the physician to the possibility of midline defects of the brain or heart. Obliteration of digits or limbs due to disruption by amniotic bands may follow a seemingly random pattern more related to the proximity of vulnerable appendages than to a specific developmental process. Anhydramnios can deform the face and limbs if it is severe and longstanding. The sequence of events leading to a grouping of anomalies has been described as either an association, an anomalad, or a sequence. If the pattern of anomalies is statistically associated but has no known etiology then the term *association* has been preferred—for example, VACTERL (vertebral abnormalities, anal atresia, tracheo-esophageal fistula and/or esophageal atresia, renal agenesis and dysplasia, and limb defects) or CHARGE (coloboma, heart disease, atresia choanae, retarded growth and retarded development and/or central nervous system anomalies, genital hypoplasia, and ear anomalies and/or deafness). If the nonrandom association follows a developmental timeline in that subsequent anomalies are caused by the first defect, then *anomalad* or *sequence* has been used—for example, in oligohydramnios sequence, the Potter facies or hypoplastic lungs are anomalads of the fetal anuria. Recognizing the pattern of defects present may suggest the specific mechanism.

ETIOLOGIC CLASSIFICATION

Correct use of the ICD-9-CM (International Classification of Diseases—Ninth Revision, Clinical Modification) codes, or proper naming of the congenital anomaly and its associations, may define the syndrome and help determine the specific etiology, prognosis, or best therapy for that individual patient. However, each of the pathogenetic processes described earlier may have a different etiology or primary cause. Single-gene disorders are inherited in predictable patterns described in mendelian genetics as autosomal dominant, autosomal recessive, and X-linked inheritance. Nonmendelian inheritance patterns include imprinting, dynamic mutations (fragile X), and mitochondrial genetics. A mutation in a specific gene for a structural protein, a signal transduction ligand, or its receptor can cause a congenital malformation. The recurrence risk for future progeny follows pedigree analysis and Mendel's Law: 25% in autosomal recessive, 50% in autosomal dominant, and so on.

Another genetic etiology intrinsic to the developing embryo is a chromosomal aberration—for example, trisomy, translocations, or deletions. The resultant imbalance of genes owing to altered chromosomal number or loss of whole segments of a chromosome is a common cause of spontaneous abortion, stillbirth, or mental retardation syndromes. Recurrence risks for chromosomal anomalies vary from 1% (or age-related if older) risk for trisomies to higher rates for specific couples with balanced translocations. Most congenital anomalies, however, have pedigree or epidemiologic evidence to support a multifactorial etiology. Multifactorial inheritance implies the interaction of some genetic susceptibility to a threshold effect for an extrinsic factor. Recurrence risks are higher in certain ethnic groups, exposure cohorts, or geographic locations. Recurrence risks vary for each specific birth defect and within the particular family. Neural tube defects (NTDs) are the classic example, being most prevalent in Celtoi in the United Kingdom but also related to episodes of famine. Indeed, epidemiology studies led to the experimental use of folate supplementation to reduce the primary occurrence and recurrence risks for NTDs in the at-risk population.

Congenital rubella heralds the ever-expanding group of infectious pathogens that can afflict the fetus. TORCH now refers to toxoplasmosis, syphilis (other), rubella, cytomegalovirus, herpes, and many other agents such as the hepatitis viruses and HIV. Parvovirus, the infectious agent in fifth disease, may cause a hematopoietic crisis in the affected fetus, leading to hydrops fetalis requiring in utero fetal transfusion, but it does not cause structural anomalies. Timing of infection with regard to the developmental ontogeny is a critical element of the natural history for such disorders. Ionizing radiation from nuclear accidental exposures or diagnostic or therapeutic x-irradiation can also result in anomalous development. The extent and type of birth defects follows dosimetry and timing of exposure. Thalidomide-induced birth defects shocked the developed world into the recognition of the potential unrecognized harm of drugs for the developing embryo. Entire texts of safe drug use in pregnancy or during lactation hold a special place on the desk of all women's health care providers.[9]

An etiologic classification system is an extremely useful tool for the understanding of teratogenic mechanisms, but, more importantly, it serves as the basis for optimal patient care. The central importance of the careful dysmorphologic assessment cannot be overstressed. Each finding should lead to the search for more abnormalities in the physical examination, selective imaging, and laboratory testing. This is the basis for the targeted ultrasound or focused examination in the genetic approach to prenatal diagnosis. Pedigree analysis and the examination of relatives may identify a specific syndrome in that family when the most common explanation would be multifactorial. One should not be surprised by a 25% recurrence of congenital diaphragmatic hernia in a family with Fryn's syndrome, even though the vast majority of congenital diaphragmatic hernias are multifactorial. Whereas the recurrence rate in fetal alcohol syndrome would be directly related to maternal abstinence from alcohol use, folate supplementation only reduces recurrence of NTDs by half. Knowing the etiology is key to avoiding the unrecognized risks of misclassification errors (e.g., congenital diaphragmatic hernia in Fryn's, or NTD in trisomy 18). These examples should highlight the critical nature of the meticulous and accurate differential diagnostic workup for each patient afflicted by a congenital anomaly to ascertain the specific etiology for their defect. Prognosis and therapeutic options follow proper etiologic classification.

HISTORY—KEY POINTS

If you do not ask the proper questions, you will not discover the obvious familial disorder or drug exposure history. The recognition that pregnancies in insulin-dependent diabetic mothers have higher anomaly rates points to the teratogenic interactions of maternal disease and fetal development (systemic lupus erythematosus and heart block; diabetes mellitus and NTDs). More importantly, discovery of that risk should lead to tight glucose control and preconception folate supplementation to decrease the risk for anomalous development.

EXAMINATION—KEY POINTS

The same concepts that inform the careful newborn examination for minor anomalies and associated major defects are essential for the obstetrician. If a minor anomaly is suspected, a consultation by a geneticist should include dysmorphologic evaluation of the newborn. For example, cleft palate should lead to a search for midline defects in the central nervous system and heart. Careful examination of the parents may reveal bifid uvula or lip pits, which would suggest a different etiologic classification and recurrence risk.

Fetal dysmorphology uses the sonographic examination of the fetus to screen for markers of anomalous development that require more advanced targeted fetal anatomic assessment and include fetal echocardiography. Recognition of associations in the differential diagnosis may alter the specific laboratory tests needed to establish the accurate diagnosis, prognosis, and therapeutic options.

LABORATORY STUDIES—KEY POINTS

Maternal serum analyte screening programs have the goal of selecting higher-risk pregnancies for advanced diagnostic methods, which may include invasive fetal testing. For many patients, the difference of screening and diagnostic tests is counterintuitive. An abnormal maternal serum α-fetoprotein (MS-AFP) does not necessarily indicate an abnormal pregnancy, but rather serves as a call for a focused fetal evaluation. Indeed, the cause of elevated MS-AFP may be maternal hepatic dysfunction. A fetal structural anomaly detected during routine fetal anatomic survey as part of an ultrasound screening program may be a marker (choroid plexus cyst), a minor anomaly (single umbilical artery), or a major anomaly (ventricular septal defect). The finding is not the diagnosis, but it is the beginning of the expanded search for associated anomalies, potential etiologies, and indicated diagnostic procedures. Comparative risk-benefit analysis and nondirective genetic counseling facilitate the medical-ethical decision-making process necessary to plan the most appropriate course for the patient. An awareness by the health care provider and patient of the accuracy of diagnostic tests and the possibility of false-positive and false-negative screening results is an important component of appropriate counseling for patients faced with such unexpected positive screening results.[6]

Careful history, meticulous examination, and the inclusion of the predictive value of screening test results can guide the optimal selection of diagnostic testing. For example, a diagnosis of fragile X is no longer based on simple cytogenetic analysis; it is important to know that special tests will be required if this diagnosis is a consideration. It is also important to know that rapid fluorescent in situ hybridization screening for aneuploidy results is an incomplete karyotype analysis that is most helpful if it is positive, but high-resolution chromosomal banding methodologies are required for some conditions. Coordination with a genetics referral laboratory before collecting specimens is prudent.

IMAGING TECHNIQUES

A discussion of the use of fetal anatomic survey terminology is in order because so much of prenatal diagnosis hinges on expert sonology. Three levels of ultrasonographic evaluations are in common use; however, the specific terms vary between governing bodies (American College of Obstetricians and Gynecologists [ACOG], AIUM). Triage, or limited scans, refers to a simple clinical assessment for fetal viability, fetal lie, or placental location. Formal fetal anatomic survey is not an expected part of such a narrowly focused clinical adjunct. Basic scans include formal fetal anatomic survey. The basic obstetric ultrasound examination is beyond the routine level of competence of most providers, requiring specialized equipment, personnel, and training. Advanced obstetrical sonography implies a significant investment in subspecialty training and expanded ability and expertise. The critical importance of an experienced registered diagnostic medical sonographer with proper training, certification, and quality assurance was highlighted by the various results reported in the RADIUS (Routine Antenatal Diagnostic Imaging with Ultrasound) studies. Liability for ultrasound misdiagnosis depends on the level of expertise and findings, not the physician's guild. The AIUM Obstetrical US Accreditation serves as a clear distinction of quality if there are questions of competency and ability for the referring physician when choosing a consulting laboratory. Examples of the types of images covered are outlined here.[2, 3]

1. First trimester
   - Presence or absence of an intrauterine gestational sac
   - Identification of embryo or fetus
   - Fetal number
   - Presence or absence of fetal cardiac activity
   - Crown-rump length
   - Evaluation of uterus and adnexal structures
2. Limited ultrasound
   - Assessment of fluid volume
   - Fetal biophysical testing
   - Ultrasonography-guided amniocentesis
   - External cephalic version
   - Confirmation of fetal life or death
   - Localization of placenta in antepartum hemorrhage
   - Confirmation of fetal presentation
3. Basic ultrasound
   - Fetal number
   - Fetal presentation
   - Documentation of fetal life
   - Placental location
   - Assessment of amniotic fluid volume
   - Survey of fetal anatomy for GROSS malformations
   - Evaluation for maternal pelvic masses
4. Comprehensive anatomy survey

Ultrasound—Key Features

Ultrasound uses high-frequency sound having no known fetal risks for the energy range used in diagnostic medical sonography. Ultrasound is ideal for serial fetal assessment, especially for growth or progression of findings. It is limited, however, by resolution and operator experience. As a tool used correctly, it has an invaluable role in obstetric care.

ETIOLOGIES

The same anomaly can have multiple etiologies. For example, transverse limb defects can be due to amniotic bands (sporadic), perinatal cocaine exposure[10] (disruption), phocomelia (thalidomide),[9] or syndromic.[7] Prognosis is critically dependent on underlying etiology, not simply on the anatomic defect.

Cleft lip and palate can be surgically repaired with great functional outcome. Long-term outcomes, however, are quite different if cleft lip and palate is part of trisomy 13, syndromic, or an isolated multifactorial occurrence. However, severe deformations may be associated with am-

niotic band syndrome (ABS): surgical outcomes may be less optimal even though the central nervous system is unaffected. Recurrence risk is also directly related to etiology: less than 5% for multifactorial, 25% for autosomal recessive syndrome, 1% or age-related for aneuploidy, and very unlikely in the case of amniotic bands. Drugs associated with increased risk for cleft lip and palate include anticonvulsants.

NTDs are most often multifactorial, but they may also be associated with trisomy 18[11] or other genetic syndromes. Definitive diagnosis may require careful fetal or neonatal dysmorphology examination and karyotype analysis. Other factors contributing to risk include ethnicity, pedigree (family history), and maternal conditions, such as epilepsy or diabetes. A positive family history is significant. For example, having a previously affected child increases the risk for a pregnancy up to 20-fold. Anticonvulsant drug therapy, such a valproate, is also associated with increased incidence of NTDs. Modes of detection include MS-AFP screening, fetal sonographic imaging, and amniotic fluid α-fetoprotein and acetylcholinesterase (open NTDs). Ultrasound findings include the visualization of the defect itself, but other signs, such as the banana sign or the lemon sign, can indicate the presence of NTDs. The combination of all available methods allows the correct diagnosis of most NTDs. Prenatal diagnosis of NTDs provides the basis for obstetric management to include planning mode, timing, and location of delivery. Optimal planning may include consideration for in utero repair, cesarean section with immediate neonatal repair, or delayed neonatal neurosurgical repair. Long-term prognosis favors early in utero detection and a coordinated obstetric-neurosurgical care plan. Recurrence can be decreased with the use of preconception folate supplementation. Primary occurrence can be decreased in the general population using a lesser dose of folate for preconception supplementation.[12] It is not surprising that folate antimetabolites (methotrexate) embryopathy includes NTDs.[7–9]

MATERNAL DISEASE–ASSOCIATED ANOMALIES

Diabetes

Anomalies associated with maternal diabetes include macrosomia, congenital heart defects, NTDs, and caudal regression. There is a direct correlation between the incidence of congenital anomalies and the degree of maternal glycemic control. Preconception counseling and tight glucose control to keep hemoglobin A_{1c} within normal ranges is very important for optimal outcomes. Folate supplementation is also indicated. Maintaining tight glucose control during pregnancy improves perinatal outcome. Fetal anatomic survey, maternal serum analyte screening, and fetal echocardiography are all important standards of care for the management of the pregnant diabetic. Preconception counseling and contraceptive options are critical for women with diabetes. There is no justification for unintended pregnancy in this high-risk group. Gestational diabetes, although associated with macrosomia, does not convey an increased risk for fetal anomalies.

Seizure Disorders

Maternal seizure disorders have an increased incidence of congenital anomalies often attributed to anticonvulsant therapy. Dilantin is associated with fetal hydantoin syndrome, which includes facial anomalies, cardiac defects, and characteristic hypoplasia of fingernails. Valproic acid has a significant risk for NTDs. Multiple medications have a higher relative risk for congenital anomalies than each single agent. However, patients with untreated epilepsy have been shown to have higher rates of congenital anomalies, such as cleft lip and palate. This exemplifies the multifactorial nature of these congenital anomalies and the importance of obtaining a full pedigree and medical history. Maternal serum analyte screening and fetal anatomic survey are critical for the early identification of these anomalies. Maternal seizures require therapy; the choice of medication should follow a risk versus benefit assessment. Preconception counseling, folate supplementation, and contraception options are required for all female patients with seizure disorders. Unintended pregnancy should be avoided in these high-risk patients.

Phenylketonuria

Maternal phenylketonuria, if untreated, is associated with intrauterine growth retardation, mental retardation, and cardiac defects. This rare condition is more prevalent owing to the successfully treated phenylketonuria patient lost to follow-up in whom diet is no longer monitored. The key factor in these unfortunate patients is the recognition of the maternal condition. Dietary therapy requires protein restriction to limit phenylalanine levels in maternal circulation. Analogous to maternal diabetes, tight phenylalanine control is associated with improved neonatal outcomes. Maternal serum analyte screening and fetal anatomic survey are critical for the early identification of these anomalies. As in all chronic maternal disease patients at risk for pregnancy, preconception counseling, normalization of maternal metabolic state, folate supplementation, and effective contraceptive options are the standards of care.

Drug Abuse

Maternal addiction or drug abuse is also a common chronic illness in women of reproductive age. One of the goals for such patients should include preconception counseling, contraceptive options, and care aimed to minimize or eliminate the risk for adverse fetal effects, such as fetal alcohol syndrome. The list of potential teratogens is too large to cover in this review. Recommended readings include useful sources to ascertain timely information pertinent to the optimal care for patients exposed to any specific agent. Table 49-1 includes a selection of known teratogens that frequently form the basis of concern. We recommend a search of the following references to familiarize the clinician with the wealth of information available in TERIS Teratogen Information System at 1-206-543-2465 or REPROTOX 1-800-525-9083, or the web site and resources listed in ACOG Technical Bulletin No. 236, April 1997 at *http://www.acog.com/publications/educational_bulletins/btb236.htm*

X-ray

Although a great concern in Chernobyl, Three Mile Island, and other nuclear disasters, most patients present after an inadvertent radiation exposure for medically indicated reasons. Risk versus benefit assessment (e.g., following maternal trauma) and careful evaluation to correlate dosimetry with timing of gestation at exposure are most helpful. It is important to contact the facility that performed the radiographic procedure to calculate the most accurate fetal dosimetry for risk counseling rather than to rely on tables of millirad estimates of average radiologic procedures. Although there is no safe radiation dose, the normal radiation dose for humans on the surface of earth is approximately 125 mrad. No fetal anomalies have been reported below 25 rad.[7]

CONCLUSION

Recognition of a patient's risk factors preconceptionally offers the best opportunity to make a real difference. There is no better therapy than prevention. Folate supplementation for all women of reproductive age to reduce the incidence of NTDs is an effective public health policy and is among the most crucial points to be made in any consideration of teratology. In addition, simply looking is not enough in the prenatal diagnosis of fetal anomalies. AIUM Obstetrical US Accreditation is a key discriminator for determining the quality of fetal imaging consultants available to a referring provider. A genetic approach to the evaluation of congenital anomalies includes pedigree analysis, a carefully detailed differential diagnostic process

Table 49-1. Teratogens

Drugs	TORCH Syndrome
Thalidomide	Toxoplasmosis
Methotrexate	Syphilis (other)
Retinoic acid	Rubella
Alcohol	Cytomegalovirus
Cocaine	Herpes and expanded TORCH:
X-Ray Exposure	hepatitis viruses, HIV, parvovirus, etc.

to determine the correct etiology for the specific congenital anomaly affecting the patient, and the most appropriate genetic/teratogenic counseling for the family.[13]

Suggestions for Future Reading

Briggs GG, Freeman RK, Yaffe SJ: Drugs in Pregnancy and Lactation, 5th ed. Baltimore, Williams & Wilkins, 1998. http://www.wwilkins.com

Chez RA, Suitor CW: Teratology (ACOG Technical Bulletin No. 236; replaces No. 233, February 1997). Washington, DC, American College of Obstetricians and Gynecologists, April 1997. http://www.acog.com/publications/educational_bulletins/btb236.htm

Evans MI (ed): Reproductive Risks and Prenatal Diagnosis. Norwalk, Conn, Appleton & Lange, 1992.

Stevenson RE, Hall JG, Goodman RM (eds): Human Malformations and Related Anomalies (Oxford Monographs on Medical Genetics No. 27). New York, Oxford University Press, 1993.

TERIS Teratogen Information System and Shepard's Catalog of Teratogenic Agents. Seattle, Wash, 1-206-543-2465 or REPROTOX 1-800-525-9083.

References

1. Wagner RK, Calhoun BC: The routine obstetric ultrasound examination. In Utilizing Sonography in a General Obstetric Practice. Obstet Gynecol Clin North Am 1998;25:451–463.
2. American College of Obstetricians and Gynecologists: Ultrasonography in pregnancy (ACOG Technical Bulletin No. 187). Washington, DC, ACOG, December, 1993. http://www.acog.com/publications/educational_bulletins/btb236.ht
3. Standards for Performance of the Antepartum Obstetrical Ultrasound Evaluation. Laurel, Md, American Institute of Ultrasound in Medicine, 1994.
4. Chez RA, Suitor CW: Teratology (ACOG Technical Bulletin No. 236; replaces No. 233, February 1997). Washington, DC, American College of Obstetricians and Gynecologists, April 1997. http://www.acog.com/publications/educational_bulletins/btb236.htm
5. Calhoun BC, Hoeldtke NJ, Hinson RM, Judge KM: Perinatal hospice: Should all centers have this service? Neonatal Network 1997;16(6):101–102.
6. Evans MI (ed): Reproductive Risks and Prenatal Diagnosis. Norwalk, Conn, Appleton & Lange, 1992.
7. Stevenson RE, Hall JG, Goodman RM (eds): Human Malformations and Related Anomalies (Oxford Monographs on Medical Genetics No. 27). New York, Oxford University Press, 1993.
8. TERIS Teratogen Information System and Shepard's Catalog of Teratogenic Agents. Seattle, Wash, 1-206-543-2465 or REPROTOX 1-800-525-9083.
9. Briggs GG, Freeman RK, Yaffe SJ: Drugs in Pregnancy and Lactation, 5th ed. Baltimore, Williams & Wilkins, 1998.
10. Hume RF, Martin LS, Bottoms SF, et al: Vascular disruption birth defects and history of prenatal cocaine exposure: a case control study. Fetal Diagn Ther 1997;12:292–295.
11. Hume RF, Drugan A, Reichler A, et al: Aneuploidy among prenatally detected neural tube defects. Am J Med Genet 1996;61:171–173.
12. Daly LE, Kirke PN, Molloy A, et al: Folate levels and neural tube defects: Implications for prevention. JAMA 1995;274:1698–1718.
13. Evans MI, Hume RF, Johnson MP, et al: Integration of genetics and ultrasound in prenatal diagnosis: Just looking is not enough. Am J Obstet Gynecol 1996;174:1925–1931.

CHAPTER

FIFTY

Universal Ultrasound Screening—Useful or a Waste?

Christine H. Comstock

Ultrasound has allowed the obstetrician to see the second patient in the pregnancy duad—the fetus—and thus has transformed modern obstetrics. There is little controversy over the use of ultrasound in cases in which dates are unknown, size too large, and so on. Since 1980 in West Germany, at least two ultrasound examinations have been offered during pregnancy. In Great Britain, the Royal College of Obstetricians and Gynaecologists also recommends screening. However, in the United States, the 1984 Consensus Conference of the National Institutes of Health concluded that the data available at that time on clinical efficacy and safety did not allow a recommendation for routine screening of low-risk women.

The issue of routine ultrasound screening of low-risk pregnancies seems to be still uniquely and strongly argued in the United States. For at least two reasons, the situation in the United States is different from the rest of the world: private insurers pay for medical care of the pregnant woman, for the most part, and care is more expensive than in other countries. Termination of pregnancy in the instance of a life-threatening anomaly is also hotly debated in the United States and is believed by some not to be a personal issue but rather one that should be regulated by the government.

In Europe, screening of low-risk pregnancies is widely accepted and is paid for by government health care. Does routine screening improve outcome or make a difference in the health of a population? This question has been repeatedly asked in both the United States and Europe since at least 1982.

The question as to whether or not screening ultrasound is useful and worth the money is not easily answered and depends on many factors: how skilled the examiner, the gestational age, whether termination of pregnancy is a possibility, cost of the examination, what outcome is being looked at and whether that outcome can be modified by altered care, the frequency of the outcome and whether or not there were enough patients in the groups to show a difference statistically. Some of these issues are discussed in this chapter. First, however, the two large studies that are most frequently referred to merit individual discussion.

THE RADIUS TRIAL

RADIUS is an acronym for Routine Antenatal Diagnostic Imaging with Ultrasound.[1, 2] This study was conducted in the United States, primarily in private offices and by radiologists in a separate office. However, some of the scans were done in university settings. The study was designed to test the hypothesis that screening ultrasound would improve perinatal outcome in low-risk pregnancies.

One of the problems in the study was that it addressed clinical problems in obstetrics for which there is no effective management (e.g., small-for-date). Another problem was that the number of anomalies missed in all but the university centers was much higher than expected. If an anomaly is not detected, then there will be no difference in outcome. There were no protocols for managing twins, premature labor, and so on, in an organized fashion, so whether or not identification of twins made a difference cannot be shown. For obstetrics practice in the United States in private offices, no improvement in neonatal morbidity or mortality was shown. The study did show that it is not possible to detect anomalies by physical examination or clinical evaluation alone because only a total of 11% were detected prenatally in the control group and only 5% before 24 weeks. Only 7.6% of all patients had no scan at all, a fact that weakened the control group. Thirty-five percent of the scans in the control group were performed outside the study and its quality-control process. (Please see Chapter 42.)

In summary, there were too many scans in the experimental group—the second scan doubling costs but adding no useful information. Many of the control group patients ended up having scans as well, making a difference between the two groups hard to demonstrate. In some cases, the outcomes were ones for which we have no effective treatment. Many anomalies were missed. Lastly, low-risk was defined so strictly that it encompassed only 40% of patients. Thus, the evaluation of usefulness addressed less than half the population.

THE HELSINKI TRIAL

During a 19-month period, 95% of all pregnant women in the Helsinki area of Finland were entered into a study to compare one-stage screening to selective screening.[3] There were approximately 4600 women in each of the two groups. There were no differences in the number of inductions or in birth weights between the two groups. Perinatal mortality was significantly lower in the screened group (4.6 per 1000 vs. 9.0 per 1000). This 49% reduction was due mainly to early detection of major malformations for which patients elected abortion. All twin pregnancies were detected in the screening group versus 76% in the control group, with perinatal mortality in the twin screened group of 27.8 per 1000 versus 65.8 per 1000 in the control group. However, the latter group was quite small. The advantage of this trial was that care of the two groups was similar, a major deficiency of the RADIUS trial. In addition, the screening was carried out in two women's hospitals where there was considerable ultrasound expertise.

This study did not separate out high- and low-risk women but scanned all women, whatever their risk factors. In reality, this is what the RADIUS trial ended up doing, despite its intent to screen only low-risk women. In the RADIUS trial, only half the women were entered into the study but many of the patients in the control group had ultrasound as well, just at a later date. The Helsinki study also had this problem because many women in the control group had ultrasound at some time. However, the difference was still marked because anomalies were detected early in the screened group and the patients elected abortion.

DATES

Correction of dates has been found to be improved with routine ultrasound in several studies. In the RADIUS study, gestational age was adjusted in 11% of patients versus 3% of those in the control group. At least four major studies have shown a reduction in the rate of induction for post-term pregnancy. In the RADIUS trial, this reduction rate was 5 per 1000 and did not result in a decrease in perinatal mortality. This may be due to the fact that there is a background high rate of induction in the United States: in the RADIUS trial, the induction rate was approximately 25%. The use of tocolysis was lower in the routine ultrasound group compared with controls, probably owing to more frequent correction of dating.

SCREENING FOR ANATOMIC DEFECTS

A number of factors affect the sensitivity of anomaly detection, including experience, how anomalies are calculated (when there is more than one per fetus), how an anomaly is defined, and the incidence within the population. Sensitivity has been reported to be as low as 15% in the RADIUS trial before 24 weeks to a high of 85% in England.[4]

The RADIUS study clearly showed that in the United States, there is a widely varying skill level and ability to detect anomalies, despite some attempt at quality control. Supervision, consisting of a later review of films on a lightboard, may work for simple and relatively stationary structures such as the liver and gallbladder, but for a small, complex, and moving subject the examiner must be very experienced, because anything not detected at the time will

not be recorded on tape or film. Proceeding in a logical, methodical manner with a check list is important so that no major structure is skipped. In evaluating structures such as the heart, good equipment with good resolution, a cine loop, B color, and harmonic imaging aid even the most experienced examiner. It was clear from the RADIUS study that scans performed in university settings detected many more abnormalities than those in private offices. Most studies have shown better results when the examinations have been performed at one site, rather than at multiple ones.

The Eurofetus, a database from ultrasound laboratories practicing routine obstetric ultrasound in 60 hospitals in 14 European countries, has recorded about 4600 congenital anomalies.[5] This registry indicates that same-laboratory improvements in detection of defects have been marked since the late 1980s, with an average now for major anomalies of 75%. In another European registry, the Eurocat,[6] bilateral renal agenesis was detected in 60% of cases in which there was routine screening ultrasound versus 4% when screening was not done. Spina bifida and also hydrocephalus were detected in only 2% of cases, respectively, without screening. Clearly, spina bifida and hydrocephalus are two defects that are detectable before 24 weeks, and about which parents would certainly want to be informed.

The sensitivity of detection depends not only on skill and equipment but also on what type of defect is being sought, what views are used, and at what gestational age. Some defects, such as cardiac, are very difficult to see before 18 weeks, whereas others, such as anencephaly and omphalocele, often are more readily seen early. For purposes of discussion here, routine scanning means evaluation at 17 to 19 weeks. As an additional example, the sensitivity of detection of small ventricular septal defects in experienced hands is well below the detection rate of other more obvious cardiac anomalies, such as hypoplastic heart or atrioventricular canal. The number of views obtained can influence sensitivity: conotruncal defects are frequently missed unless a view of the left ventricular outflow track is included in the screening examination. Transposition without a ventricular septal defect, a very serious defect with consequences within the first 3 days of life, will not be detected unless the vessel leading out of the left ventricle is evaluated for neck vessels or the right great vessel for branching.

The RADIUS study did show that most anomalies do not cause changes in the physical examination of the mother that might indicate the need for an ultrasound examination. That is, polyhydramnios, oligohydramnios, and intrauterine growth retardation do not cause changes in fundal height early enough to suggest an ultrasound evaluation in a time frame that would allow termination of pregnancy for renal agenesis, anencephaly, and so on.

Comparison of the RADIUS trial and the Helsinki study demonstrated that skill in detection, and then willingness to terminate a pregnancy, alters the usefulness of screening. No other parameters have had enough power to be shown to be improved by screening. This was confirmed by Van Dorsten et al.[7] Sensitivities in detection of anomalies are summarized by Dooley.[8]

SCREENING FOR FETAL HEART DEFECTS

As equipment has improved over the last 20 years, it is now possible to see many heart defects in the second trimester. In fact, the four-chamber view of the heart has become part of the standard screening ultrasound examination.[9] Whether or not screening for fetal heart defects changes outcome and management depends upon many factors.

The Four-Chamber View

This is an axial view, which shows the four-chamber view of the heart. An experienced observer notes the whole view and may not need to concentrate on each part, but there are many components to this view, which are not immediately apparent. The axis should be at 45 degrees to the midline, the AV valves off-set, the ventricles approximately equal in size and properly positioned in relation to the fetal side, and the atria equal-sized. Contractility and the integrity of the walls of the ventricle are also a part of this view.

How well does this view detect heart defects? The answer to this depends upon at least four factors: 1) The patient population and the incidence of diabetes and congenital heart disease, 2) the gestational age of the fetus, 3) equipment and experience, and 4) the heart defects for which screening is performed. Lower gestational age and maternal obesity and previous abdominal surgery lower the ability to obtain a complete four-chamber view. Under optimal conditions in which a complete view can be obtained the four-chamber view will detect approximately 50% to 60% of heart defects in fetuses 18 or more weeks old. The defects, which are difficult or impossible to detect on this view, are atrial septal defects (ASD), small ventricular septal defects (VSD), conotruncal defects (unless there is a large VSD), and late-appearing lesions such as pulmonary and aortic stenosis or atresia and mild or moderate coarctation.

The Aortic Root or Five-Chamber View

This view shows the aorta as it exits from the left ventricle. It is not yet considered a standard view, but definitely a desirable one. Depending on position, it can be easy or difficult or impossible to obtain. It will be abnormal in almost all conotruncal defects because they have VSDs. Even transposition of the great vessels without a VSD will be detected with this view because the pulmonary artery will be parallel to the aorta in this view. This view thus increases detection of heart defects to approximately 75% because there is the addition of conotruncal defects. The addition of conotruncal views is important because the structures can be ductal dependent—when adult circulation is attained they may not oxygenate blood. The remaining 25% of lesions, which are not detected by this view or the four-chamber view, are ASDs, small VSDs that are below the resolving ability of the equipment, and late-appearing lesions.

Effect on Outcome and Management

Whether or not the detection of a heart defect impacts patient care depends upon several factors. One of the most important of these is the attitude of the patient toward pregnancy termination. Since heart defects are a part of many syndromes and all of the major aneuploidies, in a population in which termination of pregnancy is not a usual choice, there is no change in pregnancy management in the second trimester despite detection of a heart defect.

Although most heart defects are now repairable, the outcome and number of procedures varies from defect to defect. Some parents do not wish to have their baby undergo the two or three major operations for a less than certain outcome in such defects as hypoplastic left heart. In those instances ascertainment may help the patient prepare for eventual death of the baby, but there is no change in management.

Many heart defects do not affect the newborn and no change of delivery site is necessary. However, if a fetus has a defect, which is probably ductal dependent (hypoplastic left heart, severe teratology, for example), there is conflicting information about whether delivery at a hospital with pediatric cardiac surgery is helpful. In the best-designed study there was some evidence that there is less acidemia, fewer cardiac arrests, and a shorter recovery period in the baby with a ductal dependent left heart lesion, which has been identified in utero.[10] It is really the amount of delay rather than location, which seems to be important. Another factor is ascertainment, since babies who appear to be normal at birth and have not been identified with a heart defect go to regular nurseries or to room in with the mother and may not be under observation when the ductus starts to close or a blue skin color develops. To this is added transport to another hospital, by which time acidemia may be severe.

TWINS

There were not enough twin pairs in the RADIUS study to show that routine screening, and therefore the early detection of twins, improved outcome. However, a logical analysis of twin pregnancies would lead to the conclusion that twin outcome may not be a useful one to evaluate in screening studies to begin with. Most twin pairs were eventually detected in the RADIUS study, albeit later than in the control group. Screening for anomalies in twins is problematic because many parents are not willing to take any action if one has an anomaly, even if dichorionic. Growth evaluation does not result in a change of management unless twins are likely to have mature lungs and therefore can be induced. Induction before this time may increase costs rather than reduce them. That is, prematurity poses a greater threat to twins than birth-weight discordance.[6] Severe twin-twin discordance (more than 30%), which carries a much higher risk of intrauterine death, is quite rare (4 in 100 pairs).

ALTERED MANAGEMENT OF NONLETHAL DEFECTS

There is no firm evidence that screening and subsequent identification of heart defects change the outlook of the fetus after it is born, but certainly parents have serious decisions to make if their fetus has a hypoplastic left side of the heart. In babies who have had complex repairs, there is a higher incidence of developmental lag. Although most other defects are repairable with varying degrees of ease, long-term outlook is not known in all.

Several studies have suggested that knowledge of a cardiac anomaly and transfer to surgical facilities do not improve outcome. However, there are major flaws in some of those studies: it is not clear how close the control facilities were to surgery facilities—if close, then dramatic differences in survival would be dampened.

PATIENT PREPARATION AND CHOICE

A strong argument can be made that the mother (and father) has a right to know if the child will have an anomaly, just as she has a right to view the data in her medical records. This right is particularly cogent if the discovered defect is one for which a parent might choose termination, such as anencephaly or hypoplastic heart. The right to make these decisions is priceless to many and not a question of dollars and cents.

However, in a population in which this is seen as a sinful act, screening for defects would not change medical care. This seemed to be the case in much of the population covered by the RADIUS study. Screening for anomalies is clearly not cost-effective in this group but would be informational only. If parents had more rights in the neonatal period, this would be less an issue, but in the United States many parents are essentially disenfranchised of all but a few types of decision once their child is born.

Even if termination is not chosen, it seems to be helpful to prepare patients for abnormalities they might see at birth and to help them think about decisions that might need to be made—surgery, life support, and so on.

SUMMARY

Universal screening is a complex subject. There is little question that perinatal mortality will be reduced and women will have more control over their reproductive destinies if all serious defects are detected and the termination of pregnancy is available to all patients. The efficacy of universal screening or lack thereof depends on many variables, including when, how often, by whom, how it is performed, and how much it costs. No efficacy can be shown if screening is performed at a substandard level. Efficacy of screening also depends on the outcome being evaluated and how that outcome is treated (if there is any treatment). The screening examination itself is evolving: since 1995, evaluation of the cervix in normal women, nuchal thickening, and the cardiac outflow tracks have been added to the routine scan of low-risk women by many centers but have not been added into the savings equation.

The emotional benefits are difficult to quantify. Reassurance of normality is probably the greatest benefit of screening but is impossible to express in economic terms. That most women want ultrasound and seek its reassurance is well known. Many are willing to pay out of pocket.

At present, no studies answer the question whether universal screening of low-risk women as it is performed in the best ultrasound units at the present time is cost-effective.

References

1. Lefevre M, Bain R, Ewigman B, et al: RADIUS Study Group: A randomized trial of prenatal ultrasonographic screening: Impact on maternal management and outcome. Am J Obstet Gynecol 1993;169:483–489.
2. Ewigman B, Crane J, Frigoletto F, et al: Effect of prenatal ultrasound screening on perinatal outcome. N Engl J Med 1993;329:821–827.
3. Saari-Kemppainen A, Karjalaininen O, Ylöstalo P, Hienonen O: Ultrasound screening and perinatal mortality: Controlled trial of systematic one-stage screening in pregnancy. The Helsinki Ultrasound Trial. Lancet 1990;336:387–391.
4. Luck C: Value of routine ultrasound scanning at 19 weeks: a four year study of 8849 deliveries. Br Med J 1992;304:1474–1478.
5. Grandjean H, Larroque D, Levi S: The performance of routine ultrasonographic screening of pregnancies in the Eurofetus study. Am J Obstet Gynecol 1999;181:446–454.
6. Eurocat Working Group. 1995: Surveillance of congenital anomalies in Europe, 1980–1992. European Union Project, Institute of Hygiene and Epidemiology, Brussels, Belgium.
7. Van Dorsten JP, Hulsey T, Newman R, Menard K: Fetal anomaly detection by second-trimester ultrasonography in a tertiary center. Am J Obstet Gynecol 1998;178:742–749.
8. Dooley SL: Routine ultrasound in pregnancy. Clin Obstet Gynecol 1999;42:737–748.
9. American Institute of Ultrasound in Medicine: Guidelines for performance of the antepartum obstetrical ultrasound examination. Laurel, Md, Author, 1994.
10. Chang AC, Huhta JC, Yoon GY, et al: Diagnosis, transport, and outcome in fetuses with left ventricular outflow tract obstruction. J Thorac Cardiovasc Surg 1991;102:841–848.

FIFTY-ONE

Cervical Length

Robert P. Lorenz

WHO CARES?

Who cares?

For most of a woman's life, the length of her cervix is as important to her as the history of the Heisman Trophy. However, during pregnancy, the integrity of the cervix is one of a number of critical elements necessary for successful pregnancy outcome. The problem obstetricians face is that currently we do not understand pregnancy physiology and pathophysiology sufficiently to translate information about cervical integrity into a reliable therapeutic plan to reduce the risk of preterm birth.

Prematurity is second only to birth defects as a leading cause of perinatal morbidity and mortality. There have been impressive advances in our understanding of the pathophysiology of spontaneous preterm birth and in neonatal outcomes for the very-low-birth-weight infant. Unfortunately, there has been very little impact, if any, on the rate of preterm birth or the efficacy of prolonging gestation in an at-risk pregnancy. Efforts to predict preterm birth have included uterine activity monitoring, biochemical markers, and surveillance of the length of the cervix. Reliable prediction of preterm birth is of benefit in two ways: It identifies the appropriate group for preventive and therapeutic intervention, and it allows caregivers to avoid unnecessary intervention in pregnancies that are destined to reach full term. The former benefit, unfortunately, is primarily an issue of research rather than clinical practice. We have no established method of avoiding preterm birth effectively.

Objectives

At the end of this chapter, the reader should be able to:

- Describe two methods for measurement of cervical length.
- List the range of normal for cervical length before and during each trimester of pregnancy.
- Define the strength of evidence demonstrating efficacy of therapeutic intervention based on cervical length.

DEFINITIONS AND ANATOMY

The cervix is the lower portion of the uterus extending from the isthmus of the uterus into the vagina. In the nonpregnant condition, it is a cylindrical structure composed of collagen, connective tissue, and smooth muscle, surrounding a narrow canal lined by glandular epithelium. Over the course of normal pregnancy, its structure changes biochemically and histologically to a less dense tissue that eventually is retracted away from the vagina and becomes continuous with the lower uterine segment in labor.

Definition of *normal cervical length*: A determination of the normal length of the cervix, like beauty, is in the eye of the beholder. More specifically, it is in the method of the beholder. The most popular methods of assessment of cervical length are physical examination and imaging by transabdominal, transvaginal, and perineal ultrasound.

Traditionally, *incompetent cervix* is a clinical diagnosis based on history of midtrimester pregnancy loss associated with painless dilatation before the onset of labor. A short cervix on ultrasound or physical examination is not the equivalent of an incompetent cervix. Cervices vary in their relative concentrations of muscle fibers, collagen, and stroma. Some short cervices have the strength to maintain pregnancy to term. Biopsy studies suggest that incompetent cervices may have more muscle fibers and less connective tissue than normal cervices. Imaging studies during the second trimester have revealed that some patients with a history characteristic of incompetent cervix may actually have progressive cervical shortening over a period of days or weeks before the typical clinical presentation.

Description of the cervix during pregnancy by physical examination for purposes of assessing risk of preterm birth usually is done by the *Bishop score*. Bishop[1] developed a scoring system for multigravidas to assess the likelihood of successful induction of labor at term based on the following characteristics of the cervix on physical examination: dilatation (closed = 0; 1 to 2 cm = 1; 3 to 4 cm = 2; ≥5 cm = 3), effacement (0% to 30% = 0; 40% to 50% = 1; 60% to 70% = 2; ≥80% = 3), station (−3 = 0; −2 = 1; −1 or 0 = 2; +1 or +2 = 3), consistency (firm = 0; medium = 1; soft = 2), and position of the cervix in the vagina (posterior = 0; mid = 1; anterior = 2). It was later applied to nulligravida patients for induction, and became the basis for attempts to use physical examination to predict risk of preterm birth.

Another method for assessment of the cervix on physical examination to predict risk of preterm birth is the *cervical score*. The cervical score is the length of the cervix in centimeters (0, 1, 2, or 3) minus the dilatation of the cervix in centimeters.

Assessment of the cervix by ultrasound can be done transabdominally, transvaginally, or transperineally. With ultrasound, the examiner measures the distance between the internal and the external os and may also describe changes in the cervicouterine junction (e.g., funnelling) or changes in the cervix over time or with fundal pressure. Limitations of ultrasound assessment of the cervix include the inability to assess the consistency of the cervix or the station of the presenting part and the expense of the equipment and the training required to perform the test properly. Transvaginal ultrasound is more invasive, uncomfortable, and time consuming compared with a transabdominal ultrasound. Transabdominal ultrasound has the challenge of avoiding artifactual lengthening of the cervix if the bladder is overdistended owing to the effect of the degree of bladder distention on the appearance of the cervix.

Funnelling is defined as the condition of the angle between the axis of the endocervical canal and the lower uterine segment of more than 90 degrees at the internal os. Physiologically, it reflects progressive shortening of the cervix, which usually begins at the internal os. Funnelling can be V- or U-shaped.

Using transvaginal sonography of the cervix, some authors have described a *cervical index,* which is a ratio: (1 + funnel length in cm) (endocervical length in cm).

The nonpregnant cervix of a woman of reproductive age is 2.5 to 3.0 cm long, based on studies of hysterectomy specimens.

Studies of measurements by transvaginal ultrasound of cervical length by gestational age vary in their results (Figs. 51–1 to 51–3).

RELATIONSHIP OF ABNORMAL CERVICAL LENGTH AND OUTCOME OF PREGNANCY

Cervical length may be the most reliable risk factor for spontaneous preterm birth. Cervical status may be assessed by physical examination or by ultrasound done transabdominally, transvaginally, or transperineally. Transperineal

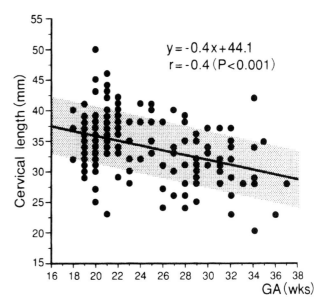

Figure 51–2. Relationship between cervical length and gestational age (GA) in the control group. (From Murakawa H, Utumi T, Hasegawa I, et al: Evaluation of threatened preterm delivery by transvaginal ultrasonographic measurement of cervical length. (Reprinted with permission from the American College of Obstetricians and Gynecologists [Obstet Gynecol 1993;82:829–832].)

measurement has not been studied extensively. It appears to be similar to transvaginal ultrasound, and is not discussed separately.

Physical Examination

Physical examination has the advantage of assessing potential risk factors for spontaneous preterm labor or

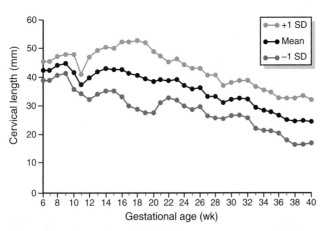

Figure 51–1. One group's findings on the relationship between cervical length and gestational age. (From Okitsu O, Mimura T, Nakayama N, et al: Early prediction of preterm delivery by transvaginal ultrasound. Ultrasound Obstet Gynecol 1992;2:402–409.)

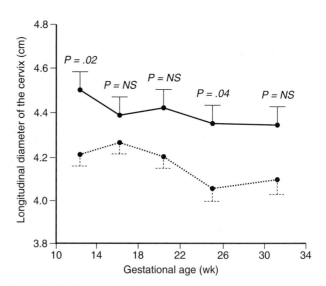

Figure 51–3. Means and standard errors of longitudinal diameters of the cervix in multiparous women (*solid line*, N = 47) and primigravidas or women with previous cesareans or first trimester abortions (*dotted line,* N = 107). (From Zorzoli A, Soliani A, Perra M, et al: Cervical changes throughout pregnancy as assessed by transvaginal sonography. (Reprinted with permission from the American College of Obstetricians and Gynecologists. [Obstet Gynecol 1994;84:960–964].)

premature rupture of membranes other than simply length. There is considerable interobserver variability in Bishop scores. If the cervix is closed and firm, physical examination can identify only the length of the cervix that protrudes into the vagina. If the cervix admits the examining finger, then a measurement of the distance to the internal os is possible.

Houlton and coworkers[2] and Neilson and associates[3] in separate studies used a "cervical score" assessed by physical examination to predict risk of preterm birth in multiple gestations. Houlton and coworkers[2] found 69% of women going into preterm labor within 14 days had a cervical score of 0 or less. Neilson and associates[3] found that 76% of twin pregnancies with a score of less than or equal to −2 before 34 weeks delivered preterm.

Transabdominal Ultrasound

The primary advantage of transabdominal sonographic assessment of the cervix is that it can be incorporated as a screening method in gestational studies done for other reasons with little additional time or equipment. The primary disadvantage of this method is that it can be limited by the effect of an overdistended bladder. If the bladder is overdistended, the length of the cervix will appear longer than in measurements with the bladder properly filled or when the cervix is measured transvaginally by ultrasound.

In a study by Smith and colleagues[4] of 72,291 obstetric ultrasounds done at less than 35 weeks' gestation in an unselected population, patients with a cervical length of less than 3.0 cm on screening transabdominal ultrasound during the second trimester had a risk of preterm birth of 30%. In that study, patients with classic risk factors for preterm birth (e.g., past history of preterm birth, multiple gestation in the index pregnancy) who also had a short cervix delivered before 37 weeks' gestation in 33% of cases. Patients with a short cervix without classic risk factors had a preterm delivery rate of 25%.

Transvaginal Ultrasound

Leitich and associates[5] reviewed 13 studies of 8463 patients, including subgroups of patients in preterm labor, and symptom-free low-risk patients studied in the second or early third trimester. For patients presenting in preterm labor (8 studies), the optimal cervical length for a marker for preterm birth ranged from 18 to 30 mm, resulting in a sensitivity rate ranging from 68% to 100% and a specificity range of 44% to 79%. Dilatation of the internal os (variously defined as a V- or U-shaped internal os, a funnel width of 5 mm or greater, or a funnel length of 3 mm) in patients presenting in preterm labor had a sensitivity range of 70% to 100% and a specificity range of 54% to 75%.

For asymptomatic low-risk patients studied between 20 and 24 weeks' gestation (7 studies), the optimal cutoff values for predicting preterm birth varied between 25 and

35 mm of cervical length, with a sensitivity range of 33% to 54% and a range of specificity of 73% to 91%. For asymptomatic low-risk patients studied between 27 and 32 weeks' gestation (6 studies), the cervical length optimal cutoff value ranged between 25 and 39 mm, with a sensitivity range of 63% to 76% and specificities varying from 59% to 69%. In asymptomatic low-risk patients, dilatation of the internal cervical os on ultrasound had a sensitivity ranging from 16% to 33% and a specificity range of 92% to 99%.

Iams and coworkers[6] studied 2915 patients at 24 weeks' gestation and determined the distribution of cervical length and then the probability of spontaneous preterm birth and the relative risk based on transvaginal sonographic cervical length measurements (Figs. 51–4 and 51–5).

Digital Examination versus Ultrasound

Assessment of the cervix for risk of preterm birth is more effective if done by ultrasound than by digital examination. Gomez and colleagues[7] compared physical examination with transvaginal ultrasound for cervical assessment to predict preterm birth in a population of patients ($N = 59$) undergoing treatment for preterm labor. They assessed ultrasound measurements of endocervical length, funnel length, and "cervical index" (defined as [funnel length + 1]/endocervical length). Using receiver operator curves and logistic regression analysis, they found that those ultrasound findings were better predictors of preterm birth than digital examination. Their optimal values for cutoffs for cervical length were 18 mm or less and cervical index 0.52 or greater.

In a similar group of patients ($N = 60$), using receiver operator curves, Iams and associates[8] found cervical sonog-

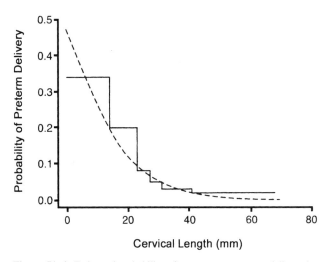

Figure 51–4. Estimated probability of spontaneous preterm delivery before 35 weeks of gestation from the logistic-regression analysis. (From Iams JD, Goldenberg RL, Meis PJ, et al: The length of the cervix and the risk of spontaneous preterm delivery. N Engl J Med 1996;334:567. Copyright © 1996 Massachusetts Medical Society. All rights reserved.)

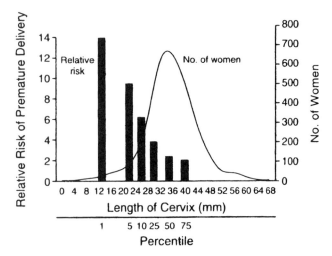

Figure 51-5. Distribution of subjects among percentiles for cervical length measured by transvaginal ultrasonography at 24 weeks of gestation and relative risk of spontaneous preterm delivery before 35 weeks of gestation according to percentiles for cervical length. (From Iams JD, Goldenberg RL, Meis PJ, et al: The length of the cervix and the risk of spontaneous preterm delivery. N Engl J Med 1996;334:567. Copyright © 1996 Massachusetts Medical Society. All rights reserved.)

raphy (length < 30 mm) superior to digital assessment of dilatation (≥2 cm) and effacement (≥50%) as a test for delivery before 36 weeks' gestation.

Berghella and coworkers[9] studied 102 singleton pregnancies serially from 14 to 30 weeks' gestation that were at high risk for preterm birth and compared ultrasound and digital assessment of the cervix. They found ultrasound measurements more predictive, with a sonographic measurement of cervical length of 25 mm the best cutoff based on receiver operator curves.

THERAPEUTIC IMPLICATIONS

Measurement of cervical length and other characteristics has potential benefits therapeutically: (1) to identify patients who may benefit from a cerclage, (2) to screen low- or high-risk women, and (3) to assess women who present in threatened preterm labor.

Cerclage

It is an unfortunate commentary on the scientific basis for obstetric interventions that cervical cerclage to improve pregnancy outcome was introduced 50 years ago, but not subject to well-designed clinical trials until 1984. In two randomized studies,[10, 11] patients at risk for preterm birth did not benefit from elective cerclage. In a multicenter randomized study by the Medical Research Council[12] of patients with possible incompetent cervix, the reduction in the rate of preterm birth with elective cerclage was only 5% versus a control group not undergoing elective cerclage.

Patients with a convincing history in a prior pregnancy for incompetent cervix may benefit from elective cerclage

at the end of the first trimester. An alternative approach to these patients would be serial transvaginal sonographic assessment of the cervix during the midtrimester and placement of a cerclage if cervical length shortens to an abnormal degree. Unfortunately, the precise cervical length at each gestational age that justifies intervention has not been determined.

Patients with a less clear history of incompetent cervix may benefit from a similar approach of serial transvaginal sonographic assessment of the cervix during the early and middle second trimester. For example, a history of a midtrimester spontaneous delivery (not preceded by an antepartum fetal death) that is not typical for an incompetent cervix may warrant such surveillance.

Screening Women at Low or High Risk for Preterm Birth

Screening all pregnant women by pelvic examination to assess risk of preterm birth has not been shown to be effective.

Women without a typical history for incompetent cervix but who are at high risk for preterm birth include, but are not limited to, those with a prior preterm spontaneous birth, multiple gestation, polyhydramnios, prior cervical conization, and prior obstetric laceration of the cervix. Most programs of preterm labor surveillance designed for women at high risk utilize assessment of the cervix by some method, either by digital examination or by ultrasound. If digital examination suggests that there is cervical effacement, change in consistency, or change in station, an ultrasound assessment demonstrating normal cervical length may be reassuring.

The dilemma in surveillance is the absence of a proven method to reduce the risk of preterm birth. If a definite change is noted, then assessment of uterine activity may lead to a diagnosis of premature labor. Management of premature labor is beyond the scope of this chapter.

Threatened Preterm Labor

A major problem in obstetrics in the United States is the overdiagnosis of threatened preterm labor, with unnecessary intervention in women who are destined to reach full-term gestation. Treatment of preterm labor involves medications and interventions that usually have few ill effects, but are potentially dangerous for the mother and fetus. Preterm labor with regular painful contractions and definite cervical dilatation does not require ultrasound assessment of the cervix. However, many patients present with symptoms, documented contractions, intact membranes, no risk factors, and minimal if any cervical change. This is the group of patients who may benefit from further assessment by biochemical markers (e.g., fetal fibronectin) or transvaginal sonographic assessment of the cervix. If either of those tests, or both if available, are reassuring, then intervention can be modified or withdrawn.

FUTURE DIRECTIONS

This chapter focused on the assessment of the cervix as a method to determine risk of preterm birth. Currently, additional research is addressing other risk assessment methods such as biochemical markers as well as interventions to reduce risk of preterm birth. Spontaneous preterm birth is incompletely understood, and probably has multiple etiologies, and therefore multiple approaches to diagnoses and therapy will emerge. For example, it appears that abnormal screening with cervicovaginal fetal fibronectin and abnormal screening with cervical length may identify separate at-risk populations. Preterm labor with intact membranes may represent a different etiologic and therapeutic group than preterm birth beginning with rupture of membranes.

Soon we will have well-defined norms for cervical length determination by various methods. The challenge remains: What therapeutic intervention is appropriate based on the assessment available—gestational age, past obstetric history, clinical risk factors for preterm birth, clinical presentation (e.g., preterm labor or asymptomatic), and cervical length measurement. Clinical trials currently under way hopefully will give us some guidance. Until then, an honest and humble approach to therapeutic intervention must admit there is no overwhelming evidence to clearly direct management of many patients who present without symptoms but with an abnormal cervix.

References

1. Bishop EH: Pelvic scoring for elective induction. Obstet Gynecol 1964;24:267.
2. Houlton MC, Marivate M, Philpott RH: Factors associated with preterm labour and changes in the cervix before labour in twin pregnancy. Br J Obstet Gynaecol 1982;89:190–194.
3. Neilson JP, Verkuyl DA, Crowther CA, et al: Preterm labor in twin pregnancies: Prediction by cervical assessment. Obstet Gynecol 1988;72:719–723.
4. Smith RS, Comstock CH, Kirk JS, et al: Cervical length assessment: A useful addition to the screening obstetric ultrasound exam. J Ultrasound Med 1998;17:S81.
5. Leitich H, Brunbauer M, Kaider A, et al: Cervical length and dilatation of the internal cervical os detected by vaginal ultrasonography as markers for preterm delivery: A systematic review. Am J Obstet Gynecol 1999;181:1465–1472.
6. Iams JD, Goldenberg RL, Meis PJ, et al: The length of the cervix and the risk of spontaneous preterm delivery. N Engl J Med 1996;334:567.
7. Gomez R, Galasso M, Romero R, et al: Ultrasonographic examination of the uterine cervix is better than cervical digital examination as a predictor of the likelihood of premature delivery in patients with preterm labor and intact membranes. Am J Obstet Gynecol 1994;171:956–964.
8. Iams JD, Paraskos J, Landon MB: Cervical sonography in preterm labor. Obstet Gynecol 1994;84:40–46.
9. Berghella V, Tolosa JE, Kuhlman K, et al: Cervical ultrasonography compared with manual examination as a predictor of preterm delivery. Am J Obstet Gynecol 1997;177:723–730.
10. Lazar P, Gueguen S, Dreyfus J, et al: Multicentred controlled trial of cervical cerclage in women at moderate risk of preterm delivery. Br J Obstet Gynaecol 1984;81:731–735.
11. Rush RW, Isaacs S, McPherson K, et al: A randomized controlled trial of cervical cerclage in women at high risk of spontaneous preterm delivery. Br J Obstet Gynaecol 1984;91:724–730.
12. Interim report of the Medical Research Council/Royal College of Obstetricians and Gynaecologists multicentre randomized trial of cervical cerclage. MRC/RCOG Working Party on Cervical Cerclage. Br J Obstet Gynaecol 1988;95:437–445.

FIFTY-TWO

Fetal Gene Therapy Update

Yuval Yaron and Avi Orr-Urtreger

With the completion of the Human Genome Project, and the overwhelming discoveries and new technologies, gene therapy for many disorders may soon become a reality. However, postnatal gene therapy may come too late in some genetic disorders owing to prenatal irreversible organ damage. For such disorders, *fetal gene therapy* (FGT) may offer a reasonable solution. In addition, FGT allows the targeting and expanding of the stem cell population that may be inaccessible later in life and may also avoid the immune response that may be mounted against the foreign therapeutic protein product.

There are still significant technical issues and ethical considerations regarding FGT, and before this mode of therapy can be applied in clinical practice, extensive research should be performed in appropriate animal models to test for efficiency and safety of both the fetus and the mother.[1, 2] Until these requirements are met, human FGT should be considered premature despite the great promise it holds for the future.[3–5]

DESIGNING THE THERAPEUTIC GENE

Loss-of-function mutations are responsible for a wide range of human diseases. Such mutations result in absence, reduction, or faulty production of an essential protein, such as an enzyme, structural protein, or membrane receptor. Restoring the lost function can theoretically be achieved by introducing the normal or wild-type gene in a manner that would facilitate the production of the missing gene-product in the affected tissues at the appropriate time and quantity. This approach appears to be the most likely to be used in FGT. Other approaches may also be considered. Primordial genes that are usually repressed may be induced to express once again. An example for this may be found in the globin system, where the fetal γ-globin is replaced by β-globin at a latter stage of development. In cases of β-thalassemia, where the β-globin genes are mutated, γ-globin production may overcome some of the serious prenatal complications associated with the disease.

In addition, foreign genes may be employed to oppose the expression of what are usually dominant genes that cause disease ranging from cancer to viral infections. This approach may also be directed to oppose the expression of genes responsible for genetic diseases caused by a mutated protein that assumes an altered function that is responsible for the disease manifestations, such as the sickling of red blood cells induced by hemoglobin S in sickle cell anemia.

DELIVERING THE THERAPEUTIC GENE TO ITS TARGET

The construction of therapeutic genes is a relatively straightforward task. In contrast, the rate-limiting step toward successful application of gene therapy, and in particular FGT, has remained the development of safe and efficient gene delivery techniques. Such techniques should bring the therapeutic gene into the target tissue where it is to be expressed at the appropriate time and quantity, in a manner that does not endanger the fetus or the mother. Most gene delivery techniques are based on various viral vectors; however, nonviral vectors are also investigated because they may be less risky.

Viral Vectors

The most widely employed techniques for gene delivery make use of viral vectors. Ideally, therapeutic genes should be exclusively expressed only in the relevant cell type and should be free of any untoward effects on healthy cells. Several different types of viral vectors have been employed for gene delivery.

Retroviruses are RNA viruses contained in a viral-encoded envelope, *env* protein, which is embedded in a lipid bilayer derived from the host plasma membrane. The viral core contains virally encoded enzymes *reverse transcriptase* and *integrase*, which are essential for viral replication and integration of the viral DNA into the host genome. Because the retroviral genome is integrated into the host genome, the transgenic cells retain the new genetic information through subsequent cell divisions, resulting in a relatively stable transgene. However, vector titers are low, require dividing cells for effective transfection to occur, and thus are unsuitable for nondividing cells like neurons or muscle cells.

Adenoviruses (AVs) are DNA viruses that do not incorporate into the host genome and generally remain within the host cell as episomes. This may limit the longevity of the expressed transgene. However, they do not require actively dividing cell lines, and high titers can be generated. Such vectors may be more suitable for targeting nondividing cells. This is especially true for the treatment of muscle cells, in particular myoblasts, because myoblasts have an abundance of β_3/β_5 integrin, which is the main component of the internalization receptor for AVs. This could contribute, among other things, to the relatively high susceptibility of myoblasts to AV infection and AV-mediated gene transduction.[6]

Adeno-associated viruses (AAVs) are nonpathogenic integrating DNA viruses from which all viral genes have been removed and helper virus cotransfection is virtually eliminated. These vectors tend to persist in infected cells for prolonged periods of time, with no significant untoward effect on the host. As with AV vectors, AAV vectors may also persist in an episomal state. Although AAV vectors may exhibit a relative preference for actively dividing cells, they do not require host cell proliferation. AAV is unique among eukaryotic DNA viruses in its ability to integrate at a specific site within the human chromosome (19q13.3-qter), and for this reason, and because it is nonpathogenic, it has become increasingly attractive as a vector for gene delivery.

Nonviral Vectors

Nonviral gene delivery techniques appear to be as safe as conventional pharmaceutical products. This results in a transient gene expression, a concept known as *gene therapeutics*. Various nonviral vectors are currently being assessed in a variety of experimental studies and clinical trials of gene therapy for a variety of disorders, including cystic fibrosis (CF), cancer, and peripheral vascular disease.[7] One such option is lipofection, in which DNA plasmids carrying the therapeutic genes are entrapped in lipid vesicles (liposomes). These liposomes act as vehicles that deliver the gene to the target cells, where they are only transiently expressed.[8] This approach is particularly promising in treatment of diseases that are manifested in the epithelial lining of various organs, making them accessible to surface delivery methods. The treatments are usually well tolerated, and no adverse respiratory, cardiac, immunologic, or other organ toxicity was detected.[9]

APPROPRIATE TIMING OF FETAL GENE THERAPY

If FGT is to prevent prenatal irreversible damage, early intervention is necessary. However, it is important to establish the optimal window of opportunity for therapy to be both beneficial and safe. Administration of FGT at various gestational ages results in different patterns of therapeutic gene expression in different tissues.[10] Early FGT may be advantageous owing to a lack of immune response and persistence of transgene expression. This suggests that fetal exposure to the foreign transgene protein and to the viral vector antigens may induce tolerance when introduced early in gestation.[11] The optimal window of opportunity for FGT in humans is still to be established.

SAFETY OF FETAL GENE THERAPY

The viral vector too may pose a theoretical danger to both mother and fetus. Studies in sheep have shown that the actual risk for accidental transfer of the viral vector into the maternal blood stream is low.[12] There is also some concern that once transfected, fetal blood-borne viral vectors may infect the placental tissue and thereby gain access to maternal circulation.[13] Further animal studies are required to fully address this issue.[4]

One of the most obvious risks to the fetus in FGT is that the viral vector itself may induce damage, either directly by its inherent pathogenic effects or secondary to an immune response mounted by the fetus causing tissue damage. Prenatal exposure to adenoviral vector in fetal sheep was associated with a high degree of pathology and mortality. Particularly, inflammatory and fibrotic responses were observed in the lungs.[14] However, in early gestation, adenoviral delivery to sheep did not seem to elicit an immune response.[15] With FGT, there is also the risk of insertional mutagenesis associated with random insertion of the therapeutic gene possibly interrupting key genetic loci that may lead to developmental disruption and even tumorigenesis. Finally, there is the theoretical risk of germ line alteration. This has not been the case in several animal studies in mice and sheep,[12, 16] but this issue needs further investigation to establish the overall incidence of germ line transmission and whether the degree of risk may be acceptable.[4]

CLINICAL TRIALS IN GENE THERAPY

Cystic Fibrosis

CF is an autosomal recessive disease caused by a mutation of the cystic fibrosis transmembrane conductance regulator (CFTCR) gene. The disease is characterized mainly by accumulation of mucus in the lung, predisposing to inflammation. Other affected organs include those in the gastrointestinal tract and the reproductive system. The first human trial of gene therapy for CF was initiated in 1993 and included four patients with CF who received the adenoviral vector (Ad-CFTCR) by instillation to their nasal or bronchial epithelium. Both the CFTCR protein and mRNA, undetectable before treatment, were observed in about 14% of one patient's epithelium cells, and mRNA alone in another patient for 1 week. However, after 10 days, no expression was found.[17] Liposome-mediated treatment has also been attempted in CF patients. The restoration rate of CFTCR activity was only 20%, peaking 3 days post-treatment, and reverting to pretreatment levels after a week.[18] Present gene delivery methods do not appear to induce permanent CFTCR gene expression. For gene therapy to be effective in CF, repeated administrations need to be performed. This would obviously limit the use of adenoviral vectors because of their potential to induce an immune response. To overcome this problem, it may be advantageous to perform FGT. To assess whether the FGT could attain a high level of organ-specific gene transfer to the fetal lung late in gestation without the immunogenic response, a recombinant adenoviral-mediated transfer of the β-galactosidase marker gene to the lung of late gestation fetal sheep was performed using a fetoscopic technique.[19] The study demonstrated that transgene expression was greatest in the distal pulmonary parenchyma, particularly in type II pneumocytes, and extended out to the pleura. There was no evidence of acute toxicity or immune response. This suggests that FGT for CF may be feasible. Further modifications in the therapeutic gene design, such as the development of transgenes with tissue specificity, may improve efficiency. In the case of CF, tissue-specific expression cassettes have been developed for airway epithelia and may prove useful in FGT.[20]

Gaucher's Disease

Gaucher's disease, a common inherited metabolic disorder, is an excellent candidate for targeted gene therapy using hematopoietic stem cells. The feasibility of introducing the human glucocerebrosidase gene into hematopoietic progenitors with long-term expression using a variety of retroviral vectors has been demonstrated in several animal models.[21] Subsequently, it was shown that glucocerebrosidase enzyme expression can be detected in peripheral blood lymphocytes more than 12 months after transplantation, with a transduction efficiency of up to 95% in hematopoietic stem cells (CD34+).[22] This provides encouraging data for the future use of gene therapy for this disease. However, the fact that therapy with the genetically engineered enzyme is adequate, and that little, if any, irreversible damage occurs prenatally in most cases, FGT may be reserved in the future for the most severe form, the acute neuronopathic type II Gaucher.

Maple Syrup Urine Disease

Maple syrup urine disease (MSUD) is an autosomal recessive disease caused by a deficiency of branched-chain keto acid dehydrogenase, a mitochondrial multienzyme complex responsible for the decarboxylation of leucine, isoleucine, and valine. The complex consists of three subunits (E1, E2, and E3) and mutations in any subunit result in MSUD. No satisfactory treatment for MSUD is currently available.[23] To assess the feasibility of gene therapy for this disease, a retroviral vector containing the human E2 cDNA was used to restore leucine decarboxylation activity in fibroblasts derived from an MSUD patient with a mutation in the E2 subunit. Decarboxylation activity in transduced cells was restored to 93% of the wild-type level. Correct targeting of the expressed wild-type E2 protein to mitochondria was demonstrated by comparing the immunofluorescent pattern of E2 and a mitochondrial marker protein. Stable expression of enzyme activity has been achieved for at least 7 weeks. These results demonstrate the capacity for phenotypic correction of a gene defect whose product is a part of a multienzyme complex.[23] Given the severity of some forms of MSUD, it may be a candidate for FGT.

Adenosine Deaminase Deficiency

Historically, the adenosine deaminase (ADA) gene was the first to be used in a postnatal gene therapy clinical trial aimed at achieving actual medical cure.[24] ADA deficiency is a severe and fatal immunodeficiency syndrome with profound T lymphocytopenia. Affected individuals have variable defects of both T and B lymphocyte function and greatly increased morbidity and mortality caused by frequent viral and bacterial infection, leading to death in early childhood. In 1990, a clinical trial was initiated using retroviral-mediated transfer of the ADA gene into the T cells of two ADA-deficient children.[24] After treatment, both children were reported to have ADA-positive circulating lymphocytes. Gene treatment ended after 2 years, but integrated vector and ADA gene expression in T cells persisted.[25, 26] Several other teams have tried similar approaches for treating ADA deficiency by gene therapy, with varying success.[27–29] Whereas FGT for this disorder would probably be successful, there is no indication that prenatal FGT would be superior to postnatal gene therapy.

The Thalassemias

Mutations at the α-globin locus are a common class of mutations in humans resulting in the various forms of α-thalassemia. Deletion of all four adult α-globin genes results in the perinatal lethal condition manifested by hydrops fetalis. It has been demonstrated that introduction of a human α-globin transgene can ameliorate the severity of the disorder in a mouse thalassemia model, providing hope for gene therapy of this disorder. To be relevant to the human disease, however, effective therapy requires FGT to avoid the severe prenatal complications.

The main pathophysiologic feature of β-thalassemia is the accumulation of unpaired α-globin chains in erythrocytes that alter membrane stability and result in early cell destruction. One option for correction of this imbalance is through the induction of fetal hemoglobin (HbF) synthesis. It has been shown that in vitro, erythropoietin increases erythroid precursors cells programmed to produce HbF in humans and to β-minor globin in mice. By introducing AAV-mediated erythropoietin gene transfer into mouse muscle, it was possible to attain robust and sustained secretion of erythropoietin in β-thalassemic mice. This resulted in a stable correction of anemia associated with improved red blood cell morphology, increased β-minor globin synthesis, and decreased amounts of α-globin chains bound to erythrocyte membranes. If this were shown to be effective in humans, then correction of the prenatal defect by FGT may bring the fetus to viability without the prenatal sequelae.[30] Another option for treatment of β-thalassemia is by increasing γ-globin gene expression, reverting to an early fetal condition where HbF predominates. The possibility of activating the γ-globin gene expression by triplex-forming oligonucleotide–directed targeted mutagenesis was recently evaluated.[31] Using a psoralen-conjugated triplex-forming oligonucleotide designed to bind to a site overlapping with an Oct-1 binding site at the -280 region of the γ-globin gene, targeted mutagenesis of the Oct-1 binding site has been achieved by transfecting the in vitro–formed plasmid-oligo complex into human normal fibroblast cells. These results suggest that targeted mutagenesis at the Oct-1 binding site can lead to a condition similar to hereditary persistence of fetal hemoglobin. This may provide a novel approach for gene therapy of β-thalassemia and sickle cell disease by FGT.[31]

Coagulation Disorders

These disorders are also potential candidates for gene therapy and FGT. Hemophilia B, a model of such coagulation disorders, is characterized by an X-linked deficiency of factor IX. It has previously been suggested that keratinocytes in the skin might provide a suitable target cell for delivery of factor IX to the systemic circulation in patients with hemophilia B. Experiments in transgenic mice demonstrated that human factor IX can be efficiently synthesized in the skin by keratinocytes and secreted across the epidermal basement membrane to reach the systemic circulation, where significant levels can be attained.[32] To evaluate the applicability of such an approach to FGT, an E1/E3-deleted adenoviral vector carrying the human coagulation factor IX gene was administered into the amniotic cavities of mid- to late-gestation mouse fetuses. The transgenic protein was found to be produced in the fetal skin, mucosae, and amniotic membranes and was shown to be present for several days after birth of healthy pups. This approach for FGT of hemophilia B may prevent hemorrhagic complications during delivery, such as intracranial bleeding.[33]

Neurologic Disorders

Treatment of central nervous system disease poses a significant challenge owing to complex functions of the nervous system and the permanent damage caused in utero in numerous genetic disorders. One of the modes of therapy that is being investigated is the potential use of central nervous system–derived neural progenitor cells. These cells would theoretically be good candidates for multiple cell-based therapies for neural diseases. Further identification of the molecules that direct the differentiation of adult neural progenitors may allow their activation in vivo to induce self-repair.[34] Experiments have shown that clones of neural stem cells isolated from human fetal telencephalon have a self-renewing capacity and give rise to all fundamental neural lineages in vitro. After these clones were transplanted into germinal zones of the newborn mouse brain, they were found to participate in all aspects of normal development, including normal migration patterns, and dissemination into various regions of the central nervous system, where they differentiated into developmentally and regionally appropriate cell types. Indeed, these cells were shown to correct genetic metabolic defects in

neurons and glia cells in vitro. It may be envisioned that such cells genetically engineered to express therapeutic genes may facilitate FGT for neurodegenerative disorders.[35]

FETAL GENE THERAPY: ETHICAL CONSIDERATIONS

Currently, FGT is still considered experimental, and ethical issues need to be established before this technique becomes clinically available. Before FGT may be considered for human clinical trials, thorough evaluation of safety and efficacy should be performed in appropriate animal models. Concern has been expressed about the possibility that FGT may lead to the uptake and expression of genetic material in cells other than those intended as the targets of gene therapy. The greatest concern is the possibility that genetic material may be incorporated into the germ line of subjects, leading to permanent changes that will be passed on to future generations.[36] The possibility of germ line transmission of the transgene may, in theory, occur inadvertently or as a deliberate action in a process termed *germ line gene therapy* (GLGT). There is a great deal of controversy concerning both the technical feasibility and the ethical acceptability of human germ line modification for the prevention of serious disease. It is argued by some that this technique constitutes a slippery slope toward the Orwellian concept of "human genetic engineering," and that GLGT has a potential for misuse in trait enhancement and "neo-eugenics."[37] Some proponents of FGT claim that its use in the form of GLGT for the purpose of trait enhancement is certainly deplorable, yet they maintain that potential future misuse should not be allowed to prevent the legitimate development of a technology that can save lives and relieve suffering. Furthermore, they suggest that the theoretical specter of germ line transfer should not deter attempts at FGT, because most proposed protocols involve second trimester fetuses, by which time all organ systems have formed. Moreover, all published data to date indicate that GLGT is highly unlikely, or may not even be possible, using present techniques.[38] A practical view is that the most likely candidates for FGT will probably not live to reproductive age, and even if they do, inadvertent germ-line transmission would likely produce an individual incapable of reproducing.[36] Others do not even eschew GLGT and view it as another form of FGT, merely taken a step further.[39] Some suggest that there is merit in continuing the discussion about human germ line intervention, so that this technique can be carefully compared with alternative strategies for preventing genetic disease.[40]

Opponents of FGT maintain that there are very few examples in which existing alternatives, such as gamete donation and preimplantation genetic diagnosis, would not allow families affected by genetic disease to have genetically related children.[41] It has been claimed that the whole issue of FGT is becoming a hypothetical one since the advent of preimplantation genetic diagnosis.[42] Given the current state of postnatal gene therapy, some would claim that it is premature to embark on a project that is more complicated and poses a risk to both the fetus and the mother. There is currently a prohibition on human GLGT, established by law in many countries. The UK Gene Therapy Advisory Committee prohibited direct injection of viral vectors into fetuses for the purpose of FGT on safety and ethical grounds. The U.S. National Institutes of Health Recombinant DNA Advisory Committee is setting up working groups to discuss various aspects of FGT and review proposed clinical trials.[43] As recently stated by Caplan and Wilson, "The real moral challenge facing fetal gene therapy is to find ways to insure that the review of protocols is adequate; that those undertaking trials are competent to do so; that adequate financing exists to permit fair access to clinical trials; and that careful procedures are worked out for insuring informed consent, equity in subject selection and adequate oversight and review for the earliest clinical studies, in which the prospect of direct benefit to the fetus is tiny or non-existent. In our view, that is where the efforts of researchers, policy makers, regulators and ethicists ought to be directed."[36]

References

1. Senut MC, Gage FH: Prenatal gene therapy: Can the technical hurdles be overcome? Mol Med Today 1999;5:152–156.
2. Douar AM, Themis M, Coutelle C: Fetal somatic gene therapy. Mol Hum Reprod 1996;2:633–641.
3. Moulton G: Panel finds in utero gene therapy proposal is premature. J Natl Cancer Inst 1999;91:407–408.
4. Zanjani ED, Anderson WF: Prospects for in utero human gene therapy. Science 1999;285:2084–2088.
5. Yang EY, Flake AW, Adzick NS: Prospects for fetal gene therapy. Semin Perinatol 1999;23:524–534.
6. Acsadi G, Jani A, Huard J, et al: Cultured human myoblasts and myotubes show markedly different transducibility by replication-defective adenovirus recombinants. Gene Ther 1994;1:338–340.
7. Ledley FD: Non-viral gene therapy. Curr Opin Biotechnol 1994;5:626–636.
8. Alton EW, Middleton PG, Caplen NJ, et al: Non-invasive liposome-mediated gene delivery can correct the ion transport defect in cystic fibrosis mutant mice. Nat Genet 1993;5:135–142.
9. Nabel EG, Yang Z, Muller D, et al: Safety and toxicity of catheter gene delivery to the pulmonary vasculature in a patient with metastatic melanoma. Hum Gene Ther 1994;5:1089–1094.
10. Schachtner S, Buck C, Bergelson J, Baldwin H: Temporally regulated expression patterns following in utero adenovirus-mediated gene transfer. Gene Ther 1999;6:1249–1257.
11. Yang EY, Kim HB, Shaaban AF, et al: Persistent postnatal transgene expression in both muscle and liver after fetal injection of recombinant adenovirus. J Pediatr Surg 1999;34:766–772.
12. Porada CD, Tran N, Eglitis M, et al: In utero gene therapy: Transfer and long-term expression of the bacterial neo(r) gene in sheep after direct infection of retroviral vectors into preimmune fetuses. Hum Gene Ther 1998;9:1571–1585.
13. Tsukamoto M, Ochiya T, Yoshida S, et al: Gene transfer and expression in progeny after intravenous DNA injection into pregnant mice. Nat Genet 1995;9:243–248.
14. Iwamoto HS, Trapnell BC, McConnell CJ, et al: Pulmonary inflammation associated with repeated, prenatal exposure to an E1, E3-deleted adenoviral vector in sheep. Gene Ther 1999;6:98–106.
15. Yang EY, Cass DL, Sylvester KG, et al: Fetal gene therapy: Efficacy, toxicity, and immunologic effects of early gestation recombinant adenovirus. J Pediatr Surg 1999;34:235–241.
16. Ye X, Gao GP, Pabin C, et al: Evaluating the potential of germ line transmission after intravenous administration of recombinant adenovirus in the C3H mouse. Hum Gene Ther 1998;9:2135–2142.
17. Crystal R, McElvaney M. Rosenfeld M, et al: Administration of an adenovirus containing the human CFTR cDNA to the respiratory tract of individuals with cystic fibrosis. Nat Genet 1994;8:42–50.
18. Caplen NJ, Alton EW, Middleton PG, et al: Liposome-mediated CFTR gene transfer to the nasal epithelium of patients with cystic fibrosis. Nat Med 1995;1:39–46.
19. Sylvester KG, Yang EY, Cass DL, et al: Fetoscopic gene therapy for congenital lung disease. J Pediatr Surg 1997;32:964–969.
20. Chow YH, O'Brodovich H, Plumb J, et al: Development of an epithelium-specific expression cassette with human DNA regulatory elements for transgene expression in lung airways. Proc Natl Acad Sci U S A 1997;94:14695–14700.
21. Wei JF, Wei FS, Samulski RJ, Barranger JA: Expression of the human glucocerebrosidase and arylsulfatase A genes in murine and patient primary fibroblasts transduced by an adeno-associated virus vector. Gene Ther 1994;1:261–268.
22. Nimgaonkar M, Bahnson A, Kemp A, et al: Long-term expression of the glucocerebrosidase gene in mouse and human hematopoietic progenitors. Leukemia 1995;9(Suppl 1):S38–S42.
23. Mueller GM, McKenzie LR, Homanics GE, et al: Complementation of defective leucine decarboxylation in fibroblasts from a maple syrup urine disease patient by retrovirus-mediated gene transfer. Gene Ther 1995;2:461–468.
24. Culver K, Anderson F, Blaese R: Lymphocyte gene therapy. Hum Gene Ther 1991;2:107–109.
25. Blaese RM, Culver KW, Miller AD, et al: T lymphocyte–directed gene therapy for ADA-SCID: Initial trial results after 4 years. Science 1995;270:475–480.
26. Kohn D, Weinberg KI, Parkman P, et al: Gene therapy for neonates with ADA-deficient SCID by retroviral-mediated transfer of the human ADA cDNA into umbilical cord CD34+ cells [abstract 1245]. Blood 1993;82(Suppl 1):315a.
27. Bordignon C, Notarangelo LD, Nobili N, et al: Gene therapy in peripheral blood lymphocytes and bone marrow for ADA-immunodeficient patients. Science 1995;270:470–475.
28. Kohn DB, Weinberg KI, Nolta JA, et al: Engraftment of gene-modified umbilical cord blood cells in neonates with adenosine deaminase deficiency. Nat Med 1995;1:1017–1023.
29. Parkman R, Weinberg K, Crooks G, et al: Gene therapy for adenosine deaminase deficiency. Annu Rev Med 2000;51:33–47.
30. Bohl D, Bosch A, Cardona A, et al: Improvement of erythropoiesis in beta-thalassemic mice by continuous erythropoietin delivery from muscle. Blood 2000;95:2793–2798.
31. Xu XS, Glazer PM, Wang G: Activation of human gamma-globin gene expression via triplex-forming oligonucleotide (TFO)–directed mutations in the gamma-globin gene 5' flanking region. Gene 2000;242:219–228.
32. Alexander MY, Bidichandani SI, Cousins FM, et al: Circulating human factor IX produced in keratin-promoter transgenic mice: A feasibility study for gene therapy of haemophilia B. Hum Molec Genet 1995;4:993–999.
33. Schneider H, Adebakin S, Themis M, et al: Therapeutic plasma concentrations of human factor IX in mice after gene delivery into the amniotic cavity: A model for the prenatal treatment of haemophilia B. J Gene Med 1999;1:424–432.
34. Shihabuddin LS, Palmer TD, Gage FH: The search for neural progenitor cells: Prospects for the therapy of neurodegenerative disease. Mol Med Today 1999;5:474–480.
35. Flax JD, Aurora S, Yang C, et al: Engraftable human neural stem cells respond to developmental cues, replace neurons, and express foreign genes. Nat Biotechnol 1998;16:1033–1039.
36. Caplan AL, Wilson JM: The ethical challenges of in utero gene therapy. Nat Genet 2000;24:107.
37. Penticuff J: Ethical issues in genetic therapy. J Obstet Gynecol Neonatal Nurs 1994;23:498–501.
38. Anderson WF: Risks inherent in fetal gene therapy. Nature 1999;397:383.
39. Resnik D: Debunking the slippery slope argument against human germ-line gene therapy. J Med Philos 1994;19:23–40.
40. Wivel NA, Walters L: Germ-line gene modification and disease prevention: Some medical and ethical perspectives. Science 1993;262:533–538.
41. King D, Shakespeare T, Nicholson R, et al: Risks inherent in fetal gene therapy. Nature 1999;397:383.
42. Pergament E, Bonnicksen A: Preimplantation genetics: A case for prospective action. Am J Med Genet 1994;52:151–157.
43. Wadman M: NIH launches discussion of in utero gene therapy. Nature 1998;395:420.

FIFTY-THREE

Multifetal Pregnancy Reduction

Mark I. Evans

The use of modern fertility techniques has enabled thousands of women, previously infertile, to have their own biologic children. Sadly, as a byproduct of this remarkable success in treatment, has come a virtual epidemic of multifetal pregnancies. The rate of twin pregnancies, commonly quoted literally for generations as 1 in 90, has now doubled to more than 1 in 45. Even since the early 1990s, twin pregnancies have risen 20%, and triplets or higher orders well over 100% (Table 53–1). The ratio of observed to expected multifetal pregnancies shows that twins are approximately twice the number expected, but that quintuplets are now more than a thousandfold over expected numbers without infertility therapies (Table 53–2).

Public fascination with multifetal pregnancies extends back to the 1930s, when the Dionne quintuplets were born in Ontario, Canada. The same fascination has existed in all the years since, but whereas in the 1980s, quintuplets would make the national news, the bar keeps getting set higher and higher for lay press interest (Fig. 53–1). In the early 1990s, sextuplets, such as the Dillys in Indiana, drew several rounds of national attention, and help from diaper companies, formula companies, crib companies, and neighbors in their small town.

The ultimate example was that of the McCaughey septuplets in Iowa, where virtually the entire town of Carlisle was marshaled to help the family deal with the rigors of so many children at once. The family was given a van by a local automotive dealer, and the state of Iowa contributed a house. Miraculously, that pregnancy lasted until about 31 weeks, and the national media reported that all was coming along well. Closer inspection, however, revealed that the presenting fetus was a transverse lie, who fundamentally blocked the cervix from opening, rather than acting as the usual wedge to cause dilatation. Unpublished assessments of the children at age 2 years reveal that two of them have cerebral palsy, a fact glossed over and ignored by the media. The Houston octuplets born a year later received much less attention. Whether this lack of attention was due to saturation of the concept of multifetal pregnancies, or to the African origin of the couple, is open for speculation. One of these fetuses died very shortly after birth, and the other seven are said to be doing reasonably well.

MULTIFETAL PREGNANCY REDUCTION

Multifetal pregnancy reduction (MFPR) is a clinical procedure that dates back to the mid-1980s when a small number of centers in both Europe and the United States began to try to ameliorate the usual tremendously adverse sequelae of multifetal pregnancies by selective reduction or reducing the number of fetuses to a more manageable number. The first European reports by Dumez and associates[1] and the first American reports by Evans and colleagues,[2] followed by a report by Berkowitz and coworkers,[3] laid out for physicians a possible dramatic approach to improve the outcome in such cases while recognizing the ethical conundrum faced by couples and physicians under such difficult circumstances. In the mid 1980s, despite poor ultrasound visualization, needles were inserted transabdominally and maneuvered into the thorax of the fetus, with either mechanical destruction or air embolization, or potassium chloride (KCl) injections. Transcervical aspirations were also tried, without much success. The most commonly used method is KCl injection. The needle is inserted into the appropriate sac and maneuvered into the fetal thorax. KCl is injected, creating a pleural effusion and cessation of cardiac activity (Fig. 53–2).

Several of the centers with the world's largest experi-

Table 53–1. Multiple Births in the United States

Year	Twins	Triplets	Quadruplets	Quintuplets and Higher Multiples
1998	110,670	6919	627	79
1997	104,137	6148	510	79
1996	100,750	5298	560	81
1995	96,736	4551	365	57
1994	97,064	4233	315	46
1993	96,445	3834	277	57
1992	95,372	3547	310	26
1991	94,779	3121	203	22
1990	93,865	2830	185	13
1989	90,118	2529	229	40
Increase from 1989–1998 (%)	**22.8**	**173.6**	**173.8**	**97.5**

Data from National Vital Statistics Report 48(3):17. U.S. Government Printing Office, 2000.

Table 53–2. Multiple Births in the United States

Births	Observed	Expected	Ratio
Twins	110,670	43,795	2.5:1
Triplets	6919	487	14.2:1
Quadruplets	627	5	125.4:1
Quintuplets and higher multiples	79	0.06	1316.7:1

Note: Total births in 1998: 3,941,553.

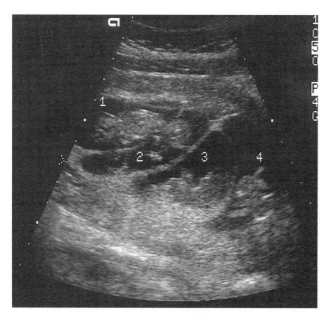

Figure 53–1. Quadruplet gestation.

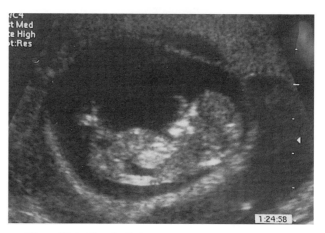

Figure 53–2. Pleural effusion after potassium chloride injection.

ence began collaborating to leverage the power of their data. The first collaborative report was published in 1993. It showed a 16% pregnancy loss rate up through 24 completed weeks, which was a big improvement compared with expectations of higher-order multiple pregnancies, particularly of quadruplets and above. Further collaborative efforts were published in 1994,[4] 1996,[5] and 2001,[6] which have revealed continued dramatic improvements in the overall outcomes of such pregnancies (Table 53–3). The most recently published collaborative data are summarized in Figure 53–3. These data show that triplets reduced to twins and quadruplets reduced to twins now perform essentially as though the fetuses started as twins. The 95% take-home baby rate for triplets and the 92% take-home baby rate for quadruplets are clearly dramatic improvements over natural statistics, even with tremendous advances in neonatal care. Not only has the pregnancy loss rate been substantially reduced, but also has the rate of very early prematurity. Both the loss and the prematurity rates continue to be a function of the starting number, showing that there is still price to be paid for overaggressive fertility therapies (Fig. 53–3). Further analysis of the data suggests that the improvements in MFPR outcomes

are a function of extensive operator experience, combined with improved ultrasound.

Historically, most observers, except those completely opposed to intervention on religious grounds, accepted MFPR with quadruplets or more and saw no need for reducing twins. The debate was over triplets. Although there are conflicting data in the literature, our experiences suggest that triplets reduced to twins do much better in terms of loss and prematurity than do unreduced triplets. Several previous papers have argued whether triplets have better outcomes "reduced" or not. In a recent paper, Yaron and associates[7] looked at triplets reduced to twins at Wayne State University, and compared these data with unreduced triplets at Wayne State and two large cohorts of twins. The data show substantial improvement of reduced twins, compared with triplets. The data from our series suggest that outcomes for pregnancies starting at triplets or even quadruplets reduced to twins do fundamentally as well as starting as twins. The data therefore support some cautious aggressiveness in infertility treatments to achieve pregnancy in tough situations. However, when higher numbers occur, good outcomes clearly diminish. We believe that if a patient's primary goal is to maximize outcome, reduction of triplets is the best course.

The demographics of patients seeking MFPR have also changed since the early 1990s. Particularly with the availability of donor eggs, the number of "older women" seeking MFPR has increased dramatically. In several programs,

Table 53–3. Multifetal Pregnancy Reduction—Losses by Years

		Losses		Deliveries			
	Total	(N) <24 Wk (%)	>24 Wk (%)	25–28 Wk (%)	29–32 Wk (%)	33–36 Wk (%)	≥37 Wk (%)
1986–1990	508	13.2	4.5	10.0	21.1	15.7	35.4
1991–1994	724	9.4	0.3	2.8	5.4	21.1	61.0
1995–1998	1356	6.4	0.2	4.3	10.2	31.5	47.4

From Evans MI, Berkowitz R, Wapner R, et al: Multifetal pregnancy reduction: Improved outcomes with increased experience. Am J Obstet Gynecol 2001;184:97–103.

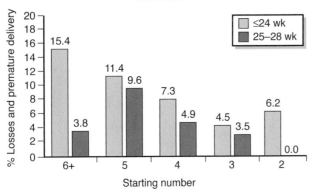

Figure 53–3. Increasing risks of pregnancy loss and extreme prematurity are a function of increasing starting number.

over 10% of all patients seeking MFPR are older than 40 years of age and using donor eggs. As a consequence of the shift to older patients, many of whom already had previous relationships and children, there is an increased desire by these patients to have only one further child. The number of experienced centers willing to do two to one reductions is still limited, but I believe it can be justified in the appropriate circumstances. Likewise, for patients who are older using their own eggs, the issue of genetic diagnosis comes into play.

There are two schools of thought about the best approach to genetic diagnosis: should it be before or after the performance of MFPR? In Detroit until the late 90's, we generally preferred to do the reduction down to twins or triplets first, at approximately 10.5 weeks, followed by chorionic villus sampling (CVS) approximately 1 week later. Published data describing performing CVS first, followed by reduction, suggested an error rate of between 1% and 2% as to which fetus was which, particularly if the entire karyotype is obtained before going on to reduction. However, in patients reducing to a singleton pregnancy, therefore putting "all their eggs in one basket," we believed the best approach is to know what is in the basket before reducing the other embryos. In these cases, we perform a CVS usually on all fetuses and do a fluorescent in situ hybridization (FISH)

analysis with probes for chromosomes 13, 18, 21, X, and Y. It is true that about 30% of anomalies seen on karyotype would not be detectable by FISH with these probes, but the absolute risk, given a normal FISH and a normal ultrasound, is about 1 in 500. We believe that the risk is lower than the increased risk from the 2-week wait necessary to get the full karyotype. Likewise, with more patients in their late 30s and 40s having their own eggs and wanting twins, it has become more common for us to do CVS first with FISH, and reduction the next day even when leaving two or three fetuses.

MFPR continues to be controversial. Feelings about MFPR do not, in our experience, follow the classic "pro-choice/pro-life" dichotomy. Nevertheless, we believe that the real debate over the next several years will not be whether or not MFPR should be performed with triplets or more. The fact is that MFPR clearly does improve outcomes. The debate will be whether or not it would be appropriate to offer MFPR routinely for twins, for whom the outcome is generally considered "good enough." Our data suggest that reduction of twins to a singleton actually improves the outcome of the remaining fetus. No consensus on this point is likely to emerge.

References

1. Dumez Y, Oury JF: Method for first trimester selective abortion in multiple pregnancy. Contrib Gynecol Obstet 1986;15:50–53.
2. Evans MI, Fletcher JC, Zador IE, et al: Selective first-trimester termination in octuplet and quadruplet pregnancies: Clinical and ethical issues. Obstet Gynecol 1988;71:289–296.
3. Berkowitz RL, Lynch L, Chitkara U, et al: Selective reduction of multifetal pregnancies in the first trimester. N Engl J Med 1988;318:1043–1047.
4. Evans MI, Dommergues M, Timor-Tritsch I, et al: Transabdominal versus transcervical and transvaginal multifetal pregnancy reduction: international collaborative experience of more than one thousand cases. Am J Obstet Gynecol 1994 Mar;17:902–909.
5. Evans MI, Dommergues M, Wapner RJ, et al: International collaborative experience of 1789 patients having multifetal pregnancy reduction: A plateauing of risks and outcomes. J Soc Gynecol Invest 1996;3:23–26.
6. Evans MI, Berkowitz R, Wapner R, et al: Multifetal pregnancy reduction: Improved outcomes with increased experience. Am J Obstet Gynecol 2001;184:97–103.
7. Yaron Y, Bryant-Greenwood PK, Dave N, et al: Multifetal pregnancy reductions of triplets to twins: comparison with nonreduced triplets and twins. Am J Obstet Gynecol 1999 May;180:1268–1271.

Emerging Psychosocial Issues in Prenatal Diagnosis

David W. Britt

Several large-scale trends are shaping prenatal diagnosis sessions and decisions throughout the world. In the developed world, there is a shift of focus away from short-term technocentric medical advances to focus on the effectiveness of prenatal care interventions on longer-term benefits for women and children's health. This is an encouraging reaction to technologic change because it is based on the fact that there are no purely technologic fixes to the quality of prenatal care with which prenatal diagnosis is associated.

There are other trends, however, about which we should be less sanguine. In the developed world, there is a progressive concentration of wealth and income among a small minority of (usually white, in the United States) individuals. This inequality-of-wealth trend is coupled with trends that have led some to estimate that, by the midpoint of the 21st century, whites will be a minority in the United States and that there will be greater segregation among whites and minorities than there is at present. Because of rapid technologic change in the United States, such shifts in wealth *may* be somewhat more rapid than in other countries, but inequality of wealth (and these related trends) is hardly a phenomenon that is limited to the United States. In short, in the United States at least, wealth appears to be becoming more and more concentrated in the hands of a small number of whites, while the country is becoming more multicultural and at risk of becoming more segregated.

Against that historical backdrop, consider that we also live in a period of astonishing growth in genetic knowledge that has powerful implications for the future of prenatal diagnosis and many other aspects of health care. Addressing questions such as who should have access to such knowledge for individuals and for what purpose and the trade-offs between fostering universal health care versus underwriting high-tech breakthroughs are continuing concerns. Such questions become more pressing to ask, but more difficult to answer, as access to resources becomes more concentrated by class. When only the wealthy or well-insured can gain access to effective prenatal diagnosis, the bias may work in both blatant and more subtle ways.

As with the birth-control movement during the 20th century, what starts out as a right for the privileged may become a duty to the poor. Because we can detect and prevent disabilities, it may become obligatory to do so. There is a difference between prevention and control over options. With regard to prenatal diagnosis, there is a difference between preventing illness and promoting informed consent with respect to options. One cannot understand the implications of the tensions between prevention and control without appreciating the power and cultural differences that exist between counselor/physician and patient in developed countries. Nor can one ignore the fact that such issues are writ large in developing countries—where, some have estimated, 95% of the world's future children will be born.

One may examine such issues on at least three levels: as community or nationwide issues of access, control, and equity; through the lens of the diagnostic counseling session; and through the context surrounding the individual woman and her family as they decide, serially, what tests to take, what counseling to seek, and what actions to take given "what is so antiseptically called a 'positive' diagnosis,"[1] but which may have a variety of meanings depending on context. In this chapter, rather than seeking to exhaustively review the many studies at these three levels, a context-sensitive perspective is presented for helping to integrate discussions across the three levels.

DESCRIBING CONTEXT

Contexts can be treated as cultural, situational, and personal-biographic factors that intersect in multiple ways, forming different configurations or combinations of contexts. At its core are elements of current and past pregnancies, the *proximate decision context*. The major sources of contextual variation that intersect with the proximate decision context are familial, cultural, technologic, and institutional. Others have discussed in some detail several of these contexts. Hence, I discuss only one of these at length: institutional context.

In seeking to understand the institutional context relevant in any given situation, one must move beyond an understanding of the role of organized groups such as health maintenance organizations (HMOs) and financial/insurance barriers that are so substantially a part of the environment within which patients and providers interact. One must move beyond the structure of laws and regulations that characterize a particular society at a given time, although these often permit a relatively subtle understanding of the possible kinds of interactions between providers and patients. It is necessary to understand in the particular environment under consideration—in which the term *envi-*

ronment serves as a shorthand way of referring to the combination of contexts within which such transactions occur and women are also making decisions—that medical professionals construct in active or passive collaboration with their patients. One aspect of this is getting a sense of how receptive the clinic is, and the general structure of the medical setting in terms of what are presented as routine tests—as opposed to more nonroutine tests requiring decisions. One should also understand the discipline and training of the medical professional (because genetic counselors tend to differ from physicians). Integral to such a discussion is the gender of these individuals in *combination with* where they are practicing. Women physicians, outside of the United States, for example, have been shown to be more pessimistic about disabilities and more willing to abort fetuses with genetic disorders than men. Three things should stand out from this example. First, many factors other than personality characteristics of individual patients are important in understanding the phenomena associated with prenatal diagnosis. Second, combinations of these factors are critical for understanding the nature of context as it affects action. Third, there is no substitute for careful, detailed, qualitative, and comparative analysis of such situations.

These contexts and their change over time may be studied on a single level or on multiple levels. So, for example, one might examine the impact of various factors on the level and/or rate of aggregate uptake in prenatal diagnostic services across countries. Some aspects of uptake are going to be a straightforward function of the extent of resource commitment at the national level. Part of the impact of resource commitment will be mediated by the level of professionalization of prenatal diagnostic services and the extent to which networks of physicians and counselors have been built. And part of the effect of national commitments will be mediated by how cost-effectively such funds are utilized. Such factors speak to a relatively rational process of implementation and development of prenatal diagnostic services. Cross-country or cross-cultural analyses, however, involve more complicated and abstract aspects of the development process. For example, cultures vary in the extent to which they can integrate scientific and nonscientific thinking. Although some work on such matters has been done, much dialogue needs to take place regarding the diffusion of prenatal diagnostic technologies and the conditions under which they may be successfully integrated into a society. All of this leaves us with the conclusion that we can say little more about collective uptake than that there will be much disagreement about what factors are important and how much progress has been made.

Successful implementation, however, is problematic in and of itself. If one were to examine the inequality of access within and across countries, or the extent of coerciveness of the system, the nature of the analysis would be quite different. For most practitioners, however, such analyses become more relevant as they embrace a level of

analysis that touches on how context shapes the ways in which individuals make a series of decisions regarding involvement in prenatal diagnostic services or how patients and counselors/physicians construct counseling sessions.

The joint consideration of the work of prediagnostic services may be reviewed on two levels of analysis: in terms of contradictions and tensions for the society as a whole and in terms of the counseling session. Two critical factors in the counseling interview are the level of trust in medical authorities and the level of education of the patients.

Trust in medical professionals is an especially complicated dimension. At the heart of the issues involved, however, is the question of how tensions regarding genetic reasoning are dealt with culturally. The existence of tension is an unavoidable consequence of advancing technical knowledge of genetics. There will be uneven development both within and across countries. Where development is more pronounced, however, there will be accompanying modes of dissemination, training, and credentializing as the medical professions whose knowledge base is being fundamentally altered by this new knowledge struggle to adapt to the sea change of information.

At the societal level, there may be considerable tension between those who want to explain health and disease, normality and abnormality, in terms of genetics and those who see such an approach as reductionist at best and controlling and hostile at worst. Lippman,[2] for example, uses the term *geneticization* to refer to a medical model couched in the language of genetics that gives priority to differences among individuals on the basis of their DNA codes. As the human genome project and its aftermath proceed, such a "scientific" position and its potential for eugenic implications may become more dominant in a society. The implications go much further than scientists and medical professionals talking to one another. One characteristic of dominant rhetorics is that they may become taken-for-granted, routine aspects of culture. This has immediate implications for prenatal diagnosis. Santalahti and his colleagues,[3] for example, ascribe the high participation rate in prenatal screening tests in Finland to the

great trust [my emphasis] *placed in Finnish maternity care, and from the general tendency to assume that whatever care is offered has been carefully considered and is the best available.*

Such trust is a double-edged sword. On the one hand, it leads to high participation in maternal care centers. On the other hand, offering serum screening as part of maternity care implies general approval for the screening process. Hence, it may decrease the chances of *active* decision making on the part of women living in such circumstances. These authors estimated that only a minority of the patients in their sample made an active decision on whether to participate in serum screening. The rest accepted it as a routine part of medical care.

At the same time, there may be strong cultural forces at

work that emphasize the gulf between "science-speaking genetics counselors and their multicultural patient populations."[1] Taken further, such a gulf might lead to what Fletcher (1998: 820)[4] has called *genicity:*

[a] public reaction to advances in human genetics, that is, fear, images of mad scientists and Nazi eugenics, and a sense that there were no longer any mystery about human beings . . . focused especially on reproduction and manipulation of genes for eugenic [my emphasis] *purposes.*

Genicity and geneticization are too complicated to be thought of as polar opposites on a single dimension. Not only are they inherently multidimensional, they also reflect a constantly changing tug of war for a dominant and legitimate position regarding genetic knowledge. Yet they do serve as convenient shorthand ways of referring to the different clusters of phenomena that should be considered as part of an assessment of trust. On one extreme, geneticization rules. Genetics is considered both legitimate and relevant for explaining disease. And the medical establishment is trusted to apply this knowledge in a carefully considered manner that puts the interests of the patient first. On the other extreme, genicity rules. Genetics is considered as a fundamental threat to humanity, and the medical establishment is not trusted to apply this knowledge for the common good.

The companion dimension that must be considered is the extent of education and general knowledge of the population of women who will be undergoing prenatal testing. The variations in both general levels of literacy and specific genetic knowledge are enormous both within and across nations and cultures. Literacy is also a proxy for how relatively powerful women are in their families, workplaces, and communities, so variation on this dimension is at least as multidimensional and complicated as is variation in trust levels. Hence, any discussion here risks oversimplification. Yet again, considering the extremes is a useful exercise. On one pole are situations in which the majority of women are educated and genetic knowledge (at least with respect to the role of genetics in their pregnancies) is relatively high. On the other pole are women with less education and with a less well developed understanding of the potential implications of genetics for their pregnancies.

Where patients are relatively well educated and informed, and where there is reasonable trust in medical authorities, the chances of a *shared collective definition* of the counseling interview are good. Genetics counselors and primary care/obstetric-gynecologic physicians will be well informed, but importantly, the gulf in knowledge between the counselor and the patient will be less pronounced than where women are less well educated and informed. Consequently, the negative consequences of such a gulf, reinforced by differences in social class and race, should be blunted. In turn, an informed discussion of information and options may be negotiated within a climate of trust and mutual respect.

The downside risk, however, lies in how fragile such *shared mutual definition* is. Its continuance rests on increasing professionalization of those medical professionals who interact with patients around medical issues not only in terms of their knowledge of genetics but also in terms of their capacities for developing rapport with their patients. As Frankel's work[5] on doctor-patient interactions has shown, as medical issues become more complicated and have more serious consequences for patients, much effort and training are required to ensure that medical personnel are able to listen, empathize, and develop rapport with their patients.

Where women are less well informed or less well educated, it is more realistic to think in terms of a *collective fiction* than a shared collective definition. Under such conditions, the legitimacy and power of the medical authorities in the situation allow them to simply impose (intentionally or unintentionally) their own definition of what is happening and what is important. Such dynamics are not peculiar to developed countries.

Consider how this becomes more complicated as cultural differences provide another element of the combinatorial context. Rapp,[1] for example, has spoken to how many elements come together as women make decisions regarding testing and other matters:

class, racial and ethnic markers, experiences with, and attitudes toward, a range of disabilities all strongly influence a woman's responses to the [amniocentesis] test. We need to insist simultaneously on the collective and individual nature of these orienting features each woman brings to her encounter [my emphasis] with prenatal testing. It matters whether one is African-American, Polish or Irish-Catholic, middle-class or working class or poor. But it also matters whether this is a first or fourth pregnancy, whether you have experienced difficulties in getting or staying pregnant, whether you had a cousin with Down syndrome or a neighbor who was hemophiliac.

Such analyses become even more complicated when features of the larger culture and *features each physician/counselor brings to the encounter* are considered. Consider the painful situation confronting physicians and patients in Argentina. After prenatal diagnosis, physicians are put in the position of telling their patients that abortion is illegal. Over 400,000 illegal abortions are performed each year, with a third of the high maternal mortality rate being attributable to the lack of safety of such procedures. Here, trust becomes a much more complicated achievement and burden, with institutional conflict between the Church and the medical establishment being played out in the counseling interview.

Training in listening skills and empathy can go only so far—even in those situations in which there exists a fundamental trust of medical authorities to act in the interest of their patients. More dramatic and longer-term solutions are required to shift what are essentially collective fictions to negotiated collective definitions. The basic concepts of access and support are not mysterious, but there needs to be innovative experimentation in different contexts to find ways of conveying the meaning of genetic information and supporting the legitimacy of choice. In some cases, this may mean using the knowledge that providers may shape how women understand and the meaning and purpose of screening to reinforce the legitimacy of choice.

Finally, there are those situations in which trust is not vested in the medical establishment, either because of a past history of untrustworthy actions (as with the Tuskeegee experiments), because of conflicts within the culture regarding scientific and nonscientific reasoning, or more locally because of past experiences of women, their friends, and families. Under such conditions, whether the patient is educated or not, the chances for hostility and distrust are high.

Short-term fixes cannot be effective in such situations. A general strategy that might be effective in some contexts is working through community institutions in which a) there is a lot of contact and b) experience with these high-contact institutions has been benign. Under such conditions, medical clinics might be able to "borrow the credibility" of their more trusted counterparts.

In summary, the interactions women have with medical personnel around prenatal diagnostic issues and their subsequent decisions are powerfully affected by contextual forces. As women become more educated, as the medical establishment becomes more professionalized and trusted, as genetics information becomes more incorporated into cultures, and as medical personnel become more sensitive to and competent regarding psychosocial issues, these sessions will be characterized by a collective definition of what is happening. On the other hand, in those situations in which women are less educated, the medical establishment is underdeveloped and not considered trustworthy, genetics information is treated with suspicion, and medical personnel are not well trained in the psychosocial aspects of medical encounters, there will be at best a collective fiction in these sessions and, at worst, outright hostility.

Suggestions for Future Reading

Novaes HMD: Social impacts of technological diffusion: Prenatal diagnosis and induced abortion in Brazil. Soc Sci Med 2000;50:41–51.

Press NA, Browner CH: Characteristics of women who refuse an offer of prenatal diagnosis. Am J Med Genet 1998;78:433–455.

Punales-Morejon D: Genetic counseling and prenatal diagnosis: A multicultural perspective. J Am Med Womens Assoc 1997;52:30–32.

References

1. Rapp R: Communicating about chromosomes: Patients, providers and cultural assumptions. J Am Med Womens Assoc 1997;52:28–29, 32.
2. Lippman A: Prenatal genetic testing and geneticization. Prenatal Diagn Ther 1993;8(suppl):175–188.
3. Santalahti P, Hemmminki E, Aro AR, et al: Participation in prenatal screening tests and intentions concerning selective termination in Finnish medical care. Fetal Diagn Ther 1999;14:71–79.
4. Fletcher J: The long view: How genetic discoveries will aid health care. J Women's Health 1998;7:817–823.
5. Frankel R: Communicating with patients: Research shows it makes a difference. Deerfield, IL, MMI Risk Management Resources, 1994.
6. Barry K, Britt DW: Outreach: Targeting high-risk women and understanding their relationships with formal institutions. Women's Health Issues (in press).

Multifetal Pregnancy Reduction: Psychosocial and Family Issues

Virginia L. Miller and Mark I. Evans

Multifetal pregnancy reduction (MFPR) has been performed since the mid 1980s as a means of improving perinatal outcome for families with higher-order multiple pregnancies. Perinatal outcomes data have been reported on large numbers of patients by the international collaborative experience.[1, 2] MFPR has been shown to be an effective method of improving perinatal outcomes in multifetal pregnancies.

The medical aspects of MFPR have been the subject of several investigations. In contrast, however, relatively little is known about the psychosocial issues associated with MFPR and its effect on the family. As more and more families seek infertility treatment, research is needed to provide the very best counseling information for families considering MFPR.

As highlighted by Souter and Goodwin,[3] the data needed to counsel families about MFPR are often incomplete. Bergh and colleagues[4] noted that the psychological reactions of parents after MFPR as well as the longer-term well-being of the children and the family has rarely been studied. Studies of this nature are immensely important, given the circumstances by which families arrive at the MFPR procedure. First, most of the women involved with MFPR have a long history with infertility. The paradox of deciding about MFPR after the stress of infertility treatment may create a psychologically high-risk situation. The decision to terminate fetuses might be very difficult and painful to reach. Second, little is known about the long-term psychosocial implications of the MFPR for the parents and the family. Third, the decision to undergo MFPR is a voluntary decision and, unlike a miscarriage or a genetic abortion, may carry with it additional grief reaction.[4]

This chapter presents an overview of the existing literature on the psychosocial and family issues associated with MFPR and proposes recommendations for a prospective program of research. The goal of a longitudinal program of research is to offer families the best counseling available based on comprehensive data.

RELATED LITERATURE

Some of the published studies regarding the emotional and psychological follow-up of families undergoing MFPR have limitations. For example, many of the studies are retrospective and the comparison groups do not include families who had not undergone an MFPR and carried a higher-order multiple pregnancy. Families choosing to not participate in follow-up studies may have more negative feelings than those participating families. It has been noted that families who miscarried after MFPR reported higher rates of depressive symptoms than those who had a successful pregnancy.[5] Further, McKinney and coworkers[5] suggested that women in the late stages of infertility treatment may be particularly "psychologically hardy." Moreover, most studies have not examined a time frame extending beyond 2 years after delivery. It may be that this length of time is too short to identify longer-term consequences. An additional limitation, as pointed out by Garel and associates,[6] is that the assessment of family relationships is often based on self-reports.

Garel and associates[6] conducted a prospective qualitative study to learn about the emotional state of women during the 2 years after an MFPR and to compare the emotional well-being and the relationship with children of women who had undergone an MFPR with those from a previous study who did not undergo MFPR and had delivered triplets. At 1 year after the delivery, one third of the women who had undergone reduction reported persistent depressive symptoms, primarily sadness and guilt. It should be noted that eight women from the original sample were not included owing to refusals, miscarriages, and relocation. At the time of the interview at 2 years, all but two women appeared to have overcome the emotional pain associated with the MFPR. Most women recalled the MFPR as a sad, but needed, intervention.[6]

In the second component of the Garel and associates'[6] study comparing mothers who had undergone a reduction with mothers of triplets at 2 years, mothers were interviewed in the home. The areas investigated included the mothers' health, the marital relationship, the families' organization of everyday life, and the relationship with the other children. Overall, in comparison with the mothers having delivered triplets, the mothers' relationship with the children and the mothers' psychological health were more satisfactory among the MFPR group.

In a study examining the psychological effects of MFPR, McKinney and coworkers[5] conducted interviews with 42 women who had undergone MFPR along with a control group of 44 women who had become pregnant after infertility evaluation or treatment, but who had not had a reduction. The interviews were completed within 1 year after the reduction, and standardized measures of psychiatric symptoms and depressive disorders were used. The results of the study suggested that MFPR does not appear to pose a significant mental health risk; however, spontaneously aborting a desired pregnancy after fertility problems places women at high risk for a depressive disorder. Seventy-five percent of the MFPR patients who spontaneously aborted the pregnancy and 60% of the control group who spontaneously aborted had symptoms of a major depressive disorder.[5] In this study, religion did not predict the emotional response to the higher-order pregnancy or the fetal reduction. Whereas religious affiliation and religiosity were not correlated with depressive episodes, the demographic factor that was linked to depression was having existing children. The women with prior living children were significantly more likely to report depressive episodes and to indicate their mood changes with the diagnosis of multifetal pregnancy and the MFPR procedure.[5] Overall, MFPR was characterized as a sad and unwelcome stress.

Each couple's decision and response to MFPR may reflect personal and family values. Decision making about MFPR is done in the context of culture, ethnicity, educational background, socioeconomic status, and existing children. Bergh and colleagues[4] studied the psychological outcomes for 13 couples who underwent MFPR as well as the outcomes of 2 couples who declined MFPR. Personal interviews along with standardized measures were conducted between 2.5 months and 4 years after delivery. The personal interviews examined the couples' experience with infertility, reaction to information regarding multiple gestation and the possibility of MFPR, feelings and thoughts before and after the MFPR, interaction between the couple, and interaction with the social surroundings.[4] When learning about the higher-order multiple pregnancy, all the couples indicated that the need for a fast decision was very stressful and they began a process of weighing the pros and cons of MFPR. The couples relayed varying degrees of difficulty in decision making ranging from easy to very difficult. At the time of the interview, all but one woman believed they had made the right decision, and all but two women indicated they would make the same decision again.

Schreiner-Engel and colleagues[7] studied the acute and persistent impact of MFPR and the women's ability to cope with fetal loss while bonding to surviving infants. Interviews took place an average of 2.7 years after the reduction. Among the 91 women included in the study, persistent depressive symptoms were mild. The most prevalent and intense feelings at the time of the interview were sadness and guilt. Twenty percent of the women had a median symptom score of mild to moderate at the time of the interview. This group, compared with the other 80%, was significantly younger, was more religious, desired larger families, had more ultrasonographic viewings, and had more severe reactions to the MFPR itself.[7] Ninety-three percent of the women who delivered would choose

MFPR again, whereas 70% of the women who miscarried would repeat MFPR.

In regard to bonding with surviving infants, Schreiner-Engel and colleagues[7] found that 43% of the women believed the MFPR made their surviving children "more special" to them. Attaching emotionally to the surviving infants after delivery was perceived to be only somewhat hindered by the fetal loss. Among the women in the study, viewing the multifetal pregnancy on ultrasound before the MFPR occurred an average of 3.8 times. Fifty-four percent of the women believed that viewing the ultrasound made them feel closer and more attached to the fetuses and made the MFPR more difficult emotionally. The frequency of viewing the fetuses on ultrasound before the MFPR was significantly related to the women's remembered emotional reactions to the MFPR and to the grief response that continued at the time of the interview.

In a follow-up study by Kanhai and coworkers,[8] 20 families who had undergone MFPR were interviewed regarding the psychological and emotional aspects of the procedure. At the time of the interview, none of the families expressed regret regarding the MFPR, but two couples reported occasional grief and mourning reactions. Eighteen of the couples discussed the MFPR with close family members and friends before and after the procedure. Moreover, most of the couples reported being able to talk to each other about their emotions during the decision-making process. The authors indicated that the initial emotional conflict with MFPR had no harmful effect on the mother's bonding with the surviving children.

Britt and associates[9] examined a socially constructed intervention with 36 couples during the MFPR procedure. The bonding intervention is intended to reduce the high level of anxiety that a woman and her partner typically experience in the MFPR process and to refocus their attention on the surviving embryos. The bonding intervention entails three stages: bringing the couple together immediately after the procedure to view the surviving embryos; taking and sharing photographs of the surviving embryos with the couple; and committing the couple to sending in baby pictures. Data were collected during the couples' final counseling session and the MFPR procedure. The bonding intervention was defined as successful based on defined criteria at each stage of the bonding intervention. Among the 36 couples who were studied, the bonding intervention was successful in 61% of the cases. The authors suggest that the success of the intervention will be best evaluated over time with regard to how the couples cope with the entire pregnancy as well as the nature of the pregnancy outcomes.

CONCLUSION

MFPR is a complex issue. The irony of addressing the decision of reducing much wanted pregnancies after the stress of infertility treatment demands careful study. Lack of comprehensive information about the longer-term psychosocial outcomes for the families should drive a prospective program of research that enrolls families before MFPR and follows them over the long term. Families who choose MFPR as well as families who decline MFPR should be enrolled in longitudinal studies. Further, the research should examine the issues comprehensively and, when possible, employ standardized measures to enhance the generalizability of results. Such research will work to ensure that families have the best counseling information available to them.

References

1. Evans MI, Dommergues M, Wapner RJ, et al: International, collaborative experience of 1789 patients having multifetal pregnancy reduction: A plateauing of risks and outcomes. J Soc Gynecol Invest 1996;3:23–26.

2. Evans MI, Berkowitz R, Wapner R, et al: Multifetal pregnancy reduction (MFPR): Improved outcomes with increased experience. Am J Obstet Gynecol 2001;184:97–103.

3. Souter I, Goodwin TM: Decision making in multifetal pregnancy reduction for triplets. Am J Perinatol 1998;15:63–71.

4. Bergh C, Moller A, Nilsson L, Wikland M: Obstetric outcomes and psychological follow-up of pregnancies after embryo reduction. Hum Reprod 1999;14:2170–2175.

5. McKinney M, Downey J, Timor-Tritsch I: The psychological effects of multifetal pregnancy reduction. Fertil Steril 1995;64:51–61.

6. Garel M, Stark C, Blondel B, et al: Psychological reactions after multifetal pregnancy reduction: A 2-year follow-up study. Hum Reprod 1997;12:617–622.

7. Schreiner-Engel P, Walther VN, Mindes J, et al: First-trimester multifetal pregnancy reduction: Acute and persistent psychologic reactions. Am J Obstet Gynecol 1995;172:541–547.

8. Kanhai HHH, de Han M, Van Zanten LA, et al: Follow-up of pregnancies, infants, and families after multifetal pregnancy reduction. Fertil Steril 1994;62:955–959.

9. Britt DW, Mans M, Risinger ST, Evans MI: Bonding and coping with loss: Examining the construction of an intervention for multifetal pregnancy reduction procedures. Fetal Diagn Ther 2001;16:158–165.

CHAPTER

FIFTY-SIX

Molecular Diagnostics in Obstetrics and Gynecology

Peter Bryant-Greenwood

The application of molecular biology to both laboratory and clinical medicine is an ongoing revolution. Nowhere is this translation more evident than in the field of obstetrics and gynecology. Obstetric-gynecologic practitioners will need to understand the issues and application of molecular technology to virtually the entire spectrum of human diagnostics:

1. Prenatal and antenatal diagnosis of inherited disease
2. Diagnosis of infectious agents
3. Accurate diagnosis and classification of neoplasia
4. Pharmacologic profiling for patient therapy customization
5. Determination of genetic susceptibility to complex genetic diseases: diabetes, hypertension, hyperlipidemia, thrombosis, cancer
6. Molecular fingerprinting for paternity, transplantation, and forensics

This chapter begins with an overview of the polymerase chain reaction (PCR)—the foundation of present molecular diagnostics. Next, alternative nucleic acid amplification techniques are discussed. I then review the tests that are directly applicable to the practice of obstetrics and gynecology. Finally, I examine some novel applications and technologies that may further accelerate the molecular renaissance.

THE STANDARD PCR

Without PCR, we would not have molecular diagnostics. Developed by Kary Mullis in the early 1980s, PCR is the *bidirectional, repetitive* synthesis of new DNA from a smaller quantity of initial template.[1-3] PCR thereby amplifies a specific sequence of DNA to the point at which it can be both detected and analyzed. PCR amplification requires two oligonucleotide primers (single-stranded stretches of DNA, usually up to 30 base pairs in length), the four deoxynucleotide triphosphates (dNTPs): G, A, T, C; magnesium ions in molar excess of the dNTPs; and a thermostable DNA polymerase to perform the actual DNA synthesis. Three distinct steps occur in a given PCR cycle: denaturation, primer annealing, and DNA synthesis.

Denaturation

Denaturation (Fig. 56–1) of the DNA occurs when the reaction mixture is heated to 92°C to 96°C. This step is

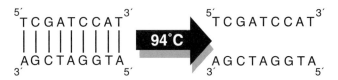

Figure 56–1. Denaturation.

necessary, not only to separate the complimentary strands of DNA but also to eliminate any secondary structure in the single strands themselves that would otherwise inhibit the following stages. This secondary structure results when there is complementarity between basepairs on a single strand of DNA—the single strand folds and binds into itself, preventing the primers from binding to their target sites. Secondary structure issues are important for primer design as well.

Annealing

Annealing (Fig. 56–2) of the oligonucleotide primers to their complementary single-strand target sequence is the next step in the PCR cycle. The temperature of this step varies from 37°C to 65°C. The temperature selected generally differs from one PCR assay to the next, and it is critical to successful PCR. The better the "match" between the primers and the target sequence, the higher the annealing temperature the reaction will allow. If the annealing temperature is too high, annealing will not take place at all. If the temperature is too low, nonspecific primer binding will take place, resulting in serious product formation. Oligonucleotide primers are present at a significantly greater concentration than the target DNA and are shorter in length (20 to 30 basepairs). This enables the primers to hybridize to the complementary target DNA faster than the time it takes for the single-stranded DNA to reanneal to each other.

5′
T C G A T C C A T T C G A T C C A T 3′
A G G T

G A T C
A G C T A G G T A A G C T A G G T A
3′   5′

Figure 56–2. Annealing.

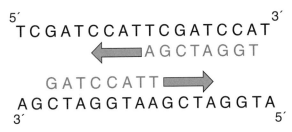

5′
TCGATCCATTCGATCCAT   3′
⟵ AGCTAGGT

GATCCATT ⟹
AGCTAGGTAAGCTAGGTA
3′   5′

Figure 56–3. DNA synthesis.

DNA Synthesis

Once the primer has annealed to its DNA target sequence, the next step is extension of the primer by thermostable polymerase (Fig. 56–3). This portion of the cycle is usually accomplished at 72°C. The time required to fully copy the template depends on the length of PCR product desired. Although longer is often better (especially if the products need to be sequenced), the quality of the initial DNA often dictates smaller products. When amplifying from formalin-fixed tissue, for example, most products are 150 to 220 base pairs in size.

These three steps allow for the exponential amplification of the target DNA sequence of interest. Each round of amplification follows the same steps: denaturation, annealing of specific oligonucleotide primers to each of the two complementary DNA strands, followed by the creation of new double-stranded DNA by a thermostable polymerase. In theory, this will double the amount of specific DNA in each round. After the third round of amplification, the specific product will start to accumulate. When the usual 30 to 40 rounds of amplification are completed, a several million–fold amplification of the specific target sequence has taken place. The amplified products can be detected by numerous methods that vary in sensitivity, accuracy, and speed. These include gel electrophoresis, Southern blot, probe capture and visualization in microtiter plates, and direct real-time detection by fluorescence. This real-time technique is specifically discussed in a following section because it not only affords rapid throughput but also allows for quantitation.

PCR's specificity, efficiency (yield), and fidelity determine the success of a particular assay. A highly specific PCR generates one and only one product. More efficient amplification generates more products with fewer cycles. A high-fidelity PCR contains a homogeneous PCR product with minimal amplification errors. Whereas an ideal PCR reaction would have high specificity, yield, and fidelity, adjusting PCR parameters for one objective may not be compatible with the needs of another. Knowing the important methods for optimizing a PCR reaction assists with the test.

Template. Template concentration directly affects reproducibility, specificity, and product yield. Excess template either inhibits the reaction altogether or increases mispriming. If too little template is used, the amplification of the higher-molecular-weight, lower-copy-number target is either less reproducible or not detectable. The initial template concentration should be optimized to achieve a balance between specificity and yield, given the expected size range of the PCR products generated. Typically, 1 μg of DNA template is used for PCR. One microgram of DNA corresponds to 3×10^5 copies of autosomal genes.

Template quality and quantity are major issues in a diagnostic laboratory. Whereas fresh, frozen, and ethanol-fixed specimens (the latter seen most often in cytology) are optimal for most reactions, PCR from formalin-fixed tissue can be difficult. Formalin crosslinks and fragments DNA. Whereas products up to 2000 base pairs have been amplified from formalin, products of 150 to 400 base pairs are more optimal.

Primers. The optimal primer length is 18 to 25 base pairs. When designing primers for amplification of regions from complex genomes, such as in the human, or of regions containing a high concentration of G and C nucleotides, increased length confers additional stability. Assuming that the nucleotide sequences of a genome are randomly distributed, the probability of finding a match using a 20–base pair primer set is 9×10^{26}—much greater than the 3×10^9 base pairs constituting the haploid human genome. However, spurious products are commonly generated from such primers. There are always some mismatched primer-target complexes that get amplified. In addition to raising the annealing temperature, several PCR techniques including Hot Start and Nested PCR have been successfully employed to eliminate these nonspecific PCR products. When amplifying a specific gene that may share significant homology with other genes in the genome, primer sequences should be chosen from the gene's intronic sequences, because such sequences are divergent even in members of tandemly repeated genes. Additionally, complementarity at the 3′ ends between the primer pairs should be avoided to prevent primer-primer annealing. Similarly, intraprimer base pair complementarity should also be avoided to prevent a primer from annealing to itself and creating a secondary structure.

To maximize amplification yield, there must be a nonlimiting amount of each primer. In a typical 100-μl reaction mixture, between 0.3 μmol and 3 μmol of each primer is used. Having such a large excess of primers ensures that once the template DNA has been denatured, it will anneal to the primers rather than to itself. The ratio between primer and template is also critical to PCR sensitivity. If the ratio is too high, PCR is prone to generate unspecific amplification products. If the ratio is too low, the efficiency or yield of amplification product will be too low.

dNTPs and MgCl₂. The number of dNTPs (G, A, C, T) should also be nonlimiting. The fraction of free dNTPs, however, depends not only on the number of PCR products generated (number of PCR cycles) but also on the length of the target sequence. For example, generation of 10^{12} copies (the maximum possible number of copies) of a

100–base pair target consumes 10^{14} dNTP molecules. On the other hand, generating 10^{12} copies of a 2000–base pair fragment consumes 2×10^{15} molecules.

The presence of divalent cations is critical to the PCR reaction, and Mg^{2+} ions have been found to be superior to magnesium and calcium. The concentration of magnesium should be optimized whenever a new combination of target and primers is first used or when the concentration of dNTPs or primers is altered. dNTPs are the major source of phosphate groups in PCR, and any change in their concentration affects the concentration of available Mg^{2+}.

Polymerase. Many different polymerase enzymes are available. These include enzymes with names such as PFU, Vent, Taq, T4, and T7. In addition to having different dNTP, pH, and Mg^{2+} requirements, and number of cycles required to obtain a standard 10^6-fold product amplification, these enzymes have different error rates as measured by error/base pair incorporated. For most applications of PCR, where a relatively homogeneous population is analyzed, for example, for sequencing, the enzyme-induced errors are of little concern. However, when PCR is used to study rare sequences in heterogeneous populations, such as the study of rare allelic polymorphisms in mRNA transcripts, it is vital that the amplified sequence is as error free as possible. Each error, once introduced, is amplified exponentially along with the original sequence during the subsequent cycles. Analyses that use small amounts of starting template are particularly prone to PCR-induced amplification error.

False-negative PCR results occur for a number of reasons. If the extraction procedure to remove the DNA or RNA from the cells of interest leaves too much contaminating protein, no or little amplification will take place, even in the presence of a large amount of template. Three to 10 copies of the specific target sequence must be in the reaction mixture to create a detectable product. One of the problems we encounter often in our laboratory is the presence of too much nonspecific DNA—samples have to be rediluted and run again. If the primers are not specific, if primer annealing temperature is not optimized, or if the concentration of the components of the reaction is not optimized, a false-negative result can occur because of inefficient or nonspecific amplification. If two primers share complementary sequences, they will bind to themselves rather than the template in the so-called primer-dimer artifact, resulting in a false-negative result. These primer-dimer interactions can also occur when the primer or enzyme concentration is too high.

False-positive PCR results occur if the primers are homologous to sequences other than the target gene or if products from previous similar PCR analyses are contaminating the reaction. The first problem can be avoided by engaging in rigorous primer design (now done with the aid of a computer program), sequence homology search in GeneBank, and by a screening test using DNA from a number of related as well as unrelated specimens (e.g.,

microorganisms, tumors). Contamination can be avoided by rational laboratory design, stringent handling techniques, and the application of carryover prevention systems already included in commercial PCR kits. This system substitutes uracil for the thymidine nucleotide in the PCR mixture, and if subsequent PCR reactions are incubated with a uracil-degrading enzyme, contaminating, but not wild-type DNA will be degraded.

PCR FROM RNA

To this point, I have been talking about the amplification of DNA. Analyzing a cell's mRNA allows us to answer questions concerning gene expression. Whereas DNA "germline" analysis can tell whether a gene has a specific mutation, it cannot tell whether a particular gene is up-regulated or down-regulated. An overview of the various methods for the amplification of RNA by PCR is shown in Figure 56–4.

A cell's total RNA is made up of a large quantity of ribosomal RNA, tRNA, and mRNA. For diagnostic considerations, we are interested in mRNA, which has a characteristic sequence that separates it from the other types. This includes a "cap" at the 3′ end consisting of blank nucleotides, and a poly A tail at the 5′ end. All of the PCR amplification methods for mRNA require an enzyme called *reverse transcriptase*. This enzyme synthesizes cDNA from mRNA. cDNA is more stable than its RNA counterpart, and can be amplified by one of the DNA polymerase enzymes mentioned previously. Because the reverse transcriptase–polymerase chain reaction (RT-PCR) depends on the reverse transcription of mRNA into cDNA, maximum conversion of RNA into cDNA is of critical importance. SuperScript and SuperScript II are Rnase H-derivatives of the Moloney murine leukemia virus (MMLV) reverse transcriptase. Other reverse transcriptase enzymes retain their inherent Rnase function—the ability to degrade the original RNA molecule while it makes cDNA. Rnase reverse transcriptases can convert a greater proportion of the RNA molecules into cDNA and can synthesize longer cDNA strands than other RNase+ enzymes. These enzymes also function at a higher temperature than their wild-type counterparts. This allows them to synthesize cDNA from mRNA molecules that may have significant secondary structure, and that therefore cannot be amplified at lower temperatures. First-strand synthesis of cDNA can be achieved with three methods (see Fig. 56–4). The relative specificity of each primer for RNA influences the amount and variety of cDNA synthesized. After first-strand synthesis, an aliquot is taken and amplified via PCR in a separate tube with fresh reagents and a thermostable DNA polymerase.

Random Hexamers. Random hexamers are the most nonspecific of the priming methods. These are useful when a particular mRNA is difficult to copy in its entirety,

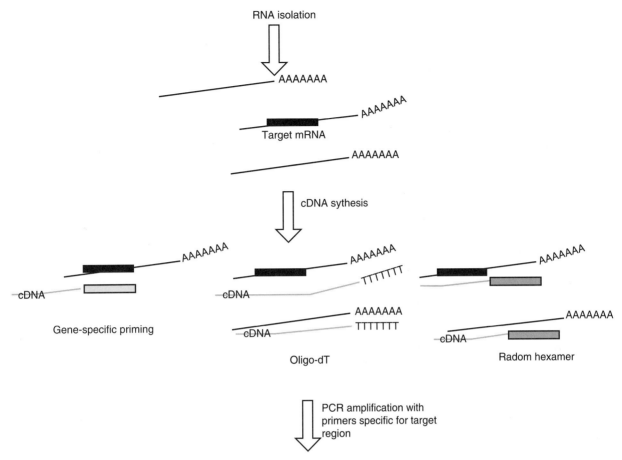

RNA isolation

Target mRNA

cDNA sythesis

Gene-specific priming

Oligo-dT

Radom hexamer

PCR amplification with
primers specific for target
region

Figure 56–4. Overview of the various methods for the amplification of RNA by polymerase chain reaction.

because of the presence of certain sequences that abort synthesis. With this method, all RNAs in a population serve as templates for first-strand cDNA synthesis, including tRNAs and ribosomal RNA molecules. The PCR primers that ''pull'' the cDNA molecule of interest are in the following amplification step. Roughly 96% of all cDNA synthesized using random hexamers is from ribosomal RNA. To maximize the size of the cDNA synthesized using random hexamers, the ratio of primers to RNA may need to be optimized for each individual reaction.

Oligo(dT). Unlike their random hexamer cousins, these primers are specific for mRNA molecules. They are specific to the 3' poly(A) tail characteristic of eukaryotic mRNA. mRNA constitutes only 1% to 4% of the RNA species in a cell. The amount and complexity of the resulting cDNA are considerably less that the products generated in the random hexamer reaction. Optimization is not necessary owing to the specific nature of these primers. Once all the mRNA has been made into cDNA, a specific cDNA of interest can be selected for and amplified in the following PCR step using specific primers.

Gene-specific Priming. This is the most specific priming method. Here, primers that are complementary to the target mRNA of interest are used. If the PCR amplification reaction also uses two specific primers to the target, the first-strand cDNA synthesis step can be primed using the same primer in the amplification step that hybridizes nearest to the 3' terminus of the mRNA. The advantage of gene-specific priming is that only the desired cDNA is produced in a more specific amplification. The disadvantage is that if a laboratory wants to assay for another mRNA, RNA has to be extracted from the source all over again and reverse transcriptase repeated, adding considerable time and cost to the subsequent assay. If, however, *all* the mRNAs in a sample have already been made into cDNA, such as in the oligo(dT) reaction, an aliquot can be taken and amplified with a second set of primers specific for another target of interest.

When measuring gene expression by RT-PCR, minute amounts of contaminating DNA can add to the signal derived from the mRNA. Two methods are used by a laboratory to deal with this problem. First is the addition of Dnase to the RNA once it has been extracted. Dnase is an enzyme that digests the DNA in the sample, leaving only RNA. The second method has to do with primer placement—when possible, PCR primers are placed on different exons within the gene. The primers are much closer to each other in the RNA form in which the intron has been spliced out. The PCR product from the DNA is significantly larger and may not produce a product. In practice, both of these methods are employed in concert to reduce the impact of contaminating DNA.

ALTERNATIVE FORMS OF DNA/RNA AMPLIFICATION

Ligase Chain Reaction

The ligase chain reaction (LCR) shares many of the same characteristics of PCR in that it amplifies a specific DNA segment of interest (Fig. 56–5). The basis of the reaction is the ligation of adjacent oligonucleotide primers that have hybridized to the target DNA. This ligation is achieved using a thermostable DNA ligase. LCR is designed to detect specific nucleic acid sequence variation and, as such, does not provide quantitative information about the sequence in question.

1. DNA is denatured at 94°C.
2. *Four* complementary oligonucleotide primers anneal to their target sequences at 65°C.
3. Ligase enzyme will covalently attach only adjacent primers that are perfectly complementary to their target.
4. The cycle is repeated as above with the product of the previous cycle becoming a target for the next round, thereby exponentially amplifying the desired product.

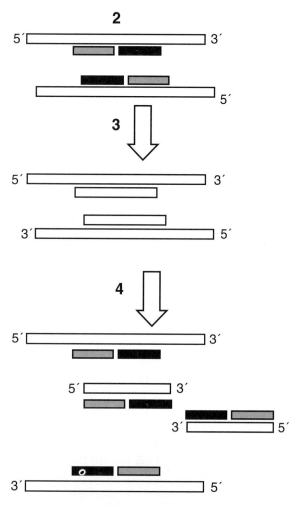

Figure 56–5. Ligase chain reaction.

If even a single base mismatch exists between the oligonucleotides and their target, efficient ligation will be prevented. If the oligonucleotides are not ligated, they cannot serve as templates for the next round.

The main problem with LCR is the high background limit of detection. This high background results from ligations even when mismatched bases exist. This background ligation process generates misprimed ligation fragments that are identical in size to the correctly primed product. To eliminate this problem, two-enzyme LCR systems have been developed. These systems couple the primer extension reaction of a 5′ to 3′ exonuclease-deficient thermostable DNA polymerase with a thermostable DNA ligase, so-called gap-LCR.

Gap-LCR uses four oligonucleotide primers with the two primers of each pair being separated by a gap of one or more consecutive bases that are specific for the target DNA. By adding only the missing deoxynucleotides to the reaction (G, A, T, C), together with a thermostable, exonuclease-deficient DNA polymerase and a thermostable DNA ligase, the gap must first be filled in the presence of the matching target before the resulting nick can be sealed by the ligase. In other words, if the gap contains a G residue and we have supplied the requisite matching C residue, the DNA polymerase will "fill the gap" with this C. If, for instance, the gap instead contains a C, A, or T, the C residue that we supplied will not fill the gap with the polymerase, and the two oligonucleotides will not be ligated together. This technique limits itself to the detection of base-pair changes from AT/TA to GC/CG or vice versa. For example, gap-LCR could not distinguish the β^A globin from β^B globin because the difference is an A to T transversion.

Another critical step to minimize target-independent ligation is close attention to primer design. The creation of primers with a single base-pair overhang, rather than having blunt ends, further limits the amount of nonspecific ligation events. The melting temperature—that is, the temperature necessary to pull the ligated primers off the target—should be within a narrow range for all four oligonucleotide primers, ideally with an absolute Tm of 70°C ± 2°C as determined by the addition of 2°C for each A or T and 4°C for each G and C in the sequence of the primer. The primers should also be designed so that one primer cannot serve as a bridging template for others. This leads to target-independent ligation and subsequent amplification and a false-positive result. False-negative results, as in PCR, can result when primers stick to each other, rather than the target sequence, or fold in half and bind to themselves. Primers should therefore be constructed so that there is little or no homology between them or within each primer. Further false-negative results can occur if there is inefficient phosphorylation of primers—unphosphorylated primers cannot be ligated together. This can be avoided by making sure enough ATP is added to the reaction mixture, and avoiding multiple freezings and thawings of the ATP, events that degrade the ATP before it is added to the mixture.

The many applications of LCR include the screening of large populations for monogenic disease polymorphisms, linkage analysis for complex genetic disorders via single nucleotide polymorphisms, determining human leukocyte antigen (HLA) haplotypes in tissue typing, and screening for multiple bacteria species after a standard PCR amplification of 16s ribosomal DNA sequences. Indeed, gap-LCR has presently been commercially applied to the detection of *Neisseria meningitidis* and *Chlamydia trachomatis*.

Self-Sustained Sequence Replication

Self-sustained sequence replication (3SR), an alternative method of amplification, is actually part of a family of related methodologies that combine three different enzyme activities at the same temperatures (42°C to 50°C): reverse transcriptase, RnaseH, and T7RNA polymerase. Other assays that use this technique are NASBA (nucleic acid–based amplification), and TAS (transcription amplification system). All three of these methods have a reverse transcriptase step as the initial reaction—the RNA template is transcribed into cDNA by an initiating downstream primer with the recognition sequence for T7RNA polymerase at its 5′ end.

The template RNA is destroyed by RNaseH activity of the reverse transcriptase as the cDNA is synthesized. This allows for the reaction to proceed in absence of a high-temperature physical denaturation step. The upstream primer will then anneal to the single-stranded cDNA, and the double-stranded DNA will be synthesized by the reverse transcriptase. After double-stranded DNA is synthesized, the T7RNA polymerase (which binds to the 5′ end of the double-stranded DNA) takes over, initiating a new round of amplification by reconverting the double-stranded DNA back into the antisense RNA, where the reverse transcriptase can begin the cycle anew.

This process continues in a self-sustained, cyclic fashion until enzymes or other components in the reaction mixture become limiting or inactivated. This technology can amplify an RNA signal more than 10^8-fold in 30 minutes. Specificity is a major issue in 3SR. Because of the relatively low temperatures, the reaction must take place, as not all the enzymes necessary for the reaction are heat stable at temperatures higher than 50°C. Despite these issues with specificity, 3SR has an enormous advantage in testing for microbiologic specimens: by using RNA as the initial template, 3SR can discriminate between dead and viable organisms.

Branched DNA Amplification

Rather than using PCR to amplify the target itself, another technique used in molecular diagnostics is the

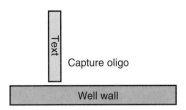

Figure 56–6. "Capture" oligonucleotides, specific for the target sequence of interest, are attached to the well walls and base of a micotiter plate.

amplification of a signal generated by the target. Branched DNA is one such method of amplification and detection.

1. "Capture" oligonucleotides, specific for the target sequence of interest, are attached to the well walls and base of a micotiter plate (Fig. 56–6).
2. Sample DNA or RNA is added to the well. The capture oligonucleotides bind to the target sequence, effectively immobilizing it on the solid surface of the well (Fig. 56–7).
3. Bivalent "detection" oligonucleotides are added to the well. These detection oliogonucleotides hybridize to the target, serving as a link between the target and the branched DNA molecules. The well is then washed to remove the unbound DNA or RNA and the unbound detection oligonucleotides (Fig. 56–8).
4. Branched DNA is added where it hybridizes to the detection oligonucleotides. Excess, unbound branched DNA is washed out of the well (Fig. 56–9).
5. "Enzyme" oligonucleotides are added to the well. These oligonucleotides stick to the branched DNA. Excess, unbound enzyme oligonucleotides are washed out of the well (Fig. 56–10).
6. Chemiluminescent substrate is added, which the enzyme activates.
7. Light output is measured on a plate reader.

A distinct advantage of the branched DNA method is the minimal risk of contamination: the target is not being amplified, only the detection signal is. Additionally, because no exponential amplification of the target sequence takes place, genuine quantification can be achieved com-

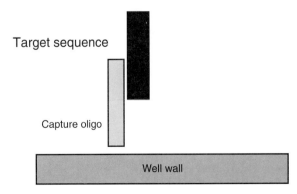

Figure 56–7. Sample DNA or RNA is added to the well. The "capture" oligonucleotides bind to the target sequence, effectively immobilizing it on the solid surface of the well.

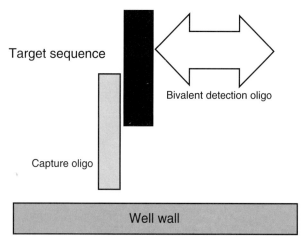

Figure 56–8. Bivalent "detection" oligonucleotides are added to the well. These detection oligonucleotides hybridize to the target, serving as a link between the target and the branched DNA molecules. The well is then washed to remove the unbound DNA or RNA and the unbound detection oligonucleotides.

pared with the semiquantitative LCR, 3SR, and most PCR techniques. There is also a distinct advantage in terms of template preparation. Because no DNA or RNA amplification is necessary, the sample can be maintained in buffers that, although offering superb protection from degradation, would otherwise inhibit any self-respecting PCR or other nucleic acid amplification technique.

The major problem with the branched DNA is its sensitivity, which is comparably lower than the other technologies described previously. At the present time, approxi-

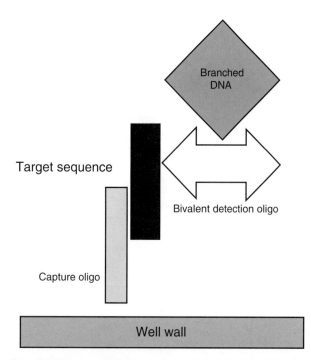

Figure 56–9. Branched DNA is added where it hybridizes to the detection oligonucleotides. Excess, unbound branched DNA is washed out of the well.

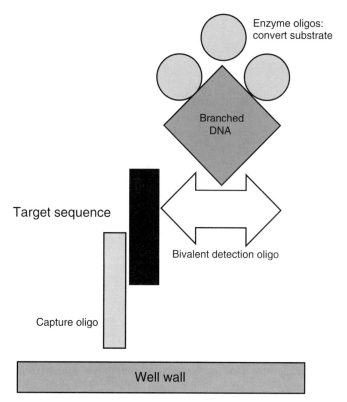

Figure 56–10. "Enzyme" oligonucleotides are added to the well. These oligonucleotides stick to the branched DNA. Excess, unbound enzyme oligonucleotides are washed out of the well.

mately at least 500 copies per milliliter are needed for reliable, reproducible detection. Such levels may be too high for specimens such as cerebrospinal fluid, bronchoalveolar lavage, or potentially, amniotic fluid. Currently, branched DNA methods have been commercially applied to detection and quantification of HIV, hepatitis C virus, hepatitis B virus, and cytomegalovirus.

Real-Time PCR

Whereas PCR has been excellent in terms of test sensitivity and specificity, quantification of target sequences has remained elusive. This is due to two important obstacles inherent to the PCR reaction. The first of these is the plateau of PCR product accumulation. PCR amplification occurs only for a finite period of time, eventually—owing to product concentration, limiting substrates, and reagents in the reaction mixture—the reaction ceases to produce further product. The reaction literally exhausts itself. At this point, the ability to quantitate results is extremely difficult. Second, because of the presence of PCR inhibitors, PCR reactions occur with variable reaction efficiencies. Whereas only rigorous technique and quality control can prevent the latter problem, several new systems have been developed to measure the products of PCR as they are produced with each sequential cycle of amplification. These include the TaqMan system, the Molecular Beacon system, and the FRET (fluorescent resonance energy transfer) system. All three of these methodologies share the same basic idea: probes with luminescent markers are added into the reaction mix, where they bind to the product as it forms. Once they bind, the luminescent properties of the probe are activated, allowing a detection device in the PCR thermocycler machine to detect their presence. The amount of lumination is correlated by the presence of product.

The FRET system involves PCR amplification and real-time detection using four oligonucleotides in each reaction (Fig. 56–11). The oligonucleotides include two unlabeled PCR primers that exponentially generate an unlabeled amplicon, a 3′ fluorescein isothiocyanate (FITC) end-labeled probe, and a 5′ LC-red 640–labeled anchor probe designed to hybridize within 1 to 3 nucleotides of the FITC probe. The PCR amplification and detection takes place in the LightCycler (Roche Molecular Biochemicals) thermocycler. The LightCycler generates incident light that excites the FITC "donor" fluorophore. This energy is then transferred to the LC-red 640 fluorophore "reporter" only when the two probes are in very close proximity—that is, have annealed to the same template molecule.

Successful primer design is critical to FRET, as well as for the other PCR quantitative methods. This is because one needs to generate both probes and primers, each of which can react with each other, rather than with the target sequence of interest. Primers should be screened for any potential secondary structure and potential primer-dimer formation. The 3′ end should have a low G + C content (usually less than three G or C in the last five base pairs of the 3′ end) to prevent nonspecific target amplification. The T_m of each primer should be as close to 76°C as possible (this effectively makes the annealing and extension temperature of 72°C the same, allowing for high stringency, and subsequent high specificity). The probes should be between 30 and 33 base pairs in length. This is again to ensure high specificity with T_ms that are 5°C to 10°C higher than the primers.

The strength of the FRET system is twofold. First, the probes can be long, 30 base pairs compared with 15 base pairs in the TaqMan system, which allows for greater specificity. This high degree of specificity allows for mutation analysis: if a probe has a single base-pair mismatch, it will stop fluorescing at a lower denaturing temperature than if it was a complete match. Second, the reporter probe fluoresces only when the probes are together, unlike the TaqMan system in which the reporter fluorophore is "loose" in the reaction mixture, sometimes imparting a high background that complicates detection. Additionally, several assays have been developed in which two different reporter probes are used, one with red 640, and the other with red 720, thereby allowing for the detection of more than one product.

APPLICATIONS OF MOLECULAR DIAGNOSTICS

Inherited Disease

The Helix database, supported through the National Library of Medicine at the National Institutes of Health (NIH), is a major genetic testing resource. As of 2001, there are over 650 diseases for which testing is available at more than 350 clinical and research testing facilities. For the obstetrician-gynecologist, many of these tests are the foundation of prenatal diagnostics, preconception counseling, and postconception management. An overview of the most requested genetic assays follows. These tests can be broadly stratified according to the type of genetic error they represent: trinucleotide expansion, point mutation, and deletions.

Trinucleotide Expansion

Fragile X syndrome is the most common cause of mental retardation, with an incidence of 1 in 1500 in males to 1 in 2000 in females. The phenotype includes floppy ears, a broad nose with prominent ridges above the eyes, and a

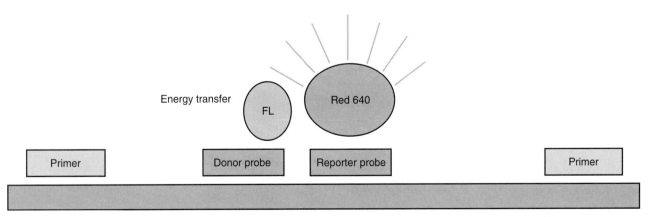

Figure 56–11. The FRET (fluorescent resonancy energy transfer) system.

long, narrow face. The patient's joints are hyperextensible, and the IQ is most often in the 50 to 75 range. Fragile X derives its name from a fragile site at Xq27.3 that is observed in the lymphocytes of affected patients cultured in folate-deficient media.[4] The gene *FMR1* was cloned in 1991.[5] The FMR1 protein was shown to be a RNA-binding protein. The protein is predominantly cytoplasmic, but it will shuttle between the nucleus and the cytoplasm. A common mutation has been identified in fragile X patients—a CCG repeat in the 5' untranslated region of the gene.[6] This form of genetic mutation was the first of its kind to be described. In *FMR1,* the number of CGG repeats varies from 6 to 50 in the normal population. In affected individuals, however, there exists an excessive expansion from several hundred to nearly a thousand. As a result of this expansion, the entire region becomes hypermethylated, rendering the gene silent.[7] Repeats in the 50 to 200 are considered to be premutations. Interestingly, as much as 35% of females with this genetic premutation are mentally retarded, whereas males not only are phenotypically normal but also fail to pass on their mutation to their offspring—the expansion to a full mutation of over 200 repeats is maternally derived.

Analysis of *FMR1* is performed by Southern blot technique. In this technique, the patient's DNA is extracted, cut with a set of restriction enzymes, and electrophoreses after radiographic labeling of the products. Different numbers of repeats present in the patient's DNA result in different-sized fragments of DNA as cleaved by the restriction enzymes. These size differences can be resolved by gel analysis. Cytogenetic methodologies have also been used to confirm the diagnosis of fragile X, but are not the method of choice owing to the technique's ability to resolve only the very largest repeat expansions. PCR is now the preferred method to be used in conjunction with the Southern blotting technique. PCR is best at determining just how many repeats an individual has—an absolute requirement for determining the relative risk of expansion in a female carrier. Southern blot is used when little or no PCR products are detected: the repeat size may be so large that efficient PCR cannot take place. This used to be a frequent occurrence, but has become less common with the application of new (see earlier section under Polymerase) polymerase enzymes that enable long-distance amplification.[8] As with all things in medicine, there are few absolutes. Point mutations and deletions in the *FMR1* gene have also been decried as having given the same phenotype.

Huntington's disease (HD) is another important hereditary disorder that, because of its adult onset, can provide special challenges in genetic and prenatal diagnostics. HD involves a CAG repeat. The disease is characterized by choreic movements, dementia, psychosis, and eventual death. The caudate is the major site of neuronal degeneration. The gene for HD is *IT15* and maps to 4p16.3, which was cloned in 1993.[9] The CAG repeats result in the translation of too many glutamine residues on the amino terminus

of the gene. Experimental evidence shows that these additional residues result in a gain in function, with resultant cell death. In the normal population, the normal number of repeats is 11 to 28. Repeats of 29 to 35 are less common and are thought to predispose to repeat expansion. Repeats of 36 to 39 are already considered pathologic, although with reduced penetrance as such repeat lengths have been observed in both affected and normal individuals. Repeats of 40 or greater are associated with full expression of HD. The greater the number of expanded repeats, the earlier HD will manifest. Unlike fragile X, paternal, rather than maternal, inheritance is associated with increased risk of acquiring HD. The diagnosis of HD is made by PCR amplification of the desired repeat region, followed by sequencing to determine the precise number of nucleotide repeats.

Deletions

Duchenne's muscular dystrophy (DMD) is an X-linked recessive progressive muscle-wasting disease with an incidence of 1 in 3500 births. Symptoms at presentation include proximal muscle weakness before the age of 5 years and serum creatine kinase levels at least 40 times the upper limit of normal. The dystrophin gene represents one of the largest genes in the human genome, spanning 2.4 million base pairs. The gene itself contains 79 exons and encodes a 14-kb mRNA molecule. The dystrophin protein is a subsarcolemmic cytoskeletal protein that forms part of a membrane-associated dystrophin-glycoprotein complex. Lack of dystrophin is thought to reduce the capacity of the plasma membrane to withstand the mechanical forces generated with repeated muscle contraction. Both DMD and Becker's muscular dystrophy (BMD), which is a milder form of DMD, result from mutations in the dystrophin gene. However, although the dystrophin gene is virtually absent in all patients with DMA, the protein is present in reduced amounts or in structurally aberrant forms in BMD.

The definite diagnosis of DMD is made on muscle biopsy. However, multiplex PCR is a cheaper, less invasive method that allows for the detection of the 18 of the most common deleted exons.[10] If a deletion is present, no amplification products are generated. Additional studies can be performed if the multiplex method is nondiagnostic. These include RT-PCR of muscle RNA with sequence analysis and single-strand conformation polymorphism SSCP.

Point Mutations

Cystic fibrosis (CF) is an autosomal recessive disease and one of the most common genetic disorders of whites of northern European ancestry, with an incidence of 1 in 2500 births.[11] The carrier frequency in the population is estimated to be 1 in 25. CF affects the patient's lungs, gastrointestinal tract, and reproductive system. There is variable phenotypic expression, with severe respiratory failure in infants to mild pulmonary symptoms in adults. The CF transmembrane conductance regulator gene (CFTR) was cloned in 1989. The CFTR protein is located within the lipid bilayer of the cell membrane, where it serves as a cAMP-activated chlorine ion channel to regulate chlorine ion conductance. Without CFTR, abnormal electrolyte transport takes place across the epithelial cell, resulting in thick, mucoid secretions that cause obstruction, secondary infection, and subsequent end-organ damage. The severity of CF depends on the type and location of the mutation within the CFTR gene. In the North American white population, 70% of affected individuals share a common 3–base pair deletion at codon 508. There are, however, some 700 other known mutations that make up the remainder.

Molecular diagnosis of CF is complicated by the heterogeneity of the mutations. One method is to combine multiplex PCR (multiple primers in the PCR mixture that generate multiple PCR products), with dot blotting. This is the so-called MASDA test—Multiplex Allele-Specific Diagnostic Assay. These products can then be blotted and probed. If no product is detected on hybridization, the inference is that either there exists a mutation in the primer annealing site, which prevented the latter from binding and subsequently amplifying, or there is a mutation somewhere in the product that prevents the probe from binding. If the precise mutation is needed, the patient's sample can be reamplified using only the primers to the particular region in question and sequenced.

The success of the MASDA technique, as well as future technologies that will allow for the amplification of each codon and rapid sequences on DNA chips, has yet to have a substantial impact on the practice of obstetrics. In 1997, the NIH issued a statement on CF testing.[12] NIH recommended that testing be offered to adults with a history of CF, partners of patients with CF, couples planning a pregnancy, and couples seeking prenatal care. General screening of the adult population and newborn infants was thankfully not recommended. In a pivotal study in Rochester, New York, the cost of screening as recommended by the NIH (at a cost of $150 per person) cost $1.3 million.[13] This amount compares favorably with the estimated cost of care of an affected patient with CF—1.0 million. The NIH recommendations, however, have not been disseminated to the obstetricians in the field: 286 private practice primary obstetricians in North Carolina failed to correctly answer basic questions about CF carrier frequency and testing.[14] Similarly, of a cohort of obstetricians in Maryland, only 18% were familiar with the NIH guidelines and the vast majority said that they never discussed CF testing with their patients who did not have a family history of CF. Clearly a more concerted effort between the NIH and the genetic community is necessary to reverse this trend, for both CF on the one hand and new tests on the other.

Factor V Leiden (R506Q) is at present the most common identifiable genetic defect in the coagulation cascade. Venous thromboembolic events are common, affecting 0.1% of the population each year.[15] These events are a major source of medical management complications and of subsequent health care cost. Unlike many other genetic tests, there are useful interventions that can clearly prevent thromboembolic events. For the practicing obstetrician-gynecologist, this includes preoperative diagnosis, postoperative management, and birth control decision making. The factor V mutation is very common; 3% to 7% of the general population is heterozygous for the mutated allele.[16] It is estimated that 20% of all thrombotic events are related to the factor V mutation and up to 50% of all recurrent events. The mutation itself causes resistance to activated protein C (APC) by the abolishment of a protein C cleavage site in the factor V procoagulant protein.[17] Although there are many methods for detecting the mutation associated with factor V, the most common is a two-step procedure: PCR followed by RFLP (restriction fragment length polymorphism). Although this test is accurate, it is labor intensive, slow, and expensive. Recently, the FRET system (see earlier under Real-Time PCR) has been applied to not only factor V Leiden but also for assays for prothrombin G20210A—the second most common thrombophilic genetic defect, and HFE C282Y (hereditary hemochromatosis).[18]

Hereditary hemochromatosis (HH) is an autosomal recessive disease of iron metabolism that results in widespread iron deposition and subsequent end-organ damage and failure. Death usually results from the cardiac manifestation of the disease, with arrhythmia and congestive heart failure being the most common, or liver failure or liver cancer. The iron itself is directly toxic to cells owing to superoxide free radical formation via the Fenton reaction, as well as nonspecific protein chelation and subsequent inactivation. HH is a common disorder with an incidence of 1 in 200 and an estimated carrier rate of 1 in 10. Two mutations in the HFE gene are responsible for 95% of affected individuals. The most common, representing roughly 85% of individuals, is a single G to A base pair mutation that results in a cysteine to tyrosine residue at the 282 amino acid position. The second most common, representing approximately another 10% of affected individuals, is also a single base pair change from C to G in exon 2 that results in a histidine to aspartate substitution. The first of these mutations abolishes HFE's usual cell surface expression, thereby preventing its normal ability to bind to the transferrin receptor and down-regulate the receptor's affinity for iron-bound transferrin. Homozygotes thus fail to normally regulate iron metabolism. This explains the usual constellation of abnormal laboratory values, including elevated serum iron, transferrin, and ferritin concentrations.

Similar to factor V Leiden, there is an effective, inexpensive therapy (phlebotomy) to prevent iron overload.

This fact, combined with the high prevalence of the mutation, may make screening desirable. However, a recent Centers for Disease Control and Prevention and National Human Genome Research Institute conference recommended that such screening would be premature owing to uncertainty regarding HFE prevalence, penetrance, proper care for asymptomatic patients, and an access issue with regard to genetic counseling.[19] These recommendations will undoubtedly change with further research. Also similar to factor V, the present molecular test for HFE includes a PCR reaction followed by RFLP, but again a higher throughput FRET assay has been developed that is both faster and cheaper.[18]

Neoplasia

To date, molecular methods have had relatively small impact on either cancer diagnosis or determination of the risk of cancer predisposition. In terms of cancer diagnosis, most molecular tests involve PCR amplification and detection of fusion transcripts common in pediatric tumors, soft tissue sarcomas, and lymphoma. Such fusion transcripts are absent in the predominantly epithelial, germ cell, and endocrine neoplasms encountered in gynecologic oncology. There are, however, some molecular diagnostic assays that may make it into clinical gynecologic practice in the very near future. These include telomerase testing, tests for minimal residual disease or circulating tumor cells, and HER-2/neu testing—the latter being presented as a paradigm for as yet undefined prognostic tumor markers in gynecologic malignancies.

Telomerase is an enzyme that maintains the tandem arrays of short TTAGGG sequences at the linear ends of chromosomes—the telomeres. These telomere structures have two functions. First, they stop natural chromosome ends behaving as random breaks or stick ends that might otherwise generate interchromosomal fusions and activate damage-induced cell cycle arrest. Second, they provide the structural basis for solving the so-called end-replication problem: the inability of DNA polymerase to completely replicate the very end of DNA duplex—sequence is lost from the end of the chromosome with each successive cell division. There is a lack of telomerase activity in somatic cells. This leads to progressive telomere shortening with every cycle.[20] Eventual end-to-end chromosomes occur and the cell undergoes apoptosis. Many human cancer cells somehow manage to restore their telomerase activity, making it a potential useful molecular marker for neoplasia, even though telomerase itself may not be necessary for carcinogenesis.[21]

Most cervical carcinomas express telomerase—76% to 100%.[22] This also includes dysplastic, preinvasive lesions. Of 10 invasive cervical cancers with expression of telomerase, 7 were also positive for high-risk human papillomavirus (HPV) 16 and 18 by PCR.[23] With the Telomeric

Repeat Amplication Protocol (TRAP), five cases of squamous intraepithelial lesions without Pap smear abnormality expressed telomerase activity, indicating that some false-negative cytologic finding could be detected by the TRAP assay.[24] This is especially tantalizing, given the more fluid-phase cervical sampling. This move facilitates not only Thin-Prep cytologic preparation but also HPV testing (discussed under Infectious Disease later), and telomerase testing. With in situ hybridization techniques, 13 of 13 invasive cervical carcinomas (6 squamous and 7 adenocarcinoma) were positive, 9 of 9 adenocarcinomas in situ, and 14 of 14 high-grade squamous intraepithelial lesions. Twenty-one normal, metaplastic, and low-grade squamous lesions exhibited weak positivity limited to the basal layer.[25] One study, however, found telomerase expression in normal ectocervical and endocervical endothelium, suggesting that a quantitation standard is necessary and that hormonally responsive epithelium may have a high level of telomerase activity as that of quiescent epithelium, but not as high as frankly neoplastic epithelium.[26] Indeed, telomerase activity has been detected in proliferative and secretory endometrium, endometrial hyperplasia, and carcinoma,[27] but was absent in atrophic, postmenopausal endometrium.[28]

Telomerase activity was detected in 33 of 41 ovarian cancers of epithelial origin, 3 of 5 tumors of low malignant potential, and none in 7 benign tumors or normal epithelium.[29] The intensity of telomerase expression is significantly higher in invasive ovarian lesions than in low malignant potential (LMP) tumors,[29] as are tumors with lymph node metastases.

The TRAP assay, as developed by Kim and coworkers,[30] consists of two steps. In the first step, telomerase present in the specimen extends an oligonucleotide trimer, which serves as a substrate for the enzyme. Note that this means a fresh specimen must be used—not very applicable to biopsy, but definitely workable with fresh cytology specimens. Second, the extended trimers serve as a new template for PCR amplification. There is also a commercial kit available, the TRAP-eze ELIZA assay that combines the first step of the TRAP with PCR followed by direct chromogenic detection of TRAP products with ELIZA. Although these techniques are accurate, they are costly and slow. Roche has recently produced a real-time, quantitative telomerase assay with its LightCycler system. This will reduce the cost of the assay and increase processing speed and accuracy. In our hands, 5-hour turnaround times can be achieved. Irrespective of the technique, however, telomerase must include cytologic and pathologic correlation: normal cells under particular circumstances may have high levels of telomerase, and telomerase is only a general marker for tumor genesis—pathologic correlation is needed to precisely determine exactly what tumor type is involved.

Minimal residual disease is an evolving concept in oncology. Molecular methods permit the detection of cells too few in number to be detected by microscopy, immunohistochemistry, and flow cytometry. RT-PCR has been applied to tumor cell detection in blood, lymph nodes, and bone marrow aspirates. Whereas what to do with positive results is presently unclear, detection of these small populations may eventually have an enormous impact on the management of gynecologic cancers.

RT-PCR for these small populations is based on the detection of an amplified product from an mRNA molecule that is uniquely expressed in a particular cell type. In the case of epithelial neoplasms, there is a real paucity of such markers. The few that exist are for breast cancer: gross cystic disease fluid protein. As yet, there are no specific epithelial markers for ovarian, cervical, endometrial, or endocervical carcinoma. We must therefore rely on general markers for epithelial cells alone, inferring that the mere presence of these cells means metastatic disease. One such marker for all gynecologic malignancies is cytokeratin.

The first step involved the use of magnetic, polystyrene beads covered with an antibody specific for epithelial cells. The sample is added to a suspension of these beads in buffer. This permits the elimination of false-positive signals from background expression of the chosen marker in nonepithelial cells, as well as enriches the specimen for the epithelial cells of interest for subsequent PCR. In our laboratory, the RT-PCR step involves primers for cytokeratin-19, a widely expressed gene in cells of epithelial origin. Primers must be carefully chosen to avoid complementarity to pseudogenes that may be present and primers must be selected at intron-exon boundaries. Without this, amplicons may be generated from traces of genomic DNA that are indistinguishable from the desired mRNA of the tumor cells. RT-PCR generates cDNA, which is amplified. These products are run on an agarose gel and stained with ethidium bromide. This is followed by probe hybridization for cytokeratin 19 via Southern blot, which increases assay sensitivity and specificity. Eventually, we would like to move to real-time PCR, which will be faster, more accurate, and quantitative. Real-time quantitative assays may make detection of minimal residual disease clinically useful.

The *HER-2/neu* gene is a member of a family of closely related growth factor receptors including epidermal growth factor. The proto-oncogene is located on chromosome 17q and encodes a transmembrane tyrosine kinase growth factor receptor. Overexpression of HER-2/neu has been identified in 10% to 34% of breast cancers. No such expression has been reliably demonstrated in gynecologic malignancies. The interest in HER-2/neu lies not with its expression in breast cancer cells, but rather with the unique prognostic and predicative value in its expression. These include identification of high-risk preinvasive lesions, prediction of response to traditional hormonal and chemotherapeutic agents, and finally, response prediction to novel therapies targeting the receptor itself.

HER-2/neu expression has been associated with ductal carcinoma in situ extent,[31] ductal carcinoma in situ type and grade,[31] increased risk of local recurrence after surgery and radiation,[32] high rate of cell proliferation, DNA aneuploidy,[33] p53 overexpression,[34] and the development of invasive disease.[33] Thus, a single marker can provide an enormous amount of clinical information and allow us for the first time to biochemically stratify preinvasive lesions. Development of such markers from gynecologic malignancies should be of the utmost importance.

The most common therapy association with HER-2/neu expression is the apparent resistance of tumors treated with hormonal therapy alone.[35, 36] Indeed, in one longitudinal study,[37] positive tumors treated with hormonal therapy alone actually had a worse outcome than tumors left alone. HER-2/neu had also been associated with increased response to Adriamycin.[37]

By far the most exciting is the development of novel therapies directed at the receptor itself. Herceptin is a monoclonal antibody that blocks the receptor. Herceptin has a favorable toxicity profile and has recently achieved an overall response rate of 15% when given alone for metastatic breast cancer.[38] Herceptin and HER-2/neu testing are now the standard of care for the management of breast cancer.

What is not standard is how to test for HER-2/neu expression. Southern blot, PCR, fluorescent in situ hybridization (FISH), and immunohistochemistry are all used to quantify HER-2/neu expression. At present, the battle is between immunohistochemistry and FISH. These two techniques have advantages in that they are cheap, have high throughput, preserve the ability of the pathologist to actually determine what type of cells are staining (e.g., ductal carcinoma in situ, invasive tumor) and have been approved by the U.S. Food and Drug Administration—which often determines reimbursement rates for such tests. However, both tests are subjective assays and depend on quality of both the specimen and the fixation technique. Real-time PCR assays of fine-needle aspiration cytology specimens will undoubtedly further confuse the issue. Although these issues apply to HER-2/neu and breast cancer, these very same issues will undoubtedly arise when similar markers for cervical, endometrial, and ovarian cancers become available.

Infectious Disease

At the present time, PCR can be considered only an adjunct to classic routine microbiologic testing. PCR is clearly inferior in terms of sensitivity to classic methods such as blood culture when fast-growing bacteria such as staphylococci are present. Moreover, although some antibiotic genes can be identified by PCR, the sequence of the gene still has to be known, whereas the classical disc method reveals susceptibility and resistance no matter whether the gene in question is plasmid or chromosomal in mechanism. PCR has been routinely applied to the detection of slow-growing bacteria, such as *Chlamydia* or

Mycobacterium species. In contrast, pathologic viruses and fungi are excellent candidates for molecular identification because present, classic techniques of culture are slow and insensitive.

The classic PCR method for detecting microorganisms is based on the amplification of a sequence of genetic material that is unique for that organism. If a broad range of pathogens is to be detected in a clinical sample, conserved genetic sequence must be utilized. The bacterial 16s ribosomal subunit contains many of these conserved regions that can be utilized for diagnosis. Indeed, analysis of some of these conserved sequences challenges the existing classification schemes that are based on shape, staining, and biochemical behavior.

Management of infectious disease is an enormous component to the practice of obstetrics and gynecology. The microorganisms that are the most important clinically and for which PCR is routinely employed are presented in Table 56–1.

HPV is the most common sexually transmitted virus, and it approaches *Chlamydia* infection as the most commonly sexually transmitted pathogen overall. More than 70 distinct viral types exist, 23 of which are specific for the genital tracts of the male and female. These latter types are often divided into two distinct sets. "Low-risk" types result in warts that usually resolve and do not progress into invasive cancer. Other, "high-risk" types are associated with malignant transformation. Indeed, it is now accepted that HPV infection not only is necessary for the development of carcinoma in situ lesions but also is universally present in carcinoma.[39, 40] HPV types 16 and 18 are present in 60% and 20% of cervical carcinomas, respectively. Worldwide, carcinoma of the cervix is the second most common malignancy in women, accounting for some 15,700 new cases and 4900 deaths in the United States each year.[41]

Whereas exfoliative cytologic examination of the cervix has made the Pap smear the best cancer screening test ever devised, we have reached a major obstacle to further decreasing the rate of cervical cancer. The reason for this lies in the very nature of the Pap smear itself: it is a screening test based on subjective observation that is vulnerable to interobserver and intraobserver variability, sampling error (80% of the cells remain of the collection device), and not-infrequent false negatives due to obscuring blood, mucus, inflammation, and collection artifact. In addition, the Pap smear is nonprognostic—we can infer biologic behavior for only the highest grade of lesions. Lastly, patient compliance is a major unresolved issue—two thirds of preventable cervical cancers occur in women who have not had a Pap test in at least 5 years.[42]

The issues previously discussed are related to the test itself. Another set of issues concerns the Bethesda system, which was devised in 1991 to correlate cytology with histology and to standardize the management approach to cervical dysplasia. The Bethesda system did succeed at standardizing nomenclature but only with the creation of several controversial categories:

1. ASCUS (atypical squamous cells of undetermined significance) is a wastebasket of uncertainty leading to overuse, unnecessary colposcopic examinations, and legal hell.
2. Incorporation of HPV koilocytosis into LSIL (low-grade squamous intraepithelial lesion), which has resulted in unnecessary treatment.
3. AGUS (atypical glandular cells of undetermined significance), see No. 1.

HPV molecular testing, as patented and offered by Digene, is now the standard of care for the management of ASCUS specimens. With the move to fluid-phase collection systems, a cytopathologist will have enough material to make a monolayer cytologic specimen (e.g., Thin-Prep) and render a visual diagnosis. If the diagnosis is ASCUS, or in even LSIL, the remainder of the specimen can be tested for HPV low-risk and high-risk types, utilizing the hybrid capture technique that is a signal amplification technique and chemiluminescent detection system similar to the branched DNA method outlined previously (with all of its advantages and disadvantages). The basis of this technology is two probe cocktails. One with probes for all the low-risk types, the other with probes to all known high-risk types. If a test is positive for the high-risk HPV type, the patient goes to colposcopy. If the test is positive for the low-grade type, the patient can be given the option of colposcopy or to be followed by repeat Pap and HPV testing. Many laboratories have dispensed with the low-risk probe cocktail altogether because of these aforementioned, ambiguous management issues. In the future, testing for telomerase, p53, and other markers may further customize or refine management for a particular patient.

The Future

The human genome has been sequenced far ahead of schedule. As of May 2001, there are still some significant

---

Table 56–1. Clinically Important Microorganisms for Which Polymerase Chain Reaction is Routinely Employed

Bacteria	Viruses
Haemophilus influenzae	HIV 1 and 2
Treponema pallidum	Herpesviruses 1 and 2
Mycoplasma genitalium	Varicella virus
Mycoplasma fermentas	Cytomegalovirus
Chlamydia trachomatis	Hepatitis viruses A/B/C/D/E/F/G
	Parvovirus B19
	Human papillomavirus

Other
Toxoplasmosis

gaps that the National Human Genome Research Institute (NHGRI) and Celera will need to fill in. What we do know is that instead of the 150,000 to 200,000 genes postulated at the beginning of the project, the human genome contains a paltry 30,000, interrupted by huge tracts of meaningless genetic material—repeats, ancient incorporated viral genomes, pseudogenes. How then do we explain both the complexity of the human organism and the myriad of diseases that afflict us? The answer lies in two places. The first is the subtle sequence changes or variations that exist between individuals. When combined with perhaps other subtle genetic sequence variations, these differences may result in profound changes in biologic behavior. The second place is at the protein level: posttranslation modification of a single transcribed gene, through either activation by phosphorylation or variant splicing, can result in a whole host of different though related proteins with each potentially involved in a different cellular pathway.

Oligonucleotide sequencing arrays may prove to be a breakthrough method for sequencing genes of interest.

Although there are several different techniques for sequencing on a DNA chip, the approach currently used the most is the loss-of-signal approach. In this technique, sequence variations are evaluated by quantitating relative losses of hybridization signal to perfect-match oligonucleotide probes in test samples relative to wild-type reference targets. Ideally, a homozygous sequence change results in complete loss of hybridization signal to perfect-match probes interrogating the region surrounding the sequence change.

For heterozygous sequence variation, a 50% loss of signal intensity relative to the wild-type target would ideally be found for perfect-match probe signal interrogating and flanking the sequence change. Loss-of-signal analysis allows for a practical screen to be set up for virtually every sequence variation. With this approach, an array designed to interrogate both target strands of N base pairs, for all possible sequence changes, minimally consists of two $2N$ overlapping probes. For example, an array of 11,000 oligonucleotides would be needed to screen the 5.5 kb of

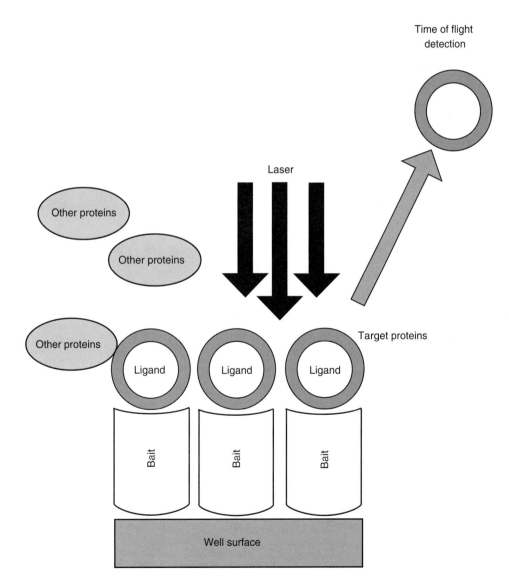

Figure 56–12. SELDI (surface-enhanced laser desorption ionization) protein chip.

BRCA1 for all possible sequence variations.[43] A disadvantage of this approach is that traditional sequencing is still required to come up with the exact genetic change. But this can be done much faster, more accurately, and for less cost, once the area has been localized. Although there are many issues unresolved at present, DNA chip technology may prove to be a powerful tool in the future.

Another potentially powerful platform for diagnostic analysis addresses the protein expression profile of a patient's specimen—the SELDI protein chip (surface enhanced laser desorption ionization). This array-type system allows proteins to be analyzed at femtomole levels directly from their native environments (e.g., amniotic fluid, ascites) (Fig. 56–12). Proteins of interest are directly applied to 1 of 24 wells on an aluminum support. These well surfaces are purchased precoated with a defined chemical "bait" matrix comprising standard chromatographic separations (e.g., hydrophobic, cationic, anionic), or, in the near future, biochemical bait molecules such as purified ligands, receptors, antibodies, or DNA oligonucleotides.

The proteins applied to the well selectively bind to the bait molecules. Unbound proteins are then washed off the well. The remaining proteins are then ionized off the surface of the well by a laser and analyzed by a time-of-flight mass spectrometer. Protein techniques have distinct advantages over their molecular counterparts. First, no amplification step is needed. Second, because the proteins are the actual affector units of a cell, we can more accurately determine what is being expressed in a given sample. Lastly, proteins are more robust than RNA, enabling better preservation and storage. Perhaps in the next edition of this book, the chapter will be entitled "Molecular Proteomics."

References

1. Mullis KB: The unusual origin of the polymerase chain reaction. Sci Am 1990; 262:36–43.
2. Saiki RK, Scharf S, Faloona F, Mullis KB: Enzymatic amplification of beta-globin genomic sequences and restriction site analysis for diagnosis of sickle cell anemia. Science 1985; 230:1350–1354.
3. Saiki RK, Gelfand DH, Stoffel S, Scharf SJ: Primer-directed enzymatic amplification of DNA with a thermostable DNA polymerase. Science 1988; 239:387–491.
4. Sunderland GR: Fragile sites on human chromosomes: Demonstration of their dependence on the type of tissue culture media. Science 1977; 197:265–267.
5. Verkerk AJMH, Pieretti M, Sutcliff JS, et al: Identification of a gene (FMR-1) containing a CCG repeat coincident with breakpoint cluster region exhibiting length variation in fragile X syndrome. Cell 1991; 65:905–914.
6. Oberle I, Rosseau F, Heitz D, et al: Instability of a 550-base pair DNA segment and abnormal methylation in fragile X syndrome. Science 1991; 252:1097–1102.
7. Sutcliff JS, Nelson DJ, Zhang F, et al: DNA methylation represses FMR-1 transcription in fragile X syndrome. Hum Mol Genet 1992; 1:397–400.
8. Hecimovic S, Barisic I, Muller A, et al: Expand long PCR for fragile X mutation detection. Clin Genet 1997; 52:147–154.
9. Huntington's Disease Collaborative Research Group: A novel gene containing a trinucleotide repeat that is expanded and unstable on Huntington's disease chromosomes. Cell 1993; 72:971–983.
10. Beggs AH, Koenig M, Boyce FM, et al: Detection of 98% of DMD/BMD gene deletions by PCR. Hum Genet 1990; 86:45–48.
11. The Cystic Fibrosis Genetic Analysis Consortium: Population variation of common cystic fibrosis mutations. Am J Hum Genet 1994; 54:443–446.
12. National Institutes of Health: Genetic testing for cystic fibrosis. (Consensus Statement No. 106). Bethesda, Md, NIH, 1997.
13. Rowley PT, Loader S, Kaplan RM: Prenatal screening for cystic fibrosis carriers: Can we afford it? Am J Hum Genet 1998; 63:A13.
14. Kuller J, Baughman R, Biolsi C: Cystic fibrosis and the NIH consensus statement: Are obstetrician-gynecologists ready to comply? Am J Hum Genet 1998; 63:A202.
15. Ridker PM, Hennekens CH, Lindpainter K, et al: Mutation in the gene encoding for coagulation factor V and the risk of myocardial infarction, stroke, and venous thrombosis in apparently healthy men. N Engl J Med 1995; 332:912–917.
16. Ridker PM, Miletich JP, Stampfer MJ, et al: Factor V Leiden and risks of recurrent idiopathic venous thromboembolism. Circulation 1995; 92:2800–2802.
17. Feder JN, Penny DM, Irrinki A, et al: The hemochromatosis gene product complexes with the transferrin receptor and lowers its affinity for ligand binding. Proc Natl Acad Sci U S A 1998; 95:1472–1477.
18. Parks SB, Popovich BW, Press RD: Real-time PCR with fluorescent hybridization probes for the detection of prevalent mutation causing common thrombophilic and iron overload phenotypes. Am J Clin Pathol 2001; 115:439–447.
19. Burke W, Thomson E, Khoury MJ, et al: Hereditary hemochromatosis: Gene discovery and its implication for population-based screening. JAMA 1998; 280:172–178.
20. Blackburn EH: Structure and function of telomeres. Nature 1991; 350:569–573.
21. Wynford-Thomas D, Kipling D: Cancer and the knockout mouse. Nature 1997; 389:551–552.
22. Shroyer KR, Thompson LC, Enomoto T, et al: Telomerase expression in normal epithelium, reactive atypia, squamous dysplasia and squamous cell carcinoma of the uterine cervix. Am J Clin Pathol 1998; 109:153–162.
23. Anderson S, Shera K, Ihle J, et al: Telomerase activation in cervical cancer. Am J Pathol 1997; 151:25–31.
24. Kyo S, Takakura M, Ishikawa H, et al: Application of the telomerase assay for the screening of cervical lesions. Cancer Res 1997; 57:1863–1867.
25. Yashima K, Ashfaq R, Nowak J, et al: Telomerase activity and expression of its RNA component in cervical lesions. Cancer 1998; 82:1319–1327.
26. Yakoyama Y, Takahasi Y, Shinohara A, et al: Telomerase activity in the female reproductive tract and neoplasms. Gynecol Oncol 1998; 68:145–149.
27. Shroyer KR, Stephens JK, Silverberg SG, et al: Telomerase expression in normal endometrium, endometrial hyperplasia, and endometrial adenocarcinoma. Int J Gynecol Pathol 1997; 16:225–232.
28. Brian TP, Kallakury BVS, Lowry CV, et al: Telomerase activity in benign endometrium and endometrial carcinoma. Cancer Res 1997; 57:2760–2764.
29. Oishi T, Kigawa J, Minagawa Y, et al: Alteration of telomerase activity associated with development and extension of epithelial ovarian cancer. Obstet Gynecol 1998; 91:568–571.
30. Kim NW, Piatyszek MA, Prowse KR, et al: Specific association of human telomerase activity in immortal cells and cancer. Science 1994; 266:2011–2015.
31. De Potter CR, Schelhout AM, Verbeeck P, et al: Neu overexpression correlates with extent of disease in large cell ductal in situ carcinoma of the breast. Hum Pathol 1995; 26:601–606.
32. Haffty BG, Brown F, Carter D, et al: Evaluation of Her-2/neu oncoprotein in expression as a prognostic indicator of local recurrence in conservatively treated breast cancer: A case control study. Int J Radiat Oncol Biol Phys 1996; 35:751–757.
33. Bower FT, Ahmed S, Tartter P, et al: Prognostic variables in invasive breast cancer: Contribution of comedo versus non-comedo in-situ component. Ann Surg Oncol 1995; 2:440–444.
34. Zafrani B, Leroyer A, Fourquet A, et al: Mammographically detected ductal in-situ carcinoma of the breast analyzed with a new classification. Semin Diag Pathol 1994; 11:208–214.
35. Archer SG, Eliopoulis SA, Spandidos D, et al: Expression of ras, p21, p53 and C-erb B2 in advanced breast cancer and response to line hormonal therapy. Br J Cancer 1995; 72:1259–1266.

36. Yu D, Liu B, Tan M, et al: Overexpression of c-erbB-2/neu in breast cancer cell lines confers increased resistance to Taxol via mdr-1-independent mechanisms. Oncogene 1996; 13:1359–1365.

37. Muss HB, Thor AD, Berry DA, et al: C erb-B2 expression and response to adjuvant therapy in women with node positive early breast cancer. N Engl J Med 1994; 330:1260–1266.

38. Baselga J, Tripathy D, Mendelsohn J, et al: Phase II study of weekly intravenous recombinant humanized anti p185 Her-2 monoclonal antibody in patients with her-2/neu over expressing metastatic breast cancer. J Clin Oncol 1996; 14:737–744.

39. Schiffman MH, Bauer HM, Hoover RN, et al: Epidemiologic evidence showing that human papillomavirus infection causes most cervical intraepithelial neoplasia. J Natl Cancer Inst 1993; 85:958–964.

40. Walboomers JM, Jacobs MV, Manos MM, et al: Human papillomavirus is a necessary cause of invasive cervical cancer worldwide. J Pathol 1998; 189:12–19.

41. Wilkinson ES, Malik S, et al: J Womens Health 1998; 7:604–605.

42. Ackerman S: The abnormal pap smear, what your gynecologist isn't telling you. Sexual Health 1997; 1:58–63.

43. Hacia JG, Brody LC, Chee MS, et al: Detection of heterozygous mutations in BRCA1 using high density oligonucleotide arrays and two color fluorescence analysis. Nature Genet 1996; 14:441–447.

Selective Estrogen Receptor Modulators in the Long-term Management of Postmenopausal Women

Ira H. Mickelson

As early as the 1950s, the process of progressive bone loss, osteoporosis, and its relationship to estrogen deficiency were identified. It was considered the medical breakthrough of the decade when it was discovered that calcium ingestion and exercise alone were insufficient and that the addition of a catalytic dose of estrogen produced a regression of the osteoporotic process. When patients began relating a cessation of vasomotor symptoms while on the medication, it was considered an unexpected beneficial side effect. It was not until the late 1970s that a causal relationship between unopposed estrogen and endometrial hyperplasia and cancer was noted. After a moratorium on the use of estrogen replacement therapy, the addition of a progestational agent for the stabilization of the endometrium became commonplace. Over the next several years, there were few major changes in the clinical management of menopause. Cyclic estrogen and progestin, along with calcium and exercise, became the standard treatment of choice.[1-3] Great advances were made in the areas of modes of delivery and patient convenience. Alternative dosing regimens were identified. Transdermal preparations of estrogens and progestins were found to be effective. Natural sources of both estrogen and progesterone became available.[4]

Despite all of this and the many documented benefits of estrogen replacement therapy, compliance remains a significant problem. Many women refuse or discontinue estrogen therapy. Studies show that less than half of all women who are potentially eligible are prescribed estrogen, less than half of all women who are prescribed estrogen fill the prescription, and less than half of all women who start estrogen are still on the medication after 1 year.[5] The primary reasons for estrogen discontinuation are perceived cancer risks (primarily breast and uterine cancer) and adverse side effects. These side effects include vaginal bleeding, return of menses, breast pain and tenderness, headaches, weight gain, nausea, bloating, and edema. Recent advances in the mechanisms of action of these hormones and their receptors may have started us down the road to solving these problems.

ESTROGEN RECEPTOR MECHANISM

Multiple target organs have estrogen and progesterone receptors, including the breast, bone, cardiovascular system, uterus, and brain. Estrogens (and progesterone) have specific positive or negative effects on each of these target organs. The specificity of the reaction on tissues of sex steroid hormones (estrogen, progesterone, and androgen) is due to the presence of specific intracellular receptor proteins. The mechanism of action includes the following:

- Unbound steroid hormones are rapidly transported across the cell membrane through simple diffusion.
- The steroid hormone binds to its specific receptor protein, causing its activation as a hormone-receptor complex.
- The hormone-receptor complex interacts with the nuclear DNA to synthesize mRNA. The amount of mRNA synthesized depends on the dose and duration of exposure to the complex.
- The mRNA is transported to the ribosome where a protein is thus synthesized in the cytoplasm that results in specific cellular activity.

Antiestrogenic agents have been around since as early as 1958. Clomiphene citrate, an antiestrogen still commonly used today, was approved in 1967 for the treatment of ovulatory dysfunction. It was not until the late 1980s, however, that an agent was found that had a paradoxical effect: lowering the risk of breast cancer while increasing the risk of uterine cancer. This sent scientists scrambling for a suitable explanation. Only one was found: whereas throughout the previous decades, it was commonly believed that the estrogen receptors in the five target organs were identical, the only logical explanation was that there were differences in these receptors and their cellular responses.

An agonist is a substance that stimulates a response. An antagonist inhibits the actions of an agonist. In the original simple model, the role of estrogen was to bind to the receptor, switching it from an inactive to an active state. More recently, however, research in this area has suggested that estrogen receptor action is far more complex. Specifically, it has now been established that there are at least two estrogen receptors, that ligands differentially alter the biochemical properties of the receptor, and that the resulting ligand-receptor complex is not recognized in the same fashion by all cells.

Two different estrogen receptors have been identified thus far, designated estrogen receptor alpha (ER-α) and estrogen receptor beta (ER-β). ER-α was discovered in

1960 and its amino acid sequence identified in 1986. Its gene is located on chromosome 14 and is in close proximity to genes related to Alzheimer's disease. ER-β was not discovered until 1995. The shape of the hormone-receptor complex helps determine the exact message transmitted to the gene. Therefore, there are different responses when hormones bind to these two different sites. Estradiol, tamoxifen, and raloxifene all bind at the same site on the two receptors, but the subsequent shape of each is not identical, which contributes to the ultimate message of agonism or antagonism. Different concentrations and expressions of the ER-α and ER-β occur in different tissues. Human ovarian follicle granulosa cells contain only beta receptors; breast contains both; and some parts of the brain contain only alpha, some only beta, and still others both. In addition, the same estrogen binding to ER-α and ER-β can produce different effects. For example, estradiol can stimulate gene transcription with ER-α and inhibit gene transcription with ER-β in the same system. Also, different steroids exhibit different affinities toward the two receptor sites. Phytoestrogens, for example, have a greater affinity for ER-β than for ER-α. Different messages can therefore be determined by the specific combination of the particular steroid, the ER-α and ER-β concentrations, and the target organ's response. The identification of a second estrogen receptor, ER-β, is considered one of the most important discoveries in the understanding and advancement of hormone therapies.

THE SELECTIVE ESTROGEN RECEPTOR MODULATORS

Our greater understanding of the estrogen receptor mechanism allows us to understand how mixed estrogen agonists-antagonists can have selective actions on specific target tissues.[6-8] These estrogen agonist-antagonists make up an exciting new class of medications called *selective estrogen receptor modulators* (SERMs).[9] By virtue of variation in conformational changes in the drug-receptor complex and the cellular context of specific tissues, SERMs can be developed to produce beneficial effects in certain target systems (such as bone) and to avoid unwanted actions (such as endometrial stimulation). This new class of drugs represents an additional option for the prevention of osteoporosis and menopausal symptoms for postmenopausal women. New agents are currently being developed in an effort to isolate desired actions from unwanted side effects. We can expect to see new agents with progressively better agonist-antagonist profiles, yielding increasingly user-friendly drugs in the future. Thus far, two major subcategories of SERMs have been identified: the triphenylethylenes and the benzothiophenes. Both display a mixed estrogen agonist-antagonist profile. They bind to estrogen receptors with the same or higher affinity than estrogen itself. Once bound, however, they elicit a specific mixed agonist-antagonist response depending on the specific end-

target organ and the SERMs' specific molecular structure. When the SERM molecule binds to the estrogen receptor, the differences in their molecular structures induce diverse conformational changes in the receptor, which in turn cause variable tissue effects. These two major subgroups of SERMs have very different molecular structures and produce very different responses on each target organ.

The triphenylethylene derivatives include clomifene citrate, tamoxifen citrate, and tamoxifen derivatives such as toremifene, droloxifene, and idoxifene citrate. The triphenylethylene derivatives act as estrogen antagonists in breast tissue, as estrogen agonists in bone remodeling and lipid metabolism, and as partial estrogen agonists in endometrial tissue. Three triphenylethylene derivatives are currently in clinical use. Clomiphene citrate (Clomid, Serophene) was approved in 1967 for ovulatory dysfunction. Tamoxifen (Nolvadex) was first approved in 1977 for the treatment of advanced breast cancer and was subsequently approved as an adjuvant therapy for both node-positive and node-negative disease; in 1998, it received expanded approval for breast cancer prevention.[10] Toremifene (Fareston) was approved in 1997 for treatment of metastatic breast cancer in postmenopausal women with estrogen receptor-positive or unknown tumors.

The most widely studied and the first clinically available benzothiophene derivative is raloxifene hydrochloride (Evista).[11] Like the triphenylethylenes, raloxifene mimics the effects of estrogen on the skeleton and on serum lipids. It inhibits bone resorption and improves lipids (although there is no effect on high-density lipoprotein-cholesterol [HDL-C]). Raloxifene, however, acts as a complete estrogen antagonist in both the breast and the endometrium. Like tamoxifen, raloxifene originally was investigated as a treatment for advanced breast cancer. In preclinical studies, raloxifene was found to have antiproliferation effects on estrogen receptor–positive human breast cancer cell lines and antitumor activity similar to that of tamoxifen. However, in a small phase-2 trial in postmenopausal women with advanced breast cancer in whom tamoxifen therapy had failed, raloxifene showed no additional antitumor effects.[12] Based on this study, further research on raloxifene as a breast cancer chemotherapeutic agent ceased. Subsequently, raloxifene was studied for its skeletal effects and was approved for osteoporosis prevention in postmenopausal women in December of 1997.

Let us examine in further detail the effect of tamoxifen and raloxifene on each of the major sex steroid target organs: breast, bone, cardiovascular system, uterus (gynecologic pelvic organs), and brain (vasomotor).

Tamoxifen

Breast

With over 25 years of study, tamoxifen has been extensively researched as a medication for treatment and prevention of breast cancer. It was initially approved in 1977 for the treatment of advanced metastatic breast cancer in postmenopausal women.[13, 14] In 1985, tamoxifen was approved as an adjuvant therapy with chemotherapy in postmenopausal patients with earlier, nonmetastatic disease,[15, 16] and, in 1986, it was approved for use alone.[17, 18] By 1989, approval was obtained for the use of tamoxifen in premenopausal women and extended to include node-negative estrogen receptor–positive breast cancer in 1990. Many studies conclusively support these claims.[19, 20] An update of a meta-analysis conducted by the Early Breast Cancer Trialists Collaborative Group studied more than 37,000 women with operable breast cancer treated with adjuvant tamoxifen therapy with a median follow-up of 10 years.[21] This review concluded that tamoxifen significantly improved survival. After 5 years of tamoxifen therapy, women with estrogen receptor–positive tumors (approximately 70% of all breast cancers) had reductions in recurrence and death with tamoxifen treatment compared with placebo by 47% and 26%, respectively. These benefits increased with duration of treatment. The results of several large clinical trials show little or no benefit in women with estrogen receptor–negative tumors.[22]

Three major studies examine the relationship between tamoxifen and the treatment and prevention of breast cancer in women. The National Surgical Adjuvant Breast and Bowel Project (NSABP) Tamoxifen Breast Cancer Prevention Trial was launched in 1992 in the United States.[23] The study enrolled 13,388 women over the age of 35 years with various stages of breast cancer and various degrees of breast cancer risk. Trial results were released in April 1998 because of the overwhelming evidence of tamoxifen's efficacy.[23] Tamoxifen was found to reduce the incidence of invasive and noninvasive breast cancer by an average of 49%. Tamoxifen also reduced breast cancer risk in women with a history of lobular carcinoma in situ by 56% and atypical hyperplasia by 86%. In addition, tamoxifen decreased the occurrence of estrogen receptor–positive tumors by 69% and reduced the risk of breast cancer in high-risk pre- and postmenopausal women. Tamoxifen had no impact on the incidence of estrogen receptor–negative tumors in this study.

Two European tamoxifen breast cancer prevention trials (the Royal Marsden Hospital Trial in the United Kingdom[24] and the Italian Tamoxifen Prevention Study[25]) were begun at approximately the same time as the NSABP study. Interestingly enough, neither study confirmed the NSABP findings for the reduction of the risk of breast cancer in high-risk pre- and postmenopausal women. After much deliberation, it was believed that there were some inherent flaws in these two European studies.[26] They were both smaller trials than the United States study, and the Italian study recruited participants from the general population with a lower overall risk of breast cancer. In addition, compliance rates in the Italian study were quite low. Despite the results of these two studies, the U.S. Food and Drug Administration approved the use of tamoxifen for the primary prevention of breast cancer in women at high risk for breast

cancer in 1998. The use of tamoxifen is limited to high-risk women because of the potentially serious side effects such as endometrial cancer and deep vein thrombosis. In order to help clinicians identify the high-risk population, the National Cancer Institute has developed a computer program that uses the Gail model to determine a woman's 5-year and lifetime risks for developing breast cancer.[27] This model takes into account nulliparity, age at menarche, age at first live birth, preexisting benign and malignant breast biopsies, and family history of breast cancer in calculating a woman's risk for breast cancer. Copies of this computer software can be obtained from the tamoxifen manufacturer.

There has been much recent debate as to the optimal length of tamoxifen therapy. Although it is easy to extrapolate that "if 5 years is good, 10 must be better," some studies have not shown this to be true.[28, 29] One must remember that tamoxifen is both an estrogen agonist and an estrogen antagonist. It appears that by 10 years of therapy, the risk of breast cancer begins to rise. For this reason, the optimal treatment duration recommended for tamoxifen at this time is 5 years.

Bone

Because the last 2 decades of tamoxifen research has primarily focused on its relationship to breast cancer, the data on its skeletal effects are more limited, coming primarily from randomized trials of breast cancer treatment or prevention.[30] Animal studies have shown that although tamoxifen has minimal effect on new bone deposition, it reduces bone resorption and overall bone turnover.[31] Several small human studies have found that women receiving tamoxifen showed a significant decrease in bone resorption as measured by pyridinoline and deoxypyridinoline levels.[32, 33] These levels returned to baseline values after therapy was discontinued.

Studies in breast cancer patients suggest that tamoxifen improves bone mineral density (BMD) by approximately 1% to 2% in the hip and spine.[34] This increase, however, is lower than the reported 4% to 8% increases in hip and spine BMD observed with estrogen. There is much debate as to whether BMD is the proper diagnostic test to assess the relative efficaciousness of estrogen, raloxifene, or tamoxifen therapy. There is a strong correlation between baseline BMD measurement before initiating therapy and fracture risk. Despite the differences in BMD, however, alendronate, estrogen, calcitonin, tamoxifen, and raloxifene all appear to reduce the risk for vertebral fractures by approximately 50% during the course of treatment. The Breast Cancer Prevention Trial (BCPT)[23] assessed the effect of tamoxifen therapy on the risk for clinically diagnosed wrist, hip, and spine fractures. In this 5-year study, hip and spine fractures were reduced by 45% and 26%, respectively. Ongoing analyses are currently seeking to clarify the relationship among reductions in bone turnover, changes in bone density, and fracture risk reduction.

Interestingly, the Framingham Study and the Prospective Study of Osteoporosis Fractures[35] found that women with lower bone density are at lower risk for breast cancer. This presumably reflects the paradoxical effects of estrogenic activity on different target organs. Theoretically, women with higher bone density have higher estriol levels, and the higher the long-term exposure to these higher circulating estriol levels, the greater the risk for breast cancer.

Cardiovascular System

As with bone density and fractures, studies of the effects of tamoxifen on the risk of coronary heart disease (CHD) primarily involved women with breast cancer.[36] Tamoxifen has been found to have a favorable impact on lipid profiles in postmenopausal women. Although most studies have shown no increase in HDL-C, many note a decrease in total serum cholesterol, fibrinogen levels, and lipoprotein(a) levels in patients treated with tamoxifen.[37]

Three large, randomized, controlled trials[38–40] found that tamoxifen used for the treatment of breast cancer also reduced the incidence of fatal and nonfatal myocardial infarction. The NSABP, the Scottish Cancer Trials Breast Group, and the Stockholm Breast Cancer Study Group conducted them.[41] Owing to a paucity of research, however, the long-term effects of tamoxifen on the cardiovascular system are still essentially unknown. In fact, meta-analysis[42] showed no significant reduction in cardiovascular mortality among patients treated with tamoxifen. Further clinical studies are needed in this area.

Uterus

Like all SERMs, tamoxifen acts as both an estrogen agonist and an estrogen antagonist, depending on the target organ receptors. Despite its use since the 1970s, however, it was not until the late 1980s that those cases of endometrial cancer in patients receiving tamoxifen were first reported.[43] Since that time, tamoxifen has been shown to have a stimulatory effect on the endometrium similar to that of estrogen in both laboratory and clinical trial studies. Clinical trials in women with breast cancer have confirmed that tamoxifen induces endometrial cellular proliferation and increases a woman's relative risk of developing uterine cancer two- to threefold.[44] This increased risk does not appear to be dose dependent, but it is time dependent. One and 2 years of tamoxifen use doubled the incidence of endometrial cancer and 5 years quadrupled the incidence.[45]

The largest study investigating the association between endometrial cancer and tamoxifen is the NSABP B-14 trial.[46] This prospective randomized trial followed over 4000 women with invasive breast cancer on either tamoxifen or placebo. Two cases of endometrial cancer occurred in the placebo group whereas 23 cases of endometrial cancer and 4 deaths due to endometrial cancer were noted in the tamoxifen group, with a relative risk of 7.5. The NSABP prevention trials confirmed those of the treatment trial in over 13,000 women at high risk for breast cancer. Several smaller studies, utilizing ultrasound, hysteroscopy, and biopsy specimens, have also found an unusually high incidence (up to 30%) of both polyps and hyperplastic changes in tamoxifen-treated women, along with the overall increase in the incidence of endometrial cancer.[47]

When the general population incidence of uterine cancer was taken into account, however, it was noted that the annual rate of endometrial cancer among tamoxifen users was still quite low: 1.6 per 1000 as compared with 1.4 per 1000 in women not on tamoxifen. During the first decade of tamoxifen use, it was estimated the cumulative risk was 2 deaths per 1000 women.[44] In addition, most studies indicated that endometrial tumors in breast cancer patients who receive tamoxifen were less aggressive than tumors in women who did not receive tamoxifen.[48, 49] From these results, the authors of the NSABP B-14 trials concluded that the net benefit of tamoxifen therapy, both therapeutically in women with breast cancer and prophylactically in high-risk women, greatly outweighs the risk for endometrial cancer.[46]

Unfortunately, data from prospective clinical trials are insufficient to provide definitive guidelines about appropriate endometrial follow-up evaluation for women taking tamoxifen. A set of recommendations was developed by the American College of Obstetricians and Gynecologists (ACOG) for breast cancer patients receiving tamoxifen therapy.[50] As of this date, there are no guidelines for the use of tamoxifen for prevention of breast cancer. The ACOG recommendations are as follows:

- Perform annual gynecologic examinations on women with breast cancer, including Pap tests and bimanual and rectovaginal examinations.
- Thoroughly evaluate abnormal bleeding, including bloody discharge, spotting, or any other gynecologic symptoms. Investigate any bleeding or spotting by biopsy.
- Be alert to the increased incidence of endometrial malignancy. Screening procedures or diagnostic tests should be performed at the discretion of the individual gynecologist.
- Closely monitor women without breast cancer who are being treated with tamoxifen within a chemopreventive trial for the development of endometrial hyperplasia or cancer.
- If atypical hyperplasia develops, discontinue use of tamoxifen and institute dilatation and curettage or other appropriate gynecologic management within an approximate interval.
- If tamoxifen therapy must be continued, consider hysterectomy in women with atypical endometrial hyperplasia.
- Tamoxifen use may be reinstituted after hysterectomy for endometrial carcinoma with consultation with the physician responsible for the woman's breast care.
- Transvaginal ultrasonography may be a useful, noninva-

sive tool for assessing endometrial pathology in women receiving tamoxifen therapy. Endometrial thickness of less than 5 mm, as assessed by this technique, has been shown to correlate with the absence of significant endometrial tissue on biopsy. Biopsy would be required only if endometrial thickness is 5 mm or greater. Saline infusion into the uterus during the procedure may increase the accuracy of transvaginal ultrasonography.

Central Nervous System/Other

One of the beneficial side effects of estrogen is its ability to relieve vasomotor symptoms. These include hot flushes, insomnia, fatigue, depression, and anxiety. Tamoxifen bears no such claim. Not only are vasomotor symptoms not relieved by tamoxifen, there also seems to be an increase in hot flushes in approximately 20% of women. This seems to be more prevalent in women who have just recently gone through the menopausal changes and significantly less common in women who are many years postmenopausal.

In addition to relieving vasomotor symptoms, estrogen tends to have beneficial side effects on vaginal lubrication, bladder irritation and urethral syndrome, and skin changes. Although the majority of these are unaffected by tamoxifen, vaginal discharge is listed as a known side effect and may have a beneficial effect on vaginal dryness.[10] On the other hand, breast swelling and tenderness, which seems to be a major complaint with estrogen, does not seem to be of significance with tamoxifen usage.

Raloxifene

Breast

Once the focus of raloxifene shifted from a medication for the treatment of breast cancer to one for the treatment of osteoporosis, the majority of raloxifene research took the same course.[51] Therefore, the majority of the data available on raloxifene details its beneficial effects on the bone.[52-54] The original and subsequent research, however, do show that raloxifene reduced the incidence of primary breast cancers.[55] In animal studies, raloxifene inhibits growth of breast cancers and antagonizes the mitogenic effects of both estrogen and tamoxifen in the uterus.[56] The Multiple Outcomes of Raloxifene Evaluation (MORE) trial[57] examined the clinical relationship between raloxifene and breast cancer.

Published in the *Journal of the American Medical Association* (JAMA) on June 16, 1999, the MORE trial[58] was a randomized, double-blind trial, in which women taking raloxifene or placebo were followed up for a median of 40 months from 1994 through 1998. A group of 7705 postmenopausal women younger than 81 years (average age, 66.5 years) with osteoporosis were followed primarily for BMD and vertebral fractures. In addition, they were

evaluated for new cases of breast cancer, endometrial abnormalities (evaluated by transvaginal ultrasound in 1781 women), deep vein thrombosis, pulmonary embolus, cognitive function, quality of life, and lipid metabolism. Thirteen new cases of breast cancer were identified in 5129 women on raloxifene as compared with 27 new cases in 2576 women on placebo. This translates to a relative risk of 0.24, or a decreased risk of estrogen receptor–positive breast cancer by 90%. There was no statistical difference in patients with estrogen receptor–negative breast cancer. There was a threefold increased risk of venous thromboembolic disease, but no increase in uterine cancer. The MORE study concluded that among postmenopausal women with osteoporosis, the risk of invasive breast cancer was decreased by 76% during 3 years of treatment with raloxifene.

Because raloxifene has not been studied directly as a breast cancer prophylactic (thus far, skeletal effects have been the primary end point in the majority of studies), several issues have yet to be addressed. Because malignant breast tumors require a relatively long period of time to progress from an abnormal cell to a clinically detectable mass, the impact of a specific drug treatment may reflect growth deceleration of a preexisting tumor, not causation or prevention. Still unknown is whether the preventive effects of raloxifene will be sustained in the long term. Because the SERMs are both agonists and antagonists and metastatic breast cancer has already been shown to develop resistance to tamoxifen after long-term exposure, the long-term breast effects of raloxifene must be determined. Other questions yet to be answered on the relationship between raloxifene and breast cancer are the efficacy of raloxifene as preventive therapy in women at increased risk for breast cancer, its effectiveness in younger postmenopausal women, and the overall risk-benefit ratio for raloxifene.

Bone

Raloxifene has been studied extensively for its skeletal effects and was approved in December 1997 for the prevention of osteoporosis.[59] Raloxifene reduces bone absorption by inhibiting the formation and action of osteoclasts and thereby decreasing overall bone turnover.[60] As stated previously, the MORE trial was primarily designed to determine whether raloxifene reduced fracture risk among women who already have osteoporosis.[61] Launched in 1994, this ongoing study is examining the effects of raloxifene (60 to 120 mg/day) on BMD and vertebral fractures in postmenopausal osteoporotic women. All the women received supplemental calcium (500 mg/day) and vitamin D (400 IU/day). When the first 2 years of data were evaluated, it was noted that the women taking raloxifene had approximately a 1% to 2% greater increase in bone density in the hip and spine than the placebo-treated women. There was also a decrease in the number of vertebral fractures by approximately 50%. This effect is similar to those reported for estrogen and alendronate sodium.

Raloxifene was associated with a reduction in vertebral fractures of nearly 50% after only 2 years of treatment. In addition, osteoporotic postmenopausal women treated with raloxifene for up to 2.5 years had significant increases in bone density.

Cardiovascular System

In both preclinical animal models and clinical studies, raloxifene has been found to exhibit favorable effects on lipid profiles, coagulation factors, and vascular endothelium similar to those of estrogen that may reduce the risk of CHD.[62, 63] In a 2-year randomized trial with monkeys,[64] raloxifene exerted no protection against coronary artery atherosclerosis despite changes in circulating lipids similar to those achieved in women. However, a combination of actions (antioxidant activity, some beneficial effects on lipids, a reduction in homocysteine levels) makes it likely that there will be some favorable impact on the human cardiovascular system. In several human clinical trials,[63, 65] raloxifene reduced serum cholesterol, lipoprotein(a), and fibrinogen levels along with low-density lipoprotein (LDL). However, unlike estrogen, which raises HDL-C and triglycerides, raloxifene has a mixed effect on both HDL-C and triglycerides. The reduction in fibrinogen level with raloxifene was greater than that observed with estrogen in the Postmenopausal Estrogen/Progestin Interventions (PEPI) Trial.[2, 3] The most serious adverse effect of raloxifene treatment is a 2% to 3% increase in the risk of DVT and pulmonary embolism.[11] This risk is comparable with that associated with postmenopausal estrogen therapy and hormone replacement therapy.

It is not yet known whether the beneficial effects of raloxifene on cholesterol, LDL, lipoprotein(a), and fibrinogen levels will translate to a reduction in myocardial infarctions and an improvement in cardiac risk for the women on the drug. Additional data regarding the long-term effects of raloxifene on CHD risk are needed before decisions regarding the benefits and risks of raloxifene therapy and its ultimate role in enhancing the cardiovascular health of postmenopausal women can be made. The Raloxifene Use for the Heart (RUTH) Trial[66] is a large, prospective, randomized cardiovascular outcomes study that will investigate the effects of raloxifene in women, both with CHD and at high risk for CHD risk factors. Beginning in 1998, approximately 10,000 postmenopausal women over age 55 years will be enrolled, with the results expected by 2005.

Uterus

Laboratory studies in rats have shown that raloxifene has minimal estrogen agonist activity in the uterus and does not cause increases in uterine weight or stimulation of endothelial cell height.[51] In fact, raloxifene actually has a unique ability to block uterine stimulation induced by estrogen and tamoxifen.[67] It can completely antagonize the uterine stimulatory effects of both estrogen and tamoxifen.

Clinical data also suggest that raloxifene's endometrial profile is significantly different from that of tamoxifen.[68] Raloxifene does not stimulate endometrial tissue or increase the risk of endometrial cancer. In contrast to estrogen and tamoxifen, multiple clinical studies show that raloxifene produces no histopathologic evidence of endometrial stimulation.[12] Raloxifene has even been shown to have less stimulatory effect on the endometrium than a combination of estrogen and progestin. Although the numbers were small, in the first 3 years of the MORE trial,[57] raloxifene did not increase the risk of endometrial cancer. Uterine cancer was found in 0.2% of the placebo group and in 0.25% of the raloxifene group. A meta-analysis from raloxifene osteoporosis prevention and treatment trials involving approximately 12,000 postmenopausal women suggested that raloxifene not only does not increase the risk of endometrial cancer but also may actually reduce the risk of the disease.[57] The overall relative risk in this analysis was 0.38. When two cases diagnosed with 1 month of randomization are excluded, the estimated relative risk is 0.13.

Central Nervous System/Other

As with tamoxifen, there is a paucity of data on the relationship between raloxifene and vasomotor symptoms. As with tamoxifen, not only are vasomotor symptoms not relieved by raloxifene, there also appears to be an increase in hot flushes in approximately 20% of postmenopausal women.[11, 69] This also seems to be more prevalent in women who have just recently gone through the menopausal changes and significantly less common in women who are several years postmenopausal.[70]

Although the primary objective of the MORE study was to study the effects of raloxifene on osteoporosis, secondary end points included quality of life, hot flushes, insomnia, fatigue, depression, and anxiety. In this study, hot flashes, flu syndromes, edema, and leg cramps were slightly higher in the raloxifene group over placebo.[57] Of the raloxifene group, 0.6% quit the medication early as compared with only 0.1% of the placebo group. Raloxifene has no effect on vaginal lubrication, bladder irritation, urethral syndrome, and skin changes.[71] Like tamoxifen, raloxifene also lists vaginal discharge as a known side effect and may have a beneficial effect on vaginal dryness. Compared with placebo, there was no change in diabetes mellitus, hypertension, hypercholesterolemia, hematuria, or bradycardia. In its favor, and of clinical importance to many postmenopausal women, raloxifene exhibits less vaginal bleeding and less breast pain, swelling, and tenderness compared with estrogen.

Comparisons of Tamoxifen and Raloxifene

Women's fear of developing breast cancer guides some of their most important health-related decisions.[72, 73] Concern about the link between estrogen and breast cancer is a primary reason why the vast majority of women in the United States never initiate postmenopausal estrogen therapy or discontinue it after they start.[74] Because of the apparent breast safety and ability to block the stimulatory effects of estrogen on the breast while preserving its favorable impact on other tissues, SERMs may prove to be an attractive and viable option for many postmenopausal women who otherwise would not use preventive hormone therapy.[75]

Despite all of the documented benefits of estrogen replacement therapy, many women refuse or discontinue estrogen therapy. Studies show that fewer than half of all women who would benefit from hormone therapy are given the medication by their health care professional, half of those who are prescribed estrogen actually fill the prescription, and fewer than half of all women who start estrogen are still on the medication after 1 year.[5] The primary reasons for estrogen discontinuation are perceived cancer risks (primarily breast and uterine cancer). The SERMs, both tamoxifen and raloxifene, have been reported to reduce the incidence of breast cancer within 2 to 3 years of treatment. In addition to the fear of malignancies, many women discontinue use of the estrogens because of the adverse side effects. These side effects include vaginal bleeding, return of menses, breast pain and tenderness, headaches, weight gain, nausea, bloating, and edema. The SERMs may therefore prove to be a more acceptable longterm choice for some postmenopausal women. Precisely how these two SERMs fit into a comprehensive strategy for disease prevention in women remains to be determined.

Currently, tamoxifen is indicated for breast cancer treatment and for prophylaxis in women at increased risk for the disease, whereas raloxifene is approved for osteoporosis prevention in postmenopausal women.[10, 11] As discussed previously, the SERMs have been noted to have various effects, both beneficial and detrimental, on most of the other estrogen receptor–positive target organs. Unfortunately, it takes years to document the effects of hormones on the various target organs in the human model. Each study proposed to bring us closer to a fuller understanding of the SERMs takes many years to propose, organize, finance, and complete. As studies begin to accumulate on the other effects of the SERMs, we note significant similarities and differences in their actions. Both appear to have similar favorable effects on the breast and the skeletal and cardiovascular systems whereas their major difference seems to be in the uterus.

Breast

Raloxifene reduced the risk of newly diagnosed invasive breast cancer by 76% during a median 40 months of treatment in the MORE trial.[57] The BCPT found that a median of 55 months of treatment with tamoxifen decreased the general risk of invasive breast cancer by nearly 50%, and of estrogen receptor–positive breast cancer by nearly 70%.[23] Although it appears that raloxifene reduces the risk of breast cancer more than tamoxifen does, these two studies cannot be directly compared. Women in the BCPT were, on average, at higher risk for breast cancer and were younger than the subjects in the MORE study. The incidence of symptoms associated with stimulatory effects on breast tissue, including pain or tenderness, among raloxifene-treated women is similar to that of tamoxifen and virtually indistinguishable from women receiving placebo. The breast effects of tamoxifen have been much more extensively studied.

One critical piece of information missing with raloxifene is its long-term effects on the breast. It was not until tamoxifen was in widespread clinical use for over 2 decades that it was noted that 5 years was the optimal time for breast cancer protection and that 10 years of therapy actually produced a breast cancer stimulatory effect and was detrimental. Tamoxifen's usefulness for cardioprotection and osteoporosis therapy is therefore limited by its recommended 5-year duration of therapy. Research and time will tell whether raloxifene is under the same longterm constraints as tamoxifen.[76]

Bone

Raloxifene and tamoxifen both improve bone density by slowing bone turnover. Research on the SERMs has focused on their effects on bone mineral densities.[59, 60] The ultimate goal of antiresorptive therapies is to prevent fractures, regardless of whether individuals being treated are at risk for osteoporosis (primary prevention of fractures) or have already been diagnosed with the disease (secondary prevention of fractures). Reports indicate that 2 years of raloxifene treatment reduces the risk for vertebral fractures by approximately 50% in women who have osteoporosis. Preliminary data on tamoxifen's effects on the bone are similar, with a 50% reduction in vertebral fractures. Longer-term treatment with SERMs might also reduce the risk for nonspine fractures. The skeletal effects of raloxifene have been more extensively studied than those of tamoxifen.

Cardiovascular System

Postmenopausal women are highly vulnerable to CHD. The heart attack rate in the United States is 1.2 per 1000 for women under the age of 40 years. This number skyrockets to 22.4 per 1000 for women over the age of 50 years.[77] As a result, optimal strategies for maintaining postmenopausal health must include CHD prevention. These strategies include both lifestyle modification and pharmacologic agents (both hormonal and nonhormonal) for control of hyperlipidemia, diabetes, and hypertension. SERMs, like the estrogens, have a favorable impact on many lipid and vascular parameters believed to contribute to cardioprotection. Clinical trial data indicate that raloxifene has a positive effect on LDL, fibrinogen, and lipoprotein(a), but no effect on HDL-C.[54] Patients treated with tamoxifen have also been found to produce a decrease in total serum cholesterol, fibrinogen levels, and lipoprotein(a) levels but no increase in HDL-C.[36]

Many questions remain unanswered. The ultimate goal of improving the cardiovascular health of postmenopausal women, however, has yet to be clarified. Large, randomized, clinical trials are currently under way to evaluate the cardioprotective value of estrogen, progestins, and the SERMs. Some of these studies are evaluating the effects of estrogen and hormone replacement therapy on CHD, whereas others are srudying tamoxifen's and raloxifene's effect on CHD.[78] The conclusive results of these trials will not be available for several years.

It is important to note that both SERMs increase the risk of thromboembolic disease similar to that of estrogen. In addition, the Heart and Estrogen/Progestin Replacement Study (HERS)[79] results have caused concern regarding the adverse effect of hormone replacement therapy on women with preexisting CHD. It is not known whether the HERS results are applicable to women without existing CHD or whether the SERMs have similar effects. Certain progestins, such as medroxyprogesterone acetate, have been found to blunt the beneficial effects of estrogen on lipid levels. The role of natural progesterone with estrogen therapy, as opposed to a progestin, has yet to be clarified. Raloxifene's ability to be used without concomitant progestin may prove to be an added advantage in its cardioprotective actions.

Uterus

Tamoxifen and raloxifene produce similar estrogen-like properties on the bone and heart. In addition, they both seem to produce antiestrogen-like properties on breast tissue. In the uterus, however, tamoxifen and raloxifene diverge in their pharmacologic effects. Tamoxifen behaves as a partial estrogen agonist, increasing the risk of endometrial cancer, whereas raloxifene acts as a complete estrogen antagonist, possibly even increasing the risk of endometrial cancer. Tamoxifen acts as both an estrogen agonist and an estrogen antagonist in the uterus. It stimulates endometrial tissue and also incompletely blocks the stimulatory effects of estrogen. As a result, tamoxifen has the potential to induce endometrial abnormalities, including adenocarcinoma. In contrast to tamoxifen, raloxifene has no significant stimulatory effect on endometrial tissue, even at high doses. It completely blocks the stimulatory effects of both estrogen and tamoxifen. Clinical trials have confirmed the safety of raloxifene in the endometrium.[80] Studies of approximately 8000 women with durations of therapy ranging from 8 weeks to 2 years showed that raloxifene, unlike unopposed estrogen, did not cause endometrial proliferation or bleeding. Raloxifene's uterine activity profile has been shown to be comparable with that of placebo. In fact,

there is even some indication that it actually may reduce the risk of endometrial cancer. For this reason, the U.S. Food and Drug Administration approved the use of raloxifene for the treatment of osteoporosis in 1979 without requiring the concomitant use of progestins.[11]

Of interest, tamoxifen was in general clinical use for over 2 decades before its adverse relationship to uterine cancer was identified. Although initial studies of raloxifene indicate a protective effect on the endometrium,[81] many more years of evaluation are needed to confirm this difference. Further data regarding the long-term uterine safety of raloxifene are needed.

Central Nervous System/Other

The beneficial side effects associated with estrogen include relief from hot flushes, insomnia, anxiety, depression, vaginal dryness, dyspareunia, libido dysfunction, memory loss, and bladder symptoms, such as incontinence, dysuria, and urethral syndrome. Neither tamoxifen nor raloxifene can make these claims. Although there is a paucity of data on the relationship between tamoxifen and raloxifene and vasomotor symptoms, both appear to increase vasomotor symptoms by as much as 20% in postmenopausal women. Again, this seems to be more prevalent in women who have just recently gone through the menopausal changes and is significantly less common in women who are several years postmenopausal. In the MORE trials on raloxifene, these side effects were not severe enough to significantly change adherence to therapy among clinical trial participants. Of the raloxifene group, 0.6% quit the medication early, compared with only 0.1% of the placebo group.[57] A threefold increase in leg cramping seems to be unique for raloxifene thus far. Of clinical importance to many postmenopausal women, tamoxifen and raloxifene both appear to exhibit less vaginal bleeding and less breast pain, swelling, and tenderness when compared with the estrogens.

Study of Tamoxifen and Raloxifene Trials

Many of these issues are expected to be resolved at the completion of the Study of Tamoxifen and Raloxifene (STAR) trials.[82] The ongoing STAR trial, which will explore these issues and investigate the comparative efficacy of these two compounds, is expected to answer many of the remaining questions regarding tamoxifen and raloxifene. This head-to-head, double-blind, randomized comparison of tamoxifen and raloxifene, sponsored by the National Cancer Institute, will be the largest breast cancer prevention study ever conducted, involving more than 300 institutions throughout the United States, Canada, and Puerto Rico. Approximately 22,000 postmenopausal women aged 35 to 59 years who are at increased risk for breast cancer and women aged 60 years and older with no additional risk factors will be assigned to receive either tamoxifen (20 mg/day) or raloxifene (60 mg/day) for 5 years. This long-term clinical trial will help determine the ultimate impact on clinical events, specifically fractures, CHD, stress incontinence, and cognition, of tamoxifen and raloxifene. The trial began in April 1999 and is expected to continue for 5 to 10 years. Preliminary results should be available by 2003.

SUMMARY

In summary, for women with breast cancer, the benefits of tamoxifen therapy unquestionably outweigh the risks of endometrial carcinoma. Whether this holds true for breast cancer prevention is unclear at this time and must be determined on a case-by-case basis. The use of the Gail model in the assessment of a woman's risk of breast cancer should help in this decision-making process.[23] It is highly unlikely that tamoxifen will be used to reduce CHD risk. Long-term therapy is necessary for effective cardioprotection, and tamoxifen therapy is currently recommended for only 5 years in the treatment or prevention of breast cancer. Further use of this medication seems to be associated with an increase in breast cancer. In addition, tamoxifen is associated with an increased risk for endometrial cancer. Raloxifene is an option for prevention of osteoporosis, especially for patients reluctant to use hormone therapy, but not as a substitute for estrogen owing to raloxifene's vasomotor side effects and lack of long-term data. Additional data are needed regarding long-term prophylaxis with both tamoxifen and raloxifene.

THE FUTURE

Despite the incredible strides hormonal therapy has made since about 1990, we have yet to find the perfect solution to the changes of menopause. Ideally, a compound or combination of compounds would be identified that significantly lowers a woman's risk of osteoporosis, heart disease, and uterine and breast cancer while at the same time relieving all the vasomotor symptoms associated with menopause. In addition, this compound would have a 20- to 30-year widespread clinical track record to ensure its long-term safety.

Several medications currently in use for the treatment of osteoporosis include alendronate (Fosamax) and calcitonin (salmon [Miacalcin]).[83–86] Both may be adjuvant therapy to hormonal regimens in the osteoporotic patient. In addition, several new SERMs are in various stages of investigation, including toremifene, nafoxidine, and tibolone.[87] Toremifene is chemically similar to tamoxifen with less apparent hepatocarcinogenicity in high doses.[88] Tibolone is a steroid related to 19-nortestosterone that is metabolized into three steroid isomers with varying estrogenic, androgenic, and progestogenic activities.[89, 90] Thus far, tibolone appears to reduce osteoporosis while suppressing the endometrial lin-

ing with a progestational effect and inhibiting breast cell proliferation. In addition, tibolone relieves hot flushes, vaginal bleeding, vaginal dryness, and dyspareunia while increasing libido. Studies are unclear as to the relationship between tibolone and the cardiovascular system. An initial study revealed an unfavorable change in lipoproteins but a favorable change in fibrinolysis and coagulation. Tibolone has been in clinical use in Europe and is scheduled for release in the United States by Organon under the brand name of Xyvion.

One fascinating option is the concomitant use of several existing medications. Vasomotor symptoms are a significant drawback to tamoxifen and raloxifene. Many individual clinicians have experimented with short-term estrogen, progestin, or progesterone "add-back therapy." There is a paucity of data on the long-term effects, benefit, and risks of estrogen in conjunction with the SERMs for the amelioration of vasomotor systems.[91] It is unknown whether the breast cancer protection of raloxifene or tamoxifen would be affected with the long-term concomitant addition of estrogen, progestin, or progesterone. Another possibility would be some sequential or combination use of tamoxifen and raloxifene. Raloxifene has been shown to inhibit the stimulatory effects on the endometrium of both estrogen and tamoxifen. Although a course of tamoxifen is presently limited to 5 years, no one knows the effects of following this with a course of raloxifene.

Combination therapies may also benefit the heart. With the evolution of the statin medications and their beneficial effects on lipid profiles and cardiovascular risk, it is yet unclear how they will function in conjunction with hormone replacement therapy and SERMs.[92] The relationship between low-dose aspirin, hormone replacement therapy and SERMs, and DVT is an open field for study. Despite the fascinating hypothetical potentials, no studies that evaluate a tibolone/statin/low-dose aspirin combination could be identified.

Until the data from these ongoing and future studies have been collected and analyzed, physicians must review each perimenopausal and postmenopausal woman's risk-benefit profile individually when advising these women on the available therapies for the treatment of menopause. Whether considering estrogen therapy, hormone replacement therapy, raloxifene or tamoxifen use, important factors to consider include the patient's age; severity of menopausal symptoms; risk for CHD, osteoporosis, and breast and uterine cancer; and the preferences and concerns of each woman. With a plethora of new treatment modalities available and on the horizon, it is the responsibility of every health care provider dealing with menopausal and perimenopausal patients to familiarize themselves with the ongoing literature in order to become more effective patient educators and advocates.

References

1. Effects of hormone therapy on bone mineral density: Results from the Postmenopausal Estrogen/Progestin Interventions (PEPI) Trial. The Writing Group for the PEPI Trial. JAMA 1996;276:1389–1396.

2. Effects of hormone replacement therapy on endometrial histology in postmenopusal women. The Postmenopausal Estrogen/Progestin Interventions (PEPI) Trial. The Writing Group for the PEPI Trial. JAMA 1996;275:370–375.

3. Effects of estrogen or estrogen/progestin regimens on heart disease risk factors in postmenopausal women. The Postmenopausal Estrogen/Progestin Interventions (PEPI) Trial. The Writing Group for the PEPI Trial. JAMA 1995;273:199–208.

4. Taylor M: Alternatives to conventional HRT: Phytoestrogens and botanical. Contemp Obstet Gynecol June 1999, pp 27–49.

5. Brett KM, Madans JH: Use of postmenopausal hormone replacement therapy: Estimates from a nationally representative cohort study. Am J Epidemiol 1997;145:536–545.

6. Speroff L, Glass RH, Kase NG (eds): Clinical Gynecologic Endocrinology and Infertility, 6th ed, Chaps 2, 16, and 17. Baltimore, Williams & Wilkins, 1999.

7. SERMs: Emerging role in the clinical setting—breast and gynecologic effects. Contemp Obstet Gynecol Suppl May 1999.

8. SERMs: Emerging role in the clinical setting—skeletal and coronary effects. Contemp Obstet Gynecol Suppl July 1999.

9. Bryant HU, Dere WH: Selective estrogen receptor modulators: An alternative to hormone replacement therapy. Proc Soc Exp Biol Med 1998;217:45–52.

10. Tamoxifen prescribing information. Wilmington, Del, Zeneca, 1998.

11. Raloxifene prescribing information. Indianapolis, Ind, Eli Lilly, 1998.

12. Boss SM, Huster WJ, Neild JA, et al: Effects of raloxifene HCl on the endometrium of postmenopausal women. Am J Obstet Gynecol 1997;177:1458–1464.

13. Henson JC: Current overview of EORTC clinical trials with tamoxifen. Cancer Treat Rev 1976;60:1463–1466.

14. Mouridsen H, Palshof T, Patterson J, Battersby L: Tamoxifen for the advanced breast cancer. Cancer Treat Rev 1978;5:131–141.

15. Controlled trial of tamoxifen as adjuvant agent in management of early breast cancer. Interim analysis at four years by Nolvadex Adjuvant Trial Organization. Lancet 1983;1:257–261.

16. Fisher B, Redmond C, Brown A, et al: Adjuvant chemotherapy with and without tamoxifen in the treatment of primary breast cancer: 5-year results from the National Surgical Adjuvant Breast and Bowel Project Trial. J Clin Oncol 1986;4:459–471.

17. Controlled trial of tamoxifen as single adjuvant agent in management of early breast cancer. Interim analysis at six years by Nolvadex Adjuvant Trial Organization. Lancet 1985;1:836–840.

18. Rutqvist LE, Johansson H, Signomklao T, et al, for the Stockholm Breast Cancer Study Group: Adjuvant tamoxifen therapy for early stage breast cancer and second primary malignancies. J Natl Cancer Inst 1995;87:645–651.

19. Fisher B, Dignam J, Wolmark N, et al: Tamoxifen in treatment of intraductal breast cancer: National Surgical Adjuvant Breast and Bowel Project B-24 Randomized Controlled Trial. Lancet 1999;353:1993–2000.

20. Jordan VC (ed): Tamoxifen for the Treatment and Prevention of Breast Cancer. Melville, NY, PRR, 1999.

21. Tamoxifen for early breast cancer: An overview of the randomized trials. Early Breast Cancer Trialists Collaborative Group. Lancet 1998;351:1451–1467.

22. Osborn CK: Tamoxifen in the treatment of breast cancer. N Engl J Med 1998;339:1609–1618.

23. Fisher B, Costantino JP, Wickerham DL, et al: Tamoxifen for prevention of breast cancer: Report of the National Surgical Adjuvant Breast and Bowel Project P-1 Study. J Natl Cancer Inst 1998;90:1371–1388.

24. Prowles T, Eeles R, Ashley S, et al: Interim analysis of incidence of breast cancer in the Royal Marsden Hospital Tamoxifen randomized chemoprevention trial. Lancet 1998;352:98–101.

25. Veronesi U, Maisonneuve P, Costa A, et al: Prevention of breast cancer with tamoxifen: Preliminary findings from the Italian randomized trial among hysterectomized women. Italian Tamoxifen Prevention Study. Lancet 1998;352:93–97.

26. DeGregorio MW, Maenpaa JU, Wiebe VJ: Tamoxifen for the prevention of breast cancer: No! Important Advances in Oncology 1995, Chap 12. Philadelphia, JB Lippincott, 1995.

27. Gail MH, Brinton LA, Bryar DP, et al: Projecting individualized probabilities of developing breast cancer for white females who are examined annually. J Natl Cancer Inst 1989;81:1879–1886.

28. Jalyesimi IA, Buzdar AU, Decker DA, et al: Use of tamoxifen for breast cancer: Twenty-eight years later. J Clin Oncol 1995;13:513–529.

29. Fisher B, Dignam J, Bryant J, et al: Five versus more than five years of tamoxifen therapy for breast cancer patients with negative lymph nodes and estrogen receptor–positive tumors. J Natl Cancer Inst 1996;21:1529–1542.

30. Wright CD, Garrenhan NJ, Stanton M, et al: The effect of long-term tamoxifen therapy on cancellous bone remodeling and structure in women with breast cancer. J Bone Miner Res 1994;9:153–159.

31. Ke H, Chen HK, Simmons HA, et al: Comparative effects of droloxifene, tamoxifen, and estrogen on bone, serum cholesterol, and uterine histology in the ovariectomized rat model. Bone 1997;20:31–39.

32. Kenny AM, Prestwood KM, Pilbeam CC, et al: The short-term effects of tamoxifen on bone turnover in older women. J Clin Endocrinol Metab 1995;80:3287–3291.

33. Grey AB, Stapleton JP, Evans MC, et al: The effect of the antiestrogen tamoxifen on bone mineral density in normal late postmenopausal women. Am J Med 1995;99:636–641.

34. Marttunen MB, Hietanen P, Tiitinen A, Ylikorkala O: Comparison of effects of tamoxifen and toremifene on bone biochemistry and bone mineral density in postmenopausal breast cancer patients. J Clin Endocrinol Metab 1998;83:1158–1162.

35. Dempster DW, Lindsay R: Pathogenesis of osteoporosis. Lancet 1993;341:797–801.

36. Thangaraju M, Kumar K, Ganghirajan R, Sachdanandam P: Effect of tamoxifen on plasma lipids and lipoproteins in postmenopausal women with breast cancer. Cancer 1994;73:659–663.

37. Grey AB, Stapleton JP, Evans MC, et al: The effect of the antiestrogen tamoxifen on cardiovascular risk factors in normal postmenopausal women. J Clin Endocrinol Metab 1995;80:3191–3195.

38. Costantino JP, Kuller LH, Ives DG, et al: Coronary heart disease mortality and adjuvant tamoxifen therapy. J Natl Cancer Inst 1997;89:776.

39. McDonald CC, Stewart HJ: Fatal myocardial infarction in the Scottish Adjuvant Tamoxifen Trial. BMJ 1991;303:435–437.

40. McDonald CC, Alexander FE, Whyte BW, et al: Cardiac and vascular morbidity in women receiving adjuvant tamoxifen for breast cancer in a randomized trial. BMJ 1995;311:977–980.

41. Rutqvist LE, Mattsson A, for the Stockholm Breast Cancer Study Group: Cardiac and thromboembolic morbidity among postmenopausal women with early-stage breast cancer in a randomized trial of adjuvant tamoxifen. J Natl Cancer Inst 1993;85:1398–1406.

42. Early Breast Cancer Trialists Collaborative Group. Tamoxifen for early breast cancer: An overview of the randomized trials. Lancet 1998;51:1451–1467.

43. Killackey MA, Hakes TB, Pierce VK: Endometrial adenocarcinoma in breast cancer patients receiving antiestrogens. Cancer Treat Rep 1985;65:237–238.

44. Gal D, Kopel S, Bashevkin M, et al: Oncogenic potential of tamoxifen on endometria of postmenopausal women with breast cancer—preliminary report. Gynecol Oncol 1991;42:120–123.

45. Barakat RR: The effect of tamoxifen on the endometrium. Oncology (Huntingt) 1995;9:129–134.

46. Fisher B, Costantino JP, Redmond CK, et al: Endometrial cancer in tamoxifen-treated breast cancer patients: Findings from the National Surgical Adjuvant Breast and Bowel Project (NASBP) B-14. J Natl Cancer Inst 1994;86:527–537.

47. Cohen I, Rosen DJ, Shapiro J, et al: Endometrial changes with tamoxifen: Comparison between tamoxifen-treated and non-treated asymptomatic, postmenopausal breast cancer patients. Gynecol Oncol 1994;52:185–190.

48. Magriples U, Naftolin F, Schwartz PE, et al: High-grade endometrial carcinoma in tamoxifen-treated breast cancer patients. J Clin Oncol 1993;11:485–490.

49. Barakat RR, Wong G, Curtin JP, et al: Tamoxifen use in breast cancer patients who subsequently develop corpus cancer is not associated with a higher incidence of adverse histologic features. Gynecol Oncol 1994;55:164–168.

50. American College of Obstetricians and Gynecologists: Tamoxifen and endometrial (ACOG Committee Opinion No. 169, February 1996). Committee on Gynecologic Practice. Int J Gynaecol Obstet 1996;53:197–199.

51. Black LJ, Sato M, Rowley ER, et al: Raloxifene (LY139481) HCl prevents bone loss and reduces serum cholesterol without causing uterine hypertrophy in ovariectomized rats. J Clin Invest 1994;93:63–69.

52. Turner CH, Sato M, Bryant HU: Raloxifene preserves bone strength

and bone mass in ovariectomized rats. Endocrinology 1994;1:135–200.

53. Draper MW, Boss SM, Huster WJ, Neild JA: Effects of raloxifene HCl on serum markers of bone and lipid metabolism—dose response relationship [abstract]. Calcif Tissue Int 1994;54:339.

54. Draper MW, Flowers DE, Huster WJ, et al: A controlled trial of raloxifene (LY139481) HCl: Impact on bone turnover and serum lipid profile in healthy postmenopausal women. J Bone Miner Res 1996;11:835–842.

55. Buzdar AU, Marcus C, Holmes F, et al: Phase 2 evaluation of LY156758 in metastatic breast cancer. Oncology 1988;45:344–345.

56. Black LJ, Masahiko S, Rowley ER, et al: Raloxifene (LY139481) HCl prevents bone loss and reduces serum cholesterol without causing uterine hypertrophy in ovariectomized rats. J Clin Invest 1994;93:63–69.

57. Cummings SR, Norton L, Eckert S, et al: Raloxifene reduces the risk of breast cancer and may decrease the risk of endometrial cancer in postmenopausal women: Two-year findings from the Multiple Outcomes of Raloxifene Evaluation (MORE) trial [abstract 3]. Proc Am Soc Clin Oncol 1998;17:2a.

58. Cummings SR, Eckert S, Krueger KA, et al: The effect of raloxifene on risk of breast cancer in postmenopausal women: Results from the MORE randomized trial. JAMA 1999;281:2189–2197.

59. Delmas PD, Bjarnason NH, Mitlak BH, et al: Effects of raloxifene on bone mineral density, serum cholesterol concentrations, and uterine endometrium in postmenopausal women. N Engl J Med 1997;337:1641–1647.

60. Ettinger B, Black D, Cummings S, et al: Raloxifene reduces the risk of incident vertebral fractures: 24-month interim analysis. Osteoporos Int 1998;(Suppl 3):11.

61. Ettinger B, Black DM, Mitlak BH, et al: Reduction of vertebral fracture risk in postmenopausal women with osteoporosis treated with raloxifene: Results from a randomized clinical trial. Multiple Outcomes of Raloxifene Evaluation (MORE) Investigators. JAMA 1999;282:637–645.

62. Bjarnason NH, Haarbo J, Byrjalsen I, et al: Raloxifene inhibits aortic accumulation of cholesterol in ovariectomized, cholesterol-fed rabbits. Circulation 1997;96:1964–1969.

63. Walsh BW, Kuller LH, Wild RA, et al: Effects of raloxifene on serum lipids and coagulation factors in healthy postmenopausal women. JAMA 1998;279:1445–1451.

64. Clarkson TH, Anthony MS, Jerome CP: Lack of effect of raloxifene on coronary artery atherosclerosis of postmenopausal monkeys. J Clin Endocrinol Metab 1997;83:721–726.

65. Kauffman RF, Bensch WR, Roudebush RE, et al: Hypocholesterolemic activity of raloxifene (LY139481) HCl: Pharmacological characterization as a selective estrogen receptor modulator. J Pharmacol Exp Ther 1997;280:146–153.

66. Eli Lilly & Company news release announcement. March 24, 1998.

67. Fuch-Young R, Magee DE, Adrian MD, et al: Raloxifene, a selective estrogen receptor modulator, inhibits the uterotrophic effect of tamoxifen over a 21-day time course. J Soc Gynecol Invest 1996;3:153A.

68. Black LJ, Jones CD, Falcone JF: Antagonism of estrogen action with a new benzothiophene-derived antiestrogen. Life Sci 1983;32:1031–1036.

69. Krueger MD, Evans TS, Echert S, et al: Characteristics of hot flushes with raloxifene in postmenopausal osteoporotic women on the MORE Trial [abstract]. Proceedings of the North American Menopause Society, 11th Annual Meeting Program 2000, p 69.

70. Khovidhunkit W, Shoback DM: Clinical effects of raloxifene HCl in women. Ann Intern Med 1999;130:431–439.

71. Glusman J, Lu Y, Huster W, et al: Raloxifene effects on climacteric symptoms compared with hormone oestrogen replacement therapy [abstract]. Proceedings of the North American Menopause Society, 8th Annual Meeting Program 1997, p 65.

72. Barrett-Connor E: Hormone replacement and cancer. Br Med Bull 1992;48:345–355.

73. Overview of Perceived and Real Health Threats. New York, Gallup Survey, 1995.

74. Colditz GA, Hankinson SE, Hunter DJ, et al: The use of estrogens and progesterones and the risk of breast cancer in postmenopausal women. N Engl J Med 1995;332:1589–1593.

75. Hol T, Cox MB, Bryant HU, et al: Selective estrogen receptor modulators and postmenopausal women's health. J Women's Health 1997;6:523–531.

76. Chlebowski RT, Collyar DE, Somerfield MR, Pfister DG: American Society of Clinical Oncology Technology Assessment on Breast Cancer Risk Reduction Strategies: Tamoxifen and Raloxifene. J Clin Oncol 1999;17:1939–1955.

77. Mosca L, Manson JE, Sutherland SE, et al: Cardiovascular disease in women: A statement for healthcare professionals from the American Heart Association. Circulation 1997;96:2468–2482.

78. Barrett-Connor E, Wegner NK, Grady D, et al: coronary heart disease in women, randomized clinical trials, HERS and RUTH. Maturitas 1998;31:1–7.

79. Hulley S, Grady D, Bush T, et al: Randomized trial of estrogen plus progestin for secondary prevention of CHD in postmenopausal women. Heart and Estrogen/Progestin Replacement Study (HERS) Research Group. JAMA 1998;280:605–613.

80. Bryant HU, Glasebrook AL, Yang NN, et al: A pharmacologic review of raloxifene. J Bone Miner Metab 1996;14:1–9.

81. Sato M, Glasebrook AL, Bryant HU: Raloxifene: A selective estrogen receptor modulator. J Bone Miner Metab 1995;12(Suppl 2):S9–S20.

82. Jordan VC: Designer estrogens. Sci Am 1998;279:60–67.

83. Black DM, Cummings SR, Harpf DB, et al: Randomized trial of effect of alendronate on risk of fracture in women with existing vertebral fractures. Lancet 1996;348:1535–1541.

84. Cummings SR, Black DM, Thompson DE, et al: Effects of alendronate on risk of fracture in women with low bone density but without vertebral fractures: Results from the Fracture Intervention Trial (FIT). JAMA 1998;280:2077–2082.

85. Silverman SL, Chestnut C, Andriano J, et al: Salmon calcitonin nasal spray (NS-CT) reduces risk of vertebral fractures in established osteoporosis and has continuous efficacy with prolonged treatment: Accrued 5-year worldwide data of The PROOF Study (Prevent Recurrence of Osteoporotic Fractures) [abstract]. ASBMR-IBMS Second Joint Meeting 1999;1108:S1754.

86. Miacalcin nasal spray (Calcitonin-salmon) prescribing information. East Hanover, NJ, Novartis, 1998.

87. Sato M, Rippy MK, Bryant HU: Raloxifene, tamoxifen, nafoxidine, or estrogen effects on reproductive and nonreproductive tissues in ovariectomized rats. FASEB J 1996;10:905–912.

88. Buzdar AU, Hortobagyi GN: Tamoxifen and toremifene in breast cancer: Comparison of safety and efficacy. J Clin Oncol 1998;16:348–353.

89. Rymer J: Tibolone as an alternative to HRT. Contemp Obstet Gynecol April 1999, pp 63–77.

90. Rymer J, Robinson J, Fogelman I: Long-term adherence with tibolone—protection of the postmenopausal female skeleton over 8 years [abstract]. Proceedings of the North American Menopause Society, 11th Annual Meeting Program 2000, p 27.

91. Pinkerton, J, Warren M, Shifren J, et al: Vaginal effect of oral raloxifene HCl v. placebo in postmenopausal women treated with estradiol 17-b vaginal ring [abstract]. Proceedings of the North American Menopause Society, 11th Annual Meeting Program 2000, p 14.

92. Mueck AO, Seeger H, Deuringer FU, et al: Additive effect of estradiol and statin in inhibiting the oxidation of human low-density lipoproteins [abstract]. Proceedings of the North American Menopause Society, 11th Annual Meeting Program 2000, p 23.

FIFTY-EIGHT

Current Issues in Premenstrual Syndrome

Robert L. Reid

Many unanswered questions about the epidemiology and pathophysiology of premenstrual syndrome (PMS) remain, yet consensus is developing about strategies for diagnosis and treatment of this condition. PMS has been defined as "a cyclic recurrence in the luteal phase of the menstrual cycle of a combination of distressing physical, psychological, and/or behavioral changes of sufficient severity to result in deterioration of interpersonal relationships and/or interference with normal activities."[1] Since the original description of "premenstrual tension," this condition has been given a number of different names. Most recently, the American Psychiatric Association, in an appendix to the fourth edition of its *Diagnostic and Statistical Manual of Mental Disorders*,[2] has included the category Premenstrual Dysphoric Disorder (PMDD) to alert physicians to the possibility that PMS can sometimes mimic other rapid-cycling bipolar disorders.

INCIDENCE

It is estimated that 30% of women have premenstrual symptomatology of sufficient distress that they seek some form of treatment, and 3% to 5% report severe or temporary disabling symptoms in the premenstrual and menstrual weeks.[3]

EPIDEMIOLOGY

PMS has been documented across races, cultures, and socioeconomic strata; however, it is less commonly reported in cultures in which pregnancy and breastfeeding maintain prolonged periods of amenorrhea.[1] The onset of PMS may be at any phase of reproductive life between puberty and menopause. Typically, it progresses over a number of years, becoming gradually more consistent and severe. It is generally ameliorated during times of hypothalamic amenorrhea, during pregnancy, and following cessation of cyclic menstrual function at menopause. Although PMS and dysmenorrhea may coexist, the variable nature of this association suggests that different pathophysiologic mechanisms are involved.[1] The prevalence and severity of dysmenorrhea fall with increasing parity, whereas the same is not true for premenstrual symptomatology.

Although it has been considered that PMS merely represents an entrainment or synchronization of a chronic mood disorder to the menstrual cycle, several lines of evidence argue against this. Psychological studies comparing women who have precisely defined PMS with unaffected controls reveal no differences between the two groups in the follicular phase yet significantly higher levels of depression in PMS subjects during the luteal phase. Comparison of psychological profiles and cortisol secretory dynamics in women with PMS and women with endogenous depression reveals distinct differences. Current evidence suggests that intercurrent (luteal-phase) treatment with selective serotonin reuptake inhibitors (SSRIs) may be effective for premenstrual symptomatology, whereas such intermittent dosing has no beneficial effect for endogenous depression.

CLINICAL MANIFESTATIONS

Women with PMS typically report many of the same premenstrual molimina that affect non–PMS-afflicted women. Rarely do sensations of breast swelling or tenderness, abdominal bloating, and constipation lead to functional impairment. Rather, it is the fatigue, emotional lability, depression, anger, and irritability that tend to impair social relationships or diminish work efficiency.[4] Typically, symptoms of PMS occur in the final 2 weeks of the cycle, at any time after ovulation, and abate several days into menstruation. For most women, the symptoms will be most intense in the final few days of the luteal phase. In some individuals, symptoms come on at ovulation and persist until the end of menstruation, resulting in only "one good week" before symptoms resume. Another PMS variant that has been recognized is the brief onset of symptoms coincident with the periovulatory drop in estradiol. In these individuals symptoms last for 24 to 48 hours at midcycle before remitting, only to return later in the cycle in the premenstrual week.

A variety of other medical conditions, such as asthma, epilepsy, and migraine, may show menstrual cycle–related changes in intensity and may respond to medical ovarian suppression.[5]

THEORIES OF PATHOPHYSIOLOGY

Many theories have been advanced to explain PMS, none of which has been entirely satisfactory. There is now general acceptance that PMS is the result of unusual individual susceptibility or sensitivity to normal hormone fluctuations of the menstrual cycle.[6]

One theory suggests that central estrogen deficiency may trigger PMS symptoms through induced changes in the activity of serotonin and other central neurotransmitters. Thus, estrogen blockade with clomiphene or the abrupt estrogen decline at ovulation can, in susceptible women, precipitate labile mood, headaches, and so on. Exposure to progesterone after ovulation may induce similar effects through depletion of central estrogen receptors, leading to gradually worsening symptoms as the luteal phase progresses (much like progestins added to menopausal hormone replacement therapy can induce PMS-like symptoms). Reduced central estrogen receptors and a decline in circulating estradiol in the final days of the cycle may account for the acute premenstrual intensification of PMS symptoms.[7, 8]

ASSESSMENT AND MANAGEMENT

Contrary to the claims made by several Internet sites with obvious commercial interests, there is no blood test that will diagnose PMS[6, 9] at this time. It is likely that individuals with PMS are manifesting an abnormal neuroendocrine response to normal reproductive endocrine changes.[6] Because a diagnosis of PMS relies on symptoms severe enough to result in social or work disruption, and because symptom severity may fluctuate slightly from month to month, diagnosis in milder cases may be problematic. Nevertheless, there is general agreement that prospective symptom records documenting the severity of symptoms in the luteal phase of recurrent cycles are a reliable way to identify individuals suffering from true PMS. Daily prospective records of symptoms and their impact on lifestyle for 1 to 2 months, accompanied by detailed history and physical examination, are the mainstay of diagnosis. An example of a prospective symptom record is the PRISM (prospective record of the impact and severity of menstrual symptoms) calendar (Fig. 58–1).

THERAPY

Charting and Counseling

Common concerns expressed by women with severe PMS include feelings of fear (that they are "losing their minds") and guilt (over the negative impact of their behavior on relationships with colleagues and family members). Embarrassment and frustration at the skepticism of the medical profession result when their concerns are not taken seriously. Validation of their symptom complex and reassurance that others share their hormonally triggered mood disorder can do much to allay these anxieties. The prospective symptom record often provides necessary reassurance that there is a cyclic pattern to symptoms consistent with a hormonally triggered disorder. As well, it allows the patient to understand that she should plan ahead to avoid stressful situations at times when she is symptomatic. Nevertheless, for women in whom symptoms occupy much of the month, an approach that tries to fit important activities into the

"good week" makes little sense. In these circumstances, interventions aimed at reducing symptoms are clearly most appropriate.

LIFESTYLE MODIFICATION

Much has been written about possible lifestyle changes that will alleviate PMS, yet few of these recommendations have been validated in properly controlled clinical trials. Communication skills may be improved with group counseling of affected women and their partners in a program supervised by a clinical psychologist.

Regular exercise is reported to reduce the severity of PMS for several hours after activity but clearly is not a cure-all for PMS unless the level of exercise is sufficient to induce amenorrhea.

Dietary changes that have been reported to alleviate PMS are reduction in caffeine (known to be a stimulant contributing to anxiety and sleep disturbance) and alcohol (often directly linked to depression and temper flares), as well as salt and refined carbohydrates (potentially linked to acute fluid shifts and edema). A small snack midmorning and midafternoon may minimize the impact of impaired cellular glucose uptake in women with PMS.[10]

MEDICATIONS

The degree of medical intervention clearly needs to be tailored to the severity of symptoms. When symptoms are multiple but of moderate severity, a range of nonspecific treatment options is available.

Vitamin B_6, 100 mg daily, has been shown to alleviate premenstrual symptomatology in many (but not all) controlled clinical trials.[11] At these doses, there need not be concern about peripheral neuropathy that has been reported with higher daily doses of vitamin B_6. Nonsteroidal anti-inflammatory drugs, such as mefenamic acid, taken in a dosage of 500 mg three times daily in the premenstrual and menstrual week, have been shown to reduce premenstrual and menstrual symptomatology. Danazol, 200 mg daily throughout the month, has been shown to reduce both menstrual bleeding and premenstrual symptomatology, whereas luteal-phase danazol may be effective for premenstrual mastalgia. Simple supplementation with calcium carbonate has been reported to alleviate premenstrual symptomatology slightly more than placebo and may be a simple, inexpensive intervention when symptoms are mild.

Oral contraceptives could be considered in individuals requiring contraception, particularly if dysmenorrhea or heavy menstrual flow are major contributors to the overall summation of symptomatology. Women presenting with severe PMS who are taking the oral contraceptive pill probably should consider a trial of an alternative form of contraception because contraceptive steroids may accentuate PMS in some individuals.

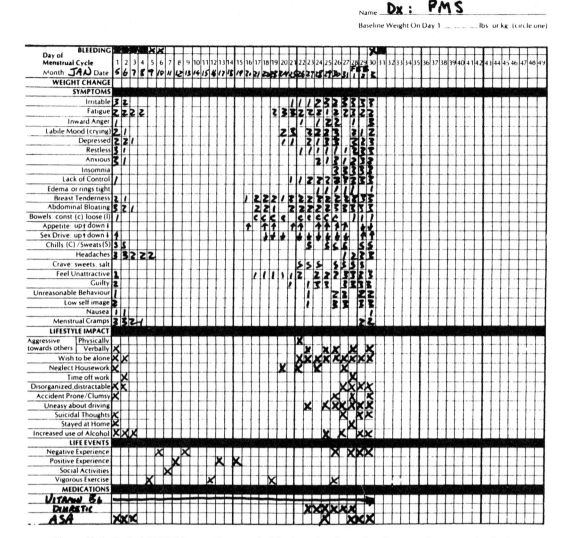

Figure 58–1. Typical PRISM (prospective record of the impact and severity of menstrual symptoms) calendar.

SPECIFIC SYMPTOMATIC THERAPIES

When specific symptoms predominate, symptom-specific therapies may be appropriate. For severe anxiety or sleep disturbance, alprazolam, 0.25 mg twice daily, or triazolam, 0.25 mg at bedtime, respectively, may be helpful. Estrogen withdrawal has been linked to menstrually related migraines, and estrogen supplementation with a 100-μg transdermal estrogen patch or the acute administration of 1 mg of estradiol sublingually at the time of migrainous aura (if these occur at menstruation) may be helpful to avert menstrual migraine.

Women with significant edema of their extremities who do not benefit by a reduction in salt or refined carbohydrates may obtain relief from a potassium-sparing diuretic such as spironolactone, 100 mg daily.

Caution must be taken with anxiolytics and medications like spironolactone because some women may come to depend on them all month rather than just for the premenstrual phase for which they were prescribed.

INTERVENTIONS FOR SEVERE PREMENSTRUAL SYNDROME

Selective Serotonin Reuptake Inhibitors

At present, the mainstay of therapy for severe or moderately severe PMS that has been unresponsive to first-line measures is to consider a trial of SSRIs. A variety of agents have been demonstrated to be highly effective for relief of PMS in controlled clinical trials, including fluoxetine, sertraline, paroxetine, and citalopram.[12] Symptom profiles may help in selecting the most appropriate agent (fluoxetine in patients in whom fatigue and depression predominate; sertraline if insomnia, irritability, and anxiety are paramount). SSRIs have been associated with loss of libido and anorgasmia, which may be particularly distressing to patients who already may experience reduced libido due to premenstrual depression. Appropriate pretreatment counseling and follow-up are essential.

Tricyclic antidepressants have not generally been effective, with the exception of clomipramine, a tricyclic antidepressant with strong serotonergic activity. Intolerance to the side effects of tricyclic antidepressants is common. Some evidence suggests that luteal-phase therapy with SSRIs may be as effective as continuous therapy.[13] In general, patients should be started on continuous therapy with SSRIs to determine the optimal benefit that is going to be achieved. After a period of 2 to 3 months, they can then reduce this to luteal-phase therapy to determine whether the same level of benefit is preserved.

MEDICAL OVARIAN SUPPRESSION

A certain percentage of women will refuse to consider SSRIs or will not tolerate their side effects. In these individuals, medical ovarian suppression with a gonadotropin-releasing hormone agonist has shown to be a highly effective means to alleviate PMS.[14] Low-dose estrogen replacement therapy averts menopause-like symptomatology while the patient is taking this medication but inevitably will lead to heavy, irregular bleeding unless a progestational agent is added. Once a progestational agent is added cyclically, it often reinduces premenstrual symptomatology. From a practical point of view, medical ovarian suppression with a gonadotropin-releasing hormone agonist and low-dose estrogen replacement therapy is often useful as a therapeutic trial. If 3 to 6 months of therapy result in complete remission of symptoms and the affected woman is convinced that this has resulted in a dramatic improvement to her quality of life, then consideration could be given to a more permanent (surgical) means of ablating ovarian activity.

SURGICAL THERAPY

When a trial of medical ovarian suppression has resulted in complete relief of PMS, this not only establishes the diagnosis clearly but also affords the affected woman the opportunity to anticipate how she would feel if she underwent surgical therapy. The cost of ongoing medical ovarian suppression is prohibitive for many women, and for others the return of PMS in conjunction with progestational therapy makes this treatment unsatisfactory. Some individuals will choose to undergo bilateral oophorectomy as a more permanent means to achieve suppression of ovarian activity. Clearly, in this circumstance, low-dose estrogen replacement therapy is required to avoid the consequences of long-term hypoestrogenism. Removal of the uterus at the time of oophorectomy avoids the need for progesta-

tional agents (and their attendant premenstrual symptomatology) in the future.[15]

SUMMARY

For most women with PMS, a judicious approach to therapy, starting with simple counseling and lifestyle modification, progressing to symptom-specific therapies or more global therapies such as SSRIs or medical ovarian suppression, can afford dramatic improvement in quality of life. In exceptional circumstances, when symptoms are severe and long-term medical therapy is unacceptable, hysterectomy and oophorectomy with subsequent estrogen replacement may provide a lasting cure.

References

1. Reid RL: Premenstrual syndrome. Curr Probl Obstet Gynecol Fertil 1985;8(2):1–51.
2. American Psychiatric Association: Diagnostic and Statistical Manual of Mental Disorders, 4th ed. Washington, DC, APA, 1994, pp. 717–718.
3. Johnson SR, McChesney C, Bean JA: Epidemiology of premenstrual symptoms in a nonclinical sample. I. Prevalence, natural history and help-seeking behavior. J Reprod Med 1988;33:340.
4. Bloch N, Schmidt PJ, Rubinow DR: Premenstrual syndrome: evidence for symptom stability across cycles. Am J Psychiatry 1997;154:1741–1746.
5. Case AM, Reid RL: Effects of the menstrual cycle on medical conditions. Arch Intern Med 1998;158:1405–1412.
6. Schmidt PJ, Nieman LK, Danaceau MA, et al: Differential behavioral effects of gonadal steroids in women with and in those without premenstrual syndrome. N Engl J Med 1998;338:209–216.
7. Reid RL: Premenstrual syndrome. Am Assoc Clin Chem 1987;5(12):1–12.
8. Rubinow DR, Schmidt PJ, Roca CA: Estrogen-serotonin interactions: Implications for affective regulation. Biol Psychiatry 1998;44:839–850.
9. Rubinow DR, Schmidt PJ, Roca CA: Hormone measures in reproductive endocrine-related mood disorders: Diagnostic issues. Psychopharmacol Bull 1998;34:289–290.
10. Diamond M, Simonson DC, DeFronzo RA: Menstrual cyclicity has a profound effect on glucose homeostasis. Fertil Steril 1989;52:204–208.
11. Wyatt KM, Dimmock PW, Jones PW, O'Brien PMS: Efficacy of vitamin B-6 in the treatment of premenstrual syndrome: Systematic review. BMJ 1999;318:1375–1381.
12. Steiner M, Judge R, Kumar R: Serotonin re-uptake inhibitors in the treatment of premenstrual dysphoria: Current state of knowledge. Int J Psychiatry Clin Prac 1997;1:241–247.
13. Wikander I, Sundblad C, Andersch B, et al: Citalopram in premenstrual dysphoria: Is intermittent treatment during luteal phases more effective than continuous medication throughout the menstrual cycle? J Clin Psychopharmacol 1998;18:390–398.
14. Freeman EW, Sondheimer SJ, Rickels K: Gonadotropin-releasing hormone agonist in the treatment of premenstrual symptoms with and without ongoing dysphoria: A controlled study. Psychopharmacol Bull 1997;33:303–309.
15. Casson P, Hahn PM, Van Vugt DA, Reid RL: Lasting response to ovariectomy in severe intractable premenstrual syndrome. Am J Obstet Gynecol 1990;162:99–105.

FIFTY-NINE

Current Therapy for Ectopic Pregnancy

Michael E. Lantz

The diagnosis of and therapy for ectopic pregnancy have undergone a revolution since the early 1990s. High-resolution endovaginal sonography and sensitive assays for the β subunit of human chorionic gonadotropin (β-hCG) have allowed for the earlier diagnosis of ectopic pregnancy and have decreased the number of patients undergoing surgery for a presumed diagnosis of this condition. The advent of diagnostic and treatment algorithms for ectopic pregnancy has resulted in a more standardized approach to patients presenting to the emergency department with symptoms of ectopic pregnancy and also has improved quality control.

Surgical treatment for ectopic pregnancy has become more conservative, with a focus on fallopian tube preservation and maintenance of fertility. Whereas it previously was reserved for patients with relative or absolute contraindications to surgery, medical therapy for ectopic pregnancy has become the treatment of choice in many institutions. This has resulted in faster recovery times for patients, lower costs, and the avoidance of complications associated with surgery and anesthesia. This chapter presents a current-day approach to the patient with a possible ectopic pregnancy and reviews the contemporary diagnosis and therapy for this condition.

EPIDEMIOLOGY

The United States has seen a progressive increase in ectopic pregnancy rates. In 1983, there were 69,600 reported cases of ectopic pregnancy, compared with 108,800 in 1992.[1, 2] Higher detection rates with current diagnostic modalities and the increased use of assisted reproductive technologies have contributed to this increase. The latter has also significantly increased the risk of heterotopic pregnancy, which is the simultaneous occurrence of two or more implantation sites. In 1965, the incidence of heterotopic pregnancy was reported as 1 in 27,500 deliveries.[3] In 1992, rates of heterotopic pregnancies after assisted reproductive technology procedures had been reported as high as 1 in 100.[4]

Another possible contributor to the increased frequency of ectopic pregnancy in the United States includes an increase in the presence of risk factors associated with this condition. Ectopic pregnancy is associated with those conditions resulting in damage to the tubal epithelium and the subsequent alteration in embryo transport through the fallopian tube.[5] Previous tubal surgery, including tubal sterilization, a prior ectopic pregnancy, known tubal disease,

and the presence of an intrauterine device are the risk factors having the strongest association with ectopic pregnancy.[6] Other known risk factors include in utero exposure to diethylstilbestrol, infertility, a history of genital infections, and multiple sexual partners.

The most common location of ectopic pregnancy is within the fallopian tube. Tubal pregnancies account for over 98% of all ectopic pregnancies.[7] The great majority of tubal pregnancies are located in the ampullary portion of the tube, followed in decreasing order by the isthmus and the fimbriated end. The interstitial part of the fallopian tube is the most proximal portion of the tube and is embodied within the muscular wall of the uterus.[8] Pregnancies within this portion of the fallopian tube traditionally have been referred to as *cornual* pregnancies and account for approximately 2% of ectopic pregnancies. Other rare locations for ectopic pregnancy include the ovary, cervix, and abdomen. The location of the ectopic gestation in a heterotopic pregnancy is most commonly the fallopian tube proper (88.3%), followed by the interstitium (6.3%).

DIAGNOSIS

The classic symptoms of ectopic pregnancy are amenorrhea, vaginal bleeding, and unilateral, lower abdominopelvic pain. Signs include adnexal tenderness and palpation of an adnexal mass. If the ectopic pregnancy has ruptured or if there is bleeding into the peritoneal cavity, orthostatic changes and rebound tenderness may be present. It is important always to include ectopic pregnancy in the differential diagnosis of a woman of reproductive age presenting with vaginal bleeding. Furthermore, if the clinical suspicion of ectopic pregnancy is high, the number of pelvic examinations should be limited and care should be taken during the examination so as not to precipitate rupture.

The assays presently employed to detect and quantify serum levels of β-hCG have sensitivities to as low as 5 mIU/mL, using the Third International Reference Standard. Furthermore, high-resolution endovaginal ultrasound can detect the presence of a gestational sac as early as 1 week after a missed menstrual period.[9] These diagnostic tests have led to increased detection rates and earlier diagnosis of both normal and abnormal pregnancies.

The β-hCG level at which an intrauterine pregnancy should be detected with endovaginal ultrasound is often referred to as the *discriminatory zone* and is dependent on the type of equipment used and operator experience. It is recommended that each institution develop and validate its own discriminatory zone when performing endovaginal sonography during early pregnancy. The discriminatory zone for high-resolution endovaginal ultrasound is usually at a β-hCG threshold of 1500 to 2000 mIU/mL.[10, 11] The combined use of endovaginal ultrasound and serial quantitative serum β-hCG levels allows for the nonsurgical detection of most ectopic pregnancies.

A consistent and well-planned approach should be taken when evaluating a patient with a possible ectopic pregnancy. A detailed history, including the presence of risk factors, and physical examination should be obtained. A quantitative level of β-hCG is obtained, and endovaginal ultrasound is performed. If the patient is hemodynamically unstable, surgical treatment is initiated. Patients who are hemodynamically stable and are found to have an ectopic pregnancy can be treated with medical therapy or surgery.

In patients in whom the quantitative β-hCG is above the discriminatory zone and ultrasound reveals no evidence of an intrauterine pregnancy, dilatation and curettage or expectant management with serial quantitative β-hCG determinations may be offered. An evaluation of patient compliance is necessary in those patients choosing expectant management. The presence of chorionic villi within the uterine curettings, as determined by gross examination when placed in saline solution or frozen section, indicates an intrauterine pregnancy.

Serial evaluations of β-hCG levels are useful if the initial level falls above or below the discriminatory zone. In normal early pregnancy, the β-hCG is expected to rise by at least 66% in a 48-hour period. Patients with normally rising β-hCG levels can be followed with repeat endovaginal sonography. If β-hCG levels do not rise or do so abnormally, diagnostic ultrasound, dilatation and curettage, or therapy can be offered.

A single progesterone level has also been used as an adjuvant to β-hCG levels and endovaginal ultrasound in discriminating between normal and abnormal early pregnancy. A serum progesterone level of greater than 25 ng/mL is associated with a continuing, normal pregnancy, whereas a level of less than 5 ng/mL is suggestive of a noncontinuing pregnancy. Levels between 5 and 25 ng/mL are inconclusive and have not been helpful in discriminating between an abnormal intrauterine pregnancy and an ectopic pregnancy.

MEDICAL THERAPY

Since about 1990, there has been a shift toward medical management of the hemodynamically stable patient with ectopic pregnancy. The first case of systemic methotrexate therapy for ectopic pregnancy was reported by Tanaka and colleagues in 1982.[12] In 1991, Stovall and associates[13] reported on their series of 100 cases of unruptured ectopic pregnancy treated with methotrexate. Since that time, methotrexate has become a first-line therapy in the treatment of ectopic pregnancy. Both single-dose therapy and multidose regimens have been employed, with an emphasis on close follow-up of quantitative β-hCG levels after treatment.

A modification of the protocol first described by Stovall and Ling[11] is outlined in Table 59–1 and is the treatment of choice for unruptured ectopic pregnancy in our institution. Patients with an ectopic pregnancy that is less than or equal to 3.5 cm in greatest diameter by endovaginal ultrasound without cardiac activity, who have a quantitative β-hCG less than 10,000 mIU/mL, and who are without evidence of hepatic dysfunction or hemodynamic instability are candidates for medical management. In addition to a quantitative β-hCG, a complete blood cell count and liver function tests are obtained before therapy. On day 1, methotrexate, 50 mg/m², is administered intramuscularly. A repeat β-hCG is obtained on day 4 and day 7. Patients with a 15% or greater decline in β-hCG levels between day 4 and day 7 are followed with weekly β-hCG titers until a negative pregnancy test is obtained. Patients not meeting this criterion are given a repeat dose of methotrexate, 50 mg/m², and the protocol is repeated. Stovall and Ling[11] reported a 94% success rate for medical therapy in their series of 120 patients.

A significant percentage of patients receiving methotrexate therapy for ectopic pregnancy will experience transient abdominal pain. Discriminating between effective therapy with the expected trophoblastic necrosis and rupture of the ectopic pregnancy can be a difficult task. Surgery should be reserved for those patients demonstrating a rising β-hCG level despite therapy and hemodynamic instability and in those with sonographic evidence of rupture of the ectopic pregnancy. There should be a low threshold for hospitalization and close observation if the diagnosis is unclear.

Other medical therapies for the treatment of ectopic

Table 59–1. Protocol for Single-dose Methotrexate for Ectopic Pregnancy

Inclusion Criteria

Patient is hemodynamically stable
Ectopic pregnancy ≤ 3.5 cm in greatest diameter
No evidence of cardiac activity
Quantitative β-hCG < 10,000 mIU/mL
No evidence of hepatic dysfunction

Day 1

Informed written consent
Complete blood cell count and liver function tests
Methotrexate, 50 mg/m² IM

Day 4

Repeat quantitative β-hCG

Day 7

Repeat quantitative β-hCG
  If ≤ 15% decline from day 4, repeat methotrexate, 50 mg/m² IM
  If > 15% decline from day 4, weekly β-hCG levels until negative

Modified from Stovall TG, Ling FW: Single-dose methotrexate: An expanded clinical trial. Am J Obstet Gynecol 1993;168:1759–1765.

pregnancy have been used with success. However, prostaglandins, hyperosmolar glucose, and potassium chloride require direct injection into the ectopic pregnancy, either by ultrasound guidance or during laparoscopic surgery.

SURGICAL THERAPY

Concurrent with the advent of medical therapy for ectopic pregnancy has come a more conservative approach in those patients requiring surgical intervention for this condition. Laparoscopic treatment has been shown to be more cost effective with less morbidity and less hospitalization time when compared with laparotomy for ectopic pregnancy.[14] Laparoscopic salpingostomy is the surgical treatment of choice in those women with ectopic pregnancy who desire preserved fertility. Using electrocautery, an incision is made along the antimesosalpinx of the fallopian tube overlying the ectopic pregnancy. Hydrodissection with an irrigating and suctioning device is used to dislodge the products of conception from the fallopian tube. The products of conception are then removed from the abdominal cavity by means of grasping forceps and sent for histologic examination. The cut margins of the incision are cauterized, and copious irrigation of the area is employed to ensure hemostasis. Closure of the fallopian tube is unnecessary and does not improve future fertility. The persistence of the ectopic pregnancy is low after this procedure[14]; however, serial β-hCG determinations are recommended to ensure complete resolution of the pregnancy.

MEDICAL VERSUS SURGICAL TREATMENT

The accepted use of both medical therapy and conservative surgery for the treatment of unruptured ectopic pregnancy has allowed for a randomized, controlled trial comparing these two treatment modalities. Hajenius and coworkers[15] reported on 100 patients randomly assigned to medical therapy with systemic, multidose methotrexate versus salpingostomy in laparoscopically confirmed tubal ectopic pregnancy. They found no significant difference in treatment success rates or ipsilateral tubal patency rates between the two groups. The subsequent fertility rates of the patients enrolled in this study are not yet available.

SUMMARY

Contemporary management of ectopic pregnancy includes a consideration of medical therapy in those meeting strict inclusion guidelines. In those patients requiring surgical intervention, an emphasis is placed on tubal conservation if future fertility is desired.

Suggestions for Future Reading

Clin Obstet Gynecol 1999;42:1–54.
American College of Obstetrics and Gynecology: Medical Management of Tubal Pregnancy (Practice Bulletin No. 3). Washington, DC, ACOG, December, 1998.

References

1. Centers for Disease Control: Ectopic Pregnancy—United States, 1981–1983. MMWR Morb Mortal Wkly Rep 1986;35:289–291.
2. Centers for Disease Control and Prevention: Ectopic Pregnancy—United States, 1990–1992. MMWR Morb Mortal Wkly Rep 1995;44:46–48.
3. Rothman A, Shapiro J: Heterotopic pregnancy after homolateral salpingo-oopherectomy. Obstet Gynecol 1965;26:718–720.
4. Goldman G, Fisch B, Ovadia J, et al: Heterotopic pregnancy after assisted reproductive technologies. Obstet Gynecol Surv 1992;47:217–221.
5. Russell JB: The etiology of ectopic pregnancy. Clin Obstet Gynecol 1987;30:181–190.
6. Pisarska MD, Carson SA, Buster JE: Ectopic pregnancy. Lancet 1998;351:1115–1120.
7. Chow W, Daling JR, Cates W, et al: Epidemiology of ectopic pregnancy. Epidemiol Rev 1987;9:70–94.
8. Lau S, Tulandi T: Conservative medical and surgical management of interstitial ectopic pregnancy. Fertil Steril 1999;72:207–215.
9. Goldstein SR, Snyder JR, Watson C, et al: Very early pregnancy detection with endovaginal ultrasound. Obstet Gynecol 1988;72:200–204.
10. Barnhart KT, Simhan H, Kamelle SA: Diagnostic accuracy of ultrasound above and below the beta-hCG discriminatory zone. Obstet Gynecol 1999;94:583–587.
11. Stovall TG, Ling FW: Single-dose methotrexate: An expanded clinical trial. Am J Obstet Gynecol 1993;168:1759–1765.
12. Tanaka T, Hayashi H, Kutzuzawa T, et al: Treatment of interstitial ectopic pregnancy with methotrexate: Report of a successful case. Fertil Steril 1982;37:851–852.
13. Stovall TG, Ling FW, Gray LA, et al: Methotrexate treatment of unruptured ectopic pregnancy: A report of 100 cases. Obstet Gynecol 1991;77:749–753.
14. Yao M, Tulandi T: Current status of surgical and nonsurgical management of ectopic pregnancy. Fertil Steril 1997;67:421–433.
15. Hajenius PJ, Engelsbel S, Mol BW, et al: Randomized trial of systemic methotrexate versus laparoscopic salpingostomy in tubal pregnancy. Lancet 1997;350:774–779.

Alternatives to Conventional Hormone Replacement

Maida Taylor

UNCERTAINTY ABOUT HORMONE REPLACEMENT THERAPY

The field of menopausal medicine is in ferment. The presumed benefits of hormone replacement therapy (HRT) are being challenged with unprecedented intensity. Since the 1940s, health providers have heavily promoted estrogen replacement therapy (ERT) as an antidote to aging and a preventive panacea. Women, however, are discontent and discouraged with the medical approach to menopause. Despite sincere, but perhaps overenthusiastic, promotion of estrogen replacement by the medical profession, fewer than 1 in 4 postmenopausal women actually take hormones. Sixty per cent to 70% of users stop their hormones within 1 to 2 years of starting, and 30% of women never get their HRT prescriptions filled. Before discussing the role of alternatives for menopause management, we need to understand the basis for the disdain and distrust engendered by HRT, in contradistinction to the widespread appeal of alternative therapies. Given a lack of consensus among health professionals coupled with a constant counterculture attack on conventional HRT, it is no wonder that only 10% to 25% of menopausal women take HRT. Of those given a prescription for HRT, only 30% get them filled. After 1 year, less than 40% of women who started HRT continue. Given that 20% of women experience few symptoms and are at low risk of cardiovascular disease or osteoporosis and may not need HRT, why it is that fewer than 1 in 4 women of the remaining 80% ever use HRT?

All of our concepts of the role of estrogen in coronary vascular disease (CVD) are based in observational studies that have been heavily tainted by selection biases, because HRT users tend to be much healthier than nonusers, and selective prescribing practices for the past 40 years have excluded most high-risk women from the pool of users. Texts and the *Physicians' Desk Reference* universally advised against the use of HRT in women with cardiovascular disease, pulmonary disease, liver and renal dysfunction, obesity, diabetes, hypertension, lipid disorders, metabolic abnormalities, family history of such, and other factors. HRT users tend to be thinner, better educated, more active, and higher in socioeconomic status, all markers of lowered disease risk.[1] "At-risk" women have not even been allowed to start taking estrogens. HRT users have been found to be better educated, to have better lipid profiles, to exercise more, and to have lower blood pressure than

nonusers.[2] Grady and associates[3] suggest that the only groups for whom ERT offers unequivocal benefits are women at very high risk of CVD or those status posthysterectomy. This unsettled and unsettling influence of estrogen on breast cancer risk has also tempered its use. A more recent analysis by Col and coworkers[4] of the impact of hormone replacement on life expectancy concluded that benefits exist for all women except those with two first-degree relatives with breast cancer. The authors state that low-risk women, those with no risk factors for CVD or osteoporosis, who also have two first-degree relatives with breast cancer, "should not receive hormone therapy." The major controversies continue to roil today and greatly affect acceptance and continuance rates for hormone use. First, all algorithms on the long-term benefits of HRT rely for their statistical validity on the assumption that HRT reduces the rate of cardiovascular mortality by 50% to 70%. When reductions attributed to estrogen are removed from the calculations, the projected benefits of HRT rapidly degrade.

Whereas the media and lay public may exaggerate the hazards of estrogen, the profession probably has overestimated the benefits of HRT. Estrogen has positive effects on at least a dozen markers of cardiovascular risk. Estrogen induces increases in high-density lipoprotein (HDL), decreases in low-density lipoprotein (LDL), LDL oxidation, and lipoprotein (a) (Lp[a]), which correlate with decreased risk of CVD. Moreover, estrogen also has salutary effects on non–lipid-mediated mechanisms, which also affect heart disease risks. These include estrogen's ability to increase insulin sensitivity, increase vasodilatation in arterial vessels, and improve endothelial function. Nonetheless, clinical studies have been less than encouraging about the effects of estrogen in recent years. Estrogen, particularly unopposed oral treatment, leads to a 20% to 30% increase in triglycerides, and more importantly, to a huge increase in postprandial triglyceride fragments, thought to represent a major risk for CVD. Estrogen also increases levels of C-reactive protein, another marker of increased risk of CVD. Recent controlled clinical trials have failed to evidence any improvements in outcome in women with preexistent coronary disease and have failed to show benefit in lowering the rate of progression of preexistent arterial lesions. The Heart and Estrogen/Progestin Replacement Study (HERS)[5] found that women with prior events evidenced no improvements in nonfatal and fatal coronary events when given hormone replacement for 4 years. The advocates for estrogen have been recalculating, reinterpreting, reanalyzing, and recounting—anything to try to explain the HERS trial away. The fact of the matter is that the cumulative mortality in both treatment and controls is the same at the end of the 4-year trial, although early attrition in the treatment arm gives the erroneous impression that death rates decline in the later years of the study.[6] The Estrogen Replacement and Atherosclerosis Study (ERA),[7] a study of 2000 women with coronary stenosis treated with placebo, conjugated estrogen, or conjugated estrogen plus medroxyprogesterone acetate, found that all groups evidenced the same degree of progression of lesions.

The role of estrogen in the development of breast cancer is still controversial. Experts are divided. Whereas the epidemiologists debate the order of magnitude of the risk, whether risks accrue with unopposed estrogen versus estrogen plus progestin,[8] or with continuous combined HRT versus sequential HRT,[9] the public and the press have made up their minds. In many lay persons' lexicon, the word *hormone* connotes *cancer*. Starting with Seaman's two books, *The Doctors' Case Against the Pill*[10] and *Women and the Crisis in Sex Hormones*,[11] and continuing with works such as *Dr. Susan Love's Hormone Book*,[12] women have been told that estrogen carries a significant measure of blame for the increased rates of breast cancer in the past 40 years. Women aged 40 to 60 years are far more fearful of disfigurement and disability imposed by a diagnosis of breast cancer than by the threat of death from myocardial infarction, because heart disease is viewed as a rather distant event. Breast cancer is a much more immediate fear because it is the leading cause of cancer death in this age group. Breast cancer is envisioned as a slow, long, lingering death, full of pain and suffering, suffering that is increased and prolonged by surgery, radiation, chemotherapy, and other horrors yet to be invented by the medical industrial establishment. Breast cancer invades and pervades the immediate consciousness of perimenopausal and menopausal women because almost all women this age have had friends and relatives diagnosed with the disease, a reality that cannot be erased with studies and statistics. One cannot obliterate terror with data.

Breast cancer is not the only cancer worry. Endometrial cancer clearly is increased with the use of unopposed estrogen. We commonly tell women that any vaginal bleeding after menopause is a possible sign of endometrial cancer. We then inform them that estrogen causes endometrial cancer if unopposed. We place them on estrogen, and add a progestin, which in turn causes withdrawal or breakthrough bleeding. Women are then told to ignore the bleeding that results, which seems like a highly paradoxical, confusing directive. Women are also told that bleeding will subside after a few short months, but the fact of the matter is quite different. Whereas most women do ultimately become amenorrheic, bleeding occurs in at least 20% of women after 2 years of HRT use.[13] For the first few months, nervous women are reassured that bleeding will stop and that the risk is nil, but after several months,

assurances are put aside and studies to "rule out" are done, rekindling fear and anxiety about cancer. Women are telling us, by their discontinuance rates, that they dislike the continued menstrual-like flow and unpredictable spotting. HRT can be quite discouraging and unsettling. Women are then driven away from the "conventional" path and out onto roads less well traveled.

ALTERNATIVE HEALTH INDUSTRY

In 1997, Eisenberg and colleagues[14] surveyed 2055 persons in the United States regarding the use of "alternative" medicine. Forty-two per cent of subjects stated that they did, in fact, seek out treatments other than those within the practice lexicon of conventional allopathic Western medicine. Alternative medicine visits exceeded visits to primary care providers, and 70% of such encounters were never discussed with the patient's regular personal physician. Present estimates are that Americans spend approximately $27 billion on alternative health services and products, more than the out-of-pocket expenditures for physician-related health care. The adherence and affection for complementary and alternative care extend across the oceans. In 1996, Australians spent 1 billion (AU) for complementary and alternative medicine (CAM), twice as much as they spent on pharmaceuticals. The European market for botanical medicines is three times larger than that in the United States. For decades, European pharmaceutical houses such as Boehringer, Boots, and Novartis produced and marketed botanical products on parallel tracks alongside their conventional pharmaceutical lines, and the use of botanicals in Europe exceeds US rates by threefold. Physicians in Germany routinely prescribe botanicals for many illnesses along with conventional prescription pharmaceuticals, with sales of over-the-counter botanicals reaching $7 billion per year. In the United States, large pharmaceutical companies, aware of the high demand for botanicals, have recently introduced over-the-counter herbs, often targeting specific health concerns: mood mixtures, prostate potions, diet draughts. The U.S. Food and Drug Administration restricts the advertising claims companies can make, but nonetheless the manufacturers, with the overt and covert cooperation with legitimate alternative practitioners and data-deficient self-styled gurus, often imply benefits far beyond those allowed in the advertising copy claims, which are supposed to center on "health maintenance." Mood implies treatment of depression, prostate health becomes therapy for benign prostatic hypertrophy, two therapeutic claims that may, in fact, be true for some botanic offerings. The line between scientific fact and fantastic fiction begins to blur as claims for appetite control become promises of weight loss without diet or exercise; wellness morphs into the capacity to reverse aging, and high-fiber laxative becomes a means to cleanse and purge the body of toxins and poisons that accumulate as a result of living in the chemically contaminated modern world.

Users of alternatives are not dissatisfied with conventional allopathic medicine. The rationales for using such therapies are manifold and complex. Astin[15] questioned over 1000 individuals about the use of alternative medicine. The highest rates of use occurred in persons aged 35 to 49 and 50 to 64 years, 42% and 44%, respectively. Predictors of use of alternatives therapies were proposed: (1) dissatisfaction with conventional medicine as ineffective, impersonal, overly technological or costly, or yielding adverse outcomes; (2) a need for personal control, viewing alternatives as less authoritarian, more empowering, and affording greater personal autonomy; or (3) philosophical congruence, a perception that alternatives are more compatible with personal values and personal ethical and religious beliefs. Users of alternatives were found to have a higher level of educational, but somewhat poorer health status. They claimed a more holistic orientation to health and were also more likely to have had a transformational experience changing one's worldview. Many respondents had chronic health conditions like anxiety, back problems, chronic pain, and urinary tract problems, problems that are often poorly addressed by conventional medical care. Certain personal cultural values and systems predicted higher rates of alternative medicine use. Individuals who held beliefs and values consistent with environmentalism, feminism, spirituality and personal growth psychology were more likely to use CAM.

Supporters of plant medicines cite the fact that the cost of bringing a new drug to market is more than $231 million and that conventional pharmaceutical manufacturers have little interest in old "plant" drugs that cannot be patented.[16] Proponents of plant medicines argue that safe and effective treatments are ignored, and physicians push more toxic, potent, "synthetic" drugs in complicity with powerful drug companies who, with gifts and trips, ingratiate and influence prescribing practices.

Consumers, trying to find preventives and remedies that are kinder and gentler, have embraced alternatives. Health food, herbal, and supplement shops exist in almost every mall in the United States and are no longer confined to bicoastal hippie communities, and complications related to the use of alternatives can show up anywhere.[17] Practitioners in every community will encounter traditional Chinese medicine, stress reduction, chiropractic manipula-

tion, homeopathy, and plant medicine practice. Much of alternative care operates outside the mazelike set of obstacles created by third-party health payers. Alternative care may actually be more widely accessible to American health consumers. The lay public often does not know what distinguishes clinically trained and licensed health professionals from alternative practitioners, some of whom do have impressive credentials, but many of whom have no formal training or licensing. Health consumers might be hard pressed to distinguish a massage therapist from a physical therapist or a homeopath from an osteopath.

Often, consumers seem not to care about training and credentialing. A large segment of the lay community has come to project that alternative providers have purer motives than medical personnel and that "natural" remedies hold fewer risks. Patients believe that commercial forces driving medical practices in the United States are subverting quality and compassion. One has only to listen to "talk radio" or attend a cancer support group to hear rhetoric damning and demeaning the mainstream. At the least, doctors are viewed as ignorant of simple things that induce wellness, like diet, supplements, and plant medicines. In the extreme, adherents of alternatives rant about medical oncologists who do not want to find a cheap and simple cure for cancer, because they make vast amounts of money by poisoning cancer victims with outrageously expensive, toxic products proffered by greedy pharmaceutical companies. When the gap is this wide, it is difficult if not impossible to cross over. Whereas a few consumers completely eschew mainstream medicine, most users of alternatives take a pluralistic tack and combine conventional medicines with botanicals and other alternatives.

Whereas alternative care may not offer medical advantages that can be proved by statistical objectification, they offer subjective superiority that patients find exceedingly appealing such as unhurried visits, comfortable settings, guarantees of success, overwhelming optimism and individualization, even when not needed for therapeutic success (Table 60–1). Whereas medical therapies must provide full, informed consent and disclosure, alternative therapies can make sweeping global claims to a wide array of unconfirmed benefits, while alleging to have no serious side effects or risks. Furthermore, alternative and complementary practitioners appear to have a vast tableau of choices:

Table 60–1. Patient Perceptions Regarding Alternative and Conventional Medicine

	Conventional	Alternative
Initial visit	Rushed, average 20–30 min	Unhurried, average 90 min
Follow-up	Often only 6–10 min	At least 20 min
Setting	Institutional	Personal, comfortable, often homelike
Symptoms	Sorted, screened, valued	Symptoms seemingly all taken at face value
Individuality	Ignored, idiosyncrasies minimized	Therapy customized for this case alone
Social issues	Often ignored	Regarded as central
Certainty	Informed consent	Treatment presented as 100% successful
Prognosis	Outcome and risk statistics presented	Usually optimistic, little downside

Modified from Buckman R, Sabbagh K: Magic or Medicine—An Investigation of Healing and Healers. Toronto, Key Porter, 1993.

nutrition, herbs, teas, foods, minerals, body therapy, meditations, and more, whereas physicians seem to have only one limited offering—hormones.

Alternative medicine encompasses a number of systematic medical practices based on physical assessments that differ from physiology as it is taught in Western medical institutions. Traditional Chinese medicine is based on balance of essential life energy called *Qi* (pronounced Chee). Acupuncture seeks to maintain wellness and to treat disease by regulating the flow of Qi along meridians that transit the body. Other medical practices commonly encountered now in the United States include Ayurveda, an ancient medical system from India, naturopathy, and homeopathy. In some regions of the United States, traditional healing systems of Native Americans, Tibetans, and other cultures may be encountered. Alternative medicine also includes mind-body interventions that are intent on pursuing health and healing using the conscious and sometimes unconscious influence of the mind over bodily processes. Manipulative and body-based treatments are commonplace, especially chiropractic, osteopathy, and massage. Meditation, hypnosis, music, and prayer are examples of mind-body practice. Studies have been done to see whether remote mind-body connections can influence health outcomes, like the influence of remote prayer by congregants unknown to the sufferer, to see if such spirituality can affect surgical morbidity and mortality. Somewhat related to mind-body medicine are so-called energy-modulating practices that seek to realign the bioelectric field of the body. Examples include therapeutic touch, Qi, Gong treatment, and magnets. The most recognizable and widely employed alternatives are biologic-based therapies like botanical medicines, dietary supplements, vitamins, minerals, and orthomolecular medicine. Every mall in America has a health food store, replete with megavitamins, herbal teas, blue-green algae powders, and the like. Every pharmacy now routinely stocks a wide array of the vitamin and mineral supplements and, oftentimes, shelves full of botanicals. Large "organic" supermarkets like Fresh Fields and Whole Foods have row after row of shelf space devoted to "natural" products ranging from kinder, gentler hair dyes to many brands of homeopathic medicines.

Expenditures for herbal medicines topped $4 billion in 1998, and the use of such preparations increased almost 400% between 1990 and 1997. As to the needs and concerns of menopausal women, according to a survey done by the North American Menopause Society in 1997, 36% of women reported using alternatives for the management of menopausal symptoms. Alternatives most commonly cited included acupuncture, herbal medicines, plant estrogens, and natural hormones, accounting for 6%, 10%, 10% and 10%, respectively.[18]

BOTANICAL MEDICINE

Whereas the term *herbal* refers to the herbaceous portions of plants, namely the leaves and stems, the term *botanical* denotes foods and supplements derived from any plant part—herbaceous plus seeds, fruits, flowers, and roots. Every country and culture has some sort of herbal or botanical tradition of healing, and at least 30% of our current pharmacopoeia is derived from old plant medicines or is still manufactured from botanical sources. America is truly a melting pot, and menopausal women are taking bits and pieces from different traditional botanical practices, taking Chinese herbs with American vitamins, Indian teas with Tibetan powders, incurring the risk of herb-herb interactions, not to mention herb-drug interactions. And patients are unlikely to report the use of botanicals unless prompted to do so, with very precise and pointed inquiry. Fortunately, most of the botanicals used to treat midlife and menstrual disorders are relatively benign and safe.

In considering the use of alternative therapies, particularly botanical medicines for menopause, one needs to be aware that different plants are used for different purposes, and different parts of the same plant may be used to different therapeutic intents. In American botanical practice, no one herbal is proffered as a panacea for menopause complaints, so that many botanical remedies for menopause are a combination of a number of herbs that claim estrogenic, progestational, androgenic, antiestrogenic, and other modes of action. Most commonly, such herbal preparations claim to be safe substitutes for estrogen, providing relief of symptoms, while avoiding hormonal stimulation of estrogen-sensitive tissues like the breast and endometrium. These types of claims usually lack substantial proof save for long-standing "folk" wisdom and experience. Much of the research on plant medicinals is not accessible via MEDLINE search, is not available in English, and is often done with less than rigorous study design, complicating our efforts to prove or disprove claims.

PHYTOESTROGENS

Phytoestrogens are defined as naturally occurring plant sterols that may exert effects similar to those of estrogen (Table 60–2). More correctly, the phytoestrogens should be called *phytoSERMs*—because they act as selective estrogen

Table 60–2. Relative Binding of Estrogens, Phytoestrogens, and Androgens to Estrogen Receptors

Compound	ERa	ERb
Estradiol	100	100
Estrone	60	37
DES	468	295
Coumestrol	94	185
Genistein	5	36
Testosterone	<.01	<.01

DES, diethylstilbestrol; ER, estrogen receptor.
From Kuiper GG, Lemmen JG, Carlsson B, et al: Interaction of estrogenic chemicals and phytoestrogens with estrogen receptor beta. Endocrinology 1997; 138:863–870.

receptor modulators (SERMs). Phytoestrogens fall into three groups: isoflavones, the most commonly consumed in human diets, and genistein and daidzein, plant sterol molecules found in soy and garbanzo beans and other legumes. Foods made from soy, such as tempeh, soy, miso, and tofu, are rich sources of genistein and daidzein. Lignans are a constituent of cell wall of plants, and become bioavailable through the action of intestinal bacteria on cereal grains. The highest amounts are found in seeds used as vegetable oil sources; flaxseed, also commonly called linseed, is one of the richest sources. Coumestans are not very important as a source of phytoestrogens for humans. High concentrations are found in red clover, sunflower seeds, and bean sprouts and are known to have estrogenic effects in grazing animals. Alternative medicine gurus often tout the phytoestrogens as replacements for pharmaceutical estrogen replacement, advancing the fantasy that soy and other isoflavone sources can provide cardioprotection, bone mineral health, and estrogenic support for symptoms while not only avoiding the risk of cancer but, supposedly, also decreasing the risk of a number of cancers—particularly sex steroid–dependent tumors.

Soy-derived phytoestrogens are abundant in traditional Asian diets. In population-based studies, research shows that in countries like China and Japan, with high dietary levels of isoflavones, the women are reputed to express few menopausal complaints and, coincidentally, also evidence a very low incidence of breast cancer. Rates of prostate cancer also are lower in men in countries with soy-rich diets. Asian women typically ingest 40 to 80 mg of isoflavones per day whereas Americans average less than 3 mg per day. In clinical trials, high intake of isoflavones depresses luteinizing hormone (LH) levels, therapy being presumed to exert some antagonistic or antiestrogenic effect. Researchers and reviewers in the field agree with Persky and Van Horn[19] that there is sufficient "epidemiologic evidence support[ing] the hypothesis that phytoestrogens inhibit cancer formation and growth in humans." But the fact remains that the outcome we seek, lowered rates of neoplasia, does not reside solely in the isoflavones. Soy-based foods exert a number of biologic effects that potentially might lower rates of cancer. Moreover, vegetarian diets in general are associated with improved health outcomes and reductions in vascular diseases and cancer. But such benefits have been described only in population-based studies in which the groups have incurred a lifetime of dietary discretion. No long-term interventional studies have been done, and most certainly none has been done in 50-year-old women, using soy or vegetarian diets as a therapeutic intervention, to see if the "typical" American can undo the damage imposed by our high-fat, high-calorie, animal protein–rich cuisine.

The health effects of soy and other isoflavone-rich foods are mediated via several proposed mechanisms. Isoflavones are often assumed to be "estrogenic" but more correctly should be thought of as SERMs, having agonist and antagonist effects and preferential binding for estrogen receptor-

beta (ERb). Soy foods modulate sex steroid metabolism by increasing sex hormone–binding globulin (SHBG) synthesis, lowering of serum E2, inhibiting aromatase activity, and by downregulating 5-alpha-reductase inhibition. They also affect other key sites of possible neoplastic degenerative change, modifying antiproliferative and apoptotic effects, inhibiting proteases, decreasing angiogenesis, and exerting antioxidant effects. But the issue of soy as a preventive is complicated by the fact that persons who eat soy-based diets are often vegetarians, and a high intake of vegetables correlates with marked reductions in vascular and neoplastic diseases. The cuisines that use soy foods also use large amounts of cruciferous vegetables like cabbage, broccoli, cauliflower, collard, kale, watercress, horseradish, turnip, radishes, bok choy, and mustard seed and umbelliferous vegetables like celery, parsley, fennel, carrot, parsnip, dill, coriander, cumin, caraway—foods that are cited over and over for effects on health outcomes. Vegetarianism is associated with lower rates of not only CVD and cancer also but with reductions in the incidence of type 2 diabetes, arthritis, gout, renal stones, osteoporosis, and macular degeneration.

Soy is commonly touted now as a safe alternative to estrogen for the treatment of menopausal symptoms and complaints and as a preventive for the major health risks associated with loss of estrogen, namely osteoporosis and cardiovascular disease. It is beyond the scope of this review to discuss the bone and vascular effects of isoflavones, but suffice it to say, the soy-based diets, either due to some direct effects on bone or through indirect effects as substitutes for high-nitrogen animal protein, appear to slow the rate of bone loss in menopause. Soy-based isoflavones do improve lipid profiles and provide a significant improvement in arterial compliance. There are, however, no long-term studies demonstrating that adding soy-based isoflavones significantly modifies the incidence of osteoporosis, nor does any research document lower rates of heart disease in a high-risk group given soy or isoflavone supplements.

Often, proponents of soy cite the fact that women in Asian societies report a much lower incidence of vasomotor symptoms than European and American women. Surveys of American women report an incidence of 85%, for Europeans 70% to 80%, but the incidence in Malaysia is 57%, and China and Singapore report 18% and 14%, respectively.[20] Such comparisons do not account for the fact that vasomotor symptoms do not figure prominently in the symptom profiles for menopause in Asian countries. Often the literature is "cherry picked," citing only references supporting this point of view. For example, in Japan, the two most common menopause complaints are fatigue and neck stiffness, occurring in over 80% of respondents, but 60% reported hot flushes of the face.[21] In considering phytoestrogens for the management of menopausal symptoms, six studies are now published in the accessible literature.

Numerous abstracts and unpublished reports exist that

cannot be reviewed in depth. The problem with the literature to date is that differing amounts and forms of isoflavones are used, and studies have been relatively short lived—usually 2 to 3 months. Representative studies include Washburn and associates,[22] who compared 20 g of soy protein with 34 mg of isoflavones with a 20-g carbohydrate complex over a 1.5-month period. There was a decrease in severity but not frequency of symptoms in the treatment group. Albertazzi and coworkers[23] treated more than 100 women with seven or more hot flushes per day for 3 months with 60 g of isolated soy protein (76 mg isoflavones) versus a casein control and reported a 45% reduction versus a 30% decrease in the control group. Murkies and colleagues[24] used a soy flour supplement in their 3-month study and found a 40% reduction versus 25% in the wheat flour–fed controls, but the differences between groups was not significant. Overall, the publications and abstracts that can be reviewed suggest that consuming around 80 mg or more of isoflavone as soy protein appears to provide relief for mild to moderate menopausal vasomotor flushing. Lesser amounts appear to be ineffective.

What remains problematic is how to get over 80 mg of active isoflavones into a typical American diet on a daily basis. An 8-ounce glass of soy milk contains between 12 and 20 mg of isoflavones, which means that to achieve a daily intake of 80 mg, one would need to drink 4 to 6 glasses per day. Soy breakfast patties contain around 10 mg of isoflavones, which means one would need to eat eight soy patties a day to get the necessary amount of isoflavones. A person eating this much soy would be getting 25% to 30% of daily calories from one food source and be in danger of developing deficiencies in other nutritional areas. An easy fix is to use soy protein powders or shake mixes. Several brands of shake mixes use isoflavone-rich varieties of soy, so that one 20-g soy shake with less than 200 calories contains 100 mg of isoflavones, an amount that reaches the "therapeutic" threshold. Long-term intake of dietary levels of isoflavones does not appear to carry any risks. Women in Japan with high dietary intake of isoflavones do not have worsened outcomes from breast cancer. But a cautionary note needs to be interjected. Many women are eating soy with abandon, taking isoflavone or clover tablets liberally, while chewing flaxseeds in an effort to avoid the risks of estrogen. Supradietary intake of phytoestrogens may impose as yet undetermined risks, and is not advisable.

When considering whether to suggest the use of phytoestrogens from soy or other foods to women in menopause, it is important to delineate the proven value of diets based on plant proteins, but not overstate the case. Whereas soy does appear to improve lipids, lipoproteins, and insulin sensitivity and to decrease progression of atherosclerosis, there are no interventional studies documenting declines in mortality from CVD when diets are altered at midlife.

Is soy truly a substitute for estrogen? Bone effects are even vague, with a slight improvement in bone mineral density with the use of a synthetic isoflavone, ipriflavone, but considerably less than that seen with ERT. Soy-based isoflavones do provide a clinically relevant improvement in vasomotor symptoms, approximately 70% to 90% of the reductions seen with ERT. The effects on cognition are unclear.[25] Thus, soy might be considered "selective estrogen light."

Soy- and Red Clover–Based Isoflavone Supplements

Soy and trifolium pratense are legumes and rich sources of a number of phytoestrogens. Whereas soy is the most common source of isoflavones in the human diet, red clover is actually the richest source of isoflavones. Isoflavones are also found in other legumes like garbanzos, lentils, and other beans. Red clover also provides large amounts of coumestans, phytochemicals with steroid-like activity responsible for degraded reproductive performance in sheep and cattle. High intake of soy-based isoflavones correlates with reduced rates of a number of diseases including cardiovascular disease and malignancies.[26]

A number of isoflavone isolates are being promoted in the United States now as "alternatives" to soy-based isoflavones from soy foodstuffs. These isolates are often made from soy or clover. The source plant material is washed with alcohol and the active isoflavones, the aglyconic forms which are alcohol soluble, are extracted. The alcohol is evaporated off and the remaining residue is packaged as a food supplement. Literature promoting these supplements often cites observational epidemiologic studies of the benefits of a high soy diet and then suggests that supplements provide similar health benefits. Randomized controlled clinical trials of isoflavone extracts as therapeutics are accumulating, and do not support these claims. Several products, like Healthy Woman from soy and Promensil from red clover, are at the center of big, expensive advertising campaigns in the United States. Technical literature on Promensil states that each 500-mg tablet contains approximately 200 to 230 mg of dried aqueous alcoholic extracted *Trifolium pratense* (red clover) and four isoflavones: biochanin A, formononetin, daidzein, and genistein in the ratios 20:12:1:1. Almost all the biochanin and formononetin are rapidly demethylated to genistein and daidzein. Conversion is incomplete, so that some residually detectable amounts of biochanin and formononetin remain in the circulation and exert mild biologic activity.

Traditional soy-based foods contain predominantly genistein and daidzein. All of the isoflavones bind to estrogen receptors, with genistein binding to ERb with 36% of the affinity of 17-beta estradiol.[27, 28] Once bound, genistein acts as an SERM, not as a true estrogen.

In an open clinical trial of menopausal women, whereas red clover effected marked improvement in systemic arterial compliance by 23%, it had no effects on plasma lipids.[29] Trials of various isoflavone isolates for hot flushes have been equivocal. Washburn and associates[22] reported in 1999 that soy supplementation in the diet of nonhypercholesterolemic, nonhypertensive, perimenopausal women resulted in significant improvements in lipid and lipoprotein levels, blood pressure, and perceived severity of vasomotor symptoms.

Red clover–derived commercial preparation containing 40 mg of total isoflavones has been studied in two controlled clinical trials and, in both instances, performed no better than placebo. Barber and associates[30] did a double-blind, placebo-controlled crossover trial of 51 women with three or more hot flushes per day. Forty-three women completed the trial comparing 40 mg/day isoflavones to placebo. The study design was a 3-month treatment followed by a washout and an additional 3-month crossover to the other arm. Hot flush frequency decreased in both groups, 18% and 20% in treatment and placebo, respectively; therefore, there was no statistically significant difference between groups. In addition, there were no differences between groups in other symptoms (Greene scale) or endometrial thickness (ultrasound). Knight and Eden[20] also studied the same product in a three-armed trial comparing isoflavone 40 mg, 160 mg, and placebo for 12 weeks. The hot flush frequency decreased in all groups by 35%, 29%, and 34%, respectively. There was no significant difference from baseline in follicle-stimulating hormone (FSH) or SHBG in any group. Serum HDL cholesterol levels increased significantly (18%) in subjects on the 40-mg dose but not in the 120-mg group. Unfortunately, total cholesterol and triglyceride were not reported. It is encouraging to know, however, that in a study of 98 women taking 40 mg of the isoflavone isolate for 12 weeks, no changes occurred in menstrual bleeding patterns or in endometrial thickness on transvaginal ultrasound. But the product does not appear to help menopausal symptoms in any clinically significant degree.

Another product, Estroven, contains 50 mg of isoflavone derived from soybean and pureria root, along with several other herbs, minerals, and vitamins including black cohosh, Kava Kava, calcium, boron, vitamin E, B_{12}, folic acid, thiamin (B_1), riboflavin (B_2), niacin (B_3), and selenium. The manufacturer reports that in consumer trials, 70% of women believed that Estroven "met or exceeded their expectations" after 14 days of use. No other documentation of efficacy can be found. Another soy-based isoflavone product, Healthy Woman, reported decreases in severity and frequency of hot flushes, but did not quite meet statistical significance at 12 weeks. The product did not affect any of the measures used to assess central or peripheral estrogenicity.[31]

Large-scale interventional studies are needed, however, to demonstrate that modifying one's diet at midlife to include large amounts of dietary isoflavones can affect the rate of myocardial infarction and breast cancer. It is very shaky logic to assume that the benefits seen in populations with a lifetime of high isoflavone food intake will accrue to recent converts, and even shakier to project that isoflavone

isolates, which clearly do not produce equivalent physiologic effects when compared with soy protein sources of phytoestrogens, will lead to significant changes in morbidity and mortality.

Botanicals Used for Menopause

Herbal and botanical products have been used for centuries to ease female suffering as a consequence of reproductive physiology and disease. Herbal interventions abound for treatment of pregnancy-related problems like labor pain, lactation, and hyperemesis and also as abortifacients. Botanical medicines have been used since ancient times to regulate menstruation, either to induce or to stem the flow. The treatment of the climacteric is a rather modern concern, because until recently most women did not live long enough to experience menopause.

The most recognizable remedy for "women's troubles" was Lydia E. Pinkham's Vegetable Compound, concocted on a stove in her basement in 1875. The compound contained unicorn root (*Aletris farinosia* [L.]), life root (*Senecio aureus* [L.]), black cohosh (*Cimicifuga racemosa* [L.] Nutt.), pleurisy root (*Asclepias tuberosa* [L.]), fenugreek seed (*Trigonella foenum-graecum* [L.]) in 18% to 19% alcohol. Lydia Pinkham's enjoyed its greatest popularity during the Prohibition era, when large amounts were imbibed by men and women with equal enthusiasm. Pleurisy root and fenugreek were supposed to have demonstrated estrogenicity in animals. The amount of black cohosh used in the compound is said to approximate the amount found in a current menopause remedy made in Germany called Remifemin.[32]

A variety of botanicals—leaves, flowers, roots—are recommended for treatment of menopausal complaints. Typically, no one herbal is used for all complaints, and therefore, menopause remedies are often "compounded" products with several botanicals used together. Often, the plants used are said to be "estrogenic" or antiestrogen and are supposed to support estrogen-dependent tissues and functions. Others are supposed to block or balance the effect of steroids other than estrogen; in some manner correcting imbalances in the reproductive endocrine system. The 1899 edition of the Merck Manual lists an interesting set of offerings for management of the climacteric (Table 60–3). Many of these substances are still in use today, in particular, belladonna, black cohosh (*Cimicifuga*), and ovarian tissue (in Rejuvex, a dong quai herbal product that also contains bovine endocrine tissues and extracts). The use of psychoactive substances like opium and cannabis informs us that mood and affective complaints have been part and parcel of menopausal medicine for the last century and likely, the last millennium.

Belladonna

Belladonna (*Atropa belladonna*, deadly nightshade) has been used to treat menopausal complaints for a century or

Table 60–3. 1899 Merck Manual's Recommendations for Management of the Climacteric

Ammonia/ammonium chloride	*Nux vomica*
Amyl nitrate	Opium
Belladonna	Ovaraden
Calabar bean	Ovariin
Camphor	Physostigma
Cannabis indica	Potassium bromide
Change of air or scene	Potassium iodide
Cimicifuga	Sodium benzoate
Eucalyptol	Stypticin
Hot spongings	Thymol
Hydrastinine hydrochlorate	Warm bath
Iron	Zinc valerianate
Methylene blue	

Data from 1899 Merck Manual. Copyright © Merck & Co., New York, 1899. Reprinted in celebration of the centennial edition by Merck Research Laboratories, a division of Merck & Co., Inc., Whitehouse Station, New Jersey, 1999.

more, alone and in combination with other medicinals. Although belladonna is listed in the German Commission E monographs on botanical medicines, it is cited for use in treatment of gastrointestinal and bile duct spasm and colic. Belladonna, ergotamine, and phenobarbital are used together in an oral preparation to treat migraine headaches, and these preparations at some time became popular for treatment of menopausal complaints. Belladonna, an anticholinergic agent containing the alkaloids hyoscyamine, atrophine, and scopolamine, is used to treat the nausea and vomiting associated with migraine headaches. Ergotamine is a cerebral arterial constrictor and helps treat the vasodilatation that appears to trigger migraine. Phenobarbital is added for its sedative effects. Long-acting and intermediate-acting barbiturates should be used in the elderly with extreme caution owing to the potential for prolonged sedation, vertigo, and increased risk of falls.

Typical of early studies of belladonna, Lebherz and French[33] found a 60% reduction in vasomotor symptoms in treated women, with a 22% reduction in control subjects. Side effects, completely predictable given the constituents, included sedation, depression, dizziness, and dry mouth. The last accessible citation, published in 1987, states that Bellergal Retard (a European version of Bellergal) did produce statistically significant improvements in symptomatology at 2 and 4 weeks, when compared with placebo. At the 8-week mark, there were no differences between the treatment and placebo arms.[34] My sense is that women taking these combination products may continue to have vasomotor symptoms, but the symptoms seemed less disturbing owing to the sedating effects of phenobarbital. Perhaps the subjects habituated to the effects of phenobarbital, and at 8 weeks or more, the sedative effects abetted so that symptoms then matched those seen in the placebo group again.

Black Cohosh

Black cohosh (*Cimicifuga racemosa* [L.] Nutt, family Ranunculaceae) is often referred to in folk medicine texts as *black snakeroot* or bugbane. Duker and coworkers[35] assert that a component of the extract binds competitively to 17-beta-estradiol receptors and lowers luteinizing hormone levels in ovariectomized rats. They also administered black cohosh (as Remifemin) to postmenopausal women for 8 weeks, and, again, LH levels fell, but FSH levels remained unchanged. The supposition was that black cohosh contained "three active compounds . . . (1) Constituents which were not ligands for the estrogen receptor but suppress LH release after chronic treatment, (2) constituents binding to the estrogen receptor and also suppressing LH release, and (3) compounds which are ligands for the estrogen receptor but without an effect of LH release." During the late 1980s, black cohosh was said to be estrogenic, but after Bergkvist and colleagues[36] published work suggesting that postmenopausal estrogen replacement might enhance the risk of breast cancer, claims regarding the estrogenicity of black cohosh became muted.

The company that manufactures Remifemin publishes a monograph containing abstracts of the clinical trials they have sponsored. Seven of the eight trials published to date did not use placebo controls, seven of the eight are available only in German, although the abstracts are accessible in English. A cursory glance at these studies gives one the impression that black cohosh offers profound palliation for the "neurovegetative" menopausal symptoms, such as anxiety, depression, and other mood disturbances, and significant reductions in Kupperman's Menopausal Index of menopausal symptoms. Some are open label, some have subjects who are premenopausal and postmenopausal, and some have no controls. But universally the studies show good benefits from black cohosh and no overt peripheral estrogenicity. Black cohosh does not appear to cause any increase in endometrial thickness, no change in maturation index of the vaginal epithelium, and no change in serum LH, FSH, estradiol, and prolactin.[37] Studies of black cohosh have been limited to 6 months' duration, and, therefore, the German Commission E recommends a 6-month maximum duration of use. The manufacturer suggests that the product can be used for 6 months, then stopped and restarted if symptoms recur. Black cohosh should not be confused with blue cohosh, *Caulophyllum thalictroides*, which has weak nicotine activity and is thought to have toxic potential. Obstetricians should be alerted to the fact that both black and blue cohosh are "prescribed" during the late third trimester of pregnancy, and are also given in enemas to stimulate desultory labor, an herbal practice that appears to be unsubstantiated.

Chasteberry Vitex

Chasteberry vitex (*Vitex agnus-castus* [L.] Verbenaceae), also known as Chaste tree, Monk's pepper, agnus castus, Indian spice, sage tree hemp, treewild pepper, and vitex, does contain hormone-like substances that competitively bind steroid receptor sites and thus exert antiandrogenic effects. Although it is promoted as a means of reducing libido in males, chasteberry is also recommended for women at menopause suffering from vaginal dryness, low libido, and depression. Its antiandrogenic effects seem antithetical to its use for symptoms of androgen deficiency in older women. Vitex has also been shown to inhibit prolactin secretion from the pituitary and has been used to treat hyperprolactinemia, mastalgia, premenstrual syndrome, and menopause symptoms. The German Commission E has approved it for the treatment of mastadynia and menstrual irregularities.

There are no studies of vitex in menopausal women. And no studies can be found to support the use of vitex to boost libido. A single in vitro study documents inhibition of secretion of prolactin by the pituitary gland with vitex extract.[38] In human studies, a single trial can be found in which 100 women with cyclic mastalgia were supposed to have quicker relief of breast pain than women treated with placebo.[38a] Another trial reported that vitex lowers prolactin levels in women with hyperprolactinemia and premenstrual syndrome (PMS), and at the same time, progesterone levels improved and luteal phase defects remitted using 20 mg daily. Two women with infertility conceived during the course of the study.[39] This paper and animal data have been cited as a reason to be cautious about the use of vitex in women undergoing fertility treatments, particularly those subject to in vitro fertilization pretreatments. Cahill and colleagues[40] reported a case of hyperstimulation during an in vitro fertilization cycle preceded by the use of vitex. This may or may not represent a true drug-herb interaction. Concern has been voiced that chasteberry might elicit drug-herb interactions with bromocriptine, dopamine, and other dopaminergic drugs, a least on a theoretical basis.

Although no studies on vitex and menopause can be found, a recent report from the United Kingdom assessed the effects of vitex on women with premenstrual syndrome, and may apply to women with similar complaints at menopause.[41] One hundred seventy women with PMS were randomly assigned to vitex versus placebo for three cycles. Women were given a self-assessment screening tool measuring menstrual symptoms. Significant improvements were seen in irritability, mood alteration, anger, headache, and breast fullness, whereas other menstrual symptoms, such as bloating, remained unchanged. Physician rating of the patient's condition also indicated significantly better effects than with placebo.

Dong Quai, Angelica Sinensis

Dong quai (aka dang gui, tang kuei [*Angelica polymorpha Maxim.*] var. *Sinensis Oliv*, aka *A. sinensis* [Oliv] Diels) is a type of angelica, whose root stock is suggested as a panacea for virtually every gynecologic ailment, including dysmenorrhea, oligomenorrhea, PMS, and menopausal syndrome. Other uses include ischemic stroke and constipation. In traditional Chinese herbal medicine, dong quai is characterized as "a warm herb that both circulates and nourishes *blood*, is also good for strengthening someone who is underweight, frail, anemic and chilly."[42] A rather interesting study of the use of a sterile 25% IV solution of dong quai root extract for stroke found improved neurologic symptoms, increased prothrombin time, and lower plasma fibrinogen.[43] Safer standardized anticoagulant therapies exist, and thus, no follow-up studies have been found.

There are no studies documenting the use of dong quai for menstrual complaints or for PMS. Dong quai is commonly said to have estrogenic activity, and is supposed to affect estradiol estrogen receptor binding in vitro. The only data supporting this assertion are evidence of increased uterine weight in ovariectomized rats mediated with dong quai. Donq quai does not increase estrogen-mediated uterine protein transcription.[44] In a placebo-controlled trial of dong quai in menopausal women, there was no evidence of estrogenicity and no palliation of menopausal symptoms over that seen with placebo, based on the Kupperman index and patients' diaries of hot flushes.[45] Critics argue that the dose of dong quai, 4.5 g, was too small to offer therapeutic benefits. In traditional practice, doses of 7 to 12 g might be used. Moreover, in traditional herbal practice, dong quai is never used alone, but rather is customarily compounded with other herbs. The combination is said to produce a synergy needed to affect biologic processes. Nonetheless, in the real world, dong quai is promoted and sold as a single botanical for menopause and menstrual disorders. Dong quai contains numerous coumarin-like substances that can act as anticoagulants and cause vasodilatory, antispasmodic, and central nervous system excitatory effects. The furocoumatin derivatives in dong quai are photosensitizing. Psoralen is also carcinogenic and mutagenic. Safrole, an oil in dong quai root, is a known carcinogen.

Given these properties of dong quai, persons on anticoagulant therapy, those with bleeding diatheses, and perhaps those taking high doses of aspirin or nonsteroidal anti-inflammatory agents should be particularly careful to avoid dong quai. One significant instance of drug-herb interaction has been reported with warfarin.[46] Given the side effect potential, lack of documented efficacy, and possible mutagenicity and teratogenicity, dong quai cannot be recommended. Note that Rejuvex, a popular and widely promoted dong quai supplement, contains bovine mammary, uterine, ovarian, adrenal, and pituitary tissue. In view of concerns about prion-related diseases, wise women who wish to remain that way might do well to consider other therapies for menopause. The use of animal organs and extracts in herbals is more common than most health professionals and laity realize.[47]

Evening Primrose

Evening primrose (evening primrose, evening star, *Oenothera biennis* [L.], family Onagraceae) is a common

Table 60–4. Suggested Uses for Evening Primrose

Acute respiratory distress syndrome	Premenstrual syndrome
Atopic dermatitis, eczema	Pruritus
Bladder dysfunction	Rheumatoid arthritis
Breast carcinoma	Sensitive or dry skin, acne
Diabetic neuropathy	Age-related changes of skin,
Hepatitis B	hair, and nails
Mastalgia and fibrocystic disease	Visual acuity
Migraine prophylaxis	Wound healing
Multiple sclerosis	

supplement source for linolenic acid, an omega-3 essential fatty acid. Alpha-linolenic acid is the main dietary omega-3 fatty acid. Sources include cold water fish, canola oil, soybean oil, and some vegetable oils. Gamma linolenic acid (GLA) comes from seed oils of currant, borage, and evening primrose. GLA alters cell activation, immune response, and inflammation and is often suggested as a therapeutic for chronic diseases. Suggested uses are listed in Table 60–4. These fatty acids are eicosanoid precursors and are part of cell membranes. The pathway for dietary GLA leads to dihomo-gamma-linolenic acid (DGLA), which in turn is converted by inflammatory cells to 15-(S)-hydroxy-8,11,13-eicosatrienoic acid and prostaglandin E_1, which has anti-inflammatory activity. GLA and DGLA appear to affect inflammatory processes by regulating T lymphocytes and GLA inhibits angiogenesis.

Evening primrose is commonly recommended as an herbal remedy for mastalgia and mastadynia and is also heavily promoted for the treatment of PMS and menopausal symptoms. Evening primrose seeds are rich in oils containing GLA plus unknown anticoagulant substances. The whole plant can be eaten and used in pickles, soups, and sautés, whereas the seeds are most often pressed to extract the oils. Commercial preparations available contain both the gamma and cis forms of linolenic acid. Typical preparations contain GLA, 45 mg, plus cis-linolenic acid, 365 mg per capsule. The recommended amounts for PMS, mastalgia, and menopausal syndrome range from 1 to 12 capsules a day. At a cost of $0.25 per capsule, the therapeutic use of evening primrose oil can be very expensive. Therefore, other cheaper sources have been developed including black currant and borage seed oils. Borage seeds contain large amounts of unsaturated pyrrolizidine alkaloids, residues of which can cause adverse reactions when large quantities are ingested. Again, these oils are a precursor to prostaglandin E_1 synthesis, and can cause prolongation of bleeding time. They also hold the potential for drug-herb anticoagulant interactions. One should be very wary of a therapy praised too loudly. GLA is touted as a ideal "miracle" fatty acid, because it is found in high concentration in breast milk and it is elaborated by the placenta. GLA is touted as a cure or preventive for a wide range of chronic disorders (see Table 60–4).

There is some support for a few of these claims, in particular for adult respiratory distress syndrome,[48] migraine,[49] rheumatoid arthritis,[50] and dermatitis.[51, 52]

Supposedly, GLA increases prostaglandin E_1, which might reduce prolactin-induced inflammation in the breast. GLA has been demonstrated to enhance the down-regulation of estrogen receptors in estrogen receptor–positive breast cancer being treated with tamoxifen.[53]

There is a single well-constructed clinical trial of evening primrose oil (EPO) for menopause. In a study of 56 women with three hot flushes per day treated for 6 months with EPO 4 g/day or placebo, EPO showed little benefit over placebo. GLA offers some interesting possibilities as an essential fatty acid, with studies suggesting a lowering of LDL cholesterol, but its clinical utility for menopause is nil.

Ginseng

Ginseng (*Panax ginseng*) is promoted for a wide array of complaints and disorders, and this is completely predictable when one realizes that the genus name, *Panax*, derives from the word *panacea*, essentially "cure all" (Table 60–5). Ginseng is supposed to be an adaptogen, helping to modulate responses to internal and external environmental stressors. Its supposed estrogen activity has led to recommendations for its use to mitigate menopausal symptoms. Ginseng is promoted to boost athletic performance and stamina, with promises of weight loss without dieting or exercise. The side effect profile of ginseng—tachycardia, irritability, insomnia, and palpitations—may not really be caused by the root itself, but occur as a consequence of the common practice of adulterating ginseng products with caffeine.

Different ginsengs have different clinical uses. Korean or Chinese ginseng is said to be a stimulant, aphrodisiac, digestive, and anabolic enhancer for the elderly. American ginseng is offered as the best "adaptogen." And Siberian ginseng, eleutherococcus, is said to be best for improving athletic performance and stamina. Unfortunately, most of the literature on eleutherococcus is not accessible in English, the research having been done in the former Soviet Union by military and Olympic trainers. The largest manu-

Table 60–5. Substances Used as "Ginseng"

***Panax* Genus**

Quinquefolium
Pseudoginseng, panaxnotoginseng
Pseudoginseng sp. *himalaicum*
Japonicus sp. *japonicum*
Trifolium
Zingeberinsis
Stipuleanatus
Vietnamensis

Others

Eleutherococcus senticosus
Rumex hymenosepalus
Pfaffia paniculata (Aramanthaceae)
Pseudostellaria heterophylla

Data from RxList—The Internet Drug Index, a HealthCentral.com Network Site, 2000 http://www.rxlist.com/cgi/alt/ginseng.htm

facturer of ginseng in the world, Ginsana, funded a large trial to investigate the effects of ginseng in menopausal women. One hundred ninety-three active treatment subjects and 191 placebo controls showed no improvement in vasomotor symptoms, but significant improvements in quality of life measures, particularly depression, general health, and well-being scores.[54]

Ginseng preparations sold in the United States vary greatly in quality and quantity of the active ingredients. Fifty-four ginseng products were found to have minimal amounts of ginseng in a study from the 1970s, with 60% of those tested having little ginseng and 25% containing no ginseng at all. Many were adulterated with high levels of caffeine.[56] Complicating matters further, *Consumer Reports 1995* tested 10 different brands of ginseng and found huge variations in potency. The active ingredient, or ginsenosides, varied from 0.2% to 7.6%. The problems continue, as reported by an independent testing agency called *Consumerlab*.[55] In their analysis, 12 of 21 recently tested ginseng products "failed" because of unacceptably high levels of pesticides or lead or inadequate concentrations of ginsenocides. Ginseng may hold some promise in treatment of fatigue, depression, immunosuppression, and other health problems, but it cannot be recommended as a menopause treatment. For its other indications, caution is advised given the poor production standards and the lack of quality evidence for the claims made.

Licorice, Liquorice

Licorice (*Glycyrrhiza glabra* [L.], leguminosae root), like ginseng, fenugreek, sarsaparilla, gotu kola, dong quai, and wild yam, supposedly has estrogen-like activity. It is used as a sweetening agent, happily in beers, and unhappily in cigarettes. Most licorice candy sold in the United States is actually anise-flavored crystallized sugar. In Europe, however, the genuine licorice made from the root stock can bought.

Prior to the synthesis of mineralocorticoids, licorice was used to treat Addison's disease. The glycyrrhizin in licorice root blocks 11-beta-dehydrogenase, which converts cortisol to cortisone. Licorice causes increased renal cortisol and, in turn, lowered amounts of renin and aldosterone. Hypertension can result from licorice ingestion and can persist for months after consumption stops. As little as 0.5 to 1.5 g of licorice taken daily for as little as 1 week may produce signs of pseudoaldosteronism: fatigue, hypertension, sodium retention, potassium wasting, and congestive heart failure in susceptible individuals.[57, 58] Removing the glycyrrhizin [deglycyrrhizinated licorice (DGL)] avoids this problem but only partially, because even DGL licorice contains 3% glycyrrhizin and holds some potential for harm.

Glycesteron in licorice has weak estrogenic activity estimated to equal 1/533th of estradiol. Compounded botanical medicines for menopause often contain licorice, but in very small amounts. There are no studies supporting or refuting

the use in menopause. A recent publication stated that licorice ingestions may lead to decreased testosterone and sperm count in men.[59] For a menopausal woman with new-onset hypertension, make especially vigorous inquiry regarding the use of supplements, herbs, infusions, and the like that might contain licorice.

St. John's Wort

St. John's wort (*Hypericum perforatum*) (SJW), although not used for treatment of symptoms classically attributed to menopause, is one of the most common herbals used by women. SJW, used for hundreds of years to treat depression, contains many constituents—hypericin, pseudohypericin, hyperforin, and flavonoids. Several mechanisms of action for the psychotropic effects of SJW have been proposed but not confirmed, possibly the inhibition of monoamine oxidase (MAO) and catechol methyl-transferase (COMT), decreasing corticotropin-releasing hormone, and then lowered levels of cortisol or affecting gamma-aminobutyric acid receptors in the brain, and serotonin receptor blockade. Hypericin does not appear to be an MAO inhibitor, and is no longer thought to be the substance responsible for the effects of SJW.[60] Preparations, previously standardized to the hypericin content, now are being standardized to contain hyperforin 0.5%, now thought to be a major active component.

Hypericum perforatum is sold in Germany as an antidepressant, and is prescribed more often than traditional antidepressants. Although products sold in Germany are manufactured to strict guidelines, in the United States, patients do not necessarily get what they pay for. As with many supplements in the United States, the labeled dose may not reflect the actual contents of the bottle. Fifteen controlled trials have been reported and assessed by meta-analysis by Linde and colleagues.[61] Combined analysis of 1757 subjects suggested that doses less than 1.2 mg per day provide a 61% decrease in mild to moderate depression, whereas doses in the 2.7-mg range yielded a 75% response. Mulrow[62] wrote a review for the Cochrane Collaborative in 1998. The information gleaned from 27 trials including 2291 patients, of which 17 with 1168 patients were placebo-controlled, yielded some proof that SJW was significantly better than placebo (rate ratio 2.47 with confidence interval 1.69 to 3.61), but that "current evidence is inadequate to establish whether hypericum is as effective as other antidepressants."

In the past, trials of SJW often have compared it with pharmacologically ineffective doses of tricyclic antidepressants, treatment options that are considered rather obsolete now that selective serotonin reuptake inhibitors have gained dominance.[63] A recent study by Woelk[64] compared SJW to an adequate dose, imipramine 75 mg bid, in a randomized controlled trial of 324 subjects with mild to moderate depression. Patients responded equally well to both interventions. In July 1999, the US National Institutes of Mental Health began a 3-year study testing SJW. Three hundred thirty-six patients have been enrolled at 12 centers, and they will receive 900 mg of extract of SJW (identical to a branded product made by Kira), sertraline, or placebo. Another very small trial with 30 patients found that SJW performed on a par with sertraline 75 mg.[65]

Although SJW does not offer better outcomes than traditional antidepressants, a large body of evidence is accumulating regarding profound drug-herb interactions with SJW. Piscitelli and associates[66] reported a 49% to 99% reduction in the protease inhibitor indinavir in healthy volunteers concomitantly taking SJW. SJW essentially lowered the protease inhibitor levels below those needed for clinical efficacy. SJW drug-herb interactions include potentiation of serotonin reuptake inhibitors and decreased bioavailability of digoxin, theophylline, cyclosporin, and phenprocoumon.[67] The effects appear to be due to potent stimulation of the cytochrome P450 system by SJW, particularly by induction of CYP3A. SJW has also been reported to lower the levels of oral contraceptives, calcium antagonists, metoprolol, propranolol, phenytoin, rifampin, midazolam, and other anesthetics. SJW induces changes in the drug efflux transport P-glycoprotein and subsequently may affect levels of drugs that are substrates for this system. Problems with SJW in particular have led anesthesiologists to request a 2- to 3-week washout of all botanicals before elective surgeries to avert complications due to drug-herb interactions. Emergencies and traumas cannot be anticipated, and The Medical Letter[68] has stated unequivocally that physicians should tell their patients not to use SJW.

Vitamin E

Although vitamin E is not an herbal, vitamin E supplementation is commonly recommended for treatment of vasomotor symptoms. Vitamin E has been suggested as a remedy for mastalgia, mastadynia, fibrocystic disease, vasomotor symptoms, venous insufficiency, and dementia, and as a cardiopreventive. First recommended for hot flushes in the 1930s, and studied during the following two decades, vitamin E is assumed to be an effective treatment for hot flushes, sweats, and mood by health professionals and laypersons alike. Barton and coworkers[69] conducted a study of 125 breast cancer survivors with 14 or more hot flushes per week. Women received vitamin E succinate 800 IU or placebo in a 4-week double-blind crossover design. Response rates for vitamin E cycles compared with the placebo cycles were 25% and 22%, respectively. Subjects experienced one less hot flush per day in the vitamin phase of study. This was statistically significant, but not "clinically" significant according to the women involved. But because vitamin E is inexpensive, it seems like a relatively benign intervention, and its use, although not strongly supported, does not warrant heavy-handed negativity by practitioners.

Wild Yam Creams

Wild yam creams are supposed to contain extract from *Dioscorea villosa* or Mexican yam and purportedly increase endogenous production of natural progesterone and other adrenal sex steroids such as dihydroepiandrosterone (DHEA). There is no pathway for conversion of *Dioscorea* to progesterone in vivo. Plants do produce sterols, called *saponins*, with structures similar to progesterone. Saponins first are hydrolyzed to sapogenins, the two principals being sarsasapogenin and diosgenin.[70] Diosgenin is used as a precursor in the commercial production of the progesterone steroid skeleton, which, in turn, can be used as the precursor for adrenal steroid synthesis.

Cutting to the chase, wild yams are neither estrogenic nor progestational because most creams on the market do not contain yam extract. Cognoscenti from conventional and alternative sides of the medical world have come to recognize the perpetration of a "wild yam scam" in the alternative medical world. Sporadic reports have surfaced suggesting that some of the over-the-counter yam creams are adulterated with progesterone, and some may even contain hidden estrogens. Any women who presents with vaginal bleeding after using rub or herbal yam, progesterone, or estrogen creams sold over the counter should be evaluated for endometrial proliferative abnormalities with appropriate biopsy and ultrasound studies.

Topical Progesterone

Sold over the counter as a cosmetic, topical progesterone cream is being actively promoted as an alternative to estrogen therapy. There is no reliable science behind the claims made, save for the articles and books written by Dr. John R. Lee, a practitioner from northern California. Dr. Lee and his disciples advocate the use of topical progesterone cream as a complete substitute for HRT, claiming that the topical use of the steroid supports estrogen and progestational and androgenic functions that decline in menopausal women. In his book, *Natural Progesterone: The Multiple Roles of a Remarkable Hormone*,[71] he cites studies that utilized a wide variety of progestins, natural progesterone, medroxyprogesterone acetate, and the C-19 nortestosterones to support his claims for progesterone. He has also published a case series using progesterone cream as treatment for osteoporosis.[72] During the 3-year study period, he states that he observed an average increase in bone mineral density in the lumbar spine of 14% in 63 women, with the greatest improvements seen in women with the worst bone density at the outset. Leonetti and colleagues[73] conducted a randomized, placebo-controlled trial trying to reduplicate these results. Of the 30 patients in the treatment arm and 26 in the placebo arm who completed the 1-year trial, no bone-sparing effects were seen. The group using progesterone cream did have a significantly greater reduction in reported vasomotor symptoms, which may explain the popular success of commercial progesterone creams. Another publication is expected in 2001 from the same group regarding the effects of topical progesterone on endometrium. At this time, no biopsy-confirmed studies exist documenting the safety of progesterone cream as a means of providing progestational opposition during exogenous estrogen administration. Studies of absorption indicate that levels are not high enough to provide endometrial protection.[74] On the other hand, cases of excessive absorption have been reported as well.[75]

Women who elect to use progesterone creams as a form of progestational opposition while taking exogenous estrogens should be regarded as if they are using unopposed estrogen and followed with annual endometrial biopsies.[76]

Conclusions

The use of alternative medicines and practices is not powered by some great driving force within the medical community, but rather from demand by consumers for a type of care that is less medicalized, less industrial, less remote. Women are using alternatives during menopause and aging because they see "natural" interventions as extensions of lifestyle and wellness endeavors. Many women eschew the notion of menopause as a disease state that requires treatment with drugs. Because we all recognize that the symptoms and diseases of the climacteric are highly variable, with only 25% of women experiencing severe symptoms, the overt need for "treatment" just is not there. The majority of women are not distressed or disturbed enough to seek medical intervention. These women are a "silent" majority. They want reassurances that they will not suffer the ravages of the degenerative processes associated with aging, but they want wise counsel and advice, not just a handful of prescriptions. The integrative approach and attitude of complementary and alternative therapies, with a focus on wellness and prevention rather than disease treatment, is very appealing. Menopause, the change of life, can be life changing. And clinicians should capitalize on the fervor and interest women show in pursuing wellness.

Herbals and botanicals are "crude," unrefined drugs and are not ineffective. But the words *natural* and *herbal* are not synonymous with *safe* and *pure*. Women need to be informed that some preparations may hold hidden risks of hepatic, hematologic, and renal toxicity, especially when taken with drugs. Contamination and adulteration are commonplace in the production of these supplements. Alternatives of proven value should be considered, especially for management of chronic problems like pain, insomnia, headache, and fatigue. In choosing therapies, each woman's personal health risks must be weighed, directing high-risk women toward medical therapeutic interventions and avoiding aggressive pressure on low-risk women to take medication assuming drugs are a shortcut to a healthy long life.

Although being challenged to justify conventional practice, conventional practitioners are also challenged to find accurate, up-to-date information about the panoply of alternative practices so popular today. With 629 million patient visits to alternative practitioners in 1997, collision is unavoidable. To practice effectively, one needs to, at the least, develop a peaceful coexistence with alternative medical practices; at best, physicians should actively interweave complementary care in their practices. It is imperative to be aware of the current complementary therapies in vogue in your community, to question patients about the use of botanicals and supplements, and to be familiar with the best data to date supporting or refuting such practices. By being empathetic to the motivation behind the use of alternative medical practices, a sensitive, caring dialogue can evolve. This dialogue is the only means of treating the whole woman—her physical, emotional, and philosophical needs—as she transits the second half of life.

Suggestions for Future Reading

Abdalla HI, Hart DM, Lindsay R, et al: Prevention of bone mineral loss in postmenopausal women by norethisterone. Obstet Gynecol 1985;66:789–792.

Buckman R, Sabbagh K: Magic or Medicine—An Investigation of Healing and Healers. Toronto, Key Porter, 1993.

Budeiri D, Li Wan Po A, Dornan JC: Is evening primrose oil of value in the treatment of premenstrual syndrome? Control Clin Trials 1996;17:60–68.

Chenoy R, Hussain S, Tayob Y, et al: Effect of oral gamolenic acid from evening primrose oil on menopausal flushing. BMJ 1994;308:501–503.

Collins A, Coleman G, Landgren BM: Essential fatty acids in the treatment of premenstrual syndrome. Obstet Gynecol 1993;81:93–98.

Gallagher JC, Kable WT, Goldgar D: Effect of progestin therapy on cortical and trabecular bone: Comparison with estrogen. Am J Med 1991;90:171–178.

Horrobin DF: Essential fatty acid metabolism and its modification in atopic eczema. Am J Clin Nutr 2000;7(Suppl 1):367S–372S.

Knekt P, Jarvinen R, Reunanen A, Maatela J: Flavonoid intake and coronary mortality in Finland: A cohort study. BMJ 1996;312:478–481.

Knight DC, Howes JB, Eden JA: The effect of Promensil®, an isoflavone extract, on menopausal symptoms. Climacteric 1999;2:79–84.

Ross RK, Paganini-Hill A, Wan PC, Pike MC: Effect of hormone replacement therapy on breast cancer risk: Estrogen versus estrogen plus progestin. J Natl Cancer Inst 2000;92:328–332.

RxList—The Internet Drug Index, A HealthCentral.com Network Site, 2000 http://www.rxlist.com/cgi/alt/ginseng.htm

References

1. Vandenbroucke JP: How much of the cardioprotective effect of postmenopausal estrogens is real? Epidemiology 1995;6:207–208.
2. Matthews KA, Kuller LH, Wing RR, et al: Prior to use of estrogen replacement therapy, are users healthier than nonusers? Am J Epidemiol 1996;15:971–978.
3. Grady D, Gebretsadik T, Kerlikowske K, et al: Hormone replacement therapy and endometrial cancer risk: A meta-analysis. Obstet Gynecol 1995;85:304–313.
4. Col NF, Eckman MH, Karas RH, et al: Patient specific decisions about hormone replacement therapy in post menopausal women. JAMA 1997;277:1140–1147.
5. Hulley S, Grady D, Bush T, et al: Randomized trial of estrogen plus progestin for secondary prevention of coronary heart disease in postmenopausal women. Heart and Estrogen/Progestin Replacement Study (HERS) Research Group. JAMA 1998;280:605–613.

6. Blakeley JA: The Heart and Estrogen/Progestin Replacement Study revisited: Hormone replacement therapy produced net harm, consistent with the observational data. Arch Intern Med 2000;160:2897–2900.
7. Herrington DM, Reboussin DM, Brosnihan KB, et al: Effects of estrogen replacement on the progression of coronary-artery atherosclerosis. N Engl J Med 2000;343:522–529.
8. Schairer C, Lubin J, Troisi R, et al: Menopausal estrogen and estrogen-progestin replacement therapy and breast cancer risk. JAMA 2000;283:485–491.
9. Ross AH, Boyd ME, Colgan TJ, et al: Comparison of transdermal and oral sequential gestagen in combination with transdermal estradiol: effects on bleeding patterns and endometrial histology. Obstet Gynecol 1993;82:773–779.
10. Seaman B: The Doctors' Case Against the Pill. New York, PH Wyden, 1969.
11. Seaman B, Seaman G: Women and the Crisis in Sex Hormones. New York, Rawson Associates, 1977.
12. Love S, Lindsey K: Dr. Susan Love's Hormone Book: Making Informed Choices About Menopause. New York, Random House, 1997.
13. Ettinger B, Li DK, Klein R: Unexpected vaginal bleeding and associated gynecologic care in postmenopausal women using hormone replacement therapy: Comparison of cyclic versus continuous combined schedules. Fertil Steril 1998;69:865–869.
14. Eisenberg DM, Davis RB, Ettner SL, et al: Trends in alternative medicine use in the United States, 1990–1997: Results of a follow-up national survey JAMA 1998;280:1569–1575.
15. Astin J: Why patients use alternative medicine: Results of a national study. JAMA 1998;279:1548–1553.
16. Lipp FJ: The efficacy, history, and politics of medicinal plants. Altern The Health Med 1996;2:36–41.
17. Koff RS: Herbal hepatotoxicity: Revisiting a dangerous alternative. JAMA 1995;273:502.
18. Kaufert P, Boggs PP, Ettinger B, et al: Women and menopause: Beliefs, attitudes, and behaviors. The North American Menopause Society 1997 Menopause Survey. Menopause 1998;5:197–202.
19. Persky V, Van Horn L: Epidemiology of soy and cancer: Perspectives and directions. J Nutr 1995;125(3 Suppl):709S–712S.
20. Knight DC, Eden JA: A review of the clinical effects of phytoestrogens. Obstet Gynecol 1996;87:897–904.
21. Aso T: The significance of the menopause in human life in the present and next century. In The Menopause in the Millennium. The Proceedings of the 9th International Menopause Society World Congresss on the Menopause. Yokohama, Japan, October 17–21, 1999.
22. Washburn S, Burke GL, Morgan T, Anthony M: Effect of soy protein supplementation on serum lipoproteins, blood pressure, and menopausal symptoms in perimenopausal women. Menopause 1999;6:7–13.
23. Albertazzi P, Pansini F, Bottazzi M, et al: Dietary soy supplementation and phytoestrogen levels. Obstet Gynecol 1999;94:229–231.
24. Murkies AL, Lombard C, Strauss BJ, et al: Dietary flour supplementation decreases post-menopausal hot flushes: Effect of soy and wheat. Maturitas 1995;21:189–195.
25. Vincent A, Fitzpatrick LA: Soy isoflavones: Are they useful in menopause? Mayo Clin Proc 2000;75:1174–1184.
26. Tham DM, Gardner CD, Haskell WL: Clinical review 97: Potential health benefits of dietary phytoestrogens: A review of the clinical, epidemiological, and mechanistic evidence. [review] J Clin Endocrin Metab 1998;83:2223–2235.
27. Kuiper GG, Carlsson B, Grandien K, et al: Comparison of the ligand binding specificity and transcript tissue distribution of estrogen receptors alpha and beta. Endocrinology 1997;138:863–870.
28. Kuiper GG, Lemmen JG, Carlsson B, et al: Interaction of estrogenic chemicals and phytoestrogens with estrogen receptor beta. Endocrinology 1997;138:863–870.
29. Nestel PJ, Pomeroy S, Kay S, et al: Isoflavones from red clover improve systemic arterial compliance but not plasma lipids in menopausal women. J Clin Endocrinol Metab 1999;84:895–898.
30. Barber RJ, Templeman C, Morton T, et al: Randomized placebo-controlled trial of an isoflavone supplement and menopausal symptoms in women. Climacteric 1999;2:85–92.
31. Upmalis DH, Lobo R, Bradley L, et al: Vasomotor symptom relief by soy isoflavone extract tablets in postmenopausal women: A multicenter, double-blind, randomized, placebo-controlled study. Menopause 2000;7:236–242.
32. http://www.remifemin.com/ Accessed August 22, 2001.
33. Lebherz TB, French L: Nonhormonal treatment of the menopausal syndrome. A double-blind evaluation of an autonomic system stabilizer. Obstet Gynecol 1969;33:795–799.
34. Bergmans MG, Merkus JM, Corbey RS, et al: Effect of Bellergal Retard on climacteric complaints: A double-blind, placebo-controlled study. Maturitas 1987;9:227–234.
35. Duker EM, Kopanski L, Jarry H, Wuttke W: Effects of extracts from Cimicifuga racemosa on gonadotropin release in menopausal women and ovariectomized rats. Planta Med 1991;57:420–424.
36. Bergkvist L, Adami HO, Persson I, et al: The risk of breast cancer after estrogen and estrogen-progestin replacement. N Engl J Med 1989;321:293–297.
37. Schaper and Brummer GmbH & Co KG: Remifemin: The Herbal Preparation for Gynecology: Scientific Brochure. Salzgitter, Germany, Schaper & Brummer, 1997. http://www.schaper-bruemmer.de
38. Halaska M, Raus K, Beles P, et al: Treatment of cyclical mastodynia using an extract of Vitex agnus-castus: Results of a double-blind comparison with placebo. Ceska Gynekol (Czech) 1998;63:388–392.
38a. Sliutz G, Speiser P, Schultz AM, et al: Agnus castus extracts inhibit prolactin secretion of rat pituitary cells. Horm Metab Res 1993;25:253–255.
39. Milewicz A, Gejdel E, Sworen H, et al: [Vitex agnus castus extract in the treatment of luteal phase defects due to latent hyperprolactinemia: Results of a randomized placebo-controlled double-blind study.] Arzneimittelforschung 1993;43:752–756.
40. Cahill DJ, Fox R, Wardle PG, et al: Multiple follicular development associated with herbal medicine. Hum Reprod 1994;9:1469–1470.
41. Schellenberg R: Treatment for the premenstrual syndrome with Agnus castus fruit extract: Prospective, randomised, placebo-controlled study. BMJ 2001;322:134–137.
42. Beinfeld H, Korngold E: Between Heaven and Earth: A Guide to Chinese Medicine. New York, Ballantine, 1991.
43. Junjie T, Huaijun H: Effects of Radix angelicae sinensis on hemorrheology in patients with acute ischemic stroke. J Tradit Clin Med 1984;4:225–228.
44. Eagon CL, Elm MS, Teepe AG, et al: Medicinal botanicals: Estrogenicity in rat uterus and liver [abstract]. Proc Annu Meet Am Assoc Cancer Res 1997;38.
45. Hirata JD, Swiersz LM, Zell B, et al: Does dong quai have estrogenic effects in postmenopausal women? A double-blind, placebo-controlled trial. Fertil Steril 1997;68:981–986.
46. Page RL II, Lawrence JD: Potentiation of warfarin by dong quai. Pharmacotherapy 1999;19:870–876.
47. Norton S: Raw animal tissues and dietary supplements. N Engl J Med 2000;343:304–305.
48. Gadek JE, DeMichele SJ, Karlstad MD, et al: Effect of enteral feeding with eicosapentaenoic acid, gamma-linolenic acid, and antioxidants in patients with acute respiratory distress syndrome. Enteral Nutrition in ARDS Study Group. Crit Care Med 1999;27:1409–1420.
49. Wagner W, Nootbaar-Wagner U: Prophylactic treatment of migraine with gamma-linolenic and alpha-linolenic acids. Cephalalgia 1997;17:127–130.
50. Zurier RB, Rossetti RG, Jacobson EW, et al: Gamma-linolenic acid treatment of rheumatoid arthritis. A randomized, placebo-controlled trial. Arthritis Rheum 1996;39:1808–1817.
51. Borrek S, Hildebrandt A, Forster J: Gamma-linolenic-acid–rich borage seed oil capsules in children with atopic dermatitis. A placebo-controlled double-blind study. Klin Paediatr 1997;209(3):100–104.
52. Whitaker DK, Cilliers J, de Beer C: Evening primrose oil (Epogam) in the treatment of chronic hand dermatitis: Disappointing therapeutic results. Dermatology 1996;193:115–120.
53. Kenny FS, Pinder SE, Ellis IO, et al: Gamma linolenic acid with tamoxifen as primary therapy in breast cancer. Int J Cancer 2000;85:643–648.
54. Wiklund IK, Mattsson LA, Lindgren R, Limoni C: Effects of a standardized ginseng extract on quality of life and physiological parameters in symptomatic postmenopausal women: A double-blind, placebo-controlled trial. Swedish Alternative Medicine Group. Int J Clin Pharmacol Rest 1999;19:89–99.
55. Consumerlab: http://www.consumerlab.com/results/ginseng.asp
56. Liberti LE, Der Marderosian A: Evaluation of commercial ginseng products. J Pharm Sci 1978;67:1487–1489.
57. Eriksson JW, Carlberg B, Hillorn V: Life-threatening ventricular tachycardia due to liquorice-induced hypokalaemia. J Intern Med 1999;245:307–310.

58. Russo S, Mastropasqua M, Mosetti MA, et al: Low doses of liquorice can induce hypertension encephalopathy. Am J Nephrol 2000;20:145–148.

59. Armanini D, Bonanni G, Palermo M: Reduction of serum testosterone in men by licorice. N Engl J Med 1999;341:1158.

60. Bennett DA, Phun L, Polk JF, et al: Neuropharmacology of St. John's Wort (*Hypericum*). Ann Pharmacother 1998;32:1201–1208.

61. Linde K, Ramirez G, Mulrow CD, et al: St. John's wort for depression—an overview and meta analysis of randomised clinical trials. BMJ 1996;313:253–258.

62. Mulrow LK: St. John's wort for depression. The Cochrane Library 1998;4:1–13 (on-line text).

63. Vorbach EU, Arnoldt KH, Hubner WD: Efficacy and tolerability of St. John's wort extract LI 160 versus imipramine in patients with severe depressive episodes according to ICD-10. Pharmacopsychiatry 1997;30(Suppl 2):81–85.

64. Woelk H: Comparison of St John's wort and imipramine for treating depression: Randomised controlled trial. BMJ 2000;321:536–539.

65. Brenner R, Azbel V, Madhusoodanan S, Pawlowska M: Comparison of an extract of *Hypericum* (LI 160) and sertraline in the treatment of depression: A double-blind, randomized pilot study. Clin Ther 2000;22:411–419.

66. Piscitelli SC, Burstein AH, Chaitt D, et al: Indinavir concentrations and St. John's wort. Lancet 2000;355:547.

67. Fugh-Berman A: Herb-drug interactions. Lancet 2000;355:134–138.

68. Drug interactions with St. John's wort. Med Lett Drugs Ther 2000;42:56.

69. Barton DL, Loprinzi CL, Quella SK, et al: Prospective evaluation of vitamin E therapy for hot flashes in breast cancer survivors. J Clin Oncol 1998;16:495–500.

70. Mirkin G: Estrogen in yams. JAMA 1991;265:912.

71. Lee JR: Natural Progesterone: The Multiple Roles of a Remarkable Hormone. Sebastopol, Calif, BLL, 1993.

72. Lee JR: Osteoporosis reversal: The role of progesterone. Intl Clin Nutr Rev 1990;10:384–391.

73. Leonetti HB, Longo S, Anasti JN: Transdermal progesterone cream for vasomotor symptoms and postmenopausal bone loss. Obstet Gynecol 1999;94:225–228.

74. Cooper A, Spencer C, Whitehead MI, et al: Systemic absorption of progesterone from Progest cream in post menopausal women. Lancet 1998;351:1255–1256.

75. Ilyia EF, McLure D, Farhat MY: Topical progesterone cream application and overdosing. J Altern Complement Med 1998;4:5–6.

76. American College of Obstetricians and Gynecologists. Hormone Replacement Therapy (Technical Bulletin No. 166). Washington, DC, ACOG, 1992.

SIXTY-ONE

Prevention and Management of Adhesions

Michael P. Diamond

Prevention of adhesions is a misnomer. Today, we cannot prevent postsurgical adhesions with any degree of consistency. Because of the problems adhesions cause, including infertility, pelvic pain, small bowel obstruction, and difficult reoperative procedures, consideration for management of adhesions should be an integral portion of the gynecologic surgical procedure. Specific choices as to surgical techniques to employ, surgical equipment, instruments, and devices and the use of adjuvants are likely to be particular to both the clinical situation encountered and, in some cases, the experience and expertise of the surgeon.

Paramount to recognition of the need for management of the problem of postoperative adhesion development is recognition of the high frequency with which adhesions develop postoperatively. It has now been demonstrated with repetitive clinical trials that adhesions develop in the vast majority of surgical procedures. In a study in the early 1980s[1] looking at the frequency of adhesion development after microsurgery for infertility performed by laparotomy, adhesions were identified to develop in over 85% of patients. Furthermore, in these patients, it was identified that not only was adhesion reformation (redevelopment of adhesions at sites of adhesiolysis) a problem, but the occurrence of de novo adhesion formation (development of adhesion at sites which did not have adhesions at the time of the initial surgical procedure) also was. In a second report conducted in the early 1990s,[2] after laparoscopic adhesiolysis, adhesion reformation was noted in 66 of 68 women (97%) at the time of a second-look procedure. Therefore, regardless of whether entry into the abdominal cavity is by laparotomy or laparoscopy, there is a tremendous need for considerations for the consequences of postoperative adhesions.

The problem of postoperative adhesion development is not limited solely to infertile women who are the subjects for most of these early studies. In a recent report among men and women undergoing colectomy for familial polyposis or ulcerative colitis,[1] adhesion development to the anterior abdominal wall incision site was identified at the time of ileostomy takedown and bowel anastomosis. By placing a laparoscope through the ostomy site in the anterior abdominal wall, it was possible to identify that 94% of the subjects had adhesions to the anterior abdominal wall. Because this series includes women who are not seeking fertility, and in fact includes men as well, it is clear that this problem of adhesion development is not limited to a small group of the population.

At this time, probably the most important contribution

to reduction of postoperative adhesions remains the surgical technique utilized to conduct this procedure. To the extent possible for the surgical procedure being performed, application of the tenets of gynecologic microsurgery appears to remain of value. These include minimization of tissue handling, preventing tissues from drying, minimizing devascularization of tissues, using less reactive and as little suture material as possible.

Other previously described tenets may not be completely accurate. For example, it is often stated that there should be avoidance of introduction of foreign material into the abdominal cavity. Whereas this remains true for items such as talc, large suture, and some other permanent devices used during surgical procedure, the only agents currently available for reduction of postoperative adhesions would also be classified as foreign materials. Currently in the United States, products approved for reductions of adhesions at laparotomy are INTERCEED (Gynecare, Somerville, NJ) and Seprafilm (Genzyme, Boston). INTERCEED is composed of oxidized regenerated cellulose, and Seprafilm is composed of modified hyaluronic acid and carboxylmethylcellulose. Each of these agents is a barrier, which is placed at the site of the surgical injury. The concept is that these barriers remain in place during the process of re-epithelialization of the underlying peritoneum. While separating the potentially opposing surfaces during the period of 3 to 5 days over which healing is thought to occur, development of adhesions bridging adjoining sites does not occur. Each of these products has been shown in randomized clinical trials to significantly reduce adhesions compared with the control group. In most of the INTERCEED trials, this represented the contralateral corresponding part of the pelvis (initially pelvic sidewalls, but, in later studies, ovaries and fallopian tube).[3, 4] In the case of Seprafilm, the control group was other patients undergoing colectomy in a general surgery trial or other patients undergoing myomectomy with wrapping of the uterus in the Seprafilm, but not the control, subjects.[5, 6] Unfortunately, even with the use of these agents, adhesions developed in many patients, thus leaving room for improvement in the ability of adjuvants to reduce postoperative adhesions. Of note, there are currently no products in the United States for reduction of adhesions after laparoscopic surgery.

A second tenet of gynecologic microsurgery, which is probably no longer applicable for purposes of reducing postoperative adhesions, is precise approximation of tissue planes. Whereas reapproximation of peritoneum at the conclusion of a surgical procedure often may aesthetically improve the appearance of the pelvis, data demonstrating that this reduces postoperative adhesion development are lacking. In fact, in animal studies such as one we conducted involving ovarian bisection bilaterally,[7, 8] the ovary, which was not sutured closed, ended up with fewer adhesions. This may represent a foreign body reaction from the suture utilized, devascularization from having placed the suture, or response to the added handling required for suture placement. Regardless, the adhesions left open, healed with fewer adhesions. It should be noted, however, that other considerations might lead a surgeon to approximate tissue planes, such as re-approximation of the bladder to the anterior abdominal wall after a bladder suspension procedure so as to avoid herniation of bowel into the space of Retzius postoperatively.

An additional caveat is that handling of tissue is obviously required to conduct a surgical procedure. However, when possible, if grasping and manipulation of tissue can be done in portions of tissue subsequently expected to be excised (as opposed to the portions that will remain in situ at the completion of the procedure), then it may be possible to minimize adhesion development at that site. Similarly, it is extremely important to achieve hemostasis when possible. However, attempts to do this should be done in manners that do not result in devascularization of large amounts of tissue, such as by tying large pedicles or extensive use of elective surgery to stop oozing. Such approaches may leave large areas that are devascularized that may then become a nidus for adhesion development.

There have been many claims in the past that use of many surgical modalities will reduce postoperative adhesions. At this point, there does not, however, appear to be any consistent findings in well-designed studies demonstrating superiority of one modality over another. In animal trials, and in comparison trials in humans, for example, it has not been possible to show that use of a CO_2 laser conveys an advantage for reduction of adhesions above and beyond that achievable with other means of conducting surgery, such as electrosurgery.[9] The choice of instrumentation and equipment thus should depend on availability in the operative suite, as well as experience and expertise of the surgeon.

Perhaps it should not be so surprising that it has been so difficult to reduce postoperative adhesion development. Teleologically, adhesions represent a means of resupplying oxygen and nutrients to tissue, that has been devascularized by pathologic processes and the surgical technique undertaken to correct it. Furthermore, with repeated surgeries, the ability of the body to adequately respond by resupplying oxygen and nutrients a second or third time to injured tissues would be expected to be limited by fibrosis and adhesions from the initial surgical procedure and from deficiencies in the reestablished vascular supply previously created. Thus, it is not surprising that it is more difficult to prevent adhesion reformation than development of adhesions in a surgical procedure.[8] This observation is consistent with a recent meta-analysis[9] that demonstrated higher frequency of adhesion development at sites of adhesiolysis than surgical sites (such as following a myomectomy or ovarian cystectomy) without adhesiolysis. It is our belief that major contributions to reduction of postoperative adhesions will likely not be made until we have a much clearer understanding of mechanisms of peritoneal healing and what is altered when an adhesion develops.[10] Once these mechanisms are identified, approaches will be able to be targeted so as to reduce (and one day prevent) postoperative adhesion development. This will not only reduce adhesion-related morbidity and mortality but will also have a significant impact on the cost of medical care, because economic consequences of gynecologic adhesions in 1 year alone have been estimated to be 1.2 to 1.3 billion, not counting time lost from work and reductions in productivity.

References

1. Diamond MP: Surgical aspects of infertility. In Sciarra JJ (ed): Gynecology and Obstetrics, vol 5. Philadelphia, Harper & Row (in press).
2. Diamond MP, Daniell JF, Johns DA, et al: Postoperative adhesion development following operative laparoscopy: Evaluation of early second look procedures. Fertil Steril 1991;55:700–704.
3. Azziz R, Cohen S, Curole DN, et al: Microsurgery alone or with INTERCEED Absorbable Adhesion Barrier for pelvic sidewall adhesion reformation. Surg Gynecol Obstet 1993;177:135–139.
4. Franklin RR, Diamond MP, Malinak LR, et al: Reduction of ovarian adhesions by the use of Interceed. Obstet Gynecol 1995;86:335–340.
5. Diamond MP, and the Seprafilm Adhesion Study Group: Reduction of adhesions after uterine myomectomy by Seprafilm (HAL-F): A blinded prospective, randomized, multicenter clinical study. Fertil Steril 1996;66:904–910.
6. Diamond MP, and the Sepracoat Adhesion Study Group: Reduction of de novo postsurgical adhesions by intraoperative precoating with Sepracoat (HAL-C) solution: A prospective, randomized, blinded, placebo-controlled multicenter study. Fertil Steril 1998;69:1067–1073.
7. Saed GM, Zhang W, Diamond MP: Molecular characterization of fibroblasts isolated from human peritoneum and adhesions. Fertil Steril 2001;75:763–768.
8. Leach RE, Diamond MP: Postoperative adhesion formation in gynecologic surgery: Etiology and treatment. In Ransom S, Dombrowski MP, McNeeley SG, et al (eds): Practical Strategies in Obstetrics and Gynecology. Philadelphia, WB Saunders, 2000; pp 709–716.
9. Diamond MP: Incidence of postoperative adhesions: In diZerega GS, DeCherney A, Diamond MP, et al (eds): Peritoneal Surgery. New York, Springer-Verlag, 2000; pp 217–220.
10. Diamond MP, Moghissi KS: Hyaluronan in the prevention of postsurgical adhesions. In Abatangelo G, Weigel PH (eds): New Frontiers in Medical Sciences: Redefining Hyaluronan. Padua, Italy, 2000; pp 333–337.

New Methods of Giving Progesterone: Are They Better?

R. Stan Williams, M.D.

Progesterone is a 21-carbon steroid hormone, primarily produced by the ovary from the corpus luteum and from the placenta during pregnancy. The production of progesterone induces secretory changes in an estrogen-primed endometrium in preparation for implantation and maintenance of pregnancy. Progesterone is also responsible for altering immune responses to the pregnancy, as well as altering myometrial and tubal contractility. The withdrawal of estrogen and progesterone in a nonpregnant menstrual cycle induces endometrial arterial spasm, with subsequent endometrial shedding. Progesterone's antiproliferative action in the endometrium is an important natural counterbalance to estrogen stimulation of mitogenesis.

The administration of progestins, synthetic and natural, has four primary indications in gynecology. First, progestins are used as antiproliferative agents in physiologic and pharmacologic unopposed estrogenic states, including chronic anovulation and estrogen replacement therapy. Second, progestins are used in steroid contraception, both in combination with estrogen in oral contraceptives and as continuous progestin-only methods, as with Depo-Provera and Norplant. Third, progestins primarily in the form of progesterone have been used in infertility therapy to supplement corpus luteal progesterone output in luteal-phase defects, to aid in the luteal support of in vitro fertilization (IVF) cycles, and for luteal-phase replacement of endogenous progesterone in donor egg IVF. Finally, progestins have been used as treatments for endometrial hyperplasia, as well as adjunctive therapy in the treatment of endometrial cancer.

Progestins may be either synthetic or natural progesterone and can be delivered in a variety of vehicles. The two primary types of synthetic progestins are (1) C21 progesterone-derived compounds, including medroxyprogesterone acetate (Provera) and megestrol (Megace) as well as other compounds, and (2) testosterone-derived (19-nortestosterone), which includes compounds such as norethindrone acetate, levonorgestrel, desogestrel, and norgestimate. Synthetic progestins have been used most extensively in the past because of the low bioavailability of orally administered progesterone. However, synthetic progestins retain some androgenic activity that may result in adverse side effects, such as fluid retention and weight gain, and may attenuate the beneficial lipid and cardioprotective effects of estrogen.

Progesterone in its natural state is now available in four pharmacologic forms. Progesterone in oil has been used for many years for intramuscular injection, resulting in very high serum levels of progesterone. Progesterone in oil (usually sesame oil) generally is given in doses of 25 to 100 mg IM daily; marked discomfort at the injection site is common and occasionally sterile abscesses form. Progesterone also has been compounded into vaginal suppositories in a variety of vehicles, including cocoa butter and glycerin. These suppositories, delivered in doses of 25 to 200 mg daily, have resulted in a wide variety of serum levels because of leakage from the vagina before absorption. Recently, two alternative delivery methods for progesterone have been approved by the U.S. Food and Drug Administration (FDA): micronized progesterone tablets and progesterone in a polycarbophil vaginal gel. This chapter discusses in detail the latter two methods of progesterone delivery, including the benefits and problems of each.

MICRONIZED PROGESTERONE

In the past, rapid metabolism and poor bioavailability have limited the use of oral progesterone. Recently, however, better absorption has been obtained through the micronization of progesterone in peanut oil (Prometrium, Solvey Pharmaceuticals, Marietta, Ga). Although only 10% of an oral dose is absorbed compared with intramuscular administration, mean plasma levels achieved with oral progesterone doses greater than 100 mg are equivalent to normal luteal-phase levels. Progesterone levels remain elevated for up to 12 hours and do not return to baseline until at least 24 hours after administration. The maximum concentration is achieved within 2 to 3 hours. With multiple dosing over 5 days, pharmacokinetic properties are unchanged, indicating no significant accumulation of progesterone. Concomitant ingestion of food with micronized progesterone results in significantly increased peak levels and enhanced absorption. Considerable individual variability has been reported in all studies of oral micronized progesterone.[1]

Orally administered progesterone is extensively metabolized in the liver to pregnanediol-3α-glucuronide, 20α-dihydroprogesterone, and 17α-hydroxyprogesterone. It is also metabolized to allopregnanolone and pregnanolone, which have sedating properties at high levels. Some women have reported significant sedative or anesthetic effects while taking high doses of oral micronized progesterone.

Micronized progesterone has been studied most extensively in the setting of hormone replacement therapy (HRT) in menopausal women. The most definitive study using micronized progesterone is the Postmenopausal Estrogen/Progestin Interventions (PEPI) trial, a randomized double-blind, placebo-controlled study conducted over 3 years at seven centers in the United States.[2–4] The PEPI trial was designed to assess the impact of HRT on four coronary artery disease risk factors: high-density lipoprotein (HDL)-cholesterol, systolic blood pressure, 2-hour serum insulin levels, and fibrinogen levels. The study randomized 875 healthy postmenopausal women from ages 45 to 64 years to one of five treatment regimens: placebo; conjugated equine estrogens (CEE), 0.625 mg/day; CEE, 0.625 mg/day + medroxyprogesterone acetate (MPA), 10 mg/day for the first 12 days per month; CEE, 0.625 mg/day + MPA, 2.5 mg/day; and CEE, 0.625 mg/day + micronized progesterone, 200 mg/day for the first 12 days per month.

The PEPI data demonstrated that all estrogen replacement regimens increased mean HDL levels and decreased mean low-density lipoprotein (LDL) levels versus placebo. Women who were in the estrogen-only group had the greatest mean increase of HDL (5.6 mg/dL). Women in the estrogen + micronized progesterone group had significantly higher HDL levels (5.1 mg/dL) when compared with the cyclic MPA (1.6 mg/dL) and the continuous MPA groups (1.2 mg/dL). All treatment groups had similar decreases in LDL. There were no significant differences in systolic blood pressure, mean 2-hour serum insulin levels, or fibrinogen levels among treatment groups. Endometrial histology showed no difference in the rates of endometrial hyperplasia among the three progestin-containing regimens when compared with placebo. Bone mineral density was also equivalent among all CEE replacement groups.

The PEPI trial provides evidence that the combination of micronized progesterone with CEE results in higher levels of HDL-cholesterol when compared with the CEE regimen containing MPA. Although in a 3-year trial, it could not be demonstrated that this higher level of HDL decreased cardiovascular disease more significantly than estrogen-containing regimens with MPA, these data are suggestive of a higher beneficial effect when extrapolated to data using HDL levels as a predictor of heart disease. One must remember, however, that it has been estimated that two thirds of the cardioprotective effect of estrogen replacement is independent of changes in lipid profiles.[5] Thus, the overall significance of the HDL differences between micronized progesterone and MPA may not significantly affect the overall cardioprotection provided in all women who take estrogen supplementation postmenopausally.

One of the primary reasons women discontinue their HRT is postmenopausal bleeding. The PEPI trial has not provided information about the incidence of bleeding, but some information is available from other, smaller studies using micronized progesterone.[6–8] Although many of these studies varied in the number of days per month patients

were administered the micronized progesterone, the amenorrhea rate after 6 months of therapy is approximately 90%. It has also been suggested that micronized progesterone may result in a decreased incidence of breast tenderness, bloating, edema, and depression when compared with MPA.[9] Further studies are warranted to investigate the exact incidence of breakthrough bleeding and side effects with the use of low-dose, continuous micronized progesterone in HRT.

Micronized progesterone has also been used in the setting of anovulatory secondary amenorrhea. Sixty women with secondary amenorrhea were randomized to receive either 200 mg or 300 mg of micronized progesterone for 10 days. Withdrawal bleeding occurred in 90% of the women who took the 300-mg dose but in only 58% of women who took the 200-mg dose.[10]

Dosing recommendations for use of micronized progesterone include 300 mg/day for 10 to 14 days for secondary amenorrhea; 200 mg/day for 12 to 14 days per month for cyclic HRT; and 100 mg/day for continuous HRT.

PROGESTERONE GEL

The vaginal delivery of progesterone has been prescribed for years, but the compounds had to be made up locally, resulting in a variety of different vehicles with unknown absorption characteristics. These vaginal suppositories also leak from the vagina once they have melted, again introducing a variability in the amount absorbed. Recently, progesterone in a polycarbophil gel (Crinone, Serono Laboratories, Norwell, Mass) has been approved by the FDA for use in the United States. This product contains progesterone as an oil-in-water emulsion contained within a bioadhesive vaginal gel. Polycarbophil gel (Replens) has previously been marketed over the counter to postmenopausal women to reduce vaginal dryness. The gel adheres to the vaginal epithelium with little if any leakage. The prolonged absorption of progesterone in polycarbophil gel results in a half-life of approximately 25 to 50 hours. The time from administration to significant serum levels is approximately 5 to 6 hours. Use of an 8% (90-mg) preparation once or twice daily by patients results in serum levels approximating luteal progesterone levels. Although serum levels of progesterone are only 25% of a comparable dose given IM, it has been demonstrated that with the vaginal application of progesterone, selective delivery to the endometrium and myometrium occurs, resulting in much higher tissue concentrations of progesterone when compared with intramuscular progesterone administration.[11]

The efficacy of Crinone was demonstrated in a donor egg IVF study.[12] Forty-eight agonadal women were randomized into the vaginal progesterone treatment group and 18 agonadal women into an intramuscular progesterone treatment group in preparation for donor eggs. Crinone 8% (90 mg) was administered twice daily, compared with intramuscular progesterone, 100 mg/day. In a mock cycle, endometrial histology was in phase for all subjects in both groups. During the treatment cycle, the ongoing pregnancy rate in the Crinone group (31%) was equivalent to that of the intramuscular progesterone group (22%), as well as being similar to their historical controls (32%). It should be mentioned, however, that these pregnancy rates appear significantly lower than the national rate of ongoing pregnancies using donor eggs, which is approximately 40%.

Crinone has also been used to supplement the luteal phase in IVF patients. One study of 283 IVF patients randomized them to receive Crinone 8% daily or micronized progesterone, 300 mg/day. Pregnancy rates (35% vs. 30%) and delivery rates (23% vs. 22%) were equivalent.[13] This study did not compare success rates of these compounds with success rates of intramuscular progesterone, the most widely used method of progesterone supplementation in IVF.

Although primarily used for infertility, Crinone has been studied in the setting of HRT. Sixty-two patients with either hypothalamic amenorrhea or premature ovarian failure were given estrogen replacement plus Crinone 4% (45 mg) every other day for 6 doses per month. Endometrial biopsies showed secretory changes in 92% of patients, and 81% of the patients experienced withdrawal bleeding.[14] Long-term studies examining hyperplasia rates have not been reported.

Dosing recommendations for use of Crinone include 8% (90 mg) twice daily for luteal-phase replacement; 8% (90 mg) once daily for luteal-phase support; and 4% (45 mg) every other day for 6 doses a month for cyclical HRT or for anovulatory amenorrhea.

Conclusion

Until recently, only synthetic progestins were widely available in the United States for HRT, and troublesome methods of progesterone administration (IM and vaginal suppositories) have been used to supplement or replace the luteal phase in infertility. Recently, two drugs have been FDA-approved, which increases the armamentarium of steroid replacement for the gynecologist. Early studies on both micronized progesterone and progesterone vaginal gel demonstrate efficacy under certain conditions. Continued studies of these compounds are warranted to examine which patients will benefit the most. One problem with all new medications is the cost when compared with existing medications, particularly when generic equivalents are available. Table 62–1 lists the average retail cost for 1 month of therapy for the most commonly used progestin in the United States, comparing it with these newer compounds. Despite cost differences, however, many patients may benefit from these newer compounds if they improve

Table 62–1. Cost Comparison of Progestins

Drug	Day's Supply for 1 Month	Average Retail Cost for 1 Month of Therapy
Provera, 10 mg	12	$13.99 ($7.69 generic)
Provera, 5 mg	12	$13.19 ($8.89 generic)
Provera, 2.5 mg	30	$18.79 ($10.99 generic)
Prometrium, 200 mg	12	$16.79
Prometrium, 100 mg	30	$20.99
Crinone 8%	12	$127.38
Crinone 4%	6	$34.19

patient compliance through a reduction of side effects and provide equivalent or better clinical outcomes.

References

1. Simon JA, Robinson DE, Andrews MC, et al: The absorption of oral micronized progesterone: The effects of food, dose proportionality, and comparison with intramuscular progesterone. Fertil Steril 1993;60:26–33.
2. PEPI Trial Writing Group: Effects of estrogen or estrogen/progestin regimens on heart disease risk factors in postmenopausal women. JAMA 1995;273:199–208.
3. PEPI Trial Writing Group: Effects of hormone therapy on bone mineral density. JAMA 1996;276:1389–1396.
4. PEPI Trial Writing Group: Effects of hormone replacement therapy on endometrial histology in postmenopausal women. JAMA 1996;275:370–375.
5. Sullivan JM: Hormone replacement therapy in cardiovascular disease: The human model. Br J Obstet Gynaecol 1996;103(Suppl 13):50–67.
6. Gillet JY, Andre G, Faguer B, et al: Induction of amenorrhea during hormone replacement therapy: Optimal micronized progesterone dose. A multicenter study. Maturitas 1994;19:103–115.
7. Hargrove JT, Maxson WS, Wentz AC, Burnett LS: Menopausal hormone replacement therapy with continuous daily oral micronized estradiol and progesterone. Obstet Gynecol 1989;73:606–612.
8. Bolaji II, Mortimer G, Grimes H, et al: Clinical evaluation of near continuous oral micronized progesterone therapy in estrogenized postmenopausal women. Gynecol Endocrinol 1996;10:41–47.
9. Fitzpatrick LA, Good A: Micronized progesterone: Clinical indications and comparisons with current treatments. Fertil Steril 1999;72:389–397.
10. Shangold MM, Tomai TP, Cook JD, et al: Factors associated with withdrawal bleeding after administration of oral micronized progesterone in women with secondary amenorrhea. Fertil Steril 1991;56:1040–1047.
11. Miles RA, Paulson RJ, Lobo RA, et al: Pharmacokinetics and endometrial tissue levels of progesterone after administration for intramuscular and vaginal routes: A comparative study. Fertil Steril 1994;62:483–490.
12. Gibbons WE, Toner JP, Hamacher P, et al: Experience with a novel vaginal progesterone preparation in a donor oocyte program. Fertil Steril 1998;69:96–101.
13. Pouly JL, Bassel S, Frydman R, et al: Luteal support after in-vitro fertilization: Crinone 8%, a sustained release vaginal progesterone gel, versus Utrogestan, an oral micronized progesterone. Hum Reprod 1996;11:2085–2089.
14. Miles MP, Ziller BMK, Shangold MM: A new clinical option for hormone replacement therapy in women with secondary amenorrhea: Effects of cyclic administration of progesterone from sustained release vaginal gel Crinone (4% and 8%) on endometrial morphologic features and withdrawal bleeding. Am J Obstet Gynecol 1999;180:42–48.

SIXTY-THREE

Advances in Surgical Technology

Robert A. Kozol

Although the laparoscope was developed early in the 20th century, laparoscopy was not a common procedure before 1960. In 1960, Kurst Semm, a German gynecologist, invented the automated gas insufflator. This opened the door for laparoscopy. During the 1970s, laparoscopy became more common in the practice of gynecology. In 1981, the American Board of Obstetrics and Gynecology established laparoscopy as a required component of residency training in obstetrics and gynecology.

The introduction of video laparoscopic cameras in the early 1980s allowed for further innovation in the field. In the late 1980s laparoscopy spilled over into general surgery and surgical subspecialties.

The application of laparoscopic techniques to cholecystectomy resulted in a paradigm shift in surgery. Laparoscopic cholecystectomy proved to be an operation easily learned by general surgeons. Suddenly, an open operation, which traditionally had a 4- to 6-day hospital stay, was converted to a minimally invasive procedure with a 1-day hospital stay. Over time, laparoscopic cholecystectomy has become a "same-day" case in many parts of the United States. This success has persuaded surgeons to apply minimally invasive techniques to multiple operations. In turn, this encouraged industry to engineer and develop better instruments for minimally invasive surgery.

As surgical scientists began to compare outcomes in minimally invasive versus traditional open procedures, some trends became evident. First, the technology was in fact applicable to many surgical situations in the abdomen, pelvis, and thoracic cavity. Second, the greatest physiologic advantages (the dampening of the neuroendocrine stress response) would be gained if major operations could be converted to minimally invasive technology. For example, inguinal hernia repair and appendectomy are readily performed laparoscopically. However, the traditional operations are not associated with big incisions, major blood loss, or significant fluid shifts. Therefore, it is not surprising that the advantages gained by minimally invasive techniques with these two operations are modest.

In contrast, consider the repair of an abdominal aortic aneurysm. The traditional open operation is accompanied by high-volume blood loss, major fluid shifts, a huge incision, and the potential for hypothermia. This operation frequently requires an intensive care stay, a hospitalization of 5 to 8 days, and a 30-day mortality of 5% to 10%, depending on the patient population. We are now in the era of endovascular aortic stenting for abdominal aortic aneurysm. This procedure avoids an open body cavity,

minimizes blood loss, and lessens both fluid shifts and core temperature changes. The endovascular procedure has cut the hospital stay by more than 50% and will undoubtedly drop the mortality to the low single digits.

So why not convert every major open operation to minimally invasive techniques? This question brings up issues of the limitations of the technology. The current major limitations are

- the requirement for airtight seals in laparoscopic surgery
- limited degrees of motion in instrumentation
- loss of tactile sense (operator cannot touch organs and tissue)
- two-dimensional optics
- difficulties with intracorporeal knot tying

Let us examine the attempts to overcome these limitations. First, in laparoscopic surgery, the peritoneal cavity is insufflated with CO_2 to allow lifting of the abdominal wall, thus affording the surgeon a field of vision. To maintain this field of vision, an airtight seal must be maintained around all trocars and instruments. This requirement resulted in the design of instruments, which are long, rigid rods, that may pass through a rubber membrane in a trocar. This design maintains the pneumoperitoneum during surgery. These instruments have strict limitations on degrees of motion (to be discussed later).

Surgeon dissatisfaction with these instruments led to efforts to allow the use of conventional surgical instruments. One concept was to replace gas insufflation with mechanical lifting of the abdominal wall. One device designed to accomplish this was the Laparolift (Guidant, Indianapolis, IN), a mechanical arm that attaches to the side of the operating table. The arm extends over the abdominal wall. A V-shaped fork is placed in the abdominal cavity through a small incision, and the Laparolift pulls the abdominal wall toward the ceiling. This in fact allows for a field of vision for a laparoscopic camera, without air insufflation. Thus the requirement for an airtight seal was eliminated. The surgeon could therefore use some conventional instruments in these operations.

Unfortunately, the field of vision with this device is tent-shaped (Fig. 63–1), as opposed to the dome-shaped field of vision obtained with pneumoperitoneum. I used this device in more than 30 major abdominal operations during the 1990s. The field of vision is inadequate for many operations. At best, it allows for "hybrid" procedures, in which the majority of the operation is completed with traditional laparoscopy and some final difficult steps, in-

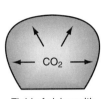
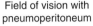

Field of vision with
pneumoperitoneum

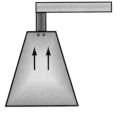

Field of vision with
Laparolift

Figure 63–1. Comparison shows superior field of vision with a pneumoperitoneum over that of a Laparolift (U.S. Surgical Corporation, Norwalk, CT).

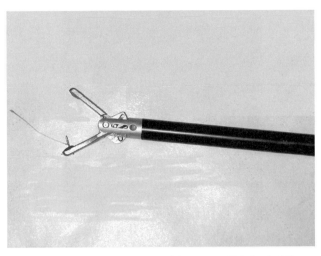

Figure 63–2. Close-up of an Endostitch instrument (U.S. Surgical Corporation, Norwalk, CT).

cluding specimen removal, are completed with strategic placement of the Laparolift. It is fair to say that this device did not gain widespread use and is unlikely to play a major role in the operating suite of the future.

The limitations of optics in minimally invasive surgery are self-evident. Two-dimensional imaging results in difficulties with depth perception. Indeed, the novice laparoscopic surgeon can be seen to be grasping at various depths when attempting to pick up tissue with an instrument. Although surgical robotics (to be discussed later) may seem like science fiction, it is not difficult to foresee the development of three-dimensional imaging (just ask Nintendo). In fact, this technology is here now but has not reached widespread utilization yet.

Surgical knot-tying in conventional surgery is taken for granted as a simple but fundamental skill. The human wrist, hand, and fingers allow for smooth and rapid knot-tying. The rigid, rodlike instruments of laparoscopy are no match for the human counterpart. Thus, suturing and knot-tying have proved to be difficult in laparoscopic surgery. This is overcome in part by the use of surgical clips, tacks, and staples to replace sutures whenever possible. The device manufacturers have created novel answers, such as the Endostitch device (U.S. Surgical Corporation, Norwalk, CT) which is somewhat like a hand-manipulated sewing machine (Fig. 63–2). Still, knot-tying with these instruments is a convoluted procedure. A second alternative is intracorporeal suturing with extracorporeal knot-tying. This is accomplished with a "knot-pusher," which pushes the knot through the trocar into the peritoneal cavity and into place. This is obviously cumbersome and time consuming. The ultimate answer to suturing and knot-tying difficulties comes with robotics.

The concept of surgical robots is not new. In fact, robots have been used to drill precise holes in bone for orthopedics since the early 1990s. Why would robotics now step to the forefront in minimally invasive surgery? The answer is that we have reached the end of what can be accomplished using rigid rods for instruments. The rigid rod instrument allows for three actions or degrees of motion. One, the instruments may be rotated. Two, the instrument may be moved up, down, left, or right by using the body wall as a fulcrum. Finally, many of the instruments

have jaws that open and close. Although acceptable for many operations, these instruments are inadequate for fine-motor applications.

The surgical robot conceptually allows for the shrinkage of the human hand. Although the robot "arm" may be a familiar look-alike to a laparoscopic rodlike instrument, the operating end of the robot arm is in fact a robot "hand." With the current systems, the surgeon sits at a console and views an image from a laparoscopic camera (Fig. 63–3). The surgeon's fingers are placed in a gauntlet at the console. The robot stands at the side of the operating table with its two arms through trocars. The magic lies in the fact that the robot duplicates the surgeon's motions—hands, fingers, and wrists (Fig. 63–4). With multiple levels of articulation, new degrees of motion are immediately available. Suturing becomes incredibly precise, and knot-tying is quite natural and can be learned by a surgeon within a few hours. Surgical robotic systems have included three-dimensional imaging plus magnification. Human physiologic tremor is eliminated on the image via computer technology. Motion tracking allows for stabilization of the

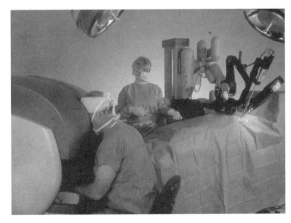

Figure 63–3. Surgeon at the console of the *da Vinci*™ Robotic Surgical System. (© 1999, Intuitive Surgical, Inc.)

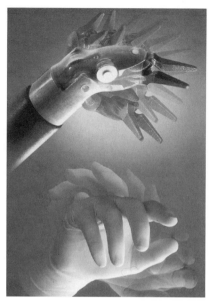

Figure 63–4. View of surgeon's hands and comparable *EndoWrist*™ (Robotic Surgical Instruments) of the *da Vinci*™ System. (© 1998, Intuitive Surgical, Inc.)

image of a moving organ, thus enabling surgery on a beating heart. Although robotics will overcome many limitations of traditional, minimally invasive surgery, at least one significant limitation remains—the lack of tactile sensation or feedback.

The loss of tactile feedback in laparoscopic surgery has been overcome in some cases with the use of "handoscopy," or a pneumo sleeve. With these devices, a small incision is made in the abdominal wall and the device is attached. These devices have two parts. The part that attaches to the abdominal wall looks like a colostomy ring. The second part is a tube made of heavy-duty "Saran-Wrap"–type material. Together, these allow the surgeon to insert the nondominant hand into the peritoneal cavity without the loss of the airtight seal needed for laparoscopy. The use of these devices allows the surgeon to feel organs and tissue planes with the nondominant hand while op-

erating laparoscopic instruments through trocars with the dominant hand. Operations performed with these devices are called *hand-assisted laparoscopy* or *laparoscopic-assisted surgery*. To some surgeons, this device is a "sell-out," in that an incision has been made, thus negating the minimally invasive concept. Advocates argue that for major procedures (e.g., colectomy), a small incision would have been required in order to remove the specimen. Nevertheless, these devices will become a historical footnote as the science of robotics moves forward.

Eventually, surgical robots will provide tactile feedback to the operator. This will be in the form of some type of haptic technology, also known as *force-feedback* technology. With this technology, the surgeon will actually sense resistance to touch, organ surface topography, tissue firmness, and so on. Robotic engineers are already using this technology in other fields; surgical applications are just around the corner.

Future robotic systems will bring imaging to a level well beyond that of the naked eye. The surgeon will be able to see an overlay field generated by magnetic resonance imaging, ultrasound, or other modalities. Thus, the live images not only will be three-dimensional and magnified but also will include imaging rivaling Superman's "x-ray vision." This has been called "augmented reality." This advance will provide undreamed of information regarding size, shape, and depth of tumors beyond the surface of any given organ.

Current and future advances in minimally invasive surgery suggest an evolution that will result in the obsolescence of conventional open surgery as we know it. The only unknown is the rate at which these changes will occur.

Suggestions for Future Reading

Ivatury RR: Laparoscopy in the new century. Surg Clin North Am 1999;79:1291–1295.

Maniscalco-Theberge ME: Virtual reality, robotics, and other wizardry in 21st century trauma care. Surg Clin North Am 1999;79:1241–1248.

Satava RM: Preparing surgeons for the 21st century. Implications of advanced technologies. Surg Clin North Am 2000;80:1353–1365.

SIXTY-FOUR

Obstetric and Gynecologic Infections

Bobby C. Howard, Gregory E. Chow, and

Mary P. Fairchok

PERINATAL AND POSTOPERATIVE GYNECOLOGIC INFECTIONS AND TREATMENT

Minimizing perinatal and postoperative gynecologic infectious morbidity is one attainable goal that is desired by all obstetricians/gynecologists. Obstetric/gynecologic physicians must possess a strong understanding of etiology, risk factors, diagnosis, and treatment of potential infectious complications associated with each procedure they perform. As with surgical procedures, practice patterns are often developed as a result of previous anecdotal experience. Certain relatively rare perinatal and postoperative infectious complications do not lend themselves well to study using prospective randomized trials, and, as is the case with all surgical specialties, treatment versus placebo arms often may be hindered by ethical considerations of "best-treatment" scenarios. Therefore, the "correct" treatment of various perinatal and gynecologic postoperative infections can, at best, be approximated by understanding the physiologic processes predisposing to these postoperative infectious sequelae and the descriptive techniques used to treat these problems. This chapter summarizes the various infectious complications associated with perinatal and major gynecologic surgical procedures and current therapies used to treat them.

Cuff Cellulitis

Cuff cellulitis is a relatively common postoperative complication associated with either abdominal or vaginal hysterectomy. Without antibiotic prophylaxis, the incidence of cuff cellulitis may be as high as 18% to 20%. The terminology of vaginal cuff cellulitis refers to a postoperative infection and inflammation of the remaining vaginal cuff following removal of the uterus. The pathophysiology of this infection involves the ascension of pathogenic microorganisms, many of which are commonly found in the vagina. Cellulitis of the vaginal cuff is polymicrobial in nature.[1] The primary organisms thought to be most responsible for this infection are the bacterial vaginosis organisms (*Bacteroides* species, *Peptostreptococcus* species, *Gardnerella vaginalis*), and *Trichomonas vaginalis*.[2, 3] However, a mixture of both aerobic and anaerobic organisms is commonly involved.

Several risk factors have been implicated in the development of cuff cellulitis. The use of prophylactic antibiotics, length of surgical time, the preoperative surgical scrub, comorbid conditions of the patient, and the technical ability of the surgeon have all been suggested to play a role in the potential development of this entity.[4] The presence of bacterial vaginosis or *Trichomonas* is probably the most significant risk factor. Administration of prophylactic antibiotic before the first incision has been shown in many studies to decrease the infectious sequelae of gynecologic surgery, particularly that of cuff cellulitis.[5] Many regimens appear to be equally efficacious for antibiotic prophylaxis at the time of hysterectomy.[6, 7] Generally, the most commonly used antibiotic agents used include second-generation cephalosporins. Repeat dosing for prophylaxis may be necessary in prolonged surgical cases or when blood losses are excessive during the procedure.[8]

The diagnosis of cuff cellulitis is made on clinical grounds. Postoperative temperature elevation (>100.4°F on 2 days subsequent to the first postoperative day) and the presence of tenderness at the vaginal cuff are necessary for the diagnosis. It may be difficult to differentiate normal postoperative discomfort from the tenderness associated with the inflammatory infectious process that occurs with cuff cellulitis. Indeed, because often the only objective evidence of this diagnosis is an elevation of temperature, other reasons for postoperative infectious morbidity must be ruled out. Cuff cellulitis is a diagnosis that is largely one of exclusion. There is some evidence that pelvic ultrasound, when used as an adjunct to clinical diagnosis, may be useful in detecting pelvic fluid collections that may be associated with an increased incidence of cuff cellulitis.[9]

Treatment of cuff cellulitis is intravenous antibiotic therapy. The most commonly used regimens include an aminoglycoside and an antibiotic with anaerobic coverage (e.g., gentamicin/clindamycin), although many other acceptable regimens are used to treat this entity.[10] In-hospital therapy with intravenous antibiotics is invariably successful in effecting treatment and recovery within 3 to 4 days. Occasionally, drainage of loculated fluid at the vaginal cuff may be necessary to obtain resolution of the patient's symptoms. Refractory symptomatology or persistent febrile morbidity suggests a misdiagnosis, and re-evaluation is necessary to ascertain the source of infection.

Pelvic Abscess

Pelvic abscess is a potentially life-threatening postoperative complication of gynecologic procedures. The incidence of pelvic abscess varies with the gynecologic procedure performed. The organisms most often found within pelvic abscesses closely parallel those that occur with cuff cellulitis and again, most frequently result in an infection that is polymicrobial in nature. The most frequent scenario leading to development of a pelvic abscess involves devitalized tissue with subsequent seeding of that necrotic tissue and debris by ascending bacteria from the vagina.

Numerous factors predispose to the formation of a pelvic abscess. Antibiotic prophylaxis decreases the potential for postoperative infectious morbidity, including the formation of a pelvic abscess.[11] However, rarely does a pelvic abscess form in the postoperative period of a completely uncomplicated procedure without significant pathology. Severe pelvic adhesive disease, endometriosis, and gynecologic malignancy often place the patient at increased risk for pelvic abscess for a number of reasons. Significant pathology of the pelvis often disrupts normal surgical planes and frequently results in a greater propensity for residual bleeding and hematoma formation. These procedures are also notable for typically being longer in duration, a factor also associated with an increased likelihood of pelvic abscess. Certainly, other comorbid conditions of the patient,[11] such as diabetes, atherosclerotic disease, obesity, smoking history, and bleeding dyscrasias, play a potentially important role in the development of postoperative pelvic abscess. Pelvic abscess can be associated with a specific organ within the pelvis (e.g., ovarian abscess, perirectal abscess) or may be discovered as a free, discrete mass that has resulted from seeding of a hematoma. In any case, the resultant inflammation that ensues may invest pelvic organs to such a degree that extirpative therapy is indicated.

The diagnosis of pelvic abscess is based on clinical symptoms that include postoperative fever, pelvic mass, and worsening abdominopelvic pain. However, even in the presence of these findings, an imaging study is almost uniformly performed to augment treatment therapies. Most commonly, ultrasound is utilized and gives excellent clinical information owing to the cystic nature of these masses. Size, complexity, location, and proximity to vital structures are important aspects of the abscess that will often assist in guiding therapy. Computed tomography may provide some other useful information in unusual, more complex circumstances of suspected bowel or ureteral involvement or fistula formation.

The most common presentation of pelvic abscess in the postoperative period usually follows an extirpative therapy such as hysterectomy. Pelvic abscess after vaginal hysterectomy is most often related to hematoma formation with resultant seeding of a walled-off hematoma cavity. Pelvic abscess after abdominal hysterectomy is most often the result of bacterial seeding of devitalized tissue following a difficult procedure. In these cases, significant pelvic pathology often mandates an abdominal approach. In either case, standard therapy involves initial treatment with broad-spectrum antibiotics (e.g., gentamicin/clindamycin/ampicillin), although alternative regimens have been used with seemingly equal efficacy.[12, 13] A broad-spectrum approach is necessary because of the polymicrobial nature of the bacteria involved. Gram-negative, anaerobic, and enterococcus organisms are significant pathogens in this disease. Resolution can be expected in a reasonable number of cases, perhaps as high as 60% to 70%.[14] A small number of patients, after initial resolution, will require further antibiotic therapy or surgical drainage. These patients are considered late failures of therapy. With improvement of symptoms and resolution of fever, no other treatment may be necessary.

When an abscess is recalcitrant to therapy, it is essential that it be drained at the earliest possible time. However, the ability to accomplish this procedure successfully may be compromised by the abscess size, location, complexity, and proximity to other vital structures. Pelvic abscesses often can be reached transabdominally, directly through the vaginal cuff, and even through a transperineal drainage approach. There have been reports of transrectal drainage for abscesses that have been inaccessible through the cuff,[15] and multiple other routes are feasible to attempt drainage.[16] Retroperitoneal abscess can be successfully drained under computed tomography guidance with a skilled interventional radiologist.

Finally, failed resolution of symptoms with these therapies requires re-exploration of the pelvis and removal of the abscess cavity.[17] Generally, laparotomy is the preferred procedure for exploration, although there have been successful reports of drainage and removal through the laparoscope.[18] Association with remaining ovaries often will require removal of these organs. Mechanical bowel preparation before surgery is advisable because, typically, dissection of the inflammatory phlegmon from the bowel is associated with a significantly higher risk for enterotomy.

Septic Pelvic Thrombophlebitis—Gynecologic

Septic pelvic thrombophlebitis (SPT) is an unusual entity, associated most frequently with obstetric surgical procedures, although it is seen after gynecologic procedures as well. When associated with a gynecologic procedure, it is most often diagnosed with concurrent pelvic infection. SPT is a diagnosis of exclusion, and the ability to diagnose this condition clinically is uncommon.

The major risk factor associated with this entity is an infectious process that is associated with the performance of a major pelvic surgical procedure and vascular injury. The pathogenesis of SPT is thought to be the result of microthrombi formed within the pelvic veins, with subsequent bacterial seeding of these thrombi. In the gynecologic setting, this is most often the result of vascular injury or compromise and it is therefore uncommon to diagnose in the absence of a surgical procedure. It is more frequently seen in puerperium or as a result of postabortal sepsis. SPT in the postpartum period should be considered whenever there is no clear etiology for fever.

The diagnosis of SPT had previously been difficult to make based on clinical examination. In fact, it was previously necessary to explore the patient surgically to establish the diagnosis of SPT firmly. Patients who develop postoperative SPT present frequently with spiking temperatures and minimal physical signs or symptoms. In fact, the majority of patients appear remarkably well, given the objective findings of fever and tachycardia. Pelvic examination is helpful in excluding other etiologies for postoperative infectious morbidity. Findings on pelvic examination are typically nondescript, with the patient reporting minimal to mild tenderness on examination. Imaging studies are performed to rule out the presence of pelvic abscess. With improvement in imaging studies such as computed tomography, the ability to diagnose SPT has improved.

Treatment of SPT involves the use of intravenous heparin therapy in conjunction with the antibiotic therapy that usually has been started at the time the diagnosis is made. Anticoagulation results in a prompt response in clinical improvement of the patient. This is manifested most notably by a sharp resolution of the fever curve. There is some debate in the literature about the need for treatment with intravenous heparin therapy, as the data failed to show a difference between treatment and nontreatment groups.[19] However, given the strength of descriptive data that have accumulated regarding the treatment of SPT, it is difficult to ignore the regimens that utilize heparin for treatment.[20–24] Randomized, controlled trials that have been performed may lack the power to determine a difference between treatment and nontreatment arms.

Wound Cellulitis

Wound cellulitis is a relatively common postoperative complication of gynecologic surgery. The incidence reported in the gynecologic literature may be as high as 5%. The postoperative morbidity resulting in a greater length of hospital stay and frequent need for wound care make this a complication taking a considerable amount of time and economic resources, which could be spared if its frequency were reduced. Gynecologic surgeons can effect a decrease in the incidence of this complication by implementing preventive measures at the time of surgery. Wound cellulitis rarely results in serious morbidity or mortality, with the exception of the development of necrotizing fasciitis.

Many risk factors are associated with wound cellulitis, most of which are associated with techniques of surgical sterility, draping, and preparation of the patient and operating surgeon. Age and nutritional status of the patient, obesity, the presence of an already existing debilitating disease state, injury to visceral organs, previous irradiation, and diabetes are other factors that play a significant role in the development of a wound cellulitis. The length of the surgical procedure is also well recognized as a predisposing factor.

The diagnosis of wound cellulitis is clinically straightforward. The patient usually presents 4 to 6 days postoperatively with low-grade fever and induration or erythema at the wound site. The patient invariably complains of wound tenderness that has been increasing over time. Examination reveals expected signs of the inflammatory response to infection and may reveal fluctuance within the wound.

Treatment of the cellulitis consists of antibiotic therapy and local wound care. The most commonly used antibiotics (e.g., synthetic penicillins) are specific for *Staphylococcus* and *Streptococcus*, because these microorganisms are the most commonly found pathogenic flora of the skin. However, because of the nature of gynecologic procedures, gram-negative organisms must also be considered. Antibiotic therapy, of course, should be tailored to suit any associated complications that may have resulted from the surgical procedure. For example, enterotomy would necessitate antibiotic coverage for enteric organisms. Additionally, if the wound is examined and noted to have a fluctuant mass in the subcuticular area, the wound should be opened to allow drainage. Granulation should be encouraged to form from the base of the wound until the wound closes. Delayed reclosure is an alternative option for treatment in these cases of wound separation with minimal risk of morbidity.[24a] Resolution of erythema and induration typically occurs rapidly with antibiotic therapy and proper wound care.

Necrotizing fasciitis, also known as Fournier's gangrene, is fortunately a rare complication of surgery that may initially present with the appearance of cellulitis. Most frequently, at risk are those patients who are severely debilitated, diabetic, morbidly obese, immunocompromised, or chronically immunosuppressed. This life-threatening infection, potentially presenting as a simple cellulitis, rapidly progresses, and survival is clearly linked to early diagnosis and immediate treatment. Its rapid progression separates it from any other clinical entity, and the hallmark of treatment is prompt, rapid, wide débridement and broad-spectrum antibiotic therapy. The most commonly involved organisms are *Bacteroides* species, *Streptococci*, *Staphylococci*, *Enterococci*, *Escherichia coli*, and other gram-negative rods, with the majority being polymicrobial.[25] The wound should be cultured, because antimicrobial therapy may need to be tailored to specific organisms responsible for the infection.

A promising new therapy in the treatment of necrotizing fasciitis is the use of hyperbaric oxygen. Hyperbaric treatment delivers oxygen directly to the infected tissue and allows free radical formation with resultant bacteriocidal activity.[26] Even under the best of circumstances, it should be considered an adjunctive treatment measure to surgical débridement and antibiotic therapy. Also, unfortunately, the use of hyperbaric therapy is limited by the fact that few centers exist with the capability and technology to administer this to a patient.

Wound Dehiscence/Evisceration

Wound dehiscence with or without subsequent evisceration is an extremely serious and life-threatening complication of gynecologic surgery. It is defined as rupture of fascial layers supporting closure of an abdominal or pelvic wound, with the potential for extravasation of bowel through this tear. Its frequency is widely variable but ranges from approximately 0.3% to as high as 3% of major pelvic procedures. Experience of the surgeon and use of appropriate suture materials are the most significant factors that may prevent wound dehiscence and evisceration.

Significant patient risk factors exist that increase the likelihood of wound dehiscence. Chronic debilitating disease, obesity, poor nutritional state, chronic corticosteroid therapy, intraperitoneal infection, diabetes, and operation for gynecologic malignancy are factors that must be considered in appropriate wound closure to prevent dehiscence.[26a] The type of abdominal incision has historically always been cited as a determining factor for wound dehiscence; vertical abdominal incisions are purported to be inferior to transverse incisions in strength. This subject still promotes some controversy.[26b] However, even with expert wound closure, the potential for dehiscence is present owing to patient factors.

Diagnosis of dehiscence and evisceration is sometimes self-evident. Most often, though, the patient complains of copious serosanguineous drainage from the wound site. The diagnosis of dehiscence is obvious if bowel loops or mesentery is seen within the wound. The surgeon can also verify dehiscence by probing the wound and noting a loss of fascial integrity. Dehiscence most often occurs in the setting of infection, so the patient should be examined and appropriately treated for any postoperative surgical sequelae.[26b]

Once the diagnosis is made, any exposed bowel should be covered with a moistened sponge and the patient taken immediately to the operating room for repair. Extruding bowel should be reduced and examined carefully for any evidence of necrosis, and any damaged areas are resected. The fascia should be primarily closed and the wound débrided as necessary. Patients who have a significant amount of fascial necrosis or infection that precludes reapproximation may have a synthetic graft to permit primary closure of the abdomen.[26c] Intravenous antibiotic therapy is administered in the preoperative and postoperative periods. Following completion of the procedure, a nasogastric tube is placed and managed postoperatively until return of bowel function is noted. The patient remains under close observation for any signs of sepsis or complications as a result of the dehiscence.

OVERVIEW OF NEW DEVELOPMENTS IN LABORATORY DIAGNOSIS AND TREATMENT OF PERINATAL INFECTIONS

Group B Streptococcal Infections

Although widespread compliance with the 1996 Centers for Disease Control and Prevention (CDC) consensus guidelines on the prevention of perinatal group B streptococcal disease[27] has led to a significant decline in the incidence of perinatal group B streptococcal infections,[28] this disease remains a leading cause of perinatal infection, premature labor, urinary tract infections during pregnancy, and chorioamnionitis. Conjugate vaccines directed against the predominant group B streptococcus serotypes responsible for perinatal disease are under development, but at the present time, antimicrobial prophylaxis of high-risk deliveries remains the mainstay of prevention. Unfortunately, prenatal cultures for group B streptococcus at 35 to 37 weeks do not always correlate with culture positivity at delivery, leading to unnecessary prophylaxis in many cases. The turnaround time for standard culturing techniques is 48 to 72 hours, which makes culturing at the time of labor onset impractical as a screen. The alternative risk factor–based approach to prophylaxis against group B streptococcus infection inevitably results in missed cases of infection as well as overtreatment.

A rapid optical immunoassay (StrepB OIA, Biostar, USA) for the detection of group B streptococcal colonization at the time of labor is available commercially, but sensitivity and specificity of the test have been variable in clinical studies. The test has the advantage of being both easy to perform and rapid, taking 30 to 45 minutes. A study published in 1996 comparing this assay to standard culturing techniques was promising, with an 82.5% sensitivity and 91.8% specificity in 962 pregnant women.[29] However, subsequent studies comparing the assay to standard cultures were less reassuring, with one study of 141 nonpregnant women finding 58.5% sensitivity and 85.7% specificity (positive predictive value [PPV] 51.5% and negative predictive value [NPV] 80.9%),[30] and another study in 524 pregnant women resulting in 47% sensitivity, 96% specificity (PPV 70%, NPV 90%).[31] The assay appears to be more sensitive with higher levels of colonization, but the variability seen in sensitivity among studies raises concern about the usefulness of this test in the clinical setting.

Recently, a study was published evaluating two polymerase chain reaction (PCR) techniques versus culture results for the detection of group B streptococcus infection in pregnant women at delivery.[32] In this study, 112 pregnant women in labor had combined anal and vaginal specimens obtained; 29.5% were positive by culture for group B streptococcus. Compared with the culture results, the two PCR assays (a conventional PCR and a more rapid fluorogenic PCR) were 97% sensitive and 100% specific (NPV 98.8% and PPV 100%). The rapid PCR assay could be completed within 30 to 45 minutes. In the future, PCR assays may become useful clinical tools at delivery, but currently the expertise and expense required for this technology are beyond the capability of most clinical laboratories, and the assay remains a research tool. (See Chapter 32 on group B streptococcus.)

HIV Infection and Pregnancy

Following publication of the AIDS Clinical Trial Group's protocol 076 results, which demonstrated a decrease in perinatal transmission of HIV infection from 25.5% in the placebo arm to 8.3% in the zidovudine-treated group,[33] it has become the standard of care in the United States to offer and encourage prenatal testing for HIV infection and to begin treatment with a zidovudine-containing regimen, ideally by 14 weeks' gestation.[34] With the advent of highly active antiretroviral (HAART) therapy, many HIV-infected pregnant women are now on combination therapy with protease inhibitors as well as nucleoside or non-nucleoside analogue reverse transcriptase inhibitors. Knowledge of the pharmacokinetics during pregnancy and potential teratogenicity of these medications is limited at the present time. The best resource for updated information on teratogenicity and safety of antiretrovirals during pregnancy is the Antiretroviral Pregnancy Registry (1-800-258-4623).

Currently, all the non-nucleoside analogues as well as all the nucleoside analogue reverse transcriptase inhibitors (NRTIs), with the exception of didanosine (ddI), are classified as category C. ddI is category B. Recently, there have been concerns that use of NRTIs during pregnancy may be associated with mitochondrial dysfunction in newborn infants. French investigators reported on eight infants exposed in utero and/or during the neonatal period to zidovudine (ZDV)/3TC or ZDV alone who developed signs of mitochondrial dysfunction. Two of these infants died.[35] A large prospective study of NRTI-exposed and unexposed infants born to HIV-infected women in the United States found no association with mitochondrial dysfunction in the neonates,[36] but further data are needed.

Recently, the U.S. Food and Drug Administration issued a new warning on the use of ddI in combination with stavudine during pregnancy. This combination has been associated with severe hepatomegaly and steatosis of the liver, as well as fatal lactic acidosis. This combination should be avoided during pregnancy unless the benefits clearly outweigh risks.

In the protease inhibitor class, all the medications are category B, other than indinavir and amprenavir, which are category C. The protease inhibitor class has also all been shown to precipitate or worsen diabetes mellitus, which is an additional concern during pregnancy.

Although combination antiretroviral therapy has dramatically reduced perinatal transmission now to only 1.5%,[37] there is also evidence that combination antiretroviral therapy with and without protease inhibitors significantly increases the risk of premature delivery in pregnant women (odds ratios of 1.82 for regimens without protease inhibitors; 2.6 with protease inhibitors).[38] The risk of premature delivery in this study was highest when therapy was started before pregnancy or during the first trimester.

In spite of the limited data on optimal antiretroviral therapy during pregnancy, the present standard of care is to treat the pregnant woman the same as if she were not pregnant, with the following exceptions: The regimen should include ZDV, and consideration should be given to withholding medications until 14 weeks' gestation if

clinically feasible. Pregnant women must be counseled about the use of antiretroviral drugs, and all exposed infants should be provided with long-term follow-up regardless of HIV infection to assess for unknown teratogenicity. A comprehensive discussion of consensus recommendations on antiretroviral therapy during pregnancy can be found in the Morbidity and Mortality Weekly Reports (MMWR) Recommendations and Reports-2 published January, 1998.[39]

In spite of the recommendation to screen all pregnant women for HIV, screening is still not universal. Additionally, screening results would not be available for women presenting without prenatal care, and such women may have a higher rate of HIV risk-taking behaviors. Also, most screening is undertaken at the first prenatal visit, thus missing women who become infected during pregnancy. Because the universal screening test is indirect serology, infected women who have not yet seroconverted also will be missed. For all these reasons, screening pregnant women late in pregnancy who have either high-risk behavior or no prior screen should be considered, because intervention to decrease perinatal infection would still be possible, especially given that approximately two thirds of perinatal infection is believed to occur during delivery. Rapid HIV serology kits are commercially available and feasible for most clinical laboratories. Use of the rapid HIV screen in this setting would be of potential benefit.

Extrapolating from studies in the developing world, potential options to reduce perinatal spread for treating women presenting late in pregnancy with the diagnosis of HIV infection would include ZDV and nevirapine. A study out of Thailand evaluating the reduction of perinatal spread of HIV compared women on placebo versus women given short-course ZDV starting at 36 weeks, followed by ZDV orally every 3 hours during labor.[40] Infants were not given any medication and no infants were breastfed. The study found 9.4% transmission in the treated group versus 18.9% in the placebo group. In the United States, it should be noted, women diagnosed with HIV infection during labor should receive ZDV intravenously during labor, and the infant should receive oral ZDV for the first 6 weeks of life as per standard recommendations. An additional potential option for treating pregnant women diagnosed with HIV at labor would be nevirapine. A recent study done in Uganda,[41] of 618 women, gave one group ZDV 600 mg at labor onset, followed by 300 mg every 3 hours to delivery and 4 mg/kg twice-daily for 7 days to the infants. The other group was given 200 mg of nevirapine at labor onset, followed by a single 2-mg/kg dose to the infant at 72 hours or hospital discharge. This study found a 13.1% transmission rate in the nevirapine group versus 25.1% in the ZDV group. The women in this study all breastfed. Thus, nevirapine at delivery in combination with ZDV for newly diagnosed women would be a potential option.

Cesarean sections have recently been shown to reduce the risk of HIV transmission to infants. In a meta-analysis of 8000 pregnant women with HIV infection,[42] transmission rates of women not on antiretrovirals were 19% for those delivering by nonelective cesarean section or spontaneous vaginal delivery versus 10% in the elective cesarean section group. For the women on the 076 ZDV treatment, transmission rates were 7% versus 2% in the elective cesarean section group. Current guidelines by the American College of Obstetrics and Gynecology recommend that HIV-infected women consider an elective cesarean section delivery at 38 weeks' gestation if the plasma HIV-1 RNA levels exceed 1000 copies/mL. Whatever the method of delivery, all efforts should be made to reduce contact of the infant with maternal secretions, including avoiding scalp electrodes and internal monitoring, advising against breastfeeding, and washing the baby prior to any invasive procedures. (See Chapter 3, Management of HIV Pregnancy.)

Cytomegalovirus Infections

Cytomegalovirus (CMV) remains the most common congenital infection in the United States, with primary infections occurring in 0.7% to 4% of pregnant women and 0.2% to 2.2% of live births. For primary infections during pregnancy, there is a 40% to 50% transmission rate to the fetus, with 90% of infants born asymptomatic. Ten percent to 15% of these infants will go on to develop sequelae, most commonly hearing loss. Of the 10% of infected infants born with symptoms, 30% die in the neonatal period, and 90% of the survivors suffer serious sequelae.[43] Currently, the "gold standard" for diagnosis of congenitally infected infants remains culture of the urine within 3 weeks of delivery.

Antenatal suspicion of the infection is usually precipitated by intrauterine growth restriction, documented primary infection in the mother, or the detection of hydrocephalus. Options for antenatal diagnostic evaluation include culture and PCR of amniotic fluid, and culture, PCR, and serology of fetal blood or tissue. Of these options, PCR of amniotic fluid from a research laboratory is likely to be the least invasive and most reliable study.

For example, in one recent study out of Belgium,[44] 237 pregnant women with documented CMV infection during pregnancy were evaluated with amniocentesis. CMV DNA PCR of the amniotic fluid was performed in 218 women, 177 had CMV DNA PCR done of fetal blood samples, 209 had fetal blood CMV immunoglobulin M (IgM) serology, and 83 had fetal blood CMV culture. At birth or abortion, all infants or fetuses underwent saliva and urine culture for CMV, with 24% having evidence of infection. The PCR of the amniotic fluid was the most sensitive test (78%), with 100% specificity and a PPV of 100% and NPV of 93%. Amniocentesis was much more sensitive after 21 weeks' gestation and after at least 7 weeks of documented maternal infection. Ultrasound was not found to be a reliable predictor of infection. Unfortunately, although infection during the first trimester carried a poorer prognosis, no reliable

prognostic indicators were found in this study, as in previous studies.

Currently, owing to toxicity of available therapies and the lack of prognostic predictors, there is no recommended therapy for pregnant women diagnosed with intrauterine CMV infection. Immunization of women in the childbearing years would be an attractive option. Possible vaccines against CMV are under investigation,[45] but presently no vaccine is available. Treatment of affected infants with ganciclovir has completed a phase II trial.[46] This trial demonstrated improved or stabilized hearing loss in 5/30 (16%) of affected infants treated with ganciclovir, suggesting that treatment may prove to be of benefit, although toxicities include neutropenia and thrombocytopenia.

Congenital Toxoplasmosis

Congenital toxoplasmosis is caused by intrauterine infection with the protozoan *Toxoplasma gondii*. In the United States, congenital toxoplasmosis is not a reportable disease, so the epidemiology of congenital infection is unknown, but the CDC estimates 400 to 4000 cases per year. Congenital toxoplasmosis is most often asymptomatic, but infections earlier in gestation are more likely to cause clinical disease,[47] including congenital hydrocephalus, intrauterine growth retardation, mental retardation, and vision-threatening chorioretinitis. Determination of primary infection with toxoplasmosis during pregnancy is important because treatment of the pregnant woman to reduce congenital infection is indicated. Currently, universal serologic screening of pregnant woman for toxoplasmosis is not recommended in the United States, but the CDC is conducting research to assess the cost-effectiveness and need for national toxoplasmosis screening of newborn infants.

For suspected cases of congenital toxoplasmosis infections, screening serology testing of the pregnant woman is recommended with IgG and IgM. Several commercially available serology screens for toxoplasmosis exist, but the IgM screening tests are hampered by unacceptable rates of high false-positivity and detectability up to 18 months after infection.[48] Therefore, confirmation of infection in fetuses or neonates of pregnant women with positive screening serology should be undertaken at a reference laboratory, such as the Palo Alto Medical Foundation (1-650-853-4828). The most reliable tools for definitive diagnosis currently are PCR of amniotic fluid, cerebrospinal fluid, and blood and culture of the placenta or blood by mouse inoculation. The placenta of neonates with suspected congenital infection should be sampled and sent to the reference laboratory for culture and also sent for pathologic examination.

Although treatment of pregnant women with primary toxoplasmosis infection is recommended to reduce transmission to the fetus, a recent meta-analysis reviewing 2591 papers found only 9 studies comparing treatment with no treatment of pregnant women with suspected primary toxoplasmosis.[49] None of these studies was randomized, and control groups were in general not comparable to treated groups. Five of the studies found treatment to be effective and four did not. Clearly, more controlled trials are needed on the efficacy of therapy in this situation. Usually, pregnant women with detected primary infection who do not have evidence of fetal infection are treated with spiramycin in an effort to decrease congenital infection. Spiramycin is an investigational drug in the United States and is available only on protocol via the U.S. Food and Drug Administration (1-301-827-2127). If the fetus is determined to be infected after 17 weeks' gestation, pregnant women are treated with sulfonamides and pyrimethamine.

The CDC recently published updated guidelines for the prevention of congenital toxoplasmosis.[50]

Lymphocytic Choriomeningitis Virus

Although congenital infection with lymphocytic choriomeningitis virus, an arenavirus carried by mice and other rodents, was first reported in the literature in 1955,[51] the disease remains unrecognized and underdiagnosed. Adults infected with lymphocytic choriomeningitis virus most often have a nonspecific febrile illness, but they can also have aseptic meningitis. Congenitally infected infants resemble infants with congenital toxoplasmosis: chorioretinitis, hydrocephalus, intracranial calcifications, and mental retardation.[52] At the present time, there is no treatment, and diagnosis is made via serology through the CDC, using immunofluorescent assay (IFA) or enzyme-linked immunosorbent assay (ELISA). Transmission to the pregnant woman can occur via aerosolization of rodent excreta, so gravidas should be counseled to avoid contact with mice, rats, and hamsters during pregnancy, and caged rodents should be kept in the garage or basement to avoid the aerosolized exposure.

Parvovirus

Parvovirus B19 is a single-stranded DNA virus identified as the cause of erythema infectiosum (fifth disease) in 1983. The disease is most common in the winter and spring months and most commonly affects children aged 5 to 14 years old. The classic "slapped-cheek" rash is most common in children; adults more typically experience fever, adenopathy, arthralgias, and a mild arthritis during the viremia. Occasionally, a morbilliform rash is seen in adults, and infection is occasionally asymptomatic. The organism is highly infectious, and the risk of infection during epidemics is high for susceptible pregnant patients exposed to infected individuals, especially in the same household. Susceptible nursery school teachers had a threefold increased risk of acute infection during epidemics in Denmark.[53] Gillespie and associates[54] observed that 20% to 30% of susceptible schoolteachers had a seroconversion during an outbreak, and 60% to 80% of susceptible household contacts acquired the infection.

The Public Health Laboratory Service Working Party on Fifth Disease[55] demonstrated a 33% transplacental infection rate in 190 women infected during pregnancy. Infection during midpregnancy was associated with a 12% fetal loss rate. The overall fetal death rate is 9%. The virus is cytotoxic to erythroid progenitor cells. A propensity for the hematopoietic system makes the fetus particularly susceptible to infection because of the rapidly expanding red blood cell volume, the short half-life of red blood cells, and an immature immune system. Diagnosis is generally confirmed by ELISA for detection of IgM and IgG antibodies. A positive IgG titer with a negative IgM titer indicates prior infection and immunoprotection, and the patient can be reassured. Patients who have positive IgM titers should be followed with ultrasound. Viral DNA has been detected in maternal and fetal sera by PCR techniques, and Dieck and colleagues[56] have shown that DNA measurement using a sensitive PCR assay is a better indicator of parvovirus B19 infection than is serology.

In a survey of members of the Society of Perinatal Obstetricians conducted in 1997, 7% of 541 respondents reported using amniocentesis for PCR and 2% reported using fetal blood sampling. Additionally, of 539 cases reported in the survey, approximately one third of the parvovirus-associated cases of nonimmune hydrops resolved spontaneously. Fetal survival in the intrauterine transfusion group was 83.5%.[57] Similarly, Schild and coworkers[58] demonstrated an 83.8% survival rate in 37 fetuses with parvovirus B19 infection who were treated with cordocentesis and intravenous transfusion. Thirty-five of the 37 had nonimmune hydrops, and even fetuses with severe anemia had a favorable outcome.

Herpes

Herpes simplex virus (HSV) infections are among the most common infections encountered in gravid women and may pose a serious threat to the fetus or neonate. In the United States, the seroprevalence of HSV-2 in persons 12 years of age or older was 21.9% from 1988 to 1994.[59] In a cohort of private patients in California, the seroprevalence of HSV-2 was 32%.[60] As many as 3% to 4% of pregnant patients have a known history of recurrent genital herpes, and maternal genital disease is present at or near term in approximately 1/1000 pregnancies. Although intrauterine fetal HSV infection has been documented, the primary mode of infection is vertical transmission through an infected maternal genital tract. Viral culture has been the most common tool for confirming HSV infection; however, new techniques such as PCR and hybridization methods have demonstrated superior sensitivity. In gravid patients who were seropositive for HSV-2, Boggess and associates[61] used PCR and demonstrated asymptomatic viral shedding in 13.8% of patients in the third trimester of pregnancy. Viral culture identified only 2.3%.

Current recommendations for management of labor and delivery in patients with HSV are based on the clinical findings of an active lesion or prodromal symptoms and primary versus recurrent lesion. Cesarean delivery should be performed on a woman who has her first genital lesion at delivery because the transmission rate exceeds 50%. The risk of neonatal infection associated with vaginal delivery at the time of a recurrent HSV lesion is much lower, estimated at 3%. The role of cesarean section in recurrent genital herpes has been challenged by some owing to the very low incidence of neonatal herpes[62]; nevertheless, because of the potentially serious nature of the disease, many experts advocate cesarean delivery for patients with active genital lesions or prodromal symptoms. In the absence of active genital lesions, cesarean delivery is not indicated despite a prior history of infection, and patients who have nongenital lesions can deliver vaginally after an occlusive dressing is applied over the lesion.[63]

Antiviral treatment is recommended for primary HSV infection during pregnancy to decrease viral shedding and enhance lesion healing.[64] Prophylactic treatment with acyclovir during the third trimester has been demonstrated to decrease the rate of recurrence, and a trend toward a lower cesarean delivery rate was noted, but it did not reach statistical significance in a study by Brockelhurst and colleagues. In a recent phase I trial, valacyclovir therapy resulted in higher plasma acyclovir levels than did acyclovir therapy. Both treatments were well tolerated, and there was no evidence of drug toxicity in the patients or neonates.[65] To date, the Acyclovir in Pregnancy Registry has found no increased rate of congenital anomalies among more than 600 fetuses exposed to acyclovir during pregnancy.[66, 67] Further trials are needed to confirm the safety and determine the efficacy of suppressive valacyclovir or acyclovir during the third trimester of pregnancy. (See Chapter 26, Herpes Infections in Pregnancy.)

ROLE OF INFECTION IN PRETERM LABOR

Prematurity is the leading cause of perinatal morbidity and mortality in the United States. Preterm delivery affects 7% to 9% of pregnancies, and this rate has not changed since 1960. Maternal medical conditions, preterm premature rupture of membranes, fetal compromise, and idiopathic preterm labor can all lead to preterm delivery. Although multiple gestations, uterine abnormalities, maternal smoking, maternal cocaine use, low prepregnancy weight, maternal age younger than 18 or older than 40 years, and low socioeconomic status are risk factors for idiopathic preterm labor, the cause is unknown in most cases.[68] Evidence suggests that upper genital tract infection and the resulting inflammatory cascade play a significant role in many cases of spontaneous preterm labor.[69] The majority of early spontaneous preterm births are associated with histologic chorioamnionitis.[70]

Cervical-vaginal fetal fibronectin has been suggested as a potential marker for increased risk of preterm delivery, and it seems to be closely linked to antenatal infection. In a study by the National Institute of Child Health and Human Development[1] Maternal Fetal Medicine Units Network, patients who delivered before 32 weeks and had positive cervical-vaginal fetal fibronectin levels all had evidence of histologic chorioamnionitis, and there was a 16-fold increase in clinical chorioamnionitis. Neonatal sepsis was also six times higher if the patient had positive fetal fibronectin levels.[71] Patients who deliver preterm have a significantly higher rate of positive amniotic fluid cultures than those who have preterm labor but do not deliver preterm.[72]

Increased levels of several markers of inflammation, including interleukin-1, tumor necrosis factor, interleukin-6, colony-stimulating factor, interleukin-8, macrophage inflammatory protein-1α, and growth-related oncogene-α (GRO-α) have been associated with an increased risk of preterm delivery. A recent study by Maymon and group[73] suggests that matrix metalloproteinase 8, an interstitial collagenase, has a role in microbial invasion of the amniotic cavity and preterm labor. In addition to the sequelae of prematurity, intra-amniotic inflammation is an independent risk factor for the development of cerebral palsy. Yoon and colleagues[74] identified a significant increase in the odds of developing cerebral palsy by age 3 years in patients exposed to intra-amniotic inflammation antenatally.

Even as the evidence for a relationship between infection and preterm birth has increased, the role of antibiotic therapy in the prevention of prematurity has not been consistently demonstrated. Group B streptococci, *Neisseria gonorrhoeae*, *Chlamydia trachomatis*, *Ureaplasma urealyticum*, *Treponema pallidum*, *Trichomonas vaginalis*, and *Gardnerella vaginalis* have all been associated with increased risk for preterm labor; however, the exact role remains unclear. Treatment of group B streptococci, *Chlamydia trachomatis*, and *N. gonorrhoeae* has not had an effect on the prevention of preterm birth.

Bacterial vaginosis is a complex alteration in the vaginal flora involving a decrease in vaginal lactobacilli and an overgrowth of organisms such as *Gardnerella vaginalis, Bacteroides* species, peptostreptococci, *Mycoplasma* species, and *Mobiluncus* species. (See Chapter 4, Implications of Bacterial Vaginosis in Obstetrics.) Bacterial vaginosis has been associated with preterm delivery.[75] Based on a Cochrane Review of five trials involving 1504 patients, current evidence does not support screening and treating all pregnant patients for bacterial vaginosis to prevent preterm birth.[76] In patients at risk for preterm delivery, however, treatment of bacterial vaginosis with metronidazole and erythromycin reduced the rate of premature delivery.[77] It is uncertain whether the decrease in rate of prematurity is due to resolution of bacterial vaginosis or whether bacterial vaginosis is merely a marker for upper genital tract infection with another organism such as *U. urealyticum* and the improved outcome is due to treatment of that organism. Although much work has been done to delineate the mechanism(s) of preterm labor, further studies are needed to identify better markers and superior interventions.

ENDOMETRITIS

Postpartum endometritis has an incidence of approximately 1% to 3% after vaginal delivery and 13% to 50% after cesarean delivery. The bacteriology generally involves multiple organisms, most commonly anaerobes such as *Peptostreptococcus* species, *Prevotella* species, *Bacteroides* species, *Mobiluncus* species, and *Clostridium* species; aerobic gram-positive cocci such as enterococci, *Staphylococcus aureus*, and groups A, B, and D streptococci; and gram-negatives such as *E. coli*, *Klebsiella* species, and *Proteus* species. The diagnosis is made clinically by postpartum fever, fundal tenderness, and foul lochia. Cesarean delivery is the greatest risk factor, and women who receive prophylactic antibiotics at the time of nonelective cesarean delivery have lower rates of endometritis and wound infections. Cefazolin or ampicillin is typically the drug of choice, and broader-spectrum antibiotics are reserved for treatment instead of prophylaxis.[78] Clindamycin is a reasonable choice in patients who are allergic to penicillin. Prophylaxis with a single dose of antibiotics is as efficacious as multiple doses.

Chorioamnionitis is also a risk factor for endometritis. In patients who receive antibiotic treatment for clinical chorioamnionitis, therapy should be continued after cesarean section until the patient has been asymptomatic and afebrile for 24 to 48 hours. After vaginal delivery, antibiotics may be discontinued if the patient defervesces. Once postpartum endometritis is diagnosed, an extended-spectrum treatment should be initiated and continued until the patient is afebrile and asymptomatic for 24 to 48 hours. Multiple regimens have been used, including gentamicin plus clindamycin; extended-spectrum cephalosporins such as cefoxitin, cefotetan, ceftizoxime, and cefotaxime; and extended-spectrum penicillins such as ampicillin/sulbactam, ticarcillin/clavulanic acid, and piperacillin/tazobactam. Based on a review of the Cochrane database, French and Smaill[79] concluded that oral antibiotics were not needed after a completed course of intravenous therapy in uncomplicated endometritis. Additionally, they found more treatment failures in other therapies compared with an aminoglycoside plus clindamycin (relative risk, 1.37). Regimens with poor activity against penicillin-resistant anaerobes had the highest risk of failure (relative risk, 1.73).

With the widespread use of cephalosporins, enterococcus is becoming a more significant pathogen. Brumfield and coworkers[80] demonstrated a 94% cure rate of puerperal infection by treatment with clindamycin and gentamicin, with the selective addition of ampicillin or vancomycin, in patients who remained febrile after 48 hours of treatment. Treatment failures included 6 patients with wound complications, 12 with suspected antimicrobial resistance, and 1 with an infected hematoma. Daily dosing of gentamicin, 4

mg/kg, and twice-daily dosing of clindamycin, 1200 mg, compares favorably with the traditional thrice-daily dosing of each, and the less frequent dosing regimen provides substantial cost savings.[81]

SEPTIC PELVIC THROMBOPHLEBITIS— OBSTETRIC

Septic pelvic thrombophlebitis (SPT) should be suspected when postpartum fever persists for 4 to 5 days despite adequate antibiotic treatment. Brown and colleagues[82] identified an incidence of 1:3000 among 44,922 patients who delivered at Parkland Hospital over a 3-year period ending March 1994. The incidence was approximately 1:9000 after a vaginal delivery and 1:800 after a cesarean delivery.

The diagnosis is made by imaging with computed tomography or magnetic resonance imaging. Ultrasound is not reliable for diagnosing SPT. Some investigators recommend empirical treatment with heparin for unresponsive fever. The previously held view that defervescence in 48 to 72 hours after initiating anticoagulation confirms the diagnosis has been challenged. In a review of 11 cases by Witlin and associates[83] the mean duration of fever after heparin initiation was 6 days (range 2 to 28). Among 14 women with puerperal SPT randomly assigned to receive continued antimicrobial therapy alone or continued antimicrobial therapy plus heparin, there was no significant difference between the responses of patients who were or were not given heparin. Patients in the heparin group were febrile for an additional 134 ± 65 hours; in the group not given heparin, patients remained febrile for 140 ± 39 hours ($P = .83$).[82] If heparin therapy is pursued, the optimal duration of anticoagulation is unknown.

References

1. Hemsell DL. Infections after gynecologic surgery. Obstet Gynecol Clin North Am 1989;16:381–400.
2. Soper DE, Bump RC, Hurt WG: Bacterial vaginosis and trichomoniasis are risk factors for cuff cellulitis after abdominal hysterectomy. Am J Obstet Gynecol 1990;163:1016–1021.
3. Spiegel CA: Bacterial vaginosis. Clin Microbiol Rev 1991;4:485–502.
4. Berman ML, Grosen EA: A new method of continuous vaginal cuff closure at abdominal hysterectomy. Obstet Gynecol 1994;84:478–480.
5. Eschenbach DA: Bacterial vaginosis and anaerobes in obstetric-gynecologic infection. Clin Infect Dis 1993;16(Suppl 4):S282–S287.
6. DeLalla F, Scalambrino S, Tassi PG, et al: Piperacillin versus cefotetan as single-dose prophylaxis in abdominal hysterectomy: A prospective, randomized, multicenter study. J Chemother 1993;5:113–118.
7. Haverkorn MJ: A comparison of single-dose and multi-dose metronidazole prophylaxis for hysterectomy. J Hosp Infect 1987;9:249–254.
8. American College of Obstetricians and Gynecologists: Antibiotics and Gynecologic Infections, 2000 Compendium (No. 237). Washington, DC, ACOG, June 1997.
9. Toglia MR, Pearlman MD: Pelvic fluid collection following hysterectomy and their relation to febrile morbidity. Obstet Gynecol 1994;83:766–770.
10. Cunningham FG, Gilstrap LC 3rd, Kappus SS: Cefamandole for treatment of obstetrical and gynecological infections. Scand J Infect Dis Suppl 1980;Suppl 25:75–82.

11. Helmsell DL: Prophylactic antibiotics in gynecologic and obstetric surgery. Rev Infect Dis 1991;13(Suppl 10):S821–S841.
12. Larson JW, Gabel-Hughes K, Kreter B: Efficacy and tolerability of imipenem-cilastatin versus clindamycin + gentamicin for serious pelvic infections. Clin Ther 1992;14:90–96.
13. Helmsell DL, Helmsell PG, Heard MC, et al: Piperacillin and a combination of clindamycin and gentamicin for the treatment of hospital and community-acquired acute pelvic infections, including pelvic abscess. Surg Gynecol Obstet 1987;165:223–229.
14. Mercer LJ, Hajj SN, Ismail MA, et al: Use of C-reactive protein to predict the outcome of medical management of tuboovarian abscesses. J Reprod Med 1998;33:164–167.
15. Nelson AL, Sinow RM, Oliak D: Transrectal ultrasonographically guided drainage of gynecologic pelvic abscesses. Am J Obstet Gynecol 2000;182:1382–1388.
16. Place C, Nolan RL, Nickel JC: Alternate approaches to pelvic abscess drainage after cystectomy. Urol Radiol 1989;11:161–164.
17. Hajj SN, Mercer LJ, Ismail MA: Surgical approaches to pelvic infections in women. J Reprod Med 1988;33(1 Suppl):159–163.
18. Reich H, McGlynn F: Laparoscopic treatment of tuboovarian and pelvic abscess. J Reprod Med 1987;32:747–752.
19. Brown CE, Stettler RW, Twickler D, et al: Pueperal septic pelvic thrombophlebitis: Incidence and response to heparin therapy. Am J Obstet Gynecol 1999;181:143–148.
20. Cohen MB, Pernoll ML, Gevirtz CM, et al: Septic pelvic thrombophlebitis: An update. Obstet Gynecol 1983;62:83–89.
21. Magee KP, Blanco JD, Graham JM: Massive septic pelvic thrombophlebitis. Obstet Gynecol 1993;82(4 Pt 2 Suppl):662–664.
22. Keough J, MacDonald D, Kelehan P: Septic pelvic thrombophlebitis: An unusual treatable postpartum complication. Aust N Z J Obstet Gynaecol 1993;33:204–207.
23. Zakut H, Achiron R: Septic pelvic thrombophlebitis as an enigmatic cause of persistent puerperal fever: Course of disease, diagnosis, and treatment. Clin Exp Obstet Gynecol 1984;11:133–135.
24. Josey WE, Staggers SR Jr: Heparin therapy in septic pelvic thrombophlebitis: A study of 46 cases. Am J Obstet Gynecol 1974;120:228–233.
24a. Walters MD, Dombroski RA, Davidson SA, et al: Reclosure of disrupted abdominal incisions. Obstet Gynecol 1990;76:597–602.
25. Elliott D, Kufera JA, Myers RA: The microbiology of soft tissue infections. Am J Surg 2000;179:361–366.
26. Clark LA, Moon RE: Hyperbaric oxygen in the treatment of life-threatening soft-tissue infections. Respir Care Clin North Am 1999;5:203–219.
26a. Helmkamp BF: Abdominal wound dehisence. Am J Obstet Gynecol 1977;128:803–807.
26b. Hendrix SL, Schimp V, Martin J, et al: The legendary superior strength of the Pfannenstiel incision: A myth? Am J Obstet Gynecol 2000;182:1446–1451.
26c. McNeeley SG Jr, Hendrix SL, Bennett SM, et al: Synthetic graft placement in the treatment of fascial dehisence with necrosis and infection. Am J Obstet Gynecol 1998;179:1430–1434.
27. Prevention of perinatal Group B streptococcal disease: A public health perspective. MMWR Morb Mortal Wkly Rep 1996;45(RR-7):1–24.
28. Schrag SJ, Zywicki S, Farley MM, et al. Group B streptococcal disease in the era of intrapartum antibiotic prophylaxis. N Engl J Med 2000;342:15–20.
29. Carroll KC, Ballou D, Varner M, et al: Rapid detection of group B streptococcal colonization of the genital tract by a commercial immunoassay. Eur J Clin Microbiol Infect Dis 1996;15:206–210.
30. Song JY, Lin LL, Shott S, et al: Evaluation of the Strep B OIA test compared to standard culture methods for detection of group B streptococci. Infect Dis Obstet Gynecol 1999;7:202–205.
31. Nguyen TM, Gauthier DW, Myles TD: Detection of group B streptococcus: Comparison of an optical immunoassay with direct plating and broth-enhanced culture methods. J Matern Fetal Med 1998;7:172–176.
32. Bergeron MG, Danbing K, Menard C, et al: Rapid detection of group B streptococci in pregnant women at delivery. N Engl J Med 2000;343:175–179.
33. Connor EM, Sperling RS, Gelbert R, et al: Reduction of maternal-infant transmission of human immunodeficiency virus type I with zidovudine treatment. Pediatric AIDS Clinical Trial Group Protocol 076 Study Group. N Engl J Med 1994;331:1173–1180.
34. Recommendations of the U.S. Public Health Service Task Force on the use of zidovudine to reduce perinatal transmission of human immunodeficiency virus. MMWR Morb Mortal Wkly Rep 1994;43(RR-11):1–20.
35. Blanche S, Tardieu M, Rustin P, et al: Persistent mitochondrial dysfunction and perinatal exposure to antiretroviral nucleoside analogues. Lancet 1999;354:1084–1089.
36. Smith M, Group USNSRW: Ongoing nucleoside safety review of HIV-exposed children in U.S. studies [abstract 096]. Second Conference on Global Strategies for the Prevention of HIV Transmission from Mothers to Infants. Montreal, Canada, September 1999.
37. Pediatric AIDS Clinical Trials Group 316, reported at the 8th Conference on Retroviruses and Opportunistic Infections, Chicago, Feb 8, 2001.
38. Thorne C, Rudin C, Newell M, et al: Combination antiretroviral therapy and duration of pregnancy. AIDS 2000;14:2913–2920.
39. Public Health Service Task Force recommendations for the use of antiretroviral drugs in pregnant women infected with HIV-1 for maternal health and for reducing perinatal HIV-1 transmission in the United States. MMWR Morb Mortal Wkly Rep 1998;47(RR-2):1–30.
40. Shafter N, Chuachoowong R, Mock PA, et al: Short-course zidovudine for perinatal HIV-1 transmission in Bangkok, Thailand: A randomized controlled trial. Bangkok Collaborative Perinatal HIV Transmission Study Group. Lancet 1999;353:773–780.
41. Guay C, Musole D, Fleming T, et al: A randomized trial of single-dose nevirapine to mother and infant versus azidothymidine in Kampala, Uganda, for prevention of mother-to-infant transmission of HIV-1 [abstract 312]. Program and Abstracts of the 7th Conference on Retrovirus and Opportunistic Infections, San Francisco, Jan 23–Feb 2, 2000.
42. The International Perinatal HIV Group: The mode of delivery and the risk of vertical transmission of HIV Type 1: A meta-analysis of 15 prospective cohort studies. N Engl J Med 1999;340:977–987.
43. Brown HL, Abernathy MP: Cytomegalovirus infection. Semin Perinatol 1998;22:260–266.
44. Lieshard C, Donner C, Francart F, et al: Prenatal diagnosis of congenital cytomegalovirus infection: Prospective survey of 237 pregnancies at risk. Obstet Gynecol 2000;95:881–888.
45. Plotkin SA: Cytomegalovirus vaccine. Am Heart J 1999;138:S484–S487.
46. Whitley RJ, Cloud G, Gruber W, et al: Gancyclovir treatment of symptomatic congenital cytomegalovirus infection: Results of a phase II study. National Institute of Allergy and Infectious Disease Collaborative Antiviral Study Group. J Infect Dis 1997;175:1080–1086.
47. Holliman RE: Congenital toxoplasmosis: Prevention, screening and treatment. J Hosp Infect Dis 1995;30(Suppl):179–190.
48. Wilson M, Remington JS, Clavet C, et al: Evaluation of six commercial kits for detection of human immunoglobulin M antibodies to *Toxoplasma gondii*. J Clin Microbiol 1997;35:311–325.
49. Wallon M, Liou C, Garner P, et al: Congenital toxoplasmosis: Systematic review of evidence of efficacy of treatment in pregnancy. BMJ 1999;318:1511–1514.
50. Preventing congenital toxoplasmosis. MMWR Morb Mortal Wkly Rep 2000;49(RR-2):57–75.
51. Komrower GM, Williams BL, Stone PB: Lymphocytic choriomeningitis in the newborn: Probable transplacental infection. Lancet 1955;1:697–698.
52. Barton LL, Peters CJ, Seaver LH, et al: Congenital lymphocytic choriomeningitis virus infection. Arch Pediatr Adolese Med 1996;150:445.
53. Valeur-Jensen AK, Pedersen CB, Westergaard T, et al: Risk factors for parvovirus B19 infection in pregnancy. JAMA 1999;281:1099–1109.
54. Gillespie SM, Cartler ML, Asch S, et al: Occupational risk of human parvovirus B19 infection for school and day-care personnel during an outbreak of erythema infectiosum. JAMA 1990;263:2061.
55. Public Health Laboratory Service Working Party on Fifth Disease: Prospective study of human parvovirus (B19) infection in pregnancy. BMJ 1990;300:1166–1170.
56. Dieck D, Schild RL, Hansmann M, Eis-Hubinger AM: Prenatal diagnosis of congenital parvovirus B19 infection: Value of serological and PCR techniques in maternal and fetal serum. Prenat Diagn 1999;19:1119–1123.
57. Rodis JF, Borgida AF, Wilson M, et al: Management of parvovirus infection in pregnancy and outcomes of hydrops: A survey of members of the Society of Perinatal Obstetricians. Am J Obstet Gynecol 1998;179:985–988.
58. Schild RL, Bald R, Plath H, et al: Intrauterine management of fetal

parvovirus B19 infection. Ultrasound Obstet Gynecol 1999;13:161–166.

59. Fleming DT, McQuillan GM, Johnson RE, et al: Herpes simplex virus type 2 in the United States, 1976–1994. N Engl J Med 1997;337:1105–1111.

60. Kulhanjian JA, Soroush V, Au DS, et al: Identification of women at unsuspected risk of primary infection with herpes simplex virus type 2 during pregnancy. N Engl J Med 1992;326:916–920.

61. Boggess KA, Watts DH, Hobson AC, et al: Herpes simplex virus type 2 detection by culture and polymerase chain reaction and relationship to genital symptoms and cervical antibody status during the third trimester of pregnancy. Am J Obstet Gynecol 1997;176:443–451.

62. Brown ZA, Benedetti J, Ashley R, et al: Neonatal herpes simplex virus infection in relation to asymptomatic maternal infection at the time of labor. N Engl J Med 1991;324:1247–1252.

63. American College of Obstetricians and Gynecologists: Management of Herpes in Pregnancy (Practice Bulletin No. 8). Washington, DC, ACOG, 1998.

64. Scott LL, Sanchez PJ, Jackson GL, et al: Acyclovir suppression to prevent cesarean delivery after first-episode genital herpes. Obstet Gynecol 1996;87:69–73.

65. Kimberlin DF, Weller S, Whitley R, et al: Pharmacokinetics of oral valacyclovir and acyclovir in late pregnancy. Am J Obstet Gynecol 1998;179:846–851.

66. Andrews EB, Yankaskas BC, Cordero JF, et al: Acyclovir in pregnancy registry: Six years' experience. Obstet Gynecol 1992;79:7–13.

67. Pregnancy outcomes following systemic prenatal acyclovir exposure—June 1, 1984–June 30, 1993. MMWR Morb Mortal Wkly Rep 1993;42:806–809.

68. American College of Obstetricians and Gynecologists: Preterm Labor (Technical Bulletin No. 206). Washington, DC, ACOG, 1995.

69. Andrews WA, Goldenberg RL, Hauth JC: Preterm labor: Emerging role of genital tract infections. Infect Agents Dis 1995;4:196–211.

70. Gibbs RS, Romero R, Hillier SL, et al: A review of premature birth and subclinical infection. Am J Obstet Gynecol 1992;166:1515–1528.

71. Goldenberg RL, Thom E, Moawad AH, et al: The preterm prediction study: Fetal fibronectin, bacterial vaginosis, and peripartum infection. Obstet Gynecol 1996;87:656–660.

72. Mazor M, Chaim W, Maymon E, et al: The role of antibiotic therapy in the prevention of prematurity. Clin Perinat 1998;25:659–685.

73. Maymon E, Romero R, Pacora P, et al: Human neutrophil collagenase (matrix metalloproteinase 8) in parturition, premature rupture of the membranes, and intrauterine infection. Am J Obstet Gynecol 2000;183:94–99.

74. Yoon BH, Romero R, Park JS, et al: Fetal exposure to an intra-amniotic inflammation and the development of cerebral palsy at the age of three years. Am J Obstet Gynecol 2000;182:675–681.

75. Hillier SL, Nugent RP, Eschenbach DA, et al: Association between bacterial vaginosis and preterm delivery of a low-birth weight infant. N Engl J Med 1995;333:1737–1742.

76. Brocklehurst P, Hannah M, McDonald H: Interventions for treating bacterial vaginosis in pregnancy (Cochrane Review). In The Cochrane Library, Issue 3, 2000; CD000262. Oxford, Update Software.

77. Hauth JC, Goldenberg RL, Andrews WW, et al: Reduced incidence of preterm delivery with metronidazole and erythromycin in women with bacterial vaginosis. N Engl J Med 1995;333:1732–1736.

78. Hopkins L, Smaill F: Antibiotic prophylaxis regimens and drugs for cesarean section (Cochrane Review). In The Cochrane Library, Issue 2, 2000; CD001136. Oxford, Update Software.

79. French LM, Smaill FM: Antibiotic regimens for endometritis after delivery (Cochrane Review). In The Cochrane Library, Issue 2, 2000; CD001067. Oxford, Update Software.

80. Brumfield CG, Hauth JC, Andrews WW: Puerperal infection after cesarean delivery: Evaluation of a standardized protocol. Am J Obstet Gynecol 2000;182:1147–1151.

81. Mitra AG, Whitten MK, Laurent SL, Anderson WE: A randomized, prospective study comparing once-daily gentamicin versus thrice-daily gentamicin in the treatment of puerperal infection. Am J Obstet Gynecol 1997;177:786–792.

82. Brown CE, Stettler RW, Twickler D, Cunningham FG: Puerperal septic pelvic thrombophlebitis: Incidence and response to heparin therapy. Am J Obstet Gynecol 1999;181:143–148.

83. Witlin AG, Mercer BM, Sibai BM: Septic pelvic thrombophlebitis or refractory postpartum fever of undetermined etiology. J Matern Fetal Med 1996;5:335–358.

SIXTY-FIVE

Adolescent Eating Disorders

Carole L. Kowalczyk

Adolescence is a trying time: puberty has initiated bodily changes that are new, normal, and yet awkward; societal pressures among teenagers have increased; and the desire to be accepted and acknowledged is ever so important during this stage. Societal influences on the "perfect thin" body image as well as the misconceived notion to be perfect may lead to adolescent anorectic and bulimic behaviors, eating disorders whose peak incidence is in adolescents. In this chapter, anorexia nervosa, bulimia, exercise-associated eating disorders, and their clinical manifestations are discussed. Complications arising from such disorders are reviewed, and therapeutic interventions are highlighted. Finally, a guide to improving the nutrient intake of adolescents is presented.

ANOREXIA NERVOSA

Anorexia nervosa is a severe and potentially life-threatening disorder that occurs in all socioeconomic classes in approximately 2% of women, with a consistent increase seen during the 1990s. The ratio of this disorder in girls to boys is approximately 20:1. This is partly due to the cultural or societal importance placed on thinness. Most patients come from success-achievement-appearance–oriented families with apparent "familial harmony," denying or avoiding any conflicts in the home. To gain control of the situation, the adolescent finds something to control—her weight through altered eating behaviors. At puberty, the normal weight gain may be perceived by the teenager as being excessive and may initiate the development of anorexia; in fact, early extreme exercise may be the first manifestation of the disease.

Anorexia nervosa has its onset between the ages of 10 and 30 years and is characterized by a weight loss of 25% or a weight 15% below normal for age and height. These patients usually have a distorted body image, with an extreme fear of being overweight. They usually hoard or mishandle their food and deny they have a problem. There are usually no identifiable medical or psychiatric disorders. Clinically, patients may present with signs and symptoms such as lanugo, bradycardia, overactivity, bulimia, self-induced vomiting, constipation, hypertension, diabetes insipidus, cold intolerance, hypercarotenemia, and amenorrhea. Anorexia manifests as a dysfunction of body mechanisms related to the hypothalamus, especially appetite, temperature, autonomic balance, and endocrine secretion. These patients usually have hypothalamic amenorrhea with low follicle-stimulating hormone, luteinizing hormone, and

relative hypothyroidism with normal thyroid-stimulating hormone and thyroxine levels but a low triiodothyronine and elevated reverse triiodothyronine. In addition, prolactin is normal and cortisol is elevated. With weight gain, all of the metabolic changes return to normal. However, 30% of patients will remain amenorrheic, implicating the possibility of an ongoing psychological conflict.

Brown and colleagues[1] highlighted some additional clues to the existence of anorexia nervosa, including:

1. Unexplained weight loss
2. Failure to gain weight in proportion to height
3. Hobbies or sports promoting weight loss
4. Feeling cold compared with peers
5. Hair loss
6. Refusing to eat with others
7. Eating slowly and cutting food into small portions
8. Eating at odd times

A potential new screening tool for eating disorders, the SCOFF questionnaire, was developed by Morgan and associates.[2] Five key questions address core features of anorexia nervosa and bulimia. The SCOFF questions include:

1. Do you make yourself *S*ick because you feel uncomfortably full?
2. Do you feel that you have lost *C*ontrol over how much you eat?
3. Have you recently lost more than *O*ne stone (14 pounds) in a 3-month period?
4. Do you believe yourself to be *F*at when others say you are too thin?
5. Would you say that *F*ood dominates your life?

Each yes answer equals 1 point; a score of 2 indicates a likely diagnosis of anorexia or bulimia. The questionnaire was administered in an eating disorders unit with 100% sensitivity and 87.5% specificity, providing potential promising quick techniques to aid in diagnosis of these syndromes. However, further testing in the general population is needed to confirm the test's efficacy.

BULIMIA

Bulimia is a syndrome marked by episodic and secret binge eating followed by self-induced vomiting, fasting, or the use of laxatives and diuretics. Bulimic behavior may be seen alone or in the presence of anorexia nervosa.

A study by Joiner and coworkers[3] compared personality

features between male and female bulimic patients. The eating disorder inventory (EDI), a 64-item questionnaire, was applied to 532 female and 221 males at Harvard University in 1982 and again in 1992. Eight subscales were measured, including drive for thinness, bulimia, body dissatisfaction, ineffectiveness, perfectionism, interpersonal distrust, interdisciplinary awareness, and maturity fears. Females scored significantly higher in the drive for thinness, whereas males scored higher for perfectionism and interpersonal distrust. The findings display very different trigger points among the genders in the initiation of the bulimic syndrome.

Stice and colleagues[4] investigated the impact of negative affect on eating disorders, using 4 measures:

1. The Dutch Restrained Eating Scale—a 10-item measure of dieting behaviors
2. The Dietary Intent Scale—a 9-item measure of dietary behavior with three subscales assessing reduced intake of food, abstention from eating, and consumption of low-calorie foods
3. The PANAS-X—the positive and negative affect schedule
4. The Revised Bulimia Test—used to assess binge eating

The results after interviewing 320 females and 311 males indicated that both dieting and a negative affect were independent risk factors for bulimic behaviors, but that negative affect may moderate the relation between dieting and binge eating.

MEDICAL CONSEQUENCES OF ANOREXIA NERVOSA AND BULIMIA

Gastrointestinal Complications

Most patients with anorexia have a prolongation of gastrointestinal transit time, causing bloating and constipation. These patients should be encouraged to eat smaller meals more frequently and increase their water intake as well as fiber; their symptoms should resolve within 2 to 3 weeks. Laxatives should be discouraged, secondary to the high incidence of their abuse in the population.

Endocrine Complications

Either primary or secondary amenorrhea is a cardinal manifestation of anorexia nervosa. Approximately 20% of patients with anorexia will experience amenorrhea before any weight loss. Menses will usually return if the patients reach approximately 90% of their ideal body weight. The hypoestrogenic state caused by the syndrome is a significant risk factor for osteoporosis and stress fractures. Because peak bone mass is attained by the late teenage years or early 20s, loss of bone at this stage will have a significant detriment on bone later in life. These patients require estrogen replacement therapy in the form of standard meno-

pausal hormone replacement therapy (less effective) or preferably low-dose oral contraceptives to reduce the risk of osteoporosis and stress fractures. In addition, adolescents require high-dose calcium (1500 mg/day) and adequate vitamin D intake (400 IU/day). Obviously, restoring body weight and resuming menses should be the ultimate goal.

Cardiac Complications

Common clinical manifestations in anorexia nervosa include bradycardia and hypertension. This is secondary to a lower basal metabolic rate and does not require treatment unless heart rates are less than 35 beats per minute. Deaths in adolescents with anorexia nervosa are caused by cardiovascular collapse. Brown and colleagues[1] reported that with progressive weight loss, there is a decrease in left ventricle mass and stroke volume; maximal work capacity is diminished; and there is an increase in sudden death. This process is manifested by prolonged QT intervals and arrhythmias secondary to electrolyte abnormalities. In postmortem studies, significant atherosclerosis has also been identified.

Anorexia nervosa is associated with the highest mortality of all psychotic disorders, ranging from 5% to 10%. This is manifested usually from cardiac complications secondary to emaciation.

EXERCISE-INDUCED AMENORRHEA

The adolescent athlete is especially at risk of developing eating disorders. The extreme need to be thin to compete in such sports as ballet and gymnastics may lead to delayed puberty if the patient is premenarchal or secondary amenorrhea develops. Caloric intake in adolescent athletes is far from adequate, with lower than recommended intakes in calcium, iron, magnesium, and folic acid. Twenty-three per cent of female gymnasts consumed less than 1500 calories a day, female cross-country runners less than 1790 calories a day, and 25% of ballet dancers consumed less than 1500 calories a day.[5] In addition, much of these calories consumed (almost 30% to 44%) were derived from so-called junk food, such as sugars, jams, jellies, and sodas. Both delayed puberty and secondary amenorrhea result, in part, from these low nutrition states. The role of critical body fat remains controversial, but probably has some impact. In addition, the strain of exercise itself affects menstrual function. Warren and associates[6] have shown that during a period of rest, dancers will have a return in menses, despite no change in body fat. The menstrual disruption is similar to the hypothalamic dysfunction seen in anorexia nervosa. Acute exercise inhibits gonadotropin-releasing hormone and decreases gonadotropins, while it increases prolactin, cortisol, ACTH, growth hormone, testosterone, and endorphins. In amenorrheic athletes, all the circulating thyroid hormones are low, including reverse triiodothyronine. The hypoestrogenic state that results increases the risk of osteoporosis, stress fractures, and cardiovascular changes in this population. Unlike the anorectic adolescent, however, the athlete with exercise-induced amenorrhea has a better understanding once the problem is explained and has the capability of self criticism. This favorably allows the physician and patients to compromise diet and exercise practices to return to a normal physiologic state.

TREATMENT

Treatment for anorexia nervosa and bulimia involves family counseling as well as individualized psychotherapy. Medications are more effective in treating bulimia as opposed to anorexia nervosa. Whereas most adolescents can be treated on an outpatient basis, hospitalization is necessary for patients with rapid weight loss or those who have lost greater than 25% of their ideal body weight, those with cardiac arrhythmias, and those nonresponsive to outpatient therapy. In treating these patients, one must be aware of a potentially harmful condition referred to as the *refeeding syndrome*. The refeeding syndrome refers to severe hypophosphatemia that produces widespread cellular changes that depress cardiac stroke volume and can subsequently lead to congestive heart failure. This syndrome can be prevented as long as refeeding is started slowly, and modest caloric increases occur during the first 2 to 3 weeks. Patients at risk of this syndrome are the chronically malnourished or those who have not eaten in approximately a week. Daily caloric intake should be increased by only 200 to 300 cal every 3 to 4 days until caloric intake is adequate. During this time period, electrolyte and phosphorus levels are checked weekly and the patient is monitored closely for tachycardia and edema.

IMPROVING NUTRITIONAL INTAKE

Recommendations for improving the nutrient intake of adolescents may include:

1. Training of health care professionals on the specific nutritional requirements of adolescents is mandatory.
2. Adequate screening and counseling of adolescents about nutrition and exercise should be incorporated into routine health care visits.
3. Nutrition educational programs specific to the needs and interests of adolescents should be introduced.
4. Affordable and convenient healthy foods should be easily available to adolescents.

5. Vitamin and mineral supplements should be used to correct any identified nutritional deficiencies.
6. Sports involvement should be monitored in relation to nutritional intake and changes in body weight and menstrual cyclicity. Adjustments in activity level should be made accordingly.
7. Because weight concerns and dietary behaviors seem to be a major factor in teenage nutrition, intake, and exercise, these topics should be discussed openly within clinical and educational settings.

SUMMARY

Eating disorders, especially anorexia nervosa and bulimia, reach their peak incidence in adolescents; increased sports and exercise activities may exacerbate the condition. As health care providers, we must continually be aware of the clinical signs and symptoms of eating disorders present in our patients. Adolescents should be counseled concerning proper diet and exercise and questioned openly about body image and well-being. If problems are identified, proper outpatient or inpatient therapy should be immediately initiated. Severe medical consequences such as amenorrhea, osteoporosis, cardiac complications and even sudden death can then be avoided.

Suggestions for Future Reading

Carpenter SE, Koehler S, Rock JA: Pediatric and Adolescent Gynecology. New York, Raven, 1992.

Speroff L, Glass RH, Kase NG: Amenorrhea. Clinical Gynecologic Endocrinology and Infertility 1999;6:421–485.

References

1. Brown JM, Mehler PS, Harris RH: Medical complications occurring in adolescents with anorexia nervosa. West J Med 2000;172:189–193.
2. Morgan JF, Reid F, Lacey JH: The SCOFF questionnaire: A new screening tool for eating disorders. West J Med 2000;172:164–165.
3. Joiner TE, Katz J, Heatherton TF: Personality features differentiate late adolescent females and males with chronic bulimic symptoms. Int J Eat Disord 2000;27:191–197.
4. Stice E, Akutagawa D, Gaggar A, Agras WS: Negative affect moderates the relation between dieting and binge eating. Int J Eat Disord 2000;27:218–229.
5. Wright K, Neumark-Sztainer D: Guidelines for adolescent female nutrition and implications for women's health. In Infertility and Reproductive Medicine (Obesity and Weight Management: Nutrition, Exercise, and Other Therapies) 2000;11(2):199–226.
6. Warren MP: Effects of exercise and physical training on menarche. Semin Reprod Endocrinol 1985;3:17.

SIXTY-SIX

Breast Disease

Vanessa D. Dance, Mary V. Krueger,

and Wendy Ma

Educational campaigns geared toward increasing the early detection of breast cancer have resulted in heightened awareness in women regarding changes in their breasts. Health care providers often encounter complaints related to the breasts and should be able to provide education, screening, counseling, and treatment for conditions of the breasts. This chapter discusses the diagnosis, management, and treatment options for common breast conditions. It also illustrates one institution's method for providing coordinated breast care for its patient population.

CLINICAL ASSESSMENT

A clinical assessment involves a thorough history of the patient's symptoms as well as an examination of the breasts. In obtaining the history, it is important to note the presence of any factors that increases the risk for breast cancer, such as previous history of breast cancer, nulliparity, early menarche (<age 12 years), late menopause (>age 53 years), delayed childbearing (>age 35 years), first-degree relatives with history of breast cancer, obesity, higher socioeconomic status, and a personal history of ductal or lobular hyperplasia (particularly with atypia) (Table 66–1).

Breast Examination

The patient should be seated comfortably on the examination table, with all upper garments removed. Inspection is done initially with the patient's arms relaxed at her sides. The breasts are then inspected for asymmetry, skin or nipple changes, and contour (Table 66–2). The patient should then raise her hands above her head and press hands on her hips; edema, skin dimpling, or nipple retraction should be noted. While the patient is seated, each breast

should be palpated. The axillary and supraclavicular areas should be palpated for enlarged lymph nodes. While the patient is supine with one arm over her head, the ipsilateral breast should be palpated for possible masses.

IMAGING TECHNIQUES

Mammography (Table 66–3) and ultrasonography (Table 66–4) are the most commonly used techniques for the detection of breast lesions. Magnetic resonance imaging may be of value in assessing a breast lesion of an indeterminate nature based on clinical and mammographic examination or in patients with breast implants.[1]

BENIGN BREAST CONDITIONS

Fibrocystic Change

Fibrocystic change of the breast has formerly been known by various terms such as fibrocystic disease, mammary dysplasia, and chronic cystic mastitis. Fibrocystic change is the most common lesion of the breast; this is an imprecise term that covers a spectrum of clinical signs, symptoms, and histologic changes (Table 66–5).[2, 3] These lesions are associated with benign changes in the breast epithelium, some of which are found so commonly in normal breast histology that they are probably normal variants.[4] The microscopic findings of fibrocystic change include cysts, adenosis, papillomatosis, fibrosis, and ductal epithelial hyperplasia. Fibrocystic change is not associated with an increased risk of breast cancer unless there is histologic evidence of epithelial proliferative changes with or without atypia.[5]

Differential Diagnosis

In trying to differentiate this condition from carcinoma and fibroadenomas, it is important to note the presence of

---

Table 66–1. Patient History—Key Points

Onset and duration of signs and symptoms
Age
Family history
Menstrual and reproductive history
Menopause
Cyclic pattern
Breastfeeding
Hormonal therapy
Dietary habits

Table 66–2. Breast Examination—Key Points

Breast shape and size
Mass size, position, surface, shape, consistency, pain, mobility
Nipple symmetry, discharge, retraction, eczema
Tenderness or pain
Nodularity
Lymph glands (axillary and supraclavicular)

Table 66–3. Mammography—Key Features

Readily available and easy to perform
Slight discomfort
Used in breast cancer screening
Limited in women younger than age 35 yr

pain, multiple lesions, and fluctuation in size. If a dominant mass is present, this merits a thorough evaluation, including a biopsy of the tissue to rule out carcinoma.

Mammography is of limited value in the evaluation of fibrocystic changes because no specific mammographic findings are diagnostic of fibrocystic changes. In young women, the breast tissue is usually too radiodense to allow for adequate visualization of the breast tissue with mammography. Breast ultrasound is useful in differentiating a solid from a cystic mass. If a dominant mass is identified, a fine-needle aspiration may be performed to determine its nature (Table 66–6).

If clear fluid is obtained and the mass disappears, it is prudent to perform a follow-up examination in 3 months. If there is a residual mass after aspiration or if bloody fluid is obtained, an excisional biopsy is indicated. A solid dominant mass not diagnosed as fibroadenoma also requires an excisional biopsy for definitive diagnosis.[6]

Treatment

The role of caffeine consumption in the development and treatment of fibrocystic changes is controversial. Dietary consumption of up to 500 mg of caffeine has been associated with an increased risk of fibrocystic change.[7] Recommendation for the discontinuation of coffee, tea, chocolate, and other caffeinated products may be helpful in reducing symptoms.

Mastalgia associated with fibrocystic changes may be treated by avoiding trauma and wearing a brassiere with good support and protection, preferably night and day.[8] Patients with fibrocystic changes should be advised to perform monthly self-breast examinations and report any changes to their health care provider.

Fibroadenoma

Fibroadenomas are the most common lesions found in women younger than age 25 years and the second most common benign lesion of the breast (Table 66–7).[6] Fibroadenomas persist throughout the menstrual years and appear

Table 66–4. Ultrasonography—Key Features

High-frequency sound used
Ideal for differentiating solid from cystic masses
Limited by resolution and operator experience

Table 66–5. Diagnosis of Fibrocystic Change— Key Points

Most common in ages 30–50 yr
Rare in postmenopausal women not using hormone replacement therapy
Associated with increased pain or size during premenstrual phase of the cycle
Pain and tenderness present, usually bilateral and most often in upper outer quadrants of the breast
Rapid fluctuation in size of masses is common

to regress in the postmenopausal period. During pregnancy, they may increase in size and infarct, causing significant pain.

Differential Diagnosis

In women older than age 30 years, cystic disease of the breast and carcinoma of the breast must be considered. Cysts can be identified by aspiration.

Treatment

The suspicion for a fibroadenoma should be confirmed by either excisional biopsy or fine-needle aspiration cytology. For women younger than age 25 years with small palpable fibroadenomas, careful observation may be considered in selected situations.[6] Complete excision of a fibroadenoma with the patient under local anesthesia can be done to treat the lesion and confirm the absence of malignancy. Large or growing fibroadenomas must be excised.[1]

Cystosarcoma Phyllodes

Cystosarcoma phyllodes is an uncommon lesion representing both epithelial and stromal proliferation (Table 66–8). Patients often report a previously stable nodule that suddenly increases in size. The clinical course of a phyllodes tumor is variable and often unpredictable.

Differential Diagnosis

Approximately 10% of phyllodes tumors contain some characteristics suggestive of a malignant process.[9] The his-

Table 66–6. Technique for Fine-needle Aspiration of a Dominant Mass

Immobilize the lesion with fingers
Use a 22- to 24-gauge needle and aspirate
If fluid present, aspirate and withdraw needle
If mass solid, make several passes through the mass while aspirating until a small amount of fluid or tissue is seen in the syringe
Place specimen on a slide for cytologic evaluation

tologic distinction between fibroadenoma, benign cystosarcoma, and malignant cystosarcoma can be very difficult.[1]

Treatment

Treatment is wide local excision.[1] Massive or large tumors in small breasts may require mastectomy; lymph node dissection is not indicated.

Superficial Thrombophlebitis

Superficial thrombophlebitis of the breast, also known as Mondor's disease, is an uncommon, benign process (Table 66–9).[10] This condition is often associated with a superficial thrombophlebitis in the thoracoepigastric vein, which drains the upper outer quadrant of the breast. Fibrosis may occur adjacent to the lesion, causing skin retraction.

Diagnosis

The diagnosis is made on the basis of predisposing conditions and a characteristic linear, tender, erythematous mass.[6]

Treatment

Superficial thrombophlebitis will resolve in 1 to 3 weeks. Treatment should consist of conservative measures, including analgesics and warm compresses.

Duct Ectasia

Duct ectasia is a condition in which the major ducts draining into the nipple become distended and filled with secretions (Table 66–10). This condition usually occurs in perimenopausal or postmenopausal women. The histologic

evaluation of the area shows dilated, distended terminal collecting ducts obstructed with inspissated, lipid-containing epithelial cells and phagocytic histiocytes.[6]

Differential Diagnosis

Duct ectasia can lead to infections, such as periductal mastitis. Periductal mastitis is a breast infection in which the major ducts draining into the nipple become distended and filled with secretions that then become infected and cause inflammation (mastitis). Patients with periductal mastitis often have nipple discharge that may be bloody. Duct papillomas are benign tumors, usually of a single major duct. They may cause bloody nipple discharge. Final diagnosis is confirmed on pathology after excision.

Treatment

Treatment consists of excisional biopsy. In the absence of infection, conservative management may include manual compression to the nipple area and wearing a support brassiere.

Fat Necrosis

Fat necrosis is associated with breast trauma in 50% of cases.[1] It is also common after breast surgery or radiation therapy. Usually the patient will present with a firm mass that may be accompanied by tenderness or ecchymosis. The mass is usually palpable and can cause skin or nipple retraction, similar to breast carcinoma.

Treatment

Needle or excisional biopsy is necessary to rule out carcinoma. If untreated, the mass associated with fat necrosis gradually disappears.

CONDITIONS OF THE BREASTS DURING PREGNANCY AND LACTATION

Pregnant and lactating women may develop not only the breast diseases encountered in their nonpregnant counterparts, but also are susceptible to problems unique to pregnancy and lactation.

Mastitis

Mastitis is characterized by fever higher than 38.5°C, chills, myalgias, systemic illness, and a tender, hot, swollen, wedge-shaped area of the breast. It is a bacterial cellulitis of the interlobar connective tissue of the breast and the mammary glands.[11] Mastitis is often due to bacterial infection, with *Staphylococcus aureus* being the most common etiologic agent. It commonly occurs in the first 3 weeks' postpartum, but can develop at any time while the mother is nursing.

Treatment

Treatment includes bed rest, frequent feeding on both breasts with the unaffected side being offered first, and oral antibiotics for 10 to 14 days. First line antibiotics that are effective and safe during breastfeeding include dicloxacillin (500 mg PO four times daily), first-generation cephalosporins, and erythromycin (for penicillin-allergic patients). Failure to treat mastitis adequately increases the risk of recurrence and breast abscesses. This should be emphasized to the patient, because most experience resolution of symptoms after 48 hours and therefore tend not to complete the full course of therapy needed to eradicate the infection.[11]

Breast Abscess

Breast abscesses usually occur within the first few months of breastfeeding and are more common in first-time mothers. They may also occur at the time of weaning, because there is stagnation of milk in the breasts, providing an excellent culture media for bacteria.

Treatment

Like most abscesses, those in the breast require drainage as well as antibiotic treatment. The drainage may be accomplished by either repeated needle aspirations or incision. If incisional drainage is performed, biopsy should be taken to rule out inflammatory carcinoma.[12] There are conflicting recommendations on whether it is advisable to continue feeding from the affected breast, but there is general agreement that it is safe to continue feeding from the unaffected breast.[13]

Galactocele

Galactocele is a cystic area with inspissated milk material believed to form secondary to ductal obstruction,[12] also known as milk retention cysts. This condition is usually seen after the abrupt termination of lactation. It may present as a tender mass, most often in the periphery of the breast. Although initially its content is normal milk, the composition soon becomes thick and oily as fluid is absorbed.

Treatment

Galactocele can be drained through needle aspiration, but it will tend to fill up again. Surgical removal can be accomplished with the patient under local anesthesia without stopping breastfeeding.[13]

Other tender lumps on the breast may be secondary to plugging of a collecting duct or system. Manual massage of the tender area in a warm shower may help to relieve the obstruction, as may hot packs applied to the breasts before feedings. Some women with high-calcium diets can actually form calcium stones that clog ducts and that will be excreted as "grains of sand." Other women with repeated obstruction may be able to express small fatty plugs before feeds. These will often resolve with the addition of 1 tablespoon of lecithin, a lipid constituent of human milk, to the daily diet.[13]

Engorgement

At 2 to 4 days' postpartum, colostrum changes to normal breast milk, and the breasts become engorged. Engorgement is due to congestion and increased vascularity of the breast tissue along with accumulation of milk and edema resulting from enlarged alveoli blocking lymphatic drainage. This engorgement may involve only the areola, only the body of the breast, or both. When engorgement affects the areola, the infant cannot latch on properly, which may lead to improper feeding and sore nipples.

Treatment

Gentle manual expression of milk by the mother before breastfeeding will often relieve some of the pressure and soften the nipple enough that the infant can then nurse effectively without causing pain. Peripheral engorgement is primarily vascular and will therefore not be relieved by mechanical pumping. Pumping may actually cause trauma and increased pain in the hypervascular breast. The mainstay of treatment is frequent, around-the-clock breastfeeding, which allows the suckling infant to most efficiently remove milk from the breast. Management is centered on relief of pain so that the mother can continue to nurse. Cold packs can be used to reduce the vascularity, particularly after a feeding. Chilled, uncooked cabbage leaves have also been shown to be effective in relieving the associated edema. The mother should be counseled to wear a supportive nursing bra 24 hours a day. A warm shower or warm packs before nursing may help with the letdown reflex and facilitate feeding. Pain medications, such as acetaminophen, ibuprofen, or codeine, may be necessary in some cases. Medication should be taken immediately before nursing, because it will then provide pain relief to the mother but will not be present in the breast milk for more than ½ hour after dosing.

Sore Nipples

The two main categories of sore nipples are trauma and irritation.

Nipple Trauma

Improper nursing position or infant suckling difficulties traumatize nipples. The nipple may be cracked, blistered, scabbed, or bleeding. Cracks and pain at the base of the nipple are specifically caused by the infant sucking its bottom lip into the mouth, which then rubs on the underside of the nipple, causing a friction burn.

Treatment. Pulling the infant's lower lip out of the mouth while it is nursing usually provides immediate pain relief for the mother. Generalized treatment for traumatized nipples starts with manual expression of breast milk before nursing to soften the nipple, making it easier for the infant to latch on. The couplet should then be observed during feeding and improper positioning corrected. The unaffected side should be offered first, leaving the affected side open to the air. In some cases, it may be necessary to manually express from the affected breast at each feeding for several days to allow the severely traumatized nipple to heal. After feeding, residual milk should be allowed to dry on the breast. The nipples should be exposed to air between feedings as much as possible. Bras should be made of cotton, and nursing pads should not contain plastic linings. Ointments may be used but can be a source of irritation. The most effective tool in management of nipple soreness is prevention. Correct breast presentation has been found to be the primary factor in preventing breast soreness, whereas prenatal breast preparation and length of time spent feeding have not been shown to have an effect on the amount of pain. Correct position involves having the infant squarely face the breast and take as much of the areola as possible into its wide-open mouth.

Irritated Nipples

Irritated nipples are red and swollen, often described as a burning pain by the mother. The irritation is usually due to dermatitis, candidiasis, or an underlying skin condition, such as impetigo or eczema. Dermatitis may result from an allergic response to a nipple cream or ointment; so it is important to ask the patient what topical medications she has been using. Candidal infection may also present with hot, shooting pains in the mother's breast, especially when initiating a feed.

Treatment. The infant should be examined for signs of oral thrush. If thrush is present, both the mother and the infant should be treated with nystatin for 14 days. Cool, wet compresses to the nipples along with the techniques described previously can help to relieve pain while the underlying cause is being treated. Impetigo may present as sore, cracked nipples that persist despite good breastfeeding technique. Impetigo should be treated with oral anti-staphylococcal antibiotics, because topical antibiotics have been shown to be ineffective and may allow progression to mastitis.[14]

Nipple Discharge

During the second and third trimesters, the lining of the ducts undergoes epithelial proliferation that may lead to bloody nipple discharge. Cytology of such discharge is usually not helpful. Initial treatment is reassurance and observation, because the condition will usually resolve soon after delivery. Bloody nipple discharge that starts after delivery is most often traced to a bleeding traumatized nipple or a benign papilloma. In either of these cases, bleeding should stop within a few days or as soon as a visible source on the nipple heals. If the discharge is present 2 months after delivery, further workup is warranted.

Women may also present with concerns about the color of their milk. Whereas the initial colostrum was a creamy, yellow color, mature breast milk may appear thin, even having a bluish tint. Breastfeeding mothers should be reassured that this does not mean their milk is weak, but just reflects a change in the composition of the milk to provide the growing infant the perfect balance of nutrients and hydration.[15] Milk may also appear green, blue, or pink, reflecting a mother's intake of certain vegetables, food colorings, or dietary supplements.

Breast Cancer in Pregnancy

Malignancy, although uncommon in pregnancy, does occur at a rate of 3 per 10,000 pregnancies.[16] Providers must be vigilant to detect malignancies early in pregnancy. The poor prognosis associated with breast cancer in pregnancy may be due to a delay in diagnosis and treatment. Seventy-five percent of women diagnosed with breast cancer in pregnancy have positive nodes, compared with 37% in nonpregnant women. When pregnant patients are matched stage for stage with controls, survival appears equivalent.[17]

Diagnosis

Detection of a distinct mass may be difficult owing to increased firmness, nodularity, and hypertrophy of the breast during pregnancy. Because of these physiologic changes, a baseline breast examination at the first obstetric visit is crucial. A persistent mass detected during pregnancy should raise suspicion and prompt a thorough evaluation. Ultrasound can be helpful in differentiating cystic from solid lesions. Most sources agree that mammography is not helpful during pregnancy owing to the increased density, vascularity, and water content of the tissues.[16]

Treatment

Masses discovered in the first or second trimester can be safely excised with the patient under local anesthesia, with particular attention to infection control and hemostasis. Complications are more common owing to hypervascularity and edema of the gravid breast.[16] Masses discovered during the first half of the third trimester should undergo fine-needle aspiration cytology, and those found during the later half of the third trimester can undergo postpartum management. There is controversy over whether a woman can breastfeed in the face of postpartum biopsy. Continued lactation carries an increased risk of milk fistula and abscess; some women prefer to accept this risk rather than discontinue breastfeeding.[18]

Once a diagnosis of breast cancer is made in the pregnant patient, surgical treatment should proceed as it would in other women of reproductive age. Generally, this involves a modified radical mastectomy with the patient under general anesthesia. Allowing the pregnancy to progress to fetal viability before undertaking surgery has not been shown to be of benefit for either the mother or the fetus. Therapeutic abortion is rarely advised.[17]

Staging studies such as bone scan, head computed tomography, or magnetic resonance imaging are usually postponed until after delivery.[12] Radiation therapy to the chest wall results in significant fetal exposure owing to internal scatter from the mother's body tissues. For this reason, radiation is most often postponed until after delivery.

Although all chemotherapeutic agents are potential teratogens, the observed incidence of malformations is small.[12] Patients who do start treatment during pregnancy should be counseled that low birth weight and prematurity are complications of chemotherapy at anytime in pregnancy. Early delivery after documentation of fetal lung maturity may be desirable to allow initiation of chemotherapy.

CONDITIONS OF THE AUGMENTED BREAST

Approximately 4 million women in America have undergone breast augmentation. Implants commonly used are made of an outer silicone shell filled with silicone gel or saline solution. During an augmentation mammoplasty, breast implants are placed under the pectoralis muscle or in the subcutaneous tissue of the breast. Fifteen percent to 25% of patients develop capsule contraction or scarring surrounding the implant. This leads to firmness, pain, and distortion of the breast. Another 5% to 10% of women will have implant rupture or bleeding of gel through the implant capsule. The conditions may require removal of the implant.[19]

CONCLUSION

The female breasts can undergo numerous changes ranging from benign conditions, including those associated with pregnancy, to malignant disease. Because of the public's heightened awareness of breast cancer, women are frequently anxious about a new breast finding. By understanding the disease processes and the diagnostic and treatment modalities, a new presenting breast complaint can be readily diagnosed and treated within the total framework of a woman's health and wellness. A breast pathway is established at our institution, which provides for timely diagnosis and a team approach to treatment. Any patient with a breast finding is referred to our breast diagnostic center, where the appropriate imaging study is performed. A multidisciplinary conference comprising members from radiology, oncology, surgery, gynecology, family practice, and nursing meets once a week to discuss any abnormal studies and provides input into a diagnostic or treatment plan. A pathway nurse then contacts the patient with the imaging study result and team recommendation for follow-up and/or treatment. This nurse then coordinates all the patient's care, serving as the case manager. The patient may receive needle biopsy through the radiology department under ultrasound or computed tomography guidance or open biopsy through the surgery department. If a diagnosis of breast cancer is made, the patient meets with another team comprising members from surgery, medical oncology, radiation therapy, physical therapy, social work services, and mental health services. This team discusses with the patient the best cancer treatment plan and follow-up care. Genetic counseling and testing are offered at our institution to patients with breast cancer and those with high risk for breast cancer.

Our institution has also established a Breast Watch Clinic, which serves patients with high risk for breast cancer, such as positive family history, prior breast biopsies with atypical hyperplasia, or a personal history of breast cancer. The Breast Watch Clinic provides close surveillance and also continuity of care for our patient population. Breast disease evaluation and treatment are facilitated by coordinating care with a multidisciplinary team approach that keeps the woman's health care as the essential priority, which offers optimal continuity of care and avoids lost therapeutic opportunity.

Suggestions for Future Reading

American College of Obstetricians and Gynecologists: Nonmalignant Conditions of the Breast. (ACOG Technical Bulletin No. 156). Washington, DC, ACOG, June 1991.

American College of Obstetricians and Gynecologists: Role of the Obstetrician-Gynecologist in the Diagnosis and Treatment of Breast Cancer. (ACOG Committee Opinion No. 186) Washington, DC, ACOG, Sept. 1997.

Berek JS, Adashi EY, Hillard PA (eds): Novak's Gynecology, 12th ed. Chapter 18. Baltimore, Williams & Wilkins, 1988.

Current Obstetric and Gynecologic Diagnosis and Treatment, 8th ed. Chapter 62. Norwalk, Conn, Appleton & Lange, 1994.

Helping Mothers Nurse Successfully, slide-lecture kit, videotape and monograph. Raritan, NJ, Ortho-McNeil Pharmaceutical.

References

1. Berek JS, Adashi EY, Hillard PA (eds): Novak's Gynecology, 12th ed. Baltimore, Williams & Wilkins, 1988.
2. Giuliano AE: Fibrocystic disease of the breast. In Cameron J (ed): Current Problems in Surgery. St. Louis, CV Mosby, 1986.
3. McDivitt RW, Stevens JA, Lee NC, et al: Histologic types of benign breast disease and the risk of breast cancer. The Cancer and Steroid Hormone study group. Cancer 1992;69:1408–1414.
4. Bland KI, Love N: Evaluation of common breast masses. Postgrad Med 1992;92:95–97.
5. Page DL, Dupont WD: Anatomic markers of human premalignancy and risk of breast cancer. Cancer 1990;66:1326–1335.
6. American College of Obstetricians and Gynecologists: Nonmalignant Conditions of the Breast. (ACOG Technical Bulletin No. 156). Washington, DC, ACOG, June 1991.
7. Boyle CA, Berkowitz GS, LiVolsi VA, et al: Caffeine consumption and fibrocystic breast disease: A case-control epidemiologic study. J Natl Cancer Inst 1984;72:1015–1019.
8. Maddox PR, Mansel RE: Management of breast pain and nodularity. World J Surg 1989;13:699–705.
9. Hart J, Layfield LJ, Trumbull WE, et al: Practical aspects in the diagnosis and management of cystosarcoma phyllodes. Arch Surg 1988;123:1079–1083.
10. Haagensen CD: Thrombophlebitis of the superficial veins of the breast (Mondor's disease). In Haagensen CD (ed): Diseases of the Breast. Philadelphia, WB Saunders, 1986, p. 379.
11. Kinlay JR, O'Connell DL, Kinlay S: Incidence of mastitis in breastfeeding women during the six months after delivery: A prospective cohort study. Med J Aust 1998;169:310–312.
12. Scott-Conner C, Schorr S: The diagnosis and management of breast problems during pregnancy and lactation. Am J Surg 1995;170:401–405.
13. Lawrence RA, Lawrence RM: Breastfeeding: A Guide for the Medical Profession, 5th ed. St. Louis, Mosby, 1999.
14. Livingstone V: The treatment of *Staphyloccocus aureus*–infected sore nipples: A randomized comparative study. J Hum Lactation 1999;15:241–246.
15. Huggins K: The Nursing Mother's Companion. Boston, Harvard Common Press, 1995.
16. Collins JC, Liao S, Wile AG: Surgical management of breast masses in pregnant women. J Reprod Med 1999;40:785–788.
17. King RM, Welch JS, Martin JK, Coulam CB: Carcinoma of the breast associated with pregnancy. Surg Gynecol Obstet 1985;160:228–232.
18. Neifert M: Breastfeeding after breast surgical procedure or breast cancer. NAACOGS Clin Issu Perinat Womens Health Nurs. 1992;3:673–682.
19. Nemecek JA, Young VL: How safe are silicone breast implants? South Med J 1993;86:932–944.

Urinary Tract Infections in Pregnancy

John W. Larsen and David M. Gorenberg

Urinary tract infections (UTIs) are relatively common in pregnancy, with a frequency of 2% to 10%.[1, 2] It has long been believed that an association exists between severe symptomatic infection and preterm labor.[3] As a derivative of this belief, protocols have been developed to prevent preterm labor by early diagnosis of both UTI and asymptomatic bacteriuria during pregnancy.

ASYMPTOMATIC BACTERIURIA

Asymptomatic bacteriuria traditionally has been defined as greater than or equal to 10^5 colony-forming units (CFUs) of bacteria per milliliter. This definition has been modified by various authors,[1-3] yet it is one original definition that is used over and over again. Some suggest that two clean-catch urine cultures should be taken on separate days in the absence of symptoms in order to improve the predictive value of the test. Alternatively, using a lower number of CFUs of bacteria as the threshold will increase the sensitivity of the measurement and thereby allow more women to be treated, implying greater benefit for the reduction of preterm labor. If the urine specimen has been obtained by an aseptic invasive method, such as a suprapubic aspiration or catheterization, then it is only necessary for more than 100 bacteria per milliliter to be present to have clinical significance. A single species of bacteria rather than several different species indicates significant colonization of the urine.

In both asymptomatic bacteriuria and symptomatic UTIs, the leading organism accounting for 80% to 90% of cases is *Escherichia coli*. The remaining cases of urinary tract colonization are due to *Klebsiella-Enterobacter, Proteus, Pseudomonas* species, and gram-positive organisms such as *Staphylococcus saprophyticus* and various streptococci (e.g., group B streptococcus and enterococcus).

Epidemiologic risk factors for an increased frequency of asymptomatic bacteriuria include age, parity, sickle cell trait, lower socioeconomic status, a history of prior UTIs, diabetes, and abnormal urinary tract anatomy.[2] It is thought that anatomic changes during pregnancy increase the likelihood of having asymptomatic bacteriuria progress to a UTI. However, the rate of changing from culture-negative to culture-positive during the course of pregnancy does not exceed 2%.[2]

Although all agree that it is proper to treat asymptomatic bacteriuria when diagnosed during pregnancy, uniform agreement regarding the method for making the diagnosis is lacking. A formal urine culture remains the traditional "gold standard" for establishing the presence of clinically significant bacteriuria.[1, 4, 5] Nonetheless, this culture is expensive and cumbersome. Many efforts have been made to devise a rapid testing system that will permit a decreased cost per patient screened. Rapid dip tests include measurements of protein, leukocyte esterase, nitrites, and blood. A dip test that contains culture medium can be used in some settings as a rapid culture screen test. Some advocate relying on a urinalysis plus dipstick test to be done at the time of the first prenatal visit. However, it should always be expected that rapid methods will be less sensitive and less expensive than a culture.[1, 2, 5] Dipstick sensitivity is reported to be approximately 50%. Clinicians who rely on a culture for screening can point to the need to do that test only once during pregnancy. The optimal time for a culture might be at 16 weeks' gestation.[2] Those who use rapid methods point to the ability to repeat the test at each office visit, thereby getting greater ascertainment through multiple testing.

In 1995, Rouse and associates[5] reported a cost-effectiveness and cost-benefit analyses of this issue. They concluded that at a 6% prevalence of asymptomatic bacteriuria, either method of screening is cost beneficial compared with no screening; however, when compared with the dipstick strategy, the culture method does not have enough incremental benefit to be cost beneficial. At a lower prevalence rate (2%), the dipstick strategy remains cost beneficial. Only if the bacteriuria rate is 9% or greater does the culture strategy become cost beneficial compared with the dipstick approach.

Antibiotic treatment of asymptomatic bacteriuria is universally advised, because if untreated, it will progress to pyelonephritis in approximately 30% of pregnant women who have it. Treatment of bacteriuria may also decrease the likelihood of preterm labor. The mechanism for effecting this treatment may not be solely through the impact on bacteria in the urine; the beneficial effect may be a result of reduction of pathogens in the cervix and vagina.

In recent years, it has become common to advise shorter courses of antibiotic treatment. Thus, the treatment for asymptomatic maternal bacteriuria typically has decreased from a 14-day course to a 7-day course to a 3-day course, and in some instances to a 1-day bolus treatment (Table 67–1). However, it is suggested that 1-day therapy may have an efficacy of only 50% to 60% compared with 70% to 80% for the 3-day or 7-day regimens.[2, 4-7]

The important issue is that the health care provider should follow the patient and determine whether the chosen

Table 67–1. Empirical Oral Antimicrobial Regimens for Asymptomatic Bacteriuria

Regimen Type	Antibiotic	Regimen
Single dose	Amoxicillin	3 g
	Ampicillin	2 g
	Cephalexin	2 g
	Nitrofurantoin	200 mg
	Sulfisoxazole	2 g
	Trimethoprim-sulfamethoxazole	320/1600 mg
3-day course	Amoxicillin	500 mg 3 × daily
	Ampicillin	250 mg 4 × daily
	Cephalexin	250–500 mg 4 × daily
	Nitrofurantoin	50–100 mg 4 × daily; 100 mg twice daily
	Sulfisoxazole	500 mg 4 × daily
7-day course	Amoxicillin	500 mg 3 × daily
	Cephalexin	250–500 mg 4 × daily
	Nitrofurantoin	50–100 mg 4 × daily; 100 mg twice daily
	Sulfisoxazole	500 mg 4 × daily
	Trimethoprim-sulfamethoxazole	160/800 mg twice daily
Treatment failures	Nitrofurantoin	100 mg 4 × daily for 21 days
Suppression	Nitrofurantoin	100 mg at bedtime
	Trimethoprim-sulfamethoxazole	160/800 mg at bedtime

therapy has been effective. This may be done with a follow-up culture performed about a week after conclusion of the attempted treatment regimen. Treatment failures should then be followed by adjustment of drug and dosing to agree with the results of culture and sensitivity testing. Individuals who have failed treatment on short-course therapy may then be candidates for a daily suppression regimen continued to the end of pregnancy. The typical continuous suppression regimen is 100 mg of nitrofurantoin daily.

Nitrofurantoin is favored for treatment of bacteriuria in pregnancy. Other effective oral regimens include ampicillin, cephalexin, sulfisoxazole, and trimethoprim-sulfamethoxazole. Although ampicillin has been used commonly over the years, the rate of resistant isolates to this drug makes it less desirable as empirical first-line treatment. The sulfa drugs probably should be avoided in the third trimester of pregnancy because of the possible risk of hyperbilirubinemia and subsequent kernicterus. Although both nitrofurantoin and sulfisoxazole possibly can cause hemolytic anemia in patients who have glucose-6-phosphate dehydrogenase deficiency, the actual occurrence of this type of hemolytic anemia is quite infrequent.

CYSTITIS

Symptoms of cystitis are dysuria, urgency, frequency, and suprapubic pain in the absence of fever. The presence of pregnancy may make the findings of urgency and frequency more difficult to interpret. Laboratory manifesta-

tions include bacteriuria, which may be identified by a microscopic examination of a fresh urine specimen. In addition to the laboratory identification of white cells and red cells, gross hematuria may be present. In a pregnant patient, the gross blood present may lead to some confusion at the time of history taking if it is not clear that the blood is restricted to the urinary tract rather than being uterine bleeding.

Cultured urine from cystitis patients generally contains 10^5 or more CFUs of a single uropathogen; however, the presence of more than 100 CFUs may be used as the threshold for treatment in order not to miss a true infection during pregnancy.[1] Treatment options for acute cystitis in pregnancy are the same as for asymptomatic bacteriuria; however, we recommend a 7-day course in order to maximize the cure rate (Table 67–2). It is important that beyond remission of symptoms, there is also remission of bacteriuria. The clinician should adjust the treatment regimen to respond to the results of culture and sensitivity testing and test the patient subsequently for continued resolution of the bacteriuric state.

PYELONEPHRITIS

Pyelonephritis is manifested by fever, chills, and costovertebral angle pain and tenderness. Pyelonephritis may coexist with and extend from clinical cystitis. In addition, patients with pyelonephritis may develop other manifestations of severe systemic illness, including abdominal pain, nausea, vomiting, and septic shock. Particularly in the last half of pregnancy, pyelonephritis may lead to an adult respiratory distress syndrome. In the preantibiotic era, pyelonephritis was a cause of maternal mortality as well as morbidity.

Laboratory findings are similar to those of patients with cystitis, with the additional finding of white blood cell casts on the microscopic examination. A urine culture and sensitivity study should be obtained and antibiotic therapy begun on an empirical basis, to be adjusted when the results are known. Some experts also recommend that a blood culture be performed, anticipating a 10% to 15% positive rate.[4, 6]

The treatment of pyelonephritis during pregnancy traditionally has been based on IV antibiotics and hydration in

Table 67–2. Empirical Oral Antimicrobial Regimens for Acute Cystitis During Pregnancy

Antibiotic	Regimen
Amoxicillin	500 mg 3 × daily for 7 days
Cephalexin	500 mg 4 × daily for 7 days
Nitrofurantoin	100 mg 4 × daily for 7 days
Sulfisoxazole	Initial 2 g dose, then 1 g 4 × daily for 7 days
Trimethoprim-sulfamethoxazole	160/800 mg twice daily for 7 days

Table 67–3. Empirical Treatment of Acute Pyelonephritis During Pregnancy

Antibiotic	Regimen
Ceftriaxone	1–2 g IV or IM q24h
Cefazolin	1 g IV q8h
If patient is clinically septic add: Gentamicin	3–5 mg/kg IV in three divided doses daily

When patient is afebrile, therapy may be switched to an oral antibiotic (selected based on culture results) to complete a 10- to 14-day course.

a hospital setting (Table 67–3).[4, 6, 7] Attempts have been made to minimize hospitalization and use oral rather than IV antibiotics when possible.[6, 7] We recommend a flexible regimen that begins with a conservative assessment for manifestations of possible septic shock. An IV cephalosporin is begun in a hospital setting. For those patients who appear septic, an aminoglycoside is added. While IV hydration is employed, the patient is monitored for respiratory insufficiency and fluid overload that could be manifested by dypsnea or hypoxemia. Because it may take 2 to 4 days for a patient with severe pyelonephritis to become afebrile, she is told to expect hospitalization initially. When pain is relieved and fever nearly resolved, it is then possible to be more flexible and continue treatment with IV antibiotic therapy at home: either daily IM therapy or an oral regimen to complete a 10- to 14-day course of antibiotics. Ceftriaxone is well suited for use on a once-a-day basis, either intravenously or as an IM injection. Any approach that involves outpatient management before the patient is completely well requires good communication and follow-up so that the patient can return promptly if complete clinical success is not being achieved in the expected manner.

Follow-up of the patient with pyelonephritis includes repeating urine cultures to allow the clinician to intervene with an additional course of antibiotic therapy to prevent relapse. An occurrence of acute pyelonephritis can be expected in 10% to 20% of cases. For that reason, it may be preferable to attempt daily suppression with a regimen such as 100 mg of nitrofurantoin rather than attempt management by intermittent cultures and courses of antibiotics.

PREVENTION

Symptomatic UTIs in pregnancy can be prevented largely by the detection and treatment of asymptomatic bacteriuria. Although the definitive method for detection of asymptomatic bacteriuria is a urine culture, indirect testing by rapid dipstick methods enjoys wide popularity in clinical practice. In addition to prevention of symptomatic disease by multiple courses of antibiotics based on some testing method, it is possible that bacteriuria can be decreased significantly by adjusting the urinary environment with a simple regimen of cranberry juice. It has been shown in elderly women that 300 mL of commercially available cranberry juice taken daily will reduce the odds of remaining bacteriuric-pyuric to 27% of the odds in a control group.[8] The mechanism of bacteriostatic action for cranberry juice is not clear, and this regimen is not intended to replace antibiotics in symptomatic patients.

Patients who have been controlling bacteriuria and UTIs by postcoital antimicrobial prophylaxis before pregnancy probably should continue the same regimen during pregnancy, provided the antibiotic used is safe for pregnancy. If the patient has been taking a sulfa drug for this purpose, then nitrofurantoin should be substituted in the third trimester. The quinolones (e.g., ciprofloxacin and norfloxacin) should not be used during pregnancy because of a possible teratogenic impact on fetal cartilage.

Because urinary tract catheterization has been shown to be associated with introducing bacteria into the bladder, unnecessary catheterization should be avoided during pregnancy. If catheterization is necessary, then prophylaxis with antibiotics should be considered to prevent significant bacteriuria and clinical illness.

References

1. MacLean AB: Urinary tract infection in pregnancy. Br J Urol 1997;80(Suppl 1):10–13.
2. Patterson TF, Andriole VT: Detection, significance and therapy of bacteriuria in pregnancy: Update in the managed health care era. Infect Dis Clin North Am 1997;11:593–608.
3. Romero R, Oyarzun E, Mazor M, et al: Meta-analysis of the relationship between asymptomatic bacteriuria and preterm delivery/low birth weight. Obstet Gynecol 1989;73:576–582.
4. Stamm WE, Hooton TM: Management of urinary tract infections in adults. N Engl J Med 1993;10:1328–1334.
5. Rouse DJ, Andrews WW, Goldenberg RL, Owen J: Screening and treatment of asymptomatic bacteriuria of pregnancy to prevent pyelonephritis: A cost-effectiveness and cost-benefit analysis. Obstet Gynecol 1995;86:119–123. Nunns D, Rouse DJ, Andrews WW: [Letter to the editor and reply.] Obstet Gynecol 1995;86:867–868.
6. Angel JL, O'Brien WF, Finan MA, et al: Acute pyelonephritis in pregnancy: A prospective study of oral versus intravenous antibiotic therapy. Obstet Gynecol 1990;76:28–32.
7. Millar LK, Wing DA, Paul RH, Grimes DA: Outpatient treatment of pyelonephritis in pregnancy: A randomized controlled trial. Obstet Gynecol 1995;86:560–564.
8. Avorn J, Monane M, Gurwitz JH, et al: Reduction of bacteriuria and pyuria after ingestion of cranberry juice. JAMA 1994;271:751–754.

SIXTY-EIGHT

The Contraceptive and Noncontraceptive Health Benefits of Oral Contraceptives: An Update

Kristin Dardano and Ronald T. Burkman

Although oral contraceptives have been shown to be extremely safe and effective for their primary use as a method of birth control, over the past several decades it has been recognized that they also have substantial numbers of noncontraceptive health benefits. It is important to recognize at the outset that much of the information indicating a protective role of oral contraceptives has been based on studies involving preparations that have higher steroid doses or different progestins than are contained in current preparations.

This chapter reviews the contraceptive effects as well as some of the major purported benefits, including reduced risk of ovarian and endometrial cancer, ectopic pregnancy, pelvic inflammatory disease, menstrual disorders, benign breast disease, ovarian cysts, and acne. In addition, their possible beneficial effects on bone mineral density, uterine myomas, colorectal cancer, and rheumatoid arthritis are reviewed. Comment is made as to whether the changes in oral contraceptive formulations are likely to influence these benefits.

CONTRACEPTIVE EFFECTS

During the development of the oral contraceptive pill in the 1950s, it was noted that a contaminant, mestranol, was present in contraceptive pills then containing progesterone only. Mestranol, a potent estrogen, added significant contraceptive effect to the developing "pill." Estrogen and progesterone act synergistically to inhibit the pituitary gland. Combined oral contraceptives suppress ovulation by diminishing the frequency of gonadotropin-releasing hormone pulses and halting the luteinizing hormone surge. They also alter the consistency of cervical mucus, affect the endometrial lining, and alter tubal transport. When taken correctly and consistently, they confer a greater than 99% effectiveness in preventing pregnancy.

Unfortunately, myths regarding increased cancer risks and problems with compliance have led to a significantly reduced use effectiveness. Incorrect pill-taking unfortunately leads to contraceptive failure, as well as to increased breakthrough bleeding and hence pill discontinuation.

Overall, the use effectiveness, because of these factors, ranges between 94% and 97%. Compliance is also one of the main factors limiting successful contraception. Compliance may be improved if patients are made aware of the noncontraceptive health benefits outlined in this review.

OVARIAN CANCER

In 1999, an estimated 22,500 women were diagnosed with ovarian cancer, and only about one half will survive for 5 years following treatment. Thus, although ovarian cancer is relatively uncommon, it has a high fatality rate. At least 22 case-control studies and 3 cohort studies[1-4] have examined the relationship between oral contraceptive use and ovarian cancer. All but two of these studies have shown a protective effect from oral contraceptives. Overall, there appears to be between a 40% and an 80% decrease in risk among users. The protection begins about 1 year after initiating use and conveys about a 10% to a 12% decrease in risk for each year of use. In addition, persistence of protection lasts between 15 and 20 years after a woman has discontinued use of oral contraceptives. It appears that this protective effect primarily involves epithelial tumors of the ovary.

Data also suggest that oral contraceptive use reduces the risk of ovarian cancer among women who are at high risk for the disease. For example, one group of investigators[5] concluded that use of oral contraceptives by nulliparous women for 5 years reduced their risk of ovarian cancer to that level experienced by parous women who had never used this form of contraception. Similarly, use for 10 years reduced the risk of ovarian cancer among women with a family history of the disorder below that experienced by never-users of oral contraception without such a family history. Preliminary data from one study[6] also suggest that oral contraceptive use may protect women carrying the BRCA1 or BRCA2 mutation. However, this study is limited by its small sample sizes.

The mechanisms by which oral contraceptives may produce their protective effects include suppression of ovulation, thus resulting in a reduced frequency of "injury" to the ovarian capsule, and suppression of gonadotropins. Although the "gonadotropin theory" is controversial, proponents cite data that high levels are associated with ovarian cancer in animals and that gonadotropins have been shown to stimulate some human ovarian cancer cell lines.[7] Finally, it is important to recognize that the majority of the data supporting this protective effect of oral contraceptives are derived substantially from studies involving oral contraceptive preparations containing 50 μg of estrogen or greater as well as higher doses of progestin than are contained in current formulations. However, if the aforementioned mechanisms are operant, the current low-dose preparations produce similar effects on ovulation and gonadotropins such that one might anticipate similar protection.

ENDOMETRIAL CANCER

In 1999, about 37,400 cases of endometrial cancer were diagnosed. However, unlike the case with ovarian cancer, the 5-year survival rates are much better. For example, among women with localized disease, survival exceeds 95%; even with distant metastasis, the 5-year survival rate is about 27%.[8] A significant risk factor is unopposed estrogen. At least 11 case-control studies and 1 cohort study[9-11] have demonstrated that use of oral contraceptives conveys protection against endometrial cancer. Overall, the studies suggest up to a 50% reduction in risk, which begins about 1 year after initiation of use. Protection appears to increase with duration of use, and there are data to indicate that the protection persists up to 20 years after oral contraceptive use is discontinued.[9] Protection has been demonstrated for adenocarcinoma, adenosquamous tumors, and adenoacanthomas. However, the strength of the protective effect varies, and appears to be different for women with potential risk factors such as obesity and nulliparity.

The purported protective mechanism is a reduction in the mitotic activity of endometrial cells by the action of the progestin component. Although most of the supporting data have been derived from data using higher-dose preparations than those used now, current low-dose preparations utilize highly potent progestins that have the same endometrial effects as older preparations.[12]

ECTOPIC PREGNANCY

Although, strictly speaking, protection against ectopic pregnancy is not a noncontraceptive health benefit, it still has important public health implications. The rate of ectopic pregnancy has shown a steady rise since 1970, so that between one and two ectopic gestations occur for every term delivery in this country. A number of epidemiologic studies show that oral contraceptives convey about a 90% reduction in risk of ectopic pregnancy.[13] The likely mechanism is through suppression of ovulation, an effect that obviously prevents all types of pregnancy. Because current low-dose oral contraceptives have this mechanism of action, it is likely that this protective effect has not been substantially altered by the changes in their dosage and formulation.

PELVIC INFLAMMATORY DISEASE

Pelvic inflammatory disease (PID), or salpingitis, continues to be a major cause of morbidity for women of reproductive age in this country. It has been reasonably well established in a number of epidemiologic studies that use of oral contraceptives will reduce the risk of upper genital tract infection (salpingitis) by 50% to 80% compared with women not using contraception or those who use a barrier method. It is interesting that there is no protective effect against the acquisition of lower genital tract sexually transmitted diseases, including *Chlamydia trachomatis* and *Neisseria gonorrhoeae* infections of the uterine cervix. The purported mechanisms by which oral contraceptives exert protection from PID include (1) progestin-induced changes to cervical mucus, making it thick and viscous so that ascent of bacteria is substantially inhibited; (2) hypomenorrhea, so that there is less retrograde menstrual flow to the fallopian tubes and less of an environment that would promote growth of bacterial organisms; and (3) possible changes in uterine contractility making ascent of organisms less probable. Because current oral contraceptives exert these effects, they likely offer a significant degree of protection against development of PID, as do the older high-dose preparations.

MENSTRUAL DISORDERS

Menorrhagia is a common complaint among women of reproductive age. Studies clearly documenting any beneficial effects of current low-dose oral contraceptives on menstrual flow and dysmenorrhea are few,[14-18] but considerable clinical experience suggests that most users of these preparations have reduced menstrual flow and reduced dysmenorrhea. Because the progestins are 19-nortestosterone derivatives, they are highly potent in respect to their endometrial activity. Thus, for most women, the hormone-free portion of the contraceptive cycle produces orderly withdrawal bleeding of reduced quantity compared with a normal menstrual cycle. The combination of estrogen and progestin in oral contraceptives essentially stabilizes the endometrium over time.

Oral contraceptives have also been recommended to treat pathologic conditions such as dysfunctional uterine bleeding and menorrhagia associated with uterine myomas. It is likely that the same mechanisms of action apply in these conditions as well. It has been estimated in some studies[19] that up to 75% of young women will experience some dysmenorrhea in spontaneous menstrual cycles, with 15% to 20% of women experiencing severe pain. Oral contraceptives reduce the pain associated with menstruation through two possible mechanisms. First, data suggest that the prostaglandin content of menstrual fluid is reduced, leading to less local endometrial vasoconstriction and ischemia. Second, it has also been shown in oral contraceptive users that there is less uterine contractile activity.[20, 21]

BENIGN BREAST DISEASE

Over 500,000 breast biopsies are performed in the United States each year. Among women younger than age 40 years, less than 10% of these biopsies reveal malignancy, whereas in women older than age 60 years, 33% of biopsies reveal malignancy. Since breast cancer is hormonally mediated, it is prudent to dispel the myths regarding oral contraceptive use in connection with breast cancer before reviewing the relationship of contraceptives to benign breast disease. The Collaborative Group on Hormonal Factors and Breast Cancer[22] has concluded that there is no evidence that oral contraceptives increase overall breast cancer risk, even with prolonged duration of use. However, there is a current user effect for approximately 10 years, similar to that associated with pregnancy. Also, since 1971, the trend in the medical literature suggests that oral contraceptives reduce the risk of benign breast disease. Benign breast conditions encompass fibrocystic change, fibroadenoma, galactorrhea, intraductal papilloma, fat necrosis, duct ectasia, lobular hyperplasia, and sclerosing/fibrosing adenosis. The results of several studies reveal a significant decrease in the incidence of benign fibrocystic conditions with oral contraceptive use, with a 30% to 50% decrease in incidence overall.[23, 24] The occurrence of fibroadenomas, specifically, is decreased among women younger than age 45 years. These effects are mainly seen in current and recent long-term users of oral contraceptives. The likely mechanism is through suppression of ovulation and, therefore, inhibition of the breast cell proliferation that normally occurs in the first half of an ovulatory menstrual cycle. This effect should continue to be seen with the estrogen doses of 30 to 35 μg, although the effect may not be as significant with the newer 20-μg pills that cause more frequent ovulatory periods. Higher doses or increased potency of progestins may improve the risk reduction. Oral contraceptive use also has been demonstrated to decrease the incidence of galactorrhea in select patients.

OVARIAN CYSTS

Ovarian cysts are a common problem among women of reproductive age. Ovarian cysts are the fourth leading cause for gynecologic admissions to hospital, with the incidence of surgery being about 40 cases per 100,000 woman-years.[25] The frequency of ovarian cysts among oral contraceptive users depends highly on the steroid dosages in oral contraceptive formulations.[25] Although the data are somewhat inconsistent, there is a suggestion that higher-dose contraceptives, for example, 50 μg or greater of ethinyl estradiol, protect against cyst formation. In contrast, current lower-dose formulations appear to have no protective effect on ovarian cyst formation.

However, it is important to recognize that many of the recent studies evaluating this issue utilize ultrasound definitions of cysts as opposed to clinical definitions in which some type of therapy might be indicated.[26] Thus, definitions of a cyst may include structures 3 or 4 cm in diameter seen by ultrasound that actually may represent partially recruited follicles rather than cysts. Furthermore, many of these "cysts" identified in such studies regress over time. Thus, it appears that current low-dose oral contraceptives reduce the frequency of ovulation but may still allow early recruitment of follicles that do not progress to the stage of ovulation. No data support the use of oral contraception in the treatment of existing cysts, although higher-dose formulations can be used as a means to prevent cyst formation for women who are plagued by recurrent symptoms owing to ovarian cyst formation.

ACNE

Over 25% of women of reproductive age are affected by acne. Furthermore, about 60% of the more than 5 million visits to health care providers for this condition are by women. It has been reasonably established that the condition is associated with excess androgen secretion, especially at the level of the pilosebaceous unit. A number of case series over the years suggest that women taking oral contraceptives show improvement in their skin. However, such studies have not controlled for placebo effects, the use of local agents in addition to oral contraceptives, nor the natural history of cyclic flare-up and remission of the disorder. Two randomized, placebo-controlled clinical trials[27, 28] conducted over a 6-month period demonstrated that about one half of women showed improvement of their acne while taking a tricyclic product containing the progestin norgestimate. (It is interesting that about 30% of women receiving a placebo preparation also showed improvement.) Overall, the response rate to the oral contraceptive in these two studies is similar to that achieved by women using topical agents, such as tretinoin or benzoyl peroxide, or systemic antibiotics.

There are several purported mechanisms of action by which oral contraceptives reduce acne. Oral contraceptives raise the levels of sex hormone–binding globulin, which in turn binds testosterone, thereby lowering the free concentration of androgen in the blood that is capable of binding to the pilosebaceous unit. They also suppress gonadotropins; both these effects lead to reduced levels of ovarian androgens. In addition, there is some evidence that adrenal output of androgens is also suppressed. Finally, some preliminary evidence suggests that various progestins may also exert effects at the level of the pilosebaceous unit to diminish the prevalence of acne.

Bone Mineral Density

An estimated 10 million Americans suffer from osteoporosis. One of every two women will experience an obvious or subclinical osteoporotic fracture during her lifetime, possibly leading to back pain, height loss, kyphosis, immobility, activity limitations, restrictive lung disease, thromboembolic complications, and even death. The lifetime risk of hip fracture in white women older than 65 years is 15%, which is approximately equal to the combined risk of breast, endometrial, and ovarian cancers. One quarter of women die within the first year after a fracture; another one fourth require long-term nursing home care, and only one third of women fully regain their prefracture level of independence.

Bone mineral density in women peaks between the ages of 20 and 25 years, stays constant for about 10 years, and then progressively declines in the later reproductive years. Accelerated bone loss then occurs in the perimenopausal/menopausal years and during all hypoestrogenic states, including natural menopause, premature ovarian failure, gonadal dysgenesis, hypothyroidism, hyperprolactinemia, anorexia nervosa, and exercise-induced amenorrhea. Other risk factors for decreased bone mineral density include smoking, family history, excessive alcohol or caffeine consumption, hyperthyroidism, white or Asian race, chronic steroid use, a thin body habitus, and a sedentary lifestyle.

Nineteen studies have revealed a positive effect on bone mineral density and 13 indicated no effect on bone mineral density among oral contraceptive users.[29] No studies have demonstrated a negative effect on bone mineral density. It appears that oral contraceptives are most effective at preventing bone loss during times of low estrogen and have a further protective effect with increased duration of use. Women who have used oral contraceptives for 5 to 10 years or longer are afforded the greatest protection. Most importantly, a population-based study revealed a 25% reduction in hip fracture risk. Oral contraceptives have a beneficial effect on bone metabolism, as demonstrated in nine studies.[30] Estrogens act on bone by increasing calcium absorption, decreasing calcium loss, and directly inhibiting bone reabsorption through inhibition of osteoclasts. These beneficial effects are not expected with the progesterone-only "minipill."

Uterine Fibroids

Leiomyomas are the most common pelvic neoplasm and are found in up to 40% of women. They may lead to pelvic pressure and pain or excessive uterine bleeding and are the major indication for women to undergo hysterectomy. One group of researchers[31] noted a reduced risk of uterine fibroids in oral contraceptive users, whereas a large case-control study from Italy found no effect.[32] Reduced estrogen states do appear to decrease the incidence of leiomyomas, although the beneficial effect may be noted only in select populations. Oral contraceptive use also has been shown to reduce menstrual blood loss in women with fibroid uteri.

Colorectal Cancer

There is growing epidemiologic evidence that oral contraceptives may protect women from developing colorectal cancer in later life. This tumor is the third most prevalent cancer in women. Colon cancer is actually more common in women than in men, although the reverse is true for rectal cancer. Several case-control studies and at least one cohort study have demonstrated a protective effect of ever-use of oral contraceptives, approaching a 40% to 50% reduction in incidence.[33] In some studies, this protective effect appears to be directly proportional to duration of use.[34] However, this relationship between duration of oral contraceptive use and protection against colorectal cancer has not been a consistent finding in all studies, and other studies have shown no effect from oral contraceptive use on the development of colon cancer.[35] The mechanism of action for this possible protective effect is essentially unknown. Furthermore, because most of these findings were related to use of higher-dose oral contraceptives, it is unclear whether users of today's preparations will experience any protective effect.

Rheumatoid Arthritis

Rheumatoid arthritis affects 2.5 million Americans and is three times more common in women than in men. Generally striking its victims between ages 20 and 50 years, this immune disorder causes joint swelling, stiffness, and pain, as well as fatigue, loss of appetite, fevers, and sweats. The joint destruction can lead to deformity and loss of function. Two studies published before 1982 suggested a 40% to 50% reduction in the risk of premenopausal rheumatoid arthritis in oral contraceptive users.[36, 37] A meta-analysis of 12 studies since that time has found no conclusive evidence of a protective effect of oral contraceptive use.[38] One study has purported to show potential prevention of polyarthritis with current oral contraceptive use.[39] The etiology of the disease is unclear, and because there are no known preventive measures the mechanism of a protective effect, if present, is unknown. Autoimmune disorders are found more commonly in women, although the exact association between sex hormones and autoimmunity has yet to be elucidated.

Summary

Since the 1960s, oral contraceptives have remained a safe and effective method of birth control. Reductions in the estrogen dose below 50 μg have significantly decreased the incidence of cardiovascular complications and deep venous thrombosis. Combined oral contraceptives inhibit ovulation; therefore, it would be expected that the majority of their noncontraceptive benefits will continue to be demonstrated with the newer formulations. A significant proportion of women believe that oral contraceptives are harmful and increase their risk for gynecologic cancers. Not only should these myths be dispelled, but also providers should outline the protective and preventive effects of oral contraceptives to their patients. Women suffering from acne, menstrual disorders, or benign breast disease who are not in need of contraception should be considered for oral contraceptive treatment. Improving patient understanding of these noncontraceptive benefits may help improve compliance.

Suggestions for Future Reading

DeCherney A: Bone-sparing properties of oral contraceptives. Am J Obstet Gynecol 1996;174:15–20.

Grimes DA, Wallach M: Modern Contraception: Updates from the Contraception Report. Totowa, NJ, Emron, 1997.

Kaunitz A: Oral contraceptive health benefits: Perception versus reality. Contraception 1999;59:29S–33S.

Mishell DR: Noncontraceptive benefits of oral contraceptives. J Reprod Med 1993;38:1021–1029.

References

1. Hankinson SE, Colditz GA, Hunter DJ, et al: A quantitative assessment of oral contraceptive use and risk of ovarian cancer. Obstet Gynecol 1992;80:708–714.
2. Piver MS, Baker TR, Jishi MF, et al: Familial ovarian cancer. A report of 658 families from the Gilda Radner Familial Ovarian Cancer Registry 1981–1991. Cancer 1993;71:582–588.
3. Risch HA, Marrett LD, Jain M, Howe GR: Differences in risk factors for epithelial ovarian cancer by histologic type. Results of a case-control study. Am J Epidemiol 1996;144:363–372.
4. Rosenberg L, Palmer JR, Zauber AG, et al: A case-control study of oral contraceptive use and invasive epithelial ovarian cancer. Am J Epidemiol 1994;139:654–661.
5. Gross TP, Schlesselman JJ: The estimated effect of oral contraceptive use on the cumulative risk of epithelial ovarian cancer. Obstet Gynecol 1994;83:419–424.
6. Narod SA, Risch H, Moslehi R, et al: Oral contraceptives and the risk of hereditary ovarian cancer. Hereditary Ovarian Cancer Clinical Study Group. N Engl J Med 1998;339:424–428.
7. Cramer EM, Breton-Gorius J, Beesley JE, Martin JF: Ultrastructural demonstration of tubular inclusions coinciding with von Willebrand factor in pig megakaryocytes. Blood 1988;71:1533–1538.
8. American Cancer Society: Cancer Facts and Figures—1999.
9. Schlesselman JJ: Risk of endometrial cancer in relation to use of combined oral contraceptives. A practitioner's guide to meta-analysis. Hum Reprod 1997;12:1851–1863.
10. Sherman ME, Sturgeon S, Brinton LA, et al: Risk factors and hormone levels in patients with serous and endometrioid uterine carcinomas. Mod Pathol 1997;10:963–968.
11. Vessey MP, Painter R: Endometrial and ovarian cancer and oral contraceptives—findings in a large cohort study. Br J Cancer 1995;71:1340–1342.
12. Key TJ, Pike MC: The dose-effect relationship between "unopposed" oestrogens and endometrial mitotic rate: Its central role in explaining and predicting endometrial cancer risk. Br J Cancer 1988;57:205–212.
13. Peterson HB, Lee NC: The health effects of oral contraceptives: Misperceptions, controversies, and continuing good news. Clin Obstet Gynecol 1989;32:339–355.
14. van Hooff MH, Hirasing RA, Kaptein MB, et al: The use of oral contraceptives by adolescents for contraception, menstrual cycle problems or acne. Acta Obstet Gynecol Scand 1998;77898–904.
15. Weng LJ, Xu D, Zheng HZ, et al: Clinical experience with triphasic oral contraceptive (Triquilar) in 527 women in China. Contraception 1991;43:263–271.
16. Milman N, Clausen J, Byg KE: Iron status in 268 Danish women agd 18–30 years: Influence of menstruation, contraceptive method, and iron supplementation. Ann Hematol 1998;77:13–19.
17. Klein JR, Litt IF: Epidemiology of adolescent dysmenorrhea. Pediatrics 1981;68:661–664.
18. Wilson CA, Keye WR Jr: A survey of adolescent dysmenorrhea and premenstrual symptom frequency. A model program for prevention, detection, and treatment. J Adolesc Health Care 1989;10:317–322.
19. Andersch B, Milsom I: An epidemiologic study of young women with dysmenorrhea. Am J Obstet Gynecol 1982;144:655–660.
20. Chan WY, Dawood MY, Fuchs F: Prostaglandins in primary dysmenorrhea. Comparison of prophylactic and nonprophylactic treatment with ibuprofen and use of oral contraceptives. Am J Med 1981;70:535–541.
21. Lalos O, Joelsson I: Effect of an oral contraceptive on uterine tonicity in women with primary dysmenorrhea. Acta Obstet Gynecol Scand 1981;60:229–232.
22. Collaborative Group on Hormonal Factors and Breast Cancer: Breast cancer and hormonal contraceptives: Collaborative reanalysis of individual data on 53,297 women with breast cancer from 54 epidemiologic studies. Lancet 1996;347:1713–1727.
23. Brinton LA, Vessey MP, Flavel R, Yeates D: Risk factors for benign breast disease. Am J Epidemiol 1981;113:203–214.
24. Charreau I, Plu-Bureau G, Bachelot A, et al: Oral contraceptive use and risk of benign breast disease in a French case-control study of young women. Eur J Cancer Prev 1993;2:147–154.
25. Westhoff C, Clark CJ: Benign ovarian cysts in England and Wales and in the United States. Br J Obstet Gynaecol 1992;99:329–332.
26. Chiaffarino F, Parazzini F, La Vecchia C, et al: Oral contraceptive use and benign gynecologic conditions. A review. Contraception 1998;57:11–18.
27. Redmond GP, Olson WH, Lippman JS, et al: Norgestimate and ethinyl estradiol in the treatment of acne vulgaris: A randomized, placebo-controlled trial. Obstet Gynecol 1997;89:615–622.
28. Lucky AW, Henderson TA, Olson WH, et al: Effectiveness of norgestimate and ethinyl estradiol in treating moderate acne vulgaris. J Am Acad Dermatol 1997;37:746–754.
29. DeCherney A: Bone-sparing properties of oral contraceptives. Am J Obstet Gynecol 1996;174:15–20.
30. Kuohung W, Borgatta L, Stubblefield P: Low-dose oral contraceptives and bone mineral density: An evidence-based analysis. Contraception 2000;61:77–82.
31. Ross RK, Pike MC, Vessey MP, et al: Risk factors for uterine fibroids: Reduced risk associated with oral contraceptives. BMJ 1986;293:359–362.
32. Parrazzini F, Negri E, La Vecchia C, et al: Oral contraceptive use and risk of uterine fibroids. Obstet Gynecol 1992;79:430–433.
33. Martinez ME, Grodstein F, Giovannucci E, et al: A prospective study of reproductive factors, oral contraceptive use, and risk of colorectal cancer. Cancer Epidemiol Biomarkers Prev 1997;6:1–5.
34. Potter JD, McMichael AJ: Large bowel cancer in women in relation to reproductive and hormonal factors: A case-control study. J Natl Cancer Inst 1983;71:703–709.
35. Fernandez E, La Vecchia C, Franceschi S, et al: Oral contraceptive use and risk of colorectal cancer. Epidemiology 1998;9:295–300.
36. Reduction in incidence of rheumatoid arthritis associated with oral contraceptives. Royal College of General Practitioners' Oral Contraception Study. Lancet 1978;1:569–571.
37. Vandenbroucke JP, Valkenburg HA, Boersma JW, et al: Oral contraceptives and rheumatoid arthritis: Further evidence for a preventive effect. Lancet 1982;2:839–842.
38. Spector TD, Hochberg MC: The protective effect of the oral contraceptive pill on rheumatoid arthritis: An overview of the analytic epidemiological studies using meta-analysis. J Clin Epidemiol 1990;43:1221–1230.
39. Jorgensen C, Picot MC, Bologna C, Sany J: Oral contraception, parity, breast feeding, and severity of rheumatoid arthritis. Ann Rheum Dis 1996;55:94–98.

SIXTY-NINE

Evaluation and Treatment of Anal Incontinence

Joseph P. Muldoon

Anal incontinence is a "silent" condition because the problem carries significant stigma. The embarrassment associated with this condition often leads to social isolation and depression. The incidence is estimated to be 0.5% to 2% of the general population and up to 36% of hospitalized elderly patients. The economic impact of fecal incontinence is not known, partly because it often goes undiagnosed.[1]

There are many reasons for fecal incontinence, and the underlying pathophysiology is often complex. General factors affecting continence include mental function, stool volume and consistency, colonic transit, rectal distensibility, anal sphincter function, anorectal sensation, and anorectal reflexes. Disturbances in a single factor, or in multiple factors, leads to fecal incontinence. Anal incontinence can result from the disruption of the sphincter muscles or neurologic dysfunction from trauma or degenerative processes. Obstetric injury may lead to both sphincter injury and pudendal nerve injury. Spinal cord injuries, multiple sclerosis, and diabetic neuropathy are examples of neurologic causes for anal incontinence. Rectal sensation is a vital component of anal continence and can be disrupted by conditions such as chronic fecal impaction or diabetes. Surgically correctable causes of fecal incontinence usually involve anal sphincter injury.

The anal sphincter complex is composed of the internal and external anal sphincter muscles. The internal sphincter represents the distal condensation of the circular muscles of the rectum. It is approximately 3 cm long and provides 80% to 85% of resting tone to the anal canal. This muscle is composed of smooth or involuntary muscle, with innervation coming from autonomic nerve branches of L5 and S2 to S4. The external sphincter muscle complex is composed mainly of striated muscle. It provides voluntary contraction in the control of defecation. The external sphincter muscle is innervated by the inferior rectal branch of the internal pudendal nerve and the perineal branch of the fourth sacral nerve.

INITIAL EVALUATION OF ANAL INCONTINENCE

Many patients with anal incontinence are undiagnosed. Patients are often embarrassed and do not offer this information, so it is up to physicians to ask the question. The incidence is higher in patients with urinary incontinence. When the condition is identified, a thorough history and physical examination often will identify the underlying cause. It is important to quantify and characterize the incontinence episodes. One must clarify whether the incontinence is due to gas, liquid stool, or solid stool. Incontinence should be differentiated from urgency secondary to diarrheal states. Patients with frequent loose stools and urgency may benefit from treatment with antidiarrheals alone or changes in the diet. Incontinence also must be distinguished from perianal leakage secondary to anal fistula, prolapsed hemorrhoids, or rectal prolapse. Patients should be asked about symptoms of concurrent urinary incontinence.

The number of incontinence episodes should be documented as well as the circumstances surrounding the events. Ask patients whether they use protective pads or need to make major adjustments in lifestyle because of the problem. These points give the examiner insight into the severity of the problem. Unfortunately, there is no standardized measuring scale for the evaluation of patients with fecal incontinence. Many scoring systems have been proposed to measure the severity of fecal incontinence, with at least 12 reported in the literature, but none have been widely accepted. This makes it difficult to measure the degree of impairment or compare the outcomes of the various treatment modalities. Generally, incontinence due to gas or liquid stool is considered partial incontinence, whereas complete incontinence is defined as the inability to control solid stool.

Past medical and surgical history may reveal the underlying cause. A history of anal surgery or obstetric trauma may point to a mechanical injury to the sphincters. Neurologic disease or diabetes may be identified as a major component. A history of inflammatory bowel disease or local radiation may contribute to decreased rectal compliance and sphincter dysfunction.

Physical examination first attempts to identify incontinence secondary to a generalized disease or neurologic disorder or whether it is a local phenomenon. Perineal examination begins with inspection for evidence of fecal soiling or pruritus. Separation of the gluteal muscles may reveal an anal gape showing lack of baseline anal sphincter tone. Evidence of hemorrhoidal or rectal prolapse can be seen either initially or after the patient is asked to strain. Scars from previous surgeries or episiotomies are noted. Simple neurologic testing includes sensation to pinprick and identifying the presence or absence of an anocutaneous reflex. The anocutaneous reflex can be elicited by gently stroking the perianal skin with a pin and observing the sphincter "wink." The loss of this reflex suggests pudendal neuropathy.

Digital examination helps assess baseline anal tone and squeeze augmentation. This is a subjective measurement, however. A crude measurement of sphincter length also can be gained. Obvious sphincter defects often can be palpated. Bidigital examination assesses the rectovaginal septum as well as the bulk of the perineal body. The examiner must also consider the possibility of rectovaginal fistula. Manual and speculum examination of the vaginal vault should be performed.

All patients with complaints of fecal incontinence should undergo anoscopic and proctosigmoidoscopic examination. These studies may reveal an inflammatory process or a neoplasm as a cause for the incontinence. The need for evaluation of the remainder of the colon should be determined on an individual basis.

After the initial office evaluation of patients presenting with complaints of fecal incontinence, many will be found to have only minimal symptoms or disease processes best treated medically. Others are evaluated further, with more specific testing to determine whether a surgically correctable problem is present.

PHYSIOLOGIC TESTING OF ANAL INCONTINENCE

Anorectal physiologic testing is often utilized in the workup of fecal incontinence. Because fecal incontinence is often multifactorial, these tests can help identify those patients who will likely benefit most from medical management versus surgical intervention. Parameters evaluated with the following tests include rectal compliance, rectal sensation, pudendal nerve latency, anal muscle morphology and defecation mechanics. In the setting of obvious traumatic injury to the anal sphincter and no suspicion of pudendal neuropathy, physiologic studies are probably unnecessary. When patients present with a more complex scenario or a subclinical injury, physiologic testing has a role in the evaluation. By collecting the information provided by these tests, the physician can offer surgery, in appropriate cases, to treat the condition.

Anorectal Manometry

Anorectal manometry measures anal canal pressures by means of a four- to eight-channel, water-perfused manometric catheter. By measuring circumferential pressures with the patient at rest and attempting to squeeze, one can evaluate anal sphincter function. Basal pressure represents mainly the internal sphincter muscle with normal resting pressures of approximately 40 mm Hg. Squeeze pressures are an estimation of external anal sphincter function. Normal squeeze pressures are generally demonstrated by doubling of a normal resting pressure. If both basal and squeeze pressures are low, patients are prone to be totally incontinent. Partial incontinence is more likely seen in patients when only the voluntary function is low.[2]

Unfortunately, manometric values do not always correlate with patient symptoms. An overlap of up to 10% is found between the manometric values obtained from incontinent and normal patients. There is no correlation between the manometric values and the severity of the incontinence.

Rectal compliance is determined during manometric studies that utilize a fluid-filled balloon. As the balloon is slowly filled with water, the catheter measures pressures and volumes at which the patient first notices sensation, the first urge to defecate, and the maximal tolerated volume. Compliance is determined by the relationship of pressure divided by the volume. Impaired rectal sensation can also be identified.

Pudendal Nerve Terminal Motor Latency

With use of a digital electrode to stimulate the pudendal nerve, the pudendal nerve terminal motor latency (PNTML) can be measured to assess function. The nerve is stimulated at the ischial spine, and the time to contraction of the external anal sphincter is recorded in milliseconds. A prolonged PNTML is consistent with pudendal neuropathy and a worse prognosis for patients undergoing an external sphincter repair procedure. This is a well-tolerated test that provides an accurate measure of pudendal nerve function.

Transanal Ultrasound

Transanal ultrasound is the most recent diagnostic test in the evaluation of anal incontinence. It provides an accurate anatomic assessment of the internal and external sphincter muscles. The internal and external sphincters can be visualized and the continuity and thickness determined by means of a 360-degree rotating ultrasound probe with a 7-MHz transducer. The internal sphincter appears as a hypoechoic band. The external sphincter is hyperechoic. This test is excellent for identifying the extent of specific sphincter defects caused by trauma. Because the test is accurate and well tolerated, it has essentially replaced electromyography in the evaluation of the anal sphincters when traumatic injury is suspected.[2]

Electromyography

Electromyography of the anal sphincter is performed by inserting concentric needles into the external anal sphincter or placing surface electrodes on the left and right of the skin overlying the external anal sphincter and measuring electrical potentials. The use of surface electrodes is better tolerated by the patient and supplies sufficient information. Electromyography can be used to map the sphincter and identify defects. It can also demonstrate re-innervation of the anal sphincter, which is indicative of pudendal neuropathy. Concentric needle or single-fiber electrodes can be used. This examination is uncomfortable for the patient and requires a high level of expertise on the part of the examiner, but it is accurate. Endoanal ultrasound has largely replaced this technology for identifying anatomic defects because of its accuracy and minimal patient discomfort.

Defecography

Defecography is a radiologic examination that demonstrates the mechanics of rectal evacuation. After the instillation of barium paste into the rectum, the patient sits on a radiolucent commode and lateral fluoroscopic images are obtained. This test quantifies puborectalis function and can identify rectocele, internal intussusception, and the length of the anal sphincter. The patient is studied while resting, straining, and evacuating. This test is most useful in the evaluation of constipation and symptoms of obstructed defecation.

TREATMENT OF ANAL INCONTINENCE

The treatment of anal incontinence commences after a complete workup to determine the etiology. The approach is influenced by the underlying cause, the severity of the symptoms, and the patient's general health.

Medical Management

In general, all patients with anal incontinence benefit from some simple dietary manipulations and the addition of fiber supplements. By avoiding foods that increase the rate of intestinal motility (i.e., caffeine, prunes, spicy foods, lactose in intolerant patients) and adding those that are constipating (i.e., cheese, yogurt, Ca^{2+}-containing antacids, bananas), the frequency of fecal incontinence usually can be decreased. Fiber supplements, such as pectins and gums, bulk the stools and have water-binding capacity. In patients with frequent loose stools or diarrhea, medications such as loperamide or diphenoxylate hydrochloride may be helpful.

For patients who do not have surgically correctable incontinence, bowel management programs can be instituted. By stimulating bowel evacuation to occur at a planned time, using enemas or suppositories, patients can improve their quality of life. Patients are encouraged to avoid fiber and to decrease stool volume. They often benefit from the use of antidiarrheals.[3]

Neuromuscular Re-education or Biofeedback Training

Biofeedback training is a method of learning through reinforcement. It is recommended for patients who have failed medical therapy, for patients who are not surgical candidates, or for those needing an adjunct to surgery. To be successful, patients must have a functional sphincter, must be able to sense rectal distention, and must be motivated.

The most commonly used method employs a three-balloon system, which provides a stimulus (rectal distention) and measures the patient's sphincter contraction in response to the stimulus. Training patients to sense impending defecation enables them to respond with sphincter contraction. The patient is shown pressure tracings to reinforce the behavior. This therapy appears to increase sphincter tone over time.

Initial studies showed promising results in patients with incontinence. Long-term results have been questioned, and studies are hard to compare. Most of the literature is composed of small, nonrandomized reports without standardized measures of incontinence or outcome. These patients may benefit from "refresher" sessions after 6 months to a year. The exact role of biofeedback training for patients with anal incontinence is unclear.

Anal Sphincter Repair and Pelvic Floor Reconstruction

Anal incontinence secondary to sphincter injury often can be corrected surgically. The most common procedures include sphincter apposition, reefing, overlapping repair of the sphincter, and pelvic floor reconstruction. The method chosen depends on the patient's anatomy and the timing of the injury.

Sphincter reefing is used for patients with sphincter thinning and incontinence. This technique involves approximation of the puborectalis muscle anteriorly and an S-shaped anterior plication of the external sphincter. The goal is to restore anterior bulk and increase sphincter tone. Initial improvement of incontinence is reported in up to 94% of patients, but long-term follow-up shows return of incontinence to gas and liquid stool in a significant number.

Postanal repair treats patients with an anatomically intact but poorly functioning anal sphincter and pelvic floor. The concept behind this repair is that it restores the anorectal angle and increases the resting tone of the anal canal. The technique involves dissection posteriorly in the intersphincteric plane, identification of the levators, then reapproximation of the levators and plication of the external sphincters. Results with this repair have not been consistent and it is rarely used in the United States, although it is used frequently in the United Kingdom.

Total pelvic floor repair is a method combining anterior levatorplasty, anterior external sphincter plication, and postanal repair. This procedure is indicated for complicated injuries to the external sphincter and puborectalis and pudendal neuropathy. The operation has been shown to improve incontinence in up to 42% of patients with neurogenic fecal incontinence. It can be performed as a single-stage or two-stage procedure.

Simple sphincter apposition is used when repair is performed at the time of injury, most commonly after birth trauma. This involves a simple re-approximation of the muscle with absorbable suture. This repair yields good results in this setting, but when delayed repair is performed, the results are inferior to overlapping sphincteroplasty.

Overlapping sphincteroplasty is the best operation for patients undergoing delayed repair of a traumatic sphincter injury. Identification and wide mobilization of the cut ends of the injured external sphincter are necessary. The ends are then overlapped and sutured with absorbable sutures. Continence to solid stool is restored in 80% of patients, with 93% reporting good or excellent results. When patients have a concurrent pudendal neuropathy, postoperative results are worse.[4]

NEW TREATMENTS FOR ANAL INCONTINENCE

Patients with anal incontinence that is not treatable by the preceding methods may be candidates for new anal encirclement procedures. These procedures are on study protocols at this time but may soon be available for use off protocol.

Gracilis muscle transposition has been used since the 1950s in the treatment of incontinence, with marginal benefit. *Dynamic graciloplasty* uses this technique, combined with placement of an electrical stimulator.[5] By chronic stimulation of the gracilis muscle over time, the characteristics of the muscle fibers change from a fast-twitch, easily fatigable type to a slow-twitch type that is slow to fatigue. The stimulator is turned off and on with a magnet to allow for defecation. The gracilis muscle is mobilized distally with preservation of the proximal neurovascular bundle. The muscle is passed around the anus and sutured to the ischial tuberosity. The electronic stimulator is then placed, through a separate abdominal incision, into the rectus sheath, and the electrodes are passed subcutaneously to the proximal muscle. The stimulator is activated after 6 weeks, and muscle training starts. The results of a dynamic graciloplasty are encouraging with a reported success rate of 73%, with a median follow-up of 2.1 years.[6] A trial has been completed recently in the United States, and the results are pending. Complications include infection, ero-

sion of the graft into the anal canal, and slippage of the wrap.

The *artificial anal sphincter* is an idea derived from the success of the artificial sphincter used in the treatment of urinary incontinence.[7] It is a three-piece silicone rubber device with an inflatable cuff that is placed around the upper anal canal. A manual pump is placed in the scrotum or labia, and the reservoir is placed in the laterovesical subperitoneal space. The system is set to produce an anal canal pressure of about 80 to 90 mm Hg when activated. Complete fecal continence can be achieved with this device. Complications include infection, erosion, and mechanical malfunction. This is not in widespread use and is used in the United States only on protocol at this time.

SUMMARY

The etiology of fecal incontinence is often complex and the clinical spectrum broad. The workup and treatment must be tailored to each patient. Thorough history and physical examination will identify patients who need further physiologic testing. Most patients benefit from medical management to some degree, but the patients with surgically correctable sphincter defects should consider operation. The role of biofeedback in the treatment of anal incontinence remains somewhat unclear. New treatments, including dynamic graciloplasty and the artificial anal sphincter, give hope to those patients whose only surgical option at present is a colostomy.

References

1. Leigh RJ, Turnberg LA: Faecal incontinence: The unvoiced symptom. Lancet 1982;1:134–151.
2. Falk PM, Blatchford GJ, Cali RL, et al: Transanal ultrasound and manometry in the evaluation of fecal incontinence. Dis Colon Rectum 1994;37:468–472.
3. Jorge JMN, Wexner SD: Etiology and management of fecal incontinence. Dis Colon Rectum 1993;36:77–97.
4. Sitzler PJ, Thompson JPS: Overlap repair of damaged anal sphincter. Dis Colon Rectum 1996;39:1356–1360.
5. Mander BJ, Wexner SD, Williams NS, et al: Preliminary results of a multicentre trial of the electrically stimulated gracilis neoanal sphincter. Br J Surg 1999;86:1543–1548.
6. Sangwan YP, Coller JA: Fecal incontinence. Surg Clin North Am 1994;74:1377–1398.
7. Lehur PA, Michot F, Denis P, et al: Results of artificial sphincter in severe anal incontinence: Report of 14 consecutive implantations. Dis Colon Rectum 1996;39:1352–1355.

Emergent Postcoital Contraception

Francisco A. R. Garcia and George R. Huggins

There are 3.6 million unplanned pregnancies in the United States each year. Fifty-three percent of these occur to fertile women not using contraception, and 47% occur as a result of contraceptive failure. It is not surprising, therefore, that women and their partners require contraceptive modalities that can be used after unplanned or unprotected exposure to pregnancy.

Postcoital or *emergent contraception* refers to therapeutic interventions designed to prevent pregnancy after unprotected intercourse. This contraceptive modality has been most commonly used after instances of rape and barrier contraceptive failure and is also made available on demand for other situations in which pregnancy is not desired after unprotected intercourse.

Postcoital contraceptive techniques can be divided into two major categories. The first category includes the most commonly used and best-studied techniques. These consist of regimens that rely on the action of combination oral contraceptive pills (COCPs), progestin-only pills (POPs), and the intrauterine device (IUD). The second category includes less frequently used and investigational methods including the use of high-dose estrogens, androgens, and progesterone inhibitors.

CATEGORY I EMERGENCY CONTRACEPTIVES

The Yuzpe Method

The method originally described by Yuzpe and Lancee[1] more than 20 years ago consists of 200 μg of ethinyl estradiol and 1.0 mg of levonorgestrel, taken in two divided doses 12 hours apart, and initiated within 72 hours of unprotected intercourse. Commonly available oral contraceptive pills containing norgestrel and levonorgestrel have been used for the same purpose.[2, 3] The American College of Obstetricians and Gynecologists[2] has published a comprehensive review and analysis of published studies in this area and has issued evidence-based practice guidelines for use of COCPs as emergency contraceptives.

The mechanism of action for postcoital contraception is incompletely understood, but it most likely involves a delay or inhibition of ovulation. Additionally, progestational atrophic histologic changes in the lining of the endometrium have been observed, and this may be sufficient in

some cases to preclude implantation. Properly timed, the Yuzpe method has been estimated to be 75% effective, but efficacy can range from 55% to 94%.

The issue of first-dose timing has been studied by various investigators. It is now clear that contraceptive efficacy does vary with timing of the first dose within the 72-hour treatment window. Pregnancy rates are lower the sooner the medication is started. Similarly, there is markedly diminished efficacy with timing of the first dose beyond the first 72 hours after exposure. It is important; however, to remember that no currently available hormonal postcoital contraceptive technique is effective once implantation has occurred.

Nausea and emesis are the most common side effects among women who take COCPs for emergency contraception (30% to 66% and 12% to 22%, respectively), and may last for up to 2 days. Nausea prophylaxis with either over-the-counter or prescription antiemetics is likely to increase both compliance with and effectiveness of the regimen. Initiation of antiemetics at least 1 hour before taking COCPs will significantly decrease the incidence of both nausea and vomiting. Mild breast tenderness has also been reported by some patients. Most women (98%) will resume menses within 21 days from the first dose, usually within 7 to 9 days.

Progestins

There is a progestin-only postcoital regimen consisting of two 0.75 mg norgestrel tablets taken in two doses 12 hours apart and initiated within 72 hours after unprotected intercourse. A randomized trial[2] comparing the levonorgestrel regimen with the Yuzpe method revealed no significant difference in failure rate between the two techniques (2.6% and 2.4%, respectively). A lower incidence of nausea and emesis was noted with levonorgestrel.

The mechanism of action of the POPs may be to inhibit ovulation by suppressing the luteinizing hormone surge in those instances when it has not yet occurred. Postovulation, levonorgestrel may impair corpus luteum function and in this way prevent pregnancy. There may also be some effect to impair implantation. POPs may be particularly useful in lactating women, women with thromboembolic disease, and others unwilling or unable to take estrogens.

Intrauterine Devices

The copper IUD, inserted within 5 days of unprotected intercourse, is an important nonhormonal postcoital contraceptive option. The failure rate of this technique is less than 1%. This user-independent method makes this an attractive choice for women desiring long-term contraception. Women who have multiple partners, active pelvic infection, increased risk for sexually transmitted disease, and nulliparas are not optimal candidates for this method. It is, however, an alternative for women in monogamous relationships that experience contraceptive failure and those with contraindications to hormonal intervention.

The mechanism of action of this method relies on two components. The primary mode of action is thought to be the sperm-toxic effect of the copper device. Additionally, the IUD stimulates an inflammatory foreign body reaction, which also decreases the likelihood of implantation. In the event of an early implantation or incorrect timing of insertion, any IUD placement has the theoretical potential to disrupt an already established pregnancy. Such considerations may make this method unacceptable to some patients.

CATEGORY II EMERGENCY CONTRACEPTIVES

Androgens

Danazol, a potent synthetic androgen used for a variety of gynecologic conditions, has also been evaluated for postcoital contraception. A regimen between 800 and 1200 mg taken in divided doses 12 hours apart has been studied. The absence of estrogen is associated with fewer gastrointestinal side effects than other hormonal methods. However, the efficacy of this technique is not well established. Although it has been reported[3] to have an efficacy similar to that of combined oral emergency contraception, other investigators have found the failure rate to be twice that of the Yuzpe method.

Progesterone Inhibitors

Mifepristone (RU-486) is a potent antiprogesterone with many potential applications in obstetrics and gynecology. It has recently been demonstrated to be useful for postcoital contraceptive use in two separate randomized control trials. No pregnancies were observed among two groups totaling 795 subjects when a single-dose treatment (600 mg) was used within 72 hours of unprotected intercourse. Significantly lower rates of nausea and vomiting were observed among mifepristone users compared with those subjects using the Yuzpe method. International multicenter studies are currently investigating the efficacy of lower dose and longer intervals after unprotected coitus. Menses have been noted to be delayed for more than 3 days; this may cause concern to both patient and practitioner.

Ironically, mifepristone is the postcoital technique that is probably best understood. Mifepristone can inhibit ovulation, as well as prevent normal endometrial maturation, and in this way render the endometrium inhospitable to implantation. After implantation, mifepristone will disrupt an existing pregnancy, hence its use as a medical abortifacient. The role of this new modality has yet to be defined.

DISCUSSION: PRESCRIBING EMERGENCY CONTRACEPTION

Traditionally, women have been required to see their practitioner in order to obtain high-dose COCP postcoital contraception. However, we believe that women receiving oral contraception should routinely be instructed on emergent contraception using their current contraceptive pill. Likewise, the anticipatory prescription and provision of COCPs for the purpose of emergency contraception should be considered for all women of reproductive age, with counseling regarding medical follow-up after its use.

Most practitioners have used the same oral contraceptive pill contraindications for this short-term therapy. This has had the effect of excluding women with a past or present history of thromboembolism, cerebrovascular disorders, coronary artery disease, breast or endometrial neoplasia, and hepatic tumors. Migraine, immobility, the puerperium, and lactation have also been suggested as physiologic states not amenable to emergency contraception. These considerations are important, but must be weighed against the risks posed by pregnancy for women with these diagnoses. The medical advisory panel of the International Planned Parenthood Federation[4] has stated that there are effectively no contraindications for the short-term use of these medications in the setting of postcoital contraception. Clearly, the only absolute contraindications for emergent contraception are pregnancy and the inability to provide informed consent.

It is vital that patients be well educated about relative efficacy, benefits, and risks of emergency contraception (Table 70–1). The emergent contraception visit is an ideal time to emphasize the need for regular, more reliable contraception. A sensitive urine pregnancy test should be used to rule out pregnancy. Women desiring a medical abortion must also be reminded that emergent contraception will most likely fail if implantation has already occurred. Method-specific side effects should be reviewed in detail with the patient, and she should be instructed to return for pelvic pain, bleeding, or nonreturn of menses within 21 days. Written material is particularly useful to reinforce these points. Thorough informed consent is the cornerstone of contraceptive practice, and the postcoital emergency is no exception.

AWARENESS

Despite the tremendous potential of this contraceptive modality, awareness and usage are generally low. A na-

Table 70–1. Comparative Efficacy of Emergency Contraceptive Modalities

Method	Estimated Efficacy (%)	Advantages and Disadvantages
COCPs (Yuzpe method)	75	Easy to obtain Nausea/emesis
POPs regimen	75	Easy to obtain Non–estrogen-containing Fewer GI side effects
IUD	~99	Long-term contraception 5-Day window of time for intervention No GI side effects
Mifepristone	~99	Fewer GI side effects Unavailable in the United States

*COCPs, combination oral contraceptive pills; GI, gastrointestinal; IUD, intrauterine device; POPs, progestin-only pills.

From Harrison PF, Rosenfeld A: Contraceptive Research and Development: Looking to the Future. Washington, DC, National Academy Press, 1996.

tional cross-sectional survey[2] of 2000 adults found that 64% of respondents were unaware of the possibility of postcoital medical intervention to prevent pregnancy. Additionally, only 25% had a substantial knowledge of emergent contraception. The level of awareness was lowest among women at greatest risk for pregnancy, including those reporting intercourse in the previous year, nonsterile women, and those younger than 45 years of age. In contrast, countries in which emergency contraception is well established report higher levels of consumer awareness, ranging from 33% to 94%. A high level of knowledge and usage is documented even among high-risk women, including adolescents and women seeking abortions. In these international settings, postcoital contraceptive practice is most effective when integrated into national family planning programs and strategies. In the United States, as in many developing countries, postcoital contraceptive interventions are not well known and are underutilized.

Provider awareness regarding emergency contraception is substantial, but prescriptive practices tend to vary by specialty. In one study,[2] 76% of gynecologists and 39% of family physicians reported prescribing emergent contraception. Among emergency room doctors, 66% reported prescribing this method, but generally restricted this practice to women who had been sexually assaulted. Among adolescent health care providers, mostly gynecologists and pedia-

tricians, 84% prescribed emergent contraception, although 80% did so infrequently.

FUTURE DIRECTIONS

New and exciting opportunities are emerging in the development of postcoital contraception. Other mifepristone-like antiprogestins have been developed. These promise to be even more effective at delaying ovulation and inducing a hostile endometrial environment. Epostane and azastene are new agents with contraceptive effects. These enzyme inhibitors prevent progesterone synthesis and have been demonstrated to be effective medical abortifacients, but they may also be useful in the immediate postcoital period. Additionally, a new class of oxytocic agents, which accelerate uterine contractility, are also being studied for this indication. Such preparations when used in combination with estrogens or with each other may make emergency contraception nearly fail safe.

SUMMARY

Nearly half of all unintended pregnancies occur among contraceptive users. Given this high rate of user failure, postcoital contraception is an appropriate adjunct to more traditional contraceptive practices. Emergent postcoital contraception is a well-established contraceptive practice that has the potential for improving the lives of many women. These interventions are safe, cost effective, and useful in decreasing the number of unwanted pregnancies and abortions currently performed. Such a goal requires a multiplicity of strategies, and postcoital interventions represent important tools to achieve that goal.

References

1. Yuzpe AA, Lancee WJ: Ethinylestradiol and dl-norgestrel as a postcoital contraceptive. Fertil Steril 1977;28:932–936.
2. American College of Obstetricians and Gynecologists: Emergency oral contraception. Washington, D.C., ACOG Practice Patterns 1996; 31:1–8.
3. Blumenthal P, McIntosh N: Emergency contraception. In Oliveras E (ed): Pocket Guide for Family Planning Service Providers, 3rd ed. Baltimore, JHPIEGO Corporation; 1996, pp. 65–72.
4. International Medical Advisory Panel of the International Planned Parenthood Federation: Statement on emergency contraception. New York, Int Planned Parenthood Med Bull 1994;26:1–2.

SEVENTY-ONE

New Advances in the Management of Endometriosis

Kamran S. Moghissi

Endometriosis is a common and frequently disabling disease that affects approximately 10% of premenopausal women. Among infertile women, the incidence may be as high as 30% to 60%. Clinical manifestations of endometriosis include pelvic pain associated with menses, dyspareunia, dysmenorrhea, and abnormal uterine bleeding. The condition commonly is associated with infertility. No satisfactory hypothesis has been advanced to explain the association of mild endometriosis with infertility when anatomic distortion of the pelvic structure is absent.

The clinical presentation and severity of symptoms of endometriosis to some degree are related to anatomic location and the extent of the disease; however, on occasion, advanced-stage endometriosis may be asymptomatic, and minimal disease may be associated with severe and disabling symptoms. Deep implants surrounded by inflammatory tissues and fibrosis usually are found in patients with pain, whereas superficial implants are most frequently associated with infertility. Endometriotic lesions usually are confined to the pelvis, but they can occur at distant sites and even outside of the abdomen. The most common sites of involvement are the ovaries, pelvic peritoneum, cul de sac, and uterosacral ligaments. Adjacent structures, such as bowel, bladder, and ureter, also may be affected. Pelvic endometriosis is suspected when pain or the characteristic symptoms and signs of the disease are present and confirmed by laparoscopy.

Major indications for the treatment of endometriosis consist of the presence of pelvic pain, pelvic pathology, and infertility. In younger women, prophylactic treatment of endometriosis should be considered to prevent future pelvic disorders associated with advanced stages of the disease (stages III and IV, American Society for Reproductive Medicine [ASRM] Revised Criteria) or to preserve reproductive function. More controversial is the need for therapy in cases of mild (stages I and II ASRM) endometriosis that are associated merely with infertility or of asymptomatic disease that is detected in the course of unrelated laparoscopy (e.g., tubal ligation).

MEDICAL MANAGEMENT OF ENDOMETRIOSIS

Several treatment modalities of endometriosis have evolved within the past few decades. The presence of advanced lesions, endometriomas larger than 2 to 3 cm, or adhesive disease requires surgical therapy. The advantage of a surgical approach is that it can be performed at the time of diagnostic laparoscopy with immediate benefit, particularly when infertility is the major symptom. There is, however, considerable evidence suggesting that all endometrial implants are not readily visible or recognized during endoscopic procedures. Thus, medical treatment, because of its generalized suppressive or pharmacologic effect, may be necessary.

Occasionally, combined medical and surgical therapy may be preferred. A short course of medical treatment may be attempted before surgical management of advanced disease to facilitate surgical excision of large endometriomas associated with severe adhesive disease. Similarly, postoperative medical therapy may be necessary after surgical management of advanced endometriosis associated with severe symptomatology to eradicate potential residual lesions.

Endometriosis may persist during the entire reproductive life of a woman for as long as functioning ovarian tissues are present. It is essential, therefore, that a concerned physician and informed patient develop a long-term management plan combining or alternating various surgical and medical treatment modalities, taking into consideration the patient's desire for fertility, family size, quality of life, and marital and professional obligations.

Analgesics

Prostaglandin synthesis by ectopic endometrium may be responsible for characteristic symptoms of endometriosis, such as pelvic pain and dysmenorrhea. Nonsteroidal anti-inflammatory drugs inhibit biosynthesis of prostaglandins and alleviate these symptoms. These drugs are well tolerated, safe, and inexpensive and are recommended as a first-line of treatment in women with mild symptoms.

Pseudopregnancy

Endometriotic lesions contain specific binding sites for estrogen, progesterone, and androgens, and their distribution is similar to that found in the endometrium from the same subject. These findings suggest that endometriotic implants respond to all three classes of steroid hormones.

Current technique involves the use of low-dose (20 to 35 µg ethinyl estradiol) oral contraceptives continuously for 6 to 9 months (that is, without scheduled withdrawal bleeding). The treatment usually is begun with 1 tablet daily and increased to 2 tablets per day only if breakthrough bleeding occurs. The administration of doses higher than 2 pills is not recommended, however, because of increasing undesirable side effects. During the initial 2 to 3 months of treatment, most patients are beset with worsening symptoms referable to the endometriosis in addition to those specifically related to the estrogen-progesterone combination. The latter side effects include abdominal swelling, depression, breast pain and tenderness, increased appetite, weight gain and edema (seen in almost all patients), breakthrough bleeding, nausea, and breast secretion. Superficial vein varicosities occasionally appear, and there is an increased risk of deep vein thrombosis. Ovulation and menstruation usually resume within 4 to 6 weeks after therapy has been discontinued.

Symptomatic relief of the disease has been reported in 75% to 100% of cases. Pregnancy rates in women who had infertility in addition to endometriosis have ranged from 10% to 58%. Several studies have shown that both danazol and surgical therapies result in greater symptomatic improvement and pregnancy rates as compared with pseudopregnancy regimens alone or in combination with surgery.

There is evidence that women who have used oral contraceptives are less likely to develop endometriosis. Also, the use of oral contraceptives in the usual cyclic fashion may delay the recurrence of the disease.

Progestins

Progestins alone have been used for the medical management of endometriosis for many years. The rationale for the use of these agents is based on the premise that sufficient endogenous circulating estrogen exists to induce progesterone receptors in both eutopic and ectopic endometrium. Progestins produce a hypoestrogenic acyclic hormonal environment by suppressing gonadotropin, inhibiting ovulation, and producing amenorrhea. In addition, progestins have a variety of effects on endometriotic tissue, characterized by acyclicity and decidualization. Progestational agents have the theoretical advantage of being better tolerated and of avoiding the complications of estrogen therapy. However, because of the increased rate of breakthrough bleeding, these agents have not been as enthusiastically received or as adequately evaluated as danazol or gonadotropin-releasing hormone (GnRH) agonists for suppression of endometrial implants.

Medroxyprogesterone acetate (MPA) is the most commonly used progestin in the United States. It may be given parenterally at a dose of 150 mg every 3 months for up to a year. A drawback to the use of depot MPA is the prolonged interval to resumption of ovulation after cessation of therapy. A better alternative to parenteral MPA is the oral route. Administration of oral MPA in doses of 30 mg/day continuously for a period of 90 days or longer has been shown to bring about amenorrhea and to suppress endometrial implants. Symptom relief occurs in almost all patients. The most prominent side effects consist of spotting, breakthrough bleeding, depression, weight gain, and bloating. Larger doses of oral MPA (50 to 100 mg/day) also have been used, but these do not seem to be more effective and are associated with a higher rate of breakthrough bleeding and other side effects. Pregnancy rates among infertility patients are similar to that of danazol or GnRH agonist therapy. Several other progestins have been used to treat endometriosis. They include megestrol acetate (40 mg/day), lynestrenol, dydrogesterone, cyproterone acetate, and gestrinone with results similar to those of MPA. Some preliminary studies indicate that antiprogestins such as RU-486 (mifepristone) may also be effective for the medical treatment of endometriosis.

Danazol

Danazol is an isoxazole derivative of the steroid 17α-ethinyl testosterone. It is well absorbed by the gastrointestinal tract and rapidly metabolized by the liver. Danazol is considered biologically to be an androgen and a glucocorticoid agonist. Danazol also binds to intranuclear progesterone receptors and appears to have a mixed agonist-antagonist activity with respect to the progesterone and estrogen receptors, but it has no estrogenic activity. In women, danazol (1) has a mild suppressive effect on basal gonadotropin secretion, (2) abolishes the luteinizing hormone surge, and (3) has an inhibitory effect on ovarian steroidogenic enzymes and the growth of normal and ectopic endometrium. Thus, the drug creates an anovulatory amenorrheic, high-androgen, low-estrogen milieu that is extremely hostile to the growth of endometriotic implants. It is known that an altered immune response may be a pathophysiologic factor in endometriosis. Therefore, danazol's immunoregulatory effect may be of an additional clinical benefit in the management of endometriosis.

When initially introduced, the standard regimen of danazol consisted of a dosage of 800 mg daily in divided doses for a period of 6 months or longer. Subsequently, it was shown that lower dosages of 400 to 600 mg/day were equally effective. At lower doses, however, the rate of breakthrough bleeding increases. For this reason, a dosage of 600 mg/day for 6 months is recommended and appears to be effective in relieving symptoms and in suppressing the endometriotic lesions. Danazol should not be administered to pregnant women because it may cause virilization of the external genitalia of the female fetus.

Danazol is highly effective in the treatment of dysmenorrhea but less effective in the management of chronic pelvic pain. Various studies have indicated symptomatic relief in 60% to 100% of cases. More than 90% of patients experience improvement or resolution of dysmenorrhea and more than 80% note relief when dyspareunia or chronic pelvic pain is the predominant symptom. Resolution of endometriotic implants occurs in almost 100% of minimal to mild cases (ASRM stages I and II) and in 50% to 70% of more advanced cases. Endometriomas greater than 1 cm in diameter, particularly those located in the ovary, respond poorly to danazol.

Side effects of danazol therapy include weight gain, acne, hirsutism, oily skin, and a decrease in breast size. Other troubling side effects include muscle cramps, flushing, mood changes, depression, and edema. Danazol has some adverse effect on lipid metabolism. It decreases high-density lipoprotein cholesterol levels and increases low-density lipoprotein cholesterol levels, but very-low-density lipoprotein levels are unchanged. Fortunately, these changes are reversible within 3 to 5 months after cessation of therapy. Hepatic dysfunction, as evidenced by reversible elevated serum enzymes or jaundice, also has been reported in patients receiving a daily dosage of danazol 400 mg or more. Thus, the drug should be used cautiously in patients with hyperlipidemia or impaired liver function, and prolonged and repeated courses of the drug should be avoided.

Gonadotropin-Releasing Hormone Agonists

GnRH is produced and released in pulsatile fashion from the arcuate nucleus and preoptic anterior hypothalamic area. It reaches the anterior pituitary through the portal system and is believed to bind to specific receptors in the anterior pituitary where it stimulates the synthesis and secretion of luteinizing hormone and follicle-stimulating hormone in both males and females. Follicle-stimulating hormone and luteinizing hormone, in turn, are essential for gonadal function. The gonadal steroids estradiol and progesterone exert modulatory effects on GnRH receptor signaling.

GnRH is rapidly degraded by peptidase and cleared by glomerular filtration. Its half-life in peripheral circulation is only 2 to 4 minutes. To increase the potency and duration of action of GnRH, analogues with agonistic or antagonistic properties have been synthesized. Substitution of an amino acid at the 6 or 10 position results in analogues with agonistic activity. Administration of GnRH agonists produces an initial stimulation of pituitary gonadotropes that results in secretion of follicle-stimulating hormone and luteinizing hormone and the expected gonadal response. Continuous or repeated administration of an agonist at nonphysiologic doses, however, produces an inhibition of the pituitary-gonadal axis. Functional changes resulting from this inhibition include pituitary GnRH receptor downregulation, gonadal gonadotropin receptor downregulation, attenuated gonadotropin secretion, and decreased steroidogenesis. The inhibitory effects of analogues are fully reversible. GnRH receptor messenger RNA also is expressed in granulosa-lutein cells of human ovary across different

Table 71–1. Gonadotropin-Releasing Hormone Agonists Studied for Gynecologic Conditions

Generic Name	Route of Administration	Dosage
Buserelin	Subcutaneous	200 µg/day
	Intranasal	300–344 µ/day × 4 days
Goserelin	Subcutaneous implant*	3.6 mg/mo or 10.8 mg/3 mo
Histrelin	Subcutaneous injection	100 µg/day
Leuprolide	Subcutaneous injection*	500–1000 µg/day
	Intranasal*	400 µg × 4 days
	Intramuscular depot*	3.75–7.5 mg/mo or 11.25 mg/mo
Nafarelin	Intranasal*	200 µg/day × 2 days
	Intramuscular depot*	3 mg/mo
Tryptorelin	Intramuscular depot	2–4 mg/mo

*Available in the United States.

functional stages, suggesting that the administration of GnRH analogues may have a direct action on the human ovary.

The ability of GnRH agonists to produce amenorrhea and anovulation has provided the basis for their use in the management of endometriosis (Table 71–1). A large number of clinical studies in the United States and European countries have demonstrated the efficacy of GnRH agonists in the management of endometriosis.

Nafarelin (Synarel), a GnRH superagonist, was the first analogue introduced in the United States for the management of endometriosis. In a parallel, double-blind study design,[1] the effect of nafarelin was compared with that of danazol. A similar degree of relief of symptoms and regression of endometrial implants was observed for both drugs. During the course of therapy, there was an initial rise of gonadotropin and estradiol levels followed by sustained hypoestrogenism, amenorrhea, and anovulation. Subsequently, a large number of randomized controlled studies were performed comparing the results of GnRH agonist therapy (see Table 71–1) with either a placebo or danazol. In almost all of these studies, a GnRH agonist was administered for 24 weeks with a period of 6 to 12 months' follow-up evaluation. These studies have clearly established the effectiveness of GnRH agonists in significantly improving the subjective symptoms of endometriosis during and after treatment and reducing endometrial implant size as determined by ASRM score.

The initial 6-month trials for GnRH were based empirically on the traditional regimen for danazol. However, more recent studies[2] indicated that there is no significant difference in relief of pain or other clinical symptoms of endometriosis when comparing 3 months versus 6 months of GnRH agonist therapy.

Recurrence of endometriosis symptoms commonly occurs within 9 to 12 months after cessation of therapy. Therefore, a repeat short course (3 months) of treatment of endometriosis with GnRH agonists or other modalities of medical treatment may be necessary to control symptoms of the disease.

Adverse reactions associated with GnRH agonists are limited to those attributable to hypoestrogenism, including hot flashes, vaginal dryness, headache, myalgia, and some loss of vertebral trabecular bone.

Pregnancy rates among infertile patients receiving GnRH agonist therapy appear to be comparable with those treated with danazol or progestins.

Prolonged treatment with GnRH agonists has a significant impact on bone metabolism. The extent to which bone loss occurs depends on the potency and dosage of the GnRH, duration of use, and, ultimately, the degree of hypoestrogenism resulting from such therapy. Bone resorption is most pronounced in sites with a high trabecular bone content. Usually, the effects of the analogues on bone metabolism are reversible and may return to pretreatment levels within 6 months after the cessation of therapy. For up to 12 months after treatment, however, a significant residual loss of trabecular bone mineral content persists. There is, therefore, some concern about the effect of repeated courses of GnRH agonist treatment on bone mineral content.

Add-Back Therapy

To obviate the undesirable effect of hypoestrogenism on bone metabolism and vasomotor symptoms, concomitant administration of a progestational agent alone or in conjunction with estrogen, along with a GnRH agonist, has been proposed. The rationale for such an approach is the notion that there may be a differential threshold of serum estradiol (E_2) level to suppress endometriosis and to maintain normal bone metabolism and calcium turnover. The optimal E_2 target to achieve this goal remains to be defined, but preliminary evidence suggests that an E_2 level in the range of 30 pg/mL may be as clinically effective as an E_2 target of 15 pg/mL for the treatment of pelvic pain caused by endometriosis. Strategies for achieving an E_2 target of 30 pg/mL might include the combination of an GnRH agonist plus E_2 add-back or adjustment of GnRH agonist dose to achieve the desired E_2 level.

Several recent studies have evaluated add-back therapy to GnRH agonists with combinations of estrogen and progestogen in women with endometriosis. The addition of an estrogen such as conjugated equine estrogen (0.3 to 0.625 mg) plus MPA (5 mg) daily beginning on day 15 of GnRH agonist therapy has been shown to significantly decrease hypoestrogenic side effect of GnRH agonist treatment while attenuating the loss of bone mineral density without altering relief of symptoms of endometriosis.[3]

SURGICAL MANAGEMENT OF ENDOMETRIOSIS

Several modalities of surgical therapy may be used for conservative management of endometriosis. These include endoscopic surgery using either fulguration with thermal cautery or ablation with laser and surgical resection and removal by laparotomy.

Laparoscopic treatment of endometriosis has several advantages. The disease can be accurately diagnosed, staged, and immediately resected or ablated all in the course of one procedure. Additionally, adhesions can be lysed and endometriomas drained or excised when indicated and possible. Electrocoagulation may be performed by using either a unipolar or a bipolar source of electrical energy. Thermal damage to peritoneum, bowel, or other adjacent structures may occasionally occur when unipolar cauterization is performed. Bipolar systems are safer than unipolar, but accidents are still possible. Ablation of endometriosis can be achieved with the CO_2 laser. The CO_2 laser beam is precise, and it causes minimal damage to adjacent tissue. The immediate and near-total tissue absorption of the CO_2 laser beam limits thermal damage to surrounding tissue. Tissue coagulation is also accomplished when using other types of laser, such as argon or KTP (potassium-titanyl-phosphate) lasers. These lasers destroy the tissue primarily by photocoagulation rather than vaporization. Although studies comparing the effectiveness of thermocoagulation or laser ablation with conservative surgery or medical therapy are not available, other studies do exist that compare the merits of some of these surgical treatment options.[4] In a randomized study of 123 infertile patients, 60.8% of those whose endometriotic implants were fulgurated conceived within 8 months after laparoscopy, whereas only 18.5% of women whose endometriotic implants were not coagulated achieved a pregnancy. Numerous publications[5] have appeared on the results achieved with laser therapy for endometriosis. Generally, these indicate a pregnancy rate of 50% to 60% in patients treated with CO_2 laser, and somewhat higher pregnancy rates when endometriosis was the only infertility factor identified. Unfortunately, the majority of these studies are uncontrolled and thus difficult to evaluate. Furthermore, whereas they provide some data on pregnancy, as an end point, they lack information relative to the relief of symptoms such as pain and recurrence. A review of the few studies containing such information indicates the following[6]:

1. The percentage of patients obtaining relief of dysmenorrhea, dyspareunia, and pelvic pain with endoscopic surgery is similar to that reported for other therapeutic modalities, including laparotomy.
2. Using newer techniques and instrumentation, the majority of cases of mild and moderate pelvic endometriosis may be managed by laparoscopic approach. Laser laparoscopy is a safe and effective treatment in alleviating pain symptoms with ASRM stages I to III endometriosis.

Surgical Excision

Removal of endometrial implants during laparoscopy is an alternative to fulguration and laser ablation. However, because of complications such as bleeding and adhesion development, as well as difficulties in removing lesions located in sites such as the bowel or ureter, laser ablation is preferred. For extensive endometriosis, conservative surgery by laparotomy is the method of choice. Laser or thermocoagulation may be used during these operations to ablate or fulgurate implants or lyse adhesions. Preoperative or postoperative medical treatment is commonly combined with conservative surgery for advanced disease. For practical purposes, mild and moderate endometriosis may be treated by a laparoscopic approach or medical therapy, whereas extensive endometriosis, particularly lesions involving bowel or urinary tract, require surgical therapy, usually through a laparotomy.

Hysterectomy with removal of ovaries should be considered in patients who have severe symptomatic disease and are no longer interested in future pregnancies.

RECURRENCE OF ENDOMETRIOSIS

Endometriosis has the potential for recurrence at any time during the reproductive age. Only menopause or hysterectomy with bilateral oophorectomy may produce a cure. Thus, the disease may reappear after all medical or conservative surgical modalities of treatment. The recurrence rate of endometriosis varies in different women and probably depends on the invasiveness of the disease, host resistance, and possibly intervening pregnancies. In some patients, a single course of medical treatment or surgical intervention may be followed by a prolonged period of relief, whereas in others, recurrences occur within a few months after termination of treatment. After a course of danazol therapy, for example, the recurrence of symptoms and lesions is approximately 5% to 20% per year. A second course of medical therapy may be provided if, in fact, the initial course resulted in a remission of disease.

References

1. Henzel M, Corson S, Moghissi KS, et al: Administration of nasal nafarelin versus oral danazol for endometriosis. A multicenter, double blind, comparative trial. N Engl J Med 1988;384:485.
2. Heinrichs WL, Henzel MR: Human issues and medical economics of endometriosis. Three versus six months GnRH agonist therapy. J Reprod Med 1988;43(suppl):299–308.
3. Moghissi KS, Schlaff WD, Olive DL, et al: Goserelin acetate (Zoladex) with or without hormone replacement therapy for treatment of endometriosis. Fertil Steril 1988;69:1056–1062.
4. Donnez J: CO_2 laser laparoscopy in infertile women with endometriosis and women with adnexal adhesions. Fertil Steril 1987;48:390–394.
5. Marcoux S, Maheux R, Bérubé S: The Canadian collaborative group on endometriosis. Laparoscopic surgery in infertile women with minimal or mild endometriosis. N Engl J Med 1997;337:217–222.
6. Roberts CP, Rock JA: Endometriosis. In Ransom SB, Dombrowski MD, Moghissi KS, et al (eds): Practical Strategies in Obstetrics and Gynecology. Philadelphia, WB Saunders, 2000, pp 709–716.

Contemporary Management of Leiomyomas

CHAPTER

SEVENTY-TWO

Joseph G. Whelan III, Nikos F. Vlahos,

and Edward E. Wallach

EPIDEMIOLOGY

Uterine leiomyomas are the most common pelvic tumors in women. Traditionally, they have been described as present in 20% of women over age 35 years, but their appearance at 50% of postmortem examinations of women suggests a much higher frequency—particularly in African American women.

PATHOLOGY

Uterine leiomyomas are generally accepted as originating from smooth muscle cells of the uterus, although in certain instances an origin from the smooth muscle of uterine blood vessels is likely. Leiomyomas are characterized microscopically by tightly interlacing bundles of benign smooth muscle cells having uniform-sized rod-shaped nuclei, arranged in a whorl-like pattern and admixed with connective tissue elements. Leiomyomas range in size from "seedlings" only millimeters in diameter to large uterine tumors that can reach up to the costal margin. These tumors may be solitary or multiple.

Malignant transformation of benign leiomyomas is extremely rare. The often-cited statistic that 0.5% of leiomyomas are malignant overstates the likelihood of malignant change. Corscaden and Singh[1] reported that malignant change developed in less than 0.13% of uterine leiomyomas. The microscopic diagnosis of a leiomyosarcoma relies on the level of mitotic activity and degree of cellular atypism. Tumors with more than 10 mitotic figures per 10 high-power fields are considered malignant.

PATHOGENESIS OF GROWTH

The growth of uterine leiomyomas is clearly related to their exposure to circulating estrogen. In contrast to the influence of estrogens on leiomyomas, progesterone and progestational compounds tend to exert an antiestrogen effect; the success of progesterone and synthetic progestogens in decreasing the size of uterine leiomyomas supports this concept. The antiprogesterone RU-486, however, has been shown to reduce the size of myomas,[2] thus demonstrating that sex hormone influence on leiomyomatous growth is certainly complex and not completely understood.

Leiomyoma growth is common during pregnancy but occurs less frequently during the cyclic use of estrogen-progestogen preparations, such as oral contraceptive pills. Enlargement of leiomyomas during pregnancy may be attributed to their dependence on estrogen as well as to the increased uterine circulation during that period.

CLINICAL MANIFESTATIONS AND DIAGNOSIS

The single most common symptom associated with myomas is prolonged or excessive bleeding associated with menstruation. Most patients with uterine leiomyomas, however, are symptom-free. When symptoms are produced, they often relate to the location of the leiomyomas, their size, or concomitant degenerative changes. Pain is most often experienced in patients with a pedunculated leiomyoma as its pedicle undergoes torsion. Pain may also be attributed to cervical dilatation by a submucous leiomyoma protruding through the lower uterine segment or to carneous degeneration associated with pregnancy.

Progressive "pressure" sensation and increased abdominal girth are more commonly encountered than pain, develop insidiously, are often less apparent, and are usually vaguely described by the patient. As leiomyomas grow, pressure is frequently exerted on adjacent viscera. Pressure on the urinary bladder usually provokes urinary frequency, especially when the leiomyoma is located in the subvesical region or when a large myomatous uterus fills the entire pelvis. When the leiomyoma is located adjacent to the urethra and bladder neck, urinary retention with overflow incontinence may occur. External compression of the pelvic portion of the ureter may lead to hydroureter and hydronephrosis. Constipation or tenesmus may also be associated with a posterior leiomyoma, representing pressure of the tumor on the rectosigmoid.

MANAGEMENT

A conservative "observational" approach may be appropriate in the management of the asymptomatic myomatous uterus. Physical examination and ultrasound studies performed initially at 1- to 2-month intervals can provide the physician with a reasonable appreciation of whether the leiomyomas are enlarging, and, if so, at what rate. If the size appears stationary, serial examinations at 3- to 4-month intervals are reasonable. Temporizing is also appropriate if

367

the patient is in the immediate premenopausal age range and can safely tolerate symptoms while awaiting menopausal regression in myoma size.

If a patient's uterine myomas are symptomatic or otherwise causing morbidity, interventional management is warranted. Intervention in the management of uterine myomas generally consists of hormonal therapy and/or surgical therapy.

Hormone Therapy

Progestins

Progestational therapy has been successfully employed using norethindrone, medrogestone, and medroxyprogesterone acetate to achieve diminution in aggregate size of the myomatous uterus. These compounds were thought to produce a hypoestrogenic effect by inhibiting gonadotropin secretion and suppressing ovarian function. Progestational compounds may also exert a direct antiestrogenic effect at the cellular level in the leiomyoma.

Gonadotropin-Releasing Hormone Analogues

Gonadotropin-releasing hormone (GnRH) analogues have been used successfully to achieve hypoestrogenism in various estrogen-dependent conditions, for example, endometriosis, precocious puberty, and uterine leiomyomas. Patients treated for uterine leiomyomas using this approach have experienced significant reduction in tumor size.[3] This approach offers great promise as a primary, although temporary, means of conservative therapy or as a preoperative adjunct to surgical myomectomy.

As a primary treatment, the effects of either progestational therapy or GnRH analogue treatment are, unfortunately, transient, and myomas will typically return to their previous size within several cycles after discontinuing medication. Preoperative therapy with a 3- to 4-month course of GnRH analogues should reduce leiomyoma size and render surgery easier, accompanied by less blood loss. Pretreatment with GnRH analogues not only facilitates the myomectomy itself but also provides an amenorrheic interval before surgery during which hemoglobin levels can be restored in the hypermenorrheic anemic patient, enabling presurgical blood donation for subsequent autotransfusion. Although there is a theoretical concern that presurgical shrinkage of small leiomyomas by GnRH analogues will render them undetectable at surgery and lead to early recurrence, there are no randomized, placebo-controlled studies to justify this concern.

Surgical Therapy

Myomectomy

Indications. Myomectomy should be considered for symptomatic myomas in patients who desire to preserve

their uterus. Desire for uterine retention cannot be underestimated in our culture. Technology today even enables the uterus of a woman lacking ovaries to serve as a gestational vehicle through the processes of in vitro fertilization, endometrial preparation with exogenous hormone therapy, and embryo donation. Furthermore, publicity regarding unnecessary hysterectomy has sensitized women in the decision-making process regarding uterine retention in the presence of benign pathology.

Infertility is infrequently a consequence of uterine leiomyomas, but when a causal relationship is suspected, the location of leiomyomas is usually the significant element interfering with establishment or maintenance of pregnancy. Locations associated with difficulties in pregnancy include the following: (1) submucosal, where leiomyomas may interfere with implantation and result in infertility or impair embryonic-fetal nutrition, giving rise to early pregnancy loss; (2) cornual, which may cause intramural obstruction of the fallopian tube; (3) a broad ligament site, where a leiomyoma can distort the anatomic relationship between the tubal ostium and the ovary; (4) supracervical, where leiomyomas can alter the position of the cervix within the vagina, thereby interfering with the opportunity for the cervical os to be bathed in the ejaculate after coitus.

Abdominal Technique. A uterus with an aggregate size larger than the equivalent of a 16-week gestation or one containing prominent broad ligament leiomyomas usually merits consideration of a vertical abdominal incision to facilitate exposure. Smaller myomatous uteri can usually be accessed easily via a low transverse abdominal incision. The general principles for myomectomy involve adequate exposure, minimization of uterine damage, meticulous hemostasis, and adhesion prevention. The uterine incision should be carefully selected so as to facilitate removal of the maximal number of myomas and to minimize the need for multiple uterine incisions. The incision into the uterus should be made as close to the midline as possible to avoid incising vascular areas of the uterus. A vertical midline incision also avoids injury to the interstitial portion of the fallopian tube. An anterior uterine incision has the advantage of minimizing the possibility of incorporating the adnexal structures in adhesions that may form postoperatively and usually adjacent to a posterior uterine incision.

Laparoscopic Myomectomy. Laparoscopic myomectomy can be carried out especially when myomas are easily accessible as superficial subserous or pedunculated myomas. The myomas can be morcellated and removed through the laparoscopic cannula or placed in the cul de sac and removed via a colpotomy incision. Laparoscopic removal of large intramural myomas has been related to reports of uterine rupture during pregnancy. This serious complication may reflect the reduced effectiveness of apposition of myometrium during laparoscopic myomectomy as compared with the thorough suturing technique afforded during open procedures.

Transvaginal Technique. Submucous leiomyomas can be surgically removed using a vaginal approach in certain instances. A pedunculated submucous tumor occasionally presents within the endocervical canal or having prolapsed through the cervix. This type of tumor can be removed transvaginally by advancing the bladder and making an anterior midline cervical incision or by vaginal hysterotomy. The pedicle of the leiomyoma is identified as high as possible, clamped close to its base, and resected. The pedicle is then oversewn with a transfixed ligature. The myoma can then be retrieved via the incisional opening or advanced through an already dilated cervix. If the pedicle of a completely prolapsed myoma is accessible vaginally, the pedicle stalk can be clamped, cut, and oversewn distal to the cervical external os. Preoperative and perioperative antibiotic therapy is essential in these cases because of the hazards of disseminating infection from the prolapsed, inflamed leiomyoma.

Hysteroscopic Technique. Hysteroscopic resection of certain submucous leiomyomas avoids the need for an abdominal incision, eliminates the necessity for hysterotomy, and reduces the length of hospital stay. Technologic advances in fiberoptic light sources offer the opportunity to visualize the endometrial cavity directly, evaluate the extent of the leiomyomas, and identify bleeding sites. The development of instruments to resect tissue have also made hysteroscopic excision of intramural/submucous leiomyomas possible. An electrocautery cutting loop is ideal for this purpose. A thorough knowledge of uterine distention media, each with its own potential for particular complications, is required on the part of the surgeon before attempting operative hysteroscopy. When extensive operative hysteroscopy is anticipated, laparoscopy should be done simultaneously to reduce the hazards of uterine perforation. During hysteroscopic resection, intravasation of distention media should be assessed by monitoring hysteroscopic input/output volume tabulations at intervals no greater than every 30 minutes. The patient and the operating team should also be prepared in each case for the possibility of laparotomy. Once the myoma has been resected, hemostasis can be achieved either directly by hysteroscopic cauterization or by insertion of a balloon catheter into the endometrial cavity. Inflation of the balloon tamponades the bleeding sites; the balloon can then can be deflated and removed several hours later if bleeding has ceased.

Laser Vaporization. The CO_2 laser has also been used as a surgical adjunct for myomectomy. During laparotomy, small leiomyomas have been directly vaporized with the laser whereas laser excision is used for medium to large leiomyomas in McLaughlin's series.[4] This series cited improved hemostasis, greater precision enabling removal of only abnormal tissue, and ability to remove leiomyomas from previously inaccessible areas as definite advantages of laser vaporization. "Myolysis" of difficult-to-reach myomas has also been described utilizing bipolar cautery, monopolar needle cautery, and cryomyolysis. These newer approaches have been associated with postoperative adhesion formation, but longer-term benefits and risks have not been established.

Hysterectomy

With few exceptions, removal of the uterus is the procedure of choice whenever surgery is indicated for leiomyomas and childbearing has been completed. If myomectomy is not technically feasible, hysterectomy should be carried out, especially in the presence of diffuse myomatosis of the uterus. Although it is unusual for myomectomy to be technically implausible, the procedure may be difficult, time-consuming, and associated with a high intraoperative blood loss and substantial postoperative complication rate. Therefore, to balance the risks of performing a difficult and potentially complicated myomectomy, sufficient indication for uterine preservation should be evident. Likewise, it is advisable that, during the preoperative consent process, the patient be made aware of the possible need to convert a complicated myomectomy procedure into a hysterectomy.

New Approaches—Uterine Artery Embolization

Originally established as a safe and effective treatment in the management of acute pelvic hemorrhage, uterine artery embolization has been recently applied in the treatment of nonacute hemorrhage due to leiomyomas.[5, 6] This procedure is performed by interventional radiologists. Through a single puncture in the groin, a small catheter is introduced in a retrograde mode up to the bifurcation of the aorta. Digital arteriogram is performed to evaluate the vasculature of the area. The uterine arteries bilateraly are catheterized and embolized using Gelfoam or polyvinylformaldahyde particles.

In several series, the method has been found successful in controling bleeding in up to 89% of the patients after 6 months.[7] A significant decrease in uterine size has also been recorded. Complications of the method include pelvic infection in 3% to 4% of the patients and target organ ischemia and nontarget embolization of the ovaries in 1% to 2% that may lead to premature ovarian failure. The overall impact of this procedure on future fertility has not been adequately evaluated.

CONCLUSION

Both observational and interventional approaches have been utilized traditionally in the management of myomatous uteri, and both approaches to this common gynecologic problem will no doubt continue to be used well into the future. Advances will certainly be made in the knowledge of the endocrine function of leiomyomas, which will prompt better methods of hormonal treatment, and surgical techniques will continue to evolve for safer and more efficient removal of myomas from otherwise normal uteri. Regardless of what advances the future may bring to the areas of interventional management, the gynecologic surgeon will always need to appreciate the safety and the logic of conservative observation when confronted with a benign myomatous uterus.

References

1. Corscaden JA, Singh BP: Leiomyosarcoma of the uterus. Am J Obstet Gynecol 1958;75:149–155.
2. Murphy AA, Kettel LM, Morales AJ, et al: Regression of uterine leiomyomata in response to the antiprogesterone RU486. J Clin Endocrinol Metab 1993;76:513–517.
3. Donnez J, Schrurs B, Gillerot S, et al: Treatment of uterine fibroids with implants of gonadotropin-releasing hormone agonist: Assessment by hysterography. Fertil Steril 1989;51:947–950.
4. McLaughlin DS: Micro-laser myomectomy technique to enhance reproductive potential: A preliminary report. Lasers Surg Med 1982;2:107–127.
5. Goodwin SC, Vedantham S, McLucas B, et al: Preliminary experience with uterine artery embolization for uterine fibroids. J Vasc Interv Radiol 1997;8:517–526.
6. Goodwin SC, Walker WJ: Uterine artery embolization for the treatment of uterine fibroids. Curr Opin Obstet Gynecol 1998;10:315–320.
7. Hurst BS, Stackhouse DJ, Matthews ML, Mashburn PB: Uterine artery embolization for symptomatic uterine myomas. Fertil Steril 2000; 74:855–869.

Hormone Replacement Therapy in Breast Cancer Survivors

Wendy R. Brewster and Philip J. DiSaia

The average woman in the United States can expect to spend at least 40% of her lifetime in the menopausal period. Attrition and aging of ovarian follicles result in the termination of the maturation of granulosa cells, which are responsible for estrogen production. There are several sources of estrogen in the premenopausal woman, including the direct production of estradiol by the ovaries in addition to the extraglandular aromatization in adipose cells of androstenedione created in the adrenal glands and ovary. The hallmark of menopause is the drop in ovarian production of estriol and testosterone. Peripheral aromatization of other steroids not produced by the ovaries is an additional source of estrogen in all women. However, this source is not sufficient in most women to prevent the symptoms characteristic of estrogen deprivation.

Thirty million women in the United States are currently in menopause. The incidence of breast cancer in the United States is the highest in the world. This diagnosis is made in 185,000 women annually, with the majority of diagnoses made among those in the postmenopausal period. Over the past few decades, the incidence of breast cancer has increased as the mortality rates from this disease have decreased. This is largely attributable to the detection of this malignancy at in situ or localized stages by the use of multimodality screening inclusive of mammography and breast examinations. Breast cancer survival is correlated with the tumor size, regional lymph node status, and disease stage at the time of diagnosis. Smaller cancers with no evidence of axillary node metastases are associated with longer survival rates.[1] Thus, a considerable number of Americans are likely to have a history of breast cancer treatment and at the same time be potential candidates for hormone replacement therapy (HRT). During the 1990s, the indications for chemotherapy as adjuvant treatment to surgery have widened and now encompass many more premenopausal women.[2] Adjuvant therapy for breast cancer includes the use of alkylating agents and other drugs that cause amenorrhea in 84% of women aged 35 to 44 years. Other studies indicate that this treatment causes permanent ovarian failure in 86% of women older than 40 years of age.[3] As a result, a larger number of women will potentially be rendered menopausal in the fourth and fifth decades of their life. These women will spend their lives in an estrogen–deficient state and are at significant risk to develop vasomotor instability cardiovascular disease,[4, 5] osteo-porosis,[6] impairment in cognitive function,[7] and fatal colorectal cancer.[8]

The major concern of many physicians in prescribing estrogen replacement therapy (ERT) to breast cancer survivors is the theory that metastatic quiescent tumor foci might be activated and the "fire" of breast cancer ignited by the estrogen "fuel." Other fears are that estrogen might cause a second primary tumor in the already environmentally or genetically primed contralateral breast or might change breast density and mask new mammographic findings.

The hesitancy to prescribe ERT to breast cancer survivors is in part based on epidemiologic studies that have demonstrated a relationship between duration of postmenopausal estrogen replacement and breast cancer.[9, 10] Estrogen has been clearly implicated as an etiologic factor in the development of breast cancer. Early menarche, late menopause, nulliparity, and prolonged HRT are breast cancer risk factors.[11] In a subset of premenopausal breast cancer patients, surgical oophorectomy is beneficial, and estrogen withdrawal has also been observed to promote regression of metastatic breast cancer lesions.[12] Breast cancer cells that maintain the function of their estrogen and progesterone receptors can be stimulated by estrogen in vitro. Obesity adversely affects prognosis presumably secondary to an increase in peripheral estrogen production.[13]

However, there is indirect evidence in support of the safety of ERT in breast cancer survivors. High-dose estrogens have been demonstrated to be effective in the treatment of advanced breast cancer. The standard treatment of premenopausal women with breast cancer does not include castration, even among those who maintain ovulatory function after cytotoxic therapy. These women are permitted normal cyclic ovarian function until menopause.

The well-substantiated benefits of ERT must be balanced against the theoretical concerns. Arguments in support of the safety of ERT are based on several natural experiments and observations that are discussed in detail later. The decision as to whether or not to take hormone replacement remains difficult for the postmenopausal woman because of conflicting risks and benefits and is even more difficult for the breast cancer survivor for whom there are even fewer data. One can therefore analyze situations in which women are inadvertently exposed to exogenous or endogenous estrogen at a time when they may have been harboring a subclinical breast cancer lesion. Does such exposure adversely affect survival outcome for these patients?

EXPOSURE TO EXOGENOUS OR ENDOGENOUS ESTROGEN DURING BREAST CANCER DEVELOPMENT

There are such situations in which women have harbored subclinical breast cancer cells at a time when they were exposed to exogenous or endogenous estrogen. Such situations include those in whom the diagnosis of breast cancer is made in postmenopausal women receiving ERT at the time of diagnosis; women in whom the diagnosis is made in pregnancy or during lactation; and those women with a history of oral contraceptive pill use around the time of diagnosis of their breast cancers.

Breast Cancer in Women on Estrogen Replacement Therapy

Bergkvist and coworkers[14] compared 261 women who developed breast cancer while on ERT to 6617 breast cancer patients who had no recorded treatment with estrogen. The relative survival rate over an 8-year period was higher in the breast cancer patients who had previously received ERT. This corresponded to a 32% reduction in excess mortality. Gambrell,[15] in a prospective study, also evaluated the effect on survival in breast cancer patients diagnosed while on ERT. The mortality was 22% among those diagnosed with breast cancer while on ERT compared with 46% among those who never received hormone replacement. Henderson and colleagues[16] observed a 19% reduction in breast cancer mortality among 4988 previous ERT users as compared with 3865 nonusers who subsequently developed this disease. It thus appears that postmenopausal women diagnosed with breast cancer while on ERT do not have an apparent deleterious effect on their cancer survival from current ERT use.

Pregnancy-Associated Breast Cancer

Only 0.5% to 4% of all breast cancers are diagnosed during pregnancy. Pregnancy coincident with, or subsequent to, breast cancer provides another excellent opportunity to evaluate the outcome of breast cancer patients inadvertently exposed to high levels of estrogen at times when they were harboring occult disease. During pregnancy, the serum levels of estriol increase 50-fold. Because the average breast cancer remains occult in the breast some 5 to 8 years prior to diagnosis, some authors include in this category the women in whom a diagnosis of breast cancer has been made within 12 months of delivery. The outcome in women with subclinical breast cancers exposed to elevated levels of progesterone and estrogen under these

circumstances could provide an insight into the influence of these hormones on the malignant disease process.

The physiologic changes and engorgement that occur in the breast during pregnancy often hinder early detection. This results in the diagnosis of breast cancer at more advanced stages in pregnant and lactating women. Comparisons with nonpregnant women matched for similar age and stage of breast cancer and reproductive capacity do not suggest a worse prognosis for the pregnant patients with breast cancer[17, 18] von Schoultz and associates[19] performed a comparison of women diagnosed with breast cancer 5 years before pregnancy with women without a pregnancy during the same time period. There was no survival disadvantage to the women who were pregnant 5 years before diagnosis of breast cancer. These and other studies have resulted in a discontinuation of the practice of prohibiting breast cancer survivors from becoming pregnant on clinical grounds.

Anderson and coworkers[20] reported their experience at The Memorial Sloan-Kettering Cancer Center with breast cancer in women younger than 30 years. Two hundred twenty-seven cases were identified, of whom 22 had pregnancy-associated breast cancer. The authors confirmed that pregnancy-associated breast cancers were usually larger and present in more advanced stages at the time of diagnosis as compared with a similar group who were not pregnant. However, the survival probability for women with early-stage disease was independent of the pregnancy status.

The experience of women who have completed term pregnancies after treatment of antecedent breast cancer is another situation that deserves analysis. The main concern regarding the possible effect of a subsequent pregnancy on breast cancer prognosis is that pregnancy may promote the growth of dormant microscopic metastatic disease and increase the risk of recurrence. Additionally, premenopausal women who are diagnosed with breast carcinoma may have special concerns regarding fertility. Inherent biases are associated with evaluation of this particular group of subjects. This cohort is representative of the young women who did well after primary breast cancer therapy, and because pregnancy data are not uniformly coded in cancer registry databases, the true denominator of post–breast cancer pregnancies is unknown. Clark and Chua[21] reported a 71% 5-year survival in a series of 136 women with pregnancies after breast cancer (stages I to III). von Schoultz and associates[19] reported equivalent survival outcomes when breast cancer patients with no subsequent pregnancy were compared with those who became pregnant within 5 years of their diagnosis. Velentgas and colleagues[22] evaluated the outcome of a cohort of population-based breast cancer survivors diagnosed with stage I or stage II. Fifty-three women who became pregnant after a diagnosis of breast cancer were matched with women without subsequent pregnancies based on stage of disease at diagnosis and a recurrence-free survival time. The age-adjusted relative risk of death associated with any pregnancy was 0.8 (95% confidence interval [CI], 0.3 to 2.3). No epidemiologic studies have suggested any adverse effect of pregnancy on survival after breast cancer.[23, 24]

Breast Cancer in Oral Contraceptive Pill Users

Given the long natural history of this neoplasm, it is certain that a large number of patients subsequently diagnosed with breast cancer have used oral contraceptive pills (OCPs) during the genesis and progression of their malignant disease process and are another group that deserve examination. Rosner and Lane[25] evaluated 347 women younger than 50 years diagnosed with breast cancer, of whom 112 were OCP users. The distribution of tumor size, estrogen receptor status, and family and reproductive history was the same between the two cohorts. There was no difference in disease-free survival or overall survival between the two groups. Women who used OCPs within a year of diagnosis of their breast cancer had a similar survival to those who had discontinued use more than 1 year before. There was no difference in survival among those who used OCPs 10 years or more before their diagnosis of breast cancer.

Schonborn and associates[26] evaluated the influence of a history of OCP use on survival. Four hundred seventy-one breast cancer patients were investigated. Two hundred ninety-seven (63%) patients used OCPs during any period of their life and 92 (20%) used them still at the time of diagnosis. Sixty months after diagnosis, the OCP users had a significantly increased overall survival ($P = .037$). Survival rates amounted to 79.5% and 70.3% in OCP users and nonusers, respectively.

Sauerbrei and coworkers[27] investigated the relationship between OCP use and standard prognostic factors and the effect of OCP use on disease-free survival and overall survival in 422 premenopausal node-positive patients from two trials of the German Breast Cancer Study Group. One hundred thirty-seven patients (32.5%) were OCP users who were younger in comparison to non-OCP users (mean age, 41.5 years vs. 45 years, respectively). Noteworthy was the fact that the percentage of patients with smaller tumors was higher in the group of OCP users. No significant effect of OCP use on either disease-free or overall survival could be demonstrated in univariate and multivariate analyses after adjustment for tumor size and other prognostic factors.

STUDIES ON ESTROGEN REPLACEMENT THERAPY IN BREAST CANCER SURVIVORS

DiSaia and colleagues[28] reported 71 breast cancer survivors who received ERT. There was no exclusion based on interval since diagnosis of breast cancer, stage, age, receptor status, or lymph node status. The subject received combination therapy with progestin only if she had not previously undergone hysterectomy. Later, DiSaia and associates[29] reported a comparison in which 41 of these ERT-using breast cancer survivors were compared with 82 non-ERT breast cancer subjects matched for age and stages of disease. Survival analysis did not indicate a significant difference between the two groups. The authors[30] now have 207 patients in their series. Analysis of 145 of these subjects who received ERT for at least 3 months after diagnosis of their breast cancer has identified 13 recurrences. The duration of use of estrogen before the diagnosis of recurrent breast cancer ranged from 4 months to 11.5 years.[30] More recently, DiSaia and coworkers[30a] performed a larger cohort analysis. One hundred twenty-five breast cancer patients received HRT after diagnosis of breast cancer was identified. Three hundred sixty-two control subjects were identified from the regional cancer registry. Matching criteria included age at diagnosis, stage of breast cancer, and year of diagnosis. Controls were selected only if they were alive at the time of initiation of HRT of the matched case. Only subjects not included in a previously reported matched analysis were selected. The median interval between diagnosis of breast cancer and initiation of HRT was 46 months (range, 0 to 401 months). The median duration of HRT was 22 months (range, 1–357 months). The risk of death was lower among the HRT survivors with an odds ratio (OR) of 0.28 (95% CI, 0.11 to 0.71).

Other authors have reported their experience of ERT in breast cancer survivors (Table 73–1). Eden and colleagues[31] reported six recurrences among the 90 women receiving ERT. These ERT users were matched 2:1 with control subjects with no history of sex steroid use after diagnosis of breast cancer. The recurrence rate in the ERT users was 7%, and 30% in the non-ERT users. Bluming and associates[32] reported 155 breast cancer patients who received ERT for between 1 to 56 months, among whom 7 recurrences were identified. Vassilopoulou-Sellin and coworkers[33] consecutively identified a group of women who were potential participants for a randomized prospective ERT trial. All subjects were observed prospectively whether or not they chose to enroll into the randomized trial. Of 319 women, 39 have received ERT for a minimum of 2 years.[34] One of the subjects receiving ERT developed a new lobular breast cancer lesion. In the control group of 280 breast cancer survivors, 14 subjects developed a new or recurrent breast cancer.

The breast cancer survivors discussed in the previous paragraph are heterogeneous with respect to breast cancer stage, the interval between diagnosis of breast cancer and initiation of ERT, the hormonal combinations prescribed, estrogen receptor status, and finally, the duration of use of estrogen. Despite these limitations, it remains obvious that the use of estrogen is not associated with a rash of recurrences. Overall, the data do not suggest that ERT has an adverse effect on breast cancer outcome.

CONCLUSION

The fear that administration of estrogen to women with a history of breast cancer will result in the activation of

Table 73–1. Estrogen Replacement Therapy in Breast Cancer Survivors—Breast Cancer Recurrence

First Author	Patients *(N)*	Stage of Disease	Duration of ERT (mo)	Recurrences
Stoll[35]	Unknown	Early stage	3–6	None
Wile[36]	25	All stages	24–82	3
Powles[37]	35	All stages	1–44	8
Eden[31]	90	Local	4–144	6
Vassilopoulou-Sellin[34]	39	I–II (≥2-yr disease-free interval)	24–71	1
Bluming[32]	155	Local	1–56	7
Brewster[30]	145	All stages	31–44	13

ERT, estrogen replacement therapy.

quiescent metastatic foci and the climate of medical litigation are the basis of much of the reluctance on the part of physicians to prescribe ERT to breast cancer survivors. The standard of care no longer supports prophylactic oophorectomy in young women who do not become amenorrheic after cytotoxic therapy. In addition, many women continue to menstruate regularly after treatment and may even complete pregnancies. If castration and pregnancy termination are not routinely recommended, then why should the replacement of estrogen at a much lower dose than is physiologic be flatly prohibited?

A 50-year-old woman has a 13% lifetime probability of developing breast cancer and a 3% probability of dying of breast cancer; she has a 46% chance of developing coronary heart disease and a 31% probability of dying of heart disease. Whereas breast cancer claims 43,000 lives per year in the United States, coronary heart disease will kill approximately 233,000 women annually. Further, nearly 65,000 women die each year from the complications of hip fracture. Both heart disease and osteoporosis are to a great extent preventable with ERT in postmenopausal women.

No guarantee can be made that ERT will be accompanied with freedom from recurrent breast cancer because some women will have recurrent disease coincident with renewed hormone exposure. However, can we continue to prohibit ERT for all patients who have survived breast cancer? Clinicians should discuss the theoretical risks and the proven evidence of benefit and allow the patient to make an informed decision about the consequences *she* will face.

References

1. Morrow M, Bland KI, Foster R: Breast cancer surgical practice guidelines. Society of Surgical Oncology practice guidelines. Oncology 1997;11:885–886.
2. Early Breast Cancer Trialists' Collaborative Group: Systemic treatment of early breast cancer by hormonal, cytotoxic, or immune therapy: 133 randomized trials involving 31000 recurrences and 24000 deaths among 75000 women. Lancet 1992;339:1–15, 71–85.
3. Mehta RR, Beattie CW, Das Gupta T: Endocrine profile in breast cancer patients receiving chemotherapy. Breast Cancer Res Treat 1991;20:125–132.
4. Stampfer MJ, Willet WC, Colditz GA: A prospective study of postmenopausal estrogen therapy and coronary artery disease. N Engl J Med 1985;313:1040.
5. Stampfer MJ, Colditz GA, Willet WC, et al: Postmenopausal estrogen therapy and cardiovascular disease. Ten year follow-up from the Nurses Health Study. N Engl J Med 1991;325:756.
6. Weiss NS, Ure CL, Ballard JH, et al: Decreased risk of fracture of the hip and forearm with postmenopausal use of estrogen. N Engl J Med 1980;303:1195.
7. Kampen DL, Sherwin BB: Estrogen use and verbal memory in healthy postmenopausal women. Obstet Gynecol 1994;83:979.
8. Calle EE, Miracle-McMahill HL, Thun MJ, et al: Estrogen replacement therapy and risk of fatal colon cancer in a prospective cohort of postmenopausal women. J Natl Cancer Inst 1995;87:517.
9. Colditz GA, Hankinson SE, Hunter DJ, et al: The use of estrogens and progestins and the risk of breast cancer in postmenopausal women. N Engl J Med 1995;332:1589–1593.
10. Stanford JL, Weiss NS, Voigt LF, et al: Combined estrogen and progestin hormone replacement therapy in relation to risk of breast cancer in middle age women. JAMA 1995;274:137–141.
11. Henderson IC: Risk factors for breast cancer development. Cancer 1993;71:2127–2140.
12. Dhodapkar MV, Ingle JN, Ahmann DL: Estrogen replacement therapy withdrawal and regression of metastatic breast cancer. Cancer 1995;75:43–46.
13. Hunter DJ, Willett WC: Diet, body size, and breast cancer. Epidemiol Rev 1993;15:110–132.
14. Bergkvist L, Adami HO, Persson I, et al: Prognosis after breast cancer diagnosis in women exposed to estrogen and estrogen progesterone replacement therapy. Am J Epidemiol 1992;130:221–228.
15. Gambrell DR: Proposal to decrease the risk and improve the prognosis in breast cancer. Am J Obstet Gynecol 1984;150:119–128.
16. Henderson BE, Paganini-Hill A, Ross RK: Decreased mortality in users of estrogen replacement therapy. Arch Intern Med 1991;151:75–78.
17. Holleb AI, Farrow JH: The relation of carcinoma of the breast and pregnancy in 283 patients. Surg Gynecol Obstet 1962;115:65.
18. Nugent P, O'Connell TX: Breast cancer and pregnancy. Arch Surg 1985;120:1221–1224.
19. von Schoultz E, Johansson H, Wilking N, Rutqvist LE: Influence of prior and subsequent pregnancy on breast cancer prognosis. J Clin Oncol 1995;13:430–434.
20. Anderson BO, Petrek JZ, Byrd DR, et al: Pregnancy influences breast cancer stage at diagnosis in women 30 years of age and younger. Ann Surg Oncol 1996;3:204.
21. Clark RM, Chua T: Breast cancer and pregnancy: The ultimate challenge. Clin Oncol R Coll Radiol 1989;1:11–18.
22. Velentgas P, Daling JR, Malone KE, et al: Pregnancy after breast carcinoma: Outcomes and influence on mortality. Cancer 1999;85:2424–2432.
23. Kroman N, Jensen M, Melbye M, et al: Should women be advised against pregnancy after breast cancer treatment? Lancet 1997;350:319–322.
24. Collichio FA, Agnello R, Staltzer J: Pregnancy after breast cancer: From psychosocial issues through contraception. Oncology 1998;12:759–765.
25. Rosner D, Lane W: Oral contraceptive use has no adverse effect on the prognosis of breast cancer. Cancer 1986;57:591–596.
26. Schonborn I, Nischan P, Ebeling K: Oral contraceptive use and the prognosis of breast cancer. Breast Cancer Res Treat 1994;30:283–292.

27. Sauerbrei W, Blettner M, Schmoor C, et al: The effect of oral contraceptive use on the prognosis of node positive breast cancer patients. German Breast Cancer Study Group. Eur J Cancer 1998 34:1348–1351.

28. DiSaia PJ, Odicino F, Grosen EA, et al: Hormone replacement therapy in breast cancer [Letter]. Lancet 1993;342:1232.

29. DiSaia PJ, Grosen EA, Kurosaki T, et al: Hormone replacement therapy in breast cancer survivors. A cohort study. Am J Obstet Gynecol 1996;174:1494–1498.

30. Brewster WR, DiSaia PJ, Grosen EA, et al: An experience with estrogen replacement therapy in breast cancer survivors. Int J Fertil 1999;44:186–192.

30a. DiSaia PJ, Brewster WR, Ziogas A, Anton-Culver H: Breast cancer survival and hormone replacement therapy: A cohort analysis. Am J Clin Oncol 2000;23:541–545.

31. Eden JA, Bush T, Wren BG: A case control study of combined continuous estrogen-progestin replacement therapy among women with a personal history of breast cancer. Menopause 1995;2:67–72.

32. Bluming AZ, Waisman JR, Dosik GM: Hormone replacement therapy (HRT) in women with previously treated primary breast cancer. Update III. Proc Am Soc Clin Oncol 1997;16A:63,131.

33. Vassilopoulou-Sellin R, Therriault R, Klein MY: Estrogen replacement therapy in women with prior diagnosis and treatment for breast cancer. Gynecol Oncol 1997;65:89.

34. Vassilopoulou-Sellin R, Asmar L, Hortobagyi GN, et al: Estrogen replacement therapy after localized breast cancer: Clinical outcome of 319 women followed prospectively. J Clin Oncol 1999;17:1482–1487.

35. Stoll BA: Hormone replacement therapy in women treated for breast cancer. Eur J Cancer Clin Oncol 1989;25:1909–1913.

36. Wile AG, Opfell RW, Margileth DA: Hormone replacement therapy in previously treated breast cancer patients. Am J Surg 1993;165:372–375.

37. Powles TP, Casey S, O'Brien M, Hickish T: Hormone replacement after breast cancer. Lancet 1993;342:60.

Intraoperative Hemorrhage

Paul Makela

A concern of all gynecologic surgeons is severe intraoperative hemorrhage that is difficult to control. These operating room events often occur suddenly, without warning, and result in extreme stress. For these reasons, all gynecologic surgeons must be familiar with anatomy as well as methods to control intraoperative bleeding. Gynecologic surgeons need to have a specific plan to control intraoperative bleeding quickly and effectively. In this chapter we discuss anatomy, treatment of vascular injuries, transfusion of blood products, and methods available to the surgeon to control intraoperative bleeding.

ANATOMY

An understanding of the anatomy of the pelvis is crucial to safe gynecologic surgery. The primary blood supply to the pelvis is the internal iliac (hypogastric) artery. The internal iliac artery divides into anterior and posterior divisions. The anterior division is the main blood supply to the pelvis. It follows a branching pattern that varies widely from patient to patient. The anterior division includes five visceral branches and three parietal branches. The visceral branches are the uterine, superior vesical, middle hemorrhoid, inferior hemorrhoidal, and vaginal. The parietal branches are the obturator, inferior gluteal, and internal pudendal. An extensive collateral circulation exists between the arterial branches in the female pelvis. Venous drainage of the pelvis parallels this arterial supply, ultimately ending in the internal iliac vein.

The posterior division of the hypogestric artery provides parietal branches to the iliolumbar, lateral sacral, and superior gluteal regions.

TREATMENT OF VASCULAR INJURIES

Arterial bleeding is generally high pressure, pulsatile, and bright red. Arterial injuries occurring during gynecologic surgery are usually injuries to branches of the internal iliac (hypogastric) artery. Repair of this type of injury generally requires ligation of the artery. Ischemic injury usually does not occur owing to the extensive collateral circulation in the female pelvis. In contrast, injury to the common iliac or external iliac arteries requires surgical repair, because these vessels supply blood to the lower extremity in the absense of collateral blood flow.

Venous bleeding is usually dark and steady. The site of venous injury can be difficult to identify owing to low pressure in the venous system. The repair of venous blood vessels can be difficult because thrombosis commonly occurs at the site of repair, creating risk for pulmonary embolism.

Treatment of vascular injuries that require repair needs a well-planned sequence of actions. The bleeding is initially controlled with packing and pressure. The anesthesiology department and the blood bank are notified. Assistance is requested, from a vascular surgeon or other experienced surgeon. The patient is stabilized with appropriate administration of fluid and blood products. Antibiotic prophylaxis is started as appropriate. The surgical incision should be re-evaluated and, if necessary, enlarged. Dissection is performed along the involved vessel to obtain control of bleeding proximal and distal to the injury, and to provide assess to the site of injury. Methods of repair include ligation, end-to-end anastomosis, or placement of grafts. General principles of vascular repair include removal of proximal and distal thrombi and use of fine synthetic sutures and small needles.

Transfusion of Blood Products

Red blood cells are replaced to correct hypotension secondary to blood loss and to increase oxygen-carrying capacity. A single unit of packed red blood cells usually will increase hemoglobin by 1 g/dL. Most people will tolerate a hemoglobin in the 6- to 7-g/L range. People with cardiac or pulmonary disease generally will require a higher hemoglobin, such as 10 g/L, because of the decreased ability to deliver oxygen to tissue. Transfusion of packed red blood cells is appropriate when a patient has a hemoglobin level of less than 6 g/L, or as indicated when they are symptomatic or have underlying disease.

Platelet transfusions are used to correct deficiencies of circulating platelets. A single unit of platelets usually will increase the platelet count in the average woman by 5000 to 10,000 mm^3. Platelets should be maintained at 50,000 mm^3 before and during surgical procedures.

Fresh frozen plasma is transfused to correct coagulopathies. Platelets may also be needed to correct coagulopathies. Coagulopathies can develop after 5 to 10 units of blood loss. Coagulation studies should be checked periodically. Fresh frozen plasma should be transfused only when indicated by a prothrombin time study or partial thromboplastin time study that is one and one-half times normal.

Cell Saver

The cell saver recycles blood lost during a surgical procedure and readministers it to the patient after the blood is harvested and cleaned. The cell saver requires 500 mL of blood for priming. The cell saver cannot be used during operations that are contaminated with bacteria, such as when the bowel or the vaginal canal is entered, or in operations involving malignancies. The cell saver is expensive to maintain and use; these costs must be balanced against the costs and risks involved in transfusion of banked blood components.

METHODS OF CONTROLLING INTRAOPERATIVE BLEEDING

Packs

Packs can be used to control bleeding quickly while preparing to repair the bleeding source permanently. Intraabdominal packs are useful in controlling diffuse bleeding that is not responding to traditional measures or when there is a component of disseminated intravascular coagulopathies. A sterile plastic bag is placed in the surgical site and packed with continuous gauze packing. The plastic bag is brought through the surgical incision or vaginal cuff. The patient is then closely monitored in the intensive care unit until returning to the operating room in 12 to 48 hours to remove the pack. In the intensive care units, the patient can be transfused with blood products to correct coagulopathies and anemia.

Thumbtacks

Stainless steel thumbtacks that have been sterilized have been used to control bleeding from the presacral plexus. Presacral blood vessels can be damaged during presacral neurectomies, abdominal sacral colpopexy, tumor debulking, and pelvic exenteration. Many reports in the literature describe the application of thumbtacks at the site of active bleeding, with immediate cessation of bleeding even after failure of other methods. Thumbtacks can be applied with a Kelly clamp, a flat instrument such as a retractor, or instruments specifically designed to place thumbtacks in bone. Thumbtacks are left in place permanently.

Hypogastric Artery Ligation

Hypogastric artery ligation is a quick and effective method to control severe pelvic hemorrhage. Bilateral internal iliac artery ligation reduces mean arterial pressure 24%,

mean blood flow 48%, and pulse pressure 85%. Decreased pulse pressure converts the high-pressure arterial system in the pelvis to a low-pressure system and can allow control of hemorrhage with pressure and packs.

The peritoneum is opened lateral to the common iliac at the level of its bifurcation. The ureter is identified and left attached to the peritoneum. The common, external, and internal iliac arteries are identified. The posterior branch of the hypogastric artery is identified on the posterior surface of the hypogastric near its origin. The hypogastric artery is dissected from the hypogastric vein, which is deep and lateral. A permanent suture is passed around the artery, just distal to its posterior branch, and tied. A second suture is usually placed. The same procedure is then performed on the opposite side of the pelvis.

Other Hemostatic Agents

Particularly useful in controlling venous oozing that has not responded to usual methods are microfibrillar collagen preparations (Avitene and Instat) oxidized regenerated cellulose (Surgicel), absorbable gelatin sponge (Gelfoam), and fibrin glue. All have the advantage of being locally applied at the site of bleeding. Their effect, if successful, is rapid.

Microfibrillar collagen preparations stimulate hemostatic activity when in contact with blood. Platelets aggregate on the collagen and release coagulation factors that, with plasma factors, form fibrin and eventually a clot. Microfibrillar collagen is applied to bleeding surfaces with pressure. The pressure is maintained for 3 to 5 minutes. Microfibrillar collagen is resorbed in 8 to 10 weeks in animal studies.

Oxidized regenerated cellulose is an absorbable local hemostatic agent. Its application does not appear to alter the normal physiologic clotting mechanism. Rather, it has a physical effect, forming a gelatinous mass when mixed with blood that helps clot formation. It is applied to oozing surfaces with pressure until hemostasis is obtained. Oxidized regenerated cellulose is bactericidal in vitro against both gram-positive and gram-negative organisms.

Absorbable gelatin sponge is a hemostatic product prepared from purified pork skin granules. It appears to work the same way as oxidized regenerated cellulose. It is also applied with direct pressure to the bleeding site. A second application can be made if necessary.

Fibrin glue forms a fibrin mass when fibrinogen, thrombin, and calcium chloride are mixed. Fibrin glue works particularly well in controlling bleeding when sutures do not work because of friable tissue or adhesions. Because fibrin glue does not rely on host clotting factors, it can be used when a coagulopathy exists. Fibrin glue is prepared by thawing cryoprecipitate, allowing it to reach room temperature, and mixing thrombin with sterile saline solution to a concentration of 1000 units/mL. Cryoprecipitate and thrombin are placed in separate syringes. The two liquids are then slowly squirted onto bleeding surfaces at the same time. A fibrin mass quickly forms, which is effective in controlling hemorrhage. Multiple applications can be made as necessary.

ARTERIAL EMBOLIZATION OF PELVIC VESSELS

Transcatheter arterial embolization of bleeding pelvic vessels is another very useful method of controlling pelvic hemorrhage. Transcatheter arterial embolization has been used in patients with bleeding from cervical pregnancies, bleeding from ectopic and abdominal pregnancies, bleeding posthysterectomy, bleeding from gynecologic malignancies, and severe obstetric hemorrhage. Numerous reports in the literature show transcatheter arterial embolization to be relatively safe, with success rates greater than 90%. Many investigators consider arterial embolization a better first choice than bilateral hypogastric artery ligation to control bleeding. Arterial embolization may be considered before surgery when it is likely that severe hemorrhage may occur, such as with abdominal pregnancies, large fibroid uteri, and gynecologic malignancies.

Embolization is performed by a percutaneous catheterization of the femoral artery with the patient under local anesthesia. The catheter is advanced in a retrograde fashion to provide access to the hypogastric artery. Angiography is performed to identify the specific vessel that is bleeding. A collateral blood vessel is used if the hypogastric artery has been ligated previously. When the site of bleeding is identified, the vessel is cannulated and embolized. A variety of materials are used for embolization, including absorbable gelatin sponge, metal coils, autologous blood, and subcutaneous tissue.

After embolization, angiography is performed, and catheters are removed when the vessel has been occluded. The patient is observed for evidence of further bleeding.

Complications of arterial embolization include pain, fever, and leukocystosis from vascular thrombosis and tissue necrosis. Occasionally, abscess formation, necrosis, or infarction of the uterus, bladder, or gluteus muscles has been reported.

SUMMARY

The management of intraoperative hemorrhage in gynecologic surgery requires knowledge and planning. The gynecologic surgeon must have knowledge of pelvic anatomy and options to control bleeding, including asking for help from other experienced surgeons. Perhaps most important is planning. Planning before surgery can be crucial to quick and effective control of bleeding during surgery.

Suggestions for Future Reading

Fehrman H: Surgical management of life-threatening obstetric and gynecologic hemorrhage. Acta Obstet Gynecol Scand 1988;67:125–128.

Finan MA, Fiorica JV, Hoffman MS, et al: Massive pelvic hemorrhage during gynecologic cancer surgery: "Pack and go back." Gynecol Oncol 1996;62:390–395.

Vedantham V, Goodwin SC, McLucas B, Mohr G: Uterine artery embolization: An underused method of controlling pelvic hemorrhage. Am J Obstet Gynecol 1997;176:938–948.

SEVENTY-FIVE

Alternatives to Hysterectomy for Abnormal Uterine Bleeding

Andrea L. Stein

Abnormal uterine bleeding is one of the most common problems seen in a general gynecologic practice and more frequently in an infertility specialist's office. It is estimated that 15% to 20% of office gynecologic visits are due to menstrual disturbances. Bleeding may be irregular, minimal or annoying; it may also be frequent or heavy, lead to anemia, or become life threatening. Appropriate treatment is dependent on accurate diagnosis of the etiology of abnormal bleeding. In past decades, treatment choices had been restricted owing to limitations in diagnostic equipment, instrumentation for surgery, and medication choices. Hysterectomies were common therapy for managing abnormal uterine bleeding. Fortunately, hysterectomies have now become a "treatment choice" rather than the mainstay of therapy for abnormal uterine bleeding.

The Centers for Disease Control and Prevention has been monitoring the statistics on hysterectomies for many years.[1] Most hysterectomies in the United States are performed with a diagnosis of uterine leiomyoma. Other frequent indications are menstrual disturbances and cervical dysplasia (women younger than age 30 years), endometriosis (30 to 34-year-olds), cancer and prolapse (older than 55 years). It is estimated that 650,000 hysterectomies were performed annually in the early 1980s and that this number has slowly declined since then owing to (1) delayed childbearing and the desire to retain fertility, (2) health care reform, and (3) new medical and surgical treatments.

DIAGNOSIS

Accurate diagnosis of the cause of abnormal uterine bleeding is imperative in order to make appropriate treatment choices. Diagnostic tests should include a beta-human chorionic gonadotropin and complete blood count. Coagulation studies are indicated with severe bleeding and in adolescents with heavy bleeding. Hormonal assays for thyroid abnormalities, hyperprolactinemia, ovulation abnormalities, perimenopause, and polycystic ovarian disease may be indicated. A pelvic examination including careful visualization of the cervix and evaluation of the uterus is necessary. An ultrasound examination is frequently helpful in the diagnosis of uterine leiomyomas and polyps—two of the most common causes of abnormal uterine bleeding. Other useful tests may include an endometrial biopsy and/or visualization of the uterus with a hysterosalpingogram, sonohysterogram, or hysteroscopy.

Etiologies of abnormal uterine bleeding may then be categorized as in Table 75–1.

TREATMENT

There have been many excellent reviews written recently on therapy for abnormal uterine bleeding and leiomyomas.[2-5] At times, more than one therapy may be most effective. Treatment alternatives are summarized.

Observation

A significant percentage of reproductive-age women have an episode of irregular bleeding each year. These episodes occur most frequently during puberty and peri-

Table 75–1. Etiologies of Abnormal Uterine Bleeding

Structural/Organic
Pregnancy and abnormal pregnancies
Endometrial or cervical polyps
Leiomyoma (especially submucosal or intracavitary)
Endometrial hyperplasia
Endometrial or metastatic cancer
Infection
Adenomyosis
Vascular abnormalities
Cervical/vaginal lesions
Endometrial atrophy

Hormonal
Anovulation
Thyroid abnormalities
Hormone-secreting ovarian cyst or tumor
Hyperprolactinemia

Systemic
Liver diseases
Malignancy (e.g., leukemia)
Coagulopathies (e.g., thrombocytopenia, factor deficiencies)

Iatrogenic
Hormone therapy
Intrauterine contraceptive device
Anticoagulation treatment (including aspirin and NSAIDs)
Other medications (e.g., phenothiazine derivatives, antidepressants)

Dysfunctional
A diagnosis of exclusion

NSAIDs, nonsteroidal anti-inflammatory drugs.

menopause. When faced with episodes of irregular bleeding such as occasional anovulatory cycles or at the reproductive "extremes," observation alone may correct the problem. Iron therapy should be initiated to prevent anemia. If the bleeding affects the woman's quality of life or becomes more persistent, hormonal therapy with oral contraceptives or progestins should be initiated if more serious causes are excluded.

Medical Therapy

Few studies adequately assess the benefits of medical therapy for abnormal bleeding owing to the difficulty in precisely measuring menstrual flow. Additionally, benefits cease soon after the discontinuation of treatment, and side effects are frequent. Nevertheless, medical treatment is often effective, inexpensive, and beneficial.

Hormonal

With heavy, acute, or prolonged bleeding with no identifiable abnormality, estrogen and progestin therapy may be used. For very serious situations, intravenous conjugated estrogens (Premarin 10 to 25 mg) is initiated. Concomitant progestin such as intramuscular progesterone-in-oil (100 mg) is frequently helpful. Nausea is a serious consequence of the high-dose estrogen. After bleeding has diminished, daily oral contraceptives with at least 30 to 35 μg ethinyl estradiol should be started to prevent recurrent bleeding. In less acute settings, oral Premarin in doses of 2.5 mg q6–12h (or its equivalent) in combination with progestins (medroxyprogesterone acetate (10 mg or norethindrone 5 mg) frequently stops or diminishes bleeding. Alternatively, three or four tablets daily of oral contraceptives (30 to 50 μg of ethinyl estradiol) can be given. Oral treatment requiring high doses of estrogen should be discontinued after 4 to 5 days and followed by a daily oral contraceptive tablet and more definitive treatment of the underlying problem.

When faced with abnormal bleeding without a structural cause, daily oral contraceptives will often regulate the bleeding pattern and diminish blood flow. In these situations, it is best to start with a monophasic, 30 to 35 μg tablet. These can be administered cyclically or continuously. Alternatively, luteal phase, monthly, or continuous oral progestin may be administered, such as with medroxyprogesterone acetate (2.5 to 10 mg), norethindrone (5 mg), or micronized progesterone (100 to 400 mg). Injectable progestins such as progesterone-in-oil (50 to 200 mg) or Depo-Provera and progestin-containing intrauterine devices are options. Unfortunately, progestin-only treatment is more often associated with the formation of ovarian cysts and endometrial atrophy that may lead to irregular bleeding. Other side effects of hormonal therapy include headaches, mood changes, bloating, breast tenderness, weight gain, cholelithiasis, or cardiovascular accidents.

Danazol (400 mg daily orally) has been used successfully to diminish uterine bleeding. Unfortunately, it is expensive, adversely affects lipid profiles, and has numerous androgenic side effects.

Use of gonadotropin-releasing hormone analogues (GnRHa) has been studied extensively, especially with abnormal bleeding caused by leiomyomas. This is a very effective treatment for inducing amenorrhea within 4 to 6 weeks. Additionally, it frequently shrinks leiomyomas and reduces uterine size in patients with adenomyosis. Unfortunately, it is expensive and causes hypoestrogenemic side effects (e.g., hot flushes, bone demineralization, vaginal dryness). Some of these problems can be minimized with progestin and/or estrogen add-back regimens. The benefits of GnRHa treatment (e.g., amenorrhea, reduction in uterine size), wear off within 2 to 6 months after stopping treatment.

In the future, there may be a role for gonadotropin-releasing hormone antagonists, mifepristone (RU-486), or other "hormones" in treating abnormal bleeding and leiomyomas.

Antifibrinolytic Drugs

There is very limited information on the use of antifibrinolytic medications (tranexamic acid and aminocaproic acid) and abnormal uterine bleeding. These medications are expensive, are associated with frequent side effects, and have a risk of vascular thrombosis.

Nonsteroidal Anti-inflammatory Drugs

Nonsteroidal anti-inflammatory drugs (e.g., ibuprofen, naproxen) have been shown to reduce blood flow in some studies.[3, 5, 6] These medications are inexpensive and well tolerated except in women with gastrointestinal disorders.

Surgery

Therapeutic and diagnostic dilatation and curettage (D&C) have been the traditional modality for treating abnormal uterine bleeding. Unfortunately, there is a very high incidence of false-negative D&Cs when used for diagnosis and a high failure rate when used alone for therapy. A D&C may be useful when the patient has severe hemorrhage or when diagnosing endometrial hyperplasia and cancer. In most other circumstances, diagnostic hysteroscopy is a better technique for accurately assessing the cause of abnormal bleeding.

Hysteroscopy

Hysteroscopic procedures can be classified as diagnostic or therapeutic; they are performed as an office procedure or in an outpatient operating room setting. The diagnostic hysteroscopy, usually with an endometrial biopsy, can frequently determine the cause of abnormal bleeding. Therapy is determined by the equipment availability and the surgeon's skill. In the office, one is limited by the size of the hysteroscope, distention media available, and anesthetic restrictions. Small polyps and pedunculated fibroids can be removed, but larger lesions are difficult to extract. Broad-based, large and/or multiple lesions are frequently better treated in an operating room setting with general or appropriate regional anesthetic. Using an operating hysteroscope or resectoscope, large polyps, leiomyoma, adhesions, retained products of conception, foreign bodies, and uterine anomalies can be removed. Complications include fluid and electrolyte imbalance, infection, thermal injuries, hematometra, bleeding, uterine perforation, and adhesion formation. There are no comparative studies for using hysteroscopic procedures versus more "traditional" approaches such as hysterectomy or abdominal myomectomy, but it is logical to conclude that there are significant cost savings and higher retention of fertility when hysteroscopy is employed.

Hysteroscopic Endometrial Ablation

In the late 1940s, Asherman[7] described amenorrhea in women after uterine trauma. Since the early 1980s, gynecologists have been reporting techniques to induce uterine trauma and amenorrhea or hypomenorrhea. Most procedures use a laser system or electrosurgical unit. Amenorrhea or hypomenorrhea is achieved in 80% to 95% of patients. It is important to rule out malignancy or unresolved hyperplasia before treatment or when bleeding occurs after ablation. Myomas and polyps should be removed before or concomitantly with the ablation procedure. Preoperative medication to thin the endometrium has been controversial, with most studies[8] showing improved success rates if medication is used. There may be a more subjective ease in performing the procedure if medications such as GnRHa are used preoperatively, and, possibly, improved outcomes if it is used postoperatively. Five-year follow-ups after ablation show a high degree of patient satisfaction but up to a 40% "failure" rate. Many of these women undergo repeat ablation or hysterectomy. Failures happen frequently when the initial cause of bleeding was multiple leiomyomas or adenomyosis. Numerous studies[2, 5, 9] have assessed the complications of ablation procedures using laser or electrosurgical equipment, with the single most important factor being operator skill.

Nonhysteroscopic Endometrial Ablation

Several new technologies are available for endometrial ablation that require far less surgical skill than those described previously. The ThermChoice thermal transfer balloon has been available for use in the United States since December 1997, with initial results similar to those of traditional endometrial ablation. It requires minimal surgical skill, takes only a few minutes to perform, and has few complications. Long-term follow-up data are still lacking. Other technologies that are still under investigation are reviewed elsewhere.[2, 5] They include cryotherapy, laser, microwaves, and phototherapy. All these systems are being developed to improve efficacy of ablation, decrease cost, present fewer complications, and lessen the need for specialized surgical skills and anesthesia.

Laparoscopic and Abdominal Myomectomy

Leiomyomas are extremely common in reproductive-age women. Problems caused by leiomyomas (especially bleeding, pain, or pressure) are the leading cause for hysterectomies in the United States. In women desiring maintenance of their fertility, myomectomies can safely be performed by laparoscopy, laparotomy, or laparoscopically assisted myomectomy.

Other

Myolysis with a laser or bipolar instrument has been effectively used to treat leiomyoma. This may be used as an adjuvant to the more traditional myomectomy procedures (especially with multiple leiomyoma) or, with experience, as the primary procedure.

Uterine artery embolization has been used to treat leiomyoma since the mid-1990s, and since the late 1970s, for serious pelvic hemorrhage. This procedure is usually performed by an interventional radiologist. This novel treatment is quite successful in managing leiomyoma, although long-term follow-up and the effects of embolization on future fertility are still unknown.

SPECIAL SITUATIONS

Pregnancy

Normal, early pregnancies often present with vaginal bleeding. Bleeding is even more common with abnormal pregnancies, such as ectopics or missed abortion. It is relatively frequent in pregnancies following controlled ovarian stimulation. Therefore, it is imperative to perform a pregnancy test on all reproductive age women with abnormal uterine bleeding. Even with a negative test, bleeding may occur with a chronic ectopic pregnancy or retained products of conception.

Severe Bleeding

Therapy for prolonged or profuse bleeding with severe anemia and/or hemostatic imbalance may require intense fluid management and blood component replacement. Correct diagnosis of the etiology of severe bleeding such as an intracavitary lesion, incomplete abortion, or cancer is very useful but frequently unsuccessful. At this time, bleeding is most appropriately stopped with hormonal therapy (discussed previously) and/or surgical intervention. Unfortunately, when heavy bleeding is present, many minimally invasive procedures (e.g., hysteroscopy) will not be useful in the diagnosis or treatment owing to limited visibility or efficaciousness. On occasion, temporary measures such as placement of an intrauterine balloon for direct pressure might be helpful.

Adolescence

Adolescence presents a unique situation, because there are frequent anovulatory cycles and stressors that might affect a young woman's menstrual pattern. When prolonged or severe bleeding is present, serious medical problems should be investigated (e.g., coagulopathies, malignancy, trauma). Other conditions to evaluate include pregnancy, hypothalamic disorders, thyroid disease, polycystic ovarian disease, infection, medications, systemic diseases, ovarian cysts, or pelvic tumors. Bleeding from anovulatory cycles are best treated either expectantly or using low-dose oral contraceptives or progestins, along with iron replacement when indicated.

Perimenopause

Few women become menopausal without experiencing some unusual bleeding. This can often be managed by reassurance and observation. Endometrial biopsies should be used to rule out hyperplasia and cancer. Transvaginal ultrasonography to identify structural abnormalities or thickened endometrium is very useful. Low-dose oral contraceptives are a safe treatment choice for "abnormal" perimenopausal bleeding.

Reproductive Age

Among the most common causes of abnormal bleeding during the reproductive years are chronic anovulation, polycystic ovarian disease, luteal phase defects, and ovarian cysts. All of these are best treated with hormonal therapy unless pregnancy is desired. Then, appropriate fertility medications are used.

Adenomyosis

Adenomyosis frequently presents with abnormally heavy uterine bleeding and/or cramps. It can be difficult to manage because treatment failures (medical and surgical) are common. GnRHa have effectively reduced uterine volume and bleeding but only temporarily. Endometrial ablation may be useful.

Tamoxifen

Abnormal bleeding in women on tamoxifen should be investigated promptly because uterine polyps, hyperplasia, and cancer are associated with the use of this medication.

Hyperplasia and Cancer

Endometrial hyperplasia and cancer frequently present with abnormal bleeding. Hyperplasias without atypia are best managed with oral contraceptives or progestins.

Dysfunctional Uterine Bleeding

Dysfunctional uterine bleeding is a diagnosis of exclusion. It is best treated with observation, medication (e.g., hormonal, nonsteroidal anti-inflammatory drugs), or endometrial ablation. Hysterectomy is a treatment choice but should not be the initial or sole method for approaching this condition.

Conclusion

A woman presenting with abnormal uterine bleeding is a common problem seen by many clinicians. Improved and sophisticated diagnostic tools allow us to identify many causes of bleeding that were previously undetected. Treatment of women with abnormal bleeding in adolescence and reproductive years involves correcting underlying pathologic conditions and hormone therapy. Improved surgical instrument in the 21st century and a wider array of medications allow women who are finished with childbearing to have many alternatives to treat abnormal bleeding. Hysterectomy should no longer be the only treatment option presented to women with abnormal uterine bleeding.

References

1. Lepine LA, Hillis SD, Marchbanks PA, et al: Hysterectomy surveillance—United States, 1980–1983. CDC Surv Summaries MMWR Morb Mortal Wkly Rep 1997;46 (SS-4):1–15.
2. Brill AI: What is the role of hysteroscopy in the management of abnormal uterine bleeding? Clin Obstet Gynecol 1995;38:319–345.
3. Chen BH, Guidice LC: Dysfunctional uterine bleeding. West J Med 1998;169:280–284.
4. Davis KM, Schlaff WD: Medical management of uterine fibromyomata. Obstet Gynecol Clin North Am 1995;22:727–738.
5. Stabinsky SA, Einstein M, Breen JL: Modern treatments of menorrhagia attributable to dysfunctional uterine bleeding. Obstet Gynecol Surv 1999;54:61–72.
6. Ylikorkala O, Pekonen F: Naproxen reduces idiopathic but not fibromyoma-induced menorrhagia. Obstet Gynecol 1986;68:10–12.
7. Asherman JG: Amenorrhea traumatica (atretica). J Obstet Gynaecol Br Emp 1948:55:23–30.
8. Brooks PG, Serden SP, Davos I: Hormonal inhibition of the endometrium for resectoscopic ablation. Am J Obstet Gynecol 1991;164:1601–1608.
9. Brooks PG: Complications of operative hysteroscopy: How safe is it? Clin Obstet Gynecol 1992;35:256–261.

Complications of Hysteroscopy: Prevention, Recognition, and Management

Rafael F. Valle

Hysteroscopy is a surgical procedure that requires manipulation of the cervix and uterus and may involve dissection and removal of intrauterine pathologic lesions; therefore, it has a potential for complications, as does any other surgical procedure. These complications may be related to the procedure itself, the distending medium used, the specific surgical procedure being performed, any additional energy modalities that may be required, and the type of anesthesia used.

PROCEDURAL COMPLICATIONS

Complications related to the procedure are similar to those that may occur during intrauterine manipulation, such as curettage. These complications are laceration of the cervix by a tenaculum, uterine perforation, bleeding, and intrauterine infection. Cervical lacerations from the tenaculum can occur when excessive traction is used during manipulation. They can be prevented by using gentle manipulation and can easily be corrected by suturing the defect. Minor lacerations can occur with placement of a tenaculum in the cervix; uterine perforation can occur at the time of uterine sounding or particularly during cervical dilatation. Bleeding can occur if the uterine walls are damaged or a pathologic tumor is disturbed. Uterine perforation is possible either during blind uterine sounding before hysteroscopy or when the hysteroscope is advanced blindly and forcibly into the uterine cavity. Perforations with the hysteroscope should not occur if the endoscope is introduced atraumatically under direct vision, following the path in front of the scope that the panoramic view has created with the distending medium. The use of a uterine sound seldom is required because the hysteroscope, guided under direct vision, follows the cervical canal into the uterine cavity.

When these complications occur, treatment varies according to the size and location of the perforation. Perforation with a uterine sound seldom requires treatment. If it occurs, the hysteroscopy should be discontinued and the patient observed for possible decompensation. However, when uterine perforation occurs with an operative hystero-scope, further evaluation may be necessary, including laparoscopy, to assess persistent bleeding or to ensure hemostasis. If perforation of the uterus occurs during operative procedures with mechanical instrumentation, usually the treatment does not vary from that for perforations with a hysteroscope. Nonetheless, when additional energy, such as electrosurgery or laser, is used and a perforation occurs with this type of surgery, further evaluation is mandatory to rule out damage to adjacent structures. If the laparoscopic evaluation is negative, the patient requires close follow-up to detect early signs of infection, intestinal injury, or delayed hemorrhage.

Infection is a possible complication from introducing an endoscope in the uterine cavity, but its occurrence is rare. With adequate precautions, such as appropriate disinfection and sterilization of instruments coupled with proper technique, this complication should be avoidable. The appropriate selection, evaluation, and preparation of patients for hysteroscopy helps prevent infection. To avoid contamination of the cervical canal and uterine cavity during hysteroscopy, sterile techniques should be maintained and the procedure performed under meticulous protocols.[1, 2]

COMPLICATIONS OF DISTENDING MEDIUM

Complications related to the distending media vary according to the medium used. When CO_2 gas exceeds the flow rate of 100 mL/min, hypercapnia, arrhythmias, acidosis, and even gas emboli may occur. These problems can be avoided by using machines specifically designed for hysteroscopy, which electronically calibrate the appropriate flow rate of delivery, about 40 to 60 mL/min, and which do not permit intrauterine pressures of more than 100 to 150 mm Hg. Other insufflators not specifically designed for hysteroscopy, particularly those used for laparoscopy, should never be used to distend the uterus.

When low-viscosity fluids are used to distend the uterine cavity during operative hysteroscopy, the most frequent complications that may be encountered are secondary to excessive fluid absorption and electrolyte imbalance, particularly if fluids devoid of electrolytes are used. It is important, therefore, to control meticulously the quantity of fluids being administered and to measure carefully the quantity of fluids recovered. When fluids with electrolytes are used, such as Ringer's lactate solution, normal saline solution, and dextrose 5% in normal saline solution, the fluid osmolality is maintained by sodium and its accompanying chloride and bicarbonate. Therefore, when excessive fluid absorption occurs, even though the patient may develop signs or symptoms of fluid overload such as pulmonary edema, hyponatremia does not occur. However, when fluids devoid of electrolytes, like dextrose 5%, glycine 1.5%, sorbitol 3%, or mannitol 5%, are used, free fluid may remain in the intravascular space, resulting in fluid overload and hyponatremia.

Glycine 1.5% is a nonelectrolytic irrigating fluid used commonly for transurethral urologic surgical procedures. It is a sterile, nonpyrogenic, hypotonic solution of the amino acid glycine. It is a nonelectrolytic solution with an osmolality of 200 mOsm/L. Its degradation will result in ammonia and oxalate crystals that can cause problems of mental confusion or precipitation of oxalate crystals in the kidneys, or both, should excessive intravascular absorption followed by degradation occur.

Sorbitol 3% solution also can be used to distend the uterus. It is a nonelectrolytic solution, electrically nonconductive, with an osmolality of 165 mOsm/L. Because it is a reduced form of dextrose, it is metabolized to carbon dioxide and water and excreted by a normally functioning kidney.

Finally, mannitol 5% is an inert substance with a 275-mOsm/L osmolality that acts as an osmotic diuretic and helps in the removal of free water if excessive amounts have been absorbed. About 6% to 10% of the absorbed mannitol is metabolized and the remainder filtered by the kidney. The half-life of mannitol in the plasma is 15 minutes. However, significant amounts of mannitol retained within the vascular space may draw fluid into this space and increase the intravascular volume as well.

High-viscosity fluids such as dextran 32% (Hyskon) were used frequently in the late 1970s and early 1980s as a medium to distend the uterine cavity. At present, their use has decreased significantly because of the poor recovery, as no continuous flow can be established with the instrumentation available. Nonetheless, it is still a good alternative as a distending medium owing to its high viscosity that requires only small amounts to perform minor hysteroscopic procedures. Be aware, however, that because of its osmotic properties, when absorbed into the vascular space via the uterus it may trigger pulmonary edema by increasing the vascular osmotic pressure. Furthermore, if excessive amounts are absorbed (more than 500 mL), it may also produce a coagulopathy with bleeding as well as changes in fibrinogen, clotting factors V, VIII, and IX, and the factor VIII—von Willebrand complex. It has been calculated that the fluid accumulated in the intravascular tree by osmotic absorption will be about ten times the amount of dextran absorbed.

Additionally, owing to its large molecular size (more than 70,000) dextran is not removed by the kidney. This contributes to its long half-life in the intravascular space (up to 6 to 7 days). As a result, on occasion, plasmapheresis has been required in cases of excessive intravascular absorption, when the fluid overload has failed to respond to appropriate ventilation and diuretics. When hysteroscopic surgery is performed with mechanical instruments or with lasers, methods that are not concerned with electrical conduction, distending fluids and electrolytes can be used. Ringer's lactate solution, normal saline solution, and dextrose 5% in normal saline solution are most appropriate in these instances. Nonetheless, even when isotonic fluids are absorbed, fluid overload may occur. Therefore, appropriate monitoring of both inflow and outflow is most important; should more than 1.5 to 2 L of intravasated fluid occur, immediate diuresis should be established to prevent pulmonary edema.[2, 3]

Three factors are taken into consideration when surgeons administer fluids into the uterus under pressure: (1) control of intrauterine pressure to no more than 100 mm Hg, so as not to exceed the mean arterial pressure, (2) expedite the procedure limiting the time to no more than 1 hour, and (3) avoid or limit extensive intramyometrial dissections.[4]

Although electronic pumps have been introduced that provide a controlled intrauterine pressure, it is important to remember that if the myometrium is dissected at a 3- to 4-mm depth from the surface, the intrauterine pressure required for intravasation will be much lower than 100 mm Hg. Therefore, these procedures should be expedited, and carried out at even lower filling pressures, and the amount of fluid infused and recovered should be accurately measured to calculate the deficit.

Because the most threatening situations of fluid overload may occur with fluid devoid of electrolytes, it is important to monitor electrolytes serially, specifically sodium, during an operation. At present, systems are available that can provide rapid results, requiring a minimal amount of whole blood to determine the level of electrolytes. These methods are most useful for operative hysteroscopy and will provide point-of-care testing for prevention rather than monitoring electrolytes for treatment, as has been traditional.

Because the threshold of toxicity is greater with fluids devoid of electrolytes, it is important to be meticulous in the monitoring of inflow and outflow. If a deficit of 1 L or more occurs, immediate monitoring of electrolytes (sodium) should be done and diuresis and electrolyte replacement instituted.

THE POST-TURP SYNDROME

The post-TURP (transurethral resection of the prostate) syndrome, or the TCRE (transcervical resection of endometrium) syndrome in gynecology, is a constellation of symptoms and signs associated with absorption of large volumes of nonelectrolytic distending media. Patients develop bradycardia and hypertension, followed by hypotension, nausea, vomiting, headache, visual disturbances, agitation, confusion, and lethargy. The symptoms are a result of hypervolemia, dilutional hyponatremia, and decreased osmolality. If unrecognized and untreated, seizures, cardiovascular collapse, and death may ensue. This syndrome is well known to urologists and anesthesiologists.

Apparently women, particularly menstruating women, are at greater risk of developing this problem, owing perhaps to some derangement of the ATPase, a brain enzyme that helps in extruding water and solutes to protect itself. The TCRE syndrome is more dangerous in these women and increases their risk of death if treatment is not provided early in its development. In fact, with chronic (greater than 48 hours) hyponatremia, the brain extrudes water in an attempt to achieve osmotic equilibrium; the desiccation and demyelination that result can be further aggravated if sodium replacement is rapid and aggressive, because the transient vascular hyperosmolality will further draw free water from tissues. In the acute state, this may be resolved by adding 1 to 2 mOsm/L of sodium per hour with a total of no more than 12 mOsm/L in 24 hours to correct acute onset of hyponatremia. No attempt should be made to normalize serum sodium rapidly, but only to achieve a level at which serious secondary problems will not occur. Therefore, 130 to 135 mOsm/L will be the goal. Patients, nonetheless, will require intensive care unit monitoring with serial determination of electrolytes and urine output. Usually, hypertonic saline solution for correction of hyponatremia is not required, and normal saline solution may be sufficient. This condition usually reverts in 12 to 24 hours.

For these reasons, when extensive dissection in the uterus is foreseen, regional anesthesia may be the anesthetic of choice, because then the patient will remain awake and the first signs of intoxication will show with some confusion, tremor and/or nausea, and headache.

When fluids devoid of electrolytes are used, if a deficit of 800 to 1000 mL occurs the operation should be stopped and the serum sodium level determined. If no lowering of the serum sodium level has occurred, the operation could proceed if it could be completed in a short period of time. If the serum sodium level is lower than normal or a prolonged operation to complete the procedure is expected, the procedure should be aborted and completed at another time. Further decompensation in the serum sodium level with fluid deficits of more than 1000 mL, should be immediately and appropriately corrected. The use of diuretics under these circumstances should be cautiously undertaken, with meticulous serial monitoring of electrolytes.

ANESTHESIA COMPLICATIONS

Complications related to the anesthetic used may occur. Local anesthetics may on occasion cause allergic reactions, but the most common complications are due to intravasa-

tion. The type of anesthetic used, that is, whether an ester or an amide, has an impact on its degradation and toxicity. The levels of toxicity of these anesthetics should be kept in mind so that they can be appropriately handled if problems of intravasation occur. Usually intravenous diazepam (Valium) helps in the correction. Anesthetics of the ester type, such as chloroprocaine (Nesacaine) and procaine, have a low toxicity, and when intravasation occurs the rapid degradation by plasma pseudocholinesterase helps in their elimination. Because the amount of local anesthetic generally required for a paracervical block is small—3 to 4 mL in each uterosacral ligament—toxicity is markedly decreased. Problems related to general anesthesia and regional anesthesia are relegated to the care of the anesthesiologist and are not discussed here.

LASER ENERGY FOR OPERATIVE HYSTEROSCOPY: POSSIBLE COMPLICATIONS

When the surgeon uses fiberoptic lasers, it is important to use either the bare fiber or only those that are of the sculpted or extruded type, avoiding coaxial fibers, which are fitted with sapphire tips. Lasers with these tips require continuous cooling by gases or fluids, and their use in the uterus has been associated with massive intravasation of the gas or air resulting in a fatal gas embolus. When using these fine fibers to operate in the uterus, perforation of the uterine wall can occur if the fiber is advanced too fast or inadvertently into the uterine wall. This should be avoided by operating at all times with these fibers under direct view and with caution. If uterine perforation occurs and the fiber is activated, the possibility of injury to other organs must always be kept in mind. Because of the reflective nature of these lasers and their attraction to pigments, the operator and assistant personnel should protect their eyes with special goggles or filters to avoid retinal injuries.

ELECTROSURGERY: COMPLICATIONS

Electrosurgery also may cause problems and complications in its use. Because monopolar current is used more frequently with hysteroscopy, the patient should be properly grounded, with an appropriate ground plate serving as a return electrode. Only insulated electrodes and probes should be used, and the machines delivering this type of energy should be properly calibrated, with display of the waveform used and the wattage selected. This energy should never be activated unless the precise and complete view of the area being treated is achieved. Finally, only fluids devoid of electrolytes should be used to distend the uterine cavity.

Recently introduced are electrosurgical electrodes that can be operated with use of saline solutions which obviates most concerns of hyponatremic complications. Although not truely bipolar, they simulate a bipolar system by passing the electrical current from one electrode to another and by increasing the current density, creating a vapor chamber that destroys the tissue by vaporization. These methods, such as the ERA sleeve, VersaPoint, and other similar electrodes that may be activated under saline solutions, are being used now in clinical practice.

It is important to remember that intravasation of excessive saline solution still may produce pulmonary edema. Furthermore, when excessive saline solutions are used and the urine output is not well monitored, the patient may excrete hypertonic urine and develop a condition called desalination. This involves the excretion of hypertonic urine made up of sodium and potassium and liberation of free water into the intravascular system that not only may contribute to pulmonary edema but also may produce a delayed hyponatremia. This process has been observed in patients who received excessive amounts of only isotonic solution like saline; later, these patients developed delayed hyponatremia and died.[5] It is therefore important to maintain similar monitoring systems as outlined earlier for fluids containing electrolytes, specifically monitoring the inflow and outflow.

It is recommended that surgeons terminate the procedure or institute active diuretic therapy when patients absorb more than 1.5 to 2 L of saline solution. Additionally, because electrocautery systems require increased power to overcome electrical dispersion by these saline solutions, proper monitoring of insulation and possible alternative pathways to electricity should be instituted.

COMPLICATIONS FROM VARIOUS HYSTEROSCOPIC PROCEDURES

Some complications are unique to the particular hysteroscopic procedure performed. The most common complications related to hysteroscopic surgery are bleeding and uterine perforation. These can occur at the time of division of uterine septa, resection of intrauterine adhesions, resection of myomas, endometrial ablation, or tubal cannulation. Perforation of the uterus may predispose the patient to injuries to other organs in the pelvic cavity. Therefore, when difficult hysteroscopic procedures are to be performed, particularly if the uterine cavity's symmetry is markedly distorted, concomitant laparoscopy must be utilized as a helpful adjunct in preventing additional injuries

to adjacent organs. Although infection from hysteroscopic procedures is uncommon, prophylactic antibiotics are selectively used in some patients, particularly those being treated to preserve fertility, such as treatment of uterine septa, treatment of intrauterine adhesions, and tubal cannulation procedures.

SUMMARY AND CONCLUSIONS

It is undeniable that the use of hysteroscopy and hysteroscopic surgery has increased since the early 1980s. This increase has been the result of gynecologists learning these techniques and the introduction of new applications for operative hysteroscopy, as well as the interest of industry in manufacturing better systems for hysteroscopy, particularly continuous-flow hysteroscopes and resectoscopes adapted with a variety of electrodes that permit electrosurgery inside the uterus. Low-viscosity fluids have become the method of choice to distend the uterine cavity during operative hysteroscopy, whether with electrolytes or devoid of electrolytes when electrosurgery is used. Because therapeutic hysteroscopic procedures usually require more time than diagnostic ones, the use of low-viscosity fluids during these procedures may result in excessive fluid absorption by patients and therefore predispose them to pulmonary edema and possible hyponatremia. It is important, therefore, to establish close monitoring of the fluids used to avoid excessive deficits. The different methods of operating with a hysteroscope should be used carefully after appropriate training of physicians. Establishment of specific protocols for all hysteroscopic procedures is of utmost importance to avoid, detect early, and appropriately treat untoward conditions when they occur.

References

1. Baggish MS: Complications of hysteroscopic surgery. In Baggish MS, Barbot J, Valle RF (eds): Diagnostic and Operative Hysteroscopy. A Text and Atlas, 2nd ed. St. Louis, Mosby, 1999, pp 367–379.
2. Valle RF: A Manual of Clinical Hysteroscopy. New York, Parthenon, 1998, pp 41–46.
3. Witz CA, Silverberg KM, Burns WN, et al: Complications associated with absorption of hysteroscopic fluid media. Fertil Steril 1993;60:745–756.
4. Garry R, Hasham F, Kokri MS, Mooney P: The effect of pressure on fluid absorption during endometrial ablation. J Gynecol Surg 1992;8:1–10.
5. Steele A, Gowelshanker M, Abrahamson S, et al: Postoperative hyponatremia despite near-isotonic saline infusion: A phenomenon of desalination. Ann Intern Med 1997;126:20–25.

SEVENTY-SEVEN

Contemporary Options in Substance Abuse Treatment for Women

Judith Fry McComish, Rivka Greenberg, and

Kimberley Shewmaker

Substance use by women is an important public health concern. The number of people who use and abuse alcohol and other drugs make it, for some observers, the primary health problem in the United States. The Institute of Medicine recommends that all patients be asked about substance use during routine health care visits, included in the assessment of other behavior and lifestyle issues. For women, the American College of Obstetricians and Gynecologists recommends that all pregnant women be asked about substance use at the first prenatal care visit, and the Substance Abuse and Mental Health Services Administration (SAMHSA) recommends that women aged 60 years and older be screened for alcohol and prescription drug use as part of routine physical examinations. Because gynecologists and obstetricians are often primary care providers for women, it is especially important to incorporate substance abuse screening and referral for treatment into routine obstetric and gynecologic practice.

PREVALENCE

Although substance use is higher among men than women, recent prevalence studies have found an increase in the use of alcohol and other drugs by women. In 1993, it was reported that approximately 200,000 women were expected to die as a result of substance-related illnesses. In the 1994 national survey on drug use from the Monitoring the Future Study (1975 to 1994),[1] the prevalence of past-month use of illicit drugs among women 19 to 32 years of age was 11.7%. Past-month use of alcohol was 61.8%. Rate of use for marijuana was 10.1%; amphetamines, 1.5%; crack/cocaine, 1%; and tranquilizers, 0.5%. Estimates from the 1995 National Household Survey on Drug Abuse[2] indicate that women account for 44.7% of reported illicit drug use. Among women of childbearing age, 15 to 44 years, 7.3%, or 4.3 million, reported past-month illicit drug use. The rate was higher among women without children (9.3%), and lower in pregnant women (2.3%). However, more than 1.6 million women who used illicit drugs were living with children.

To determine patterns of substance use among women from different age groups and ethnic backgrounds, Kandel and colleagues[3] examined data from three National Household surveys. The highest rate of alcohol use was in white women between ages 18 and 34, highest marijuana use was in white women aged 18 to 25, and highest cocaine use was in African American women aged 26 to 34 years. These data support results of earlier studies that indicate that, in general, alcohol and drug use among women is highest among white women, with an increasing trend for African American women to use crack cocaine.

Recent studies in Michigan,[4] Massachusetts,[5] and Oregon that used meconium samples to determine the prevalence of illicit drug use among *pregnant women* found higher rates of drug use than those in the National Household Survey[2] and other studies that used only self-report. The prevalence of fetal drug exposure ranged from 11.4% in Oregon, to 16.4% in Massachusetts, and 17.5% in Michigan. In the Michigan study, fetal drug exposure to marijuana was 7.6%; to opiates, 7.4%; and to cocaine, 4.9%. These studies found no associations between race or income status of the mother and illicit drug use.[4]

Among *older women*, use of illicit drugs is minimal. However, use of alcohol, prescription, and over-the-counter drugs is a major concern. Although alcohol and prescription drug misuse affects up to 17% of adults 60 years old and older, this issue had not been addressed in either the substance abuse or gerontologic research literature until recently. Therefore, this problem is believed to be underestimated and underidentified. It is estimated that 2.5 million older adults, between 1% and 3% of whom are women, have problems related to alcohol.[6] Additionally, about 21% of all hospitalized patients aged 40 years and older have alcohol-related problems,[6] and 20% of persons in nursing homes, most of whom are women, are alcoholic.[7] Among community-dwelling older adults, the prevalence of alcoholism is 2% to 15%,[8, 9] and among general medical and psychiatric inpatients, 18% to 44%.[10, 11] Furthermore, one study found that for patients aged 65 years and older,[12] the prevalence of hospitalizations for alcohol-related medical conditions and for myocardial infarction is similar.

Adults 65 years old and older consume more prescribed and over-the-counter drugs than any other group in the United States, with 30% taking eight or more prescription drugs a day. Although elderly women constitute only 11% of the population, they are prescribed more than 25% of all drugs, which is 2.5 times the number prescribed for elderly men. Given these statistics, it is not surprising that older women are more likely than their younger counterparts to misuse prescription drugs, most often benzodiazepines.

ETIOLOGY AND CONSEQUENCES OF WOMEN'S SUBSTANCE ABUSE

For women who abuse substances, alcohol or illicit drug use typically begins in adolescence. They are often introduced to alcohol or other drugs by men, usually a boyfriend or male relative, and move from substance use to substance abuse or dependence without awareness. Women use drugs in relationships and sometimes will continue to use or use at a higher rate (more frequently or higher dose) to maintain a relationship or to obliviate awareness of the negative aspects of the relationship. Physiologically, women become addicted more readily than men, becoming intoxicated with smaller quantities of alcohol and suffering negative health consequences of excessive drinking in a shorter length of time.

Most women who abuse drugs have experienced situational and emotional problems. Many come from homes in which one or both parents abused alcohol or other substances. It is estimated that as many as 75% of women who seek substance abuse treatment have a history of physical, emotional, or sexual abuse during childhood. Many others are exposed to violence or are in abusive relationships in adulthood.

Another common theme in the lives of substance-abusing women is loss with unresolved grief. Many have grown up in families in which one or both parents were either emotionally unavailable or left the family through abandonment or death. They often live in communities with high levels of chronic violence and have witnessed violent trauma, some resulting in the death of children, relatives, or significant others. Additionally, those who are mothers may have permanently lost children owing to death or judicial removal, or temporarily lost custody, with treatment as a condition for reunification. The stigma of losing custody of their children and the concomitant societal view of failure to meet maternal role expectations is a burden carried by the women. Long-term effects of nonresolution of loss or trauma are depression, low self-esteem, posttraumatic stress disorder (PTSD), and difficulty establishing healthy relationships with significant others, including their children. Thus, women who abuse drugs present in the health care setting with higher rates of depression, anxiety disorders, and PTSD.

Health Consequences

Women who abuse drugs and alcohol are at high risk for multiple adverse health consequences. As their drug dependence increases, women may have difficulty finding money to support their drug habit, which puts them at greater risk for poor nutrition, and increases the likelihood that they will not receive consistent medical or dental care, either preventive or remedial. The women are also more likely to engage in illegal behaviors, like theft or prostitution, or unsafe sexual practices to obtain drugs. These behaviors place them in situations with increased risk for violence and sexually transmitted diseases, including HIV infection and AIDS, and the health problems associated with them. Injection drug users are at high risk for infection with hepatitis C virus (HCV), through sharing of contaminated needles or equipment for snorting cocaine. Approximately 20% of the cases of HCV infection are transmitted sexually, with highest rates among persons with multiple sex partners, making this a high risk for women who engage in illicit sex or prostitution to support their drug habit. Finally, a woman with HCV may transmit the disease to her infant, and the risk increases if the woman has both HCV and HIV infection.

Among women who use heroin, needle use can cause circulatory problems, which induces risk for infection, and embolism. Many women may experience skin ulcers or osteomyelitis due to contaminated needles. Secondary effects of these infections may be severe, including amputations, endocarditis, or pneumothorax.

Effects on Fetus and Infant

The teratogenic effects of drug use during pregnancy on the developing fetus and infant are a major concern. The two addictive substances used most commonly during pregnancy are nicotine (cigarettes) and alcohol. Cigarette use during pregnancy has been associated with low birth weight (LBW) and preterm delivery. The teratogenic effects of alcohol use during pregnancy are well documented and include LBW, intrauterine growth retardation, fetal alcohol syndrome (FAS), and alcohol-related birth defects or neurodevelopmental disorders (ARBDs or ARNDs).[13–16] In the early 1990s, the Centers for Disease Control and Prevention[17] identified FAS as a leading cause of mental retardation in the United States. FAS (Table 77–1) is diagnosed when three primary characteristics occur together: growth deficiency, a characteristic pattern of abnormalities primarily observable in the face, and some manifestations of central nervous system (CNS) dysfunction. *Alcohol-related effects* is a term used if some, but not all, of the characteristics of FAS are present. Children with ARBD may exhibit a wide variety of congenital anomalies: cardiac, skeletal, renal, ocular, and auditory. Children with ARND have the CNS neurodevelopmental abnormalities or the behavioral or cognitive abnormalities listed as 1C and 3E in Table 77–1.

Among women who use illicit drugs during pregnancy, there are high rates of polydrug use, including use of tobacco, alcohol, or psychotropic drugs in combination with illicit drugs. Street drugs are rarely pure. To increase profits for drug traffickers, the illicit drug is frequently

Table 77–1. Diagnostic Criteria for Fetal Alcohol Syndrome (FAS) and Alcohol-Related Neurodevelopmental Disorders (ARNDs)

1. *FAS with confirmed maternal alcohol exposure*
   A. Confirmed maternal alcohol exposure
   B. Dysmorphic features (primarily observed in the face, such as short palpebral fissures, a pattern of flattened midface, smooth or long philtrum, and thin upper lip)
   C. Evidence of growth retardation in at least one of the following: low birth weight for gestational age, decelerating weight over time not due to nutrition, disproportional low weight to height
   D. Evidence of CNS neurodevelopmental abnormalities in at least one of the following: decreased cranial size at birth, structural brain abnormalities (e.g., microcephaly, partial or complete agenesis of the corpus callosum, cerebellar hypoplasia), neurologic hard or soft signs (as age-appropriate), such as impaired fine motor skills, neurosensory hearing loss, poor tandem gait, poor eye-hand coordination
2. *FAS without confirmed maternal alcohol exposure*
   B, C, and D as above
3. *Partial FAS with confirmed maternal alcohol exposure*
   A. Confirmed maternal alcohol exposure
   B. Evidence of some components of the pattern of characteristic facial anomalies
      Either C or D as above, or E
   C. See above
   D. See above
   E. Evidence of a complex pattern of behavior or cognitive abnormalities that are inconsistent with developmental level and cannot be explained by familial background or environment alone, such as learning difficulties, deficits in school performance, poor impulse control, problems in social perception, deficits in higher-level receptive and expressive language, poor capacity for abstraction or metacognition, specific deficits in mathematical skills, or problems in memory, attention, or judgment

From Stratton K, Howe C, Battaglia FC (eds): Fetal Alcohol Syndrome: Diagnosis, Epidemiology, Prevention, and Treatment. Washington, DC, Institute of Medicine, 1996.

combined with other substances that may also influence the effect of the drug on the developing fetus. Consequently, it is difficult to determine the effects of specific illicit drugs on developmental outcomes of infants and children. Because most research on effects of drugs on infants has been conducted on women in publicly funded treatment programs, excluding women with more economic resources, little is known about the influence of illicit drugs on infants of wealthy women. With these caveats in mind, a brief summary of recent research findings on prenatal drug exposure follows.

Like nicotine or alcohol, prenatal exposure to marijuana, heroin, methadone, and cocaine are all associated with LBW and newborn CNS problems. Common CNS problems include jitteriness, excessive crying, startle reflex abnormality, high-pitched cry, problems with attention and state regulation, and irritability. However, there is still controversy about whether these behaviors are manifestations of drug use, prematurity, or LBW.

Most infants (60% to 80%) exposed to heroin or methadone during the last trimester of pregnancy experience neonatal abstinence syndrome (NAS), which involves the central and autonomic nervous systems, gastrointestinal

system, and pulmonary system. Gastrointestinal signs include diarrhea and vomiting; CNS signs include irritability, hypertonia, hyperreflexia, poor sucking and poor feeding, and rarely, seizures (1% to 3%). Respiratory signs include tachypnea, hyperpnea, and respiratory alkalosis. Autonomic nervous system signs include lacrimation, sweating, yawning, and hyperpyrexia. If the infant is hypermetabolic, postnatal weight loss may be excessive and subsequent weight gain suboptimal.

Several studies have examined infant mortality and sudden infant death syndrome (SIDS) among drug-exposed infants, with inconclusive results. Earlier studies[18] reported a higher incidence of infant mortality among infants exposed to heroin or cocaine. However, more recent reports[19] have found no differences in rates of infant death or SIDS unless the infants were exposed to both cocaine and opiates (heroin or methadone). Common effects of drug exposure at birth are summarized in Table 77–2.

Older Women

Among older women, misuse or abuse of alcohol and prescription and over-the-counter drugs is a major concern. Physiologic, sociologic, and psychological changes all contribute to the increased prevalence of drug misuse and abuse among older women.

Age-related physiologic changes result in alterations in absorption, distribution, metabolism, and excretion of drugs. Specifically, there is an increase in body fat and a decrease in body muscle. Absorption rate is affected by a reduction in the cells in the intestine, resulting in decreased absorptive surface and a decrease in the volume of intestinal fluids. This may result in a higher concentration of water-soluble substances in older adults. With decreased absorption, reduced blood flow, and decreased total body water content, older adults accumulate substances more rapidly than younger adults; thus lower dosages of medication are needed, and standard dosages are often too high. There is also a significant decline in renal excretion, which increases the risk for multiple drug reactions or unpredictable drug reactions. Finally, a decrease in liver mass and cardiac output tends to impair liver function, increasing the risk of drug toxicity.

Table 77–2. Common Effects of Exposure to Alcohol and Other Drugs at Birth

	Alcohol	Cocaine	Heroin	Marijuana
Low birth weight	X	X	X	X
Small for gestational age	X			
Mental retardation	X			
Newborn CNS problems	X	X	X	X
Other CNS problems	X			
Neonatal abstinence syndrome			X	
Physical anomalies	X			

CNS, central nervous system.

Many psychological and sociologic life changes that accompany the aging process also contribute to drug misuse. Women live longer than men and experience multiple losses, such as loss of a spouse, children, other family members, or friends. When a spouse dies, women often face loss of income in addition to having a diminished social network. Compounding the effects of these psychological and financial changes is the phenomenon of ageism. As family members and physicians observe the losses and sociologic changes that take place in the lives of elderly women, they may inadvertently contribute to drug abuse by assuming that alcohol or drugs will make the woman "feel better." Commonly heard expressions are "Grandmother's cocktails are the only thing that makes her happy," or "What difference does it make; she won't live much longer anyway." Although well-meaning, these comments reflect lack of understanding and result in under-identification and treatment of alcoholism and drug abuse among older women.

Finally, confusion related to the many forms of dementia common among the elderly contributes to drug misuse or abuse. With changes related to dementia, women may not remember whether they have taken a prescription drug or how to do so. A concomitant factor that may contribute to continuation of drug abuse is the difficulty that physicians face in making a differential diagnosis between the signs of drug abuse and those of other age-related diseases.

As the baby boomers move into old age, the prevalence of alcoholism and marijuana use is expected to rise sharply.

Marijuana use peaked in 1978, and use of the drug has continued, with little belief that marijuana has negative long-term consequences. Some marijuana users have been reported to depict their old age as "sitting on the porch smoking weed with my children and grandchildren." This societal change in perceptions of alcohol and marijuana use leads to the prediction among experts that alcoholism and illicit drug use among older women will increase exponentially over the next decade.

IDENTIFICATION, SCREENING, AND REFERRAL

Health care providers do not routinely inquire about substance use. The reasons are many, including the discomfort of inquiring about illicit drug use, denial by physicians that their patients use substances, and the stigma of pregnant and parenting women using drugs.

The American Psychiatric Association diagnostic criteria for substance abuse and substance dependence are listed in the *Diagnostic and Statistical Manual of Mental Disorders*, fourth edition (DSM-IV) (Table 77–3). *Substance abuse* is defined as a maladaptive pattern of substance use manifested by recurrent and significant adverse consequences such as failure to meet significant role obligations, interpersonal or legal problems, or placing self or others in physically hazardous situations owing to substance use. *Substance dependence* is more severe, and there are distinct

Table 77–3. DSM-IV Diagnostic Criteria

Substance Abuse	Substance Dependence

A. Maladaptive pattern of substance use leading to clinically significant impairment or distress, as manifested by one (or more) of the following occurring within a 12-month period:
1. Recurrent substance use resulting in failure to fulfill major role obligations at work, school, or home (e.g., repeated absences or poor work performance associated with substance use; substance-related absences, suspensions, or expulsions from school; or neglect of children or household)
2. Recurrent use in situations in which it is physically hazardous (e.g., driving an automobile or operating a machine when impaired by substance use)
3. Recurrent substance-related legal problems (e.g., arrests for substance-related disorderly conduct)
4. Continued substance use despite having persistent or recurrent social or interpersonal problems caused or exacerbated by the effects of the substance (e.g., arguments with spouse about consequences of intoxication, physical fights)
B. The symptoms have never met the criteria for substance dependence for this class of substance
	A. Maladaptive pattern of substance use, leading to clinically significant impairment or distress, as manifested by three (or more) of the following occurring at any time in the same 12-month period:
	1. Tolerance, as defined by either of the following:
	  a. A need for markedly increased amounts of the substance to achieve intoxication or desired effect
	  b. Markedly diminished effect with continued use of the same amount of the substance
	2. Withdrawal, as manifested by either of the following:
	  a. The characteristic withdrawal syndrome for the substance
	  b. The same (or a closely related) substance is taken to relieve or avoid withdrawal symptoms
	3. The substance is often taken in larger amounts or over a longer period than was intended
	4. There is a persistent desire or unsuccessful efforts to cut down or control substance use
	5. A great deal of time is spent in activities necessary to obtain the substance (e.g., visiting multiple doctors or driving long distances), use the substance (e.g., chain-smoking), or recover from its effects
	6. Important social, occupational, or recreational activities are given up or reduced because of substance use
	7. The substance use is continued despite knowledge of having a persistent or recurrent physical or psychological problem that is likely to have been caused or exacerbated by the substance (e.g., current cocaine use despite recognition of cocaine-induced depression or continued drinking despite recognition that an ulcer was made worse by alcohol consumption)

From American Psychiatric Association: Diagnostic and Statistical Manual of Mental Disorders, 4th ed (DSM-IV). Washington, DC, American Psychiatric Association, 1994.

Table 77–4. Drug Withdrawal Symptoms

Nicotine	Alcohol	Marijuana	Cocaine	Opioids (e.g., Heroin, Morphine, Methadone)
Restlessness		Restlessness		Restlessness
Irritability	Irritability	Irritability		Irritability
Impatience, hostility		Mild agitation		
Dysphoria			Dysphoria	Dysphoria
Depression			Depression	
Anxiety				Anxiety
Difficulty concentrating	Sleep disturbance	Insomnia, sleep, EEG disturbance	Sleepiness, fatigue	Insomnia
	Nausea	Nausea		Nausea
		Cramping		Cramping
Decreased heart rate	Tachycardia, hypertension		Bradycardia	
	Sweating			
	Seizures			Muscle aches
				Increased sensitivity to pain
	Alcohol craving		Cocaine craving	Opioid craving
Increased appetite or weight gain	Delirium tremens*			
	Tremor			
	Perceptual disturbance			

*Severe agitation, confusion, visual hallucinations, fever, profuse sweating, nausea, diarrhea, dilated pupils.
EEG, electroencephalogram.
From O'Brien CP: Drug addiction and drug abuse. In Harmon JG, Limbird LE, Molinoff PB, et al (eds): Goodman and Gilman's The Pharmacological Basis of Therapeutics, 9th ed. New York: McGraw-Hill, 1996, pp 557–577. Reproduced with the permission of The McGraw-Hill Companies.

phases: tolerance, withdrawal, and compulsive drug-taking and drug-seeking behaviors. Withdrawal symptoms associated with abstinence from common substances of abuse are listed in Table 77–4. Because the metabolism, physiology, and life circumstances of older women are different from those of younger women, special consideration needs to be taken in applying the DSM-IV diagnostic criteria to older women with alcohol problems (Table 77–5).

Among young and middle-aged women, SAMHSA guidelines define moderate alcohol consumption as one drink (1 ounce of absolute alcohol) per day. This is the equivalent of one 4-ounce glass of wine, one 8-ounce beer, or one 1-ounce shot of liquor. For men, moderate consumption is considered to be two drinks per day.

Several tools for screening for alcohol abuse or dependence were developed in the 1970s. Among the most commonly used are the MAST (*M*ichigan *A*lcoholism *S*creening *T*ool), a shortened version of the MAST, and the CAGE (*C*ut-Down *A*nnoyed *G*uilt *E*ye-opener) questionnaire. Recently, with increased recognition of the need to screen for other drugs as well as alcohol, a six-item screener, the UNCOPE (*U*sed, *N*eglected, *C*ut-down, *O*bjected, *P*reoccupied, *E*motional discomfort) has been developed that is designed to reflect the DSM-IV criteria for substance abuse and dependence. In 1998, SAMHSA recommended that the five-item TWEAK (*T*olerance, *W*orried, *E*ye-openers, *A*mnesia, *C*ut-down) test be used for screening *pregnant women*, as it is designed for assessing alcohol abuse at lower levels, aiding in prevention of FAS, ARBD, and ARND.

The MAST, SMAST (*S*hort *MAST*), CAGE, TWEAK, CAGE-AID (*CAGE* questions *A*dapted to *I*nclude *D*rugs), and UNCOPE questionnaires are short (ranging from 4 to 24 questions) and are appropriate for use by a physician,

Table 77–5. Applying DSM-IV Diagnostic Criteria to Older Adults with Alcohol Problems

Criteria	Special Considerations for Older Adults
1. Tolerance	May have problems with even low intake due to increased sensitivity to alcohol and higher blood alcohol levels
2. Withdrawal	Many late-onset alcoholics do not develop physiologic dependence
3. Taking larger amounts over a longer period than intended	Increased cognitive impairment can interfere with self-monitoring; drinking can exacerbate cognitive impairment and monitoring
4. Unsuccessful efforts to cut down or control use	Same issues across life span
5. Spending much time to obtain and use alcohol and recover from effects	Negative effects can occur with relatively low use
6. Giving up activities because of use	May have fewer activities, making detection of problems more difficult
7. Continuing use despite physical or psychological problems caused by use	May not know or understand that problems are related to use, even after medical advice

DSM-IV, *Diagnostic and Statistical Manual of Mental Disorders,* fourth edition.
From Substance Abuse and Mental Health Services (SAMHSA), Center for Substance Abuse Treatment: Substance Abuse among Older Adults. Treatment Improvement Protocol (TIP) Series, No. 26 (DHHS Publication No. 98-3179). Washington, DC, U.S. Department of Health and Human Services, 1998.

Table 77–6. UNCOPE

U	"In the past year, have you ever drank or *used* drugs more than you meant to?" Or "Have you ever spent more time drinking or *using* than you intended to?"
N	"Have you ever *neglected* some of your usual responsibilities because of using alcohol or drugs?"
C	"Have you felt you wanted or needed to *cut down* on your drinking or drug use in the last year?"
O	"Has anyone *objected* to your drinking or drug use?" Or "Has your family, a friend, or anyone else ever told you they *objected* to your alcohol or drug use?"
P	"Have you ever found yourself *preoccupied* with wanting to use alcohol or drugs?" Or "Have you found yourself thinking a lot about drinking or using?"
E	"Have you ever used alcohol or drugs to relieve *emotional discomfort,* such as sadness, anger, or boredom?"

Scoring: Two or more positive responses indicate abuse or dependence. Four or more positive responses strongly indicate dependence.

From Zywiak WH, Hoffmann NG, Floyd AS: Enhancing alcohol treatment outcomes through aftercare and self-help groups. Med Health RI 1999;82:87–90.

nurse practitioner, or physician assistant as part of a routine medical or prenatal care examination. Questions from two of the shorter screening tools, the UNCOPE and the TWEAK, are shown in Tables 77–6 and 77–7, respectively. The UNCOPE has been selected for presentation here based on its derivation from the DSM-IV criteria for diagnosing addiction and dependence, and the TWEAK, based on the recent SAMHSA recommendation that it be used for pregnant women.

Many women who abuse alcohol or other drugs have a history of assault, rape, or incest, often as a child and over a long period of time. Because these traumas are often accompanied by symptoms of PTSD, it is important to include an assessment of PTSD in the screening process.

It is critical to assess for sexually transmitted diseases, including HIV and HCV infection and AIDS, which are prevalent among women who inject heroin or cocaine. All women who have ever injected a drug, even once, should be tested for HCV, because people in the acute phase of the disease continue to feel well. Those with symptoms experience nonspecific symptoms like anorexia, malaise,

or abdominal pain. Women should be advised to reduce alcohol intake and abstain from illicit drug use to avoid risk of progression of hepatitis C to cirrhosis.

In only 25% of patients is the HCV virus reduced significantly with treatment. The side effects of hepatitis C treatment include extreme fatigue, restless sleep, depression, suicidal behaviors, psychosis, and anemia. For pregnant women, there is increased risk for malformations or death of the fetus. Pregnancy is not recommended during treatment and for 6 months after completion for women receiving treatment and partners of men receiving treatment.

Among *older women,* misuse or abuse of alcohol, prescription, and over-the-counter drugs is a major concern. The physiologic changes that accompany the aging process decrease the amount of alcohol that can be consumed before physical effects occur. These changes also increase the risk of inadvertent alcoholism among women older than 65 years of age. Thus, SAMHSA has lowered the guidelines for alcohol consumption among the elderly: for women, the definition of moderate alcohol consumption is less than one drink per day, and for men it is one drink per day.

For these reasons, SAMHSA recommends that older women be screened not only for alcohol and other illicit drug use but also for abuse or misuse of prescription drugs. Suggested questions for screening for misuse of prescription drugs are listed in Table 77–8.

After assessing the need for further evaluation, diagnosis, or treatment, patients are referred for placement into an available treatment slot. Because only 27% of all public treatment slots are allocated to women, referral can be difficult. Many large cities and states have established centralized screening and referral centers for women with limited incomes or resources. Women with more resources can be referred directly to a private treatment program.

TREATMENT OPTIONS

Many options are available for treatment. They range from short- to long-term, outpatient and residential, and

Table 77–7. TWEAK Test

T	*Tolerance:* How many drinks can you hold?
W	Have close friends or relatives *worried* or complained about your drinking in the past year?
E	*Eye-opener:* Do you sometimes take a drink in the morning when you first wake?
A	*Amnesia:* Has a friend or family member ever told you about things you said or did while you were drinking that you could not remember?
K (C)	Do you sometimes feel the need to *cut down* on your drinking?

Scoring: A 7-point scale is used to score this test. The "tolerance" question scores 2 points if a woman reports she can hold more than five drinks without falling asleep or passing out. A positive response to the last three questions scores 1 point each. A total score of 2 or more indicates that the woman is likely to be a risk drinker.

From Russell M: New assessment tools for risk drinking during pregnancy: T-ACE, TWEAK, and others. Alcohol Health Res World 1994;18:55–61.

Table 77–8. Questions to Screen for Prescription Drug Use

1. Do you see more than one health care provider regularly? Why? Have you switched doctors recently? Why?
2. What prescription drugs are you taking? Are you having any problems with them?
3. Where do you get your prescriptions filled? Do you go to more than one pharmacy?
4. Do you use any other nonprescription medications? If so, what, why, how much, how often, and how long have you been taking them?

From Substance Abuse and Mental Health Services (SAMHSA): A Guide to Substance Abuse Services for Primary Care Clinicians. Treatment Improvement Protocol (TIP) Series, No. 24 (DHHS Publication No. 98-3257). Washington, DC, U.S. Department of Health and Human Services, 1998, p 13.

Table 77–9. Treatment Options

Pretreatment	Inpatient treatment
Outpatient	Domiciliary
Detoxification	Residential
Outpatient treatment	
Pretreatment	
Outpatient treatment	
Outpatient methadone maintenance programs	
Self-help and support groups	

include drug-specific interventions. Table 77–9 identifies the primary modalities.

Pretreatment

Pretreatment programs are designed to engage women in treatment and include harm-reduction and detoxification programs. *Outpatient pretreatment programs* are harm-reduction programs for women who are not ready to commit to treatment. Women in these programs are generally in the precontemplation or contemplation stage of change, and may be partially or completely unaware that a problem exists, or so discouraged that they are not seeking change. The programs are often focused on specialized populations of women like pregnant and parenting women or older women. They provide motivational counseling and supportive care, such as case management or referral services to prenatal care, health or dental care, and social services. Many programs also provide or refer women to support groups like Alcoholics Anonymous (AA), Narcotics Anonymous (NA), or Cocaine Anonymous (CA). The goal is to motivate women to the action stage of change, with entry into outpatient or residential treatment.

Detoxification programs, either inpatient or outpatient, are designed to address the immediate physiologic effects of drug withdrawal from alcohol, heroin or other opioids, and prescription drugs like benzodiapines or barbiturates, and to prepare women to focus on the psychological aspects of drug treatment and recovery. Programs are short, lasting from a few days to a few weeks, and the level of detoxification depends on the severity of withdrawal.

Outpatient Treatment

Programs that provide outpatient treatment range from drop-in programs to intensive involvement 5 to 6 days a week. *Traditional outpatient* programs involve individual or group therapy, or both, once a week. *Intensive outpatient* programs vary from 3 to 4 hours, three to five times per week, and generally include psychoeducation on the dynamics of addiction, and individual and group therapy. *Day treatment* generally includes the same therapeutic strategies, and is conducted four to six times per week, from 9 AM to 5 PM. Some programs also offer domicile living for those who need a safe treatment environment.

Opioid Maintenance Therapy. Opioid maintenance therapy (OMT) for users of heroin and other opiates is a component of comprehensive outpatient treatment programs that include behavior modification, psychological support and therapy, education, and social rehabilitation. Methadone maintenance therapy (MMT) is designed to reduce drug use, drug injection, and criminal activity and promote legitimate employment. Experts recommend that medical management of *pregnant heroin users* include MMT throughout pregnancy because (1) pregnant heroin users are almost impossible to detoxify; (2) maternal abstinence may produce fetal distress, which is more harmful than methadone dependence; and (3) it is believed that controlled dosages of a known drug are less harmful to the fetus than unknown dosages of street drugs. However, there is controversy about the appropriate dosage, based on potential effects of methadone on fetal health, infant birth outcomes, and neonatal withdrawal, and because no consistent relationship has been found between maternal methadone dosage and neonatal withdrawal. Several studies have demonstrated positive relationships between MMT and increased attendance at prenatal care and drug treatment programs. After birth, the treatment goal becomes detoxification.

Several new drugs are in use or being considered for OMT. These include *l*-alpha-acetyl-methadol (LAAM), which was approved by the U.S. Food and Drug Administration (FDA) in 1993, and buprenorphine, which is not yet approved.

LAAM is a long-acting alternative to methadone, with the advantage of requiring the patient to return only every 2 to 3 days for medication management. LAAM is not recommended for pregnant or breastfeeding women due to neonatal abstinence syndrome (NAS) and inadequate research on the potential effects on fetal or infant growth and development.

Buprenorphine also has the advantage of having a longer duration of action than methadone (2 to 3 days). It is less toxic than methadone and has a lower level of withdrawal and physical dependence. Several small-scale studies conducted in the United States and Austria found buprenorphine suitable for use with pregnant women. Infants were born full-term, did not have LBW, and, significantly, experienced little or no NAS. Although not yet approved by the FDA for use in the United States, the National Institute on Drug Abuse has recently recommended approval based on these studies and a large-scale clinical trail with nonpregnant adults.

Outpatient programs are usually most effective for younger women, who have not been dependent on alcohol or illicit drugs for a long period of time. Because the needs of women are so varied and complex, most outpatient programs place great emphasis on case management, including advocacy, referral, and follow-up, and include self-help groups like AA, NA, or CA. When referring women to treatment, physicians need to consider barriers to treatment such as child care and transportation, and to assess the safety of the woman's home environment, including her support system. These issues heavily influence women's success or failure.

Inpatient Options

These include domiciliary care and residential treatment. Domiciliary programs provide safe housing for women who attend outpatient treatment. Many programs provide child care and structured evening activities for the women and their children, including didactic lectures, and psycho-educational or therapy groups for the women and children.

Residential Treatment Programs. These are typically designed for a stay of 6 to 12 months, and include a comprehensive array of treatment or referral services to meet the multiple health, psychological, social, and educational needs of families (Table 77–10). A hallmark of residential programs is the high degree of structure they provide to support women and prevent relapse.

Typically, women who enter residential treatment are older (average age, 25 to 30 years) and have not succeeded in maintaining recovery in outpatient treatment. The women often have children, have a longer history of physical or sexual abuse, and frequently have some type of comorbidity (e.g., depression, PTSD, or anxiety disorder). Many enter treatment as the result of a court order mandat-ing treatment as a condition of retaining or regaining child custody.

Since the 1980's, recognizing that women need different treatment than men, women's residential treatment programs have focused on gender-specific and family issues. Typically, women's programs incorporate a treatment philosophy based on a model of women's development such as the relational model. With this model, treatment focuses not only on triggers to use or relapse but also on interpersonal issues such as relationships, major losses due to death or separation, self-esteem, and victimization. Treatment modalities include didactic lectures, psychoeducational groups, individual and group therapy, and self-help groups. On-site programming for children is often included, with child care, child, and family therapy, and parenting skills classes provided. Since the early 1990s, family-focused treatment has become the preferred model for women's treatment. This model places more emphasis on the relationship needs of the entire family and includes other family members, such as the father, as an integral part of treatment. Family-focused treatment has been shown to increase length of stay, adding to the likelihood that women will remain in recovery and that children will have improved developmental and educational outcomes. Generally, residential programs include aftercare services. These may include supportive housing for women and their families in transitional housing (e.g., halfway house) and outpatient treatment to provide continued structure and support for women as they reintegrate into mainstream society.

Considerations for Referral

When making referrals for either outpatient or inpatient programs, it is important that women be referred to programs that address their complex needs and those of their families by including the program elements listed in Table 77–10. Addressing the cultural and ethnic background of the women and their sexual orientation is also important. Many women who enter treatment have been involved in illegal activity to support their drug use, and many have legal issues to resolve. Finally, for women to return to a productive role in society, it is essential that programs address employment, by assisting women to return to high school, college, or vocational training. For women whose drug use had been long-term or who have been in abusive relationships, learning daily living skills may be a precursor of reentry into the educational system or into a vocational training program.

Treatment Programs for Older Women. These do not differ from those for younger women except in their focus on issues specific to life changes that occur with the aging process. Health care providers may not offer them treatment, based on the belief that older women will not benefit from treatment, or that it is not cost-effective because of the woman's age. SAMHSA has reported that because older women have typically not misused or abused drugs

Table 77–10. Recommended Program Elements

All Women

Health Issues	Social and Legal Issues
Detoxification	Food
Methadone maintenance	Housing
Addictions counseling	Transportation
Substance-related medical conditions	Financial management
General health care, including reproductive	Court assistance
Psychiatric care	*Educational Issues*
Dental care	High school or college
Psychological Issues	Vocational skills training
	Daily living skills
Comorbidity: depression, anxiety, post-traumatic stress disorder	*Program Philosophy*
Self-esteem, shame, guilt	Client is integral part of treatment team
Loss and grief	
Victimization: sexual, physical, or emotional abuse; family violence; relationship-imposed isolation	

Pregnant or Parenting Women	Older Women
Health	*Health Issues*
Prenatal care	Prescription drug use
Methadone maintenance	Geriatric care
Pediatric care	Geriatric mental health
Child-related Issues	*Psychological Issues*
Breastfeeding	Isolation
Child care/day care	Loss and grief
Parenting classes	Victimization
Protection from violence or victimization	
Education for children	

while young, they are actually more likely to benefit from treatment. Often, a suggestion from a physician that the woman monitor or decrease her alcohol or drug use is enough to motivate the woman to use drugs appropriately. Older people have been found to benefit from short-term treatment, motivational counseling, or age-specific AA or NA groups. It is recommended that older women be offered treatment options as soon as a problem with alcohol or drug use is identified.

CONCLUSION

Alcohol and drug abuse crosses socioeconomic boundaries and ethnic groups. It is imperative that obstetricians and gynecologists screen *all women* for substance abuse during routine health care visits. When screening for alcohol or drug use, it is especially important for physicians to be aware that many women who abuse drugs have comorbidities, including major depression or anxiety disorders. Additionally, women are prescribed more drugs than men, increasing the importance of screening for abuse or misuse of prescription drugs. Finally, two groups of women, those who are pregnant or parenting and those who are older, face unique problems related to their developmental stage in life. These women need to be referred to programs that address their special needs.

Information Resources

National Clearinghouse for Alcohol and Drug Information (NCADI)
http://www.health.org (Prevline) 1-800-729-6686
National Institutes of Health
http://www.nih.gov
The Centers for Disease Control and Prevention
http://www.cdc.gov/cdc.htm
National Mental Health Services
Knowledge Exchange Network (KEN)
http://www.mentalhealth.org 1-800-789-2647

Suggestions for Future Reading

Since treatment of women's substance abuse covers the entire adult life span, use of multiple types of drugs, and multiple treatment modalities, a few specific research articles do not provide the breadth needed for the topic. Therefore, books with compilations or a synthesis of research articles are listed here.

Substance Abuse and Mental Health Services Administration, Office of Applied Studies (SAMHSA): SAMHSA Studies: Substance abuse among women. Public Health Rep 1998; 113:13.
SAMHSA, Center for Substance Abuse Treatment: A Guide to Substance Abuse Services for Primary Care Clinicians Treatment Improvement Protocol (TIP) Series, No. 24 (DHHS Publication No. 98-3257). Washington, DC, U.S Department of Health and Human Services, 1998.
SAMHSA, Center for Substance Abuse Treatment: Substance Abuse among Older Adults. Treatment Improvement Protocol (TIP) Series,

No. 26 (DHHS Publication No. 98-3179). Washington, DC, U.S. Department of Health and Human Services, 1998.
SAMHSA, Center for Substance Abuse Treatment: Enhancing Motivation for Change in Substance Abuse Treatment. Treatment Improvement Protocol (TIP) Series, No. 35 (DHHS Publication No. 99-3354). Washington, DC, U.S. Department of Health and Human Services, 1999.
Underhill BL, Finnegan, DG (eds): Chemical Dependency Women at Risk. New York, Harrington Park Press, 1996.
Wetherington CL, Roman AB (eds): Drug Addiction Research and the Health of Women. Rockville, Md, National Institutes of Health, 1998.

References

1. National Institute on Drug Abuse: National Survey on Drug Use from the Monitoring the Future Study, 1975–1994. Washington, DC, National Institute on Drug Abuse, 1996.
2. Substance Abuse and Mental Health Services Office of Applied Studies (SAMHSA): National Household Survey on Drug Abuse. Washington, DC, SAMHSA, August 1996.
3. Kandel D, Chen K, Warner L, et al: Prevalence and demographic correlates of symptoms of last year dependence on alcohol, nicotine, marijuana and cocaine in the U.S. population. Drug Alcohol Depend 1997;44:11–29.
4. Calkins RF, Laken M, Aktan GB, Miller KS: Substance abuse and need for treatment among pregnant and postpartum women in Michigan, 1999: Final report. Lansing Mich, Michigan Department of Community Health, 1999.
5. Frank DA, McCarten KM, Robson CD, et al: Level of in utero cocaine exposure and neonatal ultrasound findings. Pediatrics 1999;104:1101–1105.
6. Schonfeld L, Dupree LW: Treatment approaches for older problem drinkers. Int J Addict 1995;30:1819–1842.
7. Kaplan HI, Sadock BJ: Pocket Handbook of Psychiatric Drug Treatment, 2nd ed. Baltimore, Williams & Wilkins, 1996.
8. Adams WL, Barry KL, Fleming MF: Screening for problem drinking in older primary care patients. JAMA 1996;276:1964–1967.
9. Gomberg ESL: Medication problems and drug abuse. In Turner FJ (ed): Mental Health and the Elderly. New York, Free Press, 1992.
10. Colsher PL, Wallace RB: Elderly men with histories of heavy drinking: Correlates and consequences. J Stud Alcohol 1990;51:528–535.
11. Saunders PA, Copeland JR, Dewey ME, et al: Heavy drinking as a risk factor for depression and dementia in elderly men: Findings from the Liverpool Longitudinal Community Study. Br J Psychiatry 1991;159:213–216.
12. Adams WL, Yuan Z, Barboriak JJ, Rimm AA: Alcohol-related hospitalizations of elderly people: Prevalence and geographic location in the United States. JAMA 1993;270:1222–1225.
13. Greene TH, Emhart CB, Ager J, et al: Prenatal exposure to alcohol and cognitive development. Neurotoxicol Teratol 1990;12:57–68.
14. Streissguth AP, Barr HM, Kogan J, Bookstein FL: Understanding the occurrence of secondary disabilities in clients with fetal alcohol syndrome (FAS) and fetal alcohol effects (FAE) (Final report, Centers for Disease Control and Prevention Grant No. RO4/CCR008515). Seattle, University of Washington School of Medicine, 1996.
15. Streissguth AP, LaDue R: Fetal alcohol: Teratogenic causes of developmental disabilities. In Schroeder SR (ed): Toxic Substances and Mental Retardation. Washington, DC, American Association on Mental Deficiency, 1987.
16. Streissguth AP, Martin DC, Martin JC, Barr HM: The Seattle longitudinal prospective study on alcohol and pregnancy. Neurobehav Toxicol 1981;3:223–233.
17. Centers for Disease Control and Prevention: Fetal alcohol syndrome: United States, 1979–1992. MMWR Morbid Mortal Wkly Rep 1993;42:339–341.
18. Robins LN, Mills JL, Krulewitch C, Herman AA: Effects of in utero exposure to street drugs. Am J Public Health 1993;83(Suppl):1–32.
19. Ostrea EM, Ostrea AR, Simpson PM: Mortality within the first 2 years in infants exposed to cocaine, opiate, or cannabinoid during gestation. Pediatrics 1997;100:79–83.

SEVENTY-EIGHT

Management of Iatrogenic Bleeding in Postmenopausal Women

David F. Archer

After menopause, there is no longer any cyclicity or regularity of uterine bleeding. This well-known fact is related to the total depletion of the follicular apparatus, consisting of the granulosa cells, theca cells, and oocytes. The postmenopausal woman should have no uterine bleeding whatsoever.

We have educated physicians and consumers to be aware of the fact that the occurrence of vaginal bleeding in a postmenopausal woman should be a cause of concern. Any vaginal bleeding requires an investigation by the physician to exclude cancer of the cervix, uterine corpus, or vagina as the etiology of the bleeding. The investigation involves simple inspection and palpation of the vagina, cervix, uterus, and adnexa, as well as obtaining a Papanicolaou smear from the cervix. The endometrium is evaluated with a biopsy using an appropriate instrument, as well as transvaginal or abdominal ultrasound, saline sonohysterography, and/or hysteroscopy as part of the diagnostic evaluation.

Hormonal therapy, consisting of a combination of estrogen and a progestin in women who have a uterus, has resulted in an increase in the occurrence of iatrogenically induced uterine bleeding. Estrogen-only therapy previously had been used in a cyclic fashion for many years. Some of the patients would indeed have a withdrawal bleeding episode, but it has been clearly shown that the use of unopposed estrogen in a woman with an intact uterus increases the woman's risk of developing cancer of the endometrium. The addition of a progestational agent to the estrogen treatment, initially in a cyclic or sequential manner, and recently as continuous combined daily estrogen and progestin, has reduced the incidence of endometrial cancer. These treatment regimens have resulted in the reinitiation of uterine bleeding. Over 85% of women who use sequential hormone replacement therapy (HRT) have been found to have a cyclic bleeding episode during or after the use of the progestational agent. The bleeding episodes are usually of 3 to 4 days' duration, consist of less blood loss than in the premenopausal years, and occur at a consistent interval based on the duration of progestin administered. Up to 50% of women who use continuous combined hormone replacement therapy (ccHRT) can have irregular unanticipated bleeding during the first 3 to 4 months after initiation of treatment.

Sequential hormone replacement therapy (sqHRT) has evolved since about 1990 from a 25-day regimen of estrogen, with the last 10 days on a progestin, to the current model of continuous estrogen and 12 to 14 days of a progestin administered monthly. As is shown later, this type of regimen is important because the duration of the progestin reduces the risk of endometrial cancer. The cyclic bleeding on this regimen is usually less in amount than what women have experienced during their reproductive years. In addition, although many physicians believe that the initiation of this withdrawal bleeding occurs on the cessation of the estrogen and progestin, fully 30% to 40% of the women who are utilizing conjugated equine estrogen with medroxyprogesterone acetate (Premphase, Wyeth-Ayerst Laboratories, St. Davids, Pa) will experience the uterine bleeding, which will begin before completion of the progestational agent.

On the other hand, individuals who are using ccHRT, whether oral or transdermal, have been found to have a 50% to 60% incidence of irregular, unanticipated uterine bleeding or spotting. The average duration of the unanticipated bleeding episode is approximately 3 days. This bleeding is not cyclic or regular. The majority of women experience spotting only, using the World Health Organization definition that "spotting" requires no sanitary protection whereas "bleeding" requires sanitary protection by the patient. Spotting is more of a nuisance than a real problem in terms of medical management. The concern is when the woman is experiencing either persistent spotting and bleeding or prolonged and heavy bleeding during the use of either sqHRT or ccHRT.

The incidence of cancer of the endometrium is one to two new cases per 1000 women per year. This incidence rises with age; in general, cancer of the endometrium is rare in women younger than age 45 years. The relative risk of carcinoma of the endometrium in estrogen replacement therapy (ERT) users has been found to be increased to a relative risk of 2.3 in a recent meta-analysis of published epidemiologic studies. The actual relative risk can vary from a low of 1.3 to a high of 10 in published reports. This increased risk is higher in women who are currently using ERT and lowers with the duration of time since cessation of ERT. Women with a uterus who have used estrogen only are still at increased risk for up to 10 to 15 years after discontinuation of ERT.

The addition of a progestational agent has been reported to reduce the incidence of cancer of the endometrium to that level found in untreated women or, in some instances, to be actually protective for the development of endometrial cancer. Three recent epidemiologic studies have indicated that the use of a progestin for less than 10 days in association with 25 days of estrogen (a standard United States treatment protocol) will result in a relative risk of 1.3 for the occurrence of endometrial cancer. This risk appears to increase after 5 years of the sequential regimen of less than 10 days of progestin. ccHRT has been found to have no increased risk or to significantly reduce the risk for endometrial cancer in these epidemiologic studies. Thus, it appears that the duration of progestin administration is more important than the dose, and that ccHRT should be the favored treatment.

The goal of ccHRT has been to obtain a state of no uterine bleeding. This "amenorrheic" state appeals to the patient, because the majority of postmenopausal women do not wish to experience any uterine bleeding whatever. It should be noted that there are women who are unable to attain this amenorrheic status. These women often experience only spotting, with occasional 1- to 2-day episodes of bleeding. The presence of uterine fibroids, even small intramural fibroids, appears to increase the incidence of irregular bleeding in women on ccHRT.

At the present time, in the United States, at least five different HRT regimens with different estrogens and progestins and with varying doses are in use. The now-classic 25 days of estrogen with 10 days of a progestin is shown as regimen *A*. A more appropriate sequential therapy is continuous estrogen with 14 days of a progestin, regimen *B*. The current continuous combined estrogen plus progestin daily is regimen *C*. A recent introduction is the cyclophasic or intermittent progestin regimen in which progestin is administered for 3 days with 3 days off, while estrogen is continuous (regimen *D*). A possible alternative is to use a continuous combined regimen for 5 days and have 2 days (the weekend) off all hormonal medication, regimen *E*. The long interval of continuous estrogen with 14 days of a progestin given every 3 months is shown as regimen *F*.

All the HRT regimens that utilize a continuous combined approach result in a 30% to 50% incidence of irregular uterine bleeding or spotting in the first 3 months. In two reports there is less bleeding in ccHRT in women who are more than 3 years from their menopausal date as opposed to those women who are more recent (less than 3 years) from the menopause. The occurrence of irregular bleeding or spotting reduces with continuous use of ccHRT.

sqHRT is thus probably best for the individual who is recently menopausal. These women could use ccHRT with appropriate counseling regarding the increased incidence of irregular bleeding/spotting and with the anticipation of no bleeding in approximately 50% of the users of ccHRT. For those women who have been on sqHRT and now wish transition to a no-bleeding regimen, simply moving them from sqHRT to ccHRT is appropriate at any time. In some instances, it may be best to wait for at least 1 to 1.5 years after the initiation of cyclic or sqHRT in order to document that there is indeed a reduced amount of bleeding without any evidence of irregularity or breakthrough bleeding.

sqHRT users should be observed carefully for changes in their withdrawal bleeding pattern or in the amount and duration of the bleeding, because these are the early sign of abnormalities in the endometrium. Reanalysis of the data from a multicenter study indicated that if women on sqHRT experience withdrawal bleeding on a specific day such as day 12 of the progestin, this pattern of withdrawal bleeding will be repeated over the subsequent cycles with a variance of plus or minus only 1 day. Thus, the regularity of withdrawal bleeding can be of reassurance to both patient and physician. The regularity of withdrawal bleeding allows the patient to anticipate the uterine bleeding episode.

ccHRT, on the other hand, because of the sporadic and unanticipated nature of the bleeding, does present a problem. Most of the studies indicate that somewhere between 70% and 90% of the women do not experience any uterine bleeding after the sixth to seventh month of ccHRT. This is important in the counseling process. A significant reduction in the incidence of bleeding/spotting occurs at 3 months after the initiation of ccHRT, which lessens with each successive cycle. If one were to remove spotting from the reports, the occurrence of bleeding in most ccHRT regimens would be somewhere between 5% and 15%.

The exact pathophysiology behind the irregularity of uterine bleeding in women on ccHRT is unknown. A variety of proposed mechanisms could be operational. All invoke the action of a progestin or the progestin withdrawal that stimulates or inhibits local cytokine or autocrine factors as well as proteinases and tissue factors. Any or all of these factors could be involved in the initiation of the bleeding episode.

Although addition of a progestin to the estrogen has clearly reduced the incidence of endometrial cancer compared with women using only estrogen, there is always the possibility that irregular bleeding on ccHRT reflects an underlying neoplasm. The reports of U.S. Food and Drug Administration–approved ccHRT regimens indicate that the progestin dose and duration will inhibit the development of endometrial hyperplasias. Simple endometrial hyperplasia will usually regress with the use of an appropriate dose and duration of progestin. Atypical hyperplasias have a different outcome, and over 50% of these patients will progress to neoplasia. Women who are experiencing irregular bleeding on ccHRT have been reported to have an atrophic or suppressed endometrium. The occurrence of hyperplasia (usually simple hyperplasia) is less than 1.0% in the reported clinical trials for these reasons, the physician who investigates continuous irregular bleeding and spotting will not find a significant occurrence of abnormal endometrial histology.

In women who are using sqHRT or ccHRT and are experiencing abnormal bleeding, principally prolonged or profuse bleeding, an appropriate investigation is warranted. The endometrium should be evaluated directly, obtaining an endometrial tissue sample through biopsy. Transvaginal or abdominal ultrasound with imaging of the endometrium can be adjunctive, but in recent publications has been shown to lack the sensitivity and specificity to exclude neoplasia. Saline infusion hysterosonography can demonstrate polyps and local lesions but is not useful for the accurate demonstration of an endometrial neoplasia. Hysteroscopy can also be utilized to evaluate the endometrium, but the most frequent finding on hysteroscopy of women on ccHRT is that of an atropic endometrium with unusual, dilated, and prominent blood vessels beneath the endometrial epithelium. In over 50% of women who have had hysteroscopy for irregular bleeding while on ccHRT, no abnormalities were found.

Management for the irregular bleeding and persistent irregular bleeding on ccHRT is not clear-cut and is often one of trial and error. One of the more intriguing approaches is to switch to another progestational agent. Progestins have been found to have various degrees of potency based on direct assay of endometrial tissue for morphologic changes, enzyme induction, and other biochemical parameters. Progesterone itself in these assays is probably the least potent, with norethindrone being the most potent. So, the approach would be to maintain the estrogen and switch to another progestin. However, there are no clinical data that this is efficacious.

A second option is to increase the dose of the progestin or the estrogen or both. The rationale is to reduce the estrogen receptor content, resulting in a reduction in the progestational receptor. In this way, the exogenous progestin has no or little potential for action. There is less bleeding on ccHRT with a higher dose of medroxyprogesterone acetate, 5.0 mg, compared with 2.5 mg. Conversely, low doses of norethindrone acetate, 0.1 mg, used with estradiol 17β, 1.0 mg, show an increased incidence of bleeding compared with estradiol, 1.0 mg with 0.5 mg of norethindrone acetate. These data indicate that a balance is needed between the estrogen and the progestin that results in no or minimal endometrial bleeding. How to determine this optimal ratio, if such a ratio exists, is difficult. Again, changing the dose of estrogen and progestin as a therapeutic trial is warranted. A minimum of 3 months' observation should ensue after each alteration of treatment.

Another intervention is to withdraw or reduce the amount of estrogen. Data have been presented that show that a lowered amount of estrogen with comparable progestin doses (5.0 to 10.0 mg medroxyprogesterone acetate) results in limited progestational morphologic changes in the endometrium of postmenopausal women. Thus, the reduction in the estrogen dose for 3 to 6 months, while maintaining the progestational agent at its previous dose and duration, may be a most effective way to reduce endometrial bleeding. After resolution of the bleeding, re-turning the estrogen dose to its initial level may be indicated, based on the individual requirements of the patient.

A third technique is to change from ccHRT to another regimen. The intermittent utilization of progestin (on 3 days, off 3 days, on 3 days, off 3 days, and so on) has been termed *cyclophasic*. This technique, in a recently introduced HRT regimen in the United States, has been found also to bring a significant amount of bleeding in some patients. However, in others it can be utilized to replace the ccHRT and reduce the bleeding/spotting. Another alternative, in terms of the administration of the progestin, is to move from continuous combined to a sequential therapy for anywhere from 3 to 6 months and then reinitiate continuous combined therapy.

Obviously, the uterine bleeding induced by the iatrogenic administration of exogenous hormones can be stopped simply by stopping the HRT. This is the final approach for some women who are tired of the bleeding and in whom control has not been obtained by the physician. It carries with it the loss of benefits from the HRT. In some instances, a respite from the bleeding may be beneficial for the patient and the physician, with plans to reinitiate therapy in the future. Many of these women will experience a return of hot flushes and other menopausal symptoms, and this is often of sufficient magnitude to cause them to reinitiate HRT.

For many women, the reinitiation of uterine bleeding and the inability to reach a no-bleeding status rapidly results in permanent discontinuation of the hormone therapy. Combined counseling and therapeutic trials of different regimens and doses for motivated women are worthwhile in establishing a therapeutic approach that has an end point of no bleeding.

SUMMARY

The iatrogenic causes of bleeding in postmenopausal women are due to the reintroduction of an estrogen alone, estrogen plus sequential progestin, or estrogen/progestin in a continuous combined or intermittent fashion in postmenopausal women. The control of this bleeding is difficult and requires a trial-and-error approach. The best results appear to be found in reducing the dose of estrogen rather than increasing the dose of progestin. An increase in the dose of progestin or changing the progestational compound itself may be of benefit in reducing the incidence of iatrogenic bleeding and spotting in some women. There is no rule of thumb for this management. It is a trial-and-error process that requires collaboration and continued commitment between the patient and the physician as an appropriate dose and route of administration of HRT are sought.

SEVENTY-NINE

Screening for Ovarian Cancer

Lawrence D. Platt, Beth Y. Karlan,

Naomi H. Greene, and Catherine A. Walla

Ovarian cancer, the leading cause of death due to gynecologic malignancy, accounts for 4% of all cancers among women. In the year 2000, approximately 23,100 new cases of ovarian cancer were estimated to develop in the United States, with an estimated 14,000 deaths occurring from this disease. With a prevalence of 30 to 50 cases per 100,000 population, the lifetime risk in a woman with no affected relatives is 1.4% (1/70). The risk increases to 5% (1/20) in a woman with one affected first-degree relative and 7% (1/14) in a woman with two or more affected first-degree relatives. Although the National Cancer Institute reported that their data showed that age-adjusted ovarian cancer mortality rates declined 9% since about 1983, the 1999 investigation by Oriel and colleagues[1] demonstrated age-adjusted ovarian cancer mortality rates that have changed little over this period. They reported a declining incidence of ovarian cancer mortality in younger women, with an increase in mortality in women 65 years of age or older during this interval.

The 5-year survival rate for all stages of ovarian cancer is 50%, but this rate varies substantially according to histologic features of the tumor, as well as how far the disease has progressed at the time of diagnosis and treatment. This rate is 95% if the carcinoma is detected and treated at stage 1; however, only 25% of all cases are detected at the localized stage. Women who have stage III or IV disease at initial presentation have a 5-year survival rate of about 28%.

In light of these statistics, the goal of ovarian cancer screening is the early diagnosis of the disease, which in turn would translate into increased ovarian cancer cure rates. It has been estimated that shifting just 10% of ovarian cancer cases from stage III to stage I by early detection would produce a greater improvement in disease survival than did the introduction of cisplatin or taxol chemotherapies. The ability to diagnose localized epithelial ovarian malignancies would have significant bearing on improving patients' survival time and quality of life, as well as reducing health care costs.

Many investigators have been focusing on detecting early disease by using ultrasound imaging or circulating tumor markers. However, these approaches are handicapped by deficiencies in knowledge of the molecular and biologic events leading to the early neoplastic changes that occur in ovarian epithelium, the lack of early clinical symptoms, and the intraperitoneal location of the ovaries.

ROLE OF ULTRASOUND IN OVARIAN CANCER SCREENING

Ultrasonography is playing a pivotal role in screening for ovarian carcinoma. The usefulness of ultrasound imaging as an ovarian cancer screening modality is based on its ability to accurately detect early morphologic changes accompanying ovarian carcinogenesis. Because the true precursor lesion to ovarian cancer remains unknown, the goal of this approach is directed toward finding presymptomatic changes in the ovary that are associated with malignancy.

Transabdominal Ultrasound

Clinical trials utilizing ultrasound techniques for ovarian cancer screening have been under way since the 1980s. In one of the earliest and most extensive studies, Campbell and associates[2] screened 5479 volunteers with transabdominal sonography (TAS) and found 326 women who had persistently abnormal ovarian findings on consecutive examinations. At laparotomy, five stage I ovarian cancers and four metastatic cancers secondarily involving the ovaries were found. A total of 255 women had "benign" ovarian cystic or solid lesions, and 62 patients who were subjected to laparotomy had "spontaneously resolved" ovarian masses. The high false-positive rate of TAS for ovarian cancer screening and the large number of women undergoing costly and potentially risky surgical procedures are unacceptable. Furthermore, TAS requires a full bladder for proper visualization of pelvic structures. The time and discomfort associated with bladder filling, and the advent of transvaginal sonography with its superior imaging have made TAS less suitable for screening.

Transvaginal Ultrasound

The introduction of the transvaginal ultrasound transducer has improved the ease and resolution of ovarian imaging. With transvaginal sonography (TVS), the transducer is placed closer to the ovaries and delivers higher-frequency (5 to 7.5 MH) ultrasound, thereby improving the image quality and tissue differentiation. Ninety-five percent of premenopausal and 85% of postmenopausal ovaries can be visualized accurately by the transvaginal approach.

Van Nagell's group,[3] who began TVS screening for ovarian cancer in 1987, have reported their results from annual TVS screening of 6470 asymptomatic postmenopausal women. Ninety (1.4%) persistent morphologic ovarian abnormalities were detected using this ultrasonographic mode. Surgical exploration of these women revealed 5 stage IA ovarian cancers (2 granulosa cell tumors, 1 adenocarcinoma, 1 serous cystadenocarcinoma, 1 endometrioid carcinoma), 1 stage IIIB ovarian cancer, and 49 benign ovarian neoplasms, of which 37 were serous cystadenomas. One false-negative case occurred in which, 11 months after a normal screen, a patient underwent a prophylactic laparoscopic oophorectomy that revealed a poorly differentiated adenocarcinoma with microscopic spread to the adjacent fallopian tube (stage IIA disease). In terms of the serous cystadenomas, the investigators proposed that these benign tumors may be premalignant and suggested that excising them may offer potential benefit to these patients and future reduction in the number of ovarian cancer cases. This hypothesis has not yet been validated owing to our limited knowledge of the true ovarian cancer precursor lesion and of the stepwise progression of events that leads to ovarian carcinogenesis.

A study utilizing follow-up data from a cohort of 5479 asymptomatic women who were self-referred for ultrasonographic screening for ovarian cancer between 1981 and 1987 was performed to assess whether the removal of persistent benign ovarian cysts was associated with a reduction in the expected number of deaths from ovarian cancer.[4] These investigators were unable to find a decrease in the proportion of expected deaths from ovarian cancer relative to other cancers.

Morphology Scoring Indices

A number of investigators[5–8] have proposed morphology scoring indices to quantify the real-time ultrasound findings and correlate them with the histopathologic diagnoses. These scoring scales include TVS findings such as ovarian volume, cyst wall structure, papillary vegetations, septation, and echogenicity to predict malignancy. Although no scoring system has been agreed on by investigators, guidance toward an optimal morphology index may be gleaned from a clinical pathologic study in which gross anatomic changes in more than 1000 ovaries examined by the surgeon were compared with a pathologist's review of the specimens' histopathology.

Papillary vegetations were the most ominous finding associated with the diagnosis of ovarian carcinoma, whereas cyst size or the presence of septations was not correlated with malignancy. The surgeons' predictions of malignancy agreed with the pathologic diagnosis 84% of the time. This percentage probably represents a realistic estimate of the limitations of ultrasound screening. Although not requiring any additional ultrasound equipment, the combination of a morphology scale with transvaginal ultrasound could improve the diagnostic accuracy of TVS in ovarian cancer screening.[3, 10]

Color Doppler Imaging

Other early detection studies for ovarian cancer have coupled conventional ultrasound techniques with color Doppler imaging (CDI) in an attempt to visualize early physiologic changes, such as angiogenesis before detectable morphologic changes in ovarian architecture. Folkman and coworkers[11] recognized that neovascularization is an obligate early event in tumor growth and neoplasia. CDI is based on the principle that fast-growing tumors contain many new blood vessels that have relatively little smooth muscle in their walls. The resistance to blood flow within these vessels is thereby less than the flow within vessels in benign lesions. CDI is thus utilized as an attempt to differentiate "malignant" blood flow patterns from physiologic or "benign" neoplastic vasculature. In theory, this technique could detect malignant neoangiogenesis before the morphologic changes in ovarian architecture detectable by real-time scanning. An early report of the use of CDI in the evaluation of adnexal masses indicated that this sonographic modality had a sensitivity of 96.4%, a specificity of 99.8%, and a positive predictive value of 98.2%.[12] Subsequent investigations have not been able to reproduce this diagnostic accuracy. In practice, clinical studies of CDI have revealed that normal physiologic changes in the premenopausal ovary near the time of ovulation have low impedance flow characteristics similar to those seen in malignancy.

Some workers believe that the evaluation of tumor vascularity confers no benefit over morphologic assessment as far as decreasing the false-positive rate is concerned. Furthermore, the relatively poor specificity precludes its use as a primary screening. Lastly, concerns regarding reproducibility, the subjective interpretation of the results, and the lack of widespread expertise and equipment further compromise the role of CDI studies as a screening modality. Questions regarding CDI, such as "Which intraovarian vessels have the greatest predictive value? Does our increasing ability to detect blood flow through smaller and smaller vessels add 'noise' to our detection systems? Which Doppler parameter and what cutoff level are the most predictive of malignancy?" reflect some of the shortcomings related to the initial promise of this technique.

CA 125 TESTING

The serum tumor marker CA 125 is an antigenic determinant detected by radioimmunoassay. It was found to be elevated in 80% to 85% of advanced epithelial ovarian cancers (stage III or IV), but only half of the patients with stage I cancers have elevated levels. Further, an elevated CA 125 is not specific for ovarian cancer. An elevated CA 125 can be found in about 1% of healthy women. Elevations in this antigen can be demonstrated not only during pregnancy and menstruation but also in a number of nongynecologic and benign gynecologic disorders (e.g., diverticulitis, pancreatitis, liver disease, renal failure, inflammatory bowel disease, endometriosis, uterine fibroids, functional ovarian cysts, and pelvic inflammatory disease) and nongynecologic cancers (e.g., pancreas, stomach, colon, and breast).

Prospectively evaluating the value of CA 125 in ovarian cancer detection, Einhorn and colleagues[13] screened 5500 asymptomatic women with serum CA 125 levels. Women with abnormal values and an equal number of age-matched controls with normal levels were followed with pelvic examinations, TAS, and serial CA 125 determinations. Of 175 women with elevated CA 125 levels, 6 ovarian cancers were identified (2, stage IA; 2, stage IIB; 2, stage IIIC). The control group had 3 cases of ovarian cancer (one, stage IA; one, stage IIIA; one, stage IIIC). Using thresholds of 30 and 35 U/mL, the specificity of a serum CA 125 level was 97% and 98.5%, respectively, in women 50 years of age and older and 91% and 94.5% respectively in women younger than 50 years.

Jacobs and associates[14] used CA 125 as a primary screening test in 22,000 postmenopausal women. Women with CA 125 levels greater than 30 U/mL were considered to have abnormal levels and were called for further testing with TAS. Abnormal ultrasound results led to surgical intervention. Of the 41 women with abnormal ultrasound examinations, 11 had ovarian cancer (3, stage I; 1, stage II; 5, stage III; 2, stage IV), whereas in 8 women with false-negative results, ovarian cancer developed during the subsequent 6 to 22 months. A specificity of 99.9% and a positive predictive value of 26.8% were achieved with this protocol.

POPULATION TO BE SCREENED

A way to improve the yield of ovarian cancer screening is to focus on high-risk female populations. At-risk groups have been targeted for screening because of the relatively low prevalence of ovarian cancer in the general population. TVS is most effective as a screening method in postmenopausal patients in whom physiologic changes in ovarian volume do not occur. Also, the prevalence of ovarian cancer is highest in women over 50 years of age. The risk of ovarian cancer increases from 15.7/100,000 at age 40 years to 54/100,000 at age 75 years.

The women at highest risk for ovarian cancer are those with a family history that is consistent with a hereditary ovarian cancer syndrome. Women with site-specific familial ovarian cancer, the breast-ovarian cancer syndrome, or Lynch syndrome II (a predisposition to develop ovarian, endometrial, and/or colon cancers) tend to have ovarian cancer at a significantly younger age than those without this genetic predisposition. Specifically, women with these familial syndromes have been reported to have ovarian cancer at the age of 30 to 40 years. Even though these three hereditary ovarian cancer syndromes account for less than 10% of ovarian cancer cases, members of these families have a lifetime risk of developing disease that approaches 50%. Many women with sporadic ovarian cancers may have other family members with ovarian cancer, yet they do not constitute hereditary ovarian cancer syndrome. It has been estimated that women with one relative with ovarian cancer have a 3.1 relative risk of ovarian cancer compared with the general population, and even when two or three members of the family are affected, the relative risk is only 4.6.

Bourne and coworkers[15] screened 1601 women with a family history of ovarian cancer, utilizing TVS as a primary screen, with CDI and morphology index used as secondary tests with persistently abnormal TVS findings. Sixty-one women (3.8%) had positive results with subsequent surgery. Six ovarian cancers (five, stage IA lesions; three with low malignant potential; one, stage III) were discovered, demonstrating a 0.69% incidence of ovarian cancer. This bimodal screening procedure had an apparent detection rate of 100%, a specificity of 99.1%, and a positive predictive value of 29%. A retrospective analysis[16] of CA 125 on stored serum samples revealed values of 5, 24, and 39 U/mL in the three cases of stage I tumors with low malignant potential, 27 and 242 U/mL in the two invasive stage I cancers, and 398 U/mL in the stage III carcinoma. This subsequent investigation also reported five additional cancers, two of which were peritoneal carcinomas identified 2 and 8 months after the last ultrasound examination.

In an on-going study initiated in 1991, a similar group of 1261 women with positive family histories has been screened for ovarian cancer with TVS, CDI, and a battery of 5 tumor markers, including CA 125.[17, 18] Each participant met with genetic counselors and had her pedigree confirmed by medical records or death certificates. Like the 1993 study of Bourne and associates,[15] a 0.81% incidence of ovarian cancer was observed. Three stage I ovarian cancers and seven cases of stage IIIC peritoneal serous papillary carcinoma were diagnosed. All the women with stage I cancers had abnormal sonographic results leading to surgical exploration; their CA 125 levels were less than 15 U/mL at the time of diagnosis. Of the seven cases of peritoneal serous papillary carcinoma, two had elevated levels of CA 125, two had abnormal ultrasound examinations, and three had abdominal symptoms 5, 6, and 15 months after screening. Genetic testing for BRCA1 and BRCA2 germline mutations was offered to 8 of the 10 surviving patients, 4 of whom accepted. Testing performed on the one stage I patient was negative whereas three patients with peritoneal serous papillary carcinoma were found to carry BRCA1 185delAG mutations. The investigators concluded that multifocal peritoneal serous papillary carcinoma may be a phenotypic variant of familial ovarian cancer. Ultrasound and CA 125 testing as screening strategies to detect early disease cannot be relied on for these women.

FUTURE DIRECTIONS

Technologic advances coupled with an improved understanding of early ovarian cancer biology will ultimately lead to the design of an optimal ovarian cancer screening modality. For example, whereas screening protocols based primarily on detecting morphologic and blood flow changes in the ovaries of women from high-risk families seem destined to fail in detecting peritoneal serous papillary carcinoma, serologic tests for shed tumor antigens might seem a logical approach. New markers, such as lysophosphatidic acid, are under development, and molecular discoveries may lead to the identification of many more.

Regarding CA 125 testing, the sensitivity of this modality may be improved by the risk of ovarian cancer (receiver-operator characteristic [ROC] curve) algorithm. Skates and colleagues[19] proposed fitting an exponential model using longitudinal data and testing for an exponential rise in the value of the marker. The ROC curve algorithm, based on mathematic modeling of CA 125 changes associated with ovarian cancer, is currently being evaluated as a primary ovarian cancer screening test.

Three-dimensional (3D) ultrasound is a likely addition as a diagnostic modality included in the armamentarium of ovarian cancer screening. With this recent development in ultrasound, three continual different planes, representing longitudinal, transverse, and horizontal sections, are displayed simultaneously. These three planes can be rotated and computer-translated to obtain accurate anatomic sections needed for diagnosis and geometric measurements such as distances, areas, and volume. An early investigation of the usefulness of 3D ultrasound in the evaluation of ovarian pathology[20] has demonstrated 3D's ability of simultaneous viewing of three orthogonal planes as well as its improved ability to define location of structures relative to one another. Additional benefits of 3D include obtaining reliable and reproducible ovarian volume measurements, closer inspection of internal cyst walls, and detailed monitoring of subtle changes over time. With high patient acceptability, the 3D scan is considered a valuable adjunct to the two-dimensional ultrasound examination.

CONCLUSIONS

Several investigators have demonstrated the feasibility of screening women using CA 125, ultrasonography, or a combination of the two modalities. There is, however, no evidence that screening reduces mortality due to ovarian cancer, even in women with hereditary ovarian cancer syndromes.

In 1994, the National Institutes of Health consensus conference on ovarian cancer screening[21] concluded that there is no evidence to support routine screening in the general population. Participation in screening trials, however, was considered to be an appropriate option. Women with hereditary ovarian cancer syndromes should be referred to a specialist to discuss the appropriate use of diagnostic testing and prophylactic surgery. Although there are no data demonstrating a reduction in mortality by screening high-risk patients, annual screening with pelvic examination, CA 125 determinations, and TVS was advised for these high-risk women.

Whereas the screening modalities in themselves pose little risk, possible risks are associated with screening for ovarian carcinoma. These include anxiety related to abnormal screening results and morbidity and mortality owing to resultant surgical procedures for nonsignificant pathology. Women undergoing oophorectomy related to false-positive screening may be placing themselves at risk for cardiovascular disease and osteoporosis. Negative results, on the other hand, may lead to a delay in the diagnosis of ovarian cancer. The limitations of testing must be recognized in order that patients and their physicians are not falsely reassured by negative screening results.

The current evidence, although encouraging, does not yet warrant the introduction of general population screening for ovarian cancer. Additional clinical screening trials are ongoing and will likely provide the data necessary to determine the true costs and effectiveness of ovarian cancer screening.

References

1. Oriel KA, Hartenbach EM, Remington PL: Trends in United States ovarian cancer mortality, 1979–1995. Obstet Gynecol 1999;93:30–33.
2. Campbell S, Bhan V, Royston P, et al: Transabdominal ultrasound screening for early ovarian cancer. BMJ 1989;229:1363–1967.
3. DePriest PD, Gallion HH, Pavlik EJ, et al: Transvaginal sonography as a screening method for the detection of early ovarian cancer. Gynecol Oncol 1997;65:408–414.
4. Crayford TJB, Campbell S, Bourne TH, et al: Benign ovarian cysts and ovarian cancer: A cohort study with implications for screening. Lancet 2000;255:1060–1063.
5. DePriest PD, Shenson BS, Fried A, et al: A morphology index based on sonographic findings in ovarian cancer. Gynecol Oncol 1993;51:7–11.
6. Timor-Tritsch IE, Lerner JP, Monteagudo A, et al: Transvaginal ultrasonographic characterization of ovarian masses by means of color flow-directed Doppler measurements and a morphologic scoring system. Am J Obstet Gynecol 1993;168:909–913.
7. Bromley B, Goodman H, Benacerraf BR: Comparison between sonographic morphology and Doppler waveform for the diagnosis of ovarian malignancy. Obstet Gynecol 1994;83:331–338.
8. Lerner JP, Timor-Tritsch IE, Federman A, et al: Transvaginal ultrasonographic characterization of ovarian masses with an improved, weighted scoring system. Am J Obstet Gynecol 1994;170:81–85.
9. Granberg S, Wikland M, Jansson I: Macroscopic characterization of ovarian tumors and the relation to the histological diagnosis: Criteria to be used for ultrasound evaluation. Gynecol Oncol 1989;35:139–144.
10. Ferrazzi E, Zanetta G, Dordoni D, et al: Transvaginal ultrasonographic characterization of ovarian masses: Comparison of five scoring systems in a multicenter study. Ultrasound Obstet Gynecol 1997;10:192–197.
11. Folkman, J, Watson K, Ingber D, Hanahan D: Induction of angiogenesis during transition from hyperplasia to neoplasia. Nature 1989;339:58–61.
12. Kurjak A, Kupasic S, Breyer B, et al: The assessment of ovarian tumor angiogenetics: What does three-dimensional power Doppler add? Ultrasound Obstet Gynecol 1998;12:136–146.
13. Einhorn N, Sjovall K, Knapp RC, et al: Prospective evaluation of serum CA 125 levels for early detection of ovarian cancer. Obstet Gynecol 1992;80:14–18.

14. Jacobs I, Davies AP, Bridges J, et al: Prevalence screening for ovarian cancer in postmenopausal women by CA125 measurement and ultrasonography. BMJ 1993;306:1030–1034.
15. Bourne TH, Campbell S, Reynolds KM, et al: Screening for early familial ovarian cancer with transvaginal ultrasonography and colour blood flow imaging. BMJ 1993;306:1025–1029.
16. Bourne TH, Campbell S, Reynolds K, et al: The potential role of serum CA 125 in an ultrasound-based screening program for familial ovarian cancer. Gynecol Oncol 1994;52:379–385.
17. Karlan BY, Raffel LJ, Crvenkovic G, et al: A multidisciplinary approach to the early detection of ovarian carcinoma: Rationale, protocol design, and early results. Am J Obstet Gynecol 1993;169:494–501.
18. Karlan BY, Baldwin RL, Lopez-Luevanos E, et al: Peritoneal serous papillary carcinoma, a phenotypic variant of familial ovarian cancer: Implications for ovarian cancer screening. Am J Obstet Gynecol 1999;180:917–928.
19. Skates SJ, Xu FJ, Yu YH, et al: Toward an optimal algorithm for ovarian cancer screening with longitudinal tumor markers. Cancer 1995;76:2004–2010.
20. Greene NH, Platt LD, Santulli TS, et al: Usefulness of three-dimensional ultrasound in evaluation of ovarian pathology. J Ultrasound Med 2000;19:S83.
21. National Institutes of Health.Consensus Development Panel on Ovarian Cancer: Ovarian cancer: Screening, treatment, and follow-up. JAMA 1995;273:491–497.

Recent Advances in the Treatment of Vulvovaginal Candidiasis

Jack D. Sobel

CANDIDA VULVOVAGINITIS

Information on the incidence and prevalence of *Candida* vulvovaginitis (VVC) is currently incomplete because VVC is a nonreportable disease. Prevalence estimates have relied mainly on self-reported histories of physician diagnosis. VVC is routinely diagnosed without the benefit of microscopy or culture, and as many as 50% of the women diagnosed with VVC may have other conditions. Published epidemiologic data have been distorted by patient selection and referral biases, and widespread use of over-the-counter (OTC) antimycotics may seriously impair future epidemiologic studies.

By the age of 25 years, 50% of all college women will have experienced at least one physician-diagnosed episode of VVC, which is rare before menarche.[1] In other age populations, at least one episode of VVC has been estimated in up to 75% of premenopausal women.[2] Although it is extremely rare before menarche, the annual incidence increases drastically toward the end of the second decade of life, peaking over the following 2 decades. VVC appears reduced in frequency in postmenopausal women, although the incidence in this subpopulation remains unstudied, as does the permissive role of estrogen replacement therapy. Although it is widely assumed that VVC is more common and difficult to eradicate during pregnancy, no recent confirmatory studies have been performed to prove this theory.

Pathogenesis

Numerous worldwide studies indicate that *Candida albicans* is responsible for 80% to 94% of episodes of VVC. Several investigators have suggested a shift of yeast pathogens with the increased frequency of non-*albicans Candida* species, particularly *Candida glabrata*.[3, 4] Only a few of these studies have provided data to support this claim. Possible reasons for the apparent increase in non-*albicans Candida* VVC include the increased use of OTC antimycotics, long-term maintenance, suppressive prophylactic regimens incorporating systemic azoles, and the use of short courses of oral or topical antifungals.

Sporadic attacks of VVC usually occur without an identifiable etiologic or precipitating factor. One explanation is recently administered antibiotic, systemic or vaginal; however, the exact mechanisms for this association and its frequency have not been adequately studied. Only a minority of women with sporadic VVC report recent antimicrobials, and only a minority of women taking antibiotics develop VVC. A prerequisite for antibiotic-induced VVC is vaginal colonization by *Candida* organisms and a readily suppressible vaginal flora; however, microbiologic data are lacking. An association between lack of or loss of vaginal lactobacilli, hydrogen peroxide production, and susceptibility to VVC has not been established in women who develop VVC while taking antibiotics. The occurrence of VVC may vary by racial and behavioral factors. VVC has been shown to be more common among black women than white women and was associated with initiation of sexual behavior in college women.[1]

Several studies have documented increased risk of VVC in women who use oral contraceptives, and the risk may be higher with use of high-estrogen–containing agents. Sexual intercourse, with the use of a diaphragm or spermicide, was found associated with a marked increase in the rate of vaginal *Candida* colonization. It has not been confirmed that there is any association between spermicide use and VVC; however, increased risk of infection is attributed to use of vaginal sponges and intrauterine devices.[2]

VVC is not considered a sexually transmitted disease, because it also occurs in women who are not sexually active, and because *Candida* is considered part of the normal vaginal flora. This does not imply that sexual transmission of *Candida* does not or cannot occur or that VVC is not sexually associated, because numerous studies have confirmed transmission of *Candida* by vaginal intercourse and other forms of sexual activity.

A self-reported history of physician diagnosis of VVC indicates a marked increase in frequency of VVC at the time most women begin regular sexual activity. Individual episodes of VVC do not appear to be related to lifetime numbers of sexual partners or frequency of coitus. Engaging in oral-genital contact appears to increase risk,[1] but sexual intercourse alone has not been shown to alter microflora or increase *Candida* colonization. With rare exceptions, dietary studies have failed to show that dietary excesses play a major role in the etiology of sporadic or recurrent VVC. However, uncontrolled diabetic patients are at high risk for VVC and for non-*albicans Candida* species.

Diagnosis

A diagnosis of VVC is readily established by the finding of normal vaginal pH (4 to 4.5) and positive microscopy,

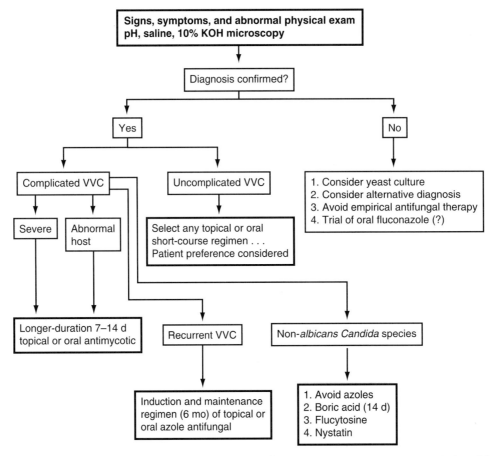

Figure 80–1. Algorithm for management of acute vulvovaginal candidiasis. KOH, potassium hydroxide; VVC, vulvovaginal candidiasis.

either saline or KOH (potassium hydroxide). Routine vaginal yeast cultures are usually unnecessary. Unfortunately, even well-trained microbiologists will miss at least 20% to 40% of cases of acute VVC, reflecting the poor sensitivity of these tests. VVC is still a possibility in patients with a compatible clinical presentation, normal pH, and negative microscopy, and a vaginal swab should then be submitted for culture.[5] In these circumstances, if symptoms are mild, antimycotic therapy can be deferred until culture results become available.

Differentiating VVC from bacterial vaginosis and trichomoniasis is simple, given the elevated pH and specific microscopy-associated features of the latter two conditions. Conditions simulating VVC are most frequently the result of hypersensitivity or allergic or chemical reactions, including contact dermatitis, and are rarely of infectious etiology. Failure to recognize the frequency of local adverse reactions may result in empirical prescription of additional topical agents, including high-potency steroids, which may further aggravate symptoms. No rapid, inexpensive diagnostic molecular techniques are currently widely available. Some studies have cast serious doubt on the accuracy of self-diagnosis of VVC and support the growing concern of OTC antimycotic abuse.[6]

Therapy

A major advance in the treatment of VVC is the acceptance of a new classification of VVC (Fig. 80–1).[3]

The majority of women with *Candida* vaginitis suffer from uncomplicated vaginitis (Table 80–1) characterized by sporadic attacks of mild to moderate severity due to *C. albicans*, that occurs in healthy adult women without any predisposing factors. In contrast, approximately 10% to 20% of women suffer from complicated *Candida* vaginitis in which attacks either are more severe, occur on a recurrent basis, or are due to non-*albicans Candida* species. Patients with complicated VVC more frequently have predisposing factors in the form of uncontrolled diabetes or other immunosuppressive conditions. Vaginitis caused by *C. glabrata* represents a complicated form of disease because of diminished yeast susceptibility to azole therapeutic agents.

Table 80–1. Complicated and Uncomplicated Vaginitis

Uncomplicated	Complicated
Mild to moderate	Moderate to severe
+	or
Infrequent/sporadic	Recurrent (>4/yr)
+	or
Pseudohyphae/hyphae	Budding yeast only
+	or
Normal host	Adverse factors:
	Pregnancy (?)
	Uncontrolled diabetes
	Immunocompromised

Uncomplicated Vulvovaginal Candidiasis

All forms of antimycotic therapy are highly effective against uncomplicated infections, and cure rates in excess of 80% can be expected[7] (Table 80–2).

No difference exists in overall in vitro activity and clinical efficacy of the various azole topical agents in the treatment of uncomplicated VVC. All the topical agents available are highly effective and can be expected to provide high cure rates. There is no evidence that any one formulation is superior to others. Selection of formulation should be based on the patient's preference. A critical issue pertains to the importance of duration of therapy versus total dose of the antimycotic agents. Historically, conventional topical therapy consisted of a 14-day regimen. In the process of shortening the course of therapy, more and more active drug was given in higher and higher concentrations. The assumption was that total dose was more important than the duration of therapy. Duration of therapy is of little significance in treating uncomplicated VVC, although longer follow-up studies (>30 days) have not been performed, and hence comparative relapse rates are unknown. Nevertheless, uncomplicated VVC responds well to all short-course regimens, including single-dose, single-day topical OTC antimycotic agents. The problem with the OTC use is not whether it is effective, because indeed it is highly effective; instead, inherent in OTC use is the fact that the patient is self-diagnosed. Unfortunately, self-diagnosis is unreliable, and abuse of OTC mycotics is possible when patients self-evaluate treatment efficacy.

Oral agents are highly effective in the treatment of acute, uncomplicated VVC.[8] These agents include flucona-zole, 150-mg single dose; ketoconazole, 400 mg daily for 5 days, and itraconazole, 200 mg twice in a single day or 200 mg daily for 3 days. Single-dose fluconazole has distinct pharmacokinetic advantages; therapeutic concentrations are present in vaginal tissue secretions for at least 72 hours. Numerous studies indicate both clinical and mycologic equivalence among single-dose fluconazole, single-day itraconazole, and multidose conventional topical azole therapy.

Complicated Vulvovaginal Candidiasis

In complicated VVC, yeast or host factors exist that have an adverse impact on the cure rate. Predisposing host factors include uncontrolled diabetes mellitus, immunocompromised and debilitated subjects, and ongoing antibiotic therapy, as well as severe local vulvovaginal inflammation and a history of recurrent VVC. Microbial determinants include non-*albicans Candida* species, particularly *C. glabrata* and *Saccharomyces cerevisiae*, which are less susceptible in vitro to azoles.[3] Women who have complicated VVC are less likely to respond to short courses of topical or systemic antimycotics and require 7 to 14 days of therapy.[9] Longer-duration initial therapy is critical in complicated patients, especially in an abnormal host. Women with severe local manifestations of VVC respond less well to abbreviated courses of topical or systemic antifungal agents. A recently completed randomized, placebo-controlled study[10] indicated that longer duration (>7 days) is necessary in women with severe VVC. Severe accompanying vulvitis may require additional topical mea-

Table 80–2. Therapy for Vaginal Candidiasis

Drug	Formulation	Dosage Regimen
Topical Agents		
Butoconazole*	2% cream	5 g × 3 d
Clotrimazole*	1% cream	5 g × 7–14 d
	100-mg vaginal tablet	1 tablet × 7 d
	100-mg vaginal tablet	2 tablets × 3 d
	500-mg vaginal tablet	1 tablet, single dose
Miconazole*	2% cream	5 g × 7 d
	100-mg vaginal suppository	1 suppository × 7 d
	200-mg vaginal suppository	1 suppository × 3 d
	1200-mg vaginal suppository	1 suppository, single dose
Econazole	150-mg vaginal tablet	1 tablet × 3 d
Fenticonazole	2% cream	5 g × 7 d
Tioconazole*	2% cream	5 g × 3 d
	6.5% cream	5 g, single dose
Terconazole	0.4% cream	5 g × 7 d
	0.8% cream	5 g × 3 d
	80-mg vaginal suppository	1 suppository × 3 d
Nystatin	100,000-U vaginal tablet	1 tablet × 14 d
Oral Agents		
Ketoconazole	200 mg	bid × 5 d
Itraconazole	200 mg	bid × 1 d
	200 mg	× 3 d
Fluconazole	150 mg	Single dose

*Over-the-counter drug.

sures, especially when oral azoles are prescribed; however, high-potency steroids may exacerbate burning.

RECURRENT VULVOVAGINAL CANDIDIASIS

Recurrent vulvovaginal candidiasis (RVVC) is defined as four or more episodes of infection during a period of 12 months. Most women categorized with RVVC have been misdiagnosed by physicians or incorrectly self-diagnosed. Among the most common reasons for misdiagnosis is that an initial *Candida* vaginitis may perpetuate itself as a nonmycotic topical contact dermatitis. In addition, hypersensitivity and clinical, irritant, and allergic reactions to topical agents and other environmental factors may produce chronic or intermittent vulvovaginal symptoms indistinguishable from those of VVC. The magnitude of culture-confirmed RVVC is unknown and is estimated at 5% to 8% of healthy women.

In a minority of women who have RVVC, including those with antibiotic-induced recurring episodes, the pathogenesis is apparent: abnormal hosts (e.g., uncontrolled diabetes) and those in whom relatively resistant non-*albicans Candida* species are responsible. Resistance among *C. albicans* is rare. Women with RVVC can develop repeated, persistent, acute attacks of symptomatic vaginitis with highly susceptible strains of *C. albicans*, proved by longitudinal DNA typing studies. The pathogenesis of RVVC, caused by *C. glabrata* and other less sensitive species of *Candida*, may be different, in that persistence of these relatively resistant strains reflects drug failure, rather than host failure.

The role of sexual transmission, and therefore reinfection with a new or identical strain of *C. albicans* in causing repeated episodes, remains unresolved. Most studies have failed to demonstrate that treatment of the male partner reduces VVC recurrence; however, Spinillo and associates,[11] in a case control study, were able to reduce recurrence rates in women whose culture-positive partners were treated with systemic antimycotics. Current views regarding pathogenesis of idiopathic RVVC, especially when due to *C. albicans*, suggest that local vaginal immune mechanisms may be responsible for the frequent relapses. A biologic susceptibility to RVVC in women, possibly related to Lewis blood group antigens and secretor status, may facilitate vaginal yeast colonization. No evidence exists that women with RVVC have a vaginal flora deficient in lactobacilli.

RVVC in an otherwise healthy adult female is not considered a justification for performing a glucose tolerance test or obtaining HIV serology tests, unless other indications are present. Following culture confirmation of diagnosis, RVVC is best managed by judicious use of antimycotics. Several controlled long-term studies have confirmed the efficacy of maintenance suppressive therapy for 6 months after an initial intensive induction regimen achieves culture-negative status. Regimens to consider include ketoconazole (100 mg/day), itraconazole (50 to 100 mg/day), fluconazole (150 mg/wk), or clotrimazole vaginal suppositories (500 mg) administered once a week for 6 months.

Vulvovaginal Candidiasis and Non-*albicans Candida* Species

There is little information regarding the clinical effectiveness of azoles against non-*albicans Candida* species. There are, however, increasing reports of clinical failures, especially with *C. glabrata*.[3] Unresponsive patients or early relapses following azole therapy remain a therapeutic challenge and frequently respond to 600 mg of intravaginal boric acid administered once or twice a day for 2 weeks, or topical flucytosine therapy. Maintenance regimens remain unavailable, presenting a major hiatus in our therapeutic armamentarium, although vaginal suppositories of the polyene agent nystatin are useful in this context.

References

1. Geiger AM, Foxman B: Risk factors for vulvovaginal candidiasis: A case-control study among university students. Epidemiology 1996;7:182–187.
2. Sobel JD: Vaginitis. N Engl J Med 1997;337:1896–1903.
3. Sobel JD: Vulvovaginitis due to *Candida glabrata*: An emerging problem. Mycoses 1998;41:18–22.
4. Horowitz BJ, Giaquinta D, Ito S: Evolving pathogens in vulvovaginal candidiasis: Implications for patient care. J Clin Pharmacol 1992;32:248–255.
5. Eckert LO, Hawes SE, Stevens CE, et al: Vulvovaginal candidiasis: Clinical manifestations, risk factors, management algorithm. Obstet Gynecol 1998;92:757–765.
6. Ferris DG, Dekle C, Litaker MS: Women's use of over-the-counter antifungal medications for gynecologic symptoms. J Fam Pract 1996;42:595–600.
7. Reef S, McNeil M, Sobel JD, Pinner R: Vulvovaginal candidiasis: A review of available therapeutic options. Infect Dis Clin Pract 1995;4:36–40.
8. Sobel JD, Brooker D, Stein GE, et al: Single oral dose fluconazole compared with conventional clotrimazole topical therapy of *Candida* vaginitis. Am J Obstet Gynecol 1995;172:1263–1268.
9. Sobel JD, Faro S, Force RW, et al: Vulvovaginal candidiasis: Epidemiologic, diagnostic, and therapeutic considerations. Am J Obstet Gynecol 1998;178:203–211.
10. Sobel JD, Kapernick PS, Zervos M, et al: Treatment of complicated *Candida* vaginitis: Comparison of single and sequential doses of fluconazole. Am J Obstet Gynecol 2001;185:363–369.
11. Spinillo A, Carratta L, Pizzoli G, et al: Recurrent vaginal candidiasis: Results of a cohort study of sexual transmission and intestinal reservoir. J Reprod Med 1992;37:343–347.

Update on Endometrial Ablation and Related Techniques

Spencer S. Richlin and John A. Rock

Six hundred thousand hysterectomies are performed yearly in the United States, costing $5 billion.[1] Of these hysterectomies, 282,000 to 292,000 are performed for dysfunctional bleeding. Endometrial ablation offers an alternative to hysterectomy in the properly chosen patient. It is well known that hysterectomy has complications including infection, hemorrhage, pain, injury to bowel or bladder, ileus, sexual dysfunction, altered pelvic support, thromboembolism, and even death (at a rate of approximately 6 per 10,000 procedures).[2] Although hysterectomy is a 100% cure for menorrhagia and postmenopausal bleeding from hormone replacement, many women have come to prefer endometrial ablation, knowing that it is less invasive but not as curative. For most patients undergoing ablation procedures, treatment success is not judged solely by amenorrhea. Avoiding major surgery with a long hospital stay and reduction in menstrual flow to eumenorrhea or less are realistic surgical end points. Dilatation and curettage (D&C) has been used in the past as the first-line surgical treatment for abnormal bleeding. The limitations of D&C are decreased menstrual flow for only a few cycles.

The goal of endometrial ablation is to remove or destroy the portion of the uterus that causes bleeding. This includes the endometrium and 2.5 to 3.0 mm of myometrium because it also contains some endometrial glands.[3] Many ablation techniques have evolved since 1975, all of which attempt to create an Ascherman syndrome. Different types of energy systems have been and are being developed, some of which utilize the hysteroscope. Newer systems are using devices placed blindly into the uterus, without dilating the cervix, as office procedures. The goal is to develop ablation procedures that are safer, cheaper, and less invasive, have a quicker recovery time, and are faster to perform than abdominal or vaginal hysterectomy.

Traditional ablation techniques using a resecting loop, rollerball cautery, and laser all require training and skill. These procedures use potentially dangerous energy sources and uterine distending mediums. Perioperative complications include uterine perforation,[4] bowel injury,[5] air embolism,[6] fluid overload,[7] hematometra,[8] fatal hyponatremic encephalopathy,[9] hyperammonemia,[10] cardiac arrest,[11] endometriosis by implantation,[12] hemorrhage,[13] necrotizing granulomatous endometritis,[14] and toxic shock syndrome.[15]

Overall complication rates range from 6% for a first ablation to 15% for a repeat procedure.[16] Thermal balloon ablation has been widely studied to treat menorrhagia and has attained similar clinical efficacy, with no intraoperative complications, when compared with other ablation procedures.[17] Balloon ablation has been touted as an alternative to hysterectomy and traditional ablation for high-risk surgical candidates.[18] Patients with bleeding disorders, obesity, pacemakers, postmenopausal bleeding, bowel disease with adhesions and ileostomies, heart-lung transplants, and cervical stenosis underwent successful balloon ablation with no intraoperative complications and a 79% success rate. In the patient with cardiac disease, balloon ablation does not pose the risk of fluid overload, because no distention medium is used. Patients with bleeding disorders can remain on warfarin (Coumadin) before surgery and not risk a thromboembolic event.

PREOPERATIVE EVALUATION AND PATIENT SELECTION

The indications for endometrial ablation include menorrhagia for greater than 6 months that does not respond to hormonal management or D&C, including refusal by the patient to use long-term hormonal treatment. Additionally, high-risk surgical patients may better tolerate a less invasive ablation procedure. Patients must have finished their childbearing. Unprotected intercourse could result in pregnancy if contraception is not used; thus, concurrent laparoscopic tubal sterilization is offered to younger patients.

Preoperative workup includes a thorough history and physical examination with pelvic examination, a complete blood count, thyroid panel, prothrombin time, partial thromboplastin time, platelet count, bleeding time, chest x-ray, and urinalysis. Uterine sampling, before ablation, with D&C, endometrial biopsy, or hysteroscope-directed biopsy is mandatory. Of these screening techniques, hysteroscopic evaluation and biopsy of the uterine cavity are preferred. Visualization of the cavity can rule out a structural cause for bleeding (e.g., myomas, polyps, endometrial cancer), which may negate the need for ablation. In the case of a small submucous or pedunculated myoma, resection could take place at the same time as ablation. Endometrial sampling is especially important in a postmenopausal patient who is spotting while on hormone replacement. Patients with endometrial carcinoma or endometrial hyperplasia (with or without atypia) should not be offered ablation.

Patients at high risk for endometrial carcinoma are not good candidates for ablation. Instead they should undergo hysterectomy. Poor surgical candidates may be offered balloon ablation. High-risk factors include obesity, unopposed estrogen therapy in the past, diabetes mellitus, hyperplasia unresponsive to progestins, late menopause, and nulliparity.[19] Eight high-risk patients in the literature developed endometrial carcinoma after ablation and had subsequent hysterectomies. With ablation, there is always the risk of "missing" an area of endometrial tissue that may later become malignant or may have been metastatic and invaded the myometrium at the time of ablation.[20] Thus, in high-risk patients, or in any patient who has vaginal bleeding after ablation, carcinoma must be ruled out. Abnormal bleeding after an ablation procedure should not be thought of as only a treatment failure—endometrial carcinoma is still part of the differential diagnosis.[21]

Partial rollerball endometrial ablation, which ablates only the anterior or posterior endometrial wall and avoids the cornual areas, has been investigated as a method to decrease postoperative adhesion formation while allowing earlier detection of endometrial cancer.[22] Because only one wall is ablated, scarring does not form. Good control of menorrhagia has been reported. Scarring, adhesions, and a hematometra, which can form with traditional anterior and posterior wall ablation, may potentially prevent vaginal bleeding (thus obscuring the first indication of endometrial cancer). This technique is still being investigated.

Informed consent before surgery includes a discussion of the surgical risks and realistic outcomes. Patients must realize that amenorrhea results in the minority of patients. Amenorrhea, oligomenorrhea, normal menses, or even no improvement in menorrhagia is possible. Success rates for all ablation procedures are about the same—amenorrhea 40% to 60%, hypomenorrhea 30% to 50%, eumenorrhea 10% to 15%. There is always a chance of treatment failure and possible need for repeat ablation. A subset of these patients will opt for a definitive hysterectomy to control their menorrhagia.

LASER, ELECTROSURGICAL, AND RESECTION TECHNIQUES

Studies are summarized in Table 81–1.

Goldrath and associates[23] first described endometrial ablation using a neodymiun: yttrium-aluminium-garnet (Nd:YAG) laser. Tissue coagulation by necrosis penetrates 4 to 5 mm in depth using a 1-mm sapphire tip at 40 to 60 watts. The touch and nontouch techniques are usually combined. Nontouch is used in the thin cornual and fundal areas, and the touch technique ablates the remaining uterus. Laser treatment (rollerball and loops) requires surgical skill with

the hysteroscope to avoid thermal injuries, perforation, cervical tears, and bleeding. Anesthesia always has risks, whereas distending media have the potential for fluid overload and electrolyte disturbances. Complications of laser are well known and tend to happen with less-experienced surgeons. The complication rate depends on the study. Garry and colleagues[24] had no major complications with 600 laser ablations. Eighty-three percent of these patients had resolution of their menorrhagia, with 28% at 16 months being amenorrheic. There was a 14% repeat ablation rate and a 7% subsequent hysterectomy rate. Baggish and Sze[25] reported on 401 laser ablations with similar low complication rates. At 4.5 years, 92% of patients had no menorrhagia. Overall success rates among studies (amenorrhea and light or normal menses) range between 80% and 90%. Phillips and coworkers[26] reported on 1000 laser ablations. Fourteen percent of patients underwent one repeat, and 0.4% two repeat ablations, with 21% projected to have a hysterectomy over a 6.5-year follow-up period.

The loop electrode, rollerball, and rollerbarrel utilizing the resectoscope for ablation have established success rates similar to those of the Nd:YAG laser. Rollerball ablation is faster, safer than laser, easier to use, and less expensive—a laser costs approximately $100,000 compared with $10,000 for rollerball or loop ablation instrumentation. O'Connor and Magos[16] followed 525 women for 5 years after endometrial resection. They utilized cutting loop combined with rollerball (rollerball coagulated the fundus and ostia). This procedure has complications similar to those of laser—thermal injury to bowel, fluid overload, and perforation. Ninety percent of their patients had resolution of menorrhagia at 1 year, and 100% at 5 years (results of only 37 patients). Nine percent underwent repeat ablations and 9% eventually had a hysterectomy. There were 10 uterine perforations, 3 postoperative bleeds needing balloon tamponade, 2 cervical tears, and 19 patients with greater than 2 L of fluid overload. In this study, there was a 6% complication rate. Overall, 80% of their patients had no gynecologic surgery during the first 5 years after resection.

Loop electrocautery uses 100 to 120 watts of blended cutting and coagulation energy. Cutting loops are available in different sizes. Resection removes 2 to 3 mm of myometrium—removing glands that are in the superficial myometium. Compared with other ablation procedures that destroy tissue, the resected strips of tissue can be sent for pathologic evaluation. Loop resection is technically difficult: an inadvertent deep resection can result in thermal injury to pelvic structures, resulting even in death.[27] Laparoscopic guidance can help orientation and decrease perforation.

Rollerball ablation has replaced loop resection as the preferred ablative technique. Through the resectoscope, the electrode end (2 to 4 mm) is dragged on the endometrium coagulating down to the basalis layer. The cutting loop produces more bleeding, resected tissue strips obscure vision, and loop resection has a higher perforation rate when compared with rollerball.[28]

Martyn and Allyn[29] resected 317 patients. All took danazol preoperatively for endometrial thinning. Laminaria were placed the day before surgery. Forty-five patients were ablated with a rollerball, 21% were ablated with a loop and rollerball, 10% had polyps removed and ablated with the rollerball, 18% underwent fibroid resection and rollerball ablation, and 4.3% had a tubal ligation with rollerball ablation. There was a 3.1% complication rate—one uterine perforation (on insertion of the scope), one fluid overload, two intraoperative hemorrhages, one postoperative deep venous thrombosis, and three postoperative hematometras. This study reported a 10% failure rate at 2 years and 27% at 5 years. A failure was defined as bleeding or a pain pattern unsatisfactory to the patient. They had a 19.2% repeat surgery rate (23 repeat ablations, 35 hysterectomies). Ninety percent of women had amenorrhea at 2 years, with a drop to 73% at 5 years.

A meta-analysis of the literature from 1981 to 1996, incorporating all three methods and 6135 patients,[28] resulted in 46% of patients being amenorrheic, 37% hypomenorrheic, and 5% eumenorrheic. Caution has to be taken when looking at the literature because many studies do not have long-term (5-year) follow-up. The MISTLETOE (Minimally Invasive Surgical Techniques—Laser, Endo-Thermal or Endoresection) study, a national survey, reviewed 10,686 endometrial resection and ablation procedures from the United Kingdom. The study evaluated perioperative, postoperative, and delayed complications by method and experience of operating surgeon. Laser and rollerball had the fewest complications, whereas loop resection had the highest complication rate.

Pretreatment thinning of the endometrium with a gonadotropin-releasing hormone (GnRH) analogue before ablation is gaining acceptance. Postmenopausal or older premenopausal patients, who are hypoestrogenic, usually have thin endometrial layers and do not need preoperative endometrial thinning. Younger patients with menorrhagia have endometrial linings that vary in thickness, depending on the phase of their menstrual cycle, from 3 to 11 mm.[31] Pretreatment with a GnRH analogue before ablation renders the endometrium uniformly thin. A thick endometrial lining makes ablation more difficult and may not allow complete ablation down to the basalis layer. Donnez and associates[32] published the first randomized, multicenter, prospective double-blind study of goserelin, 3.6 mg for 2 months, before ablation using loop resection with rollerball ablation (of the cornua) versus placebo. The endometrium was significantly thinner in the goserelin treated group—1.61 versus 3.53 mm. Amenorrhea rates at 6 months were 40% in the treated versus 26% in the placebo group. Additionally, the treated group had shorter procedures that were considered easier by the operating surgeon and absorbed less distending fluid.

THERMAL BALLOON ABLATION

Owing to the high complication rates and inherent technical difficulty with ablation techniques, thermal balloon ablation has been introduced as a safer, easier, and faster technique. Patient inclusion and exclusion criteria are the same except for the following: the uterocervical length must be less than 12 cm with no submucous myomas, and patients must not have a latex allergy. ThermaChoice (Ethicon) was approved in 1997 for use in the United States. This system has a 16-cm long by 5-mm wide catheter containing a latex balloon with a heating element at its distal end. A control unit connects to the probe and monitors pressure, temperature, and duration of ablation. Only rarely does the cervix need dilatation. Sterile 5% dextrose in water is infused into the balloon until 160 to 180 mm Hg of pressure is reached. This creates good contact between the uterine wall and the balloon. The control device will stop if pressure drops below 45 mm Hg or rises above 200 mm Hg. Fluid within the balloon is heated to 87°C for 8 minutes. Destruction is limited to the endometrium and superficial myometrium. Compared with traditional ablation techniques, balloon ablation does not use distending fluids.[1] Once it is inserted, the risk of perforation is greatly reduced.

Meyer and colleagues[17] performed a multicenter study (239 women) comparing rollerball ablation with balloon ablation, with 1 year follow-up data. Amenorrhea rates were 15% in the balloon and 27% in the rollerball group. In 91% percent of the rollerball and 85% of balloon patients, bleeding was judged by patient diary scores to be eumenorrheic or less (not statistically significant). Quality of life satisfaction rates were comparable between the groups. Patients were highly satisfied at 1 year. At 2-year follow-up,[33] 227 patients were evaluated. Quality of life questionnaires were comparable with 1-year data. Significant satisfaction of 105 (86.1%) uterine balloon–treated and 91 (86.7%) rollerball-treated patients was similar to results at 1 year. One hundred nine (89.1%) women treated with uterine balloon therapy and 95 (90.4%) of those treated by rollerball had menstrual status ranging from amenorrhea to eumenorrhea. The percentage of patients reporting amenorrhea was comparable at 1 and 2 years. Ninety-seven and one-half percent of the uterine balloon–treated patients and 99% of rollerball patients stated that they would recommend the procedure they had to others. The rollerball group had one perforation, two patients with overload, and one cervical laceration. There were no major complications in the balloon group. Minor complication rates were similar. Patients in this study did not use prethinning agents. Similar results have been reported from the Collaborative Uterine Thermal Balloon Working Group.[34]

The safety profile of balloon ablation has been studied by measuring serosal temperatures and depth of thermal injury. Safe serosal temperatures were maintained, and depth of myometrial injury was less than 3.5 mm.[35] Balloon ablation may be performed in the future under local anesthesia in an office setting.[36]

The Cavaterm thermal balloon ablation system from Switzerland is another ablation system undergoing pilot studies.[37] This system uses a disposable silicone balloon

Table 81–1. Endometrial Ablation Studies

Study	Ablations (N of Patients)	Method (N of Patients)	Mean Operating Time	Menorrhagia Resolved Short-Term (N of Patients)	Menorrhagia Resolved Long-Term (N of Patients)	Amenorrhea (%)	Additional Surgery	Complications
Garry et al[24]	600 524	Nd:YAG	25 min Range, 5–105	83% (418/501) Mean, 15 mo	No data reported	28.90	34 (6.8%) hysterectomies 75 (14.3%) repeat ablations	No major complications 2 endometritis
Baggish and Sze[25]	568 560	Ny:YAG (401) Rollerball (167)	32.5 min Range, 20–40	Not reported in this paper	92% (525/568) Mean, 4.5 yr	62 laser 46 rollerball	8 repeat ablations 2 hysterectomies	4 pulmonary edema 1 endometritis 1 posteroposterior adenocarcinoma 2 postoperative bleeding
O'Connor and Magos[16]	575 525	Wire loop/rollerball	33 min Range, 10–100	90% (472/524) 1 yr	100% (37/37) 5 yr	35 at 1 yr 40 at 5 yr	48 hysterectomies	10 perforations 3 bleeding 9 endometritis 19 >2 L fluid overload 2 cervical tears
Vilos et al[51]	800	Rollerball	27 min Range, 4–72	89% at 1 yr	No data reported	60 at 1 yr	32 (4.4%) repeat ablations 18 (18%) hysterectomies	7 perforations 8 >1.5 L fluid overload 5 bleeding 4 endometritis 1 salpingitis
Martyn and Allan[29]	317 317	Rollerball	30 min Range, 9–95	90% (data of 301) at 2 yr	73% (data of 29) at 5 yr	44 at 2 yr 42 at 5 yr	23 (7.6%) repeat ablations 35 (11.6%) hysterectomies	1 perforation 1 fluid overload 2 bleeding 2 hematometra 1 anesthesia complication 1 DVT 1 endomyometritis
Aberdeen Trials[52]	204	Hysterectomy (99) Rollerball (105)	Not reported in this paper	Not reported in this paper	Rollerball 45% (33/78) amenorrhea 13 received hysterectomy 40% (29/78) hypomenorrhea at 4 yr	33 at 4 yr	Rollerball group 20 hysterectomies 4 ablations + hysterectomy 13 repeat ablations 2 double repeat ablations	Not reported in this paper

Study	n	Device	Operative Time	Short-term Outcome	Longer-term Outcome	Follow-up	Reinterventions/Hysterectomies	Complications
Meyer et al[17]	255 255	ThermaChoice Balloon (128) Rollerball (117)	27 min (range, 16–38) 39 min (range, 25–53)	Over 2/3 in both groups had resolution of menorrhagia	2 yr [51]* 89.1% [109] balloon* 90.4% [95] rollerball*	15 at 2 yr 27 at 2 yr	Balloon—4 hysterectomies Rollerball—11 hysterectomies	Balloon—no major complication Rollerball 1 perforation 1 cervical laceration 1 hematometra
Hawe et al[37]	50 50	Cavaterm Balloon	No data reported	96% mean at 14 mo Range, 6–4 mo	No data reported	68 mean 14 mo	1 laser ablation 1 hysterectomy	No complications reported
Hodgson et al[40]	137 137	Microwaves	141 sec (mean) Range, 50–310	No data reported	3-year follow-up (n = 43) 16 (37%) amenorrhea 11 (26%) very light discharge 9 (21%) improved periods satisfied 1 (2%) improved periods not satisfied	37 at 3 yr	3 repeat microwave ablations 4 hysterectomies	No complications reported
das Dores et al[41]	26 26	Hydro ThermAblator (heated saline)	No data reported	No data reported	87% (amenorrhea/hypomenorrhea) at 18 mo (n = 8)	50% at 18 mo (n = 4)	1 hysterectomy 2 repeat ablations	No complications reported
Thijssen[49]	1280 1280	Radiofrequency	20 min (mean) Range, 15–28	77% (amenorrhea/hypomenorrhea) at 6 mo (n = 22) 88% (amenorrhea/hypomenorrhea) at 1 yr (n = 17)	78.5% (amenorrhea/hypomenorrhea) (n = 966) Mean follow-up 32 mo Range, 6–58 mo	19 at mean of 32 mo	21.5% hysterectomy rate	10 superficial skin burns 3 perforations 2 hematometra 4 pelvic infections 5 vesicovaginal fistula 1 burn right finger 1 thermal bowel injury 1 thermal injury to cervix/anterior fornix

*Numbers in brackets indicate references from the study cited.
DVT, deep venous thrombosis; Nd:YAG, neodymium:yttrium-aluminum-garnet.

catheter, with 1.5% glycine filling the balloon. It also has a central monitor, but it has the following unique features different from those of ThermaChoice: a balloon is adjustable for different-sized uterine cavities; fluid maintained in constant motion as glycine conducts heat poorly; balloon pressures are higher (180 to 220 mm Hg); the cervix must be dilated; and the heating element is within the balloon. The authors believe that higher intrauterine pressures will tamponade superficial blood flow and reduce the cooling effect of uterine circulation in the superficial myometrium. The total depth of destruction is 8 mm, with a 2- to 5-mm destruction of the superficial myometrium. Treatment time is 15 minutes. Fifty patients were followed for a mean of 14 months. Sixty-eight percent had amenorrhea, 24% had only spotting, 4% were eumenorrheic, and 4% failed the treatment. There were no major complications. Only two patients developed endometritis.

A third balloon ablation device, VestaDUB, is a 12-electrode intrauterine balloon device that uses 45 watts of electrosurgical energy.[38] Treatment lasts 4 minutes, maintaining uniform surface temperatures between 70°C and 75°C. Forty-five of 69 patients have been followed for at least 3 to 9 months. Forty percent are amenorrheic.

Balloon therapy has many advantages over other ablative techniques. Gynecologists who are inexperienced with the resectoscope can achieve results similar to those of loop resection or rollerball ablation. Supporters of balloon ablation argue that using it is as easy as placing an intrauterine device.

FUTURE DIRECTIONS

Newer techniques and technologies are being developed to further decrease the skill needed to perform ablations. These include the cryoprobe, microwaves, heated saline solution, phototherapy, radiofrequency hyperthermia, and laser interstitial therapy.

Rutherford[39] used a cryoprobe maintained at −176°C. on nine patients. General anesthesia was used in three patients and intravenous sedation in six. Seven remained amenorrheic, with two reporting normal menses 2 to 3 months postablation.

Hodgson and coworkers[40] devised an ablation technique using microwave energy as a source of thermal energy. The solid applicator has a diameter of 8 mm, producing a frequency of 9.2 GHz, which generates a maximum heating depth of 6 mm into endometrial tissue. The "principle" of microwave ablation depends on the presence of succinate dehydrogenase in viable cells. Heating by microwave causes inactivation of intracellular enzymes and cell death. One hundred thirty-seven women were treated, with at least 3 years of follow-up. Patients with fibroids and previous uterine scars were excluded. Four weeks of preoperative endometrial thinning was required. Cervical dilatation to 9 mm preceded treatment. The applicator tip is placed at the fundus and slowly withdrawn using side-to-side move-

ments. When the applicator tip has ablated an area of endometrium, a temperature drop on a control screen alerts the operator that the area has been treated and that it is time to move to an untreated area of endometrium. Throughout the procedure, the applicator is withdrawn, preventing perforations. No perforations have been noted in over 400 procedures. Forty-three women have completed 3 years of follow-up. Mean treatment time was 141 seconds. Thirty-seven percent were amenorrheic, 25% had very light periods and/or discharge, 20% reported improved periods and/or were satisfied, and one patient had improved periods but was not satisfied. There were three retreatments and four hysterectomies. No complications were reported.

Installation of heated saline solution directly into the uterus has been described using the Hydro ThermAblator and the EnAbl systems. The ThermAblator uses a cannula and hysteroscope placed into the uterine cavity after cervical dilatation. Before the heated saline solution is placed into the uterus, a room temperature "saline flush cycle" enables hysteroscopic visualization of the cavity to ensure that no pathology is present. The cervix is dilated to allow a snug fit around the cannula that is placed at the junction of the endocervix and lower uterine segment. Ablation is performed with 90°C saline solution for 10 minutes, followed by another room temperature flush. Laparoscopy, during the procedure, monitored the uterus, fallopian tubes, and cornua, while watching the fallopian tubes for fluid leakage. No evidence of fluid leakage was noted inside the peritoneal cavity.

Twenty-six patients treated with heated saline solution were followed for 18 months.[41] At 6 months ($n = 21$), 41% of patients were amenorrheic, 36% hypomenorrheic, and 18% eumenorrheic. One year of follow-up ($n = 17$) found 47% amenorrheic, 41% hypomenorrheic, and 6% eumenorrheic. Eight patients were evaluated at 18 months, 87.5% were either amenorrheic or hypomenorrheic. Data are still being collected. No patient has experienced side effects or had a complication. Advantages of this procedure over balloon ablation include the fact that it is not a blind procedure and circulating fluid fills the entire cavity, even where there are irregularities. Bustos-Lopez and associates[42] evaluated the safety of heated saline solution for ablation on 11 patients undergoing hysterectomy. Before the uterus was removed, the endometrial cavities were "exposed" to 15 minutes of 70°C to 85°C recirculating saline solution. No spill was noted from the fallopian tubes. The entire endometrium and 1 to 2 mm of myometrium were necrosed uniformly, including the cornua. The cervix was not affected because there was no leakage through it and the serosal layer did not develop dangerous temperatures. One year after the procedure, no complications were reported.

Photodynamic therapy for endometrial ablation is still in its experimental stages. Light with proper energy and wavelengths interacts with a photosensitizing "drug" to create highly reactive oxygen intermediates. These intermediates, mostly singlet molecular oxygen, irreversibly oxidize cells, causing "photodestruction" of vasculature and cells resulting in tissue necrosis.[43] Several animal models and one human uterus study[44] show future promise of this method. At present, a laser and nonlaser light probe is being studied for future photodynamic therapy.[45, 46]

Phipps and colleagues[47, 48] proposed a treatment for menorrhagia by radio frequency–induced thermal ablation. This procedure relies on hyperthermia and its interaction between tissue and an electric field that is generated around a treatment applicator. Tissue within the electric field is heated but does not penetrate much beyond the endometrium. An insulated electrode was placed around the waist of 44 patients. Their cervix was dilated to 4 mm, and a hysteroscope was placed into their uterus to look for pathology before the procedure. The cervix was redilated to 10 mm, after which the radiofrequency probe was placed into the uterus. A vaginal guard was placed for protection. Three hundred thirty kilojoules (kJ) of energy was delivered to the first 10 patients, 445 kJ to the second 10, and 660 kJ to the last 22. The 22 patients who received 660 kJ had the best response. At this point in the study, patients had been followed for 4 to 6 months. Two obese patients developed a vesicovaginal fistula because their vaginal wall and bladder were in contact with the probe. Larger vaginal guards have now been developed. A follow-up study (4 to 10 months) included 33 patients treated with the "optimal" dose of 660 kJ. Eleven of 33 (30%) were amenorrheic, and 18 of 33 (55%) had reduced flow. Modifications have been made to ensure better safety for this technique. Thijssen[49] tested the safety and efficiency of radiofrequency ablation in a multicenter trial. Twelve hundred eighty patients were followed for 6 to 58 months. Median follow-up was 32 months. The mean duration of the procedure was 20 minutes, with intrauterine temperatures reaching between 62°C and 65°C. Seventy-eight percent had a resolution of their menorrhagia. Twenty-one percent required further therapy. Complications included 10 superficial skin burns, 3 uterine perforations, 2 hematometras, and pelvic inflammatory disease in 4 patients. Major complications included five vesicovaginal fistulas, one right index finger burn with loss of the distal phalanx, one thermal injury to bowel, and one thermal injury to the cervix and anterior fornix. Hysteroscopic evaluation postoperatively revealed that the endometrium was replaced by fibrous tissue with no synechia formation. This procedure is too dangerous and carries many disadvantages when compared with other ablation procedures.

Donnez and coworkers[50] designed an intrauterine device designed for endometrial ablation by Nd: YAG laser interstitial hyperthermy. Seven of the 10 patients were followed 6 to 17 months and all are amenorrheic.

SUMMARY

Many instruments and techniques have been developed for endometrial ablation. None are as successful as hyster-

ectomy; and patients have to understand that ablation procedures are intended to improve menorrhagia, not necessarily cure it. There is no question that safer and simpler instrumentation is needed. Traditional ablative techniques, and even some of the new innovative instruments, pose too much danger to patients. Balloon thermal ablation holds promise as a safe, effective procedure, which can be performed under local anesthesia in the office setting.

References

1. Carlson KJ, Nichols DH, Schiff I: Indications for hysterectomy. N Engl J Med 1993;328:856–860.
2. Dicker RC, Greenspan JR, Strauss LT: Complications of abdominal and vaginal hysterectomy among women of reproductive age in the United States. The Collaborative Review of Sterilization. Am J Obstet Gynecol 1985; 144:841–848.
3. Reid PC, Sharp F: Nd:YAG laser endometrial ablation: Histological aspects of uterine healing. Int J Gynecol Pathol 1992;11:174–179.
4. Pittrof R, Darwish DH, Shabib G: Near fatal uterine perforation during transcervical endometrial resection. Lancet 1991;338:197–198.
5. Kivnick S, Kanter MH: Bowel injury from rollerball ablation of the endometrium. Obstet Gynecol 1992; 79:833–835.
6. Michael A: Endometrial ablation and air embolism. Anaesth Intensive Care 1993;21:475.
7. Magos A: Safety of transcervical resection. Lancet 1990;335:44.
8. Hill DJ, Maher PJ, Davison GB, Wood C: Hematometra—a complication of endometrial ablation. Aust N Z J Obstet Gynaecol 1992;32:285.
9. Allen I, Arieff AI, Ayus JC: Endometrial ablation complicated by fatal hyponatraemic encephalopathy. JAMA 1993;270:1230–1232.
10. Kirwan PH, Makepeace P, Layward E: Hyperammonaemia after transcervical resection of the endometrium. Br J Obstet Gynaecol 1993;100:603–604.
11. Eugster D: Cardiac arrest during endometrial ablation. Anaesth Intensive Care 1993;21:891–892.
12. Sorenson SS, Anderson LF, Lose G: Endometriosis by implantation: A complication of endometrial ablation. Lancet 1994;343:1226.
13. Sturdee D, Hoggart B: Problems with endometrial resection. Lancet 1991;337:1471.
14. Ferryman SR, Stephens M, Gough D: Necrotising granulomatous endometritis following endometrial ablation therapy. Br J Obstet Gynaecol 1992;99:928–930.
15. Parkin DE: Fatal toxic shock syndrome following endometrial resection. Br J Obstet Gynaecol 1995;102:163–164.
16. O'Connor H, Magos A: Endometrial resection for the treatment of menorrhagia. N Engl J Med 1996;335:151–156.
17. Meyer WR, Walsh BW, Grainger DA, et al: Thermal balloon and rollerball ablation to treat menorrhagia: A multicenter comparison. Obstet Gynecol 1998;92:98–103.
18. Aletebi FA, Vilos GA, Eskandar MA: Thermal balloon ablation to treat menorrhagia in high-risk surgical candidates. J Assoc Gynecol Laparosc 1999;6:435–439.
19. Valle RF, Baggish MS: Endometrial carcinoma after endometrial ablation: High-risk factors predicting its occurrence. Am J Obstet Gynecol 1998;179:569–572.
20. Horowitz IR, Copas PR, Aaronoff M, et al: Endometrial adenocarcinoma following endometrial ablation for post menopausal bleeding. Gynecol Oncol 1995;56:460–463.
21. Friberg B, Joergensen C, Ahlgren M: Endometrial thermal coagulation—degree of uterine fibrosis predicts treatment outcome. Gynecol Obstet Invest 1998;45:54–57.
22. McCausland AM, McCausland VM: Partial rollerball endometrial ablation: A modification of total ablation to treat menorrhagia without causing complications from intrauterine adhesions. Am J Obstet Gynecol 1999;180: 1512–1521.
23. Goldrath MH, Fuller TA, Segal S: Laser photovaporization of endometrium for the treatment of menorrhagia. Am J Obstet Gynecol 1981;140:14–19.
24. Garry R, Shelly-Jones D, Mooney P, et al: Six hundred laser ablations. Obstet Gynecol 1995;85:24.
25. Baggish MS, Sze EH: Endometrial ablation: A series of 568 patients

treated over an 11-year period. Am J Obstet Gynecol 1996;174:908–913.

26. Phillips G, Chien PF, Garry R: Risk of hysterectomy after 1000 consecutive endometrial laser ablations. Br J Obstet Gynaecol 1998;105:897–903.

27. Pittrof R, Darwish DH, Shabib G: Near fatal uterine perforation during transcervical endometrial resection. Lancet 1991;338:197–198.

28. Romer T: Benefit of GnRH analogue pretreatment for hysteroscopic surgery in patients with bleeding disorders. Gynecol Obstet Invest 1998;45 (Suppl 1): 12–20; discussion 21–35.

29. Martyn P, Allan B: Long-term follow-up of endometrial ablation. J Assoc Gynecol Laparoscop 1998;5:115–118.

30. Overton C, Hargreaves J, Maresh M: A national survey of the complications of endometrial destruction for menstrual disorders: The MISTLETOE study. Minimally Invasive Surgical Techniques—Laser, EndoThermal or Endoresection. Br J Obstet Gynaecol 1997;104:1351–1359.

31. Nicholson SL, Slade RJ, Ahmed AIH, Gillmer MDG: Endometrial resection in Oxford: The first 500 cases—a 5-year follow-up. J Obstet Gynecol 1995;15:38–43.

32. Donnez J, Vilos G, Gannon MJ, et al: Goserelin acetate (Zoladex) plus endometrial ablation for dysfunctional uterine bleeding: A large randomized, double-blind study. Fertil Steril 1997;68:29–36.

33. Grainger DA, Tjaden BL, Rowland C, et al: Thermal balloon and rollerball ablation to treat menorrhagia: Two-year results of a multicenter, prospective, randomized, clinical trial. J Am Assoc Gynecol Laparosc 2000;7:175–179.

34. Amso NN, Stabinsky SA, McFaul P, et al: Uterine thermal balloon therapy for the treatment of menorrhagia: The first 300 patients from a multicenter study. Br J Obstet Gynaecology 1998;105:517–523.

35. Shah AA, Stabinsky SA, Klusak T, et al: Measurement of serosal temperatures and depth of thermal injury generated by thermal balloon endometrial ablation in ex vivo and in vivo models. Fertil Steril 1998;70:692–697.

36. Fernandez H, Capella S, Audibert F: Uterine thermal balloon therapy under local anaesthesia for the treatment of menorrhagia: A pilot study. Hum Reprod 1997;12:2511.

37. Hawe JA, Phillips AG, Chien PF, et al: Cavaterm thermal balloon ablation for the treatment of menorrhagia. Br J Obstet Gynaecol 1999;106:1143–1148.

38. Soderstrom RM, Brooks PG, Corson SL et al: Endometrial ablation using a distensible multielectrode balloon. J Am Assoc Gynecol Laparosc 1996;3:403–407.

39. Rutherford TJ: Cryosurgery is a simple modality for endometrial ablation. J Am Assoc Gynecol Laparosc 1996; 3(Suppl):S44.

40. Hodgson DA, Feldberg IB, Sharp N, et al: Microwave endometrial ablation: Development, clinical trials and outcomes at three years. Br J Obstet Gynaecol 1999;106:684–694.

41. das Dores GB, Richart RM, Nicolau SM, et al: Evaluation of Hydro ThermAblator for endometrial destruction in patients with menorrhagia. J Am Assoc Gynecol Laparosc 1999;6:275–278.

42. Bustos-Lopez HH, Ibarra-Chavarria V, Vadillo-Ortega F, et al: Endometrial ablation with the EnAbl system. J Am Assoc Gynecol Laparosc 1996;3(Suppl):S5.

43. Wyss P, Svaasand LO, Tadir Y, et al: Photomedicine of the endometrium: Experimental concepts. Hum Reprod 1995;10:221–226.

44. Fehr MK, Madsen SJ, Svaasand LO, et al: Intrauterine light delivery for photodynamic therapy of the human endometrium. Hum Reprod 1995;10:3067–3072.

45. Tadir Y, Hornung R, Pham TH, Tromberg BJ: Intrauterine light probe for photodynamic ablation therapy. Obstet Gynecol 1999;93:299–303.

46. Krzemien AA, Van Vugt DA, Pottier RH, et al: Evaluation of novel nonlaser light source for endometrial ablation using 5-aminolevulinic acid. Lasers Surg Med 1999;25:315–322.

47. Phipps JH, Lewis BV, Roberts T, et al: Treatment of functional menorrhagia by radiofrequency induced thermal endometrial ablation. Lancet 1990;1:374–376.

48. Phipps JH, Lewis BV, Prior MV, Roberts T: Experimental and clinical studies with radio frequency–induced thermal endometrial ablation for functional menorrhagia. Obstet Gynecol 1990;76:876–881.

49. Thijssen RF: Radiofrequency-induced endometrial ablation: An update. Br J Obstet Gynaecol 1997;104:608–613.

50. Donnez J, Polet R, Mathieu PE, et al: Endometrial laser interstitial hyperthermy: A potential modality for endometrial ablation. Obstet Gynecol 1996;87:459–464.

51. Vilos GA, Vilos EC, King JH: Experience with 800 hysteroscopic endometrial ablations. J Am Assoc Gynecol Laparosc 1996;4:33–37.

52. Aberdeen Endometrial Ablation Trials Group; A randomised trial of endometrial ablation versus hysterectomy for the treatment of dysfunctional uterine bleeding: Outcome at four years. Br J Obstet Gynaecol 1999;106:360–366.

EIGHTY-TWO

Guidelines for Determining the Route of Hysterectomy

S. Robert Kovac

Gynecologic surgeons continue to use the abdominal approach for a large majority of hysterectomies that could be performed vaginally, despite well-documented evidence that vaginal hysterectomy has distinct health and economic benefits in terms of fewer complications, better postoperative quality-of-life outcomes, and reduced hospital charges. Because abdominal hysterectomy is associated with less favorable medical outcomes, evidence supports its use only when documented pathologic conditions preclude the vaginal route. However, some surgeons remain reluctant to change their practice patterns, tending to select the abdominal route for most hysterectomies without documenting that the vaginal route is contraindicated. A decision-making tree, such as the one presented in Figure 82–1, offers gynecologic surgeons a more structured approach for selecting the appropriate surgical technique. Using a formal decision process to determine the route of hysterectomy has shown that precision in diagnosis will lead to more efficacious therapy, vast improvement in operative results, and lower costs.

Because no formal practice guidelines have been formulated to clearly identify the appropriateness of a particular route of hysterectomy, a surgeon may feel justified in selecting either an abdominal or a vaginal hysterectomy when, for example, the only indication is prolapse. The American College of Obstetricians and Gynecologists (ACOG) tentatively addressed this problem by issuing a statement that vaginal hysterectomy is best performed in women with mobile uteri no larger than 12 weeks' gestational size (~280 g). ACOG continued by acknowledging that the choice of hysterectomy approach should be based on the surgical indication, the patient's anatomic condition, data supporting the chosen approach, informed patient preference, and the surgeon's expertise and training.

Historically, vaginal hysterectomy has been considered the preferred route for benign conditions confined to the uterus, such as uterine prolapse, small symptomatic leiomyomata, recurrent or severe dysfunctional uterine bleeding, and carcinoma in situ of the cervix. Vaginal hysterectomy has been regarded as contraindicated when the vaginal route is presumed to be inaccessible or when more serious pathologic conditions, such as endometriosis, pelvic adhesive disease, adnexal pathology, chronic pelvic pain, and chronic pelvic inflammatory disease, are thought to exist. In addition, many surgeons hesitate to perform vaginal hysterectomy in nulliparous women, in women who have had previous pelvic surgery (including one or more cesarean sections), in those with a moderately enlarged uterus, or when oophorectomy is to be performed concurrently.

These traditional indications and contraindications must be re-evaluated based on currently available data. For example, for many years the literature has shown that the ovaries can be removed transvaginally in most women undergoing vaginal hysterectomy. In one study, prophylactic vaginal oophorectomy without laparoscopic assistance was successfully performed in 95% of 740 patients.[1] Ovaries that descend into the vagina when the infundibulopelvic ligament is stretched are usually visible and accessible for transvaginal removal, even if the descent is partial. In 966 women undergoing vaginal hysterectomy ovaries were or could have been removed vaginally without laparoscopic assistance in more than 99%.[2] The common belief that the ovaries must be removed by the abdominal route or via operative laparoscopy is questionable if no valid contraindications to transvaginal ovarian removal can be documented.

The selection of abdominal hysterectomy for more serious pathologic conditions has been a de facto guideline that has gone largely unchallenged. Surgeons do not always select the route and method of hysterectomy based on documentation of the severity of the pathology. Rather, mere suspicion of pathology frequently dictates the approach used. Although information in the gynecologic literature comparing the preoperative diagnosis of hysterectomy with pathologic results is sparse, there is sufficient evidence that presumptive preoperative diagnosis is often inaccurate.

Continued reliance on abdominal hysterectomy despite well-documented studies disputing its efficacy has been attributed to several nonclinical factors that create a discrepancy between the state of current practice and our knowledge regarding the best standard of care. As noted earlier, formal practice guidelines have not been developed to clearly identify appropriate candidates for abdominal hysterectomy, vaginal hysterectomy, or when laparoscopic assistance is required to complete a vaginal hysterectomy. Insufficient training and experience in vaginal and laparoscopic techniques have also been cited. Misperceptions have contributed further to the confusion; another issue is the fact that many surgeons simply feel more comfortable with the abdominal route in nulliparous women, when the uterus is significantly enlarged, in the absence of uterine prolapse, or when oophorectomy is required. Physician practice styles favoring a single route or method have been allowed to go unchallenged despite the pressure for more cost-effective health care.

Two outcome-based studies[2, 3] show that vaginal hysterectomy can be successfully performed in approximately

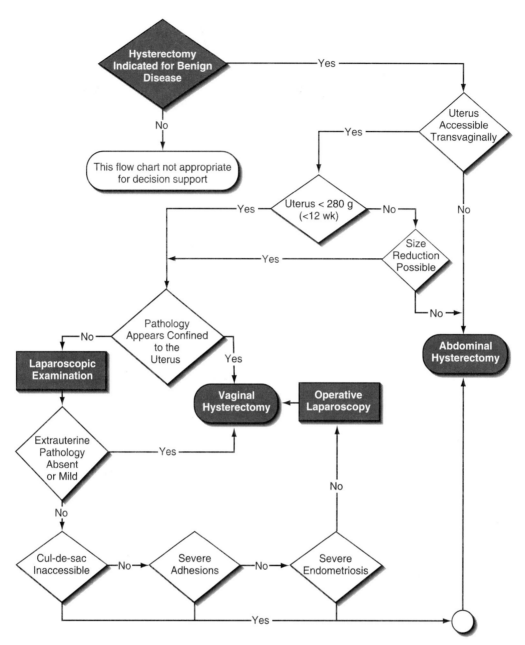

Figure 82–1. Determining the route of hysterectomy.

77% to 89% of patients with benign disease by using a formal decision-making process to determine the route of hysterectomy.

Three critical questions must be answered before selecting the surgical route of hysterectomy for patients with benign disease.

1. Can the uterus be removed transvaginally?
2. Is the pathology confined to the uterus or does it extend beyond the confines of the uterus?
3. Is laparoscopic assistance required to facilitate vaginal removal of the uterus?

TRANSVAGINAL ACCESSIBILITY

A major factor in determining the route of hysterectomy is transvaginal accessibility of the uterus. Inadequate acces-

sibility owing to a narrowed vagina at the vaginal apex makes vaginal hysterectomy technically challenging and may contraindicate vaginal hysterectomy, especially by surgeons less experienced in this procedure. However, in one study of 617 women,[3] inaccessibility was found in only 1% of patients. Two factors limit accessibility: an undescended and immobile uterus and a vagina narrower than 2 fingerbreadths, especially at the apex. Gynecologic surgeons should be alert for these indicators when examining patients. Nulliparity is not an absolute contraindication to vaginal hysterectomy. Although access to the vaginal vault may be restricted in some nulliparous women, inaccessibility cannot be assumed in all cases. In fact, there is no evidence in the literature to support the widely held belief that nulliparity makes vaginal hysterectomy difficult. If accessibility appears adequate, the woman may be a candidate for a vaginal hysterectomy with or without laparoscopic assistance.

UTERINE SIZE

Gynecologic surgeons have long considered an enlarged uterus a contraindication to vaginal hysterectomy, but the term *enlarged* has not been clearly defined. A normal-size uterus weighs approximately 70 to 125 g. ACOG and other investigators assert that vaginal hysterectomy is indicated in women with mobile uteri no larger than 12 weeks' gestational size (~280 g), although other researchers suggest that a uterus as large as 16 weeks' gestational size (~400 g) can be safely approached vaginally. However, studies show that between 80% and 90% of all uteri removed for various indications weigh 280 g or less.

When the surgeon is experienced in uterine size reduction techniques, such as coring, bivalving, and morcellation, larger uteri can be safely removed vaginally. Even though these size reduction techniques extend operative time, they are well-accepted methods of reducing an enlarged uterus so that it can be removed transvaginally. Several investigators report using pharmacologic agents to reduce the size of the uterus preoperatively. In clinical studies of patients with pretreatment uterine sizes ranging from 14 to 18 weeks' gestational size, the administration of gonadotropin-releasing hormone analogues reduced the size of symptomatic uterine leiomyomata by 30% to 50% and decreased uterine volume by approximately one third before hysterectomy, allowing physicians to perform vaginal hysterectomy in patients with enlarged uteri who would have been candidates for abdominal hysterectomy.

The size of the uterus in vivo usually can be measured by simple physical examination. If there is still a question about uterine size, transvaginal ultrasound is another option. An algebraic formula is used to determine the uterine size, expressed in weights and measurements. By multiplying the three dimensions of the uterus in centimeters (length $\times$ width $\times$ anteroposterior diameter at the fundus) by 0.52, physicians can estimate the mass of the uterus in grams in order to obtain a more accurate preoperative estimate of uterine size. (Example: 6 cm $\times$ 6 cm $\times$ 8 cm $\times$ 0.52 = 149 g.) This formula can also be used to estimate ovarian size.

EXTENT OF PATHOLOGY

Determining whether the pathology is confined to or extends beyond the confines of the uterus is critical to selecting the most appropriate route of hysterectomy for patients. According to the decision tree, a vaginal hysterectomy is indicated when pathology is confined to the uterus. When the preoperative diagnosis suggests that the pathologic condition extends beyond the confines of the uterus, further laparoscopic evaluation can help determine the severity of the condition before deciding whether to remove the uterus via the vaginal or the abdominal route.

To identify patients in whom the pathology extends beyond the confines of the uterus and might prohibit vaginal hysterectomy, the location and severity of the pathologic condition must be determined. Traditionally, gynecologic surgeons used the results of the history, physical examination, and imaging techniques, such as ultrasound and x-ray studies, to determine whether the pathology extended beyond the uterus. However, several investigators have proved that these techniques are not sufficiently accurate to adequately document the severity of those conditions, especially endometriosis, adnexal pathology, chronic pelvic pain, and pelvic inflammatory disease. When surgeons based their decision to perform an abdominal hysterectomy on the clinical history and pelvic examination without further intraoperative documentation of the severity of the patient's condition, the surgical findings often did not support the selection of the abdominal route.

When the physician suspects that the patient's pathologic condition is severe enough to warrant intra-abdominal operative intervention, a laparoscopic examination at this point can confirm the extent of the pathology and allow more accurate decision making. Not only is the laparoscope useful for accurately assessing the extent and characteristics of the disease, it is also valuable in determining the mobility of the uterus and adnexal structures. Laparoscopic examination provides a panoramic view of the pelvis and allows the surgeon to directly examine the degree of pathology and note the presence of any conditions that might contraindicate vaginal hysterectomy.

The laparoscope can prove a valuable tool of reassessing the severity of the disease process. Several investigators use a laparoscopic scoring system to determine numerically the severity of the disease based on uterine size, adnexal accessibility, and the presence or absence of adhesions, endometriosis, and other abnormalities. Three critical variables inherent in this scoring system should be assessed during the laparoscopic examination: accessibility of the cul-de-sac, severity of adhesions, and severity of endometriosis.

If the extrauterine pathology is absent or minimal on laparoscopic examination, a vaginal hysterectomy is indicated. Despite current belief, previous pelvic surgery, including cesarean section, does not preclude a vaginal hysterectomy unless extensive adhesions are observed during laparoscopy as limiting accessibility, particularly to the cul-de-sac. Patients with minimal pathology have few or no adhesions, little or no endometriosis, and an accessible cul-de-sac. If laparoscopic assessment reveals moderate pathology, including moderate adhesions or endometriosis but an accessible cul-de-sac, it is necessary to determine whether the impediments can be removed laparoscopically before proceeding to a vaginal hysterectomy. If severe endometriosis is present or the cul-se-sac is obliterated by severe adhesions, an abdominal hysterectomy is indicated.

Laparoscopically assisted vaginal hysterectomy has

compounded the decision-making dilemma in recent years. Although ACOG acknowledges that laparoscopically assisted vaginal hysterectomy is an acceptable alternative to abdominal hysterectomy, many surgeons continue to question how much laparoscopic assistance is appropriate before removing the uterus transvaginally. If operative laparoscopy is indicated, it is beneficial to convert to a vaginal hysterectomy as early as possible in the procedure, for example, after adhesiolysis. Several studies have suggested that nothing is gained by continuing the laparoscopic dissection once a vaginal hysterectomy can be performed safely, because it does little more than prolong surgery, increase costs, and increase the risk of morbidity. Although laparoscopic surgeons have proposed laparoscopically assisted vaginal hysterectomy as a replacement for abdominal and vaginal hysterectomy, its advantages over vaginal hysterectomy have not been documented in this population when there are no contraindications to the vaginal approach.

CONCLUSION

If the goal of gynecologic surgeons is to select the optimal route of hysterectomy based on the best medical outcomes, investigators need to identify the clinical factors that are valid indicators of the route to be selected. Medical standards in today's managed care environment rely on evidence-based practice guidelines that are defined by outcomes rather than subjective criteria, such as physician comfort, preference, or experience. The marked variation in health care for alternative hysterectomy procedures will likely persist until more outcome studies confirm the selec-

tion of a particular route of hysterectomy for each indication for which hysterectomy is performed.

Gynecologic surgeons must clearly demonstrate that the route of hysterectomy they choose not only benefits the patient medically but also represents a wise use of health care dollars. There is little doubt that abdominal hysterectomy should be performed in cases of documented serious disease; however, it should not be misused. Developing clinical guidelines based on physical findings is the first step in ensuring that women will receive the most appropriate route of hysterectomy that is cost-effective and meets the standard of quality care. The potential impact of the physician's decision to select the vaginal approach may be enormous in terms of decreased hospital stay, lower hospital charges, and reduced complications.

Suggestions for Future Reading

Emergency Care Research Institute: Laparoscopy in Hysterectomy for Benign Conditions. Technology Assessment Custom Report Level 2. Plymouth Meeting, Pa, The Institute, 1995.

Kovac SR: Guidelines to determine the route of hysterectomy. Obstet Gynecol 1995;85:18–23.

van den Eeden SK, Glasser M, Mathias SD, et al: Quality of life, health care utilization, and costs among women undergoing hysterectomy in a managed-care setting. Am J Obstet Gynecol 1998;178:91–100.

References

1. Dorsey JH, Holtz PM, Griffiths RI, et al: Cost and charges associated with three alternative techniques of hysterectomy. N Engl J Med 1996;335:476–482.

2. Kovac SR, Christie SJ, Bindbeutel GA: Abdominal versus vaginal hysterectomy: A statistical model for determining physician decision-making and patient outcome. Med Decis Making 1991;11:19–28.

3. Kovac SR: Hysterectomy outcomes in patients with similar indications. Obstet Gynecol 2000;95:787–793.

EIGHTY-THREE

Nonsurgical Treatments for Female Urinary Incontinence

Catherine S. Bradley and

Kristene E. Whitmore

Urinary incontinence (UI) in women is a frequent problem that is often underdiagnosed by physicians and unreported by patients. It is estimated that UI affects more than 13 million Americans, and in 1995, the annual costs of UI were estimated to be $26.3 billion.[1] A recent review of published studies reported an average prevalence of urinary incontinence in older women of 34%, and a prevalence of up to 17% with daily urinary leaking.[2] The most common types of UI in women are stress urinary incontinence (SUI) and urge incontinence or detrusor instability (DI). SUI tends to predominate in younger women, and DI is the most common etiology of UI in older women.

The choice of appropriate therapies for UI varies by the etiology of the incontinence, by individual practitioner, and by patient preference; therapies may include behavioral, pharmacologic, and surgical modalities. Surgical management of UI is common, especially SUI, which typically has surgical cure rates as high as 80% to 90%.[3] However, effective and less invasive treatments with potentially fewer adverse effects are available for the management of UI. In fact, the U.S. Agency for Health Care Policy and Research (AHCPR) recommends behavioral and pharmacologic interventions as the first-line treatments for UI.[4] Unfortunately, rigorous clinical evidence for the use of many conservative treatments is lacking, and studies in this area are frequently limited by heterogeneous study groups, inconsistencies in treatment regimens, nonstandardized outcome measurements, placebo effects, and patient compliance,[4, 5] making management decisions in these patients difficult. This chapter presents an up-to-date overview of the nonsurgical treatments available for female SUI and DI, including behavioral treatments, drug therapy, and mechanical devices (Table 83–1).

BEHAVIORAL TECHNIQUES

Behavioral therapies for UI are potentially very beneficial, pose minimal risks to the patient, and do not limit future therapy options. Behavioral therapy may include general behavioral modifications (dietary changes, a bowel regimen, scheduled fluid intake, and weight loss) as well as specific behavioral treatments, such as toileting assistance, bladder training, and pelvic floor muscle rehabilitation. These treatments may be especially useful in patients who are at greater risk for pharmacologic side effects or surgical complications, such as the elderly or those with medical illnesses.

Toileting Assistance

Toileting assistance includes habit training, timed voiding, and prompted voiding. These behavioral interventions decrease the frequency of UI and are often used for patients in nursing home environments. *Habit training* is toileting scheduled to match the patient's voiding schedule; *timed voiding* attempts to toilet patients on a regular basis (such as every 2 hours); and *prompted voiding* involves asking patients at regular intervals whether they need toileting assistance. One controlled study of habit training in nursing home residents resulted in a significant reduction in UI in 86% of the treatment group.[6] A prompted voiding protocol in another study decreased incontinence episodes in nursing home patients by up to 75%.[7]

Table 83–1. Nonsurgical Treatments for Urinary Incontinence in Women

Treatment Modality	Stress Incontinence	Urge Incontinence
Behavioral modifications (dietary changes, bowel regimen, scheduled fluid intake, weight loss)	X	X
Habit training, timed voiding, prompted voiding		X
Bladder training	X	X
Pelvic floor rehabilitation		
Pelvic muscle exercises with or without biofeedback	X	X
Pelvic muscle exercises with vaginal cones	X	
Electrical stimulation	X	X
Extracorporeal magnetic innervation	X	X
Pharmacologic therapy		
Estrogen (adjunctive therapy)	X	X
Anticholinergic/antispasmodic		X
Tricyclic antidepressants	X (imipramine only)	X
Mechanical devices	X	

Bladder Training

Bladder training is another effective behavioral therapy for UI, especially that resulting from DI. The treatment plan typically includes patient education, scheduled voiding, and positive reinforcement. A progressive, voluntary voiding schedule is used that gradually increases patients' voiding intervals over a several-week period. Bladder training is thought to improve cortical inhibition over lower urinary tract function, but its true mechanism of action is unclear. A wide range of efficacy rates for bladder training has been reported, but few controlled trials have been published. One randomized, controlled trial of bladder training found that 75% of the treatment group had at least a 50% reduction in incontinent episodes.[8] Although bladder training has traditionally been used in patients with DI, this study found it to be equally effective in patients with SUI.

Pelvic Muscle Rehabilitation

Pelvic muscle exercises (PMEs) or Kegel exercises are a behavioral therapy that improves the neuromuscular function of the pelvic floor muscle complex. These exercises are frequently recommended for women with SUI or DI. They can be performed alone or in conjunction with biofeedback or use of vaginal weights. Pelvic muscle rehabilitation can also be achieved by electrical stimulation therapy and possibly with extracorporeal magnetic innervation therapy, a recently developed treatment.

PMEs are a learned technique of contracting and relaxing the perivaginal muscles, which include the levator ani complex, in order to increase pelvic floor muscle strength and control. Contraction of these muscles exerts a closing force on the urethra and may create a learned behavior that causes inhibition of detrusor activity through a neuromuscular reflex. Studies of PMEs in the treatment of SUI have a wide range of success rates, reported to be from 51% to 96%.[9] A successful PME program requires a motivated patient and provider. Some studies have shown that success rates from PME programs are dependent on the amount of supervision and the duration of treatment provided.[10] Patients must be encouraged to continue the exercises regularly, although they may not notice an improvement in their incontinence for 6 to 8 weeks.

Electromyographic biofeedback is helpful in teaching PMEs because it aids in muscle identification and awareness, and it gives the patient immediate feedback on exercise performance. Burgio and coworkers[11] compared biofeedback-assisted PME treatment with a verbally instructed PME group in the treatment of SUI and found a significantly greater reduction in incontinence in the biofeedback group. Burgio and associates[12] published the first randomized trial to compare the effectiveness of biofeedback-assisted behavioral treatment with both a standard drug treatment (oxybutynin chloride) and a control condition (no instruction on PMEs) for patients with DI. This group found that behavioral treatment was significantly more effective in reducing incontinence episodes than the drug

treatment or control condition (mean 80.7% reduction, compared with 68.5% and 39.4% reductions, respectively), and only 14% of patients in the behavioral group wanted to change to another treatment versus 76% in each of the other groups.

The use of vaginal cones is another method of pelvic muscle rehabilitation that is effective in the treatment of SUI. A set of sequentially weighted vaginal cones can be used to train women to contract their pelvic floor muscles. Typically, patients are asked to use the cones at home for 15 minutes at a time, twice a day. When a woman can retain a particular cone within the vagina comfortably, she can progress to the next greater weight. One group[13] found a 70% subjective improvement rate in SUI and a highly significant correlation between decreased urine loss and increased retained cone weight in 30 women who completed a vaginal cones exercise program. Another study randomized patients with SUI to treatment with vaginal cones or to a traditional PME treatment program and found similar subjective improvement rates in both groups (85% and 84%).[14]

External pelvic floor electrical stimulation is also an effective muscle rehabilitation therapy for UI. Electrical stimulation of the pudendal nerves leads to reflex contraction of the pelvic floor muscles, including the striated periurethral muscles, and to a reflex inhibition of the detrusor muscle.[15] The physiology of the therapeutic effects remains unclear. Typical treatment protocols include 15 to 20 minutes of use from twice daily to once every other day, for 1 to 4 months. Few adverse effects are reported. Electrical stimulation therapy can be performed at home with portable, battery-driven stimulators connected by cable to a vaginal or anal plug electrode. Many studies have reported successful treatment of DI, SUI, and mixed UI with different methods of pelvic floor electrical stimulation. Only one prospective, randomized, controlled study has been performed in patients with genuine SUI comparing the use of an active pelvic floor stimulator with a sham device.[16] This study found a 62% objective improvement rate in UI in the treatment group versus a 19% improvement rate in the placebo group ($P = .01$).

Extracorporeal magnetic innervation therapy is a new type of pelvic muscle rehabilitation proposed for the treatment of SUI and DI. During this therapy, patients sit fully clothed on a special chair that has a magnetic field generator in the seat, which produces a rapidly changing magnetic field flux. The mechanism of the therapeutic effect is unknown, but a preliminary study performed in women with SUI reports good results: a 34% cure rate and significant decreases in patient pad weight and leak episodes per day.[17] This treatment is promising because it is noninvasive and causes little patient inconvenience; a randomized, controlled trial is under way in an attempt to confirm these outcomes.

PHARMACOLOGIC TREATMENTS

Although behavioral treatments are successful methods of managing UI, many patients are not motivated to pursue these types of treatments and will not find them successful. Drug therapy is another conservative management option for UI that is less time consuming and effort dependent for patients and providers. Table 83–2 provides a list of common pharmacologic treatments for UI.

Estrogen Therapy

Estrogen therapy has been used for many years in the treatment of UI in postmenopausal women. Although studies agree that estrogen therapy improves the irritative urinary symptoms associated with urogenital atrophy,[18] the efficacy of estrogen for treating UI is more controversial. Many uncontrolled clinical trials have reported improvements in the symptoms of SUI and DI from estrogen therapy; however, conflicting outcomes are reported in the few controlled clinical trials available. A 1994 meta-analysis that included six controlled trials of estrogen therapy in the treatment of UI in postmenopausal women concluded that estrogen treatment resulted in significant subjective improvement in UI, but there was no good evidence of an effect of estrogen on urodynamic or objective outcomes.[19] The most recent randomized, controlled trial of estrogen treatment for UI also found no improvement in clinical outcomes or quality of life variables after three months of cyclic estrogen treatment.[20] Therefore, estrogen appears to be useful in decreasing irritative urinary symptoms in postmenopausal women; however, no objective improvement in urinary SUI or DI from estrogen treatment has been consistently demonstrated in the literature. Because estrogen replacement therapy may confer other benefits or risks to each patient, the decision to treat should be made on an individual basis.

Pharmacologic Treatments for Stress Incontinence

Pharmacologic treatments for SUI function by increasing urethral outlet resistance. α-Adrenergic agents produce this effect by stimulating the α-adrenoreceptors in the bladder neck and proximal urethra to produce smooth muscle contraction. Phenylpropanolamine (PPA) is a well-studied α-agonist that has been shown to increase urethral closure

pressures and improve SUI symptoms.[21] The 1996 AHCPR Guidelines[4] reviewed seven randomized, controlled trials of PPA in the treatment of SUI and found low rates of cure (0% to 14%) but a 20% to 60% subjective improvement rate over placebo. Another α-agonist agent that may be used is pseudoephedrine, which has effects similar to those of PPA. Potential side effects of α-agonist agents include blood pressure elevation, headaches, palpitations, and cardiac arrhythmias; and recently, the use of PPA has been questioned by the Food and Drug Administration (FDA) for safety reasons. Therefore PPA and pseudoephedrine should be used with caution in patients with hypertension, cardiovascular disease, or hyperthyroidism.

Imipramine hydrochloride is a tricyclic antidepressant (TCA) medication that has some α-agonistic as well as anticholinergic effects. One uncontrolled study found that 21 of 30 women with SUI achieved continence after treatment with imipramine for 4 weeks,[22] but no controlled studies have been reported. Imipramine is recommended as an alternative pharmacologic therapy for SUI.[4]

Pharmacologic Treatments for Urge Incontinence

Pharmacologic therapy for DI is aimed at decreasing bladder contractility. Anticholinergic agents, especially oxybutynin, are the most commonly used and best-studied medications for the treatment of DI. Oxybutynin chloride has anticholinergic, antispasmodic, and local anesthetic properties. Controlled studies of oxybutynin therapy have demonstrated a 15% to 58% reduction in incontinence frequency over placebo effect.[4] Side effects from oxybutynin are common, including dry mouth, constipation, blurred vision, and change in mental status, and anticholinergic medications are contraindicated in patients with a history of closed-angle glaucoma. More recently, tolterodine, a more selective anticholinergic agent, and a once-daily, controlled-release form of oxybutynin have been developed that have comparable efficacy to oxybutynin but fewer side effects in clinical studies.[23, 24] These medications are better tolerated by patients than oxybutynin chloride, and they are becoming the most commonly prescribed medications for DI.

Table 83–2. Common Medications Used to Treat Urinary Incontinence

Type of Incontinence	Agent	Classification	Typical Dosage
Stress incontinence	Phenylpropanolamine	α-Agonist	25–100 mg (sustained-release) bid
	Pseudoephedrine	α-Agonist	15–30 mg tid
	Imipramine hydrochloride	Tricyclic antidepressant	25–75 mg qd-tid
Urge incontinence	Oxybutynin chloride	Anticholinergic/antispasmodic	2.5–5 mg bid-qid
	Controlled-release oxybutynin	Anticholinergic/antispasmodic	5–15 mg qd
	Tolterodine	Anticholinergic	1–2 mg bid
	Dicyclomine hydrochloride	Anticholinergic/antispasmodic	10–20 mg tid
	Imipramine hydrochloride	Tricyclic antidepressant	25–75 mg qd-tid

Dicyclomine hydrochloride is another agent with anticholinergic and antispasmodic properties that is used clinically to decrease bladder contractility. Studies on dicyclomine for UI are limited, and it is used primarily as an alternative to other anticholinergic agents when their side effects cannot be tolerated.

TCA agents may be useful in treating DI in selected patients. Their therapeutic effects are related to their central and peripheral anticholinergic properties and their adrenergic effects. Imipramine hydrochloride improves bladder storage by improving compliance, as well as by increasing bladder outlet resistance as discussed previously. It has been shown to decrease incontinence episodes in elderly patients with DI.[25] Because of its dual effects, it may be useful in patients with mixed incontinence. Other TCA agents, such as doxepin and amitriptyline hydrochloride, have demonstrated some effect against DI in a limited number of studies. TCA medications may cause anticholinergic side effects, as well as other serious adverse effects, such as sedation, orthostatic hypotension, and cardiac arrhythmias, so they must be prescribed with care in elderly patients and others at risk for cardiovascular disorders.

MECHANICAL AND SUPPORT DEVICES

The success rate of vaginal devices such as pessaries in the treatment of UI is not well studied. A few investigators have reported success in treating mild to moderate SUI with pessaries or a diaphragm ring. One review compared studies of three vaginal devices (contraceptive diaphragm, bladder neck prosthesis, and foam tampon) and found subjective success rates reported from 60% to 100%,[26] and a small randomized, controlled study found that 58% of women with exercise-induced SUI achieved continence with a pessary or tampon placed during exercise.[27]

Newer devices designed to treat SUI include disposable intraurethral inserts and external urethral occlusive devices. These devices function as mechanical barriers to prevent urinary leakage. The intraurethral inserts or plugs have reported success rates of 50% to 94%, require highly motivated patients, and have side effects including discomfort, urinary tract infection, and hematuria.[26] External urethral occlusive devices fit over the external urethral meatus and are held in place by suction. These devices have subjective and objective cure rates of 40% to 50%, are reusable for 1 week, and have fewer reported side effects than the intraurethral devices.[28]

CONCLUSION

UI is a frequent problem in women, and many potential treatment options are available. Nonsurgical therapy should be attempted when feasible, including behavioral techniques, pelvic floor muscle rehabilitation, pharmacologic treatment, and use of mechanical devices.

Suggestions for Future Reading

Lightner D: Conservative management of urinary incontinence. AUA Update 18(5):114, 1999.

Walters MD, Karram MM (eds): Urogynecology and Reconstructive Pelvic Surgery, 2nd ed. St. Louis, CV Mosby, 1999.

References

1. Wagner TH, Hu TW: Economic costs of urinary incontinence in 1995. Urology 1998;51:355–361.
2. Thom D. Variation in estimates of urinary incontinence prevalence in the community: Effects of differences in definition, population characteristics, and study type. JAGS 1998;46:473–480.
3. Leach GE, Dmochowski RR, Appell RA, et al: Female Stress Urinary Incontinence Clinical Guidelines Panel summary report on surgical management of female stress urinary incontinence. The American Urological Association. J Urol 1997;158:875–880.
4. Agency for Health Care Policy and Research: Urinary Incontinence in Adults: Acute and Chronic Management. Clinical Practice Guideline No. 2 (1996 Update). (AHCPR Publication No. 96-0682.) Silver Spring, Md, AHCPR, March 1996.
5. Abrams P, Larsson G, Chapple C, Wein AJ: Factors involved in the success of antimuscarinic treatment. BJU Int 1999;83(Suppl 2):42–47.
6. Colling J, Ouslander J, Hadley BJ, et al: The effects of patterned urge-response toileting (PURT) on urinary incontinence among nursing home residents. J Am Geriatr Soc 1992;39:135–141.
7. Schnelle JF: Treatment of urinary incontinence in nursing home patients by prompted voiding. J Am Geriatr Soc 1990;38:356–360.
8. Fantl JA, Wyman JF, McClish DK, et al: Efficacy of bladder training in older women with urinary incontinence. JAMA 1991;265:609–613.
9. Wells TJ: Pelvic (floor) muscle exercise. J Am Geriatr Soc 1990;38:333–337.
10. Bo K, Hagen RH, Kvarstein B, et al: Pelvic floor muscle exercise for the treatment of female stress urinary incontinence: III. Effects of two different degrees of pelvic floor muscle exercises. Neurourol Urodyn 1990;9:489–502.
11. Burgio KL, Robinson JC, Engel BT: The role of biofeedback in Kegel exercise training for stress urinary incontinence. Am J Obstet Gynecol 1986;154:58–64.
12. Burgio KL, Locher JL, Goode PS, et al: Behavioral vs drug treatment for urge urinary incontinence in older women. JAMA 1998;280:1995–2000.
13. Peattie AB, Plevnik S, Stanton SL: Vaginal cones: A conservative method of treating genuine stress incontinence. Br J Obstet Gynecol 1988;95:1049–1053.
14. Pieber D, Zivkovic F, Tamussino K, et al: Pelvic floor exercise alone or with vaginal cones for the treatment of mild to moderate stress urinary incontinence in premenopausal women. Int Urogynecol J 1995;6:14–17.
15. Bent AE, Sand PK, Ostergard DR, Brubaker LT: Transvaginal electrical stimulation in the treatment of genuine stress incontinence and detrusor instability. Int Urogynecol J 1993;4:9–13.
16. Sand PK, Richardson DA, Staskin DR, et al: Pelvic floor electrical stimulation in the treatment of genuine stress incontinence: A multicenter, placebo-controlled trial. Am J Obstet Gynecol 1995;173:72–79.
17. Galloway NT, El-Galley RE, Sand PK, et al: Extracorporeal magnetic innervation therapy for stress urinary incontinence. Urology 1999;53:1108–1111.
18. Cardozo L, Bachman G, McClish D, et al: Meta-analysis of estrogen therapy in the management of urogenital atrophy in postmenopausal women: Second report of the Hormones and Urogenital Therapy Committee. Obstet Gynecol 1998;92:722–727.
19. Fantl JA, Cardozo L, McClish D, et al: Estrogen therapy in the management of urinary incontinence in postmenopausal women: A meta-analysis. First report of the Hormones and Urogenital Therapy Committee. Obstet Gynecol 1994;83:12–18.
20. Fantl JA, Bump RC, Robinson D, et al: Efficacy of estrogen supplementation in the treatment of urinary incontinence. Obstet Gynecol 1996;88:745–749.
21. Collste L, Lindskog M: Phenylpropanolamine in treatment of female stress urinary incontinence. Urology 1987;30:398–403.

22. Gilja I, Radej M, Kovacic M, Parazajder J: Conservative treatment of female stress incontinence with imipramine. J Urol 1984;132:909–911.

23. Anderson RU, Mobley D, Blank B, et al: Once daily controlled versus immediate release oxybutynin chloride for urge incontinence. J Urol 1999;161:1809–1812.

24. Appell RA: Clinical efficacy and safety of tolterodine in the treatment of overactive bladder: A pooled analysis. Urology 1997;50(Suppl 6A):90–96.

25. Castleden CM, Renwick AB, Asher MJ: Imipramine—a possible alternative to current therapy for urinary incontinence in the elderly. J Urol 1981;125:318–320.

26. Vierhout ME, Lose G: Preventive vaginal and intra-urethral devices in the treatment of female urinary stress incontinence. Curr Opin Obstet Gynecol 1997;9:325–328.

27. Nygaard I: Prevention of exercise incontinence with mechanical devices. J Reprod Med 1995;40:89–94.

28. Versi E, Griffiths DJ, Harvey M: A new external urethral occlusive device for female urinary incontinence. Obstet Gynecol 1998;92:286–291.

EIGHTY-FOUR

Periurethral Injectables

Rodney A. Appell and J. Christian Winters

Urinary incontinence may originate at the level of the bladder or the urethra. In evaluating patients for the use of intraurethral injections as a treatment of urinary incontinence, it is essential to identify the cause(s) of incontinence in order to recommend appropriate therapy. Intraurethral injections benefit patients with incontinence occurring at the level of the urethra. Patients with intrinsic sphincteric dysfunction (ISD) commonly have had a previous surgical procedure on or near the urethra, a sympathetic neurologic injury, or myelodysplasia. Patients with ISD have poor urethral function and require procedures to increase outflow resistance. Bladder neck suspension procedures will fail in these patients owing to the poor urethral function, and these patients require pubovaginal sling procedures, artificial urinary sphincters, or periurethral injections.

In patients with ISD, the presence or absence of anatomic support will assist in directing future management. At present, patients with a lack of anatomic support (hypermobility) and ISD do best undergoing sling procedures or placement of artificial urinary sphincters. Patients with a fixed, well-supported urethra in association with ISD are excellent candidates for periurethral injection. During the multicenter investigation of collagen in the treatment of ISD, the patients selected for this treatment with anatomic incontinence did not respond as well as those selected for the treatment who had inadequate pelvic support.[1] Therefore, the recommendation has been to perform periurethral injections on patients with a poorly functioning urethra (ISD) and good anatomic support. However, more recent data suggest that intraurethral injections may be used for selected patients with anatomic stress urinary incontinence.[2]

EVALUATION AND PATIENT SELECTION

When obtaining a history from patients with urinary incontinence, it is important to elucidate whether previous surgery has been performed or an underlying neurologic disorder exists. Also, the activity precipitating urinary leakage is important. Patients who leak in the supine position, wet the bed, or leak with a sensation of urinary urgency do not have genuine stress urinary incontinence and need to be investigated for ISD. The physical examination is essential to ascertain whether concomitant urogenital prolapse and urethral hypermobility are present. The Q-tip test is used; an angle of greater than 30 degrees signifies urethral hypermobility.

Urodynamic studies are performed to evaluate possible bladder causes of incontinence (instability, decreased contractility/overflow) and to evaluate urethral function. Tests of urethral function may be performed by means of leak point pressures or urethral pressure profiles. At present, the ideal patient for periurethral injections is a patient with poor urethral function, normal bladder capacity, and good anatomic support. A clear advantage of injectables in ISD is the attainment of increased urethral closing function with only minor increases in urethral closing pressure. Patients with minimal hypermobility and high leak point pressures or elderly, less active women with anatomic incontinence may be considered for periurethral injections as well; however, it is wise to reserve this therapy for patients in this population who represent a surgical risk or have a limited mobility.

Contraindications to periurethral injections include active urinary tract infection, untreated detrusor instability, and known hypersensitivity to the agent injected. Patients who are to have intraurethral injection of collagen must undergo skin testing 1 month before the procedure to determine whether hypersensitivity to the material is present. In the collagen multicenter trial,[3] 4% of the female patients exhibited hypersensitivity during skin testing.

INJECTABLE MATERIALS

The ideal material for periurethral injection is one that is easily injected, is biocompatible, and causes little or no inflammatory reaction. Also, the substance should elicit no immunogenic response. There should be no migration of the injected material, and it should maintain its bulking effect for a long period of time.

Many agents have been used as injectables for urinary incontinence, ranging from sclerosing agents to autologous blood. Currently, the most widely used agent is cross-linked bovine collagen. Collagen (Contigen) received U.S. Food and Drug Administration approval for the treatment of ISD in male and female patients in September 1993. Autologous fat had temporarily gained acceptance in patients who demonstrated hypersensitivity to collagen, but unsatisfactory results have prevented its further usage. Polytetrafluoroethylene, or "Teflon" paste, has been removed from the United States marketplace because of concerns over its migration and safety, despite being proved as an effective method of treatment for urinary incontinence with no reports of untoward sequelae in human beings.

In September 1999, Durasphere was approved for general use in the United States, based on data equivalent to that of collagen. This material consists of nonresorbable pyrolytic carbon-coated zirconium oxide beads (212 to 500 μm in size) in a 2.8% betaglucan water-based gel. The stated theoretical advantage is that the beads encapsulate within tissue and thus retain implant bulk, as opposed to the biodegradation inherent in collagen use. If this theory becomes fact, then the efficacy obtained should be more durable over time than with collagen as the injectable agent. We believe that because these agents may be injected safely under local anesthesia and have some efficacy in patients with hypermobility, there may be additional potential for them to be used as a first line of therapy in patients with stress incontinence who are considered poor surgical risks for open surgical repairs, as well as in healthy individuals with ISD.

GLUTARALDEHYDE CROSS-LINKED BOVINE COLLAGEN (CONTIGEN)

This agent is both biocompatible and biodegradable and is currently the primary injectable agent utilized in the United States. It is a sterile, nonpyrogenic bovine dermal collagen cross-linked with glutaraldehyde and dispersed in a phosphate-buffered physiologic saline solution. The cross-linking process improves the integrity of the material for injection by increasing its resistance to collagenase as well as decreasing the antigenicity of the collagen. A minimal inflammatory response has been associated with the injection of collagen, and no granuloma formation or foreign body reaction is present. Also, no foreign body reaction occurs. Collagen begins to degrade in approximately 12 weeks; however, in this period of time, neovascularization and the deposition by fibroblasts of host collagen occur within the implant, thereby replacing the injected collagen with host collagen. The bovine collagen completely degrades within 10 to 19 months. There are no reports of particle migration of the bovine collagen material.

TECHNIQUE OF INJECTION

The technique of injection of material is not difficult; however, it is essential to perform precise placement of the material in order to ensure an optimal result. The injection can be performed either suburothelially through a needle placed directly through a cystoscope (transurethral injection) or periurethrally with a spinal needle inserted percutaneously and positioned in the urethral tissues in the suburothelial space observing the manipulation cystoscopically.

Although transurethral injections are initially easier to perform than the periurethral technique, we believe that the reduced potential for transurethral bleeding and extravasation of the injectable into the urethral lumen are worth the

steeper learning curve associated with the latter technique. After mastery of either technique is achieved, typically less injectable material is required to attain continence. We describe the technique of injection in women employing collagen, because this is currently the most widely used injectable substance. After this, we make additional comments concerning the alterations of techniques in the injection of other injectable materials.

With either approach, the woman is placed in the lithotomy position, and the introitus is anesthetized with 20% topical benzocaine. The urethra is anesthetized with topical 2% lidocaine jelly. Then, a local injection of 1% plain lidocaine is performed periurethrally at the 3 and 9 o'clock positions, using 2 to 4 mL on each side.

Periurethral Approach[4, 5]

Panendoscopy is performed with a 0- or 30-degree lens and a 22-gauge spinal needle with the obturator in place is positioned periurethrally at the 4 or 8 o'clock position, with the bevel of the needle directed toward the lumen. The needle is then advanced into the urethral muscle via the lamina propria in an entirely suburothelial plane. Once the needle is positioned in the lamina propria, it usually advances with very little force. The needle may also be placed at the 6 o'clock position, and again needle placement is fully observed endoscopically. Bulging of the tip of the needle against the lining of the urethra is observed during advancement of the needle to ensure its proper placement. When the needle tip is properly positioned just below the bladder neck, the material is injected until swelling is visible on each side, creating the appearance of occlusion of the urethral lumen. When the urethra is approximately 50% occluded, the needle is removed and reinserted on the opposite side, and additional material is injected until the urethral mucosa coapts in the midline.

Transurethral Approach[6, 7]

After cystourethroscopy, the injectable material is delivered intraurethrally by way of a transcystoscopic injection needle 1.5 to 2.0 cm distal to the bladder neck under direct vision. Needles for standard cystoscopic equipment are commercially available, as well as injector scopes. This technique is performed circumferentially, employing two to four needle placements. Material is injected until swelling of the tissue is created, with movement of the mucosa inward toward or beyond the midline. The ultimate goal, again, is to gain mucosal coaptation of the urethra in the midline.

The transcystoscopic approach is preferred for the injection of Durasphere for urinary incontinence owing to the increased viscosity of the material. As stated previously, the needle placement for the injection of collagen is into the urethral muscle; superficial injection of collagen does not compromise the procedure. However, if the needle is placed too superficially and Durasphere is injected, the Durasphere material may perforate and extrude into the urethral lumen, which can be problematic. Therefore, when injecting Durasphere, the needle is inserted at a 45-degree angle, which allows deposition of the material into the muscle. This allows for the adequate bulk-enhancing effect while minimizing the possibility of a perforation and extrusion of the injected agent into the urethra.

POSTOPERATIVE CARE

Perioperative antibiotic coverage is continued for 3 days after the procedure. Most patients are able to void easily after the procedure; however, if retention does develop, clean intermittent catheterization is begun with a 12- or 14-French catheter. Indwelling catheters are avoided in patients who have recently had injection, because this promotes molding of the material around the catheter. If long-term catheterization is needed, suprapubic cystotomy should be performed in these patients; although it is usually unnecessary.

Patients are contacted 2 weeks postprocedure to determine their continence status. Repeat injections are scheduled 1 month later as necessary.

RESULTS

In the multicenter collagen trial in which 137 female patients with ISD were studied, 96.4% did not have incontinence at 1-year follow-up.[3] In 17 patients with hypermobility of the sphincteric complex, 82.3% were either improved or completely cured. Women with ISD required approximately 2.5 injections, with an average total volume of 24.3 mL of collagen. Although the success and efficacy of collagen implantation for women with ISD have been reproduced in several series, debate exists about the efficacy of collagen material in patients with type II or anatomic stress urinary incontinence.[8-10] In 1992, Herschorn and associates[11] reported equal success rates among patients with type II or anatomic stress incontinence and patients with ISD; however, the number of injections and the amount of material injected were higher in patients with anatomic urinary incontinence. It has also been documented that elderly female patients with anatomic incontinence do well with collagen injections. The overall results with periurethral injections of collagen in women with ISD compare favorably with results obtained using slings and the artificial sphincter.[12]

COMPLICATIONS

In the multicenter U.S. clinical trial of collagen injections, transient retention developed in approximately 15% of patients.[3] With collagen, only 1% of patients experienced irritative voiding symptoms, and 5% developed a urinary tract infection. Hypersensitivity responses with collagen

are not a problem, because the possibility is assessed by skin testing for a wheal and flare response with the more immunogenic and sensitizing noncross-linked collagen before treatment.[10] Those with a positive skin test are excluded from treatment; positive skin tests were found in 11/427 patients in the multicenter US study. In addition, these patients had anticollagen antibody testing, and no significant anticollagen responses were found. There has been no evidence to link injections of bovine collagen with any disorder. Regardless of the material, the use of periurethral injections has proved to be safe, eliciting only minor complications. All complications resolve rapidly, and a serious long-term complication from the use of periurethral injections has yet to be reported.

SUMMARY

In the properly selected patient, periurethral injections offer excellent treatment results for patients with ISD. Patients with no anatomic hypermobility and ISD appear to be the most satisfactory candidates for periurethral injections. Collagen is the most widely used injectable, because it has been shown to be both biocompatible and biodegradable. There are no reports of particle migration with this material, and repeat injections can be performed safely with the patient under local anesthesia. Durasphere is an alternative injectable, particularly in patients who have had positive skin tests to the collagen material, or in our hands in those patients in whom the lack of durability of collagen has been problematic. Publications describing the use of Durasphere have yet to appear.

The treatment response in woman with these procedures is similar to those of surgical procedures to correct ISD, and the complications are minimal. Of the alternative treatments available for women with ISD, sling surgery is successful in 81% to 98%, implantation of an artificial urinary sphincter (by either abdominal or transvaginal approach) is successful in over 90%, and injection therapy successful between 64% and 95% of patients. Although long-term results (>5 years) for all these procedures are scarce in the medical literature, injected patients have been followed for only short periods of time and the data available do not take into consideration reinjection rates, which run as high as 22% with collagen at 2 years after attaining dryness. In selected elderly and less mobile female patients with anatomic incontinence, recent data suggest that collagen may be useful.[13] The use of periurethral injections in the treatment of ISD certainly has a role in treatment in the properly selected patient and allows treatment of incontinence in patients who are poor surgical candidates and may be denied other forms of therapy.

References

1. Winters JC, Appell RA: Periurethral injection of collagen in the treatment of intrinsic sphincter deficiency in the female patient. Urol Clin North Am 1995;22:673–678.
2. Herschorn S, Radomski SB: Collagen injections for genuine stress

urinary incontinence: Patient selection and durability. Int Urogynecol J 1997;8:18–24.

3. Appell RA, McGuire EJ, DeRidder PA, et al: Summary of effectiveness and safety in the prospective, open, multicenter investigation of Contigen implant for incontinence due to intrinsic sphincteric deficiency in females. J Urol 1994;151:418A.

4. Ganabathi K, Leach GE: Periurethral injection techniques. Atlas Urol Clin North Am 1994;2:101–109.

5. Smith DN, Appell RA, Winters JC, Rackley RR: Collagen injection therapy for female intrinsic sphincteric deficiency. J Urol 1997;157:1275–1278.

6. McGuire EJ, Appell RA: Transurethral collagen injection for urinary incontinence. Urology 1994;43:413.

7. O'Connell HE, McGuire EJ: Transurethral collagen therapy in women. J Urol 1995;154:1463–1465.

8. Corcos J, Fournier C: Periurethral collagen injection for the treatment of female stress urinary incontinence: 4-year follow-up results. Urology 1999;54:815–818.

9. Gorton E, Stanton S, Monga A, et al: Periurethral collagen injection: A long-term follow-up study. BJU Int 1999;84:966–971.

10. Steele AC, Kohli N, Karram MM: Periurethral collagen injection for stress incontinence with and without urethral hypermobility. Obstet Gynecol 2000;95:327–331.

11. Herschorn S, Radomski SB, Steele DJ: Early experience with intraurethral collagen injection for urinary incontinence. J Urol 1992;148:1797–1800.

12. Appell RA: Use of collagen injections for treatment of incontinence and reflux. Adv Urol 1992;5:145–165.

13. Faerber G: Endoscopic collagen injection therapy in elderly women with type I stress urinary incontinence. J Urol 1996;155:512–514.

Office Evaluation of Urinary Incontinence

Raymond Rackley

Urinary incontinence (UI) is typically defined as the involuntary loss of urine through the urethral meatus that is of sufficient magnitude to constitute a problem. Whereas prevalence rates range from 10% to 30% in young adults and from 15% to 35% in adults over the age of 65 years,[1] UI is the second leading cause of institutionalization for 1.6 million elderly American nursing home residents.[1, 2] In fact, the estimated annual cost of managing UI was 16 billion dollars in 1994.[3] Obviously, the ability to control the rising cost of managing this condition will have a direct impact on the methods of evaluating and successfully treating all female patients with UI. This chapter outlines a practical approach to the diagnosis and evaluation of female UI.

LEXICON

In conceptualizing the evaluation of patients who present with involuntary loss of urine, UI should not be considered a disease but rather a symptom or sign of an underlying problem. Physician goals are to identify causes of incontinence associated with medically treatable conditions and to triage patients who may benefit from further consultation. In many cases, especially in elderly patients, the underlying problem of multifactorial UI will require evaluation and periodic reassessment by a specialist.

Generally, the classification of UI is divided into six clinically applicable categories (Table 85–1), based on specific underlying etiologies, diagnostic evaluation, and management.

Transient incontinence is often referred to as reversible incontinence. The acute onset of transient UI, which is common in elderly or hospitalized patients, may be the result of numerous causes that also may occur in a multifactorial setting as listed in Table 85–2.[4]

Overflow incontinence results from overdistention of the bladder. Patients present with frequent or constant dribbling of urine without a normal voiding pattern. These clinical findings may result from bladder outlet obstruction (stricture or overcorrective anti-incontinence/vaginal prolapse surgery), an acontractile detrusor (diabetes, multiple sclerosis, or postpartum retention), or psychogenic retention.

Total incontinence is continuous urine leakage unrelated to any kind of activity, without sensation of bladder fullness or the urge to void. These patients may have a severe intrinsic sphincteric deficiency (ISD) of the bladder, as described later, urinary tract fistulas, congenital anomalies, or overflow incontinence.

Stress urinary incontinence (SUI) is defined as urinary leakage secondary to an increase in abdominal pressure (Valsalva maneuvers that place "stress" on the bladder and bladder support mechanisms) and is classified for treatment purposes by urologists into bladder neck/urethral hypermobility and ISD. Anterior vaginal wall relaxation with hypermobility-related stress UI (accounting for 85% of SUI) develops most commonly with aging, hormonal changes, traumatic or prolonged delivery, and pelvic surgery. Some patients with a well-supported bladder neck/urethra will still have SUI due to ISD (15% of SUI women). In these cases, ISD may be due to damage to the bladder neck after prior pelvic or anti-incontinence procedures, pelvic radiation, trauma, or neurogenic disorders resulting in bladder neck denervation.

Urge incontinence is typically described as urinary leakage associated with an abrupt desire to void (urgency) that cannot be suppressed or inhibited (referred to as an unstable bladder). Although the etiology of an unstable bladder is usually idiopathic, causes such as bacterial cystitis, bladder tumor, bladder calculus, bladder outlet obstruction, or neurologic disease can and must be excluded.

Mixed incontinence, which typically refers to the association of SUI with urge incontinence, is common in 50% to 60% of patients presenting for evaluation of SUI. Proper management requires recognition and evaluation of each contributing component of the anatomic and neurologic contributions to this form of UI.

EVALUATION

The general evaluation of all patients with UI includes a history and a fluid intake/voiding diary, physical examination, urinalysis, urine culture, and determination of a post-void residual. For selected patients who are subsequently referred for further evaluation by a specialist, the consultation may involve blood tests (urea and creatinine), urodynamic evaluation, cystoscopy, and imaging studies of the urinary tract and central nervous system.

Table 85–1. Six Types of Urinary Incontinence

Transient	Total	Urge
Overflow	Stress	Mixed

Table 85–2. Causes of Transient Urinary Incontinence

Delirium or confusional state
Infection (symptomatic)
Atrophic vaginitis or urethritis
Pharmaceuticals
Psychological disorder
Excessive urine output (congestive heart failure, hyperglycemia)
Restricted mobility
Stool impaction

HISTORY

Patient evaluation begins with a thorough history, which includes characterizing the onset, duration, evolution, progression, inciting events of leakage (e.g., Valsalva maneuvers, change of position or environment, temporal relations), and the patient's attempts at behavior modification (e.g., fluid intake, timed voiding, schedule of medications, pelvic floor exercises). The degree of incontinence can be estimated by the type and number of pads used per day and night and by assessing the effect of incontinence on the patient's daily activities and quality of life. A fluid intake/voiding diary is a useful means of obtaining information about the quantity and type of fluids consumed and a patient's unique voiding dysfunction. For instance, the diary should attempt to document the time of normal voiding, volume voided, leakage events, and the number of pads used per day. The diary gives useful information about the circumstances under which leakage occurs, determines the severity of incontinence, assesses the patient's functional bladder capacity, and serves as an objective way of documenting the clinical utility of therapeutic interventions. Environmental factors are of particular importance in the evaluation of elderly adults with urge incontinence. Such overlooked factors include access to the toilet, toilet substitutes, mobility aids, and the ease of garment removal.

In reviewing the patient's genitourinary symptoms, further questions should be asked regarding the following: urge to urinate, frequency of urination, nocturia, obstruction (low flow or double voiding), hematuria, infections, type (alcohol and caffeinated products) and amount of fluid consumed, dietary fiber, and details including hormonal status and childhood voiding patterns. Pelvic floor function can also be assessed by questions concerning the presence of prolapse, sexual function, dyspareunia, constipation, fecal impaction, or fecal incontinence.

A careful review of previous surgical interventions for incontinence and pelvic prolapse, genitourinary surgery, trauma that can affect urinary tract function, and details of the obstetric history (parity, types of delivery, difficult labor, perineal repairs, and peripartum voiding function) may provide important insights into the patient's present symptoms.

A thorough understanding of the patient's medical history will help define any conditions that may interfere with urinary output, such as renal insufficiency, diabetes, and congestive heart failure. In addition, documentation of radiation therapy and other forms of cancer treatment may reveal overlooked damage to pelvic structures and function. A neurologic review of diagnoses such as multiple sclerosis, Parkinson's disease, or cerebral vascular accidents will reveal valuable information in most patients who may have related neurologic symptoms and incontinence. All medications taken by the patient deserve review for potential side effects on the genitourinary system. Numerous over-the-counter and prescribed drugs for treatment of concurrent medical conditions have effects on the neurologic innervation and muscle function of the bladder and sphincter. These include antihypertensives, diuretics, sedatives, hypnotics, analgesics, gastric motility promoters, and antidepressants.

PHYSICAL EXAMINATION

A complete physical examination is essential for the assessment of all patients with voiding dysfunction or incontinence. Special emphasis should be placed on abdominal, genital, pelvic, and neurologic evaluations.

Abdominal examination focuses on inspection for clinical correlation of surgical scars, trauma, and obesity. Large abdominal and retroperitoneal masses or an overdistended bladder is usually evident on palpation.

Genital examination should be organized into four successive steps for completeness:

1. General appearance: Inspect for external genital abnormalities (Bartholin's cyst or scar formation, condyloma, and adhesions), overall appearance of the perineum and the introital opening for assessing pelvic floor laxity, discharge from infection, and atrophy of the vaginal epithelium (loss of rugae; shiny, thin vaginal wall).
2. Urethra: Inspect for periurethral and urethral lesions (mucosal prolapse, caruncle, condyloma, Skene's abscess, or stenosis). Palpate for scarring, fibrosis, or tenderness that suggests urethritis or urethral diverticulum. Insert a Q-tip into the urethra to the level of the bladder neck in a woman placed in the lithotomy position, then ask her to cough and strain. Deflection of the Q-tip greater than 30 degrees is a simple means of determining significant urethral hypermobility. Straight catheterization or bladder ultrasound may be used to determine a postvoid residual. Urine obtained from the straight catheterization may be sent for culture (no screens) in cases of persistent urge incontinence or difficult cases of recurrent urinary tract infections of unclear etiology. Vaginal swabs for culturing *Ureaplasma*, chlamydia, and mycoplasma are often needed for the complete evaluation of complex voiding dysfunction.
3. Provocation: By obtaining a postvoid residual urine sample with straight catheterization, the patient's bladder may then be accurately filled for further evaluation. Provocative evidence of incontinence may be easily

reproduced by filling the patient's bladder with a volume of 200 to 300 mL and asking her to cough and strain in various positions (supine, sitting, standing). Discrete, isolated leakage events indicate SUI, but in the absence of a hypermobile urethra based on the Q-tip test, ISD should be considered for patients who leak with little provocation in the supine position.[5] The diagnosis of an unstable bladder (urge incontinence) precipitated by a Valsalva maneuver will be evident when the patient leaks and is unable to restrain further urine flow or bladder emptying under inspection. Furthermore, after bladder filling, patients who demonstrate UI may be asked to practice contraction of the pelvic floor muscles before abdominal straining, standing, or coughing in an attempt to determine whether they may benefit from pelvic floor exercises. Patients who have less observable leakage (place a piece of tissue paper in front on the urethra) after this simple test are probably good candidates for initiating a pelvic floor exercise program because they demonstrate functional innervation of the pelvic floor muscles.

4. Prolapse: Inspect the anterior, posterior and apical aspects of the vaginal vault with the posterior blade of a Grave speculum and with digital palpation while the patient is asked to rest and strain her pelvic floor muscles. At this time, proper identification of the muscle groups for pelvic floor exercises may be reinforced. Determining the various components of prolapse, such as a cystocele, rectocele, enterocele, or uterine prolapse, should be evident with a systematic and proper examination.

Neurologic examination focuses on the patient's general status, perineum, and lower extremities. The general neurologic status may easily be revealed by loss of cognitive function, the presence of a tremor, weakness, or gait abnormality. Examination of the back that reveals asymmetry of bone contours, skin dimples, scar, or hair tuft suggests spinal dysraphism or tethered cord syndrome. Perineal examination involves evaluation of sensory and motor evaluation of the S2 to S4 nerve roots by testing the integrity of the external anal sphincter and touch sensation of the perineum. The bulbocavernosus reflex (a perineal striated muscle reflex: sensory limb sensation is applied to the clitoris and the motor limb demonstrates external and sphincter contraction) is present in 70% to 80% of neurologically normal women; when it is absent, this may be meaningful in conjunction with other neurologic findings. Lower extremity evaluation involves testing typical sensory patterns and evaluating deep tendon and primitive reflexes that may suggest anatomic and etiologic significance. A stocking pattern of sensory loss may indicate metabolic neuropathies such as diabetes or alcoholism. The Babinski sign (primitive reflex) and ankle clonus suggest suprasacral cord lesions. Deep tendon reflexes of the quadriceps (L4) and Achilles tendon (S1) can demonstrate segmental spinal cord function as well as suprasegmental function.

PRIMARY INVESTIGATIONS

Urinalysis is performed to exclude hematuria, pyuria, bacteriuria, glycosuria, and proteinuria. A urine culture is obtained for evidence of bacteriuria or pyuria. Urine cytology and newer diagnostic tests for basement membrane antigens of the bladder are indicated to screen for bladder cancer if there is evidence of hematuria and frequency or urgency. BUN and serum creatinine level determinations are indicated in patients with a history or findings of severe voiding dysfunction. Furthermore, the consumption of excess fluid intake may be reflected in an abnormally low level of the BUN. As mentioned earlier, urine cultures from straight catheterization and vaginal cultures for atypical bacteria are performed when indicated.

SECONDARY INVESTIGATIONS

Incontinent patients in several categories (Table 85–3) should be referred for evaluation by a specialist. These categories include patients with a history or physical findings suggestive of underlying urologic disease, prolapse, hematuria, recurrent infection, or recent history of an abdominal or pelvic procedure. The specialist often can make beneficial recommendations with minimal testing for many patients who require management of incontinence. This is especially true of patients, young and old, with multifactorial reasons for UI. The following procedures outline the indications and use of several clinical investigations the specialist can choose to employ to evaluate difficult cases of urinary incontinence.

Urodynamics (evaluating the dynamic interaction of the bladder function, levator ani muscles, and urinary sphincters) may be performed at different levels of sophistication and complexity, but it is not required for simple SUI in a women who has not had previous surgery. Whereas urodynamics aids in the confirmation of the clinical diagnosis of SUI, the primary role of testing is to identify other factors (bladder compliance, unstable bladder contractions, voiding bladder pressures) that may influence the overall management of the patient's voiding dysfunction. The following paragraph outlines the various levels of urodynamic testing used by specialists.

Initial assessment and management of UI of a female patient in a limited outpatient setting may be performed with *simple cystometrography (CMG)*, which requires only a Foley catheter, large syringe, and sterile water. With

Table 85–3. Criteria for Referral

Recent urologic or gynecologic procedure
Recurrent symptomatic urinary tract infection
Anatomic abnormality (cystocele, rectocele, uterine prolapse)
Suspecetd obstruction (straining to void, postvoid residual > 100 mL)
Urinary retention
Hematuria
Difficult management problems (consideration of permanent catheter)

specific equipment, *single-channel CMG* (one pressure transducer catheter in the bladder) records bladder compliance during filling and assesses changes in bladder pressure. *Multichannel CMG* (typically a urine flow rate channel and two catheter channels: one pressure transducer catheter in the bladder; the second pressure transducer catheter measures intra-abdominal pressure via the rectum) is necessary in the management of mixed incontinence or for failures after anti-incontinence procedures. This test documents bladder compliance and instability, as well as dynamic intrinsic sphincteric competency by determining the Valsalva pressure needed to cause urinary leakage, and measures bladder pressure during voiding. *Videourodynamics* uses a combination of fluoroscopy and multichannel urodynamics to provide simultaneous anatomic and functional assessments of the bladder. *Ambulatory urodynamic monitoring* provides continuous documentation of bladder pressure and voiding events; its use is generally restricted for research purposes and difficult cases of refractory detrusor instability. *Electromyography* measures the electrical activity of either the external urethral sphincter or the anal sphincter in order to document denervation of the pelvic floor or urinary sphincter, or abnormal coordination of the bladder and external urinary sphincter. The main indications are in patients with an abnormal neurologic examination (multiple sclerosis and spinal cord disease, injury, or surgery). *Urethral pressure profile* is the static measurement of the pressure along the length of the urethra and has very little value in determining the dynamic cause and type of female urinary incontinence. Abdominal leak point pressure is determined by having the patient perform a slow Valsalva maneuver while in the upright position to determine the level of abdominal pressure that allows urine to pass through the continence mechanism. This is an important dynamic test in the evaluation of women with SUI.

Cystoscopy has a limited role in the evaluation of patients with a straightforward clinical finding of isolated SUI. However, cystoscopy should be performed to evaluate other causes of UI or concurrent urologic diseases identified by a thorough history and physical examination, especially in those patients presenting with urge incontinence. Examination of the urethra yields information about urethral pathology, such as diverticulum, fistula, stricture, or urethritis. The bladder is inspected for mucosal or trigonal abnormalities, trabeculation, foreign bodies, and stones. Bladder neck hypermobility and ISD may be reassessed by having the patient cough or strain with the scope in the midurethra.

Urinary tract imaging has a very limited role in the evaluation of the uncomplicated case of female incontinence. Intravenous pyelography (IVP), voiding cystourethrography (VCUG), and ultrasound studies are commonly employed for evaluation of the upper and lower urinary tract but are never first-line studies in the assessment of UI. The IVP is indicated for the evaluation of female UI when the history suggests the presence of an ectopic ureter or for the workup of concurrent hematuria, recurrent urinary tract infections, and the finding of hydroureteronephrosis by ultrasound or computed tomography studies. Ultrasound studies are useful for the evaluation of the upper urinary tract, particularly to detect hydronephrosis from elevated bladder pressure in patients with neurogenic bladder sphincteric dysfunction. In addition to the study of pelvic pathology, ultrasound has been used for determining a postvoid residual volume and detecting urethral diverticula. A VCUG is a simple, safe, and reliable study to evaluate the integrity of the female lower urinary tract. The study is important when one suspects bladder or urethral pathology, such as vesicovaginal or urethrovaginal fistulas, urethral diverticulum, and bladder prolapse. Although urethral hypermobility may be detected on rest and strain views, there is a limited role for the VCUG in determining conclusive evidence of ISD because the bladder pressure is not recorded during the examination.

SUMMARY

Because of advances in both evaluation and available treatment options, the increasing incidence of female UI is becoming a recognized quality-of-life issue for patients by both the public and health care professionals. The 1992 Agency for Health Care Policy and Research has published a clinical practice guideline, *Urinary Incontinence in Adults*, which recommends that primary care practitioners take a more active role in evaluating and selecting first-line treatment options in managing UI.[6] This article reviewed the components of a comprehensive office evaluation, suggested referral criteria for consultation, and outlined the merits of secondary studies that might be considered in the office evaluation of UI.

References

1. Herzog A, Fultz N: Urinary incontinence in the community: Prevalence, consequence, management, and beliefs. Top Geriatr Rehabil 1988;3:1–12.
2. Resnick N, Yalla S, Laurino E: The pathophysiology of urinary incontinence among institutionalized elderly persons. N Engl J Med 1989;320:1–7.
3. Hu T, Gabelko K, Weis K, et al: Clinical guideline and cost implications—the case of stress urinary incontinence. Geriatr Nephrol Urol 1994;4:85–91.
4. Resnick N, Yalla S: Management of urinary incontinence in the elderly. N Engl J Med 1985;313:800–804.
5. Hsu TH, Rackley RR, Appell RA: The supine stress test: A simple method to detect intrinsic urethral sphincter dysfunction. J Urol 1999;162:406–463.
6. Urinary Incontinence Guideline Panel: Urinary Incontinence in Adults: A Patient's Guide [AHCPR Pub No. 92–0040]. Rockville, Md, U.S. Department of Health and Human Services, Public Health Service, 1992.

Perinatal Outcome after Assisted Reproductive Techniques

Charla M. Blacker

Pregnancies achieved through assisted reproductive techniques (ART) are considered "premium pregnancies," often occurring only after considerable financial and emotional investment. These pregnancies carry some risks not found in pregnancies conceived without ART. First, ART patients are usually older than those women conceiving spontaneously and thus are at increased risk for miscarriage and certain genetic disorders in the offspring. Second, ART is associated with increased risk of multifetal pregnancy with its associated complications. ART requires exposure of gametes and embryos to laboratory conditions dissimilar to those of the human fallopian tube and uterus, and potentially to invasive micromanipulative procedures. Finally, the underlying infertility problem itself may be associated with factors that increase the rate of gestational complications. Accurate factual information about potential risks of pregnancy and perinatal outcome is essential for physicians in providing care for the ART patient, with her heightened concern and emotional needs.

PREGNANCY COMPLICATIONS IN ASSISTED REPRODUCTIVE TECHNOLOGY PREGNANCIES

Infertile women experience a higher rate of complications of pregnancy than women conceiving spontaneously, regardless of the method of conception. In a prospective study of pregnancy outcome, Varma and colleagues[1] compared 500 previously infertile women with fertile women in the institution's normal obstetric population. The infertile women were significantly older, with a median age of 31.8 years compared with 23.7 years in the fertile population. Independent of history of infertility, increased maternal age is associated with a fourfold risk of preterm delivery and a fivefold risk of cesarean delivery. Chronic hypertension, a known risk for pregnancy-induced hypertension (PIH), was increased in infertile women, particularly older primigravidas. Infertile women were also at increased risk for intrauterine growth retardation and fetal distress, a finding supported by other retrospective studies. Thus, in reviewing complications in ART patients, age-corrected comparisons and use of a suitable control population (i.e., infertile women) are essential to understanding the effects of method of conception on pregnancy outcome.

Preclinical and Clinical Pregnancy Losses

The U.S. Centers for Disease Control and Prevention together with the Society for Assisted Reproductive Technology (SART) jointly publish outcome data from United States and Canadian ART programs. During 1996, 11,038 babies were born from 48,726 ART cycles, including in vitro fertilization (IVF), gamete intrafallopian transfer (GIFT), or zygote intrafallopian transfer (ZIFT) cycles. IVF was the most frequently used procedure, accounting for 92% of procedures; GIFT and ZIFT each accounted for only a small fraction (8%) of the total ART cycles. Although the methods were not directly compared, the data do not indicate that there are significant differences between pregnancies originating through these procedures. According to 1996 national statistics, pregnancies resulting from transfer of fresh embryos from nondonor eggs occurred in 33.4% of cycles for women younger than 35 years of age, 26.7% for women aged 35 to 39 years, and 13.4% for women older than 39 years, with an overall conception rate of 27%.[2] Adverse outcomes of pregnancy occurred in approximately 15% of cycles, with 12.9% resulting in spontaneous abortion, 1.5% in induced abortion, and 0.7% in stillbirth. Because the SART requires ultrasound documentation or evidence of placental tissue in aborted tissue for the diagnosis of a clinical pregnancy, the spontaneous abortion rate does not reflect "chemical pregnancies," positive β-human chorionic gonadotropin (β-hCG) tests with subsequent loss before visualization of a gestational sac. It is estimated that as many as 13% of pregnancies may be lost before they are clinically recognized.

Ectopic pregnancy is a potential risk after ART because women undergoing these procedures often have tubal damage. Although IVF "bypasses" the fallopian tubes and embryo transfer is directly into the uterine cavity, the tubal ostia are often dilated in women with tubal disease, allowing retrograde migration of the embryos into a tube incapable of normal transport. In the 1996 SART report,[2] the incidence of ectopic pregnancy in this group was 0.5%, but in previous years it ranged from 4% to 7%. Women undergoing ART are also at increased risk for heterotopic pregnancy, coexisting intrauterine and ectopic pregnancy. Heterotopic pregnancies are challenging to diagnose, because monitoring β-hCG levels is less useful, and heterotopic pregnancy cannot be treated medically. In the 1992 SART Registry,[3] 18 heterotopic pregnancies (0.1% of aspirations) occurred after ART. Heterotopic pregnancies have been reported to occur in the infertile population at a rate of about 1 in 600, not dissimilar from that reported through ART.[4] However, the rate is significantly higher than that in the general population of about 1 in 10,000 to 15,000.

Multiple Pregnancy

Both ovulation induction and ART are associated with increased risk of multifetal gestation. The incidence of multiple pregnancy is known to increase with the number of embryos transferred, whereas pregnancy rates plateau with the transfer of four or more embryos. In the 1996 SART data,[2] singleton births accounted for 52.3% of all ART-created pregnancies and multiple gestation occurred in 32.1%. Twins accounted for 26.3% of pregnancies; only 5.8% were triplets or greater. The prevalence of multifetal gestations decreased with increasing maternal age, a phenomenon opposite that observed in the general population.

Multiple gestation is a major determinant of perinatal outcome of ART pregnancies. In one study, only 17% of ART pregnancies and 27% of spontaneous multifetal pregnancies had normal course and outcome.[5] Pregnancies with three or more fetuses are more likely to abort than are singleton or twin pregnancies. Spontaneous resorption of multifetal pregnancy is not uncommon. Of patients with twins, 43% spontaneously reduce to singleton pregnancies; 70% of the triplets reduce to twins or singletons; and 80% of the quadruplets reduce to three or less. Embryo resorption is most likely during the first 7 weeks of gestation and is unlikely after the 14th week. The presence of fetal cardiac motion increases the likelihood of progression; finding three fetal heart beats is associated with a triplet delivery rate of 69%, a twin incidence of 19%, and a singleton birth rate of 12%.[6]

Compared with singleton births, fetal, neonatal, and perinatal mortality rates are 3 to 6 times higher in twins and 5 to 15 times higher in multiple births of a higher order.[7] Cerebral palsy rates among survivors are 6 times higher in twins and 20 times higher in triplets. The adverse outcomes after ART are partly due to the increased risk of multiple pregnancy and partly to preterm and low birth weight, but cannot be entirely explained by those factors alone. Selective fetal reduction (discussed elsewhere) to singleton or twins can improve outcome significantly, although controversy exists about whether the procedure results in outcomes comparable with spontaneous pregnancies.

Many of the maternal complications are also related to multiple gestation. Multiple gestation is associated with increased incidence of cesarean section and postpartum hemorrhage. Polyhydramnios and venous thrombophlebitis are increased in multifetal pregnancies. Preterm labor is observed in 86% and premature rupture of membranes in

17.5% of triplet gestations. Preeclampsia occurs in about one third of triplets. However, ART or ovulation induction may themselves have some detrimental effect on pregnancy. Nyirati and associates[8] described higher incidences of low birth weight and perinatal mortality in induced multiple gestations than in spontaneous ones. They also described a higher incidence of cervical insufficiency; increased rate of cerclage is particularly noted among triplets conceived through ART. Fetal outcome, with respect to Apgar score and umbilical cord pH, was also poorer. The occurrence of a multiple gestation places a patient at sufficient risk to warrant referral to a maternal-fetal medicine specialist.

Obstetric Outcome of Assisted Reproductive Technology Pregnancies

Many studies have attempted to evaluate the obstetric outcome of IVF and other ART procedures. Evaluation is complicated by the fact that women undergoing ART are older than the average gravida and more likely to develop diseases associated with advanced maternal age, particularly PIH and gestational diabetes mellitus, independent of route of conception. However, even when controlled for maternal age and parity, multivariate analyses show that patients who conceived by IVF or ovulation induction had approximately a twofold increased risk for gestational diabetes (odds ratio [OR], 2.0; 95% confidence interval [CI], 1.23 to 3.30) and PIH (OR, 2.1; CI, 1.04 to 4.10).[9, 10] Women conceiving through IVF are also at greater risk of cesarean section, even when corrected for multiple gestation (OR, 3.6; 95% CI, 2.44 to 5.29).

Although the rate of multiple gestation from ART is declining because of reductions in the number of embryos transferred, ART pregnancies still have poorer than normal outcome with regard to preterm birth, low birth weight, and perinatal mortality. Infants born after ART have a greater neonatal morbidity rate, including a greater requirement for assisted ventilation. To control for factors related to multifetal gestation, Tanbo[11] reported on obstetric outcome in singleton pregnancies after ART. In women conceiving through ART, the frequencies of placenta previa and PIH were increased. Pregnancies were of shorter duration with an increased incidence of preterm birth. Infants conceived through ART had a lower mean birth weight and were more likely to be delivered by elective cesarean than were spontaneously conceived babies.

Other authors have agreed that ART increases the rate of preterm births by as much as fourfold. Olivennes and coworkers[12] reported similarly increased rates of complications (i.e., prematurity, low birth weight, small for gestational age [SGA], and perinatal mortality) in patients conceiving by IVF or ovulation induction, suggesting that the increased risk is not linked to the IVF method itself but rather to a common factor (e.g., population characteristics, underlying infertile status, or ovarian stimulation). Reubinoff and colleagues,[13] however, failed to find any difference in the rate of preterm labor, low birth weight, and SGA infants in IVF singleton gestations compared with spontaneous conceptions when controlled for maternal age, parity, ethnic origin, and location of delivery. They confirmed previous findings of increased cesarean section rates among IVF patients (41.9% vs. 15.5%).

Although ART has been utilized for 2 decades, there remain few data regarding long-term consequences. In general, data are reassuring, with normal pediatric development reported in some studies with follow-up as long as 13 years after birth.[13–15] Physical growth and psychosocial development is reported as similar to those in non-IVF children. In studies evaluating mental development or school performance, children conceived through IVF performed slightly better than the comparison population,[13–16] probably resulting from their generally high socioeconomic status and the exceptional motivation of their parents.[15]

Congenital Anomalies

That there should be concern regarding congenital anomalies in ART-conceived pregnancy is natural. IVF bypasses selective mechanisms associated with in vivo fertilization, potentially allowing fertilization by genetically abnormal sperm as well as an increased possibility of polyspermic fertilization. Embryos grown in vitro are exposed to chemical and environmental perturbations that could affect subsequent development. Extensive animal data have provided reassurance concerning the probable safety of ART pregnancies. Moreover, a basic axiom of teratology suggests that insults occurring during the early embryologic stages are either lethal or result in no significant defect (the "all or none" hypothesis). Several large studies have examined the issue of congenital anomalies and in general provide reassurance about the neonates resulting from ART procedures. The malformation rate reported for neonates ranges from 0.9% to 3.15%, a figure consistent with the incidence found in the general population.[17] The most rigorous surveillance of ART pregnancies is the study of 961 children conceived through Bourn Hall and Hallam Medical Center (1978 to 1987).[18] The malformation rate was slightly higher among multiple births (2.7%) compared with singletons (2.4%), rates comparable with those detected in the first week of life from United Kingdom data. Specific congenital anomalies were considered to be comparable with those expected from maternal age–adjusted values.[17]

Although the safety of IVF with respect to congenital anomalies seems assured, questions remain about assisted fertilization techniques. Partial zona dissection (PZD) and subzonal insertion (SUZI) of spermatozoa are micromanipulative procedures that have been employed to a limited extent in the treatment of infertility. The number of children born after using these techniques is small, and at present the data are insufficient to evaluate potential genetic and teratologic risks. In one case series surveying 86 children,[19] a 5.4% rate of major malformations was reported. The corresponding rate in a historical control group was 3.7%, and the authors considered the difference to be significant. The pregnancies in the study group were achieved with PZD, SUZI, conventional IVF with hyaluronidase pretreatment, or combinations of these techniques. Because of the limited number of cases and the heterogeneous study group, the significance of the reportedly increased rate of major malformations is unclear.

Of larger concern is the effect of intracytoplasmic sperm injection (ICSI). ICSI is widely used for treatment of male infertility and involves the aspiration into a micropipet of a single spermatozoon and its consecutive direct injection into a mature oocyte. ICSI circumvents several steps in the natural fertilization process. Additionally, proteins from the sperm head are injected into the oocyte along with nuclear material, whereas the oocyte is punctured and exposed to mechanical stress. Preliminary data provide no evidence for a teratogenic effect of ICSI. The obstetric outcomes of 904 pregnancies resulting in 877 children conceived after ICSI have been compiled from American and European surveys.[20] The incidences of first trimester losses and obstetric outcome in pregnancies conceived through ICSI were similar to those of other ART procedures. In the 877 children born after ICSI, 32 (2.2%) had major congenital malformations, none of which were disproportionately frequent, and not significantly different from the rate observed in the general population.

However, there remains cause for concern. Most neonatal examinations involve only routine physical findings, and cytogenetic studies are not performed. A range of cytogenetic abnormalities is associated with impaired male fertility. Pooled data from 11 surveys of 9766 infertile men with azoospermia and oligozoospermia revealed a 5.8% incidence of chromosomal abnormalities.[21] Sex chromosome anomalies were the most common finding in azoospermic and oligozoospermic infertile men, with an incidence ranging from 1.8% to 10.8%. Azoospermic men are more likely to have sex chromosomal anomalies than oligospermic men. Autosomal anomalies have been reported in 1.5% to 3% of azoospermic or oligospermic men. The incidence is significantly increased from the reported incidence of sex chromosome and autosome anomalies in newborn screens, 0.14% and 0.25%, respectively. Additional chromosomal abnormalities associated with infertility include a variety of translocations, both robertsonian and reciprocal autosomal, X-autosome, and Y-autosome translocations. Microdeletions along the Y-chromosome have also been associated with infertility; the frequency of microdeletions within this locus in the azoospermic and severely oligozoospermic ICSI population ranges from less than 9% to 18%.[21]

Peripheral karyotype may be normal and yet offspring can be at risk of paternally transmitted genetic anomalies. Studies using fluorescent in situ hybridization (FISH) analyses of spermatozoa from oligoasthenoteratozoospermic (OAT) males demonstrated a 19.6% frequency of autosome and sex chromosome aneuploidy compared with a 1.4% frequency in fertile controls.[21] Because this analysis was only a partial screen of the complete chromosomal array, the true frequency of aneuploidy in the genomes of these sperm may be significantly higher.

Because the proportion of spermatozoa with abnormal chromosome complement is increased in men with severely abnormal sperm parameters (OAT) or nonobstructive azoospermia, the possibility that infertile fathers who undergo ICSI will transmit chromosomal abnormalities to their offspring is a major concern. Based on recent genetic surveys of obstetric outcomes, it appears that offspring conceived through ICSI for the treatment of male infertility have a 1% incidence of sex chromosome aneuploidy, significantly higher than the 0.14% to 0.19% incidence observed in non–ICSI-conceived newborns.[21] It is thought that the increased risk is secondary to the increased frequency of sperm aneuploidy rather than a result of the ICSI technique. Some authors[21] have suggested that routine karyotyping of all males before undergoing ICSI will improve detection rate; however, it must be recognized that aneuploidy may be limited to spermatozoa. Additional testing should also be considered because a variety of genetically linked diseases (e.g., cystic fibrosis, androgen insensitivity, myotonic dystrophy) may present in otherwise healthy, but infertile males. Couples who achieve a pregnancy after undergoing ICSI should be offered prenatal genetic diagnosis.

OUTCOME OF FROZEN EMBRYO PREGNANCIES

In the largest report on the outcome of frozen embryos, the French IVF registry FIVNAT reported on the results from 1987 to 1992.[22] During this time, 465 pregnancies were conceived through the transfer of frozen-thawed embryos compared with 8757 pregnancies conceived through fresh embryo transfer, resulting in 386 and 8729, babies respectively. Although the miscarriage rate was higher, the remainder of the pregnancy was normal after transfer of frozen-thawed embryos, with fewer multiple pregnancies and lower rates of preterm births and low birth weights than with other forms of ART. No difference was noted in the rate of congenital malformation between pregnancies conceived with frozen-thawed or fresh embryos, or with spontaneously occurring pregnancies. Later development likewise appears normal with no abnormalities of health or scholastic performance.[12]

SUMMARY

ART offers the opportunity for pregnancy to many couples for whom a child was once only a dream. The safety of basic ART techniques has been established over 2 decades of experience; however, perinatal outcome remains suboptimal because of complications arising from advanced maternal age and multiple gestation. There is reason to hope that the frequency of multiple gestation may decrease as laboratory developments improve outcome with single- or two-embryo transfers.

Whereas micromanipulation offers excellent pregnancy rates, there is seemingly an increased risk of genetic abnormalities in children born through ICSI. The risk of abnormality is low enough that it should not discourage most couples from attempting pregnancy; however, couples should be counseled carefully regarding risk and screened appropriately. Little is known about long-term developmental concerns, and more data are needed before these issues can be dismissed.

References

1. Varma TR, Patel RH, Bhathenia RK: Outcome of pregnancy after infertility. Acta Obstet Gynecol Scand 1988;67:115–119.
2. Society for Assisted Reproductive Technology, The American Society for Reproductive Medicine: Assisted reproductive technology in the United States: 1996 results generated from the American Society for Reproductive Medicine/Society for Assisted Reproductive Technology Registry. Fertil Steril 1999;71:798–805.
3. Society for Assisted Reproductive Technology, The American Society for Reproductive Medicine: Assisted reproductive technology in the United States and Canada. 1992 results generated from the American Fertility Society/Society for Assisted Reproductive Technology Registry. Fertil Steril 1994;62:1121–1128.
4. Correy JF, Watkins RA, Bradfield GF, et al: Assisted reproductive technology: Spontaneous pregnancies and pregnancies as a result of treatment in an in vitro fertilization program terminating in ectopic pregnancies or spontaneous abortions. Fertil Steril 1988;50:85–88.
5. Hill GA, Bryan S, Herbert CM, et al: Complications of pregnancy in infertile couples: Routine treatment versus reproduction. Obstet Gynecol 1990:75:790–794.
6. Manzur A, Goldsman MP, Stone SC, et al: Outcome of triplet pregnancies after assisted reproductive techniques: How frequent are the vanishing embryos? Fertil Steril 1995;63:252–257.
7. Frydman R, Belaisch-Allart J, Fries N, et al: An obstetric assessment of the first 100 births from the in vitro fertilization program at Clamart, France. Am J Obstet Gynecol 1986;154:550–555.
8. Nyirati I, Orvos H, Bartfai G, Kovacs L: Iatrogenic multiple pregnancy. Higher risk than a spontaneous one? J Reprod Med 1997;42:695–698.
9. Tallo CP, Vohr B, Oh W, et al: Maternal and neonatal morbidity associated with in vitro fertilization. J Pediatr 1995;127:794–800.
10. Schenker JG, Ezra Y: Complications of assisted reproductive techniques. Fertil Steril 1994;61:411–422.
11. Tanbo T: Obstetric outcome in singleton pregnancies after assisted reproduction. Obstet Gynecol 1995;86:188–192.
12. Olivennes F, Schneider ZZ, Remy V, et al: Perinatal outcome and follow-up of 82 children aged 1–9 years old conceived from cryopreserved embryos. Hum Reprod 1996;11:1565–1568.
13. Reubinoff BE, Samueloff A, Ben-Haim M, et al: Is the obstetric outcome of in vitro fertilized singleton gestations different from natural ones? A controlled study. Fertil Steril 1997;67:1077–1083.
14. Olivennes F, Kerbrat V, Rufat P, et al: Follow-up of a cohort of 422 children aged 6 to 13 years conceived by in vitro fertilization. Fertil Steril 1997;67:284–289.
15. Morin NC, Wirth FH, Johnson DH, et al: Congenital malformations and psychosocial development in children conceived by in vitro fertilization. J Pediatr 1989;115:222–227.
16. Cederblad M, Friberg B, Ploman F, et al: Intelligence and behaviour in children born after in-vitro fertilization treatment. Hum Reprod 1996;11:2052–2057.

therapy is problematic during pregnancy and oral antidiabetic agents are not approved for use in pregnant patients. These women often regain normal glucose tolerance after delivery but remain at very high risk for development of diabetes postpartum (estimated at as high as 50% during the ensuing 10 years).

WHY CARE ABOUT DIABETES?

Diabetic complications can hurt, maim, or kill. With our current knowledge, we believe we can prevent, delay, or alleviate the suffering associated with the chronic complications (owing to space constraints we do not deal here with acute complications). Diabetic complications can be simplistically divided into microvascular (those specifically occurring only in patients with diabetes) and macrovascular (which happen to all people but appear earlier and in more severe forms in persons with diabetes).

Microvascular Complications

Microvascular complications—retinopathy, nephropathy, peripheral sensory neuropathy—are tightly linked to *hyperglycemia*. Therefore, the strategies for their prevention or stabilization are aimed at achieving euglycemia (or as close as can be practically achieved in a given patient). Several large-scale trials in patients with type 1[3] and type 2 diabetes[4-6] confirmed the hypothesis. In fact, any improvement in glucose control has been associated with better outcomes when *microvascular* complications were evaluated. Most studies used glycated hemoglobin (HgbA$_{1c}$) as the "gold standard" for assessing glycemic control. The upper limit of the reference range for most laboratories using this test is 6%. There is a linear relationship between average daily glucose levels and HgbA$_{1c}$. The HgbA$_{1c}$ level typically reflects integrated glucose control over the previous 2 months. Standards of care require achieving a level under 7%. Whereas it is apparent that lowering glucose levels in a very poorly controlled patient (e.g., HgbA$_{1c}$ of 13%) even by only 1% will pay off in improved outcome, the cost-benefit ratio remains controversial for someone with only mildly elevated glucose levels (e.g., HgbA$_{1c}$ below 7%).

Macrovascular Complications

The situation is more complex for the macrovascular complications of diabetes—cardiovascular, cerebrovascular, and peripheral vascular. These account for the vast majority (by some estimates greater than 75%) of diabetic morbidity and mortality. Patients with diabetes are far more prone to these complications (ranging from 2- to 4-fold for strokes to 10-fold or higher for myocardial infarctions among diabetic women). As enunciated by Haffner,[7] the clock for microvascular complications starts ticking at the time hyperglycemia occurs. However, the macrovascular complications are present, often for decades, by the time the patient presents for the first time to his or her physician. It is clear that other known cardiovascular risk factors, such as dyslipidemia, hypertension, or hyperinsulinemia, are present long before the patient's glucose becomes diagnostic for diabetes. It is, therefore, hardly surprising that even normalization of glucose levels by our treatment does not lead to prevention or significant improvement in the macrovascular complications of diabetes.

EPIDEMIOLOGY OF DIABETES

As already pointed out, diabetes is reaching epidemic proportion in the United States. We are not alone. The World Health Organization declared diabetes a global public health concern for the 21st century. Countries, such as China, that until recently had a low prevalence of the disease, are struggling to cope with the mounting costs of diabetes to their societies. What happened? "Coca-colonization" was a term coined by Zimmet[8] to sum it up. The Westernized lifestyle is rapidly spreading along with economic advances. Increased longevity among populations expending fewer calories while taking in more high-fat, processed food has led to an explosion in the number of cases of diabetes. The unprecedented proliferation of fast-food restaurants, television and computer monitors, cell and cordless telephones, remote control and other "work-saving" devices, valet parking, elimination of sidewalks, and cutting back on mandatory physical activity in schools are just a few of the culprits responsible for the epidemic of diabetes in the United States. In many urban areas, type 2 diabetes had become the most frequent diabetic condition among children and teenagers.[9] Many pediatricians and obstetricians will have to rapidly retool in order to deal with this recent phenomenon in their practices.

Given the previously stated concern about our ability to affect the macrovascular complications of diabetes, it becomes essential that we begin to focus on the patients at risk. It has been estimated that there may be perhaps three times as many "prediabetic" people than those already affected with the disease. The 1997 classification defined two specific categories of such population: those with *impaired fasting plasma glucose* (levels between 110 and 126 mg/dL) and those with *impaired glucose tolerance* (2-hour plasma glucose after ingesting the glucose load between 140 and 200 mg/dL).[2] In some studies, those patients with impaired glucose tolerance have a three times higher incidence of fatal cardiac events than those with normal glucose status. A similar relationship between fasting glucose and cardiac events has been noted. Changes in lifestyle (smoking cessation, diet, weight control, increased physical activity) and aggressive treatment of cardiovascular risk factors (especially blood pressure and lipids) are required in order for us to significantly affect the incidence and prevalence of the deadliest diabetic complications.

This is also the most frustrating area. We believe that we already possess the means for prevention or control of diabetic complications (perhaps diabetes itself) today. However, this knowledge has not been translated into practice. Why is that? There are probably many factors responsible for this frustrating and expensive state of affairs. First, any time lifestyle changes are required to accomplish therapeutic goals, difficulties occur. Patients are led to believe that when the need arises there will be medications or procedures available to correct the situation. They also typically do not believe in the seriousness of a condition when it is asymptomatic. In order to change their lifelong habits, they have to be convinced that those changes are truly life-saving. That, in turn, implies that someone has to explain the underlying rationale and the practical implementation of these changes into a patient's specific lifestyle. Because diabetes is an incurable disease, these alterations of lifestyle have to become lifelong habits.

Diabetes is a unique disease. In contrast to the rest of the medical practice, it is the patient (and her or his family) who is in charge. The patient decides when, where, what, and how much to eat; the duration, frequency, and intensity of physical activity; and the adherence to a prescribed frequency of self–blood glucose monitoring or to drug regimen, or to smoking cessation advice. The quality of patient education largely determines the outcome of diabetes control. The problem we face is that about 95% of all ambulatory encounters of patients with diabetes take place in generalists' offices. These settings usually do not have the resources or knowledge necessary to provide the curriculum needed for optimal education of diabetic patients. If the patients do not know what they should be doing and why, it is hardly surprising that they are not doing it!

WHAT DO WE NEED TO ADDRESS IN PATIENTS WITH DIABETES?

From the previous discussion, it is clear that one should concentrate on meeting the standards of care for control of glucose, blood pressure, and lipids in order to stave off diabetic complications. The current American Diabetes Association guidelines specify $HgbA_{1c}$ under 7% as the goal for glycemic control. Further, as patients (certainly all those who are on drugs for glycemic control) with diabetes need to monitor their own blood glucose, they need to know goals for those measurements (preprandial levels between 80 and 120 mg/dL, postprandial below 160 mg/dL, and bedtime between 100 and 140 mg/dL). It has to be made clear to all practitioners and patients that guidelines for blood pressure and lipid control are more aggressive for patients with diabetes because they are presumed to already have coronary heart disease at diagnosis. Thus, blood pressure needs to be kept under 130/80 mm Hg, low-density lipoprotein (LDL) cholesterol under 100 mg/dL, triglycerides under 150 mg/dL, and high-density lipoprotein (HDL) cholesterol above 45 mg/dL. Studies are being conducted aiming to demonstrate that even tighter goals might be necessary in this high-risk population to significantly improve their outcomes.

The term *insulin-resistance syndrome* (or syndrome X, as it was originally coined by Reaven in 1988[10]) has been often used to describe the constellation of several risk factors for cardiovascular disease in a single patient. Undoubtedly, many susceptibility genes will be identified for these risk factors. The clinical phenotype of a person expressing all components would have an android habitus with abundance of central fat deposition, in combination with elevated body mass index (>27 kg/m^2), high blood pressure, dyslipidemia (typically high triglycerides and low HDL cholesterol), hyperinsulinemia, abnormal glucose tolerance, and hypercoagulable state. The fact that appropriate diet can lead simultaneously to weight loss, lower blood pressure, improved glucose and insulin levels, and better lipid profile (in absence of any drugs) supports the concept of a syndrome.

HOW DO WE ADDRESS PROBLEMS IN DIABETES?

We now have many drugs available for achieving glucose control. Those medications fall into two categories: those that elevate insulin levels and those that improve insulin action.

Drugs Elevating Insulin Levels
Insulin

For patients with insulin deficiency, in either absolute (by definition, all patients with type 1 diabetes, a proportion with type 2 or other types of diabetes) or relative terms (typically patients with type 2 diabetes), insulin itself or drugs increasing insulin secretion are used. Insulin will lower everyone's glucose level. The art of medical practice is to know which type of insulin in what amount should be given by the patients at what time and with which frequency. Again, the goal is to achieve near-euglycemia without causing significant hypoglycemia. As long as insulin is administered subcutaneously, (i.e., not physiologically), its regimen remains an imprecise science in the best of hands. Currently available insulin preparations (all synthetically made "human") in the United States include long-acting *Ultralente*; intermediate *Lente* and *NPH* (neutral protamine Hagedorn); shorter-acting *Regular;* premixed combinations (70% NPH/30% regular, 50% NPH/50% regular); rapid-acting *LisPro* and *Aspart,* insulin analogues, and its combination (75% NPLisPro/25% LisPro). A peakless insulin analogue for use as basal insulin therapy, insulin *Glargine*, was recently introduced.

Oral Medications Increasing Circulating Insulin Levels

Sulfonylureas, meglitinides (only repaglinide is approved in the United States currently), and a phenylalanine derivative nateglimide enhance insulin secretion. Thus, they are ineffective in patients with type 1 diabetes. Although there are minor differences in molecular details of their action, drugs in these three classes act similarly at the level of the beta cells to stimulate insulin release. Sulfonylureas remain the mainstay of the hypoglycemic therapy. Glyburide (1.25 to 20 mg/day), glipizide (regular 2.5 to 40 mg/day or extended-release formulation 2.5 to 20 mg/day), and glimepiride (1 to 8 mg once daily) represent the so-called second-generation sulfonylureas. Generic chlorpropamide (100 to 500 mg/day) is still the least expensive hypoglycemic agent available. Repaglinide, in contrast, is a short-acting drug that needs to be taken with meals (0.5 to 4 mg per meal, up to a maximum of 16 mg/day). Nateglimide, another mealtime insulin secretagogue, is used at 90 to 120 mg with each meal. As would be expected, the major side effect (although lowering of glucose levels is the intended effect) of these drugs is hypoglycemia.

Drugs Improving Insulin Action

Two classes of medications (biguanides and thiazolidinediones) that sensitize tissues to the effects of insulin are available. These agents do not increase insulin levels. Consequently, they are antidiabetic but not hypoglycemic when used as monotherapy. Currently, there is one approved biguanide, metformin, on the United States market. Metformin is a short-acting drug that typically needs to be taken with meals at gradually increasing doses (start with 500 mg once daily, titrate to a maximum of 2500 mg in three doses) to minimize potential gastrointestinal side effects (bloating, anorexia, flatulence, diarrhea). Metformin acts chiefly to potentiate insulin action at the level of the liver. Metformin is contraindicated in patients with renal dysfunction (to avoid potential complication of lactic acidosis), defined as serum creatinine above 1.5 mg/dL in men and 1.4 mg/dL in women. It is the only antidiabetic mediation that does not lead to weight gain. This fact can be particularly beneficial in the overweight type 2 patients.

Thiazolidinediones sensitize tissues (especially fat, skeletal muscle, liver) to the action of insulin. Results are mainly increased glucose uptake and to some degree decreased hepatic glucose production. These drugs are long acting and, among responding patients, can take up to 12 to 16 weeks to achieve their optimal effect. Currently, two are available on the United States market—rosiglitazone (2 to 8 mg/day) and pioglitazone (15 to 45 mg/day). The original representative of this class, troglitazone, was removed from the market owing to serious hepatic dysfunction among some patients. Although similar hepatic side effects have not been noted with the other two agents, serum transaminase monitoring is recommended every 2 months during the first year, and the drugs should not be initiated in patients with hepatic disease. These drugs are well tolerated, although weight gain, hemodilution, and peripheral edema have been noted in some patients.

Drugs Delaying Intestinal Glucose Absorption

Miglitol and *acarbose* are two antidiabetic agents that improve glucose control by inhibiting a small intestinal enzyme, α − glucosidase. This effect slows glucose absorption after meals and thus decreases postprandial glucose levels. Because of their mode of action, these agents cannot cause hypoglycemia if used as monotherapy. As expected, their side effects are limited to gastrointestinal ones: bloating, flatulence, and diarrhea. They are used with meals, at 25 to 100 mg each time.

Drug Combination Therapy

Having seven separate types of antidiabetic agents allows the physician to combine treatment, taking advantage of additive or even synergistic effects. α-Glucosidase inhibitors, for example, can be combined with any other agent, especially in patients whose major problem is hyperglycemia after meals. Combinations of an insulin secretagogue (sulfonylurea or repaglinide) with an insulin sensitizer make sense. In fact, one such combination is marketed in a single pill (Glucovance, combination of metformin and glyburide, 250 mg/1.25 mg, 500 mg/2.5 mg, and 500 mg/5 mg, respectively). One can also take advantage of the fact that the modes of action of the two classes of insulin sensitizers differ. Combining metformin with a glitazone has been shown to be more effective than either agent alone in those patients poorly controlled on monotherapy. Finally, combining oral agent(s) with insulin might make sense in some patients (e.g., among insulin-resistant patients on large doses of insulin, insulin dose can be decreased when metformin/glitazone is used; long-acting insulin can be used at bedtime in combination with an oral agent in patients whose major problem is fasting hyperglycemia).

CONTROL OF CARDIOVASCULAR RISK FACTORS IN DIABETES

Standards of care postulate aggressive goals for blood pressure and lipid control for patients with diabetes. To achieve them, lifestyle changes are required, as described previously. Medications will, however, need to be used in the majority of patients with hypertension and dyslipidemia.

Hypertension

Judging from the results of large-scale studies, such as the United Kingdom Prospective Diabetes Study,[11, 12] in patients with type 2 diabetes, lowering of blood pressure (goal of less than 130/80 mm Hg) regardless of agents used seems to have beneficial effects on macrovascular end points (myocardial infarction and other cardiac events, stroke). *Angiotensin-converting enzyme inhibitors* (such as captopril, enalapril, ramipril, quinapril, benazepril, trandolapril) have been first-line antihypertensive drugs among diabetes experts mainly because of their beneficial effect on diabetic nephropathy. β-Blockers, calcium channel blockers, angiotensin II receptor antagonists, thiazides (at low doses), and other drugs can be also used alone or in combination as long as they do not impair the patient's glycemic or lipid control.

Dyslipidemia

Even patients faithfully adhering to a diet plan cannot expect improvement of their LDL cholesterol levels by more than 10% to 15%. Given the current goal (less than 100 mg/dL, and it is likely that it will be lowered in the future), most patients with dyslipidemia will need to take medications to achieve it. *3-Hydroxy-3-methylglutaryl coenzyme A reductase inhibitors* or statins (e.g., lovastatin, pravastatin, simvastatin, fluvastatin, atorvastatin, cerivastatin) have been the mainstay of cholesterol-lowering therapy. Control of triglyceride levels typically requires measures on two fronts: improving glycemic control and specific drug therapy. For the latter, *fibric acid derivatives* (gemfibrozil or fenofibrate) are usually most effective.

Finally, it is recommended that all patients with diabetes (unless specifically contraindicated) use low-dose *aspirin* (81 to 162.5 mg/day) as a primary or secondary preventive for coronary heart disease. The use of folic acid in patients with elevated homocysteine levels, a biochemical marker associated with atherosclerotic disease, is also gaining popularity.

MICROVASCULAR DIABETIC COMPLICATIONS

In addition to the measures to prevent or delay macrovascular complications of diabetes, physicians taking care of these patients need to meet standards of care for dealing with the classic, microvascular complications of the disease. Diabetic retinopathy, nephropathy, and neuropathy can theoretically be prevented by meticulous glycemic control. In addition, specific diagnostic and therapeutic measures should be taken during office visits to the practitioners assuming care for diabetes. Regular visits to an eye specialist (preferably an ophthalmologist well versed in dealing with retinopathy) are required because early *retinopathy* is treatable by laser therapy. Blindness due to diabetic retinopathy is preventable. Annual screening of *renal function* by obtaining a timed 24-hour urine specimen (for creatinine clearance and albumin excretion rate) is required. Repeated random urine samples tested for albuminuria during the year can probably substitute for this requirement if a patient finds it difficult to provide the 24-hour specimen. In any case, aggressive use of angiotensin-converting enzyme inhibitors (and perhaps angiotensin II receptor antagonists) in patients with microalbuminuria (over 20 μg/min) or macroalbuminuria (over 300 μg/min), regardless of their blood pressure, can slow down or prevent development of diabetic nephropathy.

The classic peripheral sensory *neuropathy* in diabetes can take many forms. Some patients relate only "strange" sensation in their feet, especially at night ("restless leg syndrome"), often relieved by walking. Some complain of tingling, numbness, or pain. These complaints typically start in the feet, are symmetrical, and ascend with time. Many patients' feet eventually become insensate and predispose them to cuts, ulcers, infections, and gangrene, which can lead to amputations or death. It is thus essential that all patients be taught proper foot care and techniques for daily foot inspection. Further, a patient's feet have to be examined by the responsible physician during each visit. If pressure points, ulcers, calluses, infections, or any other problems are detected, referral to an experienced podiatrist is essential. It has to be kept in mind that diabetic neuropathy can take numerous forms in addition to the classic "glove and stocking" distribution. Autonomic diabetic neuropathy can also present in many different ways. Some experts believe that subtle autonomic dysfunction (especially cardiac) is present in all patients with diabetes at diagnosis if careful tests are done. For many patients, symptomatic autonomic neuropathy (gastrointestinal, vasomotor) indicates, unfortunately, a very poor prognostic finding.

FUTURE DIRECTIONS

We can expect many exciting developments in both the science and the practice of diabetes and its complications in the near future. Search is ongoing to find means to prevent both type 1 and type 2 diabetes. Genetic susceptibility not only for diabetes but also for its complications should bring us closer to an individualized approach to our populations at risk. Improved modes of delivery of insulin (e.g., by inhalation) as well as introduction of specifically designed insulin analogues and noninvasive glucose monitoring devices are on the near horizon. In addition to transplantation of the pancreas or pancreatic islets as a means of restoring endogenous insulin production in type 1 diabetes, exciting scientific developments bring a hope of gene therapy by "teaching" other human cells (most likely hepatocytes) to produce insulin in a physiologic manner. Progress in elucidating the details of insulin action will bring new generations of agents targeting specific molecular defects in our patients with type 2 diabetes. Finally, we have to figure out how to get the message out to our society that most of the misery brought on by diabetes is largely preventable by paying attention to the basic elements of healthy lifestyle, prevention of obesity, and regular exercise.

References

1. Economic consequences of diabetes mellitus in the U.S. in 1997. American Diabetes Association. Diabetes Care 1998;21:296–309.

2. Report of the Expert Committee on the Diagnosis and Classification of Diabetes Mellitus. Diabetes Care 1997;20:1183–1197.

3. The effect of intensive treatment of diabetes on the development and progression of long-term complications in insulin-dependent diabetes mellitus. The Diabetic Control and Complications Trial Research Group. N Engl J Med 1993;329:977–986.

4. Ohkubo Y, Kishikawa H, Araki E, et al: Intensive insulin therapy prevents the progression of diabetic microvascular complications in Japanese patients with non–insulin-dependent diabetes mellitus: A randomized prospective 6-year study. Diabetes Res Clin Pract 1995;28:103–117.

5. Intensive blood-glucose control with sulphonylureas or insulin compared with conventional treatment and risk of complications in patients with type 2 diabetes (UKPDS 33). UK Prospective Diabetes Study (UKPDS) Group. Lancet 1998;352:837–853.

6. Effect of intensive blood-glucose control with metformin on complications in overweight patients with type 2 diabetes (UKPDS 34). UK Prospective Diabetes Study (UKPDS) Group. 1998;352:854–865.

7. Haffner SM: Coronary heart disease in patients with diabetes. N Engl J Med 2000;342:1040–1042.

8. Zimmet P: Globalization, coca-colonization and the chronic disease epidemic: Can the Doomsday scenario be averted? J Intern Med 2001;249:301–310.

9. Type 2 diabetes in children and adolescents. American Diabetes Association. Diabetes Care 2000;23:381–389.

10. Reaven GM: Banting lecture 1938. Role of insulin resistance in human disease. Diabetes 1988;37:1595–1607.

11. UKPDS Group: Cost effectiveness analysis of improved blood pressure control in hypertensive patients with type 2 diabetes: UKPDS 40. UK Prospective Diabetes Study Group. BMJ 1998;317:720–726.

12. American Diabetes Association. Standards of Medical Care for Patients With Diabetes Mellitus. Diabetes Care 2001;24(Suppl 1):S33–S43.

EIGHTY-EIGHT

Selective Estrogen Receptor Modulators

Bruce R. Carr and Debra A. Minjarez

The menopausal state is characterized by a decrease in ovarian production of estrogens resulting in an increase in the risk of osteoporosis, cardiovascular disease, and, possibly, Alzheimer's disease. The majority of women can now expect to live well into the menopausal years, increasing the likelihood that these conditions will be the cause of significant morbidity and mortality among this group. It is estimated that a woman's risk of sustaining a hip fracture is between 10% and 20%. Thirty percent of women with hip fracture will die, and the remainder will experience significant morbidity. Furthermore, 50% of women will die as a result of cardiovascular disease. Despite a growing body of evidence supporting the use of hormone replacement therapy (HRT) to prevent and treat some of these disorders, controversy regarding an increased risk in breast cancer and uterine cancer have fueled research into other menopausal treatment modalities such as selective estrogen receptor modulators (SERMs). These compounds bind to and interact with estrogen receptors (ERs), acting as estrogen agonists in some tissue and as estrogen antagonists in others. Ideally, these compounds would mimic the effect of estrogen on the skeleton, cardiovascular system, and central nervous system, while having no estrogenic effect on the breast and reproductive system.

SERMs are a group of structurally diverse compounds with mixed agonist and antagonist activities, including the triphenylethylenes, such as clomiphene citrate (Serophene, Clomid), tamoxifen (Nolvadex), and toremifene (Fareston) and the benzothiophene derivatives, such as raloxifene (Evista). SERMs that reduce postmenopausal bone loss, exert a beneficial effect on serum lipids, and cardiovascular function, and do not stimulate the endometrium and breast tissue are currently receiving the most attention. The exact mechanism of how SERMs exert tissue-selective effects is unknown, but their mechanism of action is currently under intense investigation as the distribution of ERs and their different roles in gene regulation is elucidated.

The ER was first isolated in the 1960s. In 1996, a second ER, ERβ, was cloned from rat prostate, which had a significant amount of homology to the original ER, now termed ERα.[1] Even though conserved regions of ERα and ERβ are homologous, there are various nonconserved regions that may account for differences in action between the two receptors. It is hypothesized that individual SERMs may induce specific and unique changes in receptor conformations, accounting for their particular pharmacologic properties. Alternatively, it has been proposed that ligand binding by an SERM or an estrogen will act differently at gene transcription-activating regions. As the molecular pathways of function are identified, there will be a better understanding of how SERM action and tissue selectivity are accomplished.

The mechanism of action of clomiphene citrate to bind to and interact with ERs acting as an agonist in some tissue and an antagonist in others is a prototype of SERM compounds. Clomiphene citrate has been used widely to initiate or augment ovulation by antagonizing estrogen's action at the hypothalamus and pituitary, thereby activating negative feedback and accentuating the release of gonadotropins during the follicular phase. In addition to acting on the hypothalamus and pituitary, clomiphene citrate may act directly on the ovary. Within the endometrium, in cervical mucous-producing glands, and in mammary tissue, clomiphene citrate exerts an antiestrogenic effect.

Clomiphene citrate is typically begun at a dose of 50 mg per day for 5 days. It is given in the follicular phase on days 3 to 7 or days 5 to 9 of a spontaneous menstrual cycle or induced withdrawal bleed. Follicular ultrasound measurements or urinary luteinizing hormone kits may be used to time intercourse or insemination. If ovulation does not occur with the 50-mg dose, the dose is then increased in increments of 50 mg. If ovulation does not occur with doses of 200 to 250 mg, it is often necessary to move to alternative treatments.

Tamoxifen was synthesized and developed in the 1960s and first reported as a treatment for advanced breast cancer in the early 1970s. Currently, tamoxifen is being used in patients with invasive tumors, as well as for adjuvant therapy to surgery, radiation, and chemotherapy in earlier disease stages. In the adjuvant therapy of breast cancer, studies show that overall (25%) and disease-free (45%) survival is significantly improved versus no adjuvant therapy. Twenty milligrams of tamoxifen daily was shown to decrease the incidence of breast cancer by 45% in women at high risk compared with placebo-treated controls. Tamoxifen has also been shown to reduce the risk of development of breast cancer when given as prophylaxis to normal postmenopausal women. The optimum duration of therapy remains to be determined, however; tamoxifen is currently recommended for only 5 years.

Although primarily an estrogen antagonist, tamoxifen displays agonist properties in the skeleton, uterus, and cardiovascular system. Women receiving adjuvant tamoxifen therapy for breast cancer were found to have reductions in total cholesterol, low-density lipoprotein-cholesterol (LDL-C), and lipoprotein(a), whereas high-density lipoprotein (HDL-C) and triglycerides were essentially unchanged. These findings were similar to results in studies using tamoxifen in healthy postmenopausal women. In addition, tamoxifen was found to preserve lumbar spine and femur neck bone mineral density in postmenopausal breast cancer patients.

Overall, tamoxifen is well tolerated by patients. Side effects more commonly encountered with tamoxifen include hot flushes, nausea, and vaginal dryness. Unfortunately, tamoxifen is also associated with an increased risk of endometrial cancer by as much as six-fold over placebo. Tamoxifen stimulates proliferation of the endometrium, increasing the risk of endometrial polyps (25%), hyperplasia (50%), and cancer (6%). The majority of studies do not show a higher histopathologic grade or worse prognosis than those of other breast cancer patients not treated with tamoxifen.[2]

Tamoxifen also increases the risk of the thromboembolic events, such as deep venous thrombosis and pulmonary embolism. In one series, the incidence of thromboembolism was 0.9% for tamoxifen-treated patients compared with 0.2% for placebo-treated patients.[3] The mechanism of this increased risk of thromboembolic disease with tomoxifen has not been elucidated but may be similar to that of estrogen. Because of the risks of endometrial cancer and thromboembolic events, tamoxifen use is restricted to women with breast cancer or those in high-risk groups.

Raloxifene, a benzothiophene SERM, was initially investigated as a treatment for breast cancer based on preliminary studies showing that it binds to both ERα and ERβ with high affinity and has antagonist activity within the breast. In clinical trials, raloxifene has been shown to have beneficial effects on bone and serum lipids and proproteins without stimulating the endometrial lining of the uterus. A dose of 60 mg/day has antiresorptive effects similar to those of 0.625 mg of conjugated estrogen, with both doses resulting in bone density stabilization in postmenopausal women. This effect is reflected in a decrease in bone turnover markers such as serum levels of bone-specific alkaline phosphatase (23% decrease) and osteocalcin (15% decrease). In a more recent study, raloxifene was found to increase bone density at the hip and spine by 2%.[4] Results from the Multiple Outcomes of Raloxifene Evaluation (MORE)[5] revealed that therapy with 60 or 120 mg/day for 2 years was associated with approximately a 50% reduction in the risk of asymptomatic and symptomatic vertebral fractures compared with calcium and vitamin D therapy plus placebo alone. Findings also revealed a 2% to 3% increase in bone mineral density above baseline at the spine and hip and a reduction in the markers of bone metabolism. No significant effect was found in the risk for nonvertebral fractures, that is, hip fractures.

The beneficial effects of raloxifene on serum lipids have shown a significant reduction from baseline in LDL-C and total cholesterol. HDL-C and triglyceride levels were not significantly affected. In a 6-month randomized, placebo and HRT-control trial, raloxifene at doses of 60 and 120

mg/day decreased LDL-C by 11%, similar to that of conjugated HRT. However, raloxifene lowered lipoprotein(a) less than HRT and increased HDL-C2 (high-density lipoprotein-cholesterol 2 subfraction) only 15% to 17% compared with 33% with HRT. Because evidence suggests that increases in HDL-C2 may correlate best with a cardiovascular protective effect, this finding warrants further investigation. Furthermore, raloxifene did not change levels of plasminogen activator inhibitor 1 compared with HRT. Based on these studies, it appears that raloxifene exerts a favorable effect on serum lipids; however, physicians should not assume that SERMs have cardioprotective effects based solely on their estrogen-like effects on lipids. In fact, results of a study of raloxifene in menopausal monkeys showed no cardioprotective effect.[6]

One particular advantage of raloxifene is the lack of proliferative effect on endometrial tissue. Data have shown that raloxifene has minimal effects on the uterus and causes no significant changes in the histologic appearance of the endometrium. Two 6-month studies[4, 5] involving a total of 969 postmenopausal women showed no difference in endometrial thickness compared with women receiving placebo. Another short-term study[7] found no evidence of endometrial proliferation as measured by endometrial biopsies after 8 weeks of treatment with doses of 200 to 600 mg/day. Short-term trials appear to support the conclusion that raloxifene does not stimulate the endometrial lining; however, it is unclear whether raloxifene provides long-term protection against endometrial cancer.

Adverse effects reported by women treated with raloxifene have included hot flushes (24.6% vs. 18.3% for placebo) and leg cramps (5.9% vs. 1.9% for placebo). There was no significant uterine bleeding or breast tenderness as compared with continuous or cyclic HRT. The risk of thromboembolic events has also been studied with raloxifene, and these disorders appear more likely to occur during the first 4 months of treatment.[8] Owing to the risk of thromboembolism, it has been proposed that raloxifene be discontinued 72 hours before surgery and until the patient is fully ambulatory.

Other SERMs currently being investigated in clinical trials are droloxifene and idoxifene, both triphenyethylene derivatives. Droloxifene is currently being evaluated as a treatment for breast cancer as well as for the prevention of postmenopausal osteoporosis. It has a greater affinity for the estrogen receptor than tamoxifen and has less agonist and more antagonist activity at the uterus.[9] In the breast tissue, droloxifene has an antiestrogenic effect. It preserves bone density by reducing the formation of osteoclasts in the bone marrow through apoptosis of mononuclear precursors.[10]

Idoxifene is also being studied for the treatment of advanced breast cancer. Idoxifene has an ER-binding affinity that is twice that of tamoxifen, but is a less potent antiestrogen.[11]

SERMs are a class of drugs that help to reduce the risk of osteoporosis and breast cancer and improve serum lipids.

These medications have obvious advantages over HRT; however, more research and development are needed before this therapy becomes a mainstay. Many women who initiate HRT commonly cite relief from menopausal symptoms, such as hot flushes and night sweats. The currently available SERMs do not alleviate such symptoms and may even exacerbate them in some patients, potentially limiting their use. There are also no data to address long-term safety and efficacy questions. At this time, HRT remains the treatment of choice for osteoporosis and coronary heart disease prevention, whereas SERMs offer an alternative to only a select group of women.

References

1. Kuiper GG, Enmark E, Pelto-Huikko M, et al: Cloning of a novel estrogen receptor expressed in rat prostate and ovary. Proc Natl Acad Sci U S A 1996;93:5925–5930.
2. Assikis VJ, Jordan VC: Gynecological effects of tamoxifen and the association with endometrial cancer. Int J Gynecol Obstet 1995;49:241–257.
3. Fisher B, Constantine JP, Redmond C, et al: A randomized clinical trial evaluating tamoxifen in the treatment of patients with node-negative breast cancer who have estrogen receptor–positive tumors. N Engl J Med 1989;320:479–484.
4. Delmas P, Bjarnason N, Mitlak B, et al: Effects of raloxifene on bone mineral density, serum cholesterol concentrations, and uterine endometrium in postmenopausal women. N Engl J Med 1997;337:1641–1647.
5. Ettinger BB, Black DM, Mitlak BH, et al: Reduction of vertebral fracture risk in postmenopausal women with osteoporosis treated with raloxifene: Results from a 3-year randomized clinical trial. Multiple Outcome of Raloxifene Evaluation (MORE) Investigators. JAMA 1999;282:637–645.
6. Clarkson TB, Anthony MS, Jerone CP: Lack of effect of raloxifene on coronary artery atherosclerosis of postmenopausal monkeys. J Clin Endocrinol Metab 1998;83:721–726.
7. Draper M, Flower D, Huster W, et al: A controlled trial of raloxifene (LY 139481) HCl: Impact on bone turnover and serum lipid profile in healthy postmenopausal women. J Bone Miner Res 1996;11:835–842.
8. Weryha G, Pascal-Vigneron V, Klein M, Leclere J: Selective estrogen receptor modulators. Curr Opin Rheum 1999;11:301–306.
9. Hasman M, Rattel B, Loser R: Preclinical data for droloxifene. Cancer Lett 1994;84:101–116.
10. Grasser W, Pan L, Thompson D, et al: Common mechanism for the estrogen agonist antagonist activities of droloxifene. J Cell Biochem 1997;65:159–171.
11. Chanders S, McCague R, Lugmani Y: Pyrrolidino-4-tamoxifen and 4-iodotamoxifen, new analogues of the antiestrogen tamoxifen in the treatment of breast cancer. Cancer Res 1991;51:5851–5858.

EIGHTY-NINE

Efficient and Effective Evaluation of Infertility

Kamran S. Moghissi

Infertility is defined as failure of a couple of reproductive age to conceive after 12 months or more of regular coitus without using contraception. Infertility is considered *primary* in the absence of any previous pregnancy and *secondary* when there is a history of one or more previous pregnancies. Infertility is a disease that affects both women and men, thus, male and female infertility cannot be considered in isolation and managed independently. Physicians involved in the management of infertility must either acquire the expertise of treating the couple or work as a team member providing care for the woman as well as the man.

The contribution of men and women to infertility differs in several ways. The man must be able to develop an adequate number of good-quality sperm and deposit them in the partner's vagina. In addition to developing normal gametes (oocytes), the woman's body must be able to transport an adequate number of healthy sperm from the vagina to the distal portion of the fallopian tubes, provide an appropriate environment for fertilization of the oocyte and development of the blastocyst, transport the conceptus through the oviduct, have a receptive uterus for implantation of the blastocyst and fetal development, and, ultimately, carry a pregnancy to viability.

ETIOLOGY OF INFERTILITY

Several important factors are known to affect fertility:

- Age
- Frequency of coitus
- Nutrition
- Environmental factors
- Sexually transmitted diseases (STDs)
- Smoking
- Alcohol and drugs
- Stress

The effect of age on women's fertility has been documented repeatedly. A consistent decline in fecundity after 30 to 35 years of age has been demonstrated, with an incidence of involuntary infertility in women older than 40 years of age ranging from approximately 33% to 64%. Reduced age-related fecundity is predominantly the result of the decline in oocyte quality, enhanced follicular atresia, and an increased rate of chromosomal abnormalities in fertilized oocytes and resulting embryos. These ovarian effects are associated with a rise in basal follicle-stimulating hormone levels, indicative of reduced ovarian reserve.

With decreasing frequency of intercourse, the per-cycle probability of conception during a given interval declines.

The nutritional status of a woman appears to play an important role in her fertility. It has long been recognized that extremes of weight are associated with ovulatory disturbances and consequent infertility. At one end of the spectrum, women who significantly exceed their ideal body weight may have chronic anovulation with or without androgen excess and insulin resistance (i.e., polycystic ovarian disease). At the other end, women who are grossly below their ideal body weight experience amenorrhea and consequent infertility. Chronic deficiency of certain nutrients, such as proteins, vitamins, and trace elements, also may be a cause of reproductive failure.

Environmental and occupational factors, such as radiation, anesthetic agents, toxins, and pollutants, also may be a cause of reproductive failure, primarily via an effect on the gametes or early embryos.

STDs have a significant impact on infertility. Long-term prospective studies have shown a dose-response relationship between laparoscopically proved pelvic inflammatory disease and infertility. These data indicate that infertility occurs in 11% of women after one episode of pelvic inflammatory disease, in 23% after two episodes, and in 54% after three episodes. Both gonorrheal and chlamydial infections may lead to tubal obstruction and infertility.[1]

Approximately 25% of North American women currently smoke. Cigarette smoke contains a variety of toxins that have been shown in animal studies to affect various levels of reproductive function. The net effect is a demonstrated decrease in fertility in women smokers attempting to conceive.

Ethanol may depress the release of gonadotropin-releasing hormone from the hypothalamus by activating inhibitory endogenous pathways that are involved in gonadotropin-releasing hormone regulation. In men, alcohol affects testicular synthesis and secretion of testosterone, which can result in abnormal sperm morphology and sexual dysfunction. Chronic alcoholism in women has been associated with infertility and menstrual disorders and also may have severe consequences for the fetus. Similarly, opioids and other recreational drugs may cause an alteration of gonadotropin release and subfertility. Prescription medication may have an adverse effect in both sexes. Examples are the use of psychotropic drugs in women, which cause hyperprolactinemia and menstrual disorders, and sulfasalazine in men, which produces oligospermia.

The involvement of emotional factors in infertility has

been generally accepted. Clinicians frequently encounter menstrual irregularities, even amenorrhea, in patients who are emotionally stressed. In men, impairment of sperm density and quality may be observed after mental stress and psychic tension. Sexual activities and performance may be affected during periods of emotional stress and psychic disturbance. Decreased libido, impotence, and premature ejaculation are commonly induced psychologically. In women, vaginismus, dyspareunia, and frigidity can result from emotional trauma or strain. Conversely, psychological, sexual, and marital difficulties may also arise in the course of a lengthy infertility evaluation.

INITIAL INTERVIEW AND HISTORY

Every effort should be made to initiate the fertility survey by an interview with both partners jointly. The couple should be encouraged to appear together at the initial consultation. This visit provides an excellent opportunity for the physician to explain basic reproductive mechanisms, outline the plan of fertility treatment, allay the apprehension of the couple, and answer their questions.

Taking an in-depth and accurate patient history is the most important aspect of the initial patient evaluation. Information elicited from the patient's history should be used to focus the remainder of the infertility evaluation on optimizing the couple's chances of a successful pregnancy. The history should be obtained in an open and unbiased manner. Information regarding patient age, medical problems, medications, previous operations, hospitalizations, as well as tobacco use, should be obtained as part of any standard medical history. The gynecologic and obstetric history should include information regarding menstrual cycle length and regularity, pelvic pain, contraceptive use, hirsutism, galactorrhea, and previous pregnancies and their outcome. A thorough sexual history also should be obtained with information regarding the length of time the couple has been trying to conceive, frequency and timing of coitus, and the use of vaginal lubricants, which may be spermicidal. Any history of STDs and pelvic inflammatory disease should also be discussed. Information concerning the male partner, specifically regarding medical problems, medication use, impotence and ejaculatory dysfunction, history of STDs, and past fertility, also should be obtained. Finally, the history should include the details of any previous evaluation and treatment for infertility. When available, past medical records should be reviewed.

PHYSICAL EXAMINATION

After obtaining a complete history, a thorough physical examination is required. In women, the thyroid gland, breast, abdomen, and pelvis should be carefully examined. Cervical cultures of *Neisseria gonorrhoeae, Chlamydia trachomatis, Mycoplasma hominis*, and *Ureaplasma urealyticum* can be obtained at the time of the initial speculum

examination. In the male partner, in addition to systemic examination, the genital tract should be examined with regard to position, size, and consistency of the testes, status of the vas deferens, size and consistency of the prostate, and the presence of a palpable varicocele.

After the initial history and physical examination, the physician discusses with the couple various tests and procedures planned. Laboratory tests vary according to patient needs and suspected etiologic factors. For example, in women with irregular menstrual cycles or galactorrhea, it is helpful to order serum thyroid-stimulating hormone and prolactin levels. In women suspected of having polycystic ovarian syndrome or hyperandrogenism, serum dehydroandrosterone sulfate, 17-hydroxyprogesterone, and testosterone levels are of diagnostic value. Depending on the population, culture for *N. gonorrhoeae, C. trachomatis, M. hominis*, and *U. urealyticum* can be obtained when there is a risk of cervical colonization by these pathogens.

DIAGNOSTIC EVALUATION

Basic diagnostic and laboratory evaluations of infertility require a systematic and stepwise evaluation of various factors, including (1) documentation of ovulation, (2) tubal patency, (3) sperm–cervical mucus interaction, (4) uterine abnormalities, (5) peritoneal abnormalities, and (6) evaluation of the male factor as determined by semen analysis.

Semen Analysis

Semen analysis is an essential part of a basic infertility evaluation. The sample should be obtained, preferably by masturbation, after 2 days of abstinence, placed in a clear plastic or glass jar, and examined in a competent laboratory that uses World Health Organization guidelines. World Health Organization criteria for a normal semen analysis include a sperm count greater than 20 million sperm/mL with at least 50% motility and 30% normal morphology.

Evaluation of Female Factor

Assessment of Ovulation

Disorders of ovulation are believed to be responsible for infertility in approximately 20% to 25% of women. These disturbances of ovulation include anovulation with or without amenorrhea/oligoamenorrhea, oligo-ovulation, and luteal phase defect. Common techniques for documentation of ovulation include the following:

1. When the basal body temperature shows a biphasic pattern with a luteal phase of 12 to 14 days. The basal body temperature, however, does not predict ovulation and can be interpreted only retrospectively when the morning temperature is accurately obtained and recorded for the entire menstrual cycle.

2. Do-it-yourself kits to measure urinary luteinizing hormone are based on enzyme immunoassay techniques and are designed to be used by the patient at home once or twice per day on morning and/or afternoon urine samples, beginning several days before suspected ovulation. The tests have an accuracy of greater than 90% in their ability to detect the LH surge.
3. A measured midluteal serum progesterone level is greater than 10 ng/mL.
4. An endometrial biopsy is obtained 2 days before the onset of menses, dated by a knowledgeable pathologist, and shows a secretory pattern consistent with the day of the cycle in which it was obtained. Luteal-phase deficiency is usually diagnosed by endometrial biopsy. A short luteal phase is defined as a luteal phase of less than 10 days.

Tubal Patency Test

Hysterosalpingography (HSG) is the most common procedure to evaluate the integrity of the uterine cavity and tubal patency. The procedure is performed immediately after menses, during the follicular phase of the menstrual cycle. Initially, 2 to 3 mL of an aqueous contrast medium is injected to outline the uterine cavity. An additional 3 to 7 mL of contrast medium is then injected to determine tubal patency, which is characterized by spillage of the contrast medium into the pelvic cavity.

In addition to the diagnosis of tubal abnormalities, HSG allows for evaluation of uterine pathology. HSG may also have therapeutic benefits, for pregnancy rates have been reported to improve in the months immediately after the HSG.

Evaluation of Cervical Factor—Postcoital Test

Deposition of ejaculate in the vagina sets in motion a series of events during which healthy and vigorous spermatozoa penetrate preovulatory cervical mucus, colonize cervical crypts, and ascend into the uterine cavity and fallopian tube to meet and fertilize the ovum in the distal portion of the oviducts. Under normal circumstances, within a few minutes after coitus and for at least the next 48 hours, there is a steady upward migration of sperm reaching the site of fertilization.

The interaction of sperm with cervical mucus is assessed by the postcoital test (PCT). The test is performed within 2 days before the anticipated time of ovulation as determined by basal body temperature or a luteinizing hormone testing kit. It is customary to ask the couple to abstain from coitus for 2 days before having the PCT. The couple is instructed to have intercourse 8 to 12 hours before the PCT. The test is an office procedure during which samples of cervical mucus are obtained to assess its quality and to count the number of sperm per microscopic field in the mucus sample. Normal preovulatory cervical mucus is thin, watery, copious, and acellular, with a high spinnbarkeit (stretchability) of approximately 8 cm and a ferning pattern. More than 10 sperm per high-power field ($\times 400$) is considered normal by most authorities. Because PCT assesses only sperm transport through the cervix rather than anatomic and functional integrity of the entire reproductive tract, it is not predictive of the pregnancy rate.

Other Procedures

Laparoscopy with or without hysteroscopy is considered as part of the final steps of an infertility investigation and generally should not be performed until the noninvasive, basic workup is completed. Laparoscopy evaluates the peritoneal cavity and may detect unsuspected or unconfirmed conditions such as pelvic adhesions, particularly those involving tubes and ovaries, and endometriosis, as well as verifying tubal disease detected by HSG. Hysteroscopy is necessary for confirmation and treatment of intrauterine anomalies suspected or detected by HSG. Both these procedures may be performed earlier, during a patient's investigation if HSG shows clear abnormalities, or if other historical factors warrant.

MANAGEMENT OF INFERTILITY

With the advent of assisted reproductive technology, the treatment of infertility in both women and men has undergone a revolutionary change. Heroic measures and non–evidence-based therapies are being phased out in favor of treatment modalities with better and more predictable outcomes. However, simpler and less expensive therapeutic measures should be offered to the couple before resorting to more complex and expensive assisted reproductive techniques.

This brief review does not permit an extensive discussion of various treatment modalities required to correct complex infertility factors. However, the following abbreviated guidelines are provided to assist physicians who wish to initiate preliminary treatment or seek appropriate referral.

At the completion of basic studies, couples should be informed of the test results and their therapeutic options. They may benefit from simply being informed as to the optimal time to have intercourse or advised to avoid excessive smoking, drinking, and exposure to environmental pollutants, toxins, and injurious medication. Ovulatory disorders are initially treated with clomiphene citrate with sequential dosage increases to achieve normal ovulatory cycles. Progesterone administration may be added to support the luteal phase further. However, such treatment should not exceed more than 6 months. If pregnancy has not occurred during this period, alternative treatment such as gonadotropin stimulation is indicated. Cervical factor abnormality is often treated with intrauterine insemination using washed spermatozoa. Suspected tubal and peritoneal diseases should be confirmed by laparoscopy and may be treated, if possible, at the same time. Tuboplasty of advanced or extensive tubal disease is no longer recommended because in vitro fertilization results in better outcome with a higher pregnancy rate. Laparoscopic management of pelvic endometriosis appears to yield a higher pregnancy rate compared with medical management. Diseases of the uterus such as submucous or large intramural myomas, intrauterine adhesion, and other uterine anomalies require surgical management when adequately proved to be the cause of infertility.

In the past, oligo- or asthenospermia was treated with a variety of hormones and medications, often with dubious and unpredictable pregnancy results. With the development of intracytoplasmic sperm injection, predictable pregnancy rates similar to those of conventional in vitro fertilization may be expected. Finally, patients with unexplained infertility who have undergone extensive infertility evaluation and have no identifiable etiology for their infertility may be offered controlled ovarian hyperstimulation and intrauterine insemination or in vitro fertilization.

Reference

1. Westrom L: Incidence, prevalence and trends of acute pelvic inflammatory disease and its consequences in industrialized countries. Am J Obstet Gynecol 1980;138:880.

CHAPTER

NINETY

Male Infertility: Interpreting and Using the Semen Analysis

Kenneth A. Ginsburg

By current estimates, approximately one in six reproductive-age couples in the United States are infertile. In this group, nearly one half will be expected to have a male infertility factor that is either the sole cause or a contributing cause to the couple's reproductive difficulty. The obstetrician-gynecologist is most often the first practitioner consulted by an infertile couple. With this high probability of a male factor contributing to the couple's infertility, it is important that testing of all potentially infertile males be initiated early by those practitioners first consulted in the evaluation process. The obstetrician-gynecologist must be familiar with the basic interpretation of a semen analysis. A reproductive endocrinologist or urologist is not needed to initiate this evaluation.

This chapter briefly reviews male reproductive dysfunction and treatment options for male infertility and the use of semen analyses by the obstetrician-gynecologist to categorize male reproductive potential. Then, a decision algorithm is presented from which treatment and referral recommendations can be offered.

OVERVIEW OF THE CAUSES OF MALE INFERTILITY

In simplest terms, the testes have both basic endocrine and exocrine functions. Endocrine testicular function involves gonadotropin stimulation of the interstitial Leydig cells, which, in turn, produce testosterone. The testosterone then acts in a paracrine fashion to facilitate exocrine testicular function and also in an endocrine fashion at multiple nontesticular sites. Exocrine testicular function involves gonadotropin stimulation of the Sertoli cells of the seminiferous tubules, resulting in sperm production. Spermatozoa then leave the testis for the epididymis, where they mature and become motile before mixing with seminal plasma produced by the accessory glands (seminal vesicles, prostate) at ejaculation.

Analogous to the situation with renal failure, it is thus convenient to divide the causes of abnormal exocrine testicular and accessory gland function—semen quality—into three categories: pretesticular, testicular, and post-testicular causes. *Pretesticular* abnormalities include any endocrine disturbance that results in abnormal stimulatory control of

the testis. In this mechanism, the seminiferous tubules are not being stimulated to create mature spermatozoa. Examples include hypothalamic or pituitary disturbances, such as congenital or acquired hypogonadotropism, and prolactin-secreting pituitary adenomas. *Testicular* causes of male subfertility include congenital or acquired defects in seminiferous tubular function. Included here are examples such as gonadal dysgenesis, varicocele, environmental exposures (alcohol, tobacco, illicit drugs, pesticides, chemicals), infections (mumps virus), or iatrogenic (medications) exposures that have a deleterious effect on semen quality. *Post-testicular* causes include abnormalities of epididymal function, congenital or acquired obstruction, accessory gland dysfunction resulting in formation of abnormal seminal plasma, and ejaculatory disturbances. Arbitrarily also included here is the (inappropriate) production of antisperm antibodies by the man; when present in the ejaculate, they can cause interference with sperm migration or sperm-oocyte interaction in the female reproductive tract.

EVALUATION OF THE POTENTIALLY INFERTILE MAN

The important determinants of male fertility or infertility are semen quality and sperm function. Sperm function has been difficult to assess clinically, owing to both imperfect tests and difficulty determining a meaningful end point that defines optimal, normal, or disturbed function. The latter is true because reproductive technology has allowed us successfully to treat men with semen abnormalities that would have been deemed intractable just several years ago. For example, before approximately 1990, men with semen samples that had fewer than 1,000,000 sperm/mL would have been classified as sterile, because there was not even a reasonable expectation of fertilization in vitro. Today, these patients are routinely offered intracytoplasmic sperm injection in conjunction with in vitro fertilization (IVF), with an excellent prognosis for conception. Tests used to diagnose altered sperm function in the past include the zona-free hamster oocyte sperm penetration assay, hemizona assay, hypo-osmotic swelling test, strict morphologic evaluation, and antisperm antibody assays. A detailed discussion of these tests is beyond the scope of this chapter;

the interested reader is referred to the recommended readings for further information.

Semen analysis is the cornerstone of the evaluation of the potentially infertile man. Although the patient's historical evaluation, physical examination, results of endocrine tests, scrotal ultrasound, and so on are of potential value in explaining the *cause* or *mechanism* of subfertility, these studies do not define fertility nor test for infertility. Optimally, three semen samples are obtained at equally spaced intervals over a period of 1 to 3 months, each collected after a period of abstinence equal to the patient's usual ejaculatory interval. Complete collection is important, and if any of the sample is lost, it should not be examined. The time of ejaculation is noted, and the sample is transported to the laboratory (if not collected there) at body temperature for examination within 60 minutes. A complete semen analysis (Table 90–1) includes evaluation of seminal plasma characteristics (color, volume, pH, consistency, and liquefaction time), sperm concentration (millions of sperm per milliliter), sperm motility, sperm morphology, and evaluation of other microscopic characteristics (such as the presence of leukocytes, erythrocytes, debris, and sperm agglutination).

Sperm motility is optimally expressed as the proportion of sperm that are motile, with additionally an assessment of the quality of motility. For example, in our laboratory, the proportion of motile and nonmotile sperm is estimated by an experienced technician. The motile sperm are then further categorized into those that show movement but no forward progression; those with slow, erratic forward progression; and those with rapid, straight progression. This evaluation is done soon after the sample arrives in the laboratory, and again 2 to 6 hours later to make sure that this initial degree of motility can be maintained. When the proportion of nonmotile sperm is high, it is necessary to evaluate viability by vital stain exclusion to differentiate live nonmotile sperm from dead sperm. Sperm morphology is evaluated on a stained specimen. Spermatozoa are characterized as either normal or abnormal; those with head defects (e.g., double head, small head, large head, acrosomal abnormalities), midpiece defects, and tail abnormalities (e.g., double tails, bent tails, coiled tails) are recorded separately.

Normal values for these semen analysis parameters were defined in the past, based on actuarial expectations of spontaneous pregnancy. It must be emphasized that male fertility potential is always evaluated and defined in the context of a particular partner's fertility or infertility and the treatment employed to assist in conception. That is, certain semen analysis results might have a high probability of pregnancy with a partner at one time but a diminished probability of pregnancy with the same partner under different circumstances. On the other hand, a sample may be defined as subnormal for natural conception but acceptable for conception using IVF. Thus, if treatment is contemplated, the limit of what separates a fertile from an infertile sample is lower. The different circumstances referred to previously can include the woman's advancing age, acquired ovulatory dysfunction, tubal disease, or uterine abnormalities, or, alternatively, correction of any of these problems.

Before the advent of assisted reproductive technologies, it was generally agreed that at least 20 million spermatozoa/mL in an ejaculate of 2 to 6 mL were required for spontaneous conception, with normal motility, normal morphology, and a reproductively normal female partner (see Table 90–1). However, there has never been universal agreement regarding this concentration, and some have cited a normal limit of 60, 40, and 10 million/mL. When the sample is of this minimum quality, and the female partner has no discernible ovulatory, anatomic, or other problems, there will be an 85% to 90% probability that pregnancy will occur within 1 year of initiating unprotected intercourse. If, on the other hand, she is found to have ovulatory dysfunction, a considerably higher sperm count (in effect, compensating for her infertility) may be necessary to initiate a pregnancy. Similarly, with a normal female partner, sperm concentrations of 15 to 20 million/mL (with normal motility and morphology, an example of a borderline abnormal semen analysis) may result in pregnancy if the couple uses intrauterine insemination (IUI) or some other empirical therapy. With even lower sperm concentrations, assisted reproductive technologies (see later) would be required for conception.

In addition to the clinical context in which sperm concentration is defined, another problem in arriving at a definition of a "normal" sperm count relates to imprecision and inaccuracy in determining sperm density, motility, and morphology. The techniques commonly employed to count spermatozoa are inaccurate, with a coefficient of variation of nearly 40%. It is somewhat surprising that this inaccuracy in sperm counting is not improved with computer-assisted semen (sperm) analysis. Thus, every semen analysis must be examined with the understanding that the sperm count could vary as much as 40% in either direction. Indeed, this is one reason for the suggestion that at least

Table 90–1. Characteristics of Normal Semen Analysis

Parameter	Value
Semen volume	2–6 mL
Sperm concentration	>20 million/mL
Sperm motility	>60% with at least ⅓ of these motile sperm having rapid, straight, forward progression
Sperm morphology	>30% normal morphology
Microscopic examination	<1 million/mL white blood cells, debris or agglutination
Female partner	Reproductively normal (no ovulatory, anatomic, or other problems)

three semen analyses be obtained when evaluating someone's reproductive potential.

TREATMENT OPTIONS FOR THE COUPLE WITH MALE INFERTILITY

Depending on the severity of the semen analysis defect, the apparent etiology of the problem, and the status of the female partner, treatment of male infertility involves some combination of the following three strategies: surgical, medical, or assisted reproduction (Table 90–2). In addition, often treatment of the couple with male factor infertility involves regimens directed at the woman, in an attempt to make her more fertile and compensate for the male partner's infertility. In still other situations—owing to religious, financial, or other personal choices—the couple may elect not to pursue specific fertility treatment for the man's infertility and will elect instead to use donor insemination, adoption, or foster parenting as a means to build their family.

USING THE SEMEN ANALYSIS: REFERRAL AND MANAGEMENT RECOMMENDATIONS

The use of a semen analysis as a screening tool in the evaluation of a potentially infertile man requires understanding of the concept of fecundity. *Fecundity*, defined as the per cycle probability of pregnancy, has been determined to be 20% to 25% in normal couples. Semen abnormalities can be expected to lower a couple's fecundity, resulting in a longer time to conception and hence a diagnosis of male infertility. Identification of those individuals with semen abnormalities that give them a reasonable expectation of subnormal fertility is thus of clinical importance, because early intervention may allow pregnancy to occur sooner and with the expenditure of fewer health care resources.

Despite the aforementioned caveats regarding inaccuracy of sperm counting plus the difficulty in defining normal semen parameters and the need to consider male reproductive ability in the context of the female partner, several general recommendations can be made to the obstetrician-gynecologist who is initiating the evaluation of an infertile couple. It is hoped that these recommendations will aid the practitioner in determining the situations in which couples can be managed expectantly, those in which the couple can be treated under his or her care, or those that should be referred to a reproductive endocrinologist or urologist for additional testing and advanced therapy using medication, surgery, or assisted reproductive technologies as briefly outlined previously.

The generalist should complete four basic evaluation steps before initiating treatment of the infertile couple: (1) obtain a reproductive history and examination on both partners; (2) evaluate ovulatory function using basal body temperature charting, urinary luteinizing hormone surge detection, or follicular ultrasound; (3) evaluate tubal patency using a hysterosalpingogram; and (4) evaluate (preferably) three semen analyses over a 90-day interval. The history in the man should search for evidence of prior reproductive difficulties, hypogonadism, exposure to substances that can impair semen quality (recreational drug or alcohol use, medications, tobacco), genital tract injury, surgery or infection, and so on. The genital examination should search for evidence of hypogonadism, unilateral or bilateral testicular atrophy, or abnormalities in the spermatic cord that suggest varicocele or obstruction. The semen analyses are then used to categorize potentially infertile men as

- Those who have a reasonable expectation of *normal fertility*—no abnormalities are identified on the semen analyses or the reproductive history
- Those who have an expectation of *infertility or sterility*—either the semen analyses are abnormal or the reproductive history is abnormal or both

Based on these results, the following recommendations are advanced (Table 90–3). Semen samples are classified as either normal, borderline (with only a single abnormality such as sperm concentration, motility, morphology, or microscopic examination that varies no more than 20% from the lower limit of normal), or abnormal. As can be seen from Table 90–3, I recommend that any semen analysis abnormality (including borderline semen quality when the history is abnormal), irrespective of the evaluation of the female partner, constitutes the need to refer the couple to an infertility center with a reproductive endocrinologist or urologist. Further evaluation there would be directed toward diagnosing a problem that is amenable to medical or surgical therapy or preparing the couple for assisted reproduction using IUI, controlled ovarian hyperstimulation and IUI, IVF, or intracytoplasmic sperm injection (ICSI). The only exception to this is when semen quality has only a borderline defect, historical evaluation of the man is

Table 90–2. Treatment Strategies for Male Infertility

Treatment Strategy	Example(s)
Medical	Increase endogenous FSH using clomiphene citrate
	Directly stimulate seminiferous tubules using exogenous gonadotropins
	Correct hyperprolactinemic hypogonadotropic hypogonadism using bromocriptine
Surgical	Varicocelectomy
	Vasovasostomy, vasoepididymostomy for acquired vas deferens obstruction (vasectomy, gonococcal)
Assisted reproduction	IUI
	Controlled ovarian hyperstimulation with IUI
	IVF-ET
	Intracytoplasmic sperm injection with IVF-ET

FSH, follicle-stimulating hormone; IUI, intrauterine insemination; IVF-ET, in vitro fertilization and embryo transfer.

Table 90–3. Management Recommendations Based on the Result of the Basic Evaluation

Male Partner	Female Partner	Management Recommendations
Normal semen analysis and normal history	Normal ovulation, normal fallopian tubes, and normal history	Expectant management, or empirical therapy with clomiphene citrate (female partner) for six cycles
Normal semen analysis and normal history	Abnormal ovulation, abnormal tubal evaluation, or history suggesting other reproductive abnormality (e.g., endometriosis)	Correct abnormality and allow conception for six cycles, or Refer for further evaluation and management
Normal semen analysis and abnormal history	Normal ovulation, normal fallopian tubes, and normal history	Expectant management for three cycles, or Empirical therapy with clomiphene citrate (female partner) for three cycles
Normal semen analysis and abnormal history	Abnormal ovulation, abnormal tubal evaluation, or history suggesting other reproductive abnormality (e.g., endometriosis)	Refer for further evaluation and management
Borderline semen analysis* and normal history	Normal ovulation, normal fallopian tubes, and normal history	Empirical therapy with clomiphene citrate (female partner) for three cycles Refer for further evaluation and management
Borderline semen analysis and normal history	Abnormal ovulation, abnormal tubal evaluation, or history suggesting other reproductive abnormality (e.g., endometriosis)	Refer for further evaluation and management
Borderline semen analysis and abnormal history	Normal or abnormal ovulation, tubal evaluation, or history	Refer for further evaluation and management
Abnormal semen analysis irrespective of history	Normal or abnormal ovulation, tubal evaluation, or history	Refer for further evaluation and management

*A *borderline semen analysis* is defined as one with only a single abnormality (i.e., either an abnormal sperm concentration, motility, morphology, or microscopic examination) that varies no more than 20% from the lower limit of normal.

entirely normal, and the female partner is reproductively normal. In this case, it may be reasonable to attempt three cycles of empirical ovulation induction with clomiphene citrate with or without IUI, if the patients request a more conservative approach. Failure to conceive with this course of therapy demands that the couple be referred, as noted. In these cases, the expectation of diminished fertility in the male partner causing diminished fecundity in the couple suggests that a more aggressive treatment approach is warranted.

When the male partner has an abnormality in his history, that is, previous infertility, environmental exposures, and so on, but his semen analysis and the female partner are normal, it is appropriate to treat the couple with empirical clomiphene citrate for three cycles to stimulate multiple oocyte release. Again, some practitioners use IUI in this setting. However, in a similar situation with an *abnormal* female partner, referral is warranted without a trial of empirical therapy. Finally, when both the semen analysis and the male partner's history are normal, either an attempt is made to correct any abnormalities found in the woman and the couple are encouraged to attempt to conceive on their own or empirical treatment is offered. In this case, the assumption is that his fertility is normal and hence the couple's fecundity is not affected by male factor infertility.

Suggestions for Future Reading

Adashi EY, Rock JA, Rosenwaks Z (eds): Reproductive Endocrinology, Surgery and Infertility. Philadelphia, Lippincott-Raven, 1996.
Centola GM, Ginsburg KA (eds): Evaluation and Treatment of the Infertile Male. Cambridge, Cambridge University Press, 1996.
Lipshultz LI, Howards SS (eds): Infertility in the Male, 2nd ed. St. Louis, Mosby–Year Book, 1991.
Speroff L, Glass RH, Kase NG (eds): Clinical Reproductive Endocrinology and Infertility, 6th ed. Baltimore, Lippincott, Williams & Wilkins, 1999.

CHAPTER

NINETY-ONE

Tubal Surgery versus In Vitro Fertilization: Where Do We Draw the Line?

Michael L. Freeman and Charla M. Blacker

Infertility due to diseased or damaged fallopian tubes (termed tubal factor infertility) accounts for 30% to 40% of female infertility and approximately 20% of all infertility diagnoses. Before the advent of in vitro fertilization (IVF), which bypasses the fallopian tubes, tuboplasty was the only option available for the female patient with tubal factor infertility. Since its inception in 1978, IVF has become more refined, with improved success rates, sometimes doubling the 20% monthly conception rate afforded by nature. Today, with IVF centers easily accessible by the majority of the United States population, the role of tuboplasty in the treatment of tubal infertility has diminished. Yet, during the same interval, there have been advances in surgical therapy, including microsurgical technique, improved suture material, antiadhesive surgical adjuncts, and prophylactic antibiotics, that may make tuboplasty an appropriate option for a select group of patients. This chapter details the benefits and limitations of each therapy, patient characteristics that must be considered in the decision-making process, and newer technologies, and has a specific section on tubal re-anastomosis after elective tubal sterilization.

EVALUATION OF THE PATIENT WITH TUBAL FACTOR

When a couple has a documented tubal factor, the physician is obligated to screen thoroughly for other nontubal factors and manage those problem areas before surgery. A detailed history and physical examination of both partners can serve to guide further testing. An account of the woman's medical history should include a listing of all surgical procedures (with operative notes), contraceptive history, age of menarche, details of menstrual pattern, and frequency of appropriately timed coitus. The history should also provide information regarding the underlying etiology of her tubal infertility, for example, pelvic inflammatory disease (PID), appendiceal rupture, endometriosis, elective sterilization, and granulomatous disease. The male partner should be questioned regarding details of possible previous genital surgery such as vasectomy, vasovasostomy, varicocele repair, transurethral prostatectomy, or hypospadias repair. Information regarding medical problems, such as diabetes or other systemic disease or genital infections (prostatitis, epididymitis, mumps orchitis), should be recorded.

A thorough physical examination is performed, paying particular attention for signs of thyroid or adrenal disease. The pelvic examination should identify abnormal hair distribution, cervical motion tenderness, an immobile or tender uterus, tenderness of the uterosacral ligaments, or any enlarged adnexal masses. Documentation of ovulatory menstrual cycles and a normal semen analysis of the male partner constitute the minimal evaluation required before considering surgery, but additional testing should be considered based on the history and physical examination. If the other identified problems cannot be easily and successfully treated, IVF may be a better therapeutic choice.

Impaired ovarian function is potentially a major cause of impaired fertility. Women with World Health Organization type II anovulation will usually respond to ovulation induction; however, only about 50% of them will conceive with clomiphene citrate. The remainder require gonadotropin ovulation induction with its attendant increase in complexity, cost, and risk for multiple gestation. Decreased ovarian reserve can be a problem for women considering either tuboplasty or IVF. Women at risk for decreased ovarian reserve include those older than 35 years of age, who have a follicle-stimulating hormone level greater than 10 on cycle day 3, age similar to that of a sister or mother when they became menopausal, and poor response to ovulation induction. Scott and associates[1] used the so-called clomiphene challenge test to evaluate these women and found only 0.7% ongoing pregnancy rates among women with abnormal clomiphene challenge tests in spite of a variety of fertility therapies. Because the pregnancy rates through IVF decline with age, women older than 38 years of age may want to consider IVF instead of tuboplasty. The greatest cumulative pregnancy rates after tuboplasty occur by 2 years postoperatively; however, waiting 2 years may be a luxury women in their late 30s cannot afford. Entry into an IVF program will expedite a woman's chances of attaining a successful pregnancy.

The presence of endometriosis might impair fertility independent of tubal function, and significant adhesive disease may be an indication to consider IVF regardless of the etiology. Adjunctive indirect serologic markers may help identify high-risk patients with concomitant pathology affecting the pregnancy rates postoperatively; CA-125 titers can be elevated in endometriosis, positive chlamydial titers are suggestive of previous PID, whereas positive purified protein derivative is indicative of exposure to tuberculosis.[2]

459

Once the nontubal factors affecting fertility have been evaluated, the surgeon then accurately documents the degree of tubal disease, by either nonoperative or operative techniques. Hysterosalpingography (HSG) is an excellent preliminary test to document tubal disease, because it provides information about tubal patency, hydrosalpinges, and mucosal pattern. Intact functional tubal mucosa is a requirement for normal ovum transport to the uterus. Flattened mucosa from a longstanding hydrosalpinx or intraluminal adhesive disease from prior PID will significantly hinder proper movement of a fertilized embryo into the uterus and increase ectopic pregnancy risk. Large hydrosalpinges are associated with a poor prognosis for pregnancy after neosalpingostomy.[2] Performance of the HSG itself may be therapeutic by clearing mucus from the tubes or providing a bacteriostatic effect through the iodine in the dye; oil-based dyes are believed to be more effective than aqueous dyes in this regard. The HSG is contraindicated in women with a prior history of PID or iodine allergy. Laparoscopy is superior to the HSG primarily in the diagnosis of adhesions and other pelvic pathology such as endometriosis. The two tests offer complementary information on the overall condition of the fallopian tubes, however, with the HSG providing information on the state of the tubal mucosa and laparoscopy identifying fimbrial damage and an abnormal tubo-ovarian anatomic relationship.

Selective salpingography necessitates the use of specialized catheters that lodge into the uterine cornu to permit dye injection into each fallopian tube individually. This allows the location of the blockage in each tube to be identified, thereby decreasing the possibility of a false-positive HSG secondary to spasm or by preferential spill through one tube with a lower pressure gradient. Selective salpingography is typically performed at the same time as a hysterosalpingogram and carries the same risks; however, selective salpingography and tubal cannulation incur a greater probability of tubal perforation than does HSG. The procedure can be performed under both fluoroscopic and ultrasound guidance. Fluoroscopy is easier to utilize but has the disadvantage of additional radiation exposure to the ovaries.

Recent innovations in transcervical catheter technology have made access to the tubal lumen more feasible, allowing enhanced diagnostic and therapeutic capability. Application of coronary angioplasty techniques and linear everting catheters has aided this advancement. These procedures, however, do require extensive experience to master. Selective falloposcopy is considered the "gold standard" of tubal assessment by providing direct visualization of the tubal mucosa and endotubal pathology. This allows diagnosis of previously undetectable intratubal adhesions, mucosal abnormalities, and so on, and allows better determination of prognosis after microsurgical repair of damaged fallopian tubes. The catherization may also remove intraluminal debris or lyse intraluminal adhesions, clearing obstructions to sperm, ovum, or conceptus transport.

Falloposcopy can be performed in the same setting as hysteroscopy, with essentially the same risks. The greatest difficulties arise from negotiating the various angles and turns of the fallopian tube from cornua to fimbria. The linear everting catheter, which "unrolls" itself to deliver the falloposcope throughout the intraluminal pathway, has largely overcome this problem.[3] Laparoscopy to guide the falloposcopy and completely evaluate extraluminal distal tubal pathology may be performed concurrently. The greatest barrier to wider use of falloposcopy is the lack of generalized access to the equipment and techniques; the specialized optics required for successful visualization have improved dramatically over the last 10 years.

CONTRAINDICATIONS TO TUBAL SURGERY

Advanced maternal age and end-stage tubal disease are the two relative contraindications to tubal surgery. Tubal surgery for patients older than 40 years of age has yielded very poor results in most institutions; however, IVF delivery rates are also poor in women older than age 40 years. Oocyte donation may be a better option for these women. Absolute contraindications to both procedures include active salpingitis and medical illness making major surgery or pregnancy a risk to life.

End-stage tubal disease includes patients with *bipolar* tubal disease, that is, concomitant proximal and distal occlusion. Other factors include the degree of pelvic adhesions, the size of the hydrosalpinges, and fimbrial status. A study by Rock and colleagues[4] described prognostic factors affecting outcome after tubal surgery. Among women with dense pelvic adhesions, no visible fimbria, and hydrosalpinx greater than 30 mm in diameter, only 2 of 42 (5%) conceived after surgery. These patients would be better candidates for IVF.

RESULTS OF TUBAL SURGERY

It is generally believed that the most important factors in successful outcome of distal tuboplasty are the degree of preexisting intrinsic tubal pathology and tubo-ovarian adhesions. An ideal candidate for tuboplasty would have healthy tubal mucosa with filmy adhesions that distort the normal tubo-ovarian relationships preventing ovum pickup or that agglutinate the fimbria but once lysed allow immediate return of the proper anatomy. Studies of good-prognosis patients undergoing salpingo-ovariolysis have demonstrated cumulative intrauterine pregnancy rates ranging from 45% to 60% at 12 months postsurgery compared with 17% in untreated women. Ectopic pregnancies occurred in 5% to 10% of the treated population.[5] Although it improves reproductive outcome, adhesiolysis does not restore normal fertility even in good-prognosis patients. After 1 year of unprotected intercourse, approximately 85% of normally fertile couples can expect a pregnancy, a markedly better percentage than after tuboplasty. Obviously, even in the ideal candidate, adhesiolysis is not a perfect remedy.

Distal tubal occlusion can be associated with varying degrees of tubal involvement. The classification system of Rock and colleagues[4] categorizes tubal disease with distal fimbrial obstruction into three classes (mild, moderate, and severe) based on the size of hydrosalpinx, fimbrial condition, degree of adhesion formation, and presence of a rugal pattern on HSG. *Mild* disease includes fallopian tubes with a rugal pattern on preoperative HSG; hydrosalpinx, if present, of 15-mm diameter or less; lack of significant peritubular and periovarian adhesions; and evidence of fimbria after salpingostomy. With *moderate* involvement, there is absence of a rugal pattern on HSG; hydrosalpinx of 15- to 30-mm diameter; peritubular or periovarian adhesions without fixation; and fimbria that are difficult to identify. The *severe* category encompasses hydrosalpinx 30 mm or greater in diameter; dense pelvic or adnexal adhesions; cul-de-sac obliteration; and absence of identifiable fimbria.

Success rates for neosalpingostomy were stage dependent. The intrauterine pregnancy rate for mild disease in Rock and colleagues'[4] series ranged from 70% to 85%, whereas the pregnancy rates for moderate and severe disease were only 17% and 13%, respectively. Ectopic pregnancy rates increased with the severity of tubal disease; 7% to 10% of women with mild tubal disease undergoing neosalpingostomy developed an ectopic pregnancy, whereas about twice as many women with moderate disease (14%) had a tubal pregnancy. The relatively low rate of ectopic pregnancies (4%) among women with severe disease may be related to very poor tubal function that prevented both intrauterine and ectopic pregnancies equally.[4] Overall, most studies have demonstrated across-the-board intrauterine pregnancy rates of 20% to 35% during the first year after distal tuboplasty, corresponding to a monthly conception, or fecundation, rate of 2% to 3%.[6]

Proximal tubal disease represents a smaller proportion of tubal infertility than distal disease. It is found in 10% to 20% of HSGs performed to evaluate infertility.[2] False-positive HSGs can occur secondary to cornual spasm, accounting for approximately 15% of HSGs that demonstrate proximal occlusion. To confirm proximal obstruction, a repeat HSG with sedation, laparoscopy and chromopertubation, or selective tubal salpingography should be performed. Proximal tubal occlusion is most commonly seen in relation to sterilization and may be mechanical, such as that due to Hulka clips, Falope's rings, or segmental resection and ligation, or induced thermally or electrically by coagulation. Pathologic analyses of fallopian tubes with documented proximal obstruction not secondary to sterilization methods demonstrate obliterative fibrosis, salpingitis isthmica nodosa, endometriosis, chronic inflammation, and tubal plugging. The proximal oviduct is a microscopic structure with an inner lumen diameter of 0.4 to 1.2 mm, surrounded by well-defined muscular layers that play a major role in embryo transport. The precision with which these structures may be defined and repaired when ade-

quately magnified have made them good candidates for microtuboplasty. Excision of proximal tubal disease with microsurgical re-anastomosis has been followed by live births in well over 50% of cases in several studies.[2]

A natural extension of utilizing catheter technology for diagnosis has been therapeutic intervention. Transcervical tuboplasty using balloon dilators to diminish tubal stenosis or destroy endosalpingeal adhesions is currently available. This may be performed at the time of diagnosis of tubal stricture by either selective salpingography or falloposcopy. Sueoka and coworkers[3] achieved an 85.3% recanalization success rate using the linear everting catheter. Follow-up HSG 1 to 3 months later revealed a persistent overall patency rate of 79.4%. Other studies documented patency rates of 50% to 75% after 6 months. The subsequent pregnancy rate after treatment was 22%. The interval from surgery to conception was 2 to 26 months, with the majority of patients conceiving within 9 months. The ability to lyse endosalpingeal adhesions successfully by retrograde balloon movement did not differ significantly between proximal and distal tubal locations. Sueoka and coworkers[3] performed their series in an outpatient setting and had higher success rates when concomitant laparoscopy was not performed. Patients with hydrosalpinx were not candidates for therapy in their study. They believed that the results they attained were comparable with those produced by conventional operative tubal microsurgery. The benefits of falloposcopic tuboplasty over surgery include greatly decreased morbidity and expense, although cost was not revealed.[3] Lang and Dunaway[7] documented an intrauterine pregnancy rate of 12.8% after transcervical recanalization, with a cost of $6400 per live birth. The risk of ectopic pregnancy in both studies was low at less than 1%.

TUBAL REANASTOMOSIS AFTER ELECTIVE STERILIZATION

Tubal sterilization has become the single most utilized form of birth control in the United States today. It is not surprising that there has been a concomitant increase in the number of women desiring reversal. One percent to 10% of all women undergoing elective sterilization later express regret, although only one fifth of women considering reversal will actually progress to surgery. The desire for tubal reversal usually stems from remarriage, the loss of a child, or, occasionally, just a change of heart. Women most likely to experience regret are those whose sterilization occurred immediately postpartum, at an age younger than 25 years, or if their relationship with their partner was strained at the time of sterilization. Psychological evaluation should be strongly considered in the woman requesting reversal for the purpose of alleviating pelvic pain or depression after her sterilization.[8]

Cost and patient goals are important considerations for the patient desiring additional children after elective sterilization. The less expensive the procedure and the greater the success rate in IVF or re-anastomosis, the more attractive it becomes. For the woman who has a time constraint owing to her age or desires only one additional child, IVF may be preferable. Conversely, one benefit of a successful re-anastomosis is the ability to conceive naturally on numerous occasions without the cost or risk of multiple IVF cycles.

Many factors have an impact on the success rates of tubal reversal. In general, tubal reversals result in greater intrauterine pregnancy rates than tuboplasty for hydrosalpinx or adhesive disease, mostly owing to lack of intrinsic endotubal damage in patients electively sterilized. The following elements have been shown to affect subsequent pregnancy rates of attempted reversals: type of sterilization performed, length of remaining fallopian tube after reversal, the region(s) of destruction along the tube, and the method of reversal. The impact of the time interval from sterilization to reversal, patient age, and availability of only one or both tubes is controversial.[8]

Thorough evaluation is important when considering IVF versus re-anastomosis in a patient. As much information as possible should be collected regarding the sterilization procedure. Operative and pathology reports help determine what procedure was performed and the degree of tubal destruction. If operative and pathology reports are not available, a diagnostic laparoscopy will demonstrate the condition of the fallopian tubes. Some reproductive surgeons favor performing a minilaparotomy to visualize the tubes, then proceeding with reconstruction if they are suitable. This eliminates the additional expense of a "screening laparoscopy."

Ring and clip sterilizations are the most easily reversed, because there is little tissue damage surrounding the interruption. Fimbriectomy is generally not considered reversible, because these patients do not have an endogenous method of ovum pickup. Coagulation methods that destroy a length of the tube generally result in widespread tubal damage and are also not amenable to reconstruction. Isthmic-isthmic re-anastomoses are most optimal because they provide good muscular support to the re-anastomosis site, and luminal caliber remains relatively equal. The longer the length of the fallopian tubes after re-anastomosis, the higher the pregnancy rate and the shorter the time interval to conception. Although studies differ, a repaired tube measuring 5 cm or more is considered adequate. Normal tubes measure 8 to 12 cm. Some surgeons feel a period of greater than 5 years from sterilization to reversal reduces the likelihood of pregnancy after reversal. Microsurgical re-anastomosis, with atraumatic tissue-handling techniques, meticulous hemostasis, and a magnified field-of-view, increases live birth rates over the traditional macroscopic method.

The majority of pregnancies after successful re-anastomosis occur in the first 2 years after the procedure. Overall intrauterine pregnancy rates at the end of these 2 years, for all types of sterilization and sites of re-anastomosis, range from 55% to 85%. The corresponding rate of ectopic pregnancy is 2% to 6%. Patients not conceiving rapidly after tubal reversal or other forms of tuboplasty should be evaluated for tubal patency at 6 to 12 months postoperatively. Repeat surgery is associated with very poor pregnancy rates after tuboplasty, and patients with re-obstruction should be counseled to pursue IVF.[8]

IN VITRO FERTILIZATION

In vitro fertilization–embryo transfer (IVF-ET) has delivered children to many couples who just since 1978 would have had little hope of creating a family. Initially for treatment of tubal factor infertility, its indications have grown to include endometriosis; unexplained infertility; oligospermia, asthenospermia, or teratozoospermia; poor egg-sperm interactions; antisperm antibodies; and preimplantation genetic evaluation of potential offspring in chromosomally abnormal but otherwise fertile couples. Over the years, IVF has changed markedly, from a procedure performed with the patient under general anesthetic in an operating room to an office-based procedure performed under sedation. Retrieval by transvaginal sonography has made retrievals relatively simple for both patient and physician.

However, like any sophisticated medical technology, IVF carries certain risks and potential complications. Hemorrhage and tubo-ovarian abscesses have been reported after IVF. Ovarian hyperstimulation syndrome (OHSS) occurs in varying degrees in all women undergoing gonadotropin stimulation, with most experiencing some enlargement of the ovaries, minor weight gain, and abdominal tenderness. One percent to 2% of all women undergoing gonadotropin ovarian stimulation will develop severe OHSS that involves marked fluid shifts, ascites, pleural effusion, hypovolemia with hemoconcentration, oliguria, electrolyte disturbances, and hypercoagulability. Severe OHSS is potentially lethal, and hospitalization in an intensive care setting is usually required for these women. One currently unanswered question is whether ovaries subjected to hyperstimulation may later be at increased risk of cancer development.

The Centers for Disease Control and Prevention (CDC) and the Society for Assisted Reproductive Technology (SART) publish an annual report on assisted reproductive techniques (ARTs) success rates, including both a national summary and individual fertility clinic data. According to 1998 national statistics, pregnancies resulting from fresh embryos, nondonor eggs, occurred in 37% of initiated cycles for women younger than 35 years of age, 32% for women aged 35 to 37, 24% for women 38 to 40 years, and 13% for women older than 40 years. Singleton births accounted for 62% of all these IVF-created pregnancies; twins accounted for 32% of pregnancies, and triplets or greater for 6%. The incidence of ectopic pregnancy in this group was 0.6%. Cumulative success rates, including replacement of frozen embryos in future cycles, may be as high as 60% in some successful clinics. Good-prognosis patients undergoing IVF multiple times have been estimated to have an approximately 70% chance of conception.

To maximize the potential for pregnancy, multiple embryos are typically transferred in IVF procedures. The multiple birth rate is greatly increased over that of the normal population. Higher-order multiple gestations, triplets and above, are a very real economic and health hazard. Mothers face a high-risk pregnancy with possible OHSS, preterm labor, prolonged bed rest, and operative delivery. Prematurity and all its attendant risks affect these babies most. Varying morbidities and special health needs may follow them well into adulthood. Even a healthy, term triplet gestation presents special problems not encountered by singleton parents. Logistics of housing, food, clothing, education, transportation, vacationing, even dining out are challenges to the parents of high-order multiples.

Overcoming the problem of multiple gestations would greatly reduce the financial impact and worry associated with IVF-ET. Culture of fertilized embryos to the blastocyst stage, which improves implantation rates, is now available in mainstream IVF laboratories. This reduces the number of embryos per transfer required to achieve pregnancy, and, therefore, simultaneously decreases the risk of higher-order multiple gestations. Techniques continue to be refined, increasing success rates and decreasing side effects. Gonadotropin-releasing hormone antagonists suitable for widespread clinical use are being introduced for the first time. These drugs should shorten the stimulation phase of the IVF process, promising reduced cost and side effects and increased patient tolerance. Frozen embryo transfer success rates continue to rise, enabling a greater number of pregnancies to result from one stimulated cycle. This will reduce the need of additional stimulated cycles to have more children, diminishing expense and risk.

A specific issue getting attention in enhancing IVF-ET outcomes, especially pertinent to this discussion, is the detrimental role of hydrosalpinx. Women with hydrosalpinx have significant reductions in both implantation and pregnancy rates. There are data that the hydrosalpinx may drain potentially toxic fluid into the uterine cavity that adversely affects both embryo and endometrium. In vitro studies confirm a derangement in embryo development when exposed to hydrosalpingeal fluid, and Meyer and coworkers[9] have documented alterations of endometrial integrins implicated in implantation in women with hydrosalpinx. Improvements in outcome with IVF-ET after salpingectomy or proximal occlusion of the hydrosalpinx have been reported, with pregnancy rates doubled and a 50% reduction of miscarriage rates. These findings have prompted several investigators to perform salpingectomies or proximal ligation of hydrosalpinx routinely before IVF-ET.[10]

Proceeding with In Vitro Fertilization or Tuboplasty

Two key components to the tuboplasty versus IVF debate are expense and success. The cost per IVF cycle varies markedly across the United States, ranging from about $4000 to $12,000. Early attempts at calculating the cost-effectiveness of IVF utilized the poorer outcomes of the contemporary time periods, producing higher costs than seen today. In 1994, Neumann and coworkers[11] published figures corresponding to a cost per delivery of $66,667 if successful with the first cycle, increasing to $114,286 if six cycles were necessary. These figures are considered elevated because they include not only direct costs and costs of complications but also adjustment for nonrecurring charges and indirect costs such as lost wages. More recent analyses demonstrate a lesser expense as IVF pregnancy rates increased. In 1995, with an ongoing pregnancy rate of 27% after the first treatment cycle, the cost per delivery was $29,120 if only one cycle were required, rising to $31,590 when three cycles of IVF were needed.[12] The patient's inherent probability of pregnancy largely determined the expense, with age, ovarian status, and male factor contributing to that probability.

When stratified, a high-probability patient was younger than 33 years old with no male factor component, and her cost per delivery was $22,857. Moderate-probability patients were women younger than 40 years old with severe male factor infertility, with a corresponding cost of $34,000. The lowest-probability woman was older than 40 years of age and had a cost per delivery of $42,666. Use of donor oocytes for the older woman made economic sense, lowering cost per delivery for these patients to $35,605, including the additional expense of the donor.[11] With the SART data demonstrating yearly increases in the delivery rate, the cost of a successful IVF pregnancy should continue to decline.

Previously outlined patient selection criteria help identify those individuals most suitable for a particular therapy. Many authorities feel the monthly fecundity rate is the yardstick against which all infertility therapies should be measured.[6] Fecundity analyzed by cost of therapy yields some cost-effectiveness data; however, published reviews[13] vary in their computational methodology, differing with regard to charge versus cost, time on from work, costs of obstetric care, and so on. However, certain observations are clear. With mild distal tubal disease in the young patient, surgical repair is an acceptable form of therapy given its subsequent pregnancy rate. Isolated proximal tubal disease is probably worth ameliorating via a tubal catherization approach, because this is minimally invasive, and patency rates after dilatation are prolonged in most series. If pregnancy does not occur after 12 months following tuboplasty, progression to IVF is advisable. Women older than 39 years, patients with poor-prognosis tubal disease, or with coexisting factors such as severe ovulatory disorders or significant male factor, should be advised to consider IVF rather than tuboplasty. With a typical fecundity rate of 2% to 3.5% after tuboplasty for significant distal tubal disease, the cost of a resulting live birth after tuboplasty was anywhere from 10% to 100% higher than that achieved with IVF-ET.[12] As IVF techniques improve and pregnancy rates climb, this monetary gap will likely widen further.

Unfortunately, other factors have a heavy hand in directing what treatment modality is utilized. When insurance covers tubal surgery and not IVF, economic considerations often prevail over medical. It is hoped that education of patients and insurance carriers regarding the cost-effectiveness of appropriate therapy (or mandated insurance coverage for IVF) will ensure that in the future, medical considerations are given priority in deciding between IVF and tuboplasty.

References

1. Scott RT, Toner JP, Muasher SJ, et al: Follicle-stimulating hormone levels on cycle day 3 are predictive of in vitro fertilization outcome. Fertil Steril 1989;51:651.
2. Novy MJ: Tubal surgery or IVF—making the best choice in the 1990s. Int J Fertil Menopausal Studies 1995; 40:292.
3. Sueoka K, Asada H, Tsuchiya S, et al: Falloposcopic tuboplasty for bilateral tubal occlusion. A novel infertility treatment as an alternative for in-vitro fertilization? Hum Reprod 1998; 13:71.
4. Rock JA, Katayama KP, Martin EJ, et al: Factors influencing the success of salpingostomy techniques for distal fimbrial obstruction. Obstet Gynecol 1978; 52:591.
5. Tulandi T, Collins JA, Burrows E, et al: Treatment-dependent and treatment-independent pregnancy among women with periadnexal adhesions. Am J Obstet Gynecol 1990; 162:354.
6. Penzias AS, DeCherney AH: Is there ever a role for tubal surgery? Am J Obstet Gynecol 1996; 174:1218.
7. Lang EK, Dunaway HH: Recanalization of obstructed fallopian tube by selective salpingography and transvaginal bougie dilatation: Outcome and cost analysis. Fertil Steril 1996;66:210.
8. Leader A: Reversal of sterilization. Adv Contraception 1989; 5:213.
9. Meyer WR, Castelbaum AJ, Somkuti S, et al: Hydrosalpinges adversely affect markers of endometrial receptivity. Hum Reprod 1997;12:1393.
10. Nackley AC, Muasher SJ: The significance of hydrosalpinx in in-vitro fertilization. Fertil Steril 1998; 69:373.
11. Neumann PJ, Gharib SD, Weinstein MC: The cost of a successful delivery with in vitro fertilization. N Engl J Med 1994;331:239.
12. Trad FS, Hornstein MD, Barbieri RL: In vitro fertilization: A cost-effective alternative for infertile couples? J Assist Reprod Genet 1995;12:418.
13. Van Voorhis BJ, Stovall DW, Allen BD, et al: Cost-effective treatment of the infertile couple. Fertil Steril 1998; 70:995.

Unexplained Infertility: Management Options

Moon H. Kim

Unexplained infertility is a challenging and frustrating condition for both physicians and patients. It is a diagnosis of exclusion of apparent causes for infertility utilizing a "standard" or "complete basic" evaluation. Despite the lack of unanimity of opinion about what a standard evaluation should include, most physicians consider the following investigation as basic: semen analysis, postcoital test, evaluation of ovulation, hysterosalpingography, and possibly laparoscopy "when indicated."[1] The prevalence of unexplained infertility varies widely and is estimated to be between 5% and 30% in different studies, depending on many factors, such as the age of patients, the duration of infertility, and the extent of evaluation.

DIAGNOSTIC EVALUATION BEYOND "STANDARD INVESTIGATION"

The first step in evaluating the couple with unexplained infertility starts with a thorough review of the previous investigation for infertility. Some tests may be repeated if the results of the previous test are not clear or if many years have elapsed since those investigations. A thorough review of the history, noting particularly the age of the woman, the duration of infertility, and previous therapeutic intervention, is essential.

What further evaluation should be obtained for unexplained infertility is controversial. Some physicians may recommend various tests such as sperm antibodies, sperm penetration test (zona-free hamster egg), chlamydial testing or cervical culture, endometrial biopsy, and ultrasound monitoring of the follicles. However, no studies have shown that such tests are beneficial in the management of unexplained infertility. With new emphasis on evidence-based medicine and awareness of cost effectiveness, such additional tests should be selected carefully with a consideration of how these tests might be of help in improving the therapeutic outcome.

The workshop sponsored by the European Society of Human Reproduction[2] concluded that (1) semen analysis, (2) the tubal patency test (hysterosalpingography or laparoscopy), and (3) assessment of ovulation (midluteal progesterone) have been established to correlate with the outcome of infertility treatment. All other studies, such as sperm penetration tests, cervical culture for chlamydia or mycoplasma, sperm antibodies, and extensive endocrine evaluation including endometrial dating, have not been shown to correlate consistently with the chance of pregnancy.

Therefore, these tests are not likely to be of help in the management of unexplained infertility except for limited circumstances. Routine use of these tests should be discouraged.

In many patients, some tests previously obtained may have to be repeated. For example, an assessment of ovulation should be done when progesterone levels do not correlate with endometrial dating or when menstrual changes occur or ovulation-inducing agents are used. Semen analysis must be repeated if the male partner had an exposure to toxic substances, sexually transmitted disease, or febrile diseases since the initial evaluation. Likewise, tubal or peritoneal factors should be re-evaluated when there is a history of recent pelvic infection or surgery and if there is suspected recurrence or progression of endometriosis.

Other factors that may affect the reproductive capability must be explored. A significant psychoemotional element may exist, which could be the cause or the result of frustration and emotional turmoil from unresolved infertility. A sympathetic approach to evaluation and management is essential. Many investigators have reported that smoking in both women and men may have an adverse effect on reproduction. Smoking has been shown to compromise implantation and clinical pregnancy rates significantly. Also, smokers have a higher incidence of abnormal ovarian functional reserve based on the clomiphene citrate challenge test. Therefore, a careful history of cigarette smoking should be obtained. Also, excessive caffeine intake may have a role in unexplained infertility.

The age-related decline in ovarian function and reproductive potential has been well established, and it may be a major contributing factor to an increase in the incidence of unexplained infertility. The monthly fecundity of a 25-year-old woman declines from 25% to 15% at age 35 years.[3] Although there is no good test to evaluate ovarian functional reserve, women with advancing age, perhaps older than 35 years, and with unexplained infertility should be evaluated. A Day 3 follicle-stimulating hormone level seems to be a reasonable test. A level greater than 13 to 15 mIU/mL is suggestive of diminished ovarian function. However, this result is perhaps more important for counseling purposes than for selecting therapeutic options.

The presence of intramural or submucosal myomas may interfere with implantation because of vascular changes, local inflammation, endometrial changes owing to the myoma, or alteration of myometrial contractility. Although there have been no randomized studies, several reports suggest that myomectomy results in a better pregnancy rate and outcome.[4]

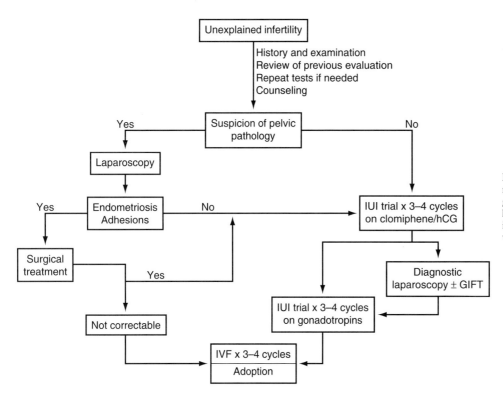

Figure 92–1. Algorithm for treatment of unexplained infertility. GIFT, gamete intrafallopian transfer; hCG, human chorionic gonadotropin; IUI, intrauterine insemination; IVF, in vitro fertilization.

PROGNOSTIC FACTORS

It is important to appropriately counsel the couple with unexplained infertility about their realistic chances of achieving pregnancy. Based on numerous studies, the following factors offer a good prognosis:

1. Age younger than 35 years
2. Duration of infertility less than 3 years
3. No history of pelvic inflammatory disease
4. Normal semen analysis and normal postcoital test

These should be discussed with the couple during the counseling process.

THERAPEUTIC OPTIONS

Patients diagnosed with unexplained infertility may indeed have subtle defects in some components of the reproductive process, which cannot be assessed currently. Thus, the treatment is largely aimed at improving the chances of conceiving through empirical approaches such as assisted reproductive technology. However, it is important to counsel couples with unexplained infertility that there is a possibility of conceiving spontaneously. There should be a thorough evaluation of the various therapeutic options and the impact of the prognostic factors mentioned previously in the context of this spontaneous conception rate.

EXPECTANT MANAGEMENT

Several studies[2, 3] report that cumulative pregnancy rates with expectant management among couples with unex-

plained infertility range from 40% to 80% after 3 years. Generally, expectant management for 12 months' duration is well justified for women younger than 30 years of age with a duration of infertility of less than 3 years. These women should expect a better than 50% chance of conceiving spontaneously. For women older than 35 years or with a longer than 3-year duration of infertility, some type of empirical therapeutic option should be considered.

EMPIRICAL THERAPY FOR UNEXPLAINED INFERTILITY

Any treatment recommended without an evidence-based outcome is as empirical one. Some practitioners consider empirical therapy inappropriate because it often raises patients' expectations unfairly, resulting in greater disappointment and frustration. However, with appropriate counseling of the couple, some type of empirical therapy may be attempted. Recent studies[5] have shown that intrauterine insemination (IUI), in conjunction with the use of either clomiphene citrate or gonadotropins, yields higher pregnancy rates compared with the control population. IUI alone on natural cycles, without the use of ovulatory stimulants, did not significantly improve pregnancy rates. On the other hand, the use of ovulatory stimulants alone, without IUI, showed some improvement in conception rate. The combination of IUI and clomiphene or gonadotropin therapy resulted in two-fold (8% per cycle) and four-fold (17% per cycle) increases in pregnancy rates, respectively. A recent randomized multicenter study[5] involving 932 couples demonstrated that IUI with gonadotropin-induced superovulation yielded a 9% pregnancy rate per insemination cycle and a 33% pregnancy rate per couple. This study included couples with mild oligospermia. The cost per treatment cycle varies widely, but generally ranges from $500 for IUI on clomiphene treatment to $1500 for IUI on gonadotropin-induced superovulation.

Assisted reproductive procedures, such as in vitro fertilization (IVF) or gamete intrafallopian transfer (GIFT), are often recommended for the treatment of unexplained infertility. These procedures have higher pregnancy rates (average, 20% to 25% for IVF or GIFT) than IUI with superovulation. There are other advantages of IVF, or GIFT combined with IVF, such as the opportunity to evaluate the fertilizing capacity of the gametes. However, average cost per treatment cycle is 6 to 10 times that of IUI with superovulation. In patients with unexplained infertility suspected of having endometriosis or pelvic adhesions requiring a laparoscopy, a GIFT procedure may be combined with a diagnostic laparoscopy. Major complications associated with the use of gonadotropins are ovarian hyperstimulation and multifetal gestation. To reduce the risk of these complications, the patients must be monitored carefully throughout the treatment. Also, the number of embryos to be transferred should be limited. Blastocyst culture and transfer may provide a significant benefit in this regard, limiting the number of embryos replaced and hence the multiple pregnancy rate, while maintaining high success rates overall.

SUMMARY

One of every 10 infertile couples will be classified as "unexplained." The age of the female partner, the duration of infertility, and the quality of semen are important prognostic factors in these patients. In younger patients or those with a duration of infertility of less than 3 years, expectant management may be appropriate. Various empirical therapeutic options should be considered when expectant management is not desired. There is no rigid algorithm for therapy. Thus, couples with unexplained infertility should be counseled about all therapeutic options and their associated costs and complications, and their realistic chances of conception, so that they can be actively involved in the decision-making process (Fig. 92–1).

Suggestions for Future Reading

Guzick DS, Sullivan MW, Adamson GD, et al: Efficacy of treatment for unexplained infertility. Fertil Steril 1998;7:207–213.
Surrey EN (ed): Unexplained infertility. Infertil Reprod Med Clin North Am 1997;8:1–194.

References

1. Committee Opinion, American Society for Reproductive Medicine, June, 2000.
2. Crosignani PJ, Collins J, Cooke ID, et al: Unexplained infertility: The recommendation of the European Society of Human Reproduction Workshop. Hum Reprod 1993;8:977–980.
3. Collins JA, Rowe TC: Age of the female partner is a prognostic factor in prolonged unexplained infertility; A multi-centered study. Fertil Steril 1989;52:15–20.
4. Vercellini P, Maddalena S, De Giorgi O, et al: Determinants of reproductive outcome after abdominal myomectomy for infertility. Fertil Steril 1999;72:109–114.
5. Guzick DS, Carlson SA, Coutifris C, et al: Efficacy of superovulation in intrauterine insemination in the treatment of infertility. N Engl J Med 1999;340:177–183.

NINETY-THREE

Management of Ovarian Cancer

John L. Currie and Leslie R. DeMars

Ovarian cancer continues to be a major health problem for women, with 23,100 new cases expected in 2000.[1] Despite decades of intensive research and eagerly anticipated therapeutic breakthroughs, over 60% of patients eventually succumb to the debilitating ravages of this disease—making it the fifth leading cause of cancer death in women.[1] The mainstays of treatment for ovarian cancer remain primary surgical intervention followed by adjuvant chemotherapy for the most common presentation of advanced disease, as there have been no real breakthroughs in early detection or prevention.

The risk for a white woman in the general population developing ovarian cancer is roughly 1 in 53 in her lifetime, whereas the lifetime risk for an African American woman is slightly lower, approximately 1 in 92. Although much media attention is focused on the hereditary aspects of ovarian cancer, fewer than 10% of cases can be linked to a hereditary pattern, such as familial breast and ovarian cancer (with defects in BRCA 1 and 2), or hereditary nonpolyposis colorectal cancer (with defects in MLH1, MSH2, and PMS2).[2, 3] Women with a BRCA 1 or 2 mutation have a 27% to 44% lifetime risk of ovarian cancer.[4] In general, however, having a single first-degree relative with ovarian cancer increases the risk from baseline to about 5%, and two such relatives may boost the risk to 10%; these cases constitute only a minority of cases.[5] Other risk factors include age, low parity, and late menopause. Oral contraceptives appear to be quite protective, with a 25% to 60% decrease in the incidence of ovarian cancer in those women who have utilized these medications in the past.[6-8] Use of oral contraceptives appears to be protective for women with BRCA 1 or 2 mutations as well.[9]

At the present time, there are no cost-effective screening methods for ovarian cancer in the general population.[10] Although multiple clinical trials suggest that the combination of pelvic examination, CA-125 determination, and particularly vaginal ultrasound of the pelvis has a high-enough positive predictive value to be of use in screening higher-risk populations, these screening tests continue to be relatively insensitive, leading to invasive procedures having a low yield of actual malignancies, while remaining relatively expensive and frequently not covered by third-party payers.[11, 12] Prevention of ovarian cancer is likewise problematic, because even prophylactic oophorectomy will not circumvent development of the virtually identical disease of primary peritoneal carcinomatosis.[13] For patients with a strong family history or BRCA 1 and 2 gene mutations, careful screening every 6 months is essential,

with oral contraceptive therapy when appropriate; strong consideration for prophylactic salpingo-oophorectomy remains the best protection.

The ovary contains totipotent cells from which any histologic cancer can arise. Epithelial ovarian cancer represents 80% of ovarian malignancies, with the histologic types of papillary serous, mucinous, and endometrioid recapitulating the epithelium of the fallopian tube, endocervix, and endometrium, respectively. About 10% of ovarian cancers are germ cell tumors, often occurring in younger women, and are best treated with fertility-sparing surgical staging and adjuvant chemotherapy. Another 5% of ovarian cancers are stromal tumors; again, surgical management is the cornerstone, and adjuvant chemotherapy depends on the stage and cell type. Finally, 5% of ovarian malignancies are secondary tumors from other sites (principally breast, gastrointestinal tract, or endometrium), sarcomas, or rare cell types from totipotent cells or vascular structures. The ensuing discussion is based on the management of epithelial tumors, although the surgical principles can apply to all ovarian malignancies.

DIAGNOSIS AND PREOPERATIVE EVALUATION

For many women, the diagnosis of ovarian cancer is made after multiple empirical treatments of nonspecific gastrointestinal complaints. Ovarian cancer has the undeserved moniker of "silent killer"; whereas early ovarian cancer is often asymptomatic, advanced ovarian cancer is heralded by multiple gastrointestinal complaints. The astute diagnostician should not be fooled by stage III or IV cancer, with its symptom complex of massive distention with ascites, early satiety or even obstructive symptoms, and usually the presence of a pelvic mass, omental "cake," or pleural effusion. When this presentation occurs, almost every health care provider has no problem recognizing the severity of the illness, and ovarian cancer is the most likely diagnosis. For early ovarian cancer, the diagnosis may be more difficult, and even serendipitous. Vague and rather common symptoms such as constipation, lower abdominal discomfort, anorexia, pelvic pressure, bloating, fatigue—the list goes on—can be early symptoms of many diseases, and unless diagnostic tests lead to surgical evaluation, the diagnosis of ovarian cancer may not be rendered until the advanced disease symptom complex occurs. Unfortunately, ovarian cancer is also frequently diagnosed intraoperatively when the surgeon is expecting other causes of the symptoms. This is most disturbing when the preoperative diagnosis includes pelvic mass and preparations are inadequate for optimal surgical management, or surgeons trained in proper staging are not available. Indeed, comparative studies have shown that the overall treatment plan for patients with ovarian cancer is better when the initial surgical procedure is performed by or with a gynecologic oncologist rather than a gynecologist or general surgeon.[14] Thus, any undiagnosed pelvic mass should prompt consideration of ovarian cancer, and diagnostic evaluation including pelvic ultrasound, abdominal/pelvic CT scan, and CA-125 determination should be done prior to surgery to enhance the opportunity for appropriate staging and debulking at the initial surgical procedure.

In postmenopausal women, the CA-125 is normally less than 35 IU/mL. A preoperative level greater than 65 in the presence of a pelvic mass is highly predictive of ovarian cancer.[15] Conversely, in premenopausal patients, the CA-125 can be elevated in a number of nonmalignant conditions, including pregnancy, endometriosis, uterine fibroids, and inflammatory conditions of the abdomen such as pelvic inflammatory disease. Unfortunately, in both premenopausal and postmenopausal women, a normal CA-125 does not exclude the possibility of malignancy. CA-125 levels can be within normal limits in 50% of patients with stage I ovarian cancer.

Patients with a suspected diagnosis of ovarian cancer should have a preoperative evaluation and preparation as follows:

1. Complete history and physical examination with appropriate laboratory testing, and consultation as indicated for treatment of comorbid illnesses.
2. Chest x-ray and other cardiac or pulmonary studies as indicated. If pleural effusion exists, consideration for thoracentesis depending on functional status.
3. Gastrointestinal tract evaluation and preparation: if colonic involvement is suspected, either colonoscopy or barium enema is helpful in planning surgical approach. Regardless, a bowel preparation is required; the magnitude and thoroughness can be tailored to the expected surgical findings and clinical picture. (It may be difficult to prepare the bowel when complete or partial obstruction exists preoperatively.)
4. Imaging of the entire abdomen will frequently diagnose disease involvement that will guide the surgical approach or infrequently weigh against a primary surgical approach. This would be the case if parenchymal liver metastasis or other upper abdominal disease would dictate a neoadjuvant chemotherapy approach initially. The most economical imaging study in most arenas is CT scan; ultrasound, MRI, or nucleotide scanning may be useful in certain circumstances.

SURGICAL APPROACH

The patient is transported to the operating room and prepared for major surgery. Prophylaxis for deep venous thrombosis using sequential compression hose is employed; heparin or low-molecular-weight heparin should be started prior to the induction of anesthesia. The anesthesia team should be prepared for a lengthy operation, which might be accompanied by major blood loss, massive fluid shifts, and dynamic changes in vital signs. Thus, appropriate measures should be entertained expectantly, including large-bore intravenous access, invasive monitoring, capability for rapid blood product transfusion, and eager anticipation of potential complications. Most gynecologic oncologists prefer that the positioning of the patient be sufficiently flexible to allow a vaginal approach or a low rectal anastomosis with the end-to-end stapler in case there is extensive disease encroaching on the pelvic sidewalls, vagina, or rectum; the majority of cases will proceed without the need to utilize the lower approach, but it would be wise to be prepared for this eventuality.

The surgical incision should almost always be lower, midline vertical to initiate the procedure. This can be extended around the umbilicus to the xyphoid if necessary to debulk upper abdominal disease, whereas any standard transverse lower abdominal incision would require a herculean effort to complete upper abdominal debulking. However, the incision may be tailored to the expected extent of disease and the patient's lifestyle and habitus; the true transverse Maylard or Cherney incisions may be used with caution. Recently, we published a film demonstrating a cosmetically appealing transverse incision that removes a layer of skin and fat and uses a vertical fascial incision to allow approaches to the upper abdomen; this approach has been used successfully for patients with large pelvic masses, including ovarian cancer, with satisfactory results.[16] The incision chosen, however, must provide adequate exposure for optimal debulking and complete surgical staging.

In patients with very large tumors and a degree of venous obstruction, the superficial abdominal wall veins may be distended and not easily controlled with electrocautery or pressure—clamping and tying may be necessary. Otherwise, standard techniques are used to enter the abdomen. When the peritoneum is encountered, care should be taken to avoid injuring the bowel, which may be adherent from previous surgery or metastatic deposits. Furthermore, the disease can present as a large ovarian cyst, and it is important to avoid entering the cyst inadvertently. Although rupture of a cystic mass is sometimes unpreventable, it nevertheless upstages the disease automatically. Thus, tedious dissection through the layers of the peritoneum to separate it from the cyst wall is worth the additional time. Usually, however, the peritoneum bulges with ascitic fluid, and a centimeter incision will allow insertion of a Poole suction tip apparatus to drain away ascites under controlled conditions. An aliquot is sent for cytologic evaluation. Because ascites is an exudative effusion, there is no limit to the amount or rate at which it can be drained, but the anesthesia team should be prepared for potential hemodynamic changes if large volumes will be drained.

Intraoperative Assessment

We hope that the operating surgeon will have anticipated the finding of ovarian cancer, and will avoid immediate reclosure of the abdomen (the "peek and shriek" procedure). If the surgeon finds herself or himself in the unenviable position of not having adequate support personnel or expertise for surgical debulking, she or he must at least carefully assess the extent of disease to aid in the treatment plans of his consultants.

The first task is to assess the resectability of the disease; this is best accomplished after dissecting adhesions away from the anterior abdominal wall. We explore the upper abdomen first, because the factors that limit the chances of optimal debulking are outside the pelvis. Whereas other surgeons have different criteria, we feel that optimal debulking is usually not safely achieved if any of the following factors are present: (1) extensive para-aortic nodes superior to the renal vessels; (2) extensive disease in the gastric mesentery along the lesser curvature of the stomach, especially with adherence to the central ligament or diaphragms; (3) extensive, small nodule involvement of the small bowel mesentery, especially near the ligament of Treitz; and (4) the presence of parenchymal liver metastases. Some surgeons add to this list involvement of the spleen, the gastrocolic omentum, or extensive diaphragmatic disease; we believe that any of these can be optimally debulked under most circumstances. Whereas it is preferred that splenectomy be avoided, it is sometimes necessary. With the standard retroperitoneal approach to the pelvic organs, optimal debulking in the pelvis is obtainable in most circumstances.

The concept of surgical debulking of epithelial ovarian cancer has strong theoretical and literature-based support, with optimal debulking associated with longer survival and longer disease-free interval.[17, 18] The definition of *optimal* varies, but the Gynecologic Oncology Group (GOG) has defined in its treatment protocols that optimal debulking means removal of all disease greater than 1 cm in maximal dimension; if disease greater than 1 cm is remaining, the surgical exercise is deemed "suboptimal." Thus, if the goal of the operation is to achieve optimal debulking, the initial assessment assumes paramount importance because removing all pelvic disease and leaving behind extensive upper abdominal tumor seem unwarranted. Hence, the surgeon who ascertains that optimal debulking is not attainable or advisable has a critical decision to make at this point: to terminate the operation after biopsy and rely on chemotherapy alone or as neoadjuvant therapy prior to further surgery or to remove as much disease as possible. In most circumstances, the removal of bulk pelvic disease and the omentum is preferable to immediate closure, usually because of the probability of pelvic bulk and bowel obstruction. It is mandatory at this point to relieve obvious small or large bowel obstruction, even if resection with or without re-anastomosis (and required ostomy) is necessary.

Surgical debulking of epithelial ovarian cancer improves gut function, decreases respiratory embarrassment from reaccumulation of ascites, decreases the likelihood of inherently resistant clones to adjuvant chemotherapy, increases the number of cancer cells sensitive to chemotherapy by increasing the growth fraction of cells within tumor nodules, and may improve immunologic response to cancer.[19]

Surgical Technique

Assuming that optimal resection is probably achievable, the surgeon can choose between the upper abdomen and the pelvis as the first task. Whereas this may be a matter of personal preference, exposure to one or the other may be limited by bulk disease, thus often the choice is dictated by the presentation. Given the choice, we prefer to eliminate upper abdominal disease first, because removal of even the largest omental "cake" can be accomplished without major blood loss, whereas massive pelvic disease may cause extensive hemorrhage to remove. As is discussed, any major debulking procedure has the risk of consumptive coagulation problems; thus, if removal of upper abdominal disease is delayed, the surgeon may be faced with defects in clotting parameters and be forced to terminate the procedure prematurely. Thus, the omentum and transverse colon are mobilized to the field and removed with a standard clamp and tie technique. We have abandoned the staple instruments for this step because omental veins seem to ooze excessively and require additional overtying. The infracolic omentum is removed first, any defects in the colon repaired, and the infracolic and subgastric disease is removed subsequently. Diaphragmatic debulking can be accomplished and the area packed with gauze pads; such pressure can remain while the pelvic portion of the operation ensues. Because suturing on the diaphragmatic area is difficult, pressure is preferred for hemostasis.

The experienced surgeon relies on the retroperitoneal approach to facilitate removal of ovarian cancer in the pelvis. It may be necessary to start at the peritoneal reflection of the ascending or descending colon and work inferiorly to encircle the disease, but usually access can be gained by incising the round and broad ligaments, opening the pelvic spaces, identifying and protecting the ureters, and dissecting the entire pelvic peritoneum off the bladder, rectum, and pelvic sidewalls. Whereas the cancer may be removed en bloc by this pelvic peritonealectomy approach, there is no therapeutic advantage for advanced disease, and removal piecemeal may be more practical. At the conclusion of the resection, hemostasis is achieved; the surfaces and integrity of the ureters, small and large bowel, and bladder are ensured before copious irrigation; reassessment of the upper abdomen, removal of pads, instruments, and retractors, and final closure of the abdomen en masse follow. We do not routinely employ closed suction drainage, but it may be useful when rapid ascites reaccumulation is anticipated, there is considerable venous ooze present in the pelvis, or an anastomosis is tenuous and the presence of a drain comforts the surgeon. Although not mandatory, some gynecologic oncologists have found that debulking and hemostasis can be improved with the use of the CUSA (Cavitron ultrasonic surgical aspirator), titanium wire loops used for excision of cervical dysplasia, or the argon beam coagulator.

Postoperative care can be challenging, with fluid management, cardiopulmonary support, and return of bowel function being the major obstacles to rapid recovery. Certainly, the patient who has undergone a massive debulking procedure for ovarian cancer is most often critically ill, and management in an intensive care unit should be strongly considered; in no circumstance should the management team consider such a patient to be in the same category as a young healthy women expected to be discharged in 24 to 72 hours after hysterectomy for benign disease.

Several surgical issues may arise in the waning moments of the operation. First, the utility and necessity for lymphadenectomy or lymph node sampling must be weighed by the status of the patient after the major portion of the procedure is completed. Whereas lymph node sampling may be required by therapeutic protocol, we perform lymphadenectomy in advanced disease when (1) there is bulk lymph node disease and removal of such is necessary to achieve optimal categorization or (2) there is absolutely no visible residual disease and lymphadenectomy is essential to complete staging. The second surgical issue is the condition of the bowel and whether splinting colostomy should be utilized. The surgeon has already made the decision whether to resect bowel to allow optimal debulking in the earlier portions of the operation, but often at the conclusion of resection, the intestine, especially the rectosigmoid colon, may be battered and abraded by the necessary dissection, and be vulnerable to postoperative disruption. In general, we favor repair without colostomy but *this is a surgical decision made with the patient's safety as the major criterion.*

Neoadjuvant Chemotherapy

The issue of neoadjuvant chemotherapy is best addressed, in our opinion, preoperatively rather than during the surgical procedure. Although somewhat controversial, the initial approach with chemotherapy rather than debulking is gaining favor in some institutions, reserving debulking surgery to a subsequent interval after chemotherapy is theoretically attractive. The GOG is studying this issue in an ongoing study, with preliminary results suggesting that optimal debulking can be achieved after neoadjuvant therapy, but survival data are not yet available. In our practice, the preoperative assessment is critical in choosing whether to proceed with surgery or to choose neoadjuvant chemotherapy after percutaneous, vaginal, or laparoscopic biopsy. In general, women who are elderly (>80 years of age), frail (performance status < 2 by GOG criteria), with lim-

iting pleural effusions, or serious preexisting medical conditions may be better served by the neoadjuvant approach. Similarly, if imaging reveals the presence of extensive upper abdominal disease as described earlier, postponing the debulking procedure until after three or four courses of chemotherapy might allow more optimal debulking at a later date. Whereas many gynecologic oncology practices or institutions have rigid prospective protocols to render these choices moot, we prefer to assess patients on a case-by-case basis. For the most part, in patients who are younger and basically healthy and have none of the limiting factors as listed, we still champion the initial surgical treatment of ovarian cancer with aggressive surgery aimed at optimal debulking.

Laparoscopy in Ovarian Cancer

With advances in endoscopic technique, many surgeons are performing complex procedures laparoscopically. A patient with an apparent stage I epithelial ovarian cancer can be approached and staged completely laparoscopically. The appropriate staging surgery should not be limited in scope by the use of the laparoscope, however, if the surgeon's expertise does not allow for all indicated biopsies, including para-aortic lymph node sampling. Although attractive for its decreased postoperative morbidity, the minimally invasive approach should be considered with caution for those women who present with a preoperative evaluation worrisome for ascites or bulky, immobile disease. Additionally, whereas there are techniques that allow extracorporeal decompression and removal of large ovarian masses, the surgeon should always keep in mind that intraperitoneal spillage of cyst content automatically upstages the patient. Although it is uncertain whether this is associated with a worsened prognosis, *it most certainly will require that the patient undergo some form of adjuvant therapy,* which may have been optional if the capsule had remained intact. Trocar site metastases have been reported in approximately 15% of patients approached laparoscopically for epithelial ovarian cancer.[20] The decision to perform a laparotomy at the time of laparoscopic diagnosis of ovarian cancer should be discussed with the patient preoperatively. Delay in definitive staging and therapy should be avoided.

Staging of Ovarian Cancer

Accurate staging of ovarian cancer usually requires intraoperative assessment unless there is disease outside the abdomen; hence, FIGO (International Federation of Gynecology and Obstetrics) stage IV, this is recognized preoperatively (e.g., thoracentesis documenting positive cytology or CT scan showing parenchymal liver metastases).[21] Stage III ovarian cancer is substaged by the presence and size of disease outside the pelvis *determined at the onset of the intraoperative assessment;* thus, if there is only microscopic disease outside the pelvis, the case is allotted to stage IIIA. If there are deposits of cancer outside the pelvis no larger than 2 cm, stage IIIB disease is determined, and patients with disease of greater than 2 cm or with lymph node metastasis are allotted to stage IIIC. Stage II disease is present when all visible disease is confined to the pelvis, and stage II disease is substaged by the presence or absence of disease in both ovaries, the other pelvic structures, or the status of peritoneal fluid, washings, or capsule integrity. Because the boundaries of the pelvis are theoretical rather than real, we believe true stage II cases are unusual. Indeed, most stage II cases are so allotted with the realization that treatment will be identical in most circumstances to stage III. Thus, distinguishing between stage II and early stage III is more academic than actual.

Strict staging is essential for patients with disease apparently confined to the ovaries. These putative stage I cases must undergo a complete intraoperative surgical staging procedure that includes: (1) thorough total abdominal inspection and palpation after obtaining four quadrant washings for cytology or removal of ascites for analysis; (2) careful (so as to avoid rupture) removal of the ovaries, tubes, and uterus (some patients may request that the cervix not be removed); (3) multiple pelvic and gutter peritoneal biopsies; (4) at least partial omentectomy; (5) diaphragmatic assessment with scraping for cytology or actual biopsy of palpable lesions; (6) thorough inspection of the small intestine from the ligament of Treitz to the cecum, including examination of both mesenteric surfaces; (7) removal of the appendix; and (8) pelvic and para-aortic lymph node sampling. Unless this exacting staging procedure is followed and pathologic examination reveals no evidence of disease outside the ovaries, cases *cannot be allotted to stage I.* Those who are not availed this evaluation but have no apparent disease outside the ovaries must be categorized as "inadequately staged, apparent stage I" cases for determining adjuvant therapy. Whereas this is a common presentation of patients for postoperative consultation, there is no definitive consensus as to whether restaging should be accomplished. Older data suggest that 30% of such patients would be upstaged with a more thorough intraoperative evaluation, but each such case should be managed individually, as circumstances vary widely.[22]

Stage I is subdivided into IA, with disease confined to one ovary; IB, with disease present in ovaries bilaterally; and IC, in which the disease is confined to one or both ovaries, but with papillary excrescences on the surface of the ovaries, intraoperative rupture of the capsule, positive peritoneal cytology, or presence of ascites.

POSTOPERATIVE THERAPY

The foundations of postoperative treatment of patients who have undergone successful surgical staging are (1) thorough, expert pathologic examination, with determination of tumor grade and histologic cell type, and consideration of in vitro chemotherapy response testing, (2) complete and accurate surgical staging reports, and (3) consensus assignment of treatment recommendations. If possible, cases should be discussed in a multidisciplinary forum that allows group evaluation of the history, physical examination, preoperative assessment, intraoperative findings, microscopic slides, and overall case summary. Certainly, after such a forum, we prefer that the patients be treated under the auspices of an approved clinical trial; whereas this is not always possible or the patient may elect not to participate, we strongly support the concept of advancing science and providing care under such a structured umbrella of cancer care.

For early-stage disease, the surgical procedure alone may be curative and adjunctive therapy may not be indicated. But for most cases of ovarian cancer, chemotherapy is indicated after surgery; whereas radiation certainly has advocates for some situations, for the most part chemotherapy is the choice of most oncologists. When a clinical trial protocol is not available or applicable, the current standard chemotherapy for ovarian cancer is a combination of paclitaxel 175 mg/m², infused over 3 hours, and carboplatin, with an AUC (area under the carboplatin plasma disappearance curve) of 5 to 7, given intravenously every 3 weeks. This regimen is well tolerated, and premedication with steroids and antiemetics allow most patients to be treated without excessive morbidity. For early stages, three cycles might be sufficient, but for advanced stage disease six cycles is recommended. Patients are followed with weekly hematologic evalutions, and biochemical markers, such as CA-125 are repeated before each course of therapy. After completion of chemotherapy, most patients will achieve clinical and biochemical remission, and close follow-up is indicated. The GOG is currently evaluating the use of additional active chemotherapeutic agents combined with carboplatin/paclitaxel in the up-front treatment of advanced ovarian cancer.

The regimen of follow-up depends on individual preference, but we prefer to examine patients every 3 months for 2 years and every 6 months for 3 years, then yearly for life. Although occasionally indicated, follow-up imaging with CT or other scans may be misleading and is quite insensitive in discovering early recurrent disease.[23] A thorough physical examination and interval history, along with a careful pelvic examination, is, in our hands, just as predictive of recurrence and is less costly, time-consuming, and energy-absorbing for the patient.

Almost all practitioners utilize serum CA-125 measurements in their management of ovarian cancer. Although valuable in the ongoing treatment of ovarian cancer, its utility in screening and follow-up is questionable. Its limited predictive value in diagnosis of pelvic masses is well established. For women with elevated levels at the time of ovarian cancer diagnosis, decline after surgery and chemotherapy is a clear indication of the success of therapy. We prefer to utilize CA-125 as follow-up with minimal emphasis on its value in prognosis; however, for many women, it remains a focus of their well-being. The treatment of patients with an asymptomatic rising CA-125 is controversial and has not been shown to improve long-term survival.

The physician facing a woman with a complete clinical remission must communicate guarded optimism. Whereas most women achieve a clinical complete response, 50% will recur within 30 months.[24] It is the high rate of failure that has prompted many investigators to seek for ovarian cancer the consolidation therapy plan that has proved successful in other malignancies. Although of unproven benefit in ovarian cancer, continuation of chemotherapy can be considered in those patients with high risk of recurrence, and certainly for those patients who never achieve complete clinical remission. We prefer to treat such patients on protocol if available; if not, consolidation therapy is prescribed on a case-by-case basis. Consolidation options used include: weekly paclitaxel, oral hexamethylmelamine, or tamoxifen; intraperitoneal radiotherapy or chemotherapy; or whole abdominal radiotherapy. Each gynecologic oncologist or medical oncologist must choose the agent(s) in which they have the most confidence.

For many years, *second-look surgery* after completion of chemotherapy was the standard of care for ovarian cancer. Today, second-look is still an important tool of assessment for some protocols, but it is utilized infrequently for nonclinical trial management. Patients should realize preoperatively that at least 50% of pathologically negative second-look procedures are falsely negative, and that even the most fastidiously performed operation cannot guarantee that no evidence of disease will translate into permanent cure. We selectively offer second-look surgery but only to fulfill these objectives: (1) There must be a surgical or therapeutic advantage to second-look, such as reversal of a colostomy or correction of partial, chronic obstruction. (2) A plan must be in place for additional therapy or consolidation therapy if the second-look operation reveals no pathologic evidence of disease. (3) There must be therapeutic options for patients who have persistent disease at the time of second-look. Intraperitoneal chemotherapy was once heralded as the answer to this problem, and it is still actively promoted by some oncologists. Further chemotherapy, hormonal therapy, and immunotherapy are other options, but most importantly, the surgeon taking a patient to second-look must be prepared to offer a secondary maximal debulking effort if disease is present.

For most patients who achieve remission with no clinical evidence of disease, and CA-125 values or other marker values (for germ cell or stromal tumors, if applicable) that are within normal range, no further therapy is the most preferred plan of action. The patient is usually physically and emotionally drained from the ordeal of surgery and chemotherapy. We encourage these patients to rebuild their lives and enjoy each day to the fullest; although we know that most of them will relapse, prediction of whom is impossible.

MANAGEMENT OF RECURRENT OVARIAN CANCER

Unfortunately, however, many patients with ovarian cancer will relapse and exhibit evidence of recurrent disease, initially by an asymptomatic elevation of the tumor marker and, ultimately, symptoms similar to their original presentations. Often, effusions are the presenting culprit, either ascites with abdominal distention or pleural effusion with concomitant shortness of breath and respiratory embarrassment. Regardless, of the presentation, however, the sad truth is that for these patients, their disease is probably incurable. The goal of therapy is to treat as aggressively as possible, and at the same time maximize the quality of their lives.

Clinically, patients with recurrent ovarian cancer fall into two broad groups: the first group usually exhibits early recurrence, usually within a year of completion of therapy, and is symptomatic, with pain, pressure, obstruction, or effusion. These patients likely never were free of disease, but rather had disease minimized by therapy to a level undetectable on examination or imaging and laboratory evaluation. The second group experiences a relatively longer period of remission, usually 1 to 3 years, but often as long as 5 to 10 years. A woman in this group is more likely to be have a slow elevation of tumor marker, the appearance and slow growth of a mass on pelvic examination, or the gradual appearance of an effusion. Although both are treated with chemotherapy, their response to chemotherapy, and their expected survival are markedly different, the former usually dying of disease within 2 years, and the latter often surviving 4 to 10 years. Although factors such as stage at original presentation, tumor grade, age, performance status, and success of original surgery are important in predicting which group patients will be in, in reality the biology of their disease individually determines outcome, and clinicians and patients together embark on treatment of recurrence with a determined but guarded attitude.

Treatment options primarily involve chemotherapy, but surgery and radiation can play a role in selected patients. When considering salvage chemotherapy, convention and experience have suggested that a patient having a "platinum-free" interval of 6 months or more prior to recurrence should again respond to platinum-based therapy, and can be retreated with carboplatin/paclitaxel or carboplatin alone. Response rates of 45% to 60% have been reported in these "platinum-sensitive" patients. Patients relapsing less than 6 months after platinum therapy or those who have progressed on platinum-based therapy are considered "platinum resistant." Chemotherapeutic options include paclitaxel, topotecan, liposomal-encapsulated adriamycin, etoposide, gemcitabine, or hormones, such as tamoxifen or progestins. Response rates differ, but in general are 15% to 20%, with a 4- to 6-month duration of response. Tamoxifen provides an excellent therapeutic index for those patients in whom it is effective. Other hormonal preparations, including gonadotropin-releasing hormone analogues have been tried with little success. Progestin therapy is usually beneficial only in palliation, but it does have some positive metabolic effects.

For those with access, entry into a clinical trial can give a patient access to novel therapies, and participation in such trials should be encouraged. In women with chemoresistant disease, third-, fourth-, or fifth-line therapy should be selected to maximize quality of life and minimize toxicity. Patients like to believe that options remain after there is failure of the one currently being used, and we find the list of useful agents to be virtually endless. In the end, the patient and the physician must decide when further therapy is futile.

Surgical therapy with secondary debulking can play an important role in carefully selected patients. Women who recur more than 12 months from prior surgery and chemotherapy, who have localized disease by CT scan, particularly a dominant mass in the pelvis, and who had a complete response to prior chemotherapy are candidates for secondary debulking. Another patient who is a candidate for a maximal debulking effort is the woman operated on for intestinal obstruction but who is found to have easily resectable disease. Those who are debulked to microscopic disease enjoy a prolonged disease-free interval, but the impact on survival is unclear. Patients can be treated with standard intravenous chemotherapy or intraperitoneal therapy after secondary debulking. It is rare, in our experience, that third-look or a second attempt at secondary debulking is worth the expected complications. Again, these situations must be approached on a case-by-case basis.

For the most part, surgery plays a limited role in the management of recurrent ovarian cancer. Surgical intervention may be indicated for intestinal obstruction. When operating on a patient with an obstruction, the surgeon encounters one of the most difficult surgical choices in existence. Frequently, such patients have been on multiple regimens and had two or more surgical interventions, and their obstructions may be chronic or partial. The obstruction may even not be mechanical, as the *carcinomatous ileus* clinical picture is well known to oncologists and may best be treated medically, with motility agents such as metoclopramide and a low-residue diet. Furthermore, the sites of obstruction are likely to be embedded in tumor mass, which may make discovery and repair impossible. The procedure in all of these circumstances will be dictated by the findings, but it is wise to be as brief and mechanical as possible and not be tempted to do too much. We often remark that the vigor with which we approach such patients depends on our most recent success or failure. In our practice, we have discovered such reoperation to be gratifying for surgeon and patient in about one in five instances. As always, extensive informed consent is mandatory.

Biologic response modifiers such as interferon have occasionally been useful. Targeted genetic therapies such as trastuzumab also have enjoyed limited success.

There are situations in which radiation therapy may be useful, but cases should be selected carefully and in conjunction with an experienced radiation oncologist. Overall, the complication rate seems to preclude radiation therapy as a routine treatment for recurrent disease.

In Vitro Chemotherapy Response Testing

For many years, investigators have tried to develop assays that will aid in the selection of chemotherapy for patients. There are no data to suggest that in vitro chemotherapy response testing has affected survival of ovarian cancer. Critics of such testing argue that tumor heterogeneity and the limited response of ovarian cancer to salvage chemotherapy make the predictive value of in vitro testing too low to be clinically useful. Proponents of in vitro testing suggest that ineffective agents can be avoided and that perhaps more effective agents can be selected earlier in the course of therapy. In our experience, we have used chemosensitivity testing to select salvage therapy with a higher likelihood of response than that predicted by the literature.

END-OF-LIFE ISSUES IN OVARIAN CANCER

The physician as a compassionate friend who practices the art of medicine is nowhere more needed than in the terminal phases of patients with ovarian cancer. It is vitally important to establish a rapport with patients that allows frank discussions about the futility of treatment well before performance status suffers to the point at which the family has to make the tough decisions. We encourage patients to have open discussions with their families, and to nominate a Durable Power of Attorney, and if desired, sign a Living Will. We always enter into a contract with our patients that we will be honest with them about their illness and when it is "time to say when." Most patients know this already, but families are more difficult to convince.

All pain and nausea medications available should be used liberally. Hospice is invaluable in the care of these patients, and dying at home is much preferred. There is a great temptation, because ovarian cancer patients' terminal dynamic is bowel failure and starvation, to utilize hyperalimentation, but the wise provider does so with caution. We limit terminal intravenous feedings to limited situations, hopefully letting the patient make the choices as to how she wants to spend her final days.

CONCLUSION

Ovarian cancer is the fifth leading cause of cancer death in women, and because of its insidious presentation and overall poor outcome, it is feared almost as much as its more common companion, breast cancer. Although early diagnosis produces high survival rates, advanced disease is present at diagnosis 75% of the time. Aggressive surgical therapy followed by combination chemotherapy offers the best survival advantage, but most patients with advanced disease will eventually succumb. Clearly, all patients with ovarian cancer will benefit from having a gynecologic oncologist involved with all aspects of their management.

References

1. American Cancer Society, Inc: Cancer Facts and Figures 2000.
2. Whittemore AS: Characteristics relating to ovarian cancer risk: Implications for prevention and detection. Gynecol Oncol 1994;55:S15.
3. Rubin SC, Blackwood MA, Bandera C, et al: BRCA1, BRCA2, and hereditary nonpolyposis colorectal cancer gene mutations in an unselected ovarian cancer population: Relationship to family history and implications for genetic tesing. Am J Obstet Gynecol 1998;178:670.
4. Frank TS: Testing for hereditary risk of ovarian cancer. Cancer Control 1999;6:327.
5. Schildkraut JM, Thompson WD: Familial ovarian cancer: A population-based case-control study. Am J Epidemiol 1988;128:456.
6. Cramer DW, Hutchinson GB, Welch WR, et al: Factors affecting the association of oral contraceptives and ovarian cancer. N Engl J Med 1982;307:1047.
7. The cancer and steroid hormone study of the Centers for Disease Control and the National Institute of Child Health and Human Development. The reduction in risk of ovarian cancer associated with oral-contraceptive use. N Engl J Med 1987;316:650.
8. The WHO collaborative of neoplasia and steroid contraceptives. Epithelial ovarian cancer and combined oral contraceptives. Int J Epidemiol 1989;18:538.
9. Narod SA, Risch J, Moslehi R, et al: Oral contraceptives and the risk of hereditary ovarian cancer. N Engl J Med 1998;339:424.
10. Trimble EL: The NIH Consensus Development Conference on Ovarian Cancer: Screening, treatment, and follow-up. Gynecol Oncol 1994;55(3 pt 2):S1–S3.
11. van Nagell JR Jr, DePriest PD, Reedy MB, et al: The efficacy of transvaginal sonographic screening in asymptomatic women at risk for ovarian cancer. Gynecol Oncol 2000;77:350.
12. Jacobs IJ, Skates SJ, MacDonald N, et al: Screening for ovarian cancer: A pilot randomised controlled trial. Lancet 1999;353:1207.
13. Tobacman JK, Tucker MA, Kase R, et al: Intra-abdominal carcinomatosis after prophylactic oophorectomy in ovarian-cancer–prone families. Lancet 1982;2:795.
14. McGowan L, Lesher LP, Norris HJ, Barnett M: Misstaging of ovarian cancer. Obstet Gynecol 1985;65:568.
15. Malkasian GD, Knapp RC, Lavin DJ, et al: Preoperative evaluation of serum CA-125 values in premenopausal and postmenopausal patients with pelvic masses: discrimination of benign from malignant disease. Am J Obstet Gynecol 1988;159:341.
16. Currie JL: The cosmetically appealing transverse incision for large pelvic masses. ACOG Film Library.
17. Hacker NF, Berek JS, Lagasse LD, et al: Primary cytoreductive surgery for epithelial ovarian cancer. Obstet Gynecol 1983;61:413.
18. Hoskins WJ, McGuire WP, Brady MF, et al: The effect of diameter of largest residual disease on survival after primary cytoreductive surgery in patients with suboptimal residual epithelial ovarian carcinoma. Am J Obstet Gynecol 1994;170:974.
19. Skipper HE: Adjuvant chemotherapy. Cancer 1978;41:936.
20. Kruitwagen RF, Swinkels BM, Keyser KG, et al: Incidence and effect on survival of abdominal wall metastases at trocar or puncture sites following laparoscopy or paracentesis in women with ovarian cancer. Gynecol Oncol 1996;60:233.
21. SGO Handbook: Staging of Gynecologic Malignancies. Washington DC, Society of Gynecologic Oncology, January 1997.
22. Young RC, Decker DG, Wharton JT, et al: Staging laparotomy in early ovarian cancer. JAMA 1983;250:3072.
23. DeRosa V, Mangoni di Stefano ML, Brunetti A, et al: Computed tomography and second-look surgery in ovarian cancer patients. Correlation, actual role and limitations of CT scan. Eur J Gynecol Oncol 1995;16:123.
24. McGuire WP, Hoskins WJ, Brady MF, et al: Cyclophosphamide and cisplatin compared with paclitaxel and cisplatin in patients with stage III and IV ovarian cancer. N Engl J Med 1996;334:1.

What Is New in the Management of Gestational Trophoblastic Disease

John O. Schorge, Donald P. Goldstein,

Marilyn R. Bernstein, and Ross S. Berkowitz

Most obstetrician/gynecologists will encounter patients with gestational trophoblastic disease (GTD). GTDs are derived from placental tissue and have varying tendencies for local invasion and spread. Partial and complete hydatidiform mole, placental-site trophoblastic tumor (PSTT), and choriocarcinoma are each histologically distinct forms of the disease. GTD is characterized by a reliable tumor marker and exquisite sensitivity to chemotherapy. However, GTD may present with widespread metastases and is potentially fatal. In this chapter, we review new developments in the evaluation and treatment of this unique condition.

COMPLETE AND PARTIAL MOLAR PREGNANCY

The reported incidence of complete molar pregnancy varies widely throughout the world from 1 per 500 pregnancies in Japan to 1 per 1000 to 1500 pregnancies in Europe and North America. Global regions with a high incidence of vitamin A deficiency and low fat content in the diet correspond to areas with a high frequency of complete molar pregnancy. Furthermore, the risk of developing a complete mole increases with advancing maternal age. The reported incidence of partial mole is about 1 per 700 pregnancies, and the risk has not been related to diet or maternal age, but is increased in women with a prior history of menstrual irregularity or spontaneous abortion.

Molar pregnancy is composed of two separate entities, complete and partial, which are distinct on the basis of histopathology, karyotype, and natural history.[1] Complete moles contain no fetal tissue and consist of diffusely hydropic chorionic villi, often described as "grapelike" vesicles, with diffuse trophoblastic hyperplasia. Partial moles are composed of a mixture of normal and hydropic, irregularly shaped villi with focal trophoblastic hyperplasia. The fetus of a partial mole generally is not viable and exhibits characteristic malformations of triploidy, including syndactyly, hydrocephalus, and growth retardation.

Complete moles have a diploid karyotype (usually 46,XX or, infrequently, 46,XY), and all chromosomes are paternally derived. In more than 90% of cases, a haploid (23,X) sperm fertilizes an anuclear ovum and then duplicates its own chromosomes. Partial moles have a triploid karyotype (69,XXX or 69,XXY) and result from fertilization of a "normal" ovum with two haploid sperm (either 23,X or 23,Y).

Persistent GTD occurs in 20% of patients with a complete mole. Patients with signs of marked trophoblastic growth, including excessive uterine size, markedly elevated human chorionic gonadotropin (hCG) levels, and theca lutein ovarian cysts, are particularly at risk of developing persistent tumor. In contrast, partial moles give rise to persistent GTD in only 3% to 4% of patients. Virtually all patients with persistent tumor after partial mole have nonmetastatic disease, whereas 4% of patients with persistent tumor after complete molar pregnancy develop metastases.

THE CHANGING NATURAL HISTORY OF COMPLETE HYDATIDIFORM MOLE

Classically, patients with complete moles were diagnosed in the second trimester. The main symptoms were heavy vaginal bleeding, hyperemesis gravidarum, theca lutein ovarian cysts, and uterine size larger than expected for dates. They frequently developed medical complications such as anemia, preeclampsia, and hyperthyroidism. Owing to the sensitivity of current diagnostic methods including ultrasound and quantitative hCG, the diagnosis of complete mole is now commonly being made during the first trimester.[2] Although the majority of patients still present with vaginal bleeding, excessive uterine size, anemia, hyperemesis and other associated symptoms are now uncommon. An hCG greater than 100,000 mIU/mL and/or ultrasonographic demonstration of an absent fetus and cystic placenta suggests the diagnosis of a complete mole. The classic "snowstorm" appearance on ultrasound may not be present during the first trimester. In some cases, the diagnosis may be made only after an evacuation for a presumed incomplete or missed abortion.[2]

Patients with partial moles usually present with vaginal bleeding and rarely exhibit any associated signs or symptoms. An elevated hCG or characteristic ultrasound appearance may suggest a molar pregnancy. In most cases, the diagnosis is based on pathologic review of curettage specimens from a presumed missed abortion.

The earlier clinical diagnosis of complete molar pregnancy can make histopathologic differentiation of complete and partial molar pregnancy and hydropic abortion more problematic. Karyotyping is a useful adjunct in these circumstances. Importantly, although complete moles are being diagnosed earlier in pregnancy, the incidence of postmolar persistent GTD has not been affected.

PLACENTAL SITE TROPHOBLASTIC TUMOR

PSTT is an uncommon variant of GTD; fewer than 100 cases were reported in the English-language literature. This tumor may arise after any type of pregnancy and is thought to derive from the intermediate trophoblasts of the placental bed. Chorionic villi are rarely present. Owing to the relative absence of syncytiotrophoblast, PSTT tends to produce low levels of hCG. Unlike in other variants of GTD, the poor correlation between tumor volume and hCG level limits the effectiveness of monitoring PSTT for a complete disease response. Surgery plays a major role in its management owing to the relative insensitivity to chemotherapy. Unfortunately, because PSTT has been recognized as a distinct entity for only a short time, the correct diagnosis is often delayed.

The majority of patients present with irregular vaginal bleeding, although other systemic symptoms, such as amenorrhea, galactorrhea, or nephrotic syndrome, may occur. When PSTT is diagnosed on endometrial curettage, a thorough metastatic workup should be performed to exclude metastatic disease. Fortunately, PSTT is usually confined to the uterus. The presence of metastases is an ominous sign. An interval longer than 2 years from the antecedent pregnancy to clinical presentation is a major adverse prognostic variable.

For nonmetastatic disease, the primary treatment should be hysterectomy. Patients with extrauterine metastases should be treated with aggressive combination chemotherapy. Recently, weekly etoposide, methotrexate, and actinomycin D alternating with etoposide and cisplatin (Platinol) (EMA/EP) has been shown to be effective in some patients with metastatic PSTT.[3]

CATEGORIES OF GESTATIONAL TROPHOBLASTIC DISEASE

Successful therapy for persistent GTD depends to a large extent on the presence of risk factors such as duration of disease, pretreatment hCG level, presence or absence of brain or liver metastases, and proper selection of chemotherapy. Classification and staging systems have been developed to help the clinician choose the most appropriate treatment. In the 1970s, Hammond and associates[4] described a clinical classification that is still commonly used (Table 94–1). The World Health Organization (WHO)[5] proposed a prognostic scoring system based on risk factors (Table 94–2) in the 1980s. More recently, the International

Table 94–1. Hammond's Clinical Classification of Gestational Trophoblastic Disease

I. Nonmetastatic
II. Metastatic
  A. Good prognosis
    1. hCG < 100,000 mIU/24 hr (urine) or < 40,000 mIU/mL (serum)
    2. Symptoms present for < 4 mo
    3. No brain or liver metastases
    4. No prior chemotherapy
    5. Antecedent pregnancy not term
  B. Poor prognosis
    1. hCG > 100,000 mIU/24 hr (urine) or > 40,000 mIU/mL (serum)
    2. Symptoms present for > 4 mo
    3. Brain or liver metastases
    4. Prior chemotherapeutic failure
    5. Antecedent term pregnancy

hCG, human chorionic gonadotropin.
Data from Hammond CB, Borchert LG, Tyrey L, et al: Treatment of metastatic trophoblastic disease. Am J Obstet Gynecol 1973;115:451–457.

Federation of Gynecology and Obstetrics (FIGO)[6] proposed a combined scoring and staging system based on both anatomic distribution of disease and risk factors (Table 94–3). Although all three systems have been in use for many years, there is still considerable disagreement on which provides the most helpful guidance. None has been shown to be clearly superior, but the majority of gynecologic oncologists still utilize Hammond and associates'[4] clinical classification.

Each of the staging systems is effective in selecting patients for single-agent chemotherapy. Appropriate candidates for single-agent chemotherapy include nonmetastatic or low-risk metastatic GTD (Hammond classification), patients with WHO scores of up to 7, and FIGO stages I, IIA, and IIIA. Single-agent chemotherapy is expected to

Table 94–2. World Health Organization Prognostic Scoring System for Gestational Trophoblastic Disease

Parameter	0	1	2	3
Age (yr)	<39	>39		
Antecedent pregnancy	Mole	Abortion	Term	
Interval†	<4	4–6	7–12	>12
Pretreatment hCG	<10^3	10^3–10^4	10^4–10^5	>10^5
Largest tumor (cm)		3–5	>5	
Site of metastases		Spleen Kidney	GI Liver	Brain
Number of metastases		1–4	4–8	>8
Prior chemotherapy failed			Single	>2

*Total score for a patient is obtained by adding the individual scores for each prognostic factor. Total score <5, low risk; 5–7, medium risk; >7, high risk.
†"Interval" is the number of months between the end of the antecedent pregnancy and the start of chemotherapy.
GI, gastrointestinal; hCG, human chorionic gonadotropin.
Data from World Health Organization Scientific Group: Gestational Trophoblastic Diseases (Technical Report Series No. 692). Geneva, WHO, 1983.

Table 94–3. International Federation of Gynecology and Obstetrics Staging System for Gestational Trophoblastic Disease

Stage

I. Disease confined to the uterus
II. Disease extending outside the uterus but limited to the genital structures (adnexa, vagina, broad ligament)
III. Disease extending to the lungs, with or without known genital tract involvement
IV. Disease at other metastatic sites

Substage

A. No risk factor
B. One risk factor
C. Two risk factors

Risk Factors

hCG > 100,000 mIU/mL
Duration from termination of the antecedent pregnancy to diagnosis > 6 mo

hCG, human chorionic gonadotropin.
Data from Goldstein DP, Zanten-Przybysz IV, Bernstein MR, Berkowitz RS: Revised FIGO staging system for gestational trophoblastic tumors. J Reprod Med 1998;43:37–43.

induce complete remission in about 80% of patients with either nonmetastatic or low-risk metastatic disease. A minority of women will require a treatment change to alternative single-agent therapy or combination chemotherapy, but eventually cure is anticipated for all patients with low-risk GTD.

Patients with high-risk metastatic GTD (Hammond classification), WHO scores of greater than 7, or FIGO stages IIB/C, IIIB/C, and IV are treated with initial combination chemotherapy with or without adjuvant radiotherapy or surgery.[6] Historically, such patients who primarily received single-agent therapy were prone to developing resistant disease and had a significantly decreased survival despite secondary treatment with combination therapy. Approximately 25% to 30% of patients with high-risk metastatic GTD will have an incomplete response to first-line chemotherapy or will relapse from remission and require secondary chemotherapy.

Treatment of Persistent Gestational Trophoblastic Disease

In patients with nonmetastatic disease, the selection of treatment for persistent GTD is based on whether the patient desires to preserve fertility.[7] Hysterectomy with adjuvant single-agent chemotherapy at the time of surgery is suitable for patients who have completed childbearing. Virtually all such patients will achieve sustained remission without further treatment. In patients with nonmetastatic GTD who desire to preserve fertility, single-agent chemotherapy is the treatment of choice. Complete sustained remission can be expected in 90% to 95% of these patients,

and the remaining patients may achieve remission with combination chemotherapy.

Methotrexate was the first chemotherapeutic drug widely used to treat GTD. Although many patients were cured, some proved to be resistant. Actinomycin D was later shown to have clinical activity in women with methotrexate-resistant GTD. Methotrexate and actinomycin D have remained the two cornerstones in the chemotherapeutic treatment of persistent GTD. The regimens utilized for single-agent chemotherapy are summarized in Table 94–4. Folinic acid is routinely used to minimize the hematologic and epithelial toxicity from methotrexate. When patients experience resistance to one drug, as determined by a plateau or re-elevation of the hCG level, or if excessive toxicity is encountered, therapy is switched to the alternative drug.

The primary multidrug regimen used as initial therapy in patients with high-risk metastatic GTD for most of the 1970s and 1980s was methotrexate, actinomycin D, and cyclophosphamide (MAC). Reported cure rates ranged from 50% to 55%. In the mid-1980s, etoposide was shown to be highly effective in GTD. During the 1990s, etoposide, methotrexate, actinomycin D, cyclophosphamide, and vincristine (Oncovin) (EMA/CO) has demonstrated a complete clinical response rate in excess of 80% in patients with high-risk metastatic GTD. However, women treated with etoposide have an increased risk of secondary tumors, including myeloid leukemia, colon cancer, breast cancer, and melanoma. Etoposide should therefore be reserved to treat patients who are likely to be resistant to single-agent chemotherapy and, in particular, patients with high-risk metastatic disease.

Patients resistant to EMA/CO may be treated with modifications, including substituting etoposide and cisplatin for cyclophosphamide and vincristine (EMA/EP). Whole-brain irradiation can be used in patients with brain metastases to prevent acute hemorrhage from tumor. Rarely, surgery is

Table 94–4. Single-Agent Chemotherapy Protocols Utilized in Treating Gestational Trophoblastic Disease

MTX

5 days: 0.4–0.5 mg/kg, IM or IV, qd × 5
Weekly: 50 mg/m², IM or IV

MTX with Folinic Acid Rescue

8 days: MTX, 1 mg/kg, IM, days: 1, 3, 5, 7
   Folinic acid, 0.1 mg/kg, PO, days 2, 4, 6, 8
12-hr infusion:
   MTX, 100 mg/m² in 250 mL normal saline solution over 30 min, then 200 mg/m², 12-hr infusion
   Folinic acid, 15 mg, PO, q12h × 4 doses (to start 24 hr after initial MTX administration)

Actinomycin D

IV bolus: 12 μg/kg, qd × 5
Weekly: 1.25 mg/m², IV bolus

MTX, methotrexate.

necessary to control acute bleeding from trophoblastic tumors in the liver, brain, or bowel. In addition, surgical resection of lung or liver tumors may be performed as an adjuvant to chemotherapy.

Patients with resistance to EMA/CO and EMA/EP may be treated with the bleomycin, etoposide, and cisplatin (BEP) or cisplatin, vinblastine, and bleomycin (PVB) protocols. The likelihood of achieving sustained remissions with BEP or PVB may be only as high as 20% with considerable hematologic toxicity, and surgical resection is often required.[8] The activity of new anticancer agents, such as paclitaxel and topotecan, needs to be assessed in cases of refractory GTD.

SUBSEQUENT PREGNANCY EXPERIENCE

After completing follow-up for a complete or partial molar pregnancy or persistent GTD, patients should be reassured that their expectation for a normal future pregnancy is about the same as that of the general population. Specifically, these patients have no increased risk for congenital anomalies or spontaneous abortion. However, after a molar pregnancy, the risk for molar gestation in a subsequent conception is increased to about 1%.

References

1. Berkowitz RS, Goldstein DP: Presentation and management of molar pregnancy. In Hancock BW, Newlands ES, Berkowitz RS (eds): Gestational Trophoblastic Disease. London, Chapman and Hall, 1997, pp. 127–142.
2. Soto-Wright V, Bernstein M, Goldstein DP, Berkowitz RS: The changing clinical presentation of complete molar pregnancy. Obstet Gynecol 1995;86:775–779.
3. Newlands ES, Bower M, Fisher RA, Paradinas FJ: Management of placental site trophoblastic tumors. J Reprod Med 1998;43:53–59.
4. Hammond CB, Borchert LG, Tyrey L, et al: Treatment of metastatic trophoblastic disease. Am J Obstet Gynecol 1973;115:451–457.
5. World Health Organization Scientific Group: Gestational Trophoblastic Diseases (Technical Report Series No. 692). Geneva, WHO, 1983.
6. Goldstein DP, Zanten-Przybysz IV, Bernstein MR, Berkowitz RS: Revised FIGO staging system for gestational trophoblastic tumors. J Reprod Med 1998;43:37–43.
7. Berkowitz RS, Goldstein DP: Chorionic tumors. N Engl J Med 1996;335:1740–1748.
8. Lurain JR: Managment of high-risk gestational trophoblastic disease. J Reprod Med 1998;43:44–52.

NINETY-FIVE

Human Papillomavirus and Genital Neoplasia

Robert T. Morris

Although the frequency of human papillomavirus (HPV) infection varies by the population examined and the method of detection, the prevalence of the virus is high among young women. Most will demonstrate no clinical evidence of HPV infection; however, HPV-mediated oncogenesis is responsible for up to 95% of squamous cell cancers of the cervix and nearly all preinvasive cervical neoplasms. Although there is currently no treatment for HPV infection, early detection and treatment of HPV-mediated neoplasia has become a cornerstone in prevention of lower genital tract cancer. This chapter briefly addresses HPV epidemiology, current techniques of detecting and treating HPV-mediated neoplasia, and future directions.

EPIDEMIOLOGY

Genital HPV infection is very common. Exact prevalence figures are difficult to obtain, but using molecular techniques, 10% to 20% of women of reproductive age will have clinical evidence of HPV genital infection and up to 50% will have evidence of HPV detectable by polymerase chain reaction.[1] Most infected people have latent or subclinical infection. Only 1% of the sexually active population will demonstrate clinically apparent genital warts. Furthermore, it is clear that the prevalence of HPV infection is higher than the prevalence of cervical dysplasia by at least one order of magnitude. It is estimated that 1 million women are diagnosed with cervical dysplasia annually in the United States. Epidemiologic data have long suggested a sexually transmitted etiology for cervical neoplasia. The risk for cervical neoplasia—and HPV infection—is higher among women with multiple sexual partners, who have first sexual intercourse at an early age, and whose partners are sexually promiscuous. It has also been suggested that immunosuppression (such as in patients with HIV, allograft transplants, lupus, or Hodgkin's disease) increases risk for HPV infection and cervical neoplasia.

Among the more than 100 different types of HPV, various clinical lesions are appreciated, as listed in Table 95–1. Types 6 and 11 are associated with condyloma acuminata, and types 16 and 18 are strongly associated with invasive cervical cancer. Molecular biologic studies provide nearly irrefutable evidence that HPV is a causative factor in lower genital tract malignancy. HPV DNA sequences can be isolated from nearly all preinvasive and invasive cervical neoplasms. Furthermore, in vitro and in vivo studies have demonstrated HPV oncoproteins capable of malignant transformation. It appears that these oncoproteins (E6 and E7) bind and inactivate the endogenous p53 and Rb tumor suppressors, respectively. Although many HPV types are capable of malignant transformation, HPV 16 and 18 oncoproteins have much higher binding affinities for the tumor suppressors. As noted in Table 95–1, the HPV types are classified according to their risk of inducing cervical neoplasia. Several types of HPV have been detected in mild dysplasia, but only a narrow spectrum of types is detected in severe dysplasia and invasive cancer. HPV types 16, 18, 31, 45, and 56 account for over 80% of invasive cervical cancers; HPV 16 is the predominant type in these lesions. Because risk can be attributed to each specific HPV type, HPV type analysis via Hybrid Capture II (Digene, Silver Spring, Md) has become clinically useful in the management of cervical neoplasia.

CERVICAL CYTOLOGIC SCREENING

Whereas the mammogram is a screening tool to detect cancer at an early, more treatable, stage of the disease, the Pap smear is a screening tool intended for cancer prevention. Such prevention is possible by detecting the preinvasive phase of the disease—namely, cervical dysplasia. Currently, the American College of Obstetricians and Gynecologists recommend initiation of Pap smears at age 18 years, or at the age of initiation of sexual activity. Annual examinations should be continued until three or more consecutive, satisfactory, normal examinations are documented; thereafter smears can be performed less frequently at the clinician's discretion. The Bethesda System for Reporting Cervical/Vaginal Cytologic Diagnoses (Table 95–2) is currently the standard for reporting. Not only does the system provide terms that correlate to histologic findings, but it also reports on specimen adequacy.

Recent criticism of the Pap smear has been focused on the rate of false-negative smears in patients with disease.

Table 95–1. Human Papillomavirus Types and Common Lower Genital Lesions

Clinical Lesion	HPV Types
Plantar wart	1
Common wart	2, 4
Genital wart	6, 11
High-risk cervical neoplasia	16, 18, 31, 45, 56
Intermediate-risk cervical neoplasia	30, 33, 35, 39, 51, 52, 58, 66
Low-risk cervical neoplasia	6, 11, 42, 43, 44, 53, 54, 55

HPV, human papillomavirus.

Table 95–2. The Bethesda System for Reporting Cervical/Vaginal Cytologic Diagnoses

Format of the report
  a. A statement on Adequacy of the Specimen for Evaluation
  b. A General Categorization that may be used to assist with clerical triage (optimal)
  c. The Descriptive Diagnosis

Adequacy of the Specimen

Satisfactory for evaluation
Satisfactory for evaluation but limited by . . . (specify reason)
Unsatisfactory for evaluation . . . (specify reason)

General Categorization (Optional)

Within normal limits
Benign cellular changes: see descriptive diagnoses
Epithelial cell abnormality: see descriptive diagnoses

Descriptive Diagnoses

Benign cellular changes
  Infection
    Trichomonas vaginalis
    Fungal organisms morphologically consistent with *Candida* species
    Predominance of coccobacilli consistent with shift in vaginal flora
    Bacteria morphologically consistent with *Actinomyces* species
    Cellular changes associated with herpes simplex virus
    Other
Reactive changes
  Reactive cellular changes associated with:
    Inflammation (includes typical repair)
    Atrophy with inflammation ("atrophic vaginitis")
    Radiation
    Intrauterine contraceptive device
    Other

Epithelial cell abnormalities
  Squamous cell
    Atypical squamous cells of undetermined significance: Qualify*
    Low-grade squamous intraepithelial lesion encompassing:
      HPV†
      Mild dysplasia/CIN 1
    High-grade squamous intraepithelial lesion encompassing:
      Moderate and severe dysplasia
      CIS/CIN2 and CIN3
      Squamous cell carcinoma
Glandular cell abnormalities
  Endometrial cells, cytologically benign, in a postmenopausal woman
  Atypical glandular cells of undetermined significance: Qualify*
  Endocervical adenocarcinoma
  Endometrial adenocarcinoma
  Extrauterine adenocarcinoma
  Adenocarcinoma, not otherwise specified (NOS)
  Other malignant neoplasms (specify)
  Hormonal evaluation (applied to vaginal smears only)
  Hormonal pattern compatible with age and history
  Hormonal pattern incompatible with age and history (specify)
  Hormonal evaluation not possible due to (specify)

*Atypical squamous or glandular cells of undetermined significance should be further qualified as to whether a reactive or a premalignant/malignant process is favored.
†Cellular changes of human papillomavirus (HPV)—previously termed koilocytosis atypia, or condylomatous atypia—are included in the category of low-grade squamous intraepithelial.
  CIN, cervical intraepithelial neoplasia; CIS, carcinoma in situ.

Despite this criticism, the screening test has proved to significantly affect the incidence and mortality of cervical cancer throughout the world. Since implementation of the screening test, the incidence of cervical cancer has decreased by 85% in British Columbia, and the mortality has decreased by 70% in the United States. Although no randomized trials are available, data such as these provide compelling evidence to support the continued use of the Pap test. In countries where screening is not available, most patients diagnosed with invasive cervical cancer have not been screened at recommended intervals. In the United States, 50% of patients diagnosed with cervical cancer have never had a Pap smear, and an additional 10% have not had one in the past 5 years. This is not always attributable to noncompliance or lack of access to medical care. Sung[2] found that 60% of women diagnosed with invasive cervical cancer in a large health maintenance organization (HMO) had not a Pap smear within 3 years, even though they were enrolled in the HMO.

Recent advances in cervical screening have become available to the clinician and are well addressed by Spitzer.[3] Although the principle of microscopic assessment of exfoliated cells from the ectocervix, endocervix, and transformation zone remains the same, new technology has been introduced to potentially reduce the false-negative rate. The rate is variable; however, most estimates place it between 15% and 25%. Half of false-negative smears are attributable to sampling error, and half are attributed to errors in interpretation. Strategies for reducing false-negative results (improving sensitivity) have targeted both of these causes of error.

Automated cytologic screening utilizes computerized image analysis and computerized rescreening of 100% of the smears. The AutoPap system (Neopath, Redmond, Wash) assigns negative smears an aggregate score indicative of the probability of being falsely negative. The top 10% of these negative slides are then selected for manual rescreening. The PapNet system (Neuromedical Systems, Sufferin, NY) records digitized images of abnormal fields on the smear, which are then reviewed by a technologist. On-screen images that are identified as abnormal or have the possibility of being falsely negative are referred to the microscope for manual review. Both systems increase the workload that a laboratory can process and, more importantly, improve the sensitivity. Automated screening will detect three to seven times the number of false-negative screenings, compared with the standard of manually reviewing only 10% of smears as mandated by law. However, automated screening identifies only 50% of the false-negative results detected if all smears were to be manually rescreened. Compared to AutoPap, PapNet appears to be more sensitive, especially in detecting smears likely to be missed by conventional screening. Whereas conventional cytologic screening remains the standard, automated cytologic screening certainly demonstrates promise in improving sensitivity.

Optimizing the collection and preparation of cells has been demonstrated to improve sensitivity as well. Two systems are clinically available that utilize fluid-based technology to create a cellular monolayer for cytologic studies. The specimen is collected and rinsed into a vial of preservation fluid. The fluid lyses fresh red blood cells, destroys bacteria, and removes most of the mucus. The sample is mixed, passed through a filter, and transferred to a slide for review. The result is an evenly dispersed monolayer of cells devoid of mucus, red blood cells, and bacteria. ThinPrep (Cytec Corporation, Boxborough, Mass) is approved by the U.S. Food and Drug Administration and has been demonstrated to have sensitivity in detecting dysplastic and malignant lesions superior to that of conventionally prepared slides. Furthermore, the frequencies of unsatisfactory slides and atypical squamous cells of undetermined significance (ASCUS) diagnosis are reduced with monolayer slides. The cost of ThinPrep may be double the cost of conventional slides and has hampered universal acceptance. Although conventional cytology remains the standard, the use of ThinPrep may be justified in certain populations. Groups with a high prevalence of HPV infection or a high rate of unsatisfactory Pap smears would be expected to benefit most from this technique.

Management Strategies for Abnormal Cervical Cytology

When an abnormal Pap smear is detected, further investigation is usually warranted. Management is primarily dictated by the cytologic findings, and in part by the patient's risk factors, compliance, and reproductive history. All patients with cytologic evidence of high-grade squamous intraepithelial lesions (HGSIL) should undergo colposcopic evaluation, with directed biopsy and endocervical curettage when indicated. Patients with low-grade squamous intraepithelial lesions (LGSIL) or with ASCUS may have more individualized management. In compliant patients without risk factors, without immunosuppression, and with no prior history of dysplasia, the Pap smear may be repeated in 3 months. In this group, cytologic screening should be repeated every 3 months until three normal consecutive results are obtained. If persistent abnormality is detected, colposcopy with directed biopsies is indicated. In patients with ASCUS or LGSIL with risk factors or who are perceived to be potentially noncompliant, colposcopy with directed biopsies should be performed at the onset.

The optimal management of ASCUS is controversial. Although the frequency of the ASCUS diagnosis should account for less than 5% of all Pap smear diagnoses, the rate is highly variable and dependent on the particular laboratory. Most data indicate that 20% of patients with ASCUS will subsequently be diagnosed with severe or moderate dysplasia. The expense burden created by the subsequent workup of the ASCUS diagnosis has resulted in strategies to manage these patients in a cost-effective manner. Most strategies have eliminated immediate colposcopic assessment either by repeating the screening Pap smear in low-risk patients or by utilizing HPV type analysis. Hybrid Capture II (Digene, Silver Spring, Md) is a highly sensitive commercial HPV DNA test that detects nine high-risk and five low-risk HPV types. Current data do not support the use of such testing as a general screen; however, it may prove effective in triaging patients with ASCUS. An ongoing trial in the United States triages patients with ASCUS to either colposcopy or repeat Pap smear according to the presence of high-risk HPV. With this strategy, 40% to 60% of patients may avoid colposcopy, depending on the prevalence of HPV in the particular population.

Patients with atypical glandular cells of undetermined significance (AGCUS) have a high frequency of severe squamous dysplasia, endocervical adenocarcinoma in situ, and invasive endocervical and endometrial cancers. Evaluation should include colposcopy, endocervical curettage, and in postmenopausal patients, endometrial biopsy. In patients with persistent AGCUS with no abnormalities with the studies previously discussed, consideration should be given to pelvic ultrasound assessment and cervical cone biopsy.

Physical Findings

HPV-mediated vulvar pathology includes condylomata, vulvar intraepithelial neoplasia (VIN), and invasive squamous cell cancer. Condyloma present as raised verrucous, hyperkeratotic papules, which are frequently pigmented. VIN lesions appear as thickened epithelium with discrete borders. They are most often white, but may also appear hyperpigmented or erythematous. Application of 5% acetic acid for 2 to 5 minutes will often make the lesions more distinguishable. The use of a colposcope in visualizing the vulva has been frequently recommended; however, the findings and histology are not as well correlated as in cervical colposcopy. Overall, little benefit is obtained by such examination. Frankly invasive cancers are fleshy and may be ulcerative or exophytic. Necrosis and marked tenderness are also features suggested of invasive cancer. Regardless of clinical impression, histologic diagnosis is necessary before initiating therapy. A 3- to 5-mm dermal punch biopsy in the most abnormal portion of the lesion provides an adequate sample. If multiple lesions are noted, several biopsies may be necessary.

Vaginal condyloma appear similar to vulvar condyloma, and vaginal intraepithelial neoplasia (VAIN) usually appears as flat or slightly raised white epithelium. Colposcopic assessment with the use of acetic acid should thoroughly evaluate the entire vaginal surface. Although nonspecific for dysplastic tissue, the use of Lugol's solution often demonstrates abnormalities missed at first inspection. Like vulvar lesions, biopsies should be obtained liberally before therapy.

Cervical neoplasia is often undetectable to the naked eye. Obvious lesions should be biopsied and considered malignant until otherwise proven. In the workup of abnormal screening cytology, the colposcope is indispensable. Biopsies should be liberally performed in abnormal areas, which should be appropriately labeled. Endocervical curettage provides highly useful information, particularly in unsatisfactory examinations and in circumstances in which colposcopic appearance is less severe than the cytologic diagnosis. Most nonpregnant patients should have an endocervical curettage at the time of colposcopic examination.

Cervical cone biopsy is indicated in patients with microinvasive disease on punch biopsy, cytologic or histologic evidence of malignant glandular epithelium (adenocarcinoma in situ), or when the cytologic and histologic diagnoses are markedly discrepant. Historically, incomplete visualization of the transformation zone and dysplasia on an endocervical curettage have been indications for cervical cone biopsy. It is the author's belief that these circumstances require individualized management. Cone biopsy may be performed by scalpel, laser, or loop electrocautery excision procedure (LEEP).

TREATMENT OF NONINVASIVE LOWER GENITAL NEOPLASIA

Condylomata of the vulva or vagina may be excised using sharp excision, cautery, or LEEP. Furthermore, they may be ablated using cautery, laser, cryotherapy, or chemical means. Commonly used chemical means include trichloroacetic acid, podophylin, and fluorouracil (5-FU). Cure rates are highly dependent on the extent of disease and patient compliance; however, overall cure rates for all methods are 40% to 60%. For small unifocal vulvar lesions, in-office excision is preferred. Multifocal vulvar and vaginal lesions are best treated with CO_2 laser vaporization. Very extensive vaginal lesions may be treated with 5-FU; however, vulvar topical 5-FU is poorly tolerated. New approaches such as vaccines and immunomodulation show promise. Imiquimod stimulates monocytes, macrophages, and keratinocytes to produce cytokines and interferon. Clinical trials of this topical treatment indicate a 70% response rate.

Treatment of preinvasive vulvar neoplastic lesions must be individualized according to size, location, and patient age. Although the previously mentioned excisional and ablative techniques are available for VIN, wide local excision using the scalpel and CO_2 laser vaporization have become the standard approaches. Cure rates for each are 80% to 90%. Excisional techniques have the benefit of providing a pathologic specimen and rapid healing; however, scar formation, deformation, and stricture may result. In contrast, laser vaporization is functionally and cosmetically superior; however, slow wound healing and lack of specimen are drawbacks. Because postmenopausal patients more frequently have invasive lesions, wide local excision is frequently preferred. Younger patients who have had representative biopsies are best managed with laser vaporization. In general, small lesions remote from the clitoris may be treated by either method in the office using local anesthetic. Any lesion greater than 2 cm or near the clitoris should be treated in an ambulatory surgery setting with adequate anesthesia. Postoperative management includes spraying the region with a handheld shower three to four times daily, blotting dry, and then drying with a handheld blow dryer on a cool setting.

Similar to vaginal condylomata, ablative and excisional approaches have been utilized in the treatment of vaginal dysplasia. The most commonly used techniques are CO_2 laser vaporization, partial vaginectomy, and intravaginal 5-FU. In any patient in whom invasion is suspected, especially patients over the age of 50 years, partial vaginectomy is indicated. The cure rate after excision (partial vaginectomy) is 90%. In younger patients who have had ample biopsies, laser ablation or intravaginal 5-FU may be considered. The cure rates for these approaches are 85% and 80%, respectively. Excision and laser ablation have the benefit of being short outpatient procedures with relatively rapid recovery. However, their use is restricted to limited disease. Very expansive lesions are best addressed by 5-FU; however, the application requires 2 weeks to 6 months, depending on the regimen. The most common regimens are every other night for 2 weeks, or 5 nights per month for 3 to 6 months. The profound sloughing of the vaginal mucosa and vulvar irritation are often poorly tolerated by elderly or sexually active patients.

The treatment of cervical intraepithelial neoplasia (CIN) is dependent on the histologic findings and the patient's age and reproductive history. The natural history of CIN is well reviewed by Oster[4] in a comprehensive review of the literature. Of patients with mild dysplasia (CIN 1), nearly 60% will regress and only 1% will progress to invasive cervical cancer. In contrast, severe dysplasia (CIN 3) regresses in only 32% of cases and progresses to invasive cancer in 12%. Such disparity in behavior mandates individualized management with consideration of the histology.

Patients who have had satisfactory colposcopic examinations and biopsies demonstrating mild dysplasia may be treated with excisional or ablative therapy, as discussed later. Patients who are considered to be compliant may also have the option of conservative management and may be followed with Pap smears and endocervical sampling every 3 months. If HGSIL is detected subsequently or if LGSIL persists for 1 year, consideration should be given to repeating the colposcopic assessment and proceeding to excisional or ablative therapy. In patients with endocervical mild dysplasia, conservative management without excision is acceptable; however, endocervical cytology and curettings should be obtained at each follow-up. If HPV typing reveals high-risk HPV, conservative therapy remains an option in motivated patients. Patients with severe dysplasia or adenocarcinoma in situ are not candidates for conservative management.

Moderate and severe dysplasias have a high rate of persistence and a significant rate of progressing to invasive cancer. These lesions are therefore best treated with excisional or ablative techniques. Both excisional and ablative approaches destroy the transformation zone, which is the most common site of disease. Ablative techniques include laser ablation, cryotherapy, and electrocautery. The most commonly used ablative technique is cryotherapy. Excisional techniques include laser excision, LEEP, and cold knife cone biopsy. Currently, LEEP is the most commonly used technique. Hysterectomy should be reserved for certain patients with recurrent severe dysplasia or those who cannot be treated with other local therapies. Cure rates for hysterectomy are similar to and perhaps slightly better than local therapy.

Cryotherapy has long been used for the treatment of cervical dysplasia. The procedure is easily performed in an outpatient setting and is well tolerated by patients. The drawback is uncontrolled destruction and the lack of a tissue specimen. Cryotherapy is performed by applying a metal probe through which compressed gases are passed. Tissue destruction occurs as a result of freezing and desiccation. The cervix is visualized through a speculum, and a probe, which covers the lesion and transformation zone, is applied. Most treat the cervix for 3 minutes, thaw, and treat again for 3 minutes to ensure that an iceball extends beyond the lesion and transformation zone. Patients may experience mild cramping abdominal pain during the procedure and a vaginal discharge (often profuse) for 2 to 4 weeks after the procedure. Cure rates approach 90%.

The CO_2 laser has been used to vaporize cervical lesions as well as to excise them. The benefit of using the laser is the ability to tailor the size and depth of the treatment according to the size and location of the lesion and the transformation zone; less thermal necrosis occurs at the treatment margin. The laser is not widely used currently owing to the expense of the equipment, the necessity for anesthesia during the procedure, and the level of expertise required to appropriately perform the procedure. Furthermore, laser vaporization does not yield a tissue specimen. Vaporization of the lesion is usually performed to a depth of 7 mm, with an additional 2 to 3 mm of depth at the endocervical canal. Laser excision or conization is performed with high-power density (25 to 50 watts with a 0.2- to 1.0-mm spot size) to reduce the thermal damage to adjacent tissue. Cure rates are 90% to 95%.

LEEP is an outpatient excisional procedure that has the benefit of producing a tissue specimen. It has become widely popular in the treatment of cervical dysplasia owing to the relative ease in performing the procedure, low cost, and minimal patient discomfort. After the cervix is visualized, an appropriate-sized loop is selected to encompass the lesion and the transformation zone. The cervix is then circumferentially infiltrated using lidocaine with epineph-

rine. The power is set at 60 to 70 watts, and cutting mode is used to excise the specimen in a single pass. Monsel's solution or cauterization is used for hemostasis. Minor bleeding is expected in the postoperative period; however, bleeding complications have been reported in approximately 5% of cases. Cure rates with LEEP are reported as 90% to 95%.

CERVICAL NEOPLASIA IN PREGNANCY

The pregnant patient with an abnormal cytologic screen represents a clinical challenge. As with the nonpregnant patient, ASCUS and LGSIL in the setting of previously normal Pap smears and no risk factors may be followed by repeating the cytology in 3 to 4 months. Patients with ASCUS or LGSIL who have risk factors such as prior abnormal Pap smears, prior sexually transmitted disease, immunocompromised state, multiple sexual partners, or uncertain medical compliance should undergo colposcopic assessment and directed biopsies. In the pregnant patient, endocervical curettage is contraindicated. All patients with HGSIL, AGCUS, and adenocarcinoma require colposcopy and directed biopsies regardless of pregnancy. Because bleeding complications are increased, care must be taken when obtaining cervical biopsies in the gravid patient. Only experienced colposcopists should approach these patients, owing to the altered appearance of the cervix in pregnancy. Furthermore, biopsies should be limited to the most severe-appearing lesions or those that appear consistent with microinvasive or frankly invasive cancer. Bleeding is usually controlled with pressure and Monsel's solution or silver nitrate; however, the clinician must be prepared to suture or pack the vagina if these measures are not successful. Histologically confirmed dysplasia may be followed conservatively throughout pregnancy with colposcopic examination and Pap smears every 3 months. Definitive treatment of dysplasia or carcinoma in situ should be delayed until the postpartum period; however, invasive or microinvasive cancer must be addressed immediately. In patients with colposcopic or histologic evidence of microinvasive cancer, cone biopsy is indicated. Cervical cone biopsies in pregnancy should be approached with great caution and are probably best referred to an expert in gynecologic oncology. Patients with invasive cancer should be referred to a gynecologic oncologist as soon as the diagnosis is made. Treatment options are based on the patient's desire to continue with the pregnancy as well as the extent of the disease.

SURVEILLANCE

After VAIN, VIN, or CIN is treated, the patient should be closely followed. Vaginal or cervical cytology should be repeated at 3-month intervals until three consecutive normal results are obtained. Thereafter, patients may resume annual screening. In patients with VIN, the vulva should be inspected with the assistance of acetic acid at 3-month intervals for the first year.

SUMMARY

Genital HPV infection is a very common infection that is responsible for cervical dysplasia and most cervical cancers. The Pap smear remains the standard for screening; however, automated screening and liquid-based monolayer preparation may improve sensitivity. HPV type analysis also promises to aid in the screening and triage of abnormal Pap smears. Fortunately, most women with mild dysplasia will spontaneously resolve, but those with severe dysplasia

have a significant rate of progressing to invasive cancer. Several methods available for the treatment of dysplasia are curative in nearly 90% of cases.

References

1. Koutsky L: Epidemiology of genital human papillomavirus infection. Am J Med 1997;102(5A):3–8.
2. Sung HY: Papanicolaou smear history and diagnosis of invasive cervical carcinoma among members of a large prepaid health plan. Cancer 2000;88:2283–2289.
3. Spitzer M: Cervical screening adjuncts: Recent advances. Am J Obstet Gynecol 1998;179:544–556.
4. Oster AG: Natural history of cervical intraepithelial neoplasia: A critical review. Int J Gynecol Pathol 1993;12:186–192.

HIV and AIDS in Cervical Neoplasia

Veronica L. Schimp and John M. Malone, Jr.

The world first became aware of HIV in 1981. Since then, there has been an explosion of new infection around the world, and AIDS continues to impose an enormous toll in both human and economic terms. In the United States, an estimated 650,000 to 900,000 people are infected with HIV, of whom more than 200,000 are unaware of their infection. Through 1998, the Centers for Disease Control and Prevention (CDC) reported 688,200 cumulative cases of AIDS and 410,800 AIDS-related deaths.[1] Despite these sobering numbers, there has been good news about AIDS. Overall, the numbers of AIDS-related deaths have decreased, primarily due to the use of protease inhibitors combined with antiretroviral agents. People infected with HIV are expected to live longer, with higher quality of life.

Unfortunately, the news about women with HIV has not been all positive. The proportion of United States cases reported among women and adolescent girls from 1985 to 1998 more than tripled, from 7% to 23%, respectively.[2] Deaths due to AIDS increased by 3% among women but decreased by 15% among men.

In the United States, the number of AIDS cases is highest among white homosexual men. The epidemiologic picture is much different among women with AIDS. Approximately 75% are nonwhite, and they acquire the disease via heterosexual intercourse (40%) or intravenous drug use (34%). Few cases of woman-to-woman transmission have been documented, but because the CDC does not recognize this as a transmission category, this low incidence may be an artifact of underreporting. The total number of homosexual female-to-female transmissions is unknown.

Women who become infected with HIV are commonly socioeconomically disadvantaged and may not seek timely medical care. Often they have been categorized unfairly as vectors (e.g., prostitutes) or vessels (e.g., pregnancy) of disease or have been invisible during the AIDS epidemic.[2]

The AIDS epidemic has affected women in other ways that are different from men. This is mostly related to the unique clinical manifestations of HIV disease. The risk of lower genital tract neoplasia is increased in women with HIV. This has been best demonstrated in cervical (squamous) intraepithelial neoplasia (CIN), but there has also been an increase in vulvar and perianal intraepithelial lesions. Although there had been a known increase in CIN among immunosuppressed patients before the HIV epidemic, the increase in these disease entities has been best explained by the alterations in the prevalence and natural course of human papillomavirus (HPV).

Frequently, HIV infection among women in the United States occurs in conjunction with behavioral and biologic risk factors for acquiring HPV and for the development of squamous intraepithelial lesions (SILs). Common factors are multiple sexual partners, young age at first intercourse, sex with men who have multiple sexual partners, low socioeconomic status, cigarette smoking, and poor compliance with recommended Papanicolaou (Pap) test screening programs. HIV-positive women are at increased risk of developing lower genital tract neoplasia on the basis of these non–HIV-related risk factors alone.[3]

WHAT IS THE HUMAN PAPILLOMAVIRUS?

HPV is a double-stranded circular DNA virus that can infect the stratified squamous epithelium of the lower genital tract. HPV can lie in a dormant state, it can replicate (usually causing genital warts), or it may transform the DNA and cause uncontrolled cell growth.[2] There are two types of HPV, low and high risk. Approximately 75% of invasive cervix cancers are associated with high-risk HPV types (subtypes 16, 18, 31, and 45) with HPV type 16 being the most common. Less than 10% of invasive cervix cancers are associated with low-risk types (subtypes 6 and 11). Thirty percent to 40% of low-grade CIN is associated with low-risk HPV subtypes, and less than 20% are associated with high-risk subtypes. HPV is a common infection, and 60% of men and women in the United States are affected. A direct relationship between certain HPV infections and CIN has been demonstrated.[3]

The association of HIV and HPV infections is not unexpected because both are sexually transmitted diseases. The increased prevalence of HPV-related neoplasia among women with HIV/AIDS is to be expected because lower genital tract neoplasia has been associated with iatrogenic immunosuppression (e.g., after organ transplantation). HIV may directly interact with HPV. As evidenced in vitro, the HIV-1 transactivator "tat" protein enhances HPV E_2-dependent transcription of HPV-16.[4] However, in vivo studies have shown that HIV and HPV do not coinfect the same cells; HIV is found in monocytes, HPV is found to infect squamous mucosal cells. Furthermore, in the absence of immunosuppression, the interaction between HIV and HPV remains unexplained. HIV and HPV appear to be interactive infections. At this point, most of the evidence suggests a difference in the course of HPV in women coinfected with HIV.[2]

Studies have found that HIV-seropositive women are at

least five times more likely to be coinfected with HPV than their seronegative controls. Among women with HPV, immunosuppression, as measured by CD4-positive cell counts of 500/mm^3 or less, results in an increased proportion of CIN and decreased proportion of latent HPV infection. The prevalence of CIN in HIV-positive women is five times greater than in the HIV-negative population, ranging from 31% to 63%. There also appears to be an increase in the severity of the CIN lesions in HIV-positive women.[5] The HIV-infected women with high-grade CIN appear to be infected with different types of HPV than are HIV-negative women. Sun and coworkers[8] demonstrated that HPV types 16 and 18 were predominant in HIV-negative women, and that among those infected with HIV, HPV subtypes 31, 33, 35, 53, and 57 were predominant. Those with HIV also expressed a higher viral load of HPV from cervico-vaginal lavage specimens.

The prevalence of disease and outcomes varies widely, depending on the degree of immunosuppression. Mandelblatt and associates[9] reviewed 21 papers published between 1986 and 1990 and identified five well-controlled studies with strict methodology. In this meta-analysis, they estimated the relative risk of CIN in HIV-positive women to be five times that of HIV-negative women. In these combined studies, 30.7% of HIV-positive women had CIN, compared with 8.3% of HIV-negative controls. The evidence suggests that HIV-positive women have about a fivefold increased risk of HPV infection and CIN lesions, mostly because HIV infections are associated with high-risk behavior that increases their risk for HPV infection. HIV-positive women who are immunocompromised are at an even higher risk of CIN. Petry and colleagues[10] studied 52 allograft recipients who were HIV-negative and discovered that without an HPV infection, even severely immunodeficient women were free of high-grade CIN. Fink and colleagues[11] discovered that among those HIV-positive women with CD4 counts of 400/mm^3 or greater, 35% had histologically confirmed CIN; of those with CD4 counts of 200/mm^3 or less, 56% had CIN. This relationship between HIV immunosuppression and the development of CIN is not completely unanticipated because an increased prevalence of CIN and cervical cancer has been demonstrated among groups of immunosuppressed patients, such as organ transplant patients.[10] This may substantiate the need to screen HIV-positive women who have CD4 counts of 400/mm^3 or less more frequently.

How Do We Detect Cervical Intraepithelial Neoplasia?

There has been some question about the adequacy of Pap smears for detecting SILs in HIV-positive women. Most studies have found Pap tests to be adequate (Table 96–1). One must keep in mind that Pap tests among the HIV-positive population may be more significant than in the HIV-negative population.[2]

Table 96–1. Sensitivity and Specificity of Pap Smears in HIV-Infected Women

Study	HIV-Positive Women (N)	Sensitivity (%)	Specificity (%)
Del Priore et al. 1995[26]	52	57	92
Korn et al, 1994[21]	52	63	84
Wright et al, 1994[5]	398	81	87

Wright and associates[5] found that 38% of HIV-positive women with SILs on Pap test had CIN on colposcopic evaluation, compared with 14% among HIV-negative women. The false-negative rate for Pap smears in the HIV-seropositive group was 19%. Because of the small number of seronegative women and their lower prevalence of CIN, Wright's group was unable to determine with any degree of accuracy the false-negative rate in the seronegative group or directly compare false-negative rates for Pap smears in the HIV-seropositive and HIV-seronegative groups. However, this false-negative rate of 19% detected in the HIV-seropositive group in the current study is within the 10% to 40% range usually reported in the general population.[5] Based on a cytologic false-negative rate of 19% and the 7.1% prevalence of high-grade CIN that was observed in this study, a single Pap test might miss high-grade lesions in 1.3% of the HIV-positive women screened. It was suggested that one way to reduce the false-negative rate would be to perform two Pap smears within a short interval after a woman initially tests HIV-positive. This approach would be less expensive and more widely available than using colposcopy as a screening tool.[12] Other studies have shown that the diagnostic sensitivity of Pap tests is not decreased in these women. The surveillance of the HIV-positive group should be based on the individual woman's risk for CIN; however, in 1993, the CDC devised guidelines for Pap smear screening in this group (Table 96–2).

Natural History

The natural history of HPV lesions in HIV-positive women is not clearly understood. There is variance between studies as to the likelihood of immunosuppressed patients with low-grade lesions and the rate of progression of CIN. Sun and colleagues[8] studied 231 HIV-negative controls versus 220 HIV-positive women and found that among women without CIN, HIV-positive women were much more likely to have HPV infection than were HIV-negative controls. Petry[10] studied the disease progression of CIN in immunocompromised patients. This study demonstrated that low-grade lesions among immunocompromised women (half were HIV-positive and half were allograft recipients) regressed less often, and progressed more often and more rapidly (6.3 months vs. 10.5 months) than immu-

Table 96–2. Centers for Disease Control and Prevention Recommendations for Papanicolaou Smear Screening of HIV-Infected Women[19, 24]

1. Women who are HIV-infected should be advised to have a comprehensive gynecologic examination, including a Pap smear, as part of their initial medical evaluation.
2. If initial Pap smear results are within normal limits, at least one additional Pap smear should be obtained in approximately 6 mo to rule out the possibility of false-negative results on the initial Pap smear.
3. If the repeat Pap smear is normal, HIV-infected women should be advised to have a Pap smear obtained annually.
4. If the initial or subsequent Pap smear shows severe inflammation with reactive squamous cellular changes, another Pap smear should be collected within 3 mo.
5. If the initial or follow-up Pap smear shows SILs (or equivalent) or ASCUS, the woman should be referred for colposcopic examination of the lower genital tract and, if indicated, colposcopically directed biopsies.

ASCUS, atypical cells of undetermined significance; SILs, squamous intraepithelial lesions.

nocompetent controls. All patients with CD4 counts of 400/mm³ or less or immunosuppression for greater than 3 years suffered progression. This study concluded that HPV-positive women must be immunocompetent to avoid progression of their CIN.

RESPONSE TO TREATMENT

Not only do untreated HIV-positive women with CIN tend to progress, but also a tendency toward recurrence and progression is seen in women treated by the known conventional methods. In a study done by Maiman and associates,[16] it was found that disease recurred in 39% of HIV-positive women who were treated by either laser vaporization, cryotherapy, or cold-knife cone biopsy, compared with 9% of HIV-negative controls. They estimated that at 12 months the recurrence rate for disease in HIV-positive women was 47% versus 7% in HIV-negative women. At 24 months, 63% of HIV-positive patients recurred versus 13% in HIV-negative patients. Forty-five percent of patients with CD4 counts of less than 500/mm³ developed recurrence compared with 18% of those with CD4 counts greater than 500/mm³. They also discovered that although cryotherapy appears to be an attractive method of therapy for HIV-positive women because of the absence of bleeding and the low risk of iatrogenic transmission of HIV, the cure rate for patients so treated was 52% versus 99% for controls. Others have confirmed this finding. The cure rates using laser therapy and cone biopsy did not differ between the HIV-positive patients and the HIV-negative control.

Another study performed by Fruchter and coworkers[22] found that 62% of HIV-positive women who were treated by a combination of ablative or excisional methods developed recurrence after 36 months compared with 18% for HIV-negative controls. A majority of recurrences occurred in the first year and reached 87% at 3 years among women with CD4 counts of less than 200/mm³, compared with 54% in less immunodeficient women. In 25% of HIV-positive women, recurrences also involved progression of CIN to a higher lesion at 36 months, compared with 2% for HIV-negative women. After a second treatment, 50% of HIV-positive women recurred and 6% of HIV-negative women recurred, with 10% of these progressing to a higher lesion. The majority of HIV-positive patients who did not recur had been treated for low-grade lesions.[15]

Clearly immunosuppressed HIV-positive women who have high-grade CIN are at an extremely high risk for recurrence and progression after treatment. As we continue to develop new medications that extend the life of these women, alternative, more aggressive surveillance, maintenance regimens, and treatment protocols should be considered for those immunosuppressed women with high-grade lesions.[16] 5-Fluorouracil (5-FU) vaginal cream has been used with limited success in the treatment of immunosuppressed women with CIN, and interferon has been used in the treatment of both CIN-related and HIV-related diseases. Currently, there are no data about the usefulness of these modalities as adjuncts to standard therapy. A recent clinical trial using 5-FU vaginal cream prophylactically every 2 weeks for 6 months after treatment for high-grade cervical disease (AIDS clinical trial group-200) has been completed. The upcoming results may offer hope for an improved outcome to immunosuppressed HIV-positive women being treated for HPV-related disease.[6]

Consideration may also be given to hysterectomy as an alternative to the prevention of recurrences, especially because of the poor prognosis for these women if they develop cervical cancer. However, there are no data using this approach. Secondarily, when considering this approach, one must remember that surgery in immunosuppressed HIV-positive men has shown to result in increased rates of infection and delayed wound healing. Finally, even though the woman's risk of cervical neoplasia will be eliminated, she is still at increased risk of vaginal, vulvar, and anal intraepithelial neoplasia and cancer.

MULTIFOCAL LOWER GENITAL TRACT NEOPLASIA

It is well known that HIV-positive women are more likely to develop multifocal lower genital tract neoplasia than their HIV-negative counterparts. In addition to intraepithelial neoplasia of the cervix, other common sites are the vagina, vulva, perineum, and anus. In one study, 90% of the HIV-positive women had lesions on the vulva or perineum.[2] In addition, vaginal intraepithelial neoplasia (VAIN) and vulvar intraepithelial neoplasia (VIN) may not be associated with CIN in HIV-infected women. Abercrombie and Korn[2] found that 15% of 52 HIV-positive women examined by colposcopy had vulvar lesions in the absence of cervical lesions.

The prevalence of VIN among HIV-positive women is difficult to estimate because many studies are small and probably exaggerate the prevalence of multifocal disease owing to selection bias. Also, most studies segregated their results by immune status. However, estimates range from 5.6% to 37%. Despite the lack of detail, evidence seems to indicate that VIN in an HIV-positive woman is a strong predictor of immune suppression. Petry and coworkers[10] found that 10 of 11 women with VIN were immunosuppressed, with CD4 counts of less than 400/mm[3], or had been taking immunosuppressive medications for greater than 10 years.

This increased risk for VIN and VAIN among HIV-positive women raises concern about the potential to develop vulvar or vaginal cancer. Cases of vulvar cancer in HIV-positive women have been documented. Pap tests alone may not be sufficient screening tools in HIV-positive women because of the increased risk of VIN or VAIN without concomitant CIN. The most efficient method of detecting these lesions may be colposcopy, especially in HIV-positive women with a history of dysplasia or with vaginal or vulvar condylomata.

The screening of HIV-positive women for anal intraepithelial neoplasia (AIN) has increased since anal cancers have been documented in HIV-positive homosexual men. Studies have shown that HIV-positive women are also at increased risk for anal dysplasia. Cytologic abnormalities of the anus were detected in 26% of 27 HIV-positive women and 6% of 6 HIV-negative women.[24] Of the smears in the HIV-positive women, 5% were low-grade AIN. There is a need to increase the evaluation of the entire lower genital tract among HIV-positive women to detect SILs and treat them early.

Unfortunately, little is known about how often HIV-positive women should be monitored for intraepithelial neoplasia with Pap smears or colposcopy. As women live longer with HIV, lower anogenital tract malignancies (especially vulvar and anal cancers) may become increasingly common. In women with iatrogenic immunosuppression after organ transplantation, a 100-fold increase in vulvar cancer has been reported, occurring after approximately 107 months.[2]

CERVICAL CANCER AND HIV

Immunosuppressed patients in general, and those infected with HIV in particular, are more predisposed to the development of cancer. Patients with AIDS have a known increased risk of developing Kaposi's sarcoma, primary central nervous system lymphoma, and non-Hodgkin's lymphoma (40,000, 3900, and 191 times higher, respectively) than the general population.[8] On January 1, 1993, the CDC expanded the surveillance case definition of AIDS to include HIV-positive women with invasive cervical cancer.

Cervical cancer may be the most common malignancy among women with AIDS. Based on the data from the CDC, the incidence of cervical cancer is approximately 10 per 100,000 among the general population, compared with 900 per 100,000 among women with AIDS. An example of a clinical setting where invasive cervical cancer is strongly associated with HIV infection is in Brooklyn, New York, where 19% of women with invasive cervical cancer were HIV-positive.[25]

Women with HIV are not only more likely to progress from CIN to cervical cancer, but also the clinical course of the disease may be worsened by concomitant infection with HIV. When compared with HIV-negative women, HIV-positive women with cervical cancer are more likely to be diagnosed at a later stage, have a poorer response to therapy, and have a higher rate of recurrent disease and a more virulent tumor. Because of this association between HIV and cervical cancer, it has been suggested that women with invasive cervical cancer be offered HIV testing if their serologic status is unknown.[2]

Despite the fact that we are not very successful in preventing recurrences, progression to invasive cancer during therapy is a rare event. We must remember to convey a positive message to women who are HIV-positive and have intraepithelial neoplasia. It is invasive cervical cancer that is life threatening, not intraepithelial neoplasia.

References

1. Fauci AS: The AIDS epidemic: Considerations for the 21st century. N Engl J Med 1999;341:1046–1050.
2. Abercrombie PD, Korn AP: Lower genital tract neoplasia in women with HIV infection. Oncology 1998;12:1735–1747.
3. Kuhn L, Sun XW, Wright TC: Human immunodeficiency virus infection and female lower genital tract malignancy. Curr Opin Obstet Gynecol 1999;11:35–36.
4. Vernon S, Hart, CE, Reeves W, et al: The HIV-1 tat protein enhances E2-dependent human papillomavirus transcription. Virus Res 1993;27:133–145.
5. Wright TC Jr, Ellerbrock RV, Chiasson MA, et al: Cervical intraepithelial neoplasia in women infected with human immunodeficiency virus: Prevalence, risk factors, and validity of Papanicolaou smears. Obstet Gynecol 1994;84:591–597.
6. Carreras R, Fuste P, Castellanos ME: Cervical intra-epithelial neoplasia in HIV-positive women and women with AIDS. Int J Gynecol Obstet 1997;58:325–326.
7. Hocke D, Leroy V, Morlat P, et al: Cervical dysplasia and human immunodeficiency virus infection in women: Prevalence and associated factors. Eur J Obstet Gynecol Reprod Biol 1998;81:69–76.
8. Sun XW, Kuhn L, Ellerbrock TV, et al: Human papillomavirus infection in HIV-seropositive women; Natural history and variability of detection. N Engl J Med 1997;337:1343–1349.
9. Mandelblatt JS, Fahs M, Garibaldi K, et al: Association between HIV infection and cervical neoplasia: Implications for clinical care of women at risk for both conditions. AIDS 1992;6:173–178.
10. Petry KU, Scheffel D, Bode U, et al: Cellular immunodeficiency enhances progress of human papillomavirus–associated cervical lesions. Int J Cancer 1994;57:836–840.
11. Fink MJ, Fruchter R, Maiman M, et al: The adequacy of cytology and colposcopy in diagnosing cervical neoplasia in HIV-seropositive women. Gynecol Oncol 1994;171:531–537.
12. Petry I: Cancers of the anogenital region in renal transplant recipients. Cancer 1986;58:611–616.
13. Wright TC Jr, Koulos J, Schnoll F, et al: Cervical intraepithelial neoplasia in women infected with the human immunodeficiency virus: Outcome after electrosurgical excision. Gynecol 1994;55:253–258.

14. Maiman M, Fruchter R, Clark M, et al: Cervical cancer as an AIDS-defining illness. Obstet Gynecol 1997;89:76–80.

15. Spitzer M: Lower genital tract intraepithelial neoplasia in HIV-infected women: Guidelines for evaluation and management. Obstet Gynecol Surv 1999;54:131–137.

16. Maiman M, Fruchter R: Cervical neoplasia and the human immunodeficiency virus. In Rubin SC, Hoskins WJ (eds): Cervical cancer and preinvasive neoplasia. Philadelphia, Lippincott-Raven, 1996, pp 405–416.

17. Wakeman R, Johnson CD, Wastell C: Surgical procedures in patients at risk of human immunodeficiency virus infection. J R Soc Med 1990;83:315–318.

18. Burke EC, Orloff SL, Freise CE, et al: Wound healing after anorectal surgery in human immunodeficiency virus–infected patients. Arch Surg 1991;126:1267–1271.

19. 1993 sexually transmitted disease guidelines. Centers for Disease Control and Prevention. MMWR Morb Mortal Wkly Rep 1993;42:1–102.

20. Petry KU, Scheffel D, Bode U, et al: Human papillomavirus is associated with the frequent detection of warty and basaloid high-grade neoplasia of the vulva and cervical neoplasia among immunosuppressed women. Gynecol Oncol 1996;60:30–34.

21. Korn AP, Autry M, DeRemer PA, Tan W: Sensitivity of the Papanicolaou smear in human immunodeficiency virus–infected women. Obstet Gynecol 1994;83:401–404.

22. Fruchter RG, Maiman M, Sillman FH: Characteristics of cervical intraepithelial neoplasia in women infected with the human immunodeficiency virus. Am J Obstet Gynecol 1994;171:531–537.

23. Chiasson MA, Ellerbrock TV, Bush TJ, et al: Increased prevalence of vulvovaginal condyloma and vulvar intraepithelial neoplasia in women infected with the human immunodeficiency virus. Obstet Gynecol 1997;89:690–694.

24. Wright TC Jr, Sun XW: Anogenital papillomavirus infection and neoplasia in immunodeficient women. Obstet Gynecol Clin North Ame 1996; 23:861–894.

25. Klevens RM, Fleming PL, Mays MA, Frey R: Characteristics of women with AIDS and invasive cervical cancer. Obstet Gynecol 1996;88:269–273.

26. Del Priore G, Maag T, Bhattacharya M, et al: The value of cervical cytology in HIV-infected women. Gynecol Oncol 1995;56:395–398.

NINETY-SEVEN

Premalignant Diseases of the Vulva and Vagina

Elizabeth Wagner and Adnan R. Munkarah

Precancerous lesions of the vulva were first described by Bowen in 1912. The lesions described in his report involved the thigh and buttock, were red and scaly, and exhibited microscopic atypia. These were later referred to as Bowen's disease and were believed to be precursors of invasive squamous cell carcinoma. Since then, other terms have been used to describe premalignant lesions of the lower genital tract, including atypia, dysplasia, carcinoma in situ, carcinoma in situ simplex, and intraepithelial carcinoma. The terms *vulvar intraepithelial neoplasia* (VIN) and *vaginal intraepithelial neoplasia* (VAIN) have been introduced to describe these precancerous lesions.

Some studies have shown an association between VIN, VAIN, and human papilloma virus (HPV) infections. Since the early 1980s, we have seen a rise in the prevalence of HPV infection of the lower female genital tract. Accurate clinical diagnosis of these infections has been made possible by the significant advances in medical and molecular technologies. Condyloma acuminatum is now the most commonly diagnosed sexually transmitted disease in the United States.

EPIDEMIOLOGY AND CLINICAL FEATURES

Vulvar Intrapithelial Neoplasia

The incidence of VIN has nearly doubled since 1980 and is currently estimated at 2.1 per 100,000 women. Risk factors associated with VIN include history of cervical dysplasia, lower genital tract infection with HPV, and smoking.

Two distinct types of VIN have been described. The first affects younger women, with the mean age at diagnosis younger than 35 years. The lesions are usually multifocal, with a high prevalence of HPV infection. The second type is usually diagnosed in women older than 50 years. Lesions are usually unifocal and have a higher risk of malignant progression. Infection with HPV is not as common in these patients as in the first group.

Patients with VIN present with a variety of symptoms, including vulvar pruritus, burning, or pain. The skin lesions may be hyperpigmented or white. Some patients may be completely asymptomatic and diagnosed incidentally at routine gynecologic examination or evaluation of an abnormal Papanicolaou (Pap) smear. It is not unusual for a woman to be treated empirically with different creams and ointments before an accurate diagnosis of VIN is made based on histologic evaluation of a biopsy specimen.

The natural history of VIN is dissimilar from that of cervical intraepithelial neoplasia. Untreated lesions are thought to progress to invasive disease only 2% to 4% of the time. Most often, regression has been documented in untreated VIN. Some investigators, however, have reported higher rates of progression. Jones and McLean followed VIN III in untreated patients for 7 to 8 years and noted progression to invasive disease in approximately 80%.

Vaginal Intraepithelial Neoplasia

VAIN is the rarest of all lower genital tract neoplasias, with an estimated incidence of 0.2 to 0.42 per 100,000 women. This incidence has not changed since 1980. VAIN, known to be a disease of postmenopausal women, is most commonly diagnosed in patients in their 50s and 60s. Few studies have reported malignant progression in VAIN; it appears that if left untreated, VAIN lesions may progress to invasive cancer in 9% to 50% of patients.

VAIN has been associated with a variety of risk factors, including low educational levels, low family income, history of a previously abnormal Pap smear, history of cervical dysplasia, and history of prior pelvic radiation.

DIAGNOSIS

The first step in the diagnosis of VIN and VAIN is a complete history and physical examination. A careful visual inspection and palpation of the vulva and vagina are essential. Any grossly suspicious lesions should be biopsied. If the patient has not had a normal Pap smear within the past year, one smear should be taken. Atypical areas should be noted on a diagram and incorporated into the medical record. Areas of thinning epithelium, coarse epithelium, discoloration, bleeding, ulceration, or mass lesions merit particular attention. After these studies, a careful colposcopic examination of the lower genital tract should be performed.

Colposcopy

In 1925, Hinselmann, a German scientist, engineered a tool to evaluate the lower genital tract. Called a colposcope, it was a microscope used to visualize surface epithelium. Today, we use the colposcope to view magnified images of the surface epithelium of the vulva, vagina, cervix, and perianal area. This evaluation is critical in the diagnosis and eventual treatment of premalignant lower genital tract disease.

The colposcope is most often a binocular microscope that is connected to a light source and attached to a mobile arm or pole. The objectives' focal length ranges from 200 to 300 mm, and the images are enlarged from 6 to 16 times. The colposcope may include accessories such as a tilting mechanism that facilitates the examination, arrangements for still and video photography that allows examinations to be reviewed and discussed with other professionals, and a green filter that absorbs red light and highlights abnormal vascular patterns.

Vulvar Examination

To improve recognition of abnormal areas, the epithelium can be treated with acetic acid. A 3% to 5% solution of acetic acid is applied by soaking a cotton sponge and laying it on the vulva for a full 5 minutes. The acetic acid temporarily coagulates the epithelial cytokeratin, causing a characteristic acetowhite change noted in abnormal epithelium.

Vulvar epithelial disease does not result in vascular changes; therefore, the green filter is not employed. Any suspicious areas should be biopsied, including areas with acetowhite discoloration.

Histologic evaluation of biopsy specimens remains the definitive diagnostic step for lower genital tract disease. The characteristic pathologic findings and treatment options are discussed later in this chapter.

Vaginal Examination

A colposcopic evaluation of the vagina is similar to the examination just described. The vagina is accessed via a speculum and initially inspected with the naked eye. The entire vagina should be visualized; the speculum should be rotated in a clockwise direction until the entire canal has been seen.

A 3% to 5% solution of acetic acid is applied via cotton-soaked swabs for 1 to 2 minutes. Acetowhite changes indicate abnormal epithelium. VAIN lesions may be associated with abnormal vasculature. A green filter is used to absorb red light waves; this filter highlights the abnormal vasculature, which is classified into one of two patterns, punctation or mosaicism.

Lugol's iodine solution applied to the vaginal canal stains normal glycogenated tissue brown. Abnormal epithelial tissue has less cytoplasm, and therefore less glycogen, and will not stain. This technique further delineates abnormal areas.

We find it is helpful to record the findings on a diagram in the medical record. Biopsy specimens of all suspicious areas should be sent for pathologic evaluation.

PATHOLOGY

Histology of Vulvar Intraepithelial Neoplasia

Histologic features characteristic of VIN include nuclear atypia, increased mitosis, loss of polarity, and pleomor-

phism. VIN lesions are usually graded based on the level of involvement of the squamous epithelium with dysplastic cells according to Richart's classification system. VIN I describes a lesion in which the abnormal cells extend to less then one third of the distance from the basement membrane to the surface epithelium. In VIN II, the cellular changes occupy greater than one third but less then two thirds of this distance, and in VIN III, the cellular changes extend to the outer third of the epithelium. Vulvar carcinoma in situ represents the most severe form of VIN III, in which the entire epithelial thickness is replaced by dysplastic cells. In all cases, however, VIN implies that dysplastic cells are confined to the epithelium and have not invaded below the basement membrane.

Histology of Vaginal Intraepithelial Neoplasia

The cytologic and histologic criteria used to diagnose and grade VAIN are similar to those used for VIN.

TREATMENT

The treatment of lower genital tract disease involves either ablation or resection of the dysplastic epithelium. Because ablative therapy destroys the tissues and does not yield a tissue specimen, one should be certain before proceeding with such therapy that invasive disease has been excluded, by means of adequate examination and diagnostic biopsies.

Vulvar Intraepithelial Neoplasia

Ablation of VIN may be accomplished through laser vaporization, cryotherapy, radiation therapy, or topical application of 5-fluorouracil (5-FU) cream.

The CO_2 laser is most accurate and effective at a power density of 600 to 800 watts/cm². The precision of destruction is exact if the right surgical techniques are applied. Four microsurgical planes can be identified at the time of laser ablation of the vulvar skin. The first plane consists of the tissue down to the epithelial basement membrane and is characterized at the time of laser destruction by "bubbles of silver opalescence beneath the surface char." The second plane extends to the upper dermis and appears as "chamois cloth yellow." The third plane includes the papillary dermis and portions of the reticular dermis. This plane is identified by the "gray-white fibers of the remaining reticular dermis." Laser vaporization beyond this third plane reveals "skin appendages that look like tiny grains of sand." Destruction to this level may require skin grafting and may result in scarring.

There are several advantages of CO_2 laser vaporization: outpatient treatment is well tolerated, multifocal disease is easily managed, scarring is limited, and success rates reach

92% in some series. The disadvantages include lack of a tissue specimen for histologic evaluation and high recurrence rates when inadequate or improper treatment is employed. As mentioned previously, laser vaporization necessitates exclusion of invasive disease before being considered.

Topical 5-FU cream prevents normal DNA synthesis, inhibiting growth of neoplastic cells. A 5% 5-FU cream may be applied twice daily for 6 weeks. The patient should be cautioned about the expected severe inflammatory reaction that occurs after 2 to 5 weeks of therapy. Local anesthetics and systemic analgesics help manage this painful response. We rarely recommend 5-FU cream treatment for VIN because of the severe skin reaction that may last for weeks and cause significant discomfort to the patient. Failure rates for 5-FU cream range from 60% to 90%; they are often due to premature termination of treatment secondary to intolerance of side effects from this inflammatory reaction.

Cryotherapy and radiotherapy offer lower success rates and no significant advantages over laser vaporization of VIN lesions and, therefore, are rarely used at present.

Surgical treatment with wide local excision or vulvectomy eliminates the dysplastic tissue while providing a surgical specimen for histologic evaluation. Histologic evaluation verifies the extent of the lesion, identifying invasion or positive surgical margins.

Wide local excision is achieved by making an elliptical incision in the direction of the skin lines around the lesion to be resected. A colposcope may be used to identify a disease-free margin of 0.5 to 1.0 cm. Surgical evaluation of these margins is critical. Disease-free margins were associated with no recurrence in some studies. On the other hand, when disease-free margins are not accomplished, recurrence rates may be as high as 32%.

Vulvectomy is reserved for difficult cases of persistent multifocal disease that has failed multiple attempts at conservative therapy (ablation or excision). It results in significant changes in the appearance of the vulva and may cause scarring and chronic pain.

Vaginal Intraepithelial Neoplasia

Therapeutic options for VAIN include topical 5-FU cream, laser, or excision. 5-FU topical cream is supplied in 25-g tubes. Recommended dosages vary from 3- to 6-g applications once or twice daily, continuing for 5 days to 1 month (Table 97–1). The dosing schedules vary from one study to the next, with little information demonstrating that one is more effective than another. This topical therapy for VAIN has a low failure rate of 12% to 15%. The patient should be cautioned about the expected severe inflammatory reaction that occurs after 2 to 5 weeks of therapy. Local anesthetics and systemic analgesics help manage this painful response. An advantage of topical therapy is no

Table 97–1. Suggested 5-Fluorouracil Dosing for Vaginal Intraepithelial Neoplasia

Twice daily for 1 mo then once per mo
Twice daily × 2 wk
Two hr daily for 5 days
Twice daily for five days/wk, × 3 wk
Five nights/mo for 1–6 mo
5 g daily for 5 days

scarring, and, when it is successful, aesthetically pleasing results are common. Disadvantages include vaginal ulcerations, at times requiring termination of therapy. We advise patients to insert a dry tampon after the intravaginal application of the cream to prevent leakage and vulvitis.

CO_2 laser destruction is a viable option for unifocal or multifocal VAIN lesions. Lesions must be clearly visible, and invasive disease must be ruled out before treatment. Power densities of 300 watts/cm² are recommended. Superficial destruction to a depth of 1 to 2 mm is all that is required. At this depth, the vaginal mucosa is destroyed to the level of the lamina propria. CO_2 laser vaporization success and failure rates are unclear. Several studies show failure rates ranging from 8% to 36%.

Surgical therapies with local excision, partial vaginectomy, or total vaginectomy have long been treatment options for VAIN. Excision offers a pathologic specimen for further evaluation, ensuring accurate identification of invasive disease. We reserve surgical excision for patients who have failed more conservative surgery and those with suspected invasive lesions. The extent of excision or vaginectomy depends on the location, size, and focality of the lesion. Vaginal reconstruction is essential after vaginectomy if greater than 50% of the upper vagina is removed. It will improve postoperative sexual function and bladder neck support. The failure rate for surgical excision is approximately 10%.

FOLLOW-UP

Post-treatment follow-up is essential to detect recurrence of VIN or VAIN. Depending on the patients' history and grade of lesion, we usually recommend follow-up visits for physical examination and Pap smear (for patients with VAIN) every 4 months. Colposcopic examinations are performed on patients with persistent symptoms, abnormal findings on physical examination, or abnormal Pap smear results. For patients who continue to be disease-free for 2 to 3 years, we extend their visits to a yearly interval.

Suggestions for Future Reading

Vulvar
Basta A, Adamek K, Pitynski K: Intraepithelial neoplasia and early stage vulvar cancer. Epidemiological, clinical and virological observations. Eur J Gynaecol Oncol 1999;20:111.

Jones RW, McLean MR: Carcinoma in situ of the vulva: A review of 31 treated and 5 untreated cases. Obstet Gynecol 1986;68:499.

Reid R: Superficial laser vulvectomy; A new surgical technique for appendage-conserving ablation of refractory condylomas and vulvar intraepithelial neoplasia. Am J Obstet Gynecol 1985;152:504.

Richart RM: Observations on the biology of cervical dysplasia. Sloane Bull 1964;75:64.

VanBeurden M, VanDer Vange N, Ten Kate FJW, et al: Restricted surgical management of vulvar intraepithelial neoplasia; Focus on exclusion of invasion and of relief of symptoms. Int J Gynecol Cancer 1998;8:73.

VanBeurden M, Ten Kate FJW, Smits HL, et al: Multifocal vulvar intraepithelial neoplasia grade III and multicentric lower genital tract neoplasia is associated with transcriptionally active human papillomavirus. Obstet Gynecol Survey 1995;50:723.

Vaginal

Cheng D, Ng T-Y, Ngan HYS, Wong L-C: Wide local excision (WLE) for vaginal intraepithelial neoplasia (VAIN). Acta Obstet Gynecol Scand 1999;78:648.

Oyakawa N, Dias AR Jr, Belotto RA, et al: Laser therapy on the vaginal intraepithelial neoplasia [abstract]. Int J Gynecol Cancer 1999;9:130.

Sillman FH, Fruchter RG, Chen Y.-S, et al: Vaginal intraepithelial neoplasia; Risk factors for persistence, recurrence, and invasion and its management. Am J Obstet Gynecol 1997;176:93.

Rhodes-Morris HE: Treatment of Vulvar Intraepithelial Neoplasia and Vaginal Intraepithelial Neoplasia. Clin Consult Obstet Gynecol 1994;6:44–53.

Singer A, Monaghan JM: Lower Genital Tract Precancer: Vaginal Intraepithelial Neoplasia. New York, Blackwell Scientific, 1994.

NINETY-EIGHT

Coding in Obstetrics and Gynecology

Philip N. Eskew, Jr.

The process of reimbursement for physician services involves coding and documentation principles. Insurance plans or managed care plans reimburse based on the submission, by the physician, of proper CPT *(Current Procedural Terminology)* and ICD-9 *(International Classification of Diseases–Ninth Edition)* codes.

CPT codes are used to record services provided by the physician. Those services include surgical procedures, hospital care, critical care, and office visits. CPT codes are five-digit numbers that indicate to the insurance company what services were provided to the patient. ICD-9 codes are three-, four-, or five-digit numbers used to define the diagnosis for the services provided.

The physician's responsibility does not end with the selection of the proper CPT and ICD-9 codes. All insurance companies require that the documentation on the patient's chart accurately reflect the physician work involved in the patient encounter. Each encounter requires the physician to document the history obtained from the patient, the amount of a physical examination performed, and the medical decision making involved in the encounter.

This process may sound simple, but most physicians have developed short cuts, abbreviated forms, and handwritten notes that do not meet documentation guidelines. In other situations, some physicians will make up a diagnosis that will allow the patient's encounter to be reimbursed by the insurer. This can be dangerous, because the patient's medical history may reflect an inaccurate diagnosis that could affect the ability of the patient to obtain health insurance in the future. Far too many physicians have been charged with fraud for falsifying insurance claims with procedures that were not performed or providing inaccurate documentation to justify the insurance claim.

The history obtained from the patient should begin at the initial visit at which the patient is required to complete a comprehensive intake history form (Fig. 98–1). Many forms are available that are comprehensive in nature and meet the requirements for a comprehensive history. It is important that the physician review the history with the patient and sign the history form, in addition to requiring the patient's signature. Several insurance companies or managed care companies inform the patient to call if they feel the physician has overcharged for the visit, and the company can request the medical records for documentation of the visit. This same comprehensive intake history form can be reviewed by the patient, signed and dated, and countersigned and dated by the physician the next year. The patient does not have to fill out a new form each year.

However, some physicians will have patients fill out an interval history form (Fig. 98–2) if they return within the year for a visit other than an annual examination. At this visit, the interval history form can simply ask the patient what changes in health, family, or medication status have taken place since the last visit. It is appropriate to put on this form, "I apologize for having you fill out this form, but most insurance companies require it." This will make up for the inconvenience and frustration that some patients feel when asked to fill out one more form.

In addition to these forms, the physician must record, on a form, by dictation, or by handwriting, the chief complaint, history of present illness, and any pertinent changes in the patient's history since the last visit that will document the reason for the encounter (Fig. 98–3). This will provide a good medical record that can be understood easily by the physician's partner and the insurance company or serve as an excellent source for the physician when the patient returns. Physicians are required to go back to basics—that is, use the history-taking methods learned in medical school and residency training—in meeting the requirements of today's insurers.

Most physicians have their own format for dictation of a complete physical examination. The physician can utilize a check-off form for the physical examination, as long as each individual item is individually checked. Some physicians prefer to dictate in order to document their physical examination, which is fine as long as they mention each body area that they actually examined. Whatever method the physician uses, the medical record must contain documentation of the clinically relevant body areas examined that relate to the patient's diagnosis.

The key for reimbursement is that the physician should perform an examination of only "clinically relevant" body areas. Performing a comprehensive physical examination will not allow the physician to be reimbursed more when the patient's diagnosis requires only an abbreviated examination. However, physicians place themselves at risk if they submit a claim for a patient encounter that does not document the physical examination required for that CPT code.

The one area of the patient's encounter that is most difficult to document is the medical decision-making component. This requires physicians to document their thought processes regarding how they are managing the patient's diagnosis, what tests they are ordering and why, prescriptions written, procedures planned, and diagnoses considered and ruled out. With each patient encounter, the physi-

GYNECOLOGIC INTAKE HISTORY

NAME:_____ BIRTH DATE:____/____/_____ DATE:____/____/____

ADDRESS:_____

CITY_____ STATE/ZIP:_____

HOME TEL:(   )_____ WORK TEL:(   )_____

EMPLOYER:_____ INSURANCE:_____

NAME OF SPOUSE/PARTNER:_____ REFERRED BY:_____

REVIEW OF SYSTEMS

PLEASE CHECK (X) IF ANY OF THE FOLLOWING APPLY TO YOU NOW, IN THE PAST OR OFTEN			
1. CONSTITUTIONAL	CURRENTLY	PAST	NOTES
Weight loss	☐	☐	
Weight gain	☐	☐	
Fever	☐	☐	
Fatigue	☐	☐	
2. EYES			
Double vision	☐	☐	
Spots before eyes	☐	☐	
Vision changes	☐	☐	
3. ENT/MOUTH			
Ear aches	☐	☐	
Ringing in ears	☐	☐	
Sinus problems	☐	☐	
Sore throat	☐	☐	
Mouth sores	☐	☐	
Dental problems	☐	☐	
4. CARDIOVASCULAR			
Painful breathing	☐	☐	
Chest pain	☐	☐	
Difficult breathing on exertion	☐	☐	
Swelling of legs	☐	☐	
Palpitations of heart	☐	☐	
5. RESPIRATORY			
Wheezing	☐	☐	
Spitting up blood	☐	☐	
Shortness of breath	☐	☐	
Cough, chronic	☐	☐	
6. GASTROINTESTINAL			
Diarrhea, frequent	☐	☐	
Bloody stool	☐	☐	
Nausea/vomiting	☐	☐	
Constipation	☐	☐	
7. GENITOURINARY			
Blood in urine	☐	☐	
Pain with urination	☐	☐	
Urgency	☐	☐	
Frequency of urination	☐	☐	
Incomplete emptying	☐	☐	
Stress incontinence	☐	☐	
Abnormal periods	☐	☐	
Painful intercourse	☐	☐	
8. MUSCULOSKELETAL			
Muscle weakness	☐	☐	

Figure 98–1. Gynecologic intake history form.

Illustration continued on following page

PLEASE CHECK (X) IF ANY OF THE FOLLOWING APPLY TO YOU NOW, IN THE PAST OR OFTEN

9. SKIN/BREAST	CURRENTLY	PAST	NOTES
Pain in breast	☐	☐	
Discharge	☐	☐	
Masses	☐	☐	
Rash	☐	☐	
Ulcers	☐	☐	

10. NEUROLOGICAL			
Dizziness	☐	☐	
Seizures	☐	☐	
Numbness	☐	☐	
Trouble walking	☐	☐	

11. PSYCHIATRIC			
Depression	☐	☐	
Crying, frequent	☐	☐	

12. ENDOCRINE			
Dry skin	☐	☐	
Abnormal thirst	☐	☐	
Hot flashes	☐	☐	

13. HEMATOLOGIC/LYMPHATIC			
Bruises, frequent	☐	☐	
Cuts do not stop bleeding	☐	☐	
Enlarged lymph nodes	☐	☐	

14. ALLERGIC/IMMUNOLOGIC			
Allergies	☐	☐	
Drugs, other	☐	☐	

PERSONAL PAST HISTORY

MAJOR ILLNESSES	YES	No		YES	NO
Asthma			Cancer		
Pneumonia			Ulcers		
Chronic Lung Disease			Depression/anxiety		
Kidney Infections/stones			Anemia/Blood transfusions		
Tuberculosis			Seizures/convulsions/epilepsy		
Venereal Disease			Bowel trouble		
Heart Trouble/murmur			Glaucoma		
Diabetes			Arthritis/joint pain		
High Blood Pressure			Fracture		
Stroke			Hepatitis/Yellow jaundice		
Rheumatic Fever			Thyroid Disease		

OPERATIONS/HOSPITALIZATIONS			
Reason	Date	Reason	Date

INJURIES/ILLNESSES			
Type	Date	Type	Date

LAST IMMUNIZATION OR TEST			
	Date		Date
Tetanus		Pneumonia	
Flu Shot		TB Skin Test	

OB/GYN HISTORY			
	Number		Number
Births		Abortions	
Miscarriages		Living children	

Figure 98–1 *Continued.*

CURRENT MEDICATIONS			
Drug Name	Dosage	Drug Name	Dosage

FAMILY HISTORY

illness	Yes	Relative	Illness	Yes	Relative
Diabetes			Drinking Problem		
Stroke			Breast Cancer		
Heart Disease			Colon Cancer		
High Blood Pressure			Ovarian Cancer		

SOCIAL HISTORY

Habits					
Smoking	Yes ☐	No ☐	Packs per day_____	Years_____	
Alcohol	Yes ☐	No ☐	Drinks per day_____	Drinks per week_____	
Drug Use	Yes ☐	No ☐			
Seat Belt Use	Yes ☐	No ☐			
Regular Exercise	Yes ☐	No ☐			

Personal Profile				
Marital Status	Married ☐	Single ☐	Widowed ☐	Divorced ☐
Number of Living Children_____				
Number of people in household_____				
School Completed	High School ☐	College ☐	Graduate Degree ☐	Other ☐
Current or most recent job_____				

PERSONAL SAFETY

Yes ☐	No ☐	Has anyone close to you ever threatened to hurt you?
Yes ☐	No ☐	Has anyone ever hit, kicked, choked, or hurt you physically?
Yes ☐	No ☐	Has anyone, including your partner, ever forced you to have sex?
Yes ☐	No ☐	Are you ever afraid of your partner?

MEDICARE "HIGH RISK" CRITERIA

Have you ever been treated for any of the following infections?
☐ Vaginosis ☐ Genital warts ☐ Chlamydia ☐ Herpes ☐ Trichomonas ☐ Gonorrhea ☐ Syphilis

Have you had a Pap smear in the last 7 years?	☐ No	☐ Yes	
Have you ever had an abnormal Pap smear test?	☐ No	☐ Yes	When?_____
Did you begin sexual activity before you were 16 years old?	☐ No	☐ Yes	
Have you had more than 5 sexual partners in your lifetime?	☐ No	☐ Yes	
Have you ever tested positive for the HIV virus?	☐ No	☐ Yes	
Did your mother take the drug DES when she was pregnant with you?	☐ No	☐ Yes	

Completed by: Patient ☐   Office Nurse   ☐   Physician   ☐

Signature of patient:_____

Date reviewed by physician with patient:_____

Physician Signature:_____

Annual Review of History

Date reviewed:_____ Physician Signature:_____

Date reviewed:_____ Physician Signature:_____

Date reviewed:_____ Physician Signature:_____

Date reviewed:_____ Physician Signature:_____

Figure 98–1 *Continued.*

INTERVAL HISTORY

Name: _____ Chart #: _____ Date: _____

Marital status: _____ Age: _____ Current home phone #: _____ Work #:_____

Please help keep us up to date by answering the following questions:

Who is your primary care physician? _____
Other physicians you see?_____

Have you had any serious illnesses, operations, injuries, or have you been hospitalized since your last appointment in our office?_____

_____

Have you discovered any additional information about your family history that we should know?_____

_____

Are you here today for a routine exam?_____ or problem? _____
If your visit is for a problem, please describe your symptoms: _____

_____

Have your medications changed in the interval since your last visit? _____
If so, list new medications or medications discontinued: _____

_____

Have you changed any habits (smoking, drinking, or drug use) or occupation since your last visit? _____

_____

Please turn over the page and circle any symptoms you are currently experiencing.

FOR OFFICE USE ONLY:
WT_____HT_____BP_____LMP_____TEMPERATURE_____

LAST PAP _____ LAST MAMMOGRAM _____

BIRTH CONTROL _____ HRT _____

Figure 98–2. Interval history form.

cian should devote a portion of the dictation or written narrative to the documentation of what conditions the patient complains of (impression) and what tests or procedures the physician is considering to help with the diagnosis and treatment of the complaint (plan).

When a patient is hospitalized, the physician must record the services performed in the hospital—surgical or medical care—and submit that information to the office billing clerk. Each patient has a hospital fact sheet with insurance information on which the physician should record the date(s) of service along with the appropriate CPT and ICD-9 codes for each day of hospitalization.

Each physician should take the time to become involved in the coding and billing portion of her or his practice. This means that the physician should meet regularly (weekly or biweekly) with the insurance or billing person in the office. Discussions as to why claims were questioned, denied, or returned for more information by the insurer will help educate the physician in the documentation phase of the patient's encounter. Several medical journals and subscription newsletters regularly publish helpful hints regarding coding, billing, and documentation information. Physicians should read these and share them with office personnel. Attendance at coding postgraduate courses by physicians

REVIEW OF SYSTEMS

Are you currently experiencing any of the following symptoms?

Constitutional:		Gynecological:	
	Fever		
	Chills		Bleeding or pain with intercourse
	Sweats		Unusual vaginal discharge or odor
	Weight change - gain or loss		Vulvar or vaginal itching or burning
	Weakness		Pelvic pain
	Fatigue		
		Urinary:	
Eyes:			Painful urination
	Change in vision		Frequent urination
			Urinary urgency
Ears, Nose, Mouth, Throat:			Blood in urine
	Change in hearing		Urinary incontinence
	Nose bleeds		Getting up at night to urinate
	Sore throat		
	Dry mouth	Musculoskeletal:	
			Back pain
Cardiovascular:			Weakness
	Dizziness		Joint pain, stiffness, swelling
	Shortness of breath		
	Chest pain	Integumentary / Breast:	
	Loss of consciousness		Nodules
	Palpitations		Change in moles, freckles
			Change in hair - growth, loss, texture
Respiratory:			Breast lumps
	Chest pain		Breast nipple discharge
	Cough - productive or dry		Breast pain
	Shortness of breath		
	Wheezing	Neurological / Psychiatric:	
			Memory change
Gastrointestinal:			Depression
	Abdominal pain		Anxiety
	Nausea, vomiting		Mood swings
	Change in bowel habits		Numbness or tingling
	Change in appetite		
	Dark or bloody stool	Endocrine:	
	Indigestion		Weight change
	Constipation or diarrhea		Excessive thirst, urination
			Tremor
Hematologic / Lymphatic:			Cold or heat intolerance
	Swollen lymph glands		
	Easy bruisability		

Thank you for taking the time to answer these questions. Most insurance companies now require this information to be updated at every visit.

Figure 98–3. Review of systems form.

and office staff is very valuable in helping everyone understand the importance of coding and documentation.

How accurately physicians code each patient encounter can affect the amount of money earned in practice. Some practices divide the financial profits based on a productivity principle. Each physician's productivity is based on the relative value units assigned to each procedure and each office encounter. The relative value unit total for the individual physician's work determines his or her productivity for that time period. If a physician incorrectly records a lower level office visit than is actually documented, the relative value unit total will be affected when profits are split.

Each year CPT and ICD-9 publish a new book with updates that add, delete, or edit several codes. The physician and the office staff need to obtain new books each year and review the changes. Several publications summarize these changes in articles or newsletters, and physicians can share this information at the regular office staff or business meetings. The practice of medicine now requires that the physician learn not only about new procedures and techniques but also about how to document the appropriate amount of history, physical examination, and medical decision making with each patient encounter.

Your Practice and the United States Congress

Lucia DiVenere

The United States Congress may seem like it is a world away, but it is really right in your examination room. Every obstetric-gynecologic practitioner that cares about patients and practice needs to care about what happens in Congress. Here is why.

Congress is making decisions that will affect

- Who you can treat
- How you can treat them
- The safety of your practice and patients
- Whether or not doctors have leverage with health maintenance organizations (HMOs)
- How many obstetric-gynecologic doctors there will be tomorrow
- What kinds of research will be conducted
- What kinds of treatments will be available in the future

In short, Congress is making decisions that will affect your future and the future of your profession. And, unlike state legislatures that can fix problems only one state at a time, the United States Congress can address problems nationwide.

This chapter examines issues of importance to obstetrician-gynecologists and how they were debated in the 106th Congress (1999 to 2000).

THE BIGGEST OBSTETRIC-GYNECOLOGIC ISSUES BEFORE THE 106TH CONGRESS

The 106th Congress was a complex, ever-changing, loosely knit body—unable to lay aside the highly partisan weapons of the 105th Congress but pressured to get on with the nation's business. This Congress was born in the aftermath of rapid turnover in the House leadership, leadership that prided itself on creating a revolutionary vision, not on the relatively mundane task of passing bills and keeping federal programs operating.

House Speaker Dennis Hastert (R-IL) and Senate Majority Leader Trent Lott (R-MS) both presided over thin majorities. The House was composed of 222 Republicans, 211 Democrats, and 2 Independents, one of whom usually voted Democratic, giving Hastert a 9-vote majority. Lott presided over 54 Republicans and 46 Democrats. His 8-vote margin could evaporate even more quickly than in the House, because, in the Senate, even one unhappy member of the minority can derail a major bill.

Members of Congress weigh and reweigh the political benefits and costs of every legislative maneuver before taking any action. Even good proposals can be burnt to ash in the crucible of election-year politics.

A broad array of congressional issues directly affects obstetricians-gynecologists, their practices, and their patients. Some issues require an offensive lobbying strategy, in which an organization or individual will try to make a positive change or take a program in a new-direction. Defensive strategies are used to prevent harmful proposals from becoming law. Ensuring that Congress takes no action is sometimes your biggest victory.

Many critical obstetric-gynecologic issues rest in Congress' hands. Let us take a look at the most important.

DIRECT ACCESS

There was a major battle in Congress over patient rights in managed care organizations, a battle that outlived the 106th Congress. Physicians were fighting an offensive war on the Patients' Bill of Rights, trying to create new protections and rights for physicians and patients. For insurers, it was a largely defensive fight—trying to prevent as much congressional action as possible.

A broad array of physicians' groups were actively involved in many of the issues in this mammoth bill, the most controversial of which was patients' rights to sue their HMOs to enforce patient protections, including direct access to obstetric-gynecologic physicians.

But what could be more important than ensuring that your patients can see you when they need to? Managed care companies all across America regularly put roadblocks between women and their obstetrician-gynecologists and the Patients' Bill of Rights offered the real possibility of strong federal direct-access legislation.

A 1999 survey of the nation's obstetrician-gynecologists showed that managed care plans keep women from the health care they need and the providers they want. Sixty percent of all obstetrician-gynecologists in managed care plans reported that their gynecologic patients are either limited or barred from seeing their physicians without first getting permission from another physician. Twenty-eight percent reported that their pregnant patients must first receive another physician's permission before seeing their obstetrician-gynecologists. Nearly 75% of obstetrician-gynecologists surveyed reported that their patients have to return to their primary care physicians for permission before they can be provided necessary follow-up care.

On the other hand, Americans overwhelmingly support direct access to obstetrician-gynecologists. A 1998 survey found that 82% of Americans support federal legislation to require health plans to provide direct access. Sixty-three percent support it even if it means higher health insurance premiums.

Whereas 40 state laws (including the District of Columbia) guarantee women in managed care plans various forms of direct access to their obstetrician-gynecologists, women in federally regulated (Employee Retirement Income Security Act [ERISA]) plans and women who reside in other states do not have this protection. Approximately 70% of the health insurance sold in the United States is purchased through employer-based plans, the great majority of which are subject to ERISA.

Only federal legislation can guarantee all women in managed care plans strong requirements for direct access to obstetric-gynecologic care. Women must have direct access to their obstetrician-gynecologists not only for the first visit but for referrals to subspecialists and needed follow-up care, too.

In 1999, the United States House and Senate passed separate managed care bills that included different direct access to obstetric-gynecologic care provisions. The House bill included the strongest direct access provision to date, guaranteeing women direct access to obstetric-gynecologic providers for all covered obstetric-gynecologic care and related follow-up care. The House bill also covered women in all managed care plans, not just federally regulated (ERISA) plans. The Senate bill covered only ERISA plans and included a number of loopholes, which weakened this protection.

A small group of House and Senate members worked to reconcile the differences between the House and the Senate bills, to no avail.

HEALTH INSURANCE COVERAGE FOR PREGNANT WOMEN

Do low-income pregnant women in your area have health care coverage for their prenatal and obstetric care? In most areas of the country, they do not, putting millions of women and their babies at risk.

In fact, in 1997, approximately 465,000 pregnant women—13.7% of all pregnancies—were uninsured. Women aged 18 to 24 years are most likely to be uninsured. Nearly one in five women of childbearing age (15 to 44 years), totaling 11.8 million women, were uninsured in 1997, accounting for 25% of all uninsured Americans. Nearly two thirds (61%) of these women had family incomes below 200% of the federal poverty line.

Medicaid, the Nation's health care program for low-income individuals, helps. Medicaid is key for pregnant women, covering more than 1.5 million births (39% of all births) in 1995 and insuring 10.6% of childbearing women in 1997. Nonetheless, a large majority (77%) of uninsured women are eligible for, but not enrolled in, Medicaid.

The new State Children's Health Insurance Program (SCHIP) offers even more promise. Under SCHIP, the federal and state governments fund programs that provide health insurance to low-income uninsured children up to age 19 years. Congress can extend this coverage to pregnant women of all ages who meet the program's income eligibility requirements and guarantee direct access to obstetric-gynecologic care for women and adolescent enrollees. Six bills were introduced in the 106th Congress to allow states to cover pregnant women under SCHIP.

BREAST AND CERVICAL CANCER TREATMENT

Early detection and treatment is crucial to women with breast and cervical cancer. But uninsured women cannot afford treatment.

In 1990, a new program was created under which uninsured women could be screened for breast and cervical cancer through the Centers for Disease Control and Prevention (CDC). Unfortunately, no funding was available to *treat* women identified with cancer under this program.

The House of Representatives passed legislation to allow states to provide Medicaid coverage for women suspected of having breast or cervical cancer under the CDC screening program. The Senate Finance Committee approved its own version of this important bill.

Good legislation can be coupled with problematic legislation—legislation that is fought through defensive lobbying strategies.

Congressman Tom Coburn (R-OK) added amendments to the House bill that might have led the federal government to develop a mandatory reporting system for human papillomavirus (HPV) and would have required condom labels that read "Condoms do not effectively prevent the transmission of human papillomavirus and such virus can cause cervical cancer."

A broad array of women's health care groups strenuously opposed these amendments and worked to defeat them.

The CDC estimates that 75% of all adult Americans will contract some form of HPV in their lives. Although millions of women yearly are infected with HPV, HPV will lead to cervical cancer in only a tiny percentage of these women. Many public health advocates are concerned that the Coburn condom warning label (1) would contradict public health messages that encourage individuals to use condoms to protect themselves from sexually transmitted diseases (STDs), including HIV/AIDS, (2) is highly misleading, suggesting that all HPVs lead to cervical cancer, and (3) does nothing to help educate women about the importance of regular Papanicolaou (Pap) examinations to screen for HPV or to explain treatment options.

Those advocates argued that making HPV a reportable diseases is also the wrong approach, because there are many variations of this disease that affect women in many different ways. Some women diagnosed with HPV will have no sign of the disease 6 months later, or even ever again. Some public health advocates argued that the government should not be in the business of collecting this information on vast numbers of women.

Ultimately, both houses of Congress passed the Breast and Cervical Cancer Treatment Act, without the troublesome Coburn amendment, and President Clinton signed the measure into law in October 2000.

CONTRACEPTIVE COVERAGE

Many insurance plans cover prescription drugs but not prescription contraceptive drugs, devices, or services. Nearly half (49%) of United States health care plans that cover prescription drugs do not cover any of the five most commonly used prescription contraceptives (oral contraceptive pills, injectable and implant hormone products, intrauterine devices [IUDs], and diaphragms), only one third cover birth control pills, and only 15% cover all five. Only 18% of all Preferred Provider Organizations (PPOs) and 33% of all point-of-service networks routinely cover all five methods.

At the same time, women aged 15 to 44 years—the prime childbearing years—have out-of-pocket expenditures for health care services that were 68% higher than those of men of the same age: $573 and $342, respectively. The annual cost for oral contraceptives, IUDs, and condoms were about $300, $500, and $50 each in 1993.

Twelve states and the District of Columbia have passed laws requiring insurers that cover prescription drugs also to cover prescription contraceptives. But why change laws one state at a time?

Congress can require all insurance plans that cover prescription drugs to cover contraceptive drugs, devices, and services, as well. Bipartisan legislation was introduced in the House and the Senate to require contraceptive coverage of all insurance plans that cover prescription drugs. Congress indicated a strong desire to include "conscience clauses" in this legislation, which would allow religious-based employers to opt out of this requirement.

Congress, since 1998, has required contraceptive coverage for government employees in the Federal Employees Health Benefits Plan (FEHBP), which serves as a model for other health care plans.

VIOLENCE AGAINST OBSTETRICIAN-GYNECOLOGISTS AND PATIENTS

It is a terrible reality. Obstetrician-gynecologists, their staff, and patients can be in jeopardy of violence at health care clinics and even at home. This violence must be stopped, and those who commit these crimes must be held responsible for their actions.

Since its passage in 1994, the Freedom of Access to Clinic Entrances (FACE) Act has helped make women's health clinics safer for patients and health care providers. But under a loophole in the bankruptcy laws, criminals found guilty of FACE crimes have avoided paying court-ordered fines simply by filing for bankruptcy. Some of this nation's worst FACE criminals have filed for bankruptcy protection to avoid paying FACE crime fines.

It is time Congress closed this gaping loophole. The Senate overwhelmingly approved Senator Charles Schumer's (D-NY) effort to do just that, voting 80 to 17 in favor of his amendment to the bankruptcy reform bill. President Clinton added his strong support to Senator Schumer's effort. Ultimately, the bankruptcy reform bill was left unfinished, and poised for action in the 107th Congress.

COLLECTIVE BARGAINING

It used to be so much simpler. You, the doctor, would decide what was best for your patient and how to manage your practice. Now managed care plans call the shots, micromanage your every decision, and seem to have all the leverage.

Doctors can reclaim their authority, level the playing field, and put patients first again. Today's antitrust laws prevent most physicians from joining together to bargain with insurers. But Congress had the opportunity to change the law and let doctors bargain collectively with health insurers by passing the Quality Health Care Coalition Act of 2000, sponsored by Representative Tom Campbell (R-CA).

This bill, one of the most hotly debated health care bills in Congress, had 220 House cosponsors, but faced fierce opposition from insurers, business groups, and health professionals.

In the summer of 1999, after much delay, the House passed the Campbell bill in modified form with a vote of 276 to 136. A companion bill was never introduced in the Senate and the bill did not become law.

GRADUATE MEDICAL EDUCATION

Every obstetrician-gynecologist has to complete a residency training program successfully before attaining his or her MD degree. The federal government, through the Medicare and Medicaid programs, provides most of the funds for these important programs—$6 billion from Medicare and $3 billion from Medicaid every year. These funds enable teaching hospitals to stay open, and they pay salaries and other costs integral to residency programs.

Congress may dramatically change the way the nation funds medical residency programs, including obstetrics-gynecology, throwing the very future of the specialty into question.

Teaching hospitals provide basic health services to their

communities and clinical education for all types of health professionals. These hospitals, which on average serve sicker patients with more complex health care needs, often have higher patient costs than other hospitals.

Medicare pays these hospitals more for the care they provide under the prospective payment system (PPS), through a payment known as the indirect medical education (IME) add-on.

States vary widely in payments to graduate medical education (GME) as a percentage of their state Medicaid in-patient payments (0% to 19.6%.) Five states, for example, do not fund any GME. In nearly half of all states, Medicaid GME spending amounts to less than 7% of their in-patient hospital costs, with only six states spending more than 15%. New York disburses nearly one third of all Medicaid GME spending. Overall, states spend about 7% of their Medicaid dollars on GME, compared with their in-patient hospital spending, the same proportion of Medicare GME spending as a percent of its in-patient payments.

The 106th Congress considered a new proposal to change dramatically how the nation pays for GME. In August 1999, the Medicare Payment Advisory Commission (MedPAC) sent a report to Congress called "Rethinking Medicare's Payment Policies for Graduate Medical Education and Teaching Hospitals," recommending a new way for Medicare to pay teaching hospitals.

Among other elements of its proposal, MedPAC is recommending that Congress pay residency programs based only on the portion of care provided to Medicare beneficiaries and make federal GME payments part of the annual appropriations process, removing it from the regular and reliable Medicare payment process. Here is what these proposals could mean to obstetrician-gynecologists.

First, every year, each residency program would report to a federal agency the number of Medicare beneficiaries it treated and the conditions for which these patients were treated. Each obstetric-gynecologic residency program would be funded only to the extent that its residents treat Medicare beneficiaries for Medicare-covered services.

Second, residency program chairs would have no certainty about how much funding their programs would receive each year, or even when they would receive the funds. By law, Congress must appropriated funds to run the federal labor and health care programs by September 30 every year—the end of the federal fiscal year. The last year that Congress met this legal deadline was 1993. Congress is habitually late in passing these important bills, and funding for federal programs is often delayed until well into the next year.

Third, residency programs could be forced to compete for funding with other residency programs and with other federal programs, like National Institutes of Health (NIH).

Hospital and physician organizations are working to restore the deep GME cuts Congress enacted in 1997 and to ensure adequate federal funding of GME, including obstetric-gynecologic residency programs, in the future. The 106th Congress agreed to restore some funds to

GME, but did not tackle the larger issue of reforming the way America pays for physician training programs.

Women's Health Research Funding

The Federal government funds millions of dollars in health care research, but how much goes to fund research into women's health?

NIH funding for women's health research has not kept pace with increases in NIH funding overall. Whereas federal funding for NIH continues to grow, the percent of NIH dollars funding women's health research has fallen steadily since fiscal year (FY) 1997. In FY97, 15.53% of all NIH dollars were spent on women's health research, falling to 15.28% in FY98, 14.86% in FY99, and 14.57% in FY2000.

Similarly, the National Institute of Child Health and Human Development (NICHHD), which funds the majority of research in obstetrics and gynecology, has traditionally received the lowest percentage funding increases of all the NIH institutes. Although overall NIH funding increased by 46.8% from FY94 to FY99, NICHHD funding rose only 36.3%, the lowest percentage funding of NIH's 20 major institutes

NICHHD's legal mission statement indicated that the Institute conducts research only into maternal health problems, ignoring the health research needs of women not of childbearing age. In reality, NICHHD's research affects the reproductive and gynecologic health of women of all ages.

NICHHD supports, for example, research on pelvic prolapse and urinary incontinence—conditions that affect as many as one third of all adult women in America and women of all ages. In fact, although urinary incontinence affects as many as 30% of all women ages 60 years and older, it also affects as many as 25% of all women younger than 65 years.

The 106th Congress recognized the importance of NICHHD's research into women's health issues, including and beyond maternal issues. This recognition, in turn, may help Congress realize the importance of this research and its relevance to millions of American women and families.

The Senate NIH funding bill highlighted women's health research at NIH and included "gynecologic," as well as maternal health, in NICHHD'S mission statement. The final bill expanded the mission statement to include "gynecologic health."

Be a Part of the Solution

Clearly, many elements of your practice, and your life, are in Congress' hands. All kinds of health care professionals and other citizens actively educate and communicate with Congress every day.

Nurses, nurse midwives, pediatricians, family physicians, patient and "disease" groups, insurers, and drug companies all actively lobby Congress in Washington and at home on health care issues. Congress considers their points of view, and many others, on issues that affect you directly. Obstetrician-gynecologists are in the congressional game, too.

You have a responsibility to your patients and your practice to get involved with Congress. You are your patients' best advocate. You are uniquely qualified to participate in national health care debates and to explain the effect that congressional proposals will have on your ability to care for your patients. Your participation is vital.

IT HAS NEVER BEEN EASIER

Working with Congress can be fascinating, frustrating, and incredibly rewarding. Fortunately, it has also never been easier to get involved.

There are many ways to get involved and be a part of the solution. Washington lobbying, grassroots lobbying, and involvement in political campaigns are all important bases to touch as you pursue a legislative victory. You can

- Write, call, or e-mail your senators and United States representative about issues that are important to you. See Sources at the end of this chapter for more information.
- Write a letter to the editor of your local newspaper on an issue about which you care. Members of Congress use this forum to keep track of what issues people are talking about at home.
- Place a petition to your representative and senators at your reception desk.
- Attend town meetings and voice your concerns.
- Meet with your member of Congress when he or she is in town, or extend an invitation to tour your clinic or health care facility.
- Offer to serve as a health advisor for your representative on legislative proposals.
- Host or attend a fundraising reception for your member of Congress or senator. You will definitely have her or his ear. See the section on Political Fundraisers for the rules and logistics of holding a political fundraiser.

YOU ALREADY ARE A CONGRESSIONAL HEALTH POLICY EXPERT

Obstetrician-gynecologists are located in nearly every United States Congressional District. And members of Congress are often very eager to hear from knowledgeable constituents who can advise them on the sometimes complex health initiatives before them. After all, every member of Congress has to vote, but very few sit on the health committees or even have staff with expertise on these issues.

It is easier to be an expert than you might think. Your member of Congress does not expect you to know statute or precedents or underlying law. He or she needs you to tell what you already know—the needs of your patients, problems you have found with health care programs, how insurance companies and government agencies affect your ability to treat your patients.

These are health policy problems in everyday clothes. And you are on the educated front lines, better situated than anyone else to speak with authority on what you see and experience every day.

POLITICAL FUNDRAISERS

It is a fact: Money makes the political world go around. Does this mean money buys votes and congressmen are taking bribes? No, but it does highlight an interesting dynamic.

It costs a lot to run successfully for Congress. At the same time, every member of Congress is besieged with requests to fix a problem, introduce a bill, or help clear a bureaucratic hurdle.

Here is how this dynamic between the high cost of elections and overwhelming demands often translates:

- If a representative has only 2 hours in the District office to meet with constituents before flying back to Washington, the member of Congress is much more likely to make time for a supporter.
- If a representative receives two conflicting invitations to speak, she or he is much more likely to speak to the group that supports her or him.
- And when the chairman of a committee gives a representative the opportunity to add only two items to a major bill, the representative is much more likely to offer items that his or her supporters have brought to him or her.

Members of Congress view financial donors as supporters and friends—individuals and organizations committed to helping them. Contributors gain attention and support for their causes, often over other equally virtuous needs of nonsupporters.

The Rules

The world of fundraisers is very simple and straightforward. As citizens, you, your colleagues, friends, and family can participate in fundraisers to the fullest extent of the law. The Federal Election Commission (FEC) makes the rules governing individuals very clear and easy to follow.

- You can give a maximum of $1000 per election to a federal candidate or the candidate's campaign committee. This maximum applies to each election, that is, $1000 for the primary, $1000 for a runoff election, $1,000 for the general election, and so on.
- Your spouse can also contribute up to $1000 per election, even if you are the sole source of income.
- You can host a fundraising party, dinner, or reception in your home. The use of your home itself is not considered a contribution. Neither are the costs of invitations, food, or drinks, as long as the total cost is below $1000 ($2000

if your spouse is participating). Any amount spent in excess of these dollar amounts counts as part of your monetary contribution to the candidate and toward your $1000 ($2000 for a couple) per election contribution limit.

- You can host a fundraiser at your church or in a community room where you live, as long as the community room is regularly made available for noncommercial purposes without regard to party affiliation. Any nominal fee you pay for use to the room is not considered a contribution and does not count toward your contribution limit.
- You should make your monetary contribution by personal check, made out to the candidate's campaign committee. It is helpful, but not necessary, for you to indicate the election (primary, general) on the memo line. **This is your only reporting requirement**. The campaign committee has to do all the rest of the paperwork and meet all other reporting requirements.

The Logistics

- Contact your candidate's campaign committee and offer to hold a fundraiser. They will be your new best friends.
- Work out the date, time, location, invitees, and contribution level. You may want to hold a small cocktail party in your home and invite 30 key friends, each contributing $100. Or you might want to make it a big informal gathering, hot dogs and lemonade, for $25 a person.
- Issue invitations along these lines:

  Let us elect a great candidate! You are invited to an evening of cocktails and conversation with John Doe, candidate for Congress.

  At my home, 123 Pleasant Street, 6:30 PM on Friday, August 1.

  Please make your checks payable to John Doe for Congress. Suggested contributions are $50 per individual, $100 per couple.

- Nametags and markers at an entry table make it easy for the candidate to remember names and faces.
- Talk to the candidate about issues that are on your mind.
- Give the candidate a chance to address the crowd. He or she probably will not need much prodding.

You will notice that you did not buy any votes. Instead, what you gained was access—a representative's time and attention to your issues. It does not guarantee a legislative success. You still have to use your other lobbying tools. But you have just touched one very important base.

Sources

American College of Obstetrics and Gynecology's Federal Legislative Action Center
http://congress.nw.dc.us/acog/
For up-to-the-minute Congressional news, summaries of top legislative issues, and to e-mail your Members of Congress and Senators. It's free and as easy as a click of your mouse.

United States Congress
http://thomas.loc.gov
An easy site to navigate, THOMAS is a resource for the legislative novice as well as the most advanced legislative guru. This site contains information about current and past legislation, committees, current Members of Congress, basic information on the legislative process, and more.

United States House of Representatives
http://www.house.gov
This website provides information about Members of Congress, committees, and the leadership of the United States House of Representatives. Find out about updates on current legislation, as well as how your Member voted on important bills.

United States Senate
http://www.senate.gov
Find out about the senators, committees, and leadership of the United States Senate. Contact you senators automatically by entering your home state. Research current legislation and how your senators voted.

White House
http://www.whitehouse.gov
Your entry to the Executive Branch.

National Institutes of Health
http://www.nih.gov
You can find everything you want to know about NIH and more at this site. Along with the latest health information from A to Z, they offer access to home pages for all 25 of the institutes and centers that make up NIH.

National Institute of Child Health and Human Development
http://www.nichd.nih.gov/
The National Institute of Child Health and Human Development is the part of the National Institutes of Health that conducts and supports research on the reproductive, neurobiologic, developmental, and behavioral processes that determine and maintain the health of children.

Women's Health Initiative
http://www.nhlbi.nih.gov/whi/index.html
The NIH established the Women's Health Initiative (WHI) in 1991 to address the most common causes of death, disability, and impaired quality of life in postmenopausal women, including cardiovascular disease, cancer, and osteoporosis. The WHI is a 15-year multimillion dollar endeavor and one of the largest American prevention studies of its kind.

Office of Research on Women's Health
http://www4.od.nih.gov/orwh/
The Office of Research on Women's Health (ORWH) serves as a focal point for women's health research at the NIH. The ORWH promotes and supports efforts to improve the health of women through biomedical and behavioral research.

Department of Health and Human Services Office on Women's Health
http://www.4women.gov/owh/index.htm
The Office on Women's Health coordinates women's health research, policy, and education across HHS, collaborating with other government organizations and consumer and health care professional groups.

National Women's Health Information Center
http://www.4woman.gov
The National Women's Health Information Center provides a gateway to federal and other women's health information resources.

Centers for Disease Control and Prevention
http://www.cdc.gov
The goal of the Centers for Disease Control and Prevention is to promote health and quality of life by preventing and controlling disease, injury, and disability.

Health Care Finance Administration
http://www.hcfa.gov
HCFA provides health insurance for over 74 million Americans through Medicare, Medicaid, and Child Health.

The Official Medicare Website
http://www.medicare.gov
Administered by the Health Care Financing Administration, the site provides an overview of the Medicare system, including everything from health plan options to Medicare publications.

Medicare Payment Advisory Commission
http://www.medpac.gov
The Medicare Payment Advisory Commission (MedPAC) advises Congress on issues affecting the Medicare program.

Implementing Quality Improvement in Obstetric and Gynecologic Practice

Scott B. Ransom

The science of clinical improvement has developed since about 1980 owing to academic institutions and health care organizations searching for ways to reduce costs while improving quality. Whereas the origins of clinical improvement can be traced to industrial quality improvement approaches, leading health care organizations have expanded these foundations to include sophisticated tools focused on clinical practices. This chapter focuses on four contemporary techniques to improve obstetrics and gynecology clinical practice: physician-specific performance measures, clinical information systems, clinical pathways, and considerations in leading quality improvement programs.

PHYSICIAN PERFORMANCE MEASURES

Physician-specific performance measures have been used successfully in many clinical practices and hospitals to improve clinical quality. Other terms used to describe physician-specific performance measurement have included: "practice profiling," "report cards," and "best practices." The contemporary use of these measurement programs has focused on reducing excess resource consumption while improving quality. Although the origins of these tools were from the managed care industry's attempt to cut costs, leading physicians and hospitals have learned that giving physicians continuous feedback on their clinical practice can and will have a major impact on physician behavior, leading to superior clinical care.

Practice profiling enables comparisons between current and expected performance of individual physicians. It is designed to assist physicians to become more proactive in their own clinical practices and improve quality for their patients. Individual physicians and hospitals may choose to benchmark their performance to leading peers, hospital standards, and nationally accepted standards of quality. The goal is to provide the individual physician with information regarding his or her quantitative performance to facilitate better quality.

The best physician performance measurement systems focus on a variety of complementary measures of performance: patient satisfaction, clinical quality, resource consumption, and patient access. It is important to observe performance from a variety of perspectives to provide the physician with proper and balanced feedback. It is rare to find an individual physician who simultaneously excels in all areas of performance. A balanced measurement program may allow the physician to more clearly appreciate all aspects of clinical practice. For example, Physician A is very proud of his very low length of stay when compared with his peer group; however, his readmission rate is very high and patient satisfaction rate is very low. Does this physician have an optimal practice? Although Physician B has excellent patient satisfaction and clinical quality measures, her length of stay and ancillary resource consumption are the highest in the community. Physician B is resulting in a substantial financial loss for the hospital and physician-owned managed care organization, which is placing her employment in jeopardy. Does this physician have an optimal practice? The best physician profiling systems will observe an individual physician's practice from a variety of perspectives to provide a balanced perspective of quality.

One obvious question that must be considered in these programs is "why profile?" Profiling provides a quantitative system to show an individual physician's practice performance. Although physicians often have a general idea of their personal cesarean section rate, vaginal birth after cesarean rate, blood transfusion frequency, readmission rate, frequency of appropriate use of antibiotics, patient satisfaction rate, length of time to schedule a patient for an office visit, and frequency of ordering appropriate tests on patients, the busy physician is often blind to reality. Performance profiling will provide the practicing physician a quantitative measure of quality versus a perception of qualitative quality.

There are many examples of performance measurement programs leading to improved quality. A multidisciplinary committee at Hutzel Hospital developed and implemented a clinical pathway for cesarean section. The committee identified the community standard of care by recommending the routine use of prophylactic antibiotics immediately following the delivery of the baby at the time of cesarean section. Outcome measures were collected for the department and individual physicians, indicating the percent of patients that received a prophylactic antibiotic. The department initially provided prophylactic antibiotics to only 42% of patients. Whereas most physicians perceived that most of their patients received antibiotics with cesarean, the data spoke volumes for their individual practices. The clinical pathway committee reviewed the specific processes and found 22 individual steps required to provide prophylactic antibiotics at the time of cesarean. The committee developed a new process that included only 4 steps, which increased the pathway compliance to over 94%. Thus, the performance measure showed a problem that was treated with a thoughtful and proactive process to improve all physicians' practice in providing antibiotics at the time of cesarean. Further, the physician-specific performance measures providing individual provider's data on their performance improved acceptance and compliance with the new processes, which led to better patient quality.

Thus, physician-specific performance measures can provide the physician with quantitative information regarding patient care quality. The information can be used by individual physicians to review their personal clinical practices or for an entire group to improve processes leading to superior performance.

CLINICAL INFORMATION SYSTEMS

The use of clinical information systems can dramatically improve clinical quality. The Institute of Medicine (IOM) and other studies have shown that adverse events occur in 2.9% to 3.7% of hospitalizations leading to 44,000 to 98,000 deaths annually. These hospital errors are responsible for more annual deaths in the United States than motor vehicle accidents (43,458), breast cancer (42,297), or AIDS (16,516). These errors can largely be classified as "an error in planning" or "an error in execution." The identification of these errors encourages health care leaders to build safety into the processes of care as an effective way to reduce errors and to improve quality. A functional clinical information system can provide an effective tool to reduce the potential for medical errors through such modalities as physician order entry and a longitudinal medical record.[4]

An electronic medical record (EMR) can significantly reduce the potential for medical errors. First, traditional paper records have many problems, such as being at the wrong location, allowing only one user at a time, being poorly organized, and requiring substantial space for storage. The EMR can eliminate many problems associated with a paper chart by providing fingertip access to the right information at the right place and time. Second, electronic order entry can reduce the potential for errors due to reducing the need for a clerk to read poor handwriting, reducing the potential for transcription errors, and provide an immediate feedback to the physician through alerts and insights.[2]

Alerts can be very helpful to the clinician by highlighting probable errors in clinical care or judgment. For example, a physician that orders a cephalosporin for a penicillin-allergic patient would be warned of the potential problem by the information system. Similarly, electronic standard order sets can be used by the clinician to save valuable time and reduce the potential to forget important orders. These electronic order sets can be a valuable tool

in reducing the potential for physician memory lapses in care such as providing a prophylactic antibiotic, ordering a time-sensitive laboratory test such as an α-fetoprotein at an appropriate gestational age, and assuring appropriately dosed medications such as methotrexate in treating an ectopic pregnancy.

Clinical information systems can be an extremely valuable aid to facilitate the care process. Specifically, the care management process can be facilitated through information systems by providing an affordable way to do the following: collect clinically detailed data needed for quality and outcome measures, incorporate up-to-date scientific evidence into daily practice, carry out multiple clinical practice improvement projects over time, and promote teamwork for clinical and administrative tasks. These systems can provide improved efficiency in many ways such as providing an automatic page or e-mail to notify the physician regarding results for a critical laboratory or radiology test. Through Palm and wireless technologies, a physician can be immediately notified of important clinical facts. These technologies reduce the time required for unnecessary phone calls by the physician to the nurse, the nurse to the pharmacist, and the pharmacist to the laboratory. Instead, the care providers are simultaneously notified of important test results to better coordinate care and reduce the potential for duplication of services and errors.[3]

The information system can be an invaluable aid in retrieving patient information at remote sites. For example, a patient calls the physician over the weekend regarding the use of her antibiotic treatment. The physician may retrieve the entire medical record at her home through wireless or Internet access to the information system. This allows the physician immediate access to the patient's medical record as well as provides the physician the opportunity to document the phone conversation with the patient. The immediate access to the medical record clearly improves the quality of the recommendations made to the patient.

These information systems can improve the billing effectiveness for most physician practices. Specifically, the billing office has direct access to on-line charting, operative notes, and discharge summaries to facilitate accurate billing. Similarly, the physician may access all hospital information through Palm technologies or Internet access to facilitate accuracy and timeliness of billing. The days of the billing manager waiting for the physician to bring the "medical record face sheet" are gone with the use of these information technologies.

CLINICAL PATHWAYS AND PROTOCOLS

Clinical pathways and protocols were originally proposed as a remedy for irrational medical practice. Dr. Wennberg and associates[1] demonstrated that patients with similar medical conditions were treated differently depending on the community in which they received care.

Similarly, investigators have highlighted substantial patient care variation for similar conditions at the same hospital depending on the physician. These findings lead to obvious questions. Does variation in treatment lead to equal patient quality care or could some patients be receiving more optimal care than others? Why do some physicians appear to have consistently very low and others very high caesarean section rates for similar patient populations? Clinical pathways provide a mechanism to thoughtfully consider the optimal care process for patients given current medical practice, research findings, technological advances, and local expertise.[5]

The development of high-quality clinical pathways can facilitate quality patient care. The preferred development of pathways occurs locally by multidisciplinary teams of physicians and ancillary personnel perceived to have the highest standards in patient care. The pathway team may adapt nationally accepted pathways to their local situation; however, any national guideline must be integrated into the local hospital culture and service availability. Conversely, the pathway team may create a new pathway based on best practices and evidenced-based literature. Further, the local pathway team must consider ways to measure clinical practices to ensure and continually improve the process. For example, a pathway includes the use of a regular diet as tolerated immediately following a hysterectomy as published in recent literature; however, a number of the physicians on the pathway team are very reluctant to accept the current literature on this subject. Thus, the pathway process can be tested through specific outcome measures comparing postoperative complications before and after the implementation of regular diet as a routine part of postoperative care to prove quality. That is, the team may oversee the clinical pathway through specific outcome measures to continually update and improve the care process.

The implementation of clinical pathways may reduce medical-legal risk. Recent research was completed to determine the medical-legal risk reduction potential by the use of clinical pathways in obstetrics. A retrospective study identified "closed" obstetric malpractice claims filed over 10 years against a large health system consisting of four hospitals delivering over 12,000 babies annually. The research reviewed 236 cases and found that 81 of these cases were directly related and 21 other cases were secondarily related to not completing the clinical pathway standard. Thus, 34.3% of the filed obstetric claims were primarily related and 43.2% were primarily or secondarily related to not completing the clinical pathway's standard of care. Thus, the study found that many obstetric malpractice cases were directly related to not following the "standard of care."[6] The study randomly selected patients that did not file a medical-legal claim to determine if variations in the clinical pathway existed for this population. Of the 240 control patients that did not file a medical-legal claim at this health system, the study found 28 (11.7%) patients with variations of care from the clinical pathway. Thus, whereas the rate of variation for the standard clinical path-

way resulted in a higher potential for a medical-legal claim, many patients do not sue despite the care being less than optimal. Clinical pathway utilization may provide a mechanism to reduce clinical variation, improve clinical quality, and reduce medical-legal risk in obstetrics.[6]

LEADING QUALITY IMPROVEMENT

Comparing health care to other industries' performance provides a telling picture. Federal Express shows an error rate of approximately 1 per million whereas medical record error rates are commonly 5% to 10%. Banking transactions present an error rate of approximately 1 per 10 million whereas hospital billing departments typically have error of over 2%. Airline landings and takeoffs showed 1 error per million whereas medication administration errors are typically 7% to 10%. This does not present the very high cost of advice for health care when compared with other industries. For example, Home Depot will provide advice from a master craftsman for a $3 purchase versus a $500 office visit with frequently little advice from the physician. These examples present a challenge to health care organizations and physicians to improve processes to force the elimination of errors.

Unfortunately, many physicians and health care leaders do not recognize obvious problems with patient care and suggest our current practices are as good as they have always been. Fortunately, other physicians and health care leaders are forcing substantial improvement to drive improved patient quality and reduced potential for medical errors. One issue is that quality and performance have not always been carefully defined in health care. As is the case in many professions, quality and performance have been treated as a matter to be judged by the practitioner, and specifically not by the patient, client, or customer. Better performance data collected on individual hospitals and providers will force leaders to develop better processes leading to better care.

Obstetrics and gynecology is an area of clinical practice that provides a challenging, but fruitful, area to lead quality improvement. The American College of Obstetrics and Gynecology has been a leader in improving clinical practice in obstetrics and gynecology through technical bulletins, practice forms, patient handouts, continuing medical education programs, and other publications. In addition, the process of care tends to be progressive and generally systematic for many obstetric and gynecologic patients allowing the use of clinical pathways, standard order sets, comprehensive outcome measures, and benchmarking. Thus, the implementation of process improvement programs leading to improved patient quality should be an integral part of any high-quality obstetrics and gynecology service.

Some of the challenges in improving health care performance include many overuse, underuse, and misuse issues in patient care. Overuse can be shown in circumstances where the potential for harm exceeds the possible benefits, such as completing an inappropriate hysterectomy. Underuse presents a failure to provide a health service when it would have produced a favorable outcome, such as using prophylactic antibiotics for cesarean section. Misuse is shown when an appropriate service is selected but a preventable complication occurs, such as using a new laparoscopic cautery device to control bleeding but simultaneously injuring the bowel due to incorrectly using the instrument.

Routine excellent performance in obstetrics and gynecology requires more than outstanding provider performance—it requires leadership. Leadership must be highly visible in the organization, leading to a systematic review of performance and seeking opportunities to improve clinical practice. Similarly, strong leadership must emphasize communication across the organization, including physician leaders, practicing clinicians, nursing, pharmacy, housekeeping, administration, and others. A performance improvement effort to increase operating room efficiency may require a large multidisciplinary team to identify specific problems and develop optimal processes. Whereas some physicians may be reluctant to work with unskilled hospital staff, such as housekeeping, the success of the performance improvement program may hinge on that group's functionality. Further, it is important to ensure standardized definitions when comparing outcomes. For example, a large hospital system compared operative time for gynecologic procedures to find that Hospital B has a much longer operative time than Hospital A with a medical staff that utilizes both hospitals. On closer review, the definitions for operative time were different at each of the two hospitals. Hospital A measured operative time from the beginning of the operative procedure at "incision time" until the procedure was completed; conversely, Hospital B measured operative time from when the patient entered the operating room to the patient's removal from the operative room. Thus, it is important to ensure that the definitions and methodologies are the same when benchmarking outcome measures within the organization or when comparing clinical practice to outside "best practices" organizations.

Excellent clinical performance requires the development of a high-performance environment with training and retraining programs for skilled and unskilled staff. Training should include programs to align culture, strategy, and the structure of the organization and emphasize leadership development. The high-performance environment provides a clear vision and objectives for all members of the team to unite and create effective partnerships. It is particularly helpful to provide recognition and rewards for projects well done to further stimulate teamwork and enthusiasm for improvement.

Physician leaders particularly require a clear understanding of expectations. The physician must perceive the time spent in performance improvement programs as highly valuable for continued support. A physician may be encouraged to support performance improvement programs by outcome measurement and continuous feedback. Fortunately, most physicians are highly competitive and will work toward performance improvement if measurement programs are meaningful and reliable. Further, leaders must maintain a nonconfrontational and nonthreatening style in working with physicians in performance improvement. When physicians and other individuals perceive threats, those individuals will generally not work toward improvement but will work toward protecting themselves. Thus, effective leadership is a complex and delicate set of skills and attitudes, including listening, planning, communicating, managing conflict, giving feedback, and encouraging others.

Successful leaders are able to learn from failure and go on to the next initiative. They have a passion for their work with an ability to see the roadblocks and power struggles in the environment. Leaders are willing to take risks and devote great energy to reach their objectives and drive the initiative to success. Thus, the leadership to drive performance improvement in an organization is absolutely critical to success.[7]

CONCLUSION

The goal of this chapter was to focus on four contemporary techniques to improve obstetrics and gynecology clinical practice: physician-specific performance measures, clinical information systems, clinical pathways, and leading quality improvement programs. Through these and other techniques, performance improvement can be effectively introduced to most organizations and physician practices; however, the willingness and focus to drive measurable high quality must be a passion throughout the organization. The top leader must actively encourage the leadership and enthusiasm to improve clinical quality, patient satisfaction, and financial performance in obstetrics and gynecology.

References

1. Wennberg J: The Dartmouth Atlas of Health Care in the United States. Chicago, American Hospital Association, 1996.
2. Howe R: Physician and Technology: Evaluating the impact of technology and information systems. Practice Pointers: Physicians and Technology 1999;491:1–6.
3. Weber J: Computer Patient Records that improve health care. Healthcare Information Management Winter 1997;11(4):1–4.
4. Berwick D: A primer on leading the improvement of systems. BMJ 1996;312:619–622.
5. Bodenheimer T: Disease management—promises and pitfalls. N Engl J Med 1999;340:1202–1205.
6. Ransom SB, Dombrowski MP, Evans MI: Reduced medical legal risk by optimal clinical pathway implementation: A case control trial. Presented to the Central Association of Obstetrics and Gynecology Annual Meeting, October 2000.
7. Kotter J: Leading change: Why transformation efforts fail. Harv Business Rev 1995;73:59.

The History, Impact, and Future of the Medicare Fee Schedule

Cynthia A. Brown

The 1980s witnessed the beginning of a steady erosion in payments for specialty care under Medicare and other insurance plans. It all started with targeted Medicare payment reductions for selected high-volume procedures, and culminated in 1989 with federal legislation that fundamentally restructured the methods used to determine physician payments—not only under Medicare but also by the increasing number of payers who subsequently adopted the federal system. For the most part, this sweeping change had the most detrimental impact on payments for surgical services and other procedures typically provided in facility settings. Now, federal policy makers say it is time to consider new proposals to fundamentally reform the entire Medicare program. How did we get to this point? What was the plan? Thinking about how we got here, what does it say about where we are going?

MEDICARE PHYSICIAN PAYMENT "REFORMS"

Until the early 1990s, Medicare's physician payment system relied on a historical charge-based methodology—specifically, a system of "customary, prevailing, and reasonable" (CPR) fees based on the payment practices of most private health insurers. It was widely believed at the time that Medicare payments for evaluation and management (E&M) services—or patient visits—were generally too low, whereas payments for procedures were generally too high. This presumption was based, at least in part, on the belief that the CPR system resulted in "sticky" pricing for new technology. In other words, the charge-based system provided no incentive for physicians to reduce what was generally billed for new, complex procedures once the knowledge and resources required to provide them became more widely available; Medicare (and other insurers) would continue to pay for these services at the rates physicians were charging.

At the same time, federal and state governments and businesses that provide health benefits for their employees were alarmed by health care costs that were projected to consume an ever-increasing portion of their operating budgets. These concerns were heightened by studies concluding that the intensity of health care services provided in a given community is related to the size of the local population of specialists—who were said to provide more

costly, but not necessarily more effective, care. Finally, projections of an undersupply of primary care physicians in a health care system growing increasingly dependent on managed care gave weight to arguments that the current payment structure was "unfair" and unwisely encouraged medical students to pursue careers in better-paying specialties.

In 1989, President George H. Bush signed into law the Omnibus Budget Reconciliation Act (OBRA 89), requiring Medicare to implement today's physician payment system. It relies on a national fee schedule constructed according to a "resource-based relative value scale" (RBRVS).* In that fee schedule, relative value units (RVUs) have been assigned to each physician service based on the resources required from physicians to provide them. RVUs have been developed for three distinct components of each physician service listed in the American Medical Association's *Current Procedural Terminology* manual:

- A work component that is intended to reflect the relative amounts of physician time and intensity involved;
- A practice expense component to account for direct and overhead costs incurred by the physician; and
- A malpractice expense component to cover the physician's liability insurance premium costs.

Each of these components, in turn, is adjusted to reflect geographic variations in costs. Finally, to determine the actual dollar amount to be paid for each service, the sum of the geographically adjusted RVUs for the three service components is multiplied by a dollar conversion factor.†

---

*The OBRA 89 payment reforms were described as a "three-legged stool." In addition to mandating the use of a national fee schedule, the law imposed limits on the amounts that physicians may bill Medicare patients above the program's allowed payment (phased down to the current limit of 115% of the fee schedule amount). The intent was to prevent lower reimbursement rates from encouraging physicians to offset their losses by shifting additional costs to their patients. OBRA 89 also established Medicare volume performance standards (MVPSs), which linked annual inflation adjustments to the fee schedule conversion factors with service volume. Again, policy makers were concerned that lower payments could provide an incentive for physicians to increase the volume of services they provide; the MVPSs provided a mechanism for the federal government to keep overall Medicare spending in check if aggregate expenditures exceeded the amount determined by formula to be appropriate.

†At the time the fee schedule took effect on January 1, 1992, the conversion factor was set at what was calculated to be a "budget neutral" figure of $31.00. For 2000, the conversion factor was $36.61.

$$(RVW \times GAF_{work}) \times (RVPE \times GAF_{pe})$$
$$\times (RVMP \times GAF_{mp}) \times \text{Conversion factor}$$
$$= \text{Allowed fee schedule amount}$$

where RVW is the relative value for physician work (work); GAF is the geographic adjustment factor; RVPE is the relative value for practice expenses (pe); and RVMP is the relative value for malpractice (mp).

The new system, hailed by most (nonsurgeons) as "rational" and "fair," produced the expected results. Generally speaking, procedure-oriented specialties that practice primarily in facility settings experienced the most severe Medicare payment and income reductions—neurosurgeons and thoracic, vascular, and general surgeons among them. On the other hand, physicians and other practitioners who rely primarily on office-based services for their income, particularly those specialties that perform procedures in the office, experienced the most significant payment increases. These included optometrists, chiropractors, family physicians, and dermatologists. Of course, the impact of the new payment system varied widely for those physicians who subspecialize, those who practice in multiple settings, and those who may provide a broad mix of procedural and E&M services. Otolaryngologists, ophthalmologists, urologists, orthopedic and plastic surgeons, and obstetrician-gynecologists fall into the category of physicians for whom Medicare's calculation of an increase in payments for the specialty as a whole often did not hold true for the individual practitioner.

THE REDISTRIBUTION CONTINUES

At the time the fee schedule was established, studies had been conducted that purported to show the relative amounts of physician work involved in providing each service, but no one had ever determined the relative amounts of practice and malpractice expenses involved. Consequently, OBRA 89 required the RVUs for these two service components to be established according to formulas that took into account payments made under the old CPR system. Lingering concerns about the "fairness" and rationality of the new payment system, though, led Congress to pass legislation in 1994 that required the development of resource-based practice expense RVUs for incorporation into the fee schedule in 1998.

The preliminary results of this effort were released early in 1997. Serious methodological flaws were evident, accompanied by predictions of severe payment reductions for many of the same specialties affected most severely by the fee schedule's initial implementation. This launched an intense lobbying effort by both medical and surgical specialties that ultimately convinced Congress to revise its plan. The Balanced Budget Act of 1997 (BBA 97) included a 1-year delay in the implementation of new practice expense RVUs (to January 1, 1999) as well as a 3-year transition period. To appease primary care physicians, how-

ever, the BBA 97 included a "down payment" to the E&M services that were expected to experience payment increases with the movement to new practice expense RVUs. BBA 97 also required the development of resource-based RVUs for the third and final fee schedule component—malpractice expenses.*

Unfortunately, whereas certain improvements in the methodology were made and the initial payment reductions have been less severe than originally projected, the goal of developing a "fair" Medicare payment system is not applied evenly. For example, when faced with choices to make in the methodology (e.g., whether and how to average cost estimates and what costs to allow for specific services), regulators frequently opt for the path that inflates payments for primary care services at the expense of specialty care. The negative impact of any individual methodological decision is often quite small, but there is growing concern that the cumulative impact of the many contested choices, and of the data refinements not yet made, may compound the negative impact on payment for procedural services.

Perhaps the simplest illustration of this can be found in the methodology used to develop resource-based RVUs for the malpractice expense component of the fee schedule. Although the specialty-specific premium data appear to be of good quality, the use of weighted averages in allocating RVUs to individual services is troubling. For example, when a high-volume service, such as an office visit, is provided by all specialties—but overwhelmingly by generalists who pay low malpractice premiums—using a weighted premium average drains money from the high-risk specialty "pools" and causes a systematic overpayment of the malpractice expenses incurred by low-risk specialties. In other words, the payment made to a family physician who sees a patient for an upper respiratory infection reflects, to a small degree, the malpractice premiums paid by neurosurgeons, obstetrician-gynecologists, orthopedic surgeons, and other high-risk specialties.

Conversely, for a high-risk service such as obstetric care, which is provided by both obstetrician-gynecologists and family physicians, the lower premium paid by family physicians deflates the RVUs assigned to the service. This results in a systematic underpayment of the premium costs incurred by the specialty that provides the service most often and to the most medically complicated patients.

Malpractice RVUs, on average, account for only 3% of physician payments under the Medicare fee schedule. So, ultimately, the true financial impact of this bias in the methodology is small. Practice expense RVUs, however, account for nearly half the average fee schedule payment and are intended to reimburse physicians for a wide range of costs that are extremely difficult to define and allocate. Therefore, the risk of inappropriately severe payment reductions (or inappropriately inflated payments) flowing from unwise methodological choices for this component of

*Resource-based malpractice RVUs were incorporated into the fee schedule in 1999, with no transition.

the fee schedule is very real—and apparently underappreciated by federal policy makers.

IMPACT ESTIMATES

The cumulative impact of all these Medicare payment changes for obstetrician-gynecologists can be seen in the historical and projected payments shown in Table 101–1 for some of their key services. Once again, it is generally true that procedural services provided in facility settings have experienced net payment reductions since the CPR system was abandoned in 1992, whereas office-based services (and those that include a significant office-based E&M component such as obstetric care) are receiving higher payments.

Interestingly, in a system purportedly based on "fairness," charges have been made that the Medicare fee schedule practices its own kind of sex discrimination. According to research originally conducted in 1996,[1] physicians are paid more under the Medicare fee schedule for gender-specific procedures performed on men than they are for comparable procedures involving women.

Whereas payment numbers for individual services are interesting, the real impact of the Medicare fee schedule may be much more subtle and difficult to ascertain. Federal advisory panels have reviewed frequency data for some of the hardest-hit specialty services and concluded that no decline in the elderly's access to these procedures resulted from sharp payment reductions. Yet, anecdotal evidence is emerging that for some specialties, significant changes may

be occurring in their practice "culture." More frequently, the American College of Surgeons receives telephone calls from surgeons who are no longer willing to accept on-call responsibilities at their hospitals. Others take call but come to the emergency room for only the most serious patients; those with less-threatening ailments are given a referral and told to set up an office appointment the following day. Some surgeons also say that they limit the number of patients they see for certain conditions, or that they refer Medicare patients to others in their specialty if an especially unprofitable procedure is needed. So, federal studies purporting to prove that access has been unaffected apparently are not asking the right questions.

OUTLOOK

OBRA 89 mandates a comprehensive review of fee schedule RVUs every 5 years so adjustments can be made to reflect changes in resource requirements arising from technologic innovations, new practice patterns, and so forth. The second 5-year review of physician work values is under way, and any changes that result are scheduled to be implemented in 2002—the same year that the phase-in to resource-based practice expense RVUs will conclude. Otherwise, no known efforts loom on the horizon that are anticipated to cause another significant redistribution of payments away from specialty care.

It is important to keep in mind, however, that none of the payment cuts experienced by specialists in recent years has contributed to reducing federal spending for health

Table 101–1. Payment History for Selected Obstetrics and Gynecology Services

Service Code	Service	1989*	1992†	2000 (F)‡	2000 (NF)	2002 (F)§	2002 (NF)
56351	Hysteroscopy; biopsy	n/a	n/a	$260.32	$283.02	$254.10	$299.50
57160	Insert pessary and/or other device	$21.66	$38.75	$43.94	$62.98	$47.23	$80.55
57240	Repair bladder and vagina	$426.09	$478.04	$445.85	n/a	$387.74	n/a
57250	Repair rectum and vagina	$380.74	$473.08	$403.85	n/a	$348.20	n/a
57260	Repair vagina	$652.87	$591.81	$582.52	n/a	$495.02	n/a
57265	Extensive repair of vagina	$754.11	$626.53	$750.21	n/a	$679.55	n/a
57282	Repair of vaginal prolapse	$670.38	$610.72	$611.08	n/a	$526.51	n/a
57454	Vagina examination and biopsy	$103.68	$89.59	$71.03	$103.62	$67.74	$108.74
58100	Biopsy of uterus lining	$55.35	$49.29	$39.91	$61.88	$38.08	$69.20
58120	Dilatation and curettage	$249.84	$188.94	$224.08	$247.51	$211.99	$258.86
58150	Total hysterectomy	$970.39	$805.10	$923.40	n/a	$864.82	n/a
58260	Vaginal hysterectomy	$949.75	$769.44	$770.72	n/a	$687.24	n/a
58262	Vaginal hysterectomy	n/a	n/a	$853.83	n/a	$783.17	n/a
58720	Removal of ovary and/or tube(s)	$581.64	$500.67	$702.62	n/a	$656.12	n/a
59400	Obstetric care	$633.13	$809.13	$1,511.05	n/a	$1,459.06	n/a
59410	Obstetric care	$489.97	$438.04	$934.75	n/a	$839.92	n/a

*1989 payments are national averages under the CPR system.
†1992 was the first year that Medicare payments were made under the RBRVS physician fee schedule.
‡With the transition to resource-based practice expense RVUs, specific site-of-service payment differentials have been implemented.
§2002 payment calculations are based on proposed future RVUs published in the Health Care Financing Administration's proposed rule for the 2001 Medicare fee schedule, issued July 17, 2000 (65 FR 44176). The conversion factor was held constant at the current 2000 amount of $36.61.
CPR, customary, prevailing, and reasonable; (F), payments for services provided in facility settings; n/a, not applicable; (NF), payments for services provided in nonfacility (office) settings; RBRVS, resource-based relative value scale; RVUs, relative value units.

care; all the money lost was redistributed. As a result, in the legislators' view, physicians as a group have been treated rather favorably! BBA 97, for example, imposed steep payment reductions for teaching hospitals, home health agencies, and other provider groups—but no budget-driven cuts were imposed on physicians. It would be prudent, therefore, for physicians and their specialty societies to question how long this "favorable" treatment will last amid calls to ensure Medicare's solvency for the baby boom generation's retirement, as well as to expand its benefits to include costly preventive services and prescription drugs.

Reference

1. Goff B: Is Adam worth more than Eve? Gynecol Oncol 1997;66:313–319.

What Are Employers and Payers Looking at in Obstetric/Gynecologic Practice?

Peter Dews and Scott B. Ransom

Employers (health care purchasers) are becoming increasingly assertive about performance-based health care purchasing. Consistent with this movement, employers are actively engaged in efforts to define and better measure quality, as well as to identify inappropriate costs. In recent years, several employers and purchasing coalitions have begun to assimilate data and create the information required to make more informed health care purchasing decisions. Some of the forerunners of this movement include The Pacific Business Group on Health (PBGH), General Motors, The Dallas–Fort Worth Business Group on Health, The Chicago Business Group on Health (CBGH), and The Gateway Purchasing Association.[1]

To date, most evaluation has targeted health plans, largely because health plans have been the level of contracting for most employers. Increasingly, however, efforts and methods are developing to assess quality at the levels of the health system, hospital, physician, and even the patient's condition. For example, the CBGH's Preferred Provider Organization (PPO) used quality measures to screen hospitals for inclusion in a network available to member employers, and the Dallas–Fort Worth Business Group on Health is collecting data to assess the quality of office-based as well as inpatient obstetric care. Several of these employers are using differential premium contributions to motivate employees to enroll in plans that have scored higher on quality assessments. This chapter outlines the rationale and methods used by one large employer, Ford Motor Company, to meet its current and future health care quality and outcome measurement objectives.

Employers Care about (But Not Just about) Costs

As they are for the nation, health care costs are a major concern for employers. National health expenditures have recently been estimated at $1.035 trillion, or approximately 13.6% of the (1996) gross domestic product, increased from $699.5 billion and 12.2% in 1990.[2] This trend was mirrored at the employer level. In 1996, employer spending on private health insurance totaled $262.7 billion, up from $61.0 billion in 1980. Business health spending as a percentage of total compensation increased from 3.7% in 1980 to a high of 6.6% in 1993, and declined to 5.9% in 1996.[3]

In the United States, the great majority of nonelderly individuals (younger than age 65 years) with private health insurance obtain their coverage through the workplace, either directly through their own employment or indirectly through a family member.[3] Consequently, large employers/purchasers of health care, like Ford Motor Company, currently exert considerable power in the health care marketplace and will continue to do so. An analysis of Ford's 1998 American health care experience revealed that 637,800 people (employees, dependents, and retirees) received health care benefits from Ford. Blue Cross/Blue Shield plans alone paid health care claims on Ford's behalf to over 2500 hospitals and over 142,500 physicians; Ford Motor Company contracted with 92 health maintenance organizations (HMOs), five PPOs, two third-party administrators, and five service-specific HMOs (e.g., vision, prescription drug, foot care). For 1998, Ford's United States health care cash payments totaled $1.5 billion.

A basic problem for purchasers (employers) today is that they are paying for "pieces" of health care. They are paying for a visit, they are paying for an operation, and they are paying for a prescription. They are paying for use of a device, implantation of a device, and so on. What purchasers really want, and are not getting, is to optimize the health of the patient and therefore the productivity of the employee. That is the whole idea behind health benefits. Outcome measurement is the linkage between what purchasers really want and what they are getting today. Purchasers need to be able to evaluate what happens as a result of these pieces of medicine being applied to the patient. Until employers are able to make this connection in a consistent, appropriate way, they will continue to suffer from the escalating cost, lack of control, and related problems that purchasers have today in managing health benefits.

The ability to make health care purchasing decisions, with purchasers equipped with credible knowledge of the relationship between the quality of health care (including patient outcomes and health status) and dollars spent, has been dubbed "value-based purchasing." Although the concept of value-based purchasing seems quite reasonable and has been implemented, albeit on a limited basis, its full

Table 102–1. Why Are We So Interested in Health Care Quality?

Health-care dollars are not limitless and must be spent wisely.
Employees, retirees, and their families depend on us to structure the best health care plan options.
There is a great deal of unexplained variation in the utilization and cost of services.

potential still awaits evolution in the science and policy of performance measurement.

There is almost universal agreement that quality measurement is feasible and valuable (Table 102–1). There is also a general acknowledgment that quality of care measurement is complex and currently suffers from technical and other limitations, such as inadequate information systems and lack of funding. Health plans are frustrated by seemingly incessant requests for information, yet there currently is no agreed on "core set" of quality measures that employers want or need. Some employers, like Ford, have invested in and desire to accelerate the advancement of quality measurement science. Conversely, not all employers or purchaser coalitions have the expertise, staff, or will to make optimal use of the quality of care information currently available to them.[4]

What Is Quality?

Provider performance measurement initiatives at Ford have embodied the classic "structure, process, outcomes" conceptualization of quality. *Structure* refers to whether the opportunity for good care exists in the organization, and whether it has the capability to meet the demands of its customers. Measures of structural quality often involve determining whether an organization has the right type and number of professionals, amenities, and access hours. *Process of care* refers to the technical and humanistic competence of an organization. Measures of process quality can include screening rates for early detection of disease, correct diagnosis (e.g., recognition of pregnancy-induced hypertension), and effective treatment (e.g., prophylactic antibiotic use for cesarean section), continuity of care, and effective patient communications. The third and most talked about dimension of quality is outcomes. *Outcomes* are the end-results of medical care: what happened to the patient in terms of palliation, control of illness, cure, or rehabilitation.[5]

The "structure, process, outcomes" framework for quality measurement does not explicitly state the appropriate "unit of analysis." That is, at what level should quality measurement be directed? At the health plan level, or provider level (hospital, individual physician) (Table 102–2)? For a number of reasons, most evaluation by employers has focused on health plans. Focusing on health plans may seem a disadvantage in that health plans are a layer (or two) removed from the actual providers of care: hospitals,

physicians, nurses, and other health care providers. However, a health plan focus does provide several advantages. First, most employers contract with health plans and not individual providers (although this may change as provider groups consolidate and increasingly overlap). Second, a health plan focus allows employers to aggregate the performance of many individual providers, to create statistically meaningful information. Third, the science to measure and compare the performance of individual providers (physicians), although improving, is still in its methodological adolescence.[6]

Three national organizations are currently involved in developing and disseminating standardized methods of performance measurement: The Foundation for Accountability (FACCT), The National Committee for Quality Assurance (NCQA), and The Joint Commission on Accreditation of Health-care Organizations (JCAHO). A shared objective of each of these organizations has been to advance the science of quality and outcome measurement, and to inform purchasers and consumers, yet each has had its own philosophy and focus.[7] Ford's quality strategy involves collaborating with and capitalizing on the experience of each organization, while building the capacity to address Ford-specific objectives.

QUALITY MEASUREMENT INITIATIVES

Ford is doing outcomes measurement because it needs to be done, and currently no one can do it the way Ford wants it done. So, Ford has taken on the job for itself. Perhaps one day Ford will either sell the service or buy parts of it from someone else. However, Ford's expectation is that because they have invested in infrastructure and have initiatives under way, they will remain in the business of quality and outcomes measurement. Ford does not believe that the issue of performance measurement is going to just go away. Ford senses that purchasers, health plans, and providers are at the beginning of a huge market that is about to develop in health services evaluation, and that the Association for Health Services Research (AHSR) is moving from the academic phase into the industrial phase.

Health Plan Evaluation

In keeping with its objective to make informed purchasing decisions and help employees become informed con-

Table 102–2. Quality Is Critical: Dimensions of Provider Performance

Efficacy	Was the treatment administered correctly?
Effectiveness	Did the patient get better?
Appropriateness	Is this the best type of care for this patient?
Availability	Are providers there when the patient needs them?
Timeliness	Is care given when it can do the most good?
Continuity	Is there coordination between physicians?
Safety	Is there compliance with infection control and other regulatory activities?

Table 102–3. Health Plan Evaluations: What Ford Found

Plan Name	ACCR	Consumer Satisfaction	Access to Care	Staying Healthy	GBLWI
Blue Care Network, Mid Michigan	1	★★	★★★	★★★	★★
Blue Care Network—Southeast	1	★★	★★	★★	★★
Blue Care Network—East	1	★★	★★	★★	★★★
Blue Care Network—West	1	★★	★★	★★	★★
Health Alliance Plan	1	★★	★★	★★	★★★
M-Care	1	★★★	★★	★★★	★★
Medical Value Plan	1	★★★	★★★	★★	★★
Omnicare	1	★★	★	★	★★
Care Choices—HMO/Mercy Health Plans	1	★★	★★	★★	★★

★★★ Significantly above average; ★★ average; ★ significantly below average.

1, Accredited by the National Committee for Quality Assurance; ACCR, accredited; GBLWI, Getting Better and Living with Illness; HMO, health maintenance organization.

sumers, Ford collaborates with unions, other employers, and experts from Rand, FACCT, and NCQA on the Health Plan Evaluation Project. The primary product of this ongoing project is a "report card" that provides employees with standardized information with which to compare HMOs (Table 102–3). All HMOs that Ford or other participating employers contract with are evaluated. Results are presented in five "domains":

- NCQA accreditation status
- *Consumer satisfaction*: a summary of the overall satisfaction of HMO members with their HMO, including how much they were helped by the care received, whether or not they would recommend the plan to family or friends, and whether they plan to re-enroll
- *Access and service*: a summary score of what HMO members say about their experiences with the plan in choosing doctors, making appointments, and obtaining desired care, including specialty referrals and resolving problems
- *Staying healthy*: measures how well the health plan helps people avoid illness through preventive care, reduction in health risks, and early detection of serious illnesses
- *Getting better and living with illness*: measures how well the health plan helps people recover when they're sick or injured, and how well it helps the quality of life of people with chronic conditions, such as diabetes or asthma

Because many purchasers and potential enrollees may see these results, plans with relatively low scores feel pressure to improve. These plans can also use the results to target specific areas for improvement, which is an important aspect.

Dissemination of comparative information on health plans is one of the mechanisms employed to support "value-based *pricing*" of health plans. The value-based pricing framework motivates employees, through lower cost sharing, to enroll in health plans with higher-quality ratings. Value-based pricing represents a step in the evolution toward "value-based *purchasing*." With the advent of

value-based purchasing, quality and outcome information will be used not only to determine cost sharing for employees but also to decide which health plans to offer, to negotiate contract price, and even to put provider payments at risk based on achieving certain outcomes.

Hospital Evaluation

Increasing hospital care costs, mounting evidence that procedure rates varied dramatically for employees and retirees in different areas of the country (even when patient characteristics were factored in), and little assurance that dollars were spent on care of high quality prompted Ford to take action. In 1986, Ford founded The Hospital Profiling Project. Ford hired a vendor to use claims data to generate quality and cost measures for local hospitals and began annual visits to show chief executive officers (CEOs) of large local hospitals their results.

A decade later, seven other large area employers and the United Automobile Workers (UAW) joined the effort. In 1997, General Motors (GM) and Daimler-Chrysler (Chrysler) began distributing the results to employees and retirees in southeast Michigan. That same year, the project was staffed with clinical and health service research expertise, and local physicians and hospital administrators were invited to help retool and improve the scientific rigor and the consumer usability of the Profiles.

Research has clearly shown that, even when adjustments are made for patient characteristics, rates of procedures and outcomes of hospital care vary, often dramatically, in different regions of the United States.[8] Even within a single region, the costs and clinical outcomes of hospital care for the same procedure often vary substantially, depending on where a patient is hospitalized. For example, the cost of a colon resection procedure at 46 hospitals in the Detroit area varied more than twofold (from $10,872 to $25,920). Unexpected complication rates for lower joint replacement showed even more variability among hospitals.[9]

Other national efforts, such as the NCQA's Health Plan

Table 102–4. Hospital Profiling: "What Patients Say" about Medical Care

Teaching Hospitals	Indicators of Medical Care						
	Respect for Patients	Care Coordin.	Information and Education	Comfort and Pain Management	Emotional Support	Involvement of Family and Friends	Discharge Preparation
Botsford General Hospital—Farmington Hills	★★	★★	★★	★★	★★	★★	★★
DMC Harper Hospital—Detroit	Low volume	—	—	—	—	—	—
DMC Hutzel Hospital—Detroit	★★	★★★	★★★	★★	★★	★★	★★★
DMC Sinai Hospital—Detroit	Low volume	—	—	—	—	—	—
Henry Ford Hospital—Detroit	★	★	★★	★★	★★	★★	★★
Mt. Clemens General Hospital	★★	★★	★	★★	★★	★★	★★
North Oakland Medical Center—Pontiac	★	★★	★	★	★	★★	★
Oakwood Hospital & Medical Center—Dearborn	★★	★	★	★★	★	★★	★★
Pontiac Osteopathic Hospital	★★	★★	★★	★★	★★	★★	★★
Providence Hospital & Medical Center—Southfield	★★	★★	★★	★★	★★	★★	★★

★★★, Significantly above average; ★★, average; ★, significantly below average.
DMC, Detroit Medical Center. "Low volume" in the "Respect for Patients" column means that too few patients reported on this indicator for significant evaluation.

Data and Information Set (HEDIS) reporting and the Health Care Financing Administration's (HCFA) Consumer Assessment of Health Plan Performance (CAHPP) project, supply information that consumers can use to make decisions about *health plans.* They do not, however, allow consumers to make informed choices once they have selected a health plan and are faced with choosing a hospital or physician.

The few comparative reports that are available (e.g., HealthcareReportCards.com; The Healthcare Investment Analysts [HCIA] Hospital Rankings; U.S. News and World Report Annual Listing) suffer from severe limitations: lack of joint provider/purchaser/labor/consumer support, omission of out-of-pocket costs to consumers, or lack of "open" methodology.[9]

The Hospital Profiling Project distributed information to retirees and employees about how hospitals perform on measures of patient-centeredness, quality, and cost in several major metropolitan regions in the United States. The Project 1998 "beta test" resulted in the distribution of over 500,000 hospital profiles in southeast Michigan.

Technical quality was assessed by measuring unexpected death rates and unexpected complications of surgical care. All outcomes were risk adjusted for patient differences between hospitals. Diagnosis-Related Groups and the Risk-Adjusted Complication Index[10, 11] were risk adjustment methods used. Because there is no "gold standard" for risk adjustment, test measures with alternative systems (Refined DRGs and the Iezzoni Complications Profiler) will be added in future profiles.

To measure patient centeredness, The Picker Inpatient Survey was used to collect patient reports of care experiences. The Picker Inpatient Survey, developed in 1989, focuses on assessment of interpersonal quality.[12] Surveys were sent to 200 patients from each hospital. Patients were randomly selected from medical units, surgical units, and maternity units. Survey questions are based on key clinical

events that patients can observe and report on and that clinicians find important and actionable for quality improvement.

The cost indicator reflects purchaser payment for service. The cost indicator was calculated as the average payment for services in each condition or disease category. In 1999, a new approach that focuses on using audited hospital financial statements as the source of information was included as a test measure.

Efforts like the Hospital Profiling Project (Table 102–4) that provide a longitudinal assessment of quality, cost, and outcomes such as the extent of patient-centeredness will be invaluable to Ford and other purchasers in achieving their goal of rewarding providers based on performance. It is important to note that health plans (or purchasers) can also use these results in direct contracting and network selection considerations.

Physician Profiles

There is little doubt that substantial variation in health care utilization exists. It exists at the geographic level[8] and also has been described at the level of race and socioeconomic status.[13] The finding that health care utilization can and does vary with factors other than the severity of illness of the population receiving (or not receiving) services has been attributed by many to irrational or inconsistent physician decision making. Despite ongoing debate regarding the validity of this attribution, health care policy makers and administrators (in the face of escalating costs and undetermined quality) have developed and implemented (profiling) tools intended to highlight the contribution of physicians to this "unexplained" variation and make them accountable. Opinions on the utility of profiling range from those who believe that it is essential to those who believe that it is dangerous. Ford Healthcare Management believes that physician profiling and evaluations are essential tools in their quest for quality care.

What Is Profiling?

No currently accepted standard definition of physician profiling exists. This factor alone contributes to confusion over what a profile is, what its intended uses should be, and who the intended audience for profiles is. In its broadest sense, physician profiling involves using data extracted from administrative databases (largely), clinical databases, and patient surveys to derive summary measures of processes of care, resource utilization, and outcomes of care provided by an individual physician. A given physician's performance can then be compared with a normative standard, other peer group physicians, or achievable benchmarks.

Just as they have for health plans and hospitals, purchasers have demanded comparative information on individual physicians. That all physicians are not created equal is a basic tenet for many purchasers (this does not mean that C and D players cannot become A and B players, given appropriate assistance and incentives). Ford believes that all suppliers, be they suppliers of automotive components or health care, should compete on quality, and this competition requires comparative information. This analogy may seem overly simplistic to some, but certainly it is not irrational. It is simply an acknowledgment that variations in quality exist (even at the physician level) and that these variations should be identified and improved upon.

Physician profiling may provide information to multiple other constituents apart from purchasers. Physicians themselves, consumers, and health plans also have wants, needs, and potential uses for information on the comparative performance of physicians. Because public release of profiles for health plans and hospitals has already occurred, disclosure of physician profiles to consumers of health care seems only a logical extension of this trend. In fact, physician profiles have been considered an essential component of proposed health care consumers bills of rights and responsibilities.[14] Health plans and hospitals have begun to incorporate individual physician profiles into their credentialing processes. Physician groups who have entered into capitated payment arrangements are profiling the resource utilization of their own physicians.[15] A central issue, however, is whether currently available data and methods can support all the current and proposed uses of physician profiles.

Cautious proponents of physician profiles, conscious of the potential misuses (intended or not) of physician profiles, favor a cooperative approach to development and release of profiles. This cooperative approach involves all constituents (purchasers, physicians, health plans, hospitals, and consumer representatives) participating in the development of profiling tools, reaching consensus on issues like parameters for public release of profiles, and the degree of accuracy expected or required for each planned use of profiles. This more deliberate approach to physician profiling is based on the very real concern that not all, or perhaps not even very much, of the observed variation in utilization is due to physician effect, but rather due to chance or unaccounted-for differences in severity of illness.[16]

Increasing physician accountability through profiling is a worthy endeavor. But if physician effect for utilization variation (process) is indeed small, and measures based on health outcomes are too rare, confounded, and uncontrollable to be dealt with practically or analytically, what aspects of care should be profiled? Perhaps patient reports of care and measures of patient-centeredness will replace or deemphasize "case-mix indexes" and "efficiency ratios" in future iterations of physician profiles.

Ultimately, the utility of profiles will depend on their validity and reliability. Limitations of current profiling methods include inadequate risk-adjustment methodologies, small numbers of patients for individual providers, and attribution of patients who see multiple providers. In its most benign and defensible application, physician profiling is an action tool directed toward quality improvement. Profiles used in an educational context have been shown to change (reduce) resource utilization patterns.[17] However, the ability of profiles to produce change in physician resource utilization behavior may be more a function of the fact that they remind physicians that they are "being watched" and less a result of any education, explanatory power, or new light shed by the profiles themselves. This phenomenon is known as the *Hawthorne effect* and it alone will likely serve as sufficient rationale for health care policy makers and administrators to continue to implement, and employers to demand, physician profiling.

Information and Analytic Strategy

Significant obstacles for purchasers in their quality and outcome measurement efforts have been limited staffing or expertise or both in the health services assessment and clinical areas, and availability of credible data. To address these issues, Ford has taken innovative steps by the creation of a Data Warehouse and formation of the Ford Healthcare Quality Consortium (FHQC) (Fig. 102–1).

Data Warehouse

The backbone of all outcome measurement is data. However, we are quickly approaching an era in health services research (and life!) in which the potential wealth of data is staggering, and the options for analyzing and presenting these data to decision makers are innumerable. And, although it is an essential managerial (and physician) skill to extract lessons from ambiguous data to guide action, it is far more desirable to have access to reliable, consistent data.

Quality evaluation and outcomes measurement on any

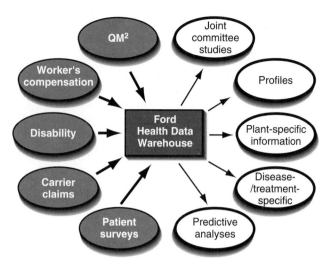

Figure 102–1. Ford health information strategy. QM², quality management.

level require data from multiple, disparate sources. Ford's Data Warehouse will provide or have the potential to provide "one-stop shopping" for information about providers (health plans, hospitals, and physician/provider groups) and beneficiaries (employees, dependents, and retirees). The warehouse will have the capability to create the numerators and denominators required to address quality measurement at all levels (health plan, hospital, and physician), within all the previously described dimensions of quality (structure, process, and outcome), and to derive risk-adjusted population-based measures. The Data Warehouse will also incorporate plant-specific data such as injury rates, occupational health and safety data, workers' compensation-disability claims, and periodic health examination results. Finally, the Data Warehouse will maintain these data, linked in informative, flexible, but *not person-identifiable*, formats.

In addition to being comprehensive and secure, the Data Warehouse is being constructed with an eye toward accommodating multiple types of users. The Data Warehouse will provide data and metadata (data about data) to meet the information needs of the manager, who, on a quarterly basis, just wants reassurances that all process criteria are being met. Similarly, the warehouse will satisfy the financial analyst, who wants to know the cost per member per month ("$PM/PM") for a recently introduced drug, and the health services researcher who needs all the administrative claims data and demographic information for a consistent population determined by a disease-specific case definition.

Quality Consortium

In 1998, Ford convened the Ford Healthcare Quality Consortium. The FHQC is a new Ford entity consisting of Ford Healthcare Management leadership, external health services analysis partners, provider association partners,

and key Ford health care suppliers. Its mission is to measure the quality of the health care services offered to and utilized by Ford employees, retirees, and their dependents.

Why a Consortium?

The evaluation of health care quality requires clinical, statistical, financial, and management expertise. Few large companies (and none outside the health services delivery and pharmaceutical industries) possess all the talent necessary to measure health care quality effectively. Because expertise is in high demand, Ford Healthcare Management decided to emulate a model that has worked well in other segments of the company: creation of partnerships with key suppliers.

Formation of the FHQC has several advantages for both Ford and consortium members. By creating the consortium, Ford gains access to expertise from the academic and provider sectors to better assist its health care management team in measuring overall quality and clinical outcomes. The consortium allows Ford (and other similarly motivated purchasers) a mechanism to accomplish outcome and quality measurement objectives without creating a measurement enterprise that is outside their core business. For consortium members with health services research interests, the opportunity to work with a large, national administrative database and its considerable potential for original research is very appealing. For providers (physicians, hospitals, and health plans), participation in the consortium represents an opportunity for constructive feedback and exchange on performance.

The FHQC consists of an oversight committee, a managing director, and a working body. The oversight committee consists of members of Ford Healthcare Management and leaders within key Ford health care supplier organizations, who individually possess recognized expertise and commitment to quality evaluation. The working body consists of individuals or centers with health services research expertise, from health care organizations that provide a substantial amount of health care services to Ford beneficiaries. The consortium has grown to include also some external analysis partners from academic and other health care quality sectors.

Anticipated uses of work from the consortium are multiple. The work of the consortium will be used to evaluate health services research priorities/opportunities within Ford, provide input into Ford health care supplier evaluation processes, review (for scientific and statistical validity) disease-specific and population-based studies conducted by or for Ford Healthcare Management, and create or distill information to be made available to Ford employees, retirees, and dependents, informing them on issues relating to individual health and provider performance.

Initial consortium projects will build on the existing work of Ford Healthcare Quality Management, which has identified cardiovascular health, mental health, and growth in pharmaceutical costs as important areas of concern for Ford. Determining patterns of utilization for individual health care services, and an assessment of population (workforce) health status, are also targets for early evaluation by the consortium.

SUMMARY

Employers can and will leverage their market power to influence health care delivery. Whereas there is legitimate debate regarding issues like privacy/confidentiality, accuracy of profiling tools, and whether employers have an obligation, or a right, to be involved in shaping the face of health care delivery, the bottom line is that it is already happening. Unique initiatives like the FHQC and Data Warehouse represent employer innovations and investment that will enable translational research (the real world application of health services research), and, it is hoped, hasten the advancement of outcomes measurement. However, Ford and other pioneers of purchaser-based quality and outcomes measurement will not consider their efforts successful until the science of health care quality measurement permits them to reliably differentiate, and reward, health care providers based on performance. Implicit in this success are employees who are well informed on quality measures for their individual provider, health plan, and/or delivery system; observable relationships between employee health status and employee productivity; and the elimination of non–value-added health care services and costs.

References

1. Agency for Health Care Policy and Research: Theory and reality of value-based purchasing: Lessons from the pioneers (AHCPR Pub. No. 98-0004). Rockville, Md, AHCPR, Nov 1997.
2. Levit KR, Lazenby BR, Braden J, National Health Accounts Team: National health spending trends in 1996. Health Affairs 1998;17:35–51.
3. Fronstin P: Features of employment-based health plans. EBRI Issue Brief 1998;201:1–21.
4. The operation of business health purchasing coalitions. AHSR FHSR Annu Meet Abstr Book 1996;13:5–6.
5. Lohr KN: Outcome measurement: Concepts and questions. Inquiry Spring 1988;25:37–50.
6. Eddy DM: Performance measurement: Problems and solutions. Health Affairs 1998;17(4):8–25.
7. Details can be found at www.NCQA.org; www.FACCT.org; www.JCAHO.org.
8. Wennberg DE: Variation in the delivery of health care: The stakes are high [editorial]. Ann Intern Med 1998;128:866–868.
9. Bechel D, Myers WA: Connecting the New Healthcare Consumer. Chicago, McGraw-Hill (in press).
10. Details can be found at www.3MHIS.com.
11. DesHarnais S, McMahon LF Jr, Wroblewski R: Measuring outcomes of hospital care using multiple risk-adjusted indexes. Health Serv Res 1991;26:425–445.
12. Donabedian A: Institutional and professional responsibilities in quality assurance. Qual Assur Health Care 1989;1:3–11.
13. Ford ES, Cooper RS: Racial/ethnic differences in health care utilization of cardiovascular procedures: A review of the evidence. Health Serv Res 1995;30:Part II 237–252.
14. Gauging quality regulation's impact on premium costs. Med Health 1997;51:1.
15. Kerr EA, Mittman BS, Hays RD, et al: Managed care and capitation in California: How do physicians at financial risk control their own utilization? Ann Intern Med 1995;123:500–504.
16. Hofer TP, Hayward RA, Greenfield S, et al: The unreliability of individual physician "report cards" for assessing the costs and quality of care of a chronic disease. JAMA 1999;281:2098–2105.
17. Bennett G, McKee W, Kilberg L: Case study in physician profiling. Manag Care Q 1994;2:60–70.

Cost-Benefit and Decision-Making Analyses in Obstetrics and Gynecology

Ira H. Mickelson and Scott B. Ransom

This chapter examines and discusses two separate research techniques. Both are poorly understood at best and dangerously utilized at worst in our medical literature. Yet, it is imperative to command a working knowledge of both in order for our specialty of obstetrics-gynecology to develop further as a science. They are cost-effectiveness analysis (CEA) (or cost-benefit analysis [CBA]) and decision-making analysis (DMA).

COST-EFFECTIVENESS ANALYSIS AND COST-BENEFIT ANALYSIS

For any nation, regardless of size or level of prosperity, the resources available to meet the demands for health care are limited. As a nation, we are forced to decide how to allocate these limited resources and exactly how they will be divided. What procedures will and will not be covered by insurances, inpatient versus outpatient, lengths of stay, and prior authorizations by gatekeepers are but a few of the difficult decisions already being made on a daily basis.

CEA and CBA are economic techniques that originated in the business literature as tools to improve resource allocation policy choices. Since about 1980, these terms have been increasingly common in the medical literature and have become basic tools in the evaluation of health care practices. Unfortunately, because of the lack of standardization and the widespread disparities in methods that investigators employ, interpretation and evaluation of data become difficult, if not impossible. Many of these disparities arise from a misunderstanding of the principles and misapplication of the practices of CEA and CBA. A review of CEA articles in the obstetrics and gynecology literature since 1980 reveals little improvement in the application of these principles over time.[1] For this reason, experts in the field of cost effectiveness in health and medicine have attempted to educate the medical academic community about the principles of CEA and to develop specific minimum requirements that should be achieved in all CEA research. Decision makers charged with resource allocation would then have a point of reference for comparability with other analyses in the medical literature.

CBA and CEA are similar but not exactly the same. CEA compares the net monetary costs of a health care intervention with some measure of clinical effectiveness. In the medical literature, CEA is a method for evaluating the health outcomes and resource costs of health interventions. Its primary function is to demonstrate the relative value of alternative interventions for improving health. CBA compares the cost of a health care intervention as well. In a CBA, the costs of a health care intervention are assessed in the same way as in CEA. The difference between the two is that, in CBA, measures of clinical outcomes or effectiveness are converted into monetary units in some standardized fashion as well. CBA makes comparisons in terms of monies lost to pay for a health care intervention compared with monies gained from the use of the intervention. The key distinction is that CBA must value all outcomes in economic terms, including lives or years of life and morbidity, whereas CEA serves to place priorities on alternative expenditures without requiring that the dollar value of life and health be assessed. The major disadvantage of CBA is the requirement that human life and quality of life be valued in dollars. CEA requires only that health outcomes be expressed in commensurate units, such as quality-adjusted life years. CEA tends to be more tolerable to physicians.

The first publications in the medical literature on the principles of CEA were presented over 20 years ago. In 1977, Weinstein and Stason,[2] from the Center for the Analysis of Health Practices, Harvard School of Public Health, wrote the first comprehensive article on the foundations and prerequisites for CEA for health and medical practices. The science of CEA/CBA began to take place. Many investigators have subsequently expounded and delved deeper into the field, but Weinstein's and Stason's[2] original article still stands as valid and creates a solid base. The goal was to develop a set of criteria that would be applied to all CEA/CBA research in order to achieve some level of academic standards and consistency.

Weinstein and Stason[2] proposed a set of three standards, or prerequisites, for useful CEA, which follow:

1. **A cost-effectiveness ratio between all net increases in health costs to all net changes in enhanced life expectancy and quality of life**. Total costs were divided into four groups:
   a. Direct and indirect costs of hospitalization, physician and nursing time, medications, counseling, laboratory, and ancillary services.
   b. All health care costs of adverse side effects of treatment.

c. Costs of treating diseases that would not have occurred if the patient had not lived longer as a result of the original treatment.

d. Subtract the savings in health care, rehabilitation, and other costs due to the prevention of the disease.

Net health effectiveness is significantly more difficult, but not impossible, to quantify. It must include a health status index formula that assigns a quality of life severity weight from 0 to 1 for each definable health status, ranging from death or coma to disability and discomfort to full health. This is multiplied by the number of years spent in this status and the probability of that status occurring. CEA and CBA should be presented as a summary measurement to explicitly express the incremental gains versus costs for the evaluation. The evaluation should calculate a ratio of the net benefits in terms of the measurable outcomes to the net increase or decrease of costs. The greater the ratio, the greater the value of performing the procedure, technique, or program.

2. **Present value analysis, or discounting of future costs and health benefits**. Basic principles of finance teach that a dollar today is not the same as a dollar in the future.[3] Two factors change the value of a dollar over time. On one hand, a dollar not spent now can be invested to yield a larger number of dollars in the future. On the other hand, a dollar not spent now lessens in value because of the effects of inflation. Economists speak about current, or nominal, dollars versus constant, or real, dollars. Using the Consumer Price Index to estimate average inflation, and average interest rates over time, most researchers assume a real rate of return of 5%. Therefore, in order to calculate the present value of X dollars spent in N years, X dollars should be divided by 1.05 to the N power. To perform a valid CEA, calculations must use real dollars, with proper discounting of future costs and health benefits. The consideration of present and future health benefits and costs should be completed to adjust for these temporal discrepancies. For example, preventive programs often have all costs immediate but the health benefits in the future. An appropriate methodology must be completed to assess the differential timing of cost and benefit through discounting techniques.

3. **The investigators explicitly present and test all assumptions leading to the study's conclusions (sensitivity analysis)**. Unfortunately, unlike many areas of manufacturing, estimates of the risks and benefits of health practices, in terms of mortality and morbidity probabilities, are rarely known with certainty. The human body is far too complex with far too many variables. It is necessary that investigators make assumptions to conduct a CEA or CBA. The assumptions should be stated to reflect the best opinions of the investigator through the scientific literature or other means; however, the study should verify the validity of the study's conclusions by calculating potential differences in the as-

sumptions. For example, the availability of quantitative measures to prove the benefit outcomes are often unknown or approximate. A quality CEA should consider potential variations in the assumptions to improve the study's meaningfulness through this process known as sensitivity analysis. (This concept is discussed further when we discuss DMA.) For the sake of a CEA, this uncertainty must be accounted for. The most easily applied method to deal with uncertainty is sensitivity analysis. In this method, the assumptions and areas of greatest uncertainty must first be identified and acknowledged. They are then varied one at a time over a chosen range of possible values. If the basic conclusions change with variations in certain assumptions, further research about that particular variable should be considered before making health care allocation decisions. If the basic conclusions do not change, confidence in the conclusion increases.

Weinstein determined four criteria that should be addressed. First, although society as a whole bears all the cost, the varying objectives of the organizations or individuals that actually make resource-allocation decisions should be identified. Second, the measures of effectiveness of health practices used in the analysis should be outcome oriented. Third, the uncertainties surrounding the estimates used in the analysis, based on the data available at the time of analysis, should be explicitly identified. Fourth, the trade-offs between present and future health benefits and costs must be considered. Although Weinstein and Stason[2] recognize that the major disadvantage of the benefit-cost framework is the requirement that human lives and quality of life be valued in dollars, they note that the principal value of formal CEA is that it forces one to be explicit about the beliefs and values that underlie allocation decisions.

This paper of Weinstein and Stason[2] marks the introduction of CEA and CBA principles as a standardized, academic discipline.

Since 1977, many articles have revisited and expounded on Weinstein and Stason's original principles.[4–9] It is interesting to note that their basic concepts have held up over time. In 1992, Udvarhelyi and associates[4] reviewed all CEAs and CBAs in the general medicine, general surgical, and medical subspecialty literature between 1978 to 1980 and 1985 to 1987 to determine how well the papers had adhered to the basic analytic principles set down by Weinstein and Stason in 1977. By reviewing "widely cited" textbooks describing the methods for performing economic analyses and by selecting the methods "universally recommended," Udvarhelyi and associates[4] expanded the basic principles to six. These six criteria are the minimum requirements for CEA research, determined by reviewing recommendations cited in articles that proposed appropriate methods for conducting a CEA and the economic evaluation of health care practices. These criteria should not be considered an inclusive set of methods necessary to perform cost-effectiveness evaluations. In fact, many additional techniques and methods may be completed, depending on the purpose of the evaluation.

The six specific criteria Udvarhelyi and associates[4] derived from the literature follow:

- Principle 1: If costs and benefits accrue during different periods, discounting should be used to adjust for the differential timing.
- Principle 2: Sensitivity analyses should be done to test important assumptions.
- Principle 3: A summary measurement of efficiency, such as a cost-benefit or cost-effectiveness ratio, should be calculated and preferably expressed in marginal or incremental terms unless one alternative or strategy is dominant.
- Principle 4: An explicit statement of a perspective for the analysis should be provided.
- Principle 5: An explicit description of the benefits of the program or technology being studied should be provided.
- Principle 6: Investigators should specify what types of costs were used or considered in their analysis.

Udvarhelyi and associates'[4] Principles 1, 2, and 3 are virtually identical to those set forth by Weinstein and Stason.[2] Let us look a little more closely at Principles 4, 5, and 6.

Principle 4. **The perspective of the CEA was explicitly stated in the article.** The evaluation may consider a variety of perspectives, including overall society: a specific Health Maintenance Organization (HMO), Managed Care Organization, or hospital; an individual department or practice; and others. These perspectives must be stated in the paper to achieve this objective.

Principle 5. **The manuscript explicitly stated the potential benefits of the technique, evaluation, program, or procedure being evaluated.** The specific benefits to an individual patient or society must be expressed to objectively reflect a measurable outcome change by using the program being evaluated. The article should reflect previous scientific proof or evidence that the program derives a specified outcome in the evaluation.

Principle 6. **The paper explicitly stated the types and methods for determining the costs used in the evaluation.** The introduction of specific cost parameters must be included in the evaluation to present the methodology for assessing cost, such as an activity-based cost model, charge proxy to approximate cost, specific cost to the provider or organization, or allocated expenses to complete the program.

Keeler,[5] in 1994, applied Weinstein and Stason's criteria of CEA and CBA to *decision-tree analysis* of specific

problems in obstetrics and gynecology. He reviewed Shepard and Thompson's[6] five steps for performing a CEA. These steps include, first, select the programs to be evaluated and define them precisely. Second, compute the net cost, which includes the gross program costs minus the cost savings, including discounting. Third, choose a measure of effect and calculate net health effects in economic terms, with discounting of future gains. Fourth, calculate the effectiveness to cost ratios by dividing net effects by net costs. Fifth, perform a sensitivity analysis.

In October 1996, Weinstein and colleagues[7–9] completed a three-part series consensus statement for the Panel on Cost-effectiveness in Health and Medicine, on the roles, reporting methods, and recommendations for CEA in health and medicine.

In Part one of the series, the panel addressed the nature and limits of CEA and defined a reference case. A reference case CEA is a standard set of methods to serve as a point of comparison across studies, conducted from a societal perspective and accounting for benefits, harms, and costs to all parties.

In Part two of the series, similar to the methodology of Udvarhelyi and associates,[4] the panel divided CEAs into six basic categories. They discussed detailed recommendations for each of these categories. The categories follow:

- Category 1: Components belonging in the numerator and denominator of a cost-effectiveness (C/E) ratio.
- Category 2: Measuring resource use in the numerator of a C/E ratio.
- Category 3: Valuing health consequences in the denominator of a C/E ratio.
- Category 4: Estimating effectiveness of interventions.
- Category 5: Incorporating time preference and discounting.
- Category 6: Handling uncertainty.

In Part three of the series, Weinstein and colleagues[9] recognized that differences in reporting complicated the user's ability to find, interpret, and adapt information, and that a standardization of reporting methods was needed. To facilitate comparisons of interventions, they produced a checklist for reporting the reference case CEA.

As can be seen, the development of a set of standards for CEA has been an evolutionary process. When a compilation of the various forms of the six criteria were applied to the obstestrics and gynecology literature, several areas of uncertainty and limitations were still noted.

First, the interpretation of a study of CEA must begin with an evaluation of the perspective of the study. Many articles that were reviewed mentioned the setting as a particular hospital or HMO. This was enough to meet compliance for criterion one. We must decide, as the health care decision makers, whether it would assist our decision-making ability by requiring CEA researchers also to apply their data to resource allocations as it applies to the society as a whole.

Second, discounting for the time value of costs and

benefits was not always applicable. In many studies, in particular those comparing one medication with another, there are no temporal discrepancies. Decision makers must be acutely aware of whether discounting was done when applicable. It would probably assist our decision-making ability to require CEA researchers to address the discounting issue even when not applicable.

Third, in the application of testing all assumptions that lead to the study's conclusions, there is confusion which and to what extent specific assumptions have to be addressed for the CEA study to be considered valid. In addition, sensitivity analysis should be applied to each assumption. Of all the factors that can affect the validity of a CEA, failure to address an important assumption is the most common and hardest to detect.

Fourth, all six criteria are being applied equally. In the evaluation of a CEA for compliance with the six principles, the decision maker might get a better interpretation of the value of the analysis if the six criteria are given different weights. For example, a paper may be considered of less value if it leaves out major assumptions or a sensitivity analysis than if it neglects to state the types and methods for determining the costs used in the evaluation. Under the present system, both CEA papers would be graded equally. One idea for future study would be to experiment with standardized different weights for each criterion.

Although some reviewers would suggest that assigning different weights to the criteria would make for a better grading system of the CEA literature, it has been repeatedly noted throughout this chapter that the six criteria developed are the minimum required for effective CEA research. These criteria represent the basic minimal requirements that should be addressed in any medical CBA/CEA. Unfortunately, these principles of CEA research have poorly and inconsistently filtered their way into the literature and often cannot be applied to the practice of CEA research on a regular basis. Udvarhelyi and associates[4] noted an 82% increase in the number of articles in the MEDLINE database that had any mention of cost-effectiveness or cost-benefit over their targeted time periods. Of the 77 articles reviewed, only 3 (4%) were consistent with all six of the basic principles, 15 (19%) used five of the six principles, and the median number of principles to which the analyses adhered was three. No clear trends of improvement were noted over the 10-year time period. The median number of principles adhered to in both groups was three. In the review of the CEA articles in the obstetrics and gynecologic literature over a 10-year span by Ransom and co-workers,[1] only 12% of the articles were fully compliant, with no significant improvement over time. The concepts that researchers had the most difficulty with were the discounted time value of costs and benefits and the testing assumptions through sensitivity analysis.

Based on these studies, if full compliance were deemed necessary for acceptance, only 12% of the obstetrics and gynecology CEA literature and 4% of the medical and surgical CEA literature would have been published. This level of compliance is still unacceptably low. It renders the CEA data in the literature virtually worthless to resource allocation decision makers. Regardless of review board acceptance, CEA authors should be thoroughly familiar with the consensus statement of the Panel on Cost-effectiveness in Health and Medicine on the roles, reporting methods, and recommendations for CEA. Every cost-effectiveness paper should address these six criteria at a minimum.

With the explosion of CEA/CBA articles in the obstetrics and gynecology literature since the early 1990s, and the increasing need for standardized, consistent data by resource allocation decision makers, there appears to be an imminent need for trained cost-effectiveness experts and reviewers. At present, manuscripts are often first reviewed by a content expert (e.g., perinatologist, gynecologic oncologist, reproductive endocrinologist) for factual data and then reviewed by a statistician for statistical review. For publication acceptance, perhaps a CEA expert should review all CEA/CBA manuscripts after acceptance by the content experts and the statistician.

DECISION-MAKING ANALYSIS

What makes medical decisions so difficult? The answer is the extreme number of variables and consequences, the degree of variability, and the uncertainty of outcomes. What helps one patient may harm another. Successful treatment must consider more than just survival rates. Hundreds of different degrees of morbidity must be taken into account. There are also trade-offs. Obstetricians must factor in the health of both the mother and the baby. Screening policies lead to trade-offs between future health and present expenditures. Even though early detection of a malignancy may benefit an individual patient tremendously, the resources involved in detecting the single cancer may have been more productively utilized elsewhere. In addition, some health care decisions involve a series of interrelated events, each with their own degrees of uncertainty.

DMA utilizes models to help make decisions. Models are a simplified representation of reality to help the decision maker gain insight and help make the decision-making process easier. The types of models include mental, visual, physical, scale, and mathematical models. Models tend to be less expensive and more timely, allowing us to examine things that would be impossible in reality and to gain insight and understanding about the problem under investigation. Modeling can lead a decision maker to the wrong conclusion if it is not a valid model. A valid model is one that accurately represents the relevant characteristics of the object or decision problem being studied.

DMA does not guarantee the best outcome. It is a technique that uses a logical structure on a series of choices to help a decision maker choose the best alternative. The method is designed to handle uncertainty, multiple variables and consequences, complex linked interrelated events, and trade-offs. The structure of the decision is laid out in a diagram called a *decision tree*. Choice nodes indicate situations in which the decision maker can choose between two or more alternative actions. The subsequent branches of the tree correspond to potential outcomes. Probabilities for the occurrence of each branch are added in parentheses.

This model has many applications. It can be applied directly to management decisions, such as mode of delivery, choosing between several different medications, or when to induce labor. It can be used to clarify diagnostic workup decisions, deciding how much information to obtain on a patient before initiating treatment. It can be used to make prophylactic health care screening decisions, such as amniocentesis, Pap smears, and mammograms.

Simple decisions with few branches, in which consequences of treatments are immediate, often can be diagrammed with pen and paper. The more complex medical models tend to require the utilization of relatively easy-to-use computer spreadsheet programs. One such decision analysis program is Solver, located under Tools in Microsoft Excel. Although not the first, Solver is one of the most efficient in handling complex spreadsheet programs, with many built-in analytic capabilities. This program has the ability for linear and nonlinear programming, network modeling, sensitivity, regression and time series analysis, handling conflicting objectives, optimization, risk assessment, and trade-offs, along with models for simulation, flow, queuing, and project management.

Let us summarize some of these functions and see how they apply to medical decisions.

Mathematical programming is a field of management science that finds the optimal, or most efficient, way of utilizing resources to achieve a specific objective. Linear programming is a type of mathematical programming that involves creating and solving optimization problems with linear objectives and linear constraints. It is a very powerful tool that can be applied to many medical decision situations. By setting an objective function, with dependent and independent variables, and limiting constraints, complex medical decisions can be better understood and an optimal range of solutions may be identified. It is not uncommon for a medical decision to have thousands of constraints, nearly impossible to solve without the use of a computer modeling program.

This optimization process is extremely useful in designing screening programs such as Pap smears, mammography, or group B streptococcus screening while optimizing the use of limited health care resources. Another example of a medical linear programming problem is calculating ranges of radiation or chemotherapeutics agents in various combination and dose regimens, with optimization of remission and cure rates and constraints of minimizing costs and side effects. This same modeling process could be applied to antibiotic combinations and dosages set to optimize clinical response to therapy while minimizing costs and side effects.

Network modeling is a form of linear programming that optimizes flow through a series of complex networks and describes or displays them in a graphic form. Several types of network flow problems include trans-shipment, shortest path, maximizing flow, and transportation/assignment problems. Utilizing supply and demand nodes and arcs, along with flow constraints, this technique may be used to calculate the most efficient way patients are directed through a hospital or emergency room. In addition, it can be used to determine the most effective clinical pathways to approach a specific medical problem, such as the workup of an ectopic pregnancy, pelvic pain, or a pelvic mass.

Variations on linear programming include integer linear programming, goal programming, and multiple objective optimization. In integer linear programming, some or all the variables in the formulation must assume only integer values. This is needed because human beings generally cannot be divided into subunits. It is also helpful in adding resource availability constraints or when medication trials are to be studied over specific amounts of time. The branch-and-bound tree analysis is a specific type of integer program that eliminates the need to enumerate explicitly all the integer-feasible solutions and selects the best of the optimal solutions.

Here is an example of an integer linear program problem: The emergency services coordinator for a county is interested in locating the county's 10 ambulances to maximize the number of residents that can be reached within 3 minutes in emergency situations. The county is divided into 10 regions, and the average time to travel from one region to another is calculated. The population of each region is known. Calculate where the ambulances should be optimally placed.

Goal programming involves solving problems that contain not one specific objective but a collection of goals that we would like to achieve. Multiple objective optimization also applies to problems that contain more than one objective, with multiple goal constraints. In medicine, different groups of patients frequently pursue different objectives, and these objectives may be linked. Case in point: the needs of the mother versus the needs of the fetus. A particular treatment regimen may be studied not only for response rates and cost of treatment but also for convenience to the patient or side effects on other organ systems. Goals for determining an optimal diet for a diabetic pregnant patient may include varying objectives of cost, calorie and nutritional makeup, patient convenience and compliance, and fetal response, to name a few. These various objectives may be in direct conflict with one another. Problems with multiple objectives require analyzing the trade-offs among the different objectives and setting target values for each objective. It is often necessary to solve several variations of the problem with various trade-offs before we find an acceptable solution.

Nonlinear programming is similar to linear programming, but objective functions and constraints cannot be modeled adequately using linear functions of the decision variables. It can be used in all the aforementioned types of problems that linear programming can handle, but it is more complex and requires a computer modeling program such as Solver. In complex nonlinear relationships, even one's starting point of reference may influence the optimal solution. A local optimal solution may be determined when a more satisfactory global solution may exist. Solver assists with this process. It also helps use calculus to determine areas under a curve, define decision variables, link multiple constraints and objectives, and use risk aversion to handle conflicting objectives in complex nonlinear relationships.

Solver and other similar computer programs can make predictions and determine the accuracy of these predictions, as well as calculate the effects of influencing factors based on several built-in powerful statistical analyses programs.

Regression analysis is a modeling technique for analyzing the relationship between a continuous (real-valued) dependent variable and one or more independent variables. The goal in regression analysis is to identify a function that describes as closely as possible the relationship between these variables so that we can predict what value the dependent variable will assume given specific values for the independent variables. By knowing a few specific remission responses to specific chemotherapeutic agents in specific combinations and doses, Solver can extrapolate and calculate a complex nonlinear relationship between these two! It can then use sensitivity, regression (for two variables), and multiple discriminant (when three or more variables exist) analyses to evaluate the degree of fit, standard error, and confidence intervals, and to test the assumptions of the proposed nonlinear relationships.

Time series analysis is a set of observations on a quantitative variable collected over a period of time. It can be used to forecast future values of a time series variable. Just as this technique takes into effect future trends and competition to help business forecast expected levels of sales, costs, profits, inventory, and back orders, time analysis can help physicians predict future trends in health care costs and forecast long-term drug responses. By using computer model programming that calculates weighted moving averages, and adjusted trend predictors with calculated and predicted seasonal indices, we are provided a powerful prognosticating tool to benefit health care decision making.

Medical decision making is fraught with uncertainty and variability. In dealing with human lives and quality of life, risk assessment is mandatory in helping the decision maker with the variability of the performance measure. Simulation modeling is a powerful technique that measures and describes various characteristics of the bottom-line performance measure of a model when one or more values for the independent variables are uncertain. If any independent variables in a model are random variables, the dependent variable also represents a random variable. The objective

in simulation is to describe the distribution and characteristics of the possible values of the dependent variables, given possible values and behavior of the independent variables.

The idea behind simulation is similar to the notion of playing out many what-if scenarios. Solver uses a variety of specific random number function generators that allow us to generate random numbers from distributions with a wide variety of shapes. It uses these random number generators to instantly construct frequency distributions to estimate the range over which the performance might vary, to estimate the performance measure mean and variance, and to estimate the probability that the actual value of the performance measure will be greater or less than a particular value. All these measurements provide a greater insight into the risk associated with a given decision than a single value that is calculated based on the expected values for the uncertain independent variable. It then allows us to analyze the risk with a wide range of statistical and data analyses, including confidence intervals.

In conclusion, resources available to meet the demands for health care are always limited, and the science of medical asset allocation is still in its infancy. CEA and CBA are economic techniques that, when properly applied, are used to improve resource allocation policy choices. Experts in the field of cost-effectiveness in health and medicine have attempted to educate the medical academic community about the principles of CEA and develop specific minimum requirements that should be achieved in all CEA research. Decision makers charged with resource allocation would then have a common standard and a point of reference for comparability with other analyses in the literature. Proper utilization of these techniques and further advancement in this new field of science will help ensure efficient health care management in the future.

References

1. Ransom SB, Mickelson IH, Mekela P, et al: The quality of cost-effectiveness and cost-benefit analysis in the obstetrics and gynecology literature [abstract]. The Annual Meeting of the Central Association of Obstetricians and Gynecologists, Kapalu, Hawaii, 1999.
2. Weinstein MC, Stason WE: Foundations of cost-effectiveness analysis for health and medical practices. N Engl J Med 1977;296:716–721.
3. Brealey RA, Meyers SC: Principles of Corporate Finance, Chap. 3, pp. 34–56. New York, McGraw-Hill, 1996.
4. Udvarhelyi IS, Colditz GA, Rai A, Epstein AM: Cost-effectiveness and cost-benefit analyses in the medical literature. Are the methods being used correctly? Ann Intern Med 1992;116:238–244.
5. Keeler EB: Decision analysis and cost-effectiveness analysis in women's health care. Clin Obstet Gynecol 1994;27:207–215.
6. Shepard DS, Thompson MS: First principles of cost-effectiveness analysis in health. Public Health Rep 1979;94:535–543.
7. Russell LB, Gold MR, Siegel JE, et al: The role of cost-effectiveness analysis in health and medicine. JAMA 1996;276:1172–1177.
8. Siegel JE, Weinstein MC, Russell LB, Gold MR: Recommendations for reporting cost-effectiveness analysis. JAMA 1996;276:1339–1341.
9. Weinstein MC, Siegel JE, Gold MR, et al: Recommendations on the panel on cost-effectiveness in health and medicine. JAMA 1996;276:1253–1258.

How to Give a Deposition

Louis Weinstein

The practice of medicine is both a stressful and a very rewarding profession. A patient dying while under the care of the physician and an unexpected adverse outcome of the care are two of the most stressful events in the practice of medicine. An equally stressful event occurs when a physician is notified that a medical malpractice action has been initiated, often without evidence of a medical negligent act having occurred. Most physicians do not understand the legal process and are ignorant of the procedures that occur in the legal operating room. The vocabulary is often foreign to the physician, and the anatomy of the case is poorly understood by the physician being sued. Assuming that medical negligence did not occur, to have a successful defense the physician must understand the process and be an active and knowledgeable participant.

In the field of obstetrics and gynecology, 80% of physicians have been sued at least once and 25% four or more times. Some of the reasons given for the proliferation of malpractice cases is the plethora of attorneys, the fact that every adverse outcome must have a cause, and the lottery mentality that is so prevalent in our society. The real reason for many of these medical malpractice cases is *medical malpractice*. It is my opinion that a patient who has been injured by a medical negligent act should be compensated in a fair and rapid manner.

When a malpractice action has been filed and negligent medical care is *absent*, the likelihood of a successful defense can be increased by the following four keys. The first is to have a clear, well-documented medical record that relates a total story, with a beginning explaining the problems of the patient, a middle that relates what and why things were done to the patient, and an end that completes the medical odyssey with documentation of outcome. The second is a clear description that the injured patient gave adequate informed consent with knowledge of alternatives for what was done. The third is to have a competent, knowledgeable, experienced attorney who is working solely on your behalf. Fourth is the need for the defendant physician to give a strong and solid deposition performance in order for the opposing attorney to understand the facts and appreciate the quality of the defendant physician. It is this process, in which a large number of mistakes occur, that may result in the plaintiff having a successful outcome to the malpractice action.

The deposition process is a performance in which you are the lead actor. The prime function of the person being deposed is to be *completely honest*. Many things are to be done before, during, and after the deposition that will result in a successful performance, and each of these is discussed individually. It is your case, your reputation, and your physical and mental well being that are at stake, and nothing less than your total effort should be expended.

Before the deposition, numerous things must be done. Learn everything you can about the deposition process by reading any of the good references about medical malpractice depositions. Have several predeposition meetings with your attorney. It is your job to educate your attorney about medicine and the attorney's job to educate you about the process. During these meetings, "depose" your attorney to be sure he or she has the right demeanor for you, has spent appropriate time reviewing the case, understands the medical facts, and has the necessary legal and trial experience to represent you adequately. You must be comfortable that the attorney is representing you and not the insurance company. If there is any doubt in your mind about the attorney, request another attorney from the insurance company. If that request is denied, hire your own attorney to look out for your interests. An excellent choice for your personal attorney is usually one of the prominent attorneys in your area who does malpractice litigation for the plaintiff.

It is critical that you review the complete medical record. This includes any care received by the patient prior to your care and especially that received after your care. You must have knowledge of how the patient is currently doing. It is not necessary to memorize facts, but you must be conversant with accurate details of all the medical events. You have the right to set the location, date, and time of the deposition, but you must be reasonable. If the deposition cannot be finished during the allotted time or you become tired, the deposition can be continued, with the plaintiff's attorney having the right to convene the deposition at a later date. You should never give a deposition after a day in the office or the operating room or after a night on call. You must be physically and mentally prepared to give the performance you need to prove your case.

A medical record is *never* to be altered. If a late entry was made in the record, you must be prepared to explain both when and why it occurred. It is critical that all notes be dated, timed, and signed at the time of entry. If the record is difficult to read, have the records transcribed and put in an orderly fashion. The medical record can easily be the best friend you will have during the malpractice process, but if it is of poor quality, it can become your worst enemy.

Before the deposition, review all the previous depositions in the case, with particular attention to that of the plaintiff and her or his expert witnesses. You have a right to be present at all depositions in your case, and it is critical that you attend those of the patient and the expert witnesses. You are not allowed to speak at these depositions, but you can give your attorney advice about inaccurate facts presented or specific questions that your attorney can ask that may benefit your case.

Review the pertinent literature before your deposition. It is important not to cite specific references unless you are totally conversant with what is contained in the article or text. An authoritative article means that you agree with everything contained within it and that you understand everything that it says. You may bring specific materials with you to the deposition, but the opposing attorney will have access to them. You should understand the basics of what has been published, but you are not the expert witness and you must not try to win the battle of egos with the opposing counsel.

There are many practices that you must follow during your actual deposition. When asked questions, you should speak slowly and clearly and give short, truthful answers. A common mistake is to answer beyond the question that is being asked. You should respond only to the specific question asked and never volunteer any information. Always pause before you answer to give your attorney time to object or instruct you about the answer. Pausing also allows you to formulate your thoughts and decrease the nervousness that most people experience. If you believe that the question asked is vague, misleading, or ambiguous, you have the right and obligation to yourself to request that the question be rephrased. Do not be afraid to question the questioner. Remember that only you are under oath, and anything you say can be brought back at a later time and may be used against you. Be careful of the tricky question, such as "Is there anything else I should have asked but that I forgot to ask?" Your answer should be, "I cannot think of anything at this moment in time."

Your behavior at the deposition will be carefully observed. You must never be arrogant, hostile, or condescending. Your appearance should be professional but not flashy. This is not the place to flaunt your financial or societal success. Both attorneys will observe how you react to stress while being questioned, which will predict how you might react to a jury. The plaintiff's attorney will also observe how you react to your own attorney, which will demonstrate your respect for and comfort with your own counsel. The opposing attorney will determine your knowledge about the patient and the subject being discussed, which will enter into the plaintiff's decision to pursue the legal matter.

After your deposition, you have the right to review it and correct any mistakes. It is critical that you do this and sign the deposition with corrections. You must realize that the possibility exists that you will be questioned about any changes made and why you made them. Never waive the right to review and sign your deposition.

Discuss your deposition performance with your attorney and ask for ways to improve your performance for your trial appearance. Carefully listen to any suggestions made, because they are for your benefit. Keep involved in the case after your deposition and continue to attend any other depositions. Your attorney should discuss with you on a timely basis any activity in your case.

The deposition process is critical to the outcome of your legal case. There are many traps to be avoided during this process to have a successful performance and satisfactory outcome to any defensible case in which you are involved.

1. Everything that is said during the deposition will be recorded and can be used either for or against you at trial. If your deposition testimony contradicts the testimony at trial, you will lose credibility in the eyes of the jury, who are the ultimate deciders of your fate.
2. Give short, crisp, concise answers and do not volunteer any information. Everything you say gives the opposing counsel the opportunity to ask further questions.
3. If you cite an article or textbook, you must be totally conversant with the material. If you agree that something is authoritative, the implication is that you agree with everything that it contains.
4. Keep control of your ego. It is perfectly correct to state that you do not know or do not remember something. This is not the time to try to impress someone with how knowledgeable you are.
5. Always keep control of your emotions, no matter how difficult it might be.
6. Understand the language and rules of the legal operating room.

In general, physicians act in the best interests of their patients, and the public has faith and confidence in the profession. Medical negligence does occur, and the patient should be compensated in a fair and rapid manner if this is the case. Our profession is not perfect, and adverse outcomes do occur that are not medical negligence. These situations can and should be vigorously defended. With proper preparation and a strong performance at the deposition, your chances of a favorable outcome are markedly increased.

Suggestions for Future Reading

American College of Obstetrics and Gynecology: Common Sense Glossary of Medical-Legal Terms. Washington, DC, Department of Professional Liability, American College of Obstetricians and Gynecologists, 1997.

B-Lynch C, Coker A, Dua JA: A clinical analysis of 500 medico-legal claims evaluating the causes and assessing the potential benefit of alternative dispute resolution. Br J Obstet Gynaecol 1996;103:1236–1242.

Hickson GB, Clayton EW, Entman SS, et al: Obstetricians' prior malpractice experience and patients' satisfaction with care. JAMA 1994;272:1583–1587.

Symonds EM, Senior EO: The anatomy of obstetric litigation. Curr Opin Obstet Gynecol 1991;1:241–243.

Weinstein L: Understanding medical-legal issues in obstetrics and gynecology. In Ransom SB, McNeeley G, Munkarah AR, et al: (eds): Practical Strategies in Obstetrics and Gynecology. Philadelphia, WB Saunders, 1999.

Medical Legal Risk Management in Obstetrics

Charles W. Fisher and Carol Ann Tarnowsky

True risk management in obstetric cases requires knowledge of multiple specialities, including family practice, obstetrics, maternal-fetal medicine, pediatrics, neonatology, genetics, pediatric neurology, pediatric neuroradiology, orthopedics, and all those specialties that assist in medically managing babies that have disabilities far into the future. Unfortunately, risk managers are often asked not only to survey the situation in terms of the obstetric factors and the nursery factors but also to read monitor strips and understand these sophisticated areas of medicine, hypoxic ischemic nursery course data, ultrasound, computed tomography scan and head scan reports and/or films. Even *more importantly, risk management has a role in controlling the immediacy of a situation and making specific recommendations for follow-up investigation that may reveal causal elements of children who are born depressed and either die or are neurologically disabled.*

Because most risk managers have limited medical training, it is highly recommended that a *team approach* be developed in such risk management investigations. Such a team would consist of an obstetrician, a neonatologist, and perhaps a pediatric neurologist along with the risk manager and the hospital attorney. These members should be *previously* appointed and prepared to move as quickly as possible in terms of conferencing and suggesting follow-up.

PROTECTING YOUR INVESTIGATION

During a lawsuit, the discovery process opens many doors to relevant and even nonrelevant information. Plaintiff's attorneys are acutely aware of such things as incident reports, committee reviews, morbidity and mortality committees, grand rounds discussions, and so on. Any and all information regarding a particular incident will likely be requested, and the defense attorney will have to present a reason as to why a particular document, investigation, and the like is somehow privileged, and not subject to court disclosure.

Hospitals have various methods of reviewing incidents, from the simple incident report, to the quality-assurance meeting, peer review, attorney investigation, and of course, risk management investigation. The methodology of investigating may or may not attach with it a privilege that prevents its disclosure during a lawsuit. *Methods to protect presuit investigations should be verified with your hospital attorney.*

The various methods that may be available to protect the investigational process include the following:

1. Directives from the quality-assurance committee to perform such reviews
2. Directives from the peer review committee to perform such reviews
3. Attorney-client communications and investigations

Education regarding the importance of maintaining confidentiality should be addressed at all levels of the organization, including employees, medical staff members, independent contractors, and board members. In order to maintain confidentiality of legally protected information, it is imperative that policies and procedures be established, complied with, and enforced. Requests to produce information and subpoenas will likely increase as adverse parties continue to become more aware of the existence of the information and computer databases make maintaining the information easier.

PRESERVATION AND SEQUESTRATION OF THE RECORD

For reasons that are quite obvious, absent or missing records are perceived as "hiding evidence" by juries. In fact, most jurisdictions have adopted an instruction such as the following:

The defendant in this case has not produced the fetal monitor strips. As this evidence was under the control of the defendant . . . you may *infer* that the evidence would have been adverse to the defendant.[1]

Many lost medical documents in obstetric cases involve lost fetal monitor strips. Because a significant portion of baby case litigation involves a claim of fetal distress during labor, monitor strips are the key and critical element in those cases. *From a purely medical standpoint, monitor strips provide no real medical value to the management of the patient during the next pregnancy.* However, the American College of Obstetrics and Gynecology has adopted the policy that monitor strips should be saved.[2]

With respect to lost monitor strips, attempts have been made to argue that if the nurse or doctor concurrently documented heart tones and interpretation of the strip in the medical record, this is equivalent evidence, and therefore the absence of the monitor strip could not be argued as a "cover-up" or a "negative inference."[3] Even when the fetal monitor strips are saved, plaintiff's experts often detect "ominous findings" that cannot be perceived by other physician experts.

The risk manager should take it upon himself or herself to collect all of the records and place them in a safe environment. This is not to say that the physician who has not yet completed a discharge summary or a particular report cannot complete that and place it in the medical records; however, because the defendants face a negative inference instruction if anything is missing, the records should not be left for access by anyone other than the risk manager, or specifically identified individuals.

Before any copies of the medical records are made for anyone, the records should be collected and sequestered by risk management. Occasionally, records are forwarded to the plaintiffs without discharge summaries or operative reports, which follow thereafter. The claim then can be made that the records were altered or added to after the fact.

ADDENDUMS TO THE RECORD

It is inevitable that subsequent to an abnormal outcome, difficult delivery, depressed baby, shoulder dystocia, and so on, there is a great temptation to add notes to clarify what occurred. Most hospitals have adopted specific practices and methods for how this should be accomplished, including noting it as a late entry and dating it on the day it was *entered* as opposed to the day of the treatment.

It is this attorney's advice, however, that no addendums, no late entries, and no record additions be made at any time after the fact. No matter how accurate those entries may be, or how well intended the entry was, or even if the addition has nothing to do with the outcome, such entries will detract from the management of a defensible lawsuit. No matter what the entry is, jurors tend to perceive such entries as cover-up, admissions of guilt, attempts to explain away inadequate treatment, and sometimes outright fraud. Unfortunately, even when the entry addresses something that does not deal with the specific claims of medical malpractice, the jury often perceives it as a reflection on the overall integrity of the health care provider.

In situations in which one is tempted to place an addendum in the record, the better approach is to simply testify to what was done due to "recollection." An important adjunct to supporting this "recollection," of course, is the testimony of other witnesses, such as nurses, administrative personnel, and, even, on occasion, other family members who are present.

If one believes that in spite of the consequences, it is absolutely mandatory to add something to the record, such as a piece of historical data, it is best done as part of a follow-up progress note, rather than a specific addendum. That is, on a follow-up visit with the patient, write an extensive note including a detailed history of the events preceding that note, the current examination, and prognosis. In that note, include information that the health care provider remembers but that may not have been specifically documented previously.

INVESTIGATIONS OF CAUSAL CONNECTION

The relationship between birth events and perinatal morbidity and mortality is actually extraordinarily low. In babies who have acidosis at birth (even with a pH below 7.0), the correlation with poor neurologic outcome is extremely small.[4, 5] Thus, one can rightfully conclude that babies who have neurologic problems most likely have them for reasons other than birth asphyxia, birth trauma, or other birthing events, *if an adequate investigation is performed to discover the alternative cause.*

Cord gases should be done routinely regardless of the claimed cost effectiveness. One good cord gas can make the difference of a million dollars or more in a lawsuit. Some health care providers express concern that a cord gas may be lower than expected even though there was no acute injury. However, this argument carries little weight or logic. If a baby is depressed and there is no cord gas obtained, it is easy to argue that there was acidosis. If a baby was not depressed at all, had normal Apgar scores and a normal nursery course, the cord blood gas, even if suggesting acidosis, certainly does not suggest recent acute injury.

The second immediate item for investigation at delivery is the placenta. Although the placenta, in and of itself, cannot ordinarily establish proximate cause, it can, in conjunction with other factors, confirm prenatal insult. Placentas, in high-risk legal cases, should be sent to a specialist in placental pathology *prior* to a lawsuit. This is not to suggest that the placenta should not also be examined by the regular hospital pathologist, but in cases in which the outcome is poor, second opinions by subspecialists are quite helpful.

Serial laboratory testing is crucial in baby cases in which there is a claim of hypoxic ischemic insult because these tests, especially kidney function tests, can help rule out multiple organ insult.[6] Laboratory tests for infection, such as blood cultures, urinalysis, and cerebrospinal fluid, are also appropriate in circumstances in which infection may be the cause of a child's depression and/or injury.

Routine laboratory tests, such as complete blood count differential and urinalysis, done early on may raise issues of whether or not there was evidence of chronic insult. Particularly important and suggestive are high counts of nucleated red blood cells and reticulocytes, which are often correlated in conjunction with other findings to chronic intrauterine hypoxia and stress that occurred before labor and delivery.[7]

Sequential ultrasounds, magnetic resonance imaging, and computed tomography scans are some of the biggest tools for the defense in hypoxic cases. Early identification of lesions that took days to develop can raise complete defenses to claims of labor and delivery hypoxia.

It should be remembered that the function and primary interest of the neonatologist is to treat the immediate condition, and although many neonatologists are skilled at recognizing abnormalities that may relate to prenatal insult or

been a call for federal regulation of the fertility industry by one of the country's leading medical ethicists, comparing the need for regulation of fertility medicine to the regulation of transplant medicine.[10] These are the types of far-reaching proposals of which physicians must be aware and prepared to present appropriate counterarguments, as appropriate.

Another case demonstrated the extent to which disappointed patients will go when their expectations are not met by their physician.[11] In a 1998 case, the patients underwent a procedure whereby the sperm of the husband was mixed with that of an anonymous donor and used to fertilize, in vitro, the eggs of his wife. The alleged expressed purpose of the couple was to have at least the option of believing that the resulting child was genetically related to the father. As reported in the case, there was a difference in testimony as to whose choice the selection of the final donor sperm would be—the patient's or their physician's. Either way, when the child was born, its physical appearance was not similar to that of the parents, and subsequent blood work demonstrated that the donor sperm was not that of the donor allegedly selected by the patients. The patients sued, claiming improper sperm selection by the doctor had deprived them of the ability to believe and represent that the husband was the true, biologic father of the child, and that this failure caused them great emotional harm.

The appellate court upheld the lower court's dismissal of the case and stated that the patients had not shown that there existed any issue of fact regarding the question of their suffering any type of bodily harm. The court furthermore indicated that the type of negligence alleged in this matter was not of the type that would cause mental distress in a person normally constituted. The court significantly noted that the patients were basically claiming that the doctor's alleged malpractice had merely caused the destruction of a fictitious belief and that the exposure to the truth about a situation could not be considered to be a recoverable injury. This case clearly shows the physician that a disappointed patient may go to great degrees to seek redress from the doctor who allegedly caused the disappointment and that the physician must be ever aware of this possibility.

CONCLUSION

Since the 1980s, there have been incredible advances in obstetrics and gynecology and their related subspecialty areas. These have also caused lawyers, courts, and ethicists to look closely at these scientific advances and their significance to society. The issues raised in this chapter have most certainly not been completely resolved, and it is even more certain that in the not-too-distant future, issues about which we now cannot even conceive will become just as controversial.

As we enter the 21st century, it is becoming more and more obvious that obstetrics and gynecology and their related subspecialty areas have a great future. The advances in these fields will likely improve the quality of life for patients. However, one must be constantly aware of the legal and ethical issues that will arise from our advances. By forearming both physicians and patients with information, the number of ethical and legal conflicts in fertility treatment should be greatly decreased.

Suggestions for Future Reading

Evans MI, Dixler AO: Human in vitro fertilization: Some legal issues. JAMA 1981;245:2324.
Gianelli DM: New York panel urges stricter controls over fertility clinics. Am Med News, May 18, 1998.
Hollinger JH: From coitus to commerce: Legal and social consequences of noncoital reproduction. U Mich J L Rev 1985;18:865.
Jones HW: History of in vitro fertilization. In Keye WR, Chang RJ, Rebar RW, Soules MR (eds): Infertility: Evaluation and Treatment. Philadelphia, WB Saunders, 1995, pp. 736–744.
Roe v Wade, 410 US 113 (1973).
Shamma FN, De Cherney AH: Infertility: A historical perspective. In Keye WR, Chang RJ, Rebar RW, Soules MR (eds): Infertility: Evaluation and Treatment. Philadelphia, WB Saunders, 1995, pp. 1–7.
Steptoe PC, Edwards RG: Birth after the reimplantation of a human embryo. Lancet 1978;2:366.

References

1. *Davis v Davis,* 842 SW2d 588 (Tn 1992).
2. *Kass v Kass,* 235 A.D.2d 150, 663 NYS2d 581 (1997).
3. *Gardner v Pawliw,* 696 A.2d 599, 150 NJ 359 (1997).
4. Parrish D, Christensen K: O.C. lawsuit charges embryo theft. Orange County Register, Sept. 6, 1995.
5. Christensen K: Asch target of second San Diego fertility suit. Orange County Register, Dec. 9, 1995.
6. Biologist Testifies There Were Ethical Violations At Fertility Clinic. Orange County Register. Feb. 29, 1996.
7. Kelleher S: Woman sues hospital, UCI, saying her eggs were misused. Orange County Register, March 5, 1998.
8. Another fertility-scandal lawsuit. Orange County Register, Sept. 11, 1998.
9. Hust SA: The need for regulation in the fertility industry. 35 U of Louisville J of Fam L 555 (Summer 1996, 1997).
10. Annas G: The shadowlands—secrets, lies, and assisted reproduction. N Engl J Med 1998;339:935–939.
11. *Harnicher v University of Utah,* 962 P. 67 (1998).

INDEX

Note: Page numbers followed by f refer to figures; those followed by the letter t refer to tables.

Angelica sinensis, for postmenopausal patient, 307

Angelman's syndrome, 218
  genetics of, 218

Annealing, in polymerase chain reaction, 264, 264f

Anorectal manometry, 355

Anorexia nervosa, 335
  amenorrhea associated with, 336
  complications of, 336

Anovulation, treatment of. *See* Ovulation, induction of.

Anticoagulation. *See also* Heparin; Warfarin.
  during pregnancy, 138–139, 142–145

Anticonvulsants, 116t
  pharmacokinetics of, 117t
  teratogenic potential of, 116, 139

Anti-D immune globulin
  eligibility for, 66–67
  hepatitis in recipients of, 68
  monoclonal, 68

Antifungals, for vulvovaginal candidiasis, 407, 407t, 408

Antihypertensives
  for diabetic patient, 446
  for patient with preeclampsia, 47, 48t
  for pregnant patient, 139

Antimicrobials
  for asymptomatic bacteriuria, in pregnant patient, 345, 346t
  for bacterial vaginosis in pregnant patient, equivocal effects of, on preterm delivery, 19, 19t, 20t
  for cellulitis of breast, in nursing patient, 341
  for cellulitis of surgical wound, 325
  for cystitis, in pregnant patient, 346t
  for endometritis, in postpartum patient, 182, 182t, 331
  for mastitis, in nursing patient, 341
  for opportunistic infections, in pregnant patient with AIDS, 14
  for perinatal streptococcal infections, 148–151, 149f, 150t, 150f
  for postpartum endometritis, 182, 182t, 331
  for preterm premature rupture of membranes, 172–173
  for pyelonephritis, in pregnant patient, 347t
  for urinary tract infections, in pregnant patient, 346t, 347t

Antiphospholipid antibody syndrome, 144, 184–187
  preeclampsia as complication of, 185
  pregnancy loss associated with, 184
  thromboses occurring in, 184, 185

Antiretroviral agents, for AIDS, 10, 11t
  cross-resistance to, 16
  in nonpregnant patient, 9, 10
    early therapy with, pros and cons of, 10t
  in pregnant patient, 9–10, 14–16, 141, 327
    changing regimens of, 16
    continuation of, during labor, 16
    relative safety of, 10t
    risk of premature delivery associated with, 327
    temporary discontinuation of, in presence of hyperemesis, 11–12
    triple therapy with, 11
      indications for, 11, 11t

Antiretroviral agents *(Continued)*
  side effects of, 11t

Antivirus software, 175

Arterial embolization. *See* Embolization.

Arthritis, rheumatoid, in users of oral contraceptives, 352

Artificial anal sphincter, 357

ASCUS (atypical squamous cells of undetermined significance), in cervix, 276, 483
  follow-up on, in pregnant patient, 485

Aspiration, fine-needle, of breast mass, 339, 339t

Aspirin
  for coronary artery disease, in diabetic patient, 446
  for pregnant patient, problems with, 145

Assisted reproductive technology, 435. *See also* Infertility, treatment of.
  complications associated with, 435–438

Asthma, in pregnant patient, 95–100
  control of, 95–100
    allergen avoidance in, 95–96, 96t
    bronchodilators in, 97–98
    corticosteroids in, 96t, 96–97
    emergency management in, 100, 100t
    home-based approach to, 99, 99t
    management of labor and delivery in, 100
    peak flowmeter values in, 99, 99t
    stepwise approach to, 98, 98t
  reported complications of, 95t
  severity of
    classification of, 96t
    intensity of fetal surveillance in relation to, 99

Asthma triggers, avoidance of exposure to, 95–96, 96t

Asymptomatic bacteriuria, 345
  antimicrobials for, in pregnant patient, 345, 346t
  cranberry juice for, 347
  in pregnancy, 345–346
    antimicrobials for, 345, 346t

Ataxia, spinocerebellar, type 1, 220
  genetics of, 220

Athletes, amenorrhea in, 336–337

Atropa belladonna, for postmenopausal patient, 305–306

Atrophy, muscular, spinal and bulbar, 220
  genetics of, 220

Atypical squamous cells of undetermined significance (ASCUS), in cervix, 276, 483
  follow-up on, in pregnant patient, 485

Augmentation, breast, sequelae of, 343

Auscultatory findings, in pulmonary edema, 133

Azidothymidine (AZT). *See* Zidovudine.

Azithromycin, for *Mycobacterium avium* complex infection, in pregnant patient with AIDS, 14

AZT (azidothymidine). *See* Zidovudine.

Bacterial vaginosis, 18–21, 330
  intra-amniotic infection associated with, 20, 20t
  preterm delivery associated with, 18, 19t, 330

Bacterial vaginosis *(Continued)*
  persistence of risk of, despite antimicrobial therapy, 19, 19t, 20t
  risk of spontaneous pregnancy loss associated with, 20

Bacteriuria, asymptomatic, 345
  antimicrobials for, in pregnant patient, 345, 346t
  cranberry juice for, 347
  in pregnancy, 345–346
    antimicrobials for, 345, 346t

Balloon ablation, of endometrium, 411, 413t, 414

Beckwith-Wiedemann syndrome, 218
  genetics of, 218

Beclomethasone, for asthma, in pregnant patient, 96t, 97

Behavioral modifications, in management of urinary incontinence, 421

Belladonna, for postmenopausal patient, 305–306

Beta-agonists, for asthma, in pregnant patient, 98

Beta-mimetics, for preterm labor, 33, 123–124

Bethesda system nomenclature, for Papanicolaou test results, 482t

Biofeedback training
  in pelvic muscle exercise, to limit urinary incontinence, 422
  in sphincter contraction, to limit fecal incontinence, 356

Biomarker(s), of preterm labor or delivery, 4–7, 6f
  cervical length as, 245f, 245–246, 246f
  fetal fibronectin levels as, 5, 5t
  indications for assessment of, 246–247
  salivary estriol levels as, 5t, 6

Biopsy, cervical, indications for, in pregnant patient, 485

Birth defects, 233–238
  potentiation of risk of, 233. *See also* Teratogen(s).
  with assisted reproductive technology, 437–438

Bishop score, 243

Black cohosh, for postmenopausal patient, 306

Bladder, inflammation/infection of, in pregnancy, 346
  antimicrobials for, 346t

Bladder training, in management of incontinence, 422. *See also* Incontinence, urinary.

Bleeding
  fetal-maternal, 65, 130
  heparin-induced, 144
  intraoperative, 376–378
  pelvic
    embolization for, 166, 378
    hypogastric artery ligation for, 377
  postpartum, 165
    arterial embolization for, 166, 167
    arterial ligation for, 165
  presacral plexus, thumbtacks in control of, 377
  uterine
    dysfunctional, 379
      causes of, 379t
      diagnosis of, 379

Cefotetan, for endometritis, in postpartum patient, 182t

Cefoxitin, for endometritis, in postpartum patient, 182t

Ceftizoxime, for endometritis, in postpartum patient, 182t

Ceftriaxone, for pyelonephritis, in pregnant patient, 347t

Cellulitis
of breast, in nursing patient, 341
of surgical wound, 325
of vaginal cuff remaining after hysterectomy, 323

Centers for Disease Control and Prevention (CDC)
approach of, to intrapartum prophylaxis against GBS, 149, 149f, 150f
recommendations of, regarding Pap testing in HIV-positive patient, 489t

Cephalexin
for asymptomatic bacteriuria, in pregnant patient, 346t
for cystitis, in pregnant patient, 346t

Cerclage, 27–30, 246
preterm premature rupture of membranes following, management of, 30
results of, 27, 28t
suture placement in, 29, 29f, 30
maneuvering of fetal membranes out of way of, 29, 29f

Cerebral palsy
in infants positive for thrombophilias, 55–56
in very-low-birth-weight infants, 111
reduced risk of, in cases of fetal exposure to magnesium sulfate, 111–112, 112t

Cervical cancer, 276
human immunodeficiency virus infection and, 490
human papillomavirus infection and, 276, 487
treatment of, insurance coverage of, 504

Cervical factor infertility, postcoital test for, 453

Cervical index, 244

Cervical intraepithelial neoplasia (CIN)
human papillomaviruses as cause of, 487
Papanicolaou test for, in HIV-positive patient, 488, 488t
CDC recommendations regarding, 489t
risk of, in HIV-positive patient, 488
treatment of, 484
in HIV-positive patient, 489
recurrence following, 489

Cervical length, 243–247
as predictor of preterm delivery, 245f, 245–246, 246f

Cervical pregnancy, management of, uterine artery embolization in, 168

Cervical ripening. *See* Labor, induction of.

Cervix, 243. *See also* Cervical *entries.*
atypical squamous cells of undetermined significance (ASCUS) in, 276, 483
follow-up on, in pregnant patient, 485
biopsy of, indications for, in pregnant patient, 485
cryotherapy for lesions of, 485
funnelling of, 244
incompetent, 243

Cervix *(Continued)*
cerclage of, 27–30, 246
preterm premature rupture of membranes following, management of, 30
results of, 27, 28t
suture placement in, 29, 29f, 30
maneuvering of fetal membranes out of way of, 29, 29f
intra-amniotic infection and, 28
laser therapy for lesions of, 485
loop electrosurgical excision of lesions of, 485
Papanicolaou smear of. *See* Papanicolaou test.
ultrasonography of, 243–244

Cesarean section
endometritis following, 181, 331
in patient with herpes simplex virus infection, 120, 121
in patient with HIV infection, 12, 327–328
perimortem, 130–131
platelet transfusion during, in patient with preeclampsia, 91
potential shoulder dystocia as indication for, 205–206
septic pelvic thrombophlebitis following, 331
vaginal delivery after, 63–64
complications of, 64
factors favorable to, 63, 63t

Chasteberry vitex, for postmenopausal patient, 306–307

Chemosensitivity testing, in patients with ovarian cancer, 474

Chemotherapy
for gestational trophoblastic disease, 479t, 479–480
for ovarian cancer
salvage, 473–474
surgery combined with, 471, 472
testing for sensitivity to, 474
for ovarian cancer recurrence, 473–474

Chest x-ray, in diagnosis of pulmonary edema, 133, 133f, 135

Chlorpropamide, for diabetes mellitus, 445

Chorioamnionitis. *See* Amniotic cavity, infection of.

Choriomeningitis, lymphocytic, 329

Chorionic villus sampling, 208–209, 211–212

Chromosomal mosaicism, 219
in material sampled from chorionic villi, 209

Cimicifuga racemosa, for postmenopausal patient, 306

CIN (cervical intraepithelial neoplasia)
human papillomaviruses as cause of, 487
Papanicolaou test for, in HIV-positive patient, 488, 488t
CDC recommendations regarding, 489t
risk of, in HIV-positive patient, 488
treatment of, 484
in HIV-positive patient, 489
recurrence following, 489

Clindamycin
for perinatal streptococcal infections, 150t
for postpartum endometritis, 182t
for vaginosis in pregnancy, equivocal effects of, on preterm delivery, 18–19, 19t

Clinical information systems, in improvement of patient care, 510

Clinical pathways/protocols, in reduction of medicolegal risk, 511

Clomiphene citrate, 190, 448
induction of ovulation with, 190–191, 448

Clotrimazole, for vulvovaginal candidiasis, 407t, 408

Coding, of services provided by obstetricians-gynecologists, 496, 500, 502

Coitus
cervical factor infertility test following, 453
contraception following, 160–161, 359–361, 361t

Collagen injections, periurethral, in management of urinary incontinence, 427–429

Color Doppler imaging, of ovarian neoangiogenesis, in detection of cancer, 400

Colorectal cancer, in contraceptive users, 352

Colposcopy, 492–493

Combination oral contraceptive pills, postcoital use of, 160, 359, 361t

Complete molar pregnancy, 477–478

Complex-partial seizures, 115

Computers, for obstetricians-gynecologists, 175–179

Condom(s), patterns of use of, in 1990s, 159, 160, 160t

Condyloma(ta)
vaginal, 483, 484
vulvar, 483, 484

Congenital anomalies, 233–238
potentiation of risk of, 233. *See also* Teratogen(s).
with assisted reproductive technology, 437–438

Congenital toxoplasmosis, 328

Congressional issues, physicians' involvement in, 503–508

Consent, informed, of pregnant patient undergoing ultrasonography, 201

Consumer perceptions, of alternative vs. conventional medicine, 301, 301t

Contigen injections, periurethral, in management of urinary incontinence, 427–429

Continuous combined hormone replacement therapy, postmenopausal, 396
uterine bleeding due to, 396, 397, 398

Contraception, 158–160
adolescents' use of, 155
cost-effectiveness of, 161
insurance coverage of, 505
patterns of, in 1990s, 160, 160t
postcoital, 160–161, 359–361
availability of, public unawareness of, 161, 361
efficacy of, 361t
preparations used in, health benefits of, 349–353

Contributions, by physicians, to Congressional candidates, 507–508

Copper IUD, contraception with, postcoital, 360

Cordocentesis, 212–213
diagnostic value of, in fetal hemolytic disease, 68

Coronary artery disease, in diabetic patient, 75

Neurotoxicity, of vitamin B$_6$, 138
Nevirapine
  for newborn exposed to HIV, 327
  for pregnant patient with HIV infection, 327
Newborn
  alcohol-related neurodevelopmental disorders in, 388, 389t
  alloimmune thrombocytopenia in, 93–94
  brachial plexus injury in, shoulder dystocia and, 50, 204. *See also* Shoulder dystocia.
  cytomegalovirus infection in, 328
  extremely-low-birth-weight, 41–42. *See also* Newborn, very-low-birth-weight.
    survival rates for, 41, 41t
  group B streptococcal infection in, 147
    antimicrobial prophylaxis against, 149, 149f
  hemolytic anemia in, 65
  herpes simplex virus infection in, 120
  HIV transmission to, reduction of risk of
    with cesarean section, 327–328
    with nevirapine, 327
  injury to, from delivery complicated by shoulder dystocia, 50, 204. *See also* Shoulder dystocia.
  low-birth-weight, 152–153. *See also* Newborn, extremely-low-birth-weight; Newborn, very-low-birth-weight.
  thrombocytopenia in, alloimmune, 93–94
  very-low-birth-weight. *See also* Newborn, extremely-low-birth-weight.
    cerebral palsy in, 111
      reduced risk of, in cases of fetal exposure to magnesium sulfate, 111–112, 112t
Nifedipine, for patient with preeclampsia, 48t
Nipples
  discharge from, during or after pregnancy, 342
  irritation of, from breast-feeding, 342
  trauma to, from breast-feeding, 342
Nitrofurantoin
  for asymptomatic bacteriuria, in pregnant patient, 346t
  for cystitis, in pregnant patient, 346t
Nitroprusside, for patient with preeclampsia, 48t
Noncardiogenic pulmonary edema, 134
Non-nucleoside reverse transcriptase inhibitors. *See also* Antiretroviral agents.
  for AIDS, 10, 11t
    cross-resistance to, 16
    side effects of, 10, 11t
Nonsteroidal anti-inflammatory drugs
  for dysfunctional uterine bleeding, 380
  for endometriosis, 362
  for premenstrual syndrome, 293
Nonviral vectors, in gene therapy, 250
Norgestrel, contraception with, postcoital, 359
Nuchal translucency, in screening for Down syndrome, 225
Nucleoside analogues. *See also* Antiretroviral agents.
  for AIDS, 10, 11t
    combined use of, in pregnant patient, 11
    side effects of, 11t

Nursing patient
  breast abscess in, 341
  breast engorgement in, 341–342
  breast presentation by, 342
  galactocele in, 341
  herpes simplex lesions in, care of, 121
  mastitis in, 341
  nipple irritation and trauma in, 342
Nystatin, for vulvovaginal candidiasis, 407t

Obstetricians-gynecologists
  computers for, 175–179
  contributions by, to Congressional candidates, 507–508
  decision-making by
    analysis of, 527–529
    outcomes of, costs vs. benefits of. *See* Cost-effectiveness analysis.
  diagnostic services provided by
    coding of, 496, 500, 502
    molecular technology–based, 264–278
      PCR in. *See* Polymerase chain reaction (PCR).
  Internet resources for, 177, 178t
  lawsuits against, 531
    approaches to settlement of, 535
    deposition process in, 531–532
    infertility treatments at issue in, 538, 539
  legislative issues of concern to, 503–506
  performance of
    expectations of. *See* Health care purchasers, expectations of.
    productivity as measure of, relative value units for, 501–502
    quality of, methods of improving, 509–512
  politicking by, 503–508
  profiling of, 509, 521
  reimbursement of
    diagnostic and procedural coding in, 496, 500, 502
    Medicare fee schedules and, 513–516, 515t
    patient history documentation required for, 496, 497f–500f
    review-of-systems documentation required for, 501f
  violence against, 505
Oenothera biennis, as herbal remedy, 308t
  for use by postmenopausal patient, 308
Office evaluation, of urinary incontinence, 431–434
Ofloxacin, for endometritis, in postpartum patient, 182t
Oligohydramnios
  as isolated finding, 37
    management implications of, 37–39
  as side effect of tocolysis with indomethacin, 35
  perinatal outcomes associated with, 38t
Opioid maintenance therapy, 393
Opportunistic infections, in pregnant patient with AIDS
  antimicrobials for, 14
  screening for, 13
  vaccines for, 13
Optical density, of lamellar bodies, as index of fetal lung maturity, 109

Oral contraceptives
  health benefits of, 349–353
  patterns of use of, in 1990s, 160, 160t
  postcoital use of, 160, 359
    efficacy of, 361t
Oral hypoglycemics, for diabetes mellitus, 445
Osmotic derangement, and pulmonary edema, 133, 134t
Osteoporosis. *See also* Bone.
  and fractures, 352
  in contraceptive users, 352
  in patients receiving heparin, 145
  in postmenopausal patients, raloxifene for, 285, 449
Outlet forceps delivery, 78t. *See also* Vaginal delivery.
Outpatient treatment programs, for substance abusers, 393
Ovarian cancer, 468–475
  chemotherapy for
    salvage, 473–474
    surgery combined with, 471, 472
    testing for sensitivity to, 474
  diagnosis of, 468–469
  recurrent, management approaches to, 473–474
  risk factors for, 468
    contraceptive use and, 349
  screening for, 399–402
  staging of, 471–472
  surgery for, 469–471
    chemotherapy combined with, 471, 472
    evaluation preceding, 469
    in cases of recurrence, 474
    optimal debulking in, 470
    preparation for, 469
    second-look, 473
  terminal, management approaches to, 474
  types of, 468
Ovarian cysts, in users of oral contraceptives, 351
Overflow urinary incontinence, 431
Ovulation
  documentation of, in infertility therapy, 452–453
  induction of, 189–194
    candidates for, 189–190
    clomiphene citrate in, 190–191, 448
    gonadotropin-releasing hormone in, 193–194
    gonadotropins in, 191–192
Oxybutynin, for urinary incontinence, 423, 423t
Oxygen therapy, for pregnant patient with pulmonary edema, 134
Oxytocin, induction of labor with, 81–82, 82t

Paclitaxel, for ovarian cancer, 472
Pain, menstrual, oral contraceptives for, 350
Palsy, cerebral
  in infants positive for thrombophilias, 55–56
  in very-low-birth-weight infants, 111
    reduced risk of, in cases of fetal exposure to magnesium sulfate, 111–112, 112t
Panax ginseng
  for postmenopausal patient, 309
  substances used as, 308t